CLASSIC TEACHINGS IN CLINICAL CARDIOLOGY

a tribute to W. Proctor Harvey, M.D.

Volume I

Edited by
Michael A. Chizner, M.D.

Director, Broward General Heart Institute
Broward General Medical Center
Fort Lauderdale, Florida
Cardiologist, The Greater Fort Lauderdale Heart Group
Clinical Professor of Medicine
University of Miami School of Medicine
Miami, Florida
Clinical Professor of Medicine
University of Florida College of Medicine
Gainesville, Florida

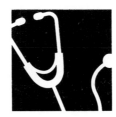

Laennec Publishing, Inc.
Cedar Grove, New Jersey

Classic Teachings in Clinical Cardiology: A Tribute to W. Proctor Harvey, M.D.
© 1996 by Laennec Publishing, Inc.
First Edition
All rights reserved. Printed in the United States of America. No part of this text may be reproduced, stored, in a retrieval system, or transmitted in any form or by any means, electronic, mechanical, photocopying, recording, or otherwise without the prior written permission of Laennec Publishing, Inc. Reviewers may quote brief passages in a review. For information, please write Laennec Publishing, Inc., 218 Little Falls Rd., Cedar Grove, NJ 07009-1231

Library of Congress Cataloging-in-Publication Data

Classic Teachings in Clinical Cardiology: A Tribute to W. Proctor Harvey, M.D.
Edited by Michael A. Chizner, M.D.
        p.   cm.
        Includes bibliographical references and index.
        ISBN: 1-886128-06-5
        1. Cardiovascular System — Diseases.   2. Cardiology
  I. Chizner, Michael A.
Library of Congress Number: 95-077138

For Laennec Publishing:
    Managing Editor: Andrew J. McCarthy
    Art Director: Mary Wright
    Typography: Graphic Connections, Inc., Melville, New York
              Chuck Albano, Pat Albano, Mary Albano
    Proofreader: Eda Levy

Printed by Edwards Brothers, Inc., Ann Arbor, Michigan

Classic Teachings in CLINICAL CARDIOLOGY

W. Proctor Harvey

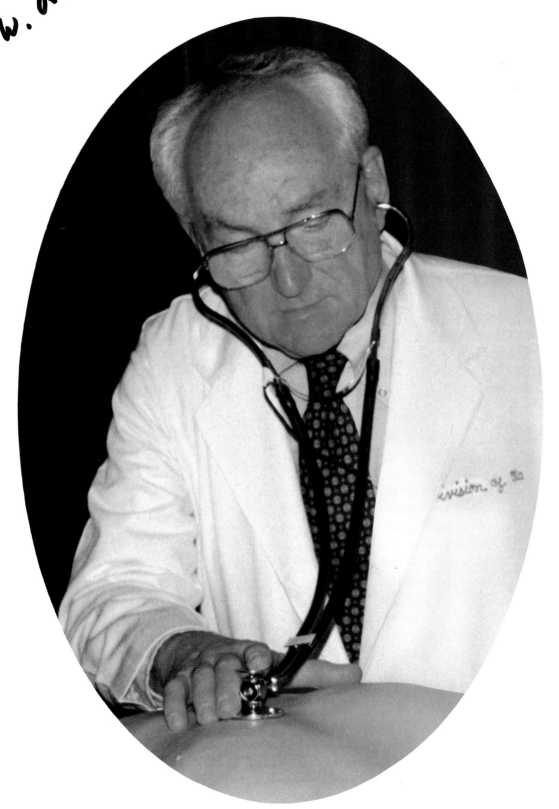

A Tribute to
W. Proctor Harvey, M.D.

This unique text pays tribute to, and is an extension of, the philosophy and practice of Dr. W. Proctor Harvey, world renowned Cardiologist, Professor of Medicine, and former Director of the Division of Cardiology at Georgetown University Medical Center in Washington, D.C., a position he held for more than thirty-five years. The value of Dr. Harvey's unceasing efforts to champion the importance of the clinical art of cardiovascular diagnosis and his exceptional ability to teach it, have been acknowledged in the numerous prestigious awards and commendations he has received. These include the Gifted Teacher Award of the American College of Cardiology, the Distinguished Teacher Award, Laureate Award and Mastership of the American College of Physicians, the Distinguished Clinical Teacher Award of the Alpha Omega Alpha National Medical Honor Society, the Gold Heart and James B. Herrick Awards of the American Heart Association, and the Distinguished Service Award of the World Congress of Cardiology. He serves or has served as a Consultant in Cardiology to the U.S. Department of State, Walter Reed Army Medical Center, Andrews Air Force Base Hospital, U.S. Naval Hospital, and the National Heart, Lung, and Blood Institute, and has held such high offices as President of both the American Heart Association and the Association of University Cardiologists.

Dr. Harvey has been lauded for his effective, highly practical, and creative manner of bedside teaching in the grand tradition, and his annual conferences on "Clinical Auscultation of the Heart" and "Cardiac Pearls" have been referred to as post-graduate and continuing medical education at its finest. In refining the teaching of Clinical Cardiology, he has pioneered the use of audiovisual aids including multimedia programs using wireless infrared stethophones, high fidelity tape recordings, audio and video cassettes, film strips, and "text boxes" of cardiac pathology specimens with clinical correlation incorporated. As medical innovator, Dr. Harvey has designed a stethoscope with three chest pieces, the Harvey Triple-Head, to enable superior and accurate auscultation. To make clear to his students the various heart sounds and murmurs, Georgetown's foremost authority on auscultation has learned to mimic the myriad acoustic findings with his voice and his hands, tapping his knuckles or fingers against a hard surface. The art of cardiac auscultation, as we know it today, is virtually synonymous with the name W. Proctor Harvey. Dr. Harvey's enormous literary talent is evident in his prolific writing and editing of books, journals, and articles that have become "classics" and help set the standard for quality medical education on cardiovascular diagnosis, evaluation, and care.

Once in a lifetime there comes an individual who leaves an indelible mark in his field. Such a man is W. Proctor Harvey, and such has been his inestimable contributions to the annals of Cardiology. His untiring dedication as a clinician, extraordinary talent as an educator and communicator, exceptional creativity as a medical innovator, keen vision as a builder of the Cardiology program at Georgetown, deep concern for excellence in patient care, and self-sacrificing commitment to the practice and teaching of Clinical Cardiology, have earned him a legendary place in the history of medicine. Although honors and awards for these outstanding achievements have come his way in abundance, Dr. Harvey's greatest reward is the affection, admiration, and esteem of generations of medical students, house officers, and Fellows who have learned so much from his thoroughly human and caring approach to medicine. Throughout his long and illustrious career he has been blessed, above all, with the unfailing support, encouragement, and understanding of his gracious partner, loving companion, and kindred spirit, his wife Irma.

Dr. Harvey has coined the term "Cardiac Pearl," which he defines as a "fact or finding" in the clinical evaluation of the patient that provides a clue that leads to, or makes, the diagnosis. Like a pearl, it does not lose its luster over time. It "stands the test of time." The "finding" we, his Fellows and students, have come to recognize as "fact" is that the most precious cardiac pearl of all is Dr. Harvey himself.

We use this vehicle as a means of expressing our indebtedness and profound gratitude to our mentor for the knowledge and skill he has imparted to us, and the great impact he has had on our professional development and personal lives. From the passion for cardiology that he has instilled in us springs the inspiration to pass along this rich legacy and to carry on the teaching tradition that is his. On behalf of all of us who have learned and benefitted so much from this gifted and giving teacher, master clinician, and consummate role model, we hereby affectionately dedicate (from our heart to his heart) these "Classic Teachings in Clinical Cardiology" to Dr. W. Proctor Harvey.

Michael A. Chizner, M.D.

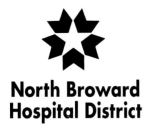
Foreword

"Classic Teachings in Clinical Cardiology" pays tribute to a living legend in clinical medicine, W. Proctor Harvey, M.D. The authors of this text book, all renowned leaders in clinical and academic cardiology, in honor of their mentor, have prepared a legacy for humanity. Dr. Harvey, who in dedicating his life to teaching and communicating the art of cardiovascular diagnosis to the caregivers, has nurtured the hearts of mankind.

The North Broward Hospital District is proud to sponsor this landmark text in clinical cardiology and commends the editor, Michael A. Chizner, M.D., Medical Director of the Broward General Medical Center Heart Institute for his dedication, commitment, vision and leadership in this outstanding effort to further medical education and enhance the quality of patient care.

As the fourth largest not-for-profit health care system in the country, the North Broward Hospital District includes four medical centers and over 1600 physicians on staff. As a model health care system for the advancement of academic excellence in a community setting, the District is affiliated with the University of Florida and Nova Southeastern University and supports research and innovation in Cardiovascular Services.

Richard J. Stull II

Richard J. Stull, II
Past President/CEO

✷ Broward General Medical Center　✷ North Broward Medical Center　✷ Imperial Point Medical Center　✷ Coral Springs Medical Center

303 S. E. 17th Street　·　Ft. Lauderdale, FL 33316　·　(305) 355-4400

Preface

We are on the threshold of a new century when closer scrutiny and growing concern over the issues of escalating health care costs and appropriate allocation and conservation of resources impact our daily lives in medicine. In this changing climate of health care reform, modern cardiology, with its rapidly advancing technologies, has become increasingly more expensive and complex. Today's physician, therefore, faces the difficult challenge and compelling responsibility of developing cost-effective management strategies while maintaining optimal, high quality patient care. The burgeoning array of elaborate "high tech" procedures and instrumentation, although useful and necessary in selected cases, results in added time, expense, potential risk, and may not be needed in the diagnosis of all patients. The astute clinician must remain in command of, not become overly dependent on, the powerful new diagnostic testing methods. These sophisticated invasive and non-invasive techniques should serve to complement and supplement, rather than supplant, the role of careful, perceptive observation and sound clinical judgment at the bedside (the "art of medicine"). The unfortunate trend to order costly, time-consuming laboratory tests, when similar information can be obtained or inferred by simpler clinical methods of examination, cannot be justified and only further taxes the financial resources of the patient and the health care system.

At no time in the history of medicine has the need been greater than it is today for the physician to learn and apply the clinical art of cardiovascular diagnosis. This ancient, virtually lost art can be acquired and mastered through experience, continued practice and patience. Despite the current emphasis on technology, it is still true that the vast majority of patients with cardiovascular disease can be diagnosed in the office or at the bedside by employing the basics of the so-called "Five Finger Approach" espoused by Dr. W. Proctor Harvey. This orderly and systematic method includes a careful detailed history, physical examination, electrocardiogram, chest x-ray, and specialized laboratory tests. The proper step-wise application of this balanced approach remains the cornerstone to an accurate clinical working diagnosis. It helps direct the patient to the appropriate selective utilization of the available technology and guide our clinical decision-making in the everyday practice of medicine.

In an age of increasing instrumentation, cost containment and managed care, this book is a timely reminder to the practicing physician of the primary importance of clinical skills in the diagnosis and evaluation of the cardiac patient. The current role of technology, its clinical indications and practical applications in the "Five Finger Approach" to data acquisition and clinical problem solving will be stressed. A broad spectrum of disease states encountered in cardiology practice will be emphasized with the patient as the central focus of teaching. Pathophysiologic mechanisms and morphologic aspects of heart disease of clinical relevance to the practicing physician will be integrated with the information derived from a complete clinical cardiovascular evaluation. Therapeutic concepts and considerations, as they relate to the clinical management of the patient with cardiovascular disease, will be discussed. Dr. Harvey's teachings, comments and timeless "Cardiac Pearls," selected and interspersed throughout the text provide the common thread that serves to emphasize and highlight the message, tying all the chapters together.

This informative reference source in clinical cardiology is designed for the practicing Cardiologist, Internist, and Primary Care Physician. Physicians-in-training, medical students, and all other disciplines involved in the care of the cardiac patient will also find much that is useful in this comprehensive "state of the art" treatise. It is written in a highly instructive, personalized and practical style based on the respective author's extensive clinical experience and expertise. Each carefully selected contributor, renowned for his or her talents in clinical cardiology and teaching, is a former Fellow or student during Dr. Harvey's tenure as Director of Cardiology at Georgetown. This fraternity of distinguished alumni, a veritable "Who's Who" in Cardiology, are among the most outstanding clinicians, teachers, and researchers in Medicine today. Many occupy important positions of leadership and are Chiefs of the Divisions of Cardiology and Medicine in the various medical schools and hospital centers throughout the United States and abroad. Despite their extremely busy schedules, these dedicated "givers" found the time to come together to honor their mentor, and provide a thoughtful, erudite discussion on their respective subject matter. We hope this book on the clinical diagnosis, evaluation and care of the patient with cardiovascular disease will prove to be a valuable and effective educational tool in the armamentarium of present and future generations of practicing physicians.

Michael A. Chizner, M.D.

Acknowledgments

I want to express my deepest appreciation to the individuals whose help was invaluable in the preparation of this text. I owe a great debt of gratitude to Dr. Henry R. Cooper, my colleague, mentor, and cherished friend, for his sage guidance and constant encouragement from the inception to the completion of this project. I am also particularly grateful to Dr. Robert A. O'Rourke and Dr. Donald F. Leon who provided me with invaluable assistance and wise counsel throughout this undertaking. I especially want to thank my associates, Drs. Carroll L. Moody, Harold Altschuler, Jeffrey S. Dennis, Alan L. Niederman, and John W. Lister, of The Greater Fort Lauderdale Heart Group, with whom I have had the pleasure and privilege to work, for their helpful suggestions and support.

I wish to acknowledge the efforts of Ms. Norma Lloyd, former Director of Special Projects for the North Broward Hospital District, Mrs. Kathy B. Novak, Executive Director of The Greater Fort Lauderdale Heart Group, Mrs. Miriam Chuang, Director of the Cardiac Care Center at Broward General Medical Center, and the many talented nurses and technical staff of the Broward General Heart Institute and The Greater Fort Lauderdale Heart Group, who have helped me in so many ways and to whom I am most appreciative. To the many dedicated physicians and medical students, too numerous to mention by name, who have made my professional life so stimulating, challenging and rewarding, and to all my patients and friends who have profoundly influenced me, I am also extremely grateful. Special thanks and recognition are due, as well, to Ms. Lee Whiteside, Medical Librarian at Broward General Medical Center for her diligent assistance in conducting literature searches, Ms. Sandra M. Hitchcock for her innovative strategic planning, and Mrs. Addie Mueller, Mrs. Mary Ellen Francis, Mrs. Sandy Kelley, Mrs. Joanne Falzone, Mrs. Olympia Caracostas, Ms. Tosca Lanzana, and Mrs. Allison Scott whose able organizational, secretarial and typographical skills and faithful support were most helpful to the completion of this project.

I sincerely appreciate the helpful assistance and cooperation of Mr. David Canfield, Mr. Douglas Canfield, Mr. James McCarthy and Mr. Andrew McCarthy of the Laennec Publishing Company. I particularly want to express my special thanks to Mr. Andrew McCarthy for his enthusiasm, dedication, commitment and professional expertise which were so essential to bringing this project to fruition. His patient understanding and willingness to extend every courtesy and indulgence has made the relationship between publisher and editor a warm and responsive partnership.

I am also extremely grateful to Mrs. Helene K. Soref and the late Mr. William C. Frogale for their kind and most generous support. To my dear friend Mr. Frogale, whose recent unexpected death has been such a great personal loss, I owe more than he would have cared to have me mention.

It is with deep and everlasting gratitude and appreciation that I acknowledge Mr. Richard J. Stull II, Past President and Chief Executive Officer of the North Broward Hospital District, Mr. Wil Trower, President and Chief Executive Officer of the North Broward Hospital District, Ms. Ruth Eldridge, Administrator of Broward General Medical

Center and Mr. T. Ed Benton, Dr. Rosalyn Y. Carter, Mrs. Ana I. Gardiner, Mr. R. Emmett McTigue, Mr. Amadeo Trinchitella, Mrs. Annie L. Weaver, and Mr. Harold Wishna of the Board of Commissioners of the North Broward Hospital District for their commitment to academic excellence and the advancement of medical education.

To my family, I owe more than words can express. I am and always will be deeply grateful to my late father, Bernard, for his guiding principles and unstinting devotion; to my beloved mother, Sybil, for her inspirational support and steadfast encouragement; and to my devoted and loving wife, Susan, and our children, Kevin, Ryan, and Blair, for their enduring patience and understanding sacrifice through the many long hours spent in the preparation of this text. I could not have accomplished this task without them.

Finally, as editor, it has been my distinct pleasure to associate with so distinguished a roster of contributing physicians. Each author contributor has been most gracious, diligent and responsive in his/her efforts to accomplish our mutual goal in such a timely manner, and has my deepest respect, admiration and gratitude. Their enthusiasm and unselfish sacrifice of considerable time and energy from their extremely busy schedules bespeaks their devotion to Dr. Harvey and dedication to this undertaking. For me, editing this textbook as a tribute to Dr. W. Proctor Harvey has been a special privilege, an honor and truly a "labor of love."

Michael A. Chizner, M.D.

Contributors

Jonathan Abrams, M.D.
Professor of Medicine (Cardiology)
University of New Mexico School of Medicine
Albuquerque, New Mexico

Mark M. Applefeld, M.D.
Director, Division of Cardiology
Mercy Medical Center
Associate Professor of Medicine
University of Maryland School of Medicine
Baltimore, Maryland

David C. Booth, M.D.
Professor of Medicine
Acting Chief of Cardiology
University of Kentucky Medical Center
Lexington, Kentucky

Michael A. Chizner, M.D.
Director, Broward General Heart Institute
Broward General Medical Center
Fort Lauderdale, Florida
Cardiologist, The Greater Fort Lauderdale
  Heart Group
Clinical Professor of Medicine
University of Miami School of Medicine
Miami, Florida
Clinical Professor of Medicine
University of Florida College of Medicine
Gainesville, Florida

Guillermo B. Cintron, M.D.
Professor of Medicine
University of South Florida College of Medicine
Chief, Cardiology Service
James A. Haley Veterans Administration Hospital
Tampa, Florida

Paul T. Cochran, M.D.
Clinical Professor of Medicine
University of New Mexico School of Medicine
President, Southwest Cardiology Association
Albuquerque, New Mexico

Modestino G. Criscitiello, M.D.
Professor of Medicine
Tufts University School of Medicine
Senior Physician, New England Medical Center
  Hospital
Boston, Massachusetts

Antonio C. de Leon, Jr., M.D.
Medical Director, Cardiovascular Institute
Director of Medical Education
St. John Medical Center
Tulsa, Oklahoma

Albert A. DelNegro, M.D.
Clinical Assistant Professor of Medicine
Georgetown University School of Medicine
Washington, D.C.

Robert DiBianco, M.D.
Director, Cardiology Research Risk Factor
  Reduction Center and Heart Failure Clinic
Washington Adventist Hospital
Takoma Park, Maryland
Associate Clinical Professor of Medicine
Georgetown University School of Medicine
Washington, D.C.

W. Bruce Dunkman, M.D.
Associate Professor of Medicine
University of Pennsylvania School of Medicine
Director, Non-Invasive Cardiac Laboratories
Department of Veterans Affairs Medical Center
Philadelphia, Pennsylvania

R. Curtis Ellison, M.D.
Professor of Medicine in Public Health
Chief, Section of Preventive Medicine
  and Epidemiology
Boston University School of Medicine
Boston, Massachusetts

Robert L. Engler, M.D.
Associate Chief of Staff for Research
V.A. Medical Center
Professor of Medicine
University of California School of Medicine,
  San Diego
San Diego, California

Gordon A. Ewy, M.D.
Director, University Heart Center
Professor of Medicine
Chief, Section of Cardiology
University of Arizona College of Medicine
Tucson, Arizona

Ross D. Fletcher, M.D.
Chief, Cardiology Section
Veterans Administration Medical Center
Associate Professor of Medicine
Georgetown University School of Medicine
Washington, D.C.

Edward D. Frohlich, M.D.
Alton Ochsner Distinguished Scientist
Vice President of Academic Affairs
Alton Ochsner Medical Foundation
Professor of Clinical Medicine and Adjunct
  Professor of Pharmacology
Tulane University School of Medicine
Professor of Medicine and Physiology
Louisiana State University School of Medicine
New Orleans, Louisiana

Julius M. Gardin, M.D.
Professor of Medicine
Chief, Division of Cardiology
University of California, Irvine Medical Center
Orange, California
President, American Society of Echocardiography

Bruce J. Genovese, M.D.
Medical Director, Coronary Care Unit
St. Joseph Mercy Hospital
Clinical Instructor in Medicine (Cardiology)
University of Michigan School of Medicine
Ann Arbor, Michigan

Steven A. Goldstein, M.D.
Director, Non-Invasive Cardiac Laboratory
Department of Cardiology
Washington Hospital Center
Washington, D.C.

Michael S. Gordon, M.D., Ph.D.
Professor of Clinical Medicine (Cardiology)
Director, Medical Training and Simulation
  Laboratory
University of Miami School of Medicine
Miami, Florida

Bertron M. Groves, M.D.
Professor of Medicine and Radiology
Director, Cardiac Catheterization Laboratories
University of Colorado Health Science Center
Denver, Colorado

Jeffrey M. Isner, M.D.
Professor of Medicine and Pathology
Tufts University School of Medicine
Chief, Cardiovascular Research
St. Elizabeth's Hospital
Boston, Massachusetts

Hanjörg Just, M.D.
Medical Director
Division of Cardiology
Professor of Medicine
University of Freiberg
Freiberg, Germany

Joel S. Karliner, M.D.
Professor of Medicine, University of California
  San Francisco School of Medicine
Chief, Cardiology Section
Ft. Miley Veterans Administration Hospital
San Francisco, California

Richard J. Katz, M.D.
Professor of Medicine
Division of Cardiology
Director, Echocardiography Laboratory
George Washington University School of Medicine
Washington, D.C.

Donald M. Knowlan, M.D.
Team Physician
Washington Redskins
Professor of Medicine
Georgetown University School of Medicine
Washington, D.C.

Bernard D. Kosowsky, M.D.
Professor of Medicine
Tufts University School of Medicine
Chief, Division of Cardiovascular Medicine
St. Elizabeth's Hospital
Boston, Massachusetts

Edward G. Lakatta, M.D.
Professor of Medicine
Johns Hopkins School of Medicine
Professor of Physiology
University of Maryland School of Medicine
Chief, Laboratory of Cardiovascular Science
National Institutes of Health
National Institute of Aging
Gerontology Research Center
Visiting Physician
Francis Scott Key Medical Center
Baltimore, Maryland

Louis Larca, M.D.
Co-Director, Echocardiography Laboratory
Washington Adventist Hospital
Takoma Park, Maryland
Clinical Instructor of Medicine
Georgetown University School of Medicine
Washington, D.C.

Donald F. Leon, M.D.
Office of the Medical Director
Dean of Clinical Affairs
Professor of Medicine
Georgetown University School of Medicine
Washington, D.C.

James J. Leonard, M.D.
Professor and Chairman
Department of Medicine
F. Edward Herbert School of Medicine
Uniformed Services University of the
    Health Sciences
Bethesda, Maryland

Keith M. Lindgren, M.D.
Clinical Associate Professor of Medicine
Georgetown University School of Medicine
Washington, D.C.
Co-Director, Department of Cardiology
Washington Adventist Hospital
Takoma Park, Maryland

Frank I. Marcus, M.D.
Distinguished Professor of Medicine (Cardiology)
University of Arizona College of Medicine
Director, Electrophysiology Services
University of Arizona Health Science Center
Tucson, Arizona

C. Edwin Martin, M.D.
Clinical Associate Professor of Medicine
University of Pennsylvania School of Medicine
Chief, Division of Cardiology
York Hospital
York, Pennsylvania

Joseph R. McClellan, M.D.
Assistant Professor of Medicine
University of Pennsylvania School of Medicine
Director, Cardiac Care Unit and Nuclear
    Cardiology
Hospital of University of Pennsylvania
Philadelphia, Pennsylvania

Michael A. Nagel, M.D.
Medical Director, Division of Cardiology
Good Samaritan Hospital of Santa Clara Valley
San Jose, California

William P. Nelson, M.D.
Medical Director, Cardiovascular Services
Saint Joseph Hospital
Denver, Colorado

Robert A. O'Rourke, M.D.
Charles Conrad Brown Distinguished Professor
    in Cardiovascular Disease
Director of Cardiology
The University of Texas Health Sciences Center
    at San Antonio
San Antonio, Texas

David L. Pearle, M.D.
Professor of Medicine and Pharmacology
Georgetown University School of Medicine
Washington, D.C.

Richard B. Perry, M.D.
Clinical Professor of Medicine
Georgetown University School of Medicine
Governor, American College of Physicians
Washington, D.C.

Nathaniel Reichek, M.D.
Director, Division of Cardiology
Professor of Medicine
Medical College of Pennsylvania
Allegheny Campus
Pittsburgh, Pennsylvania

James A. Ronan, Jr., M.D.
Clinical Professor of Medicine
Georgetown University School of Medicine
Washington, D.C.
Co-Director, Division of Cardiology
Washington Adventist Hospital
Takoma Park, Maryland

Thomas J. Ryan, M.D.
Professor of Medicine
Boston University School of Medicine
Senior Consultant in Cardiology
Boston University Medical Center Hospital
Boston, Massachusetts

Bernard L. Segal, M.D.
Clinical Professor of Medicine
University of Pennsylvania
Director, Philadelphia Heart Institute
Presbyterian Medical Center
Philadelphia, Pennsylvania

Jack P. Segal, M.D.
Clinical Professor of Medicine
Georgetown University School of Medicine
Washington, D.C.

Donald H. Singer, M.D.
Clinical Professor of Medicine (Cardiology)
University of Illinois
Chicago, Illinois

John F. Stapleton, M.D.
Professor of Medicine, Emeritus
Georgetown University School of Medicine
Washington, D.C.

R. Barrett Steelman, M.D.
Clinical Professor of Medicine
University of Texas Southwestern Medical Center
Senior Partner and Founder, North Texas
  Heart Center
Attending Physician, Presbyterian Hospital
  of Dallas
Dallas, Texas

James V. Talano, M.D.
Lester B. and Frances T. Knight Professor
  of Medicine
Northwestern University Medical School
Director, Cardiac Graphics
Northwest Memorial Hospital
Chicago, Illinois

Cynthia M. Tracy, M.D.
Assistant Professor of Medicine
Georgetown University School of Medicine
Director of Cardiac Arrhythmia Services
Division of Cardiology
Georgetown University Hospital
Washington, D.C.

Ron J. Vanden Belt, M.D.
Attending Cardiologist
Michigan Heart and Vascular Institute
St. Joseph Mercy Hospital
Clinical Assistant Professor of Medicine
  (Cardiology)
University of Michigan School of Medicine
Ann Arbor, Michigan

Bruce F. Waller, M.D.
Clinical Professor of Medicine and Pathology
Indiana University School of Medicine
Director, Cardiovascular Pathology Registry
St. Vincent Hospital
Cardiologist, Nasser, Smith, Pinkerton
  Cardiology Inc.
The Indiana Heart Institute
Indianapolis, Indiana

Richard A. Walsh, M.D.
Mabel S. Stonehill Professor of Medicine
Director, Division of Cardiology and
  Cardiovascular Center
University of Cincinnati College of Medicine
Cincinnati, Ohio

Alan M. Weintraub, M.D.
Clinical Professor of Medicine
Georgetown University School of Medicine
Washington, D.C.

CLASSIC TEACHINGS IN CLINICAL CARDIOLOGY
a tribute to
W. PROCTOR HARVEY, M.D.

C O N T E N T S

VOLUME I

Part I
Clinical Evaluation of the Cardiac Patient:
The "Five-Finger Approach" of Dr. W. Proctor Harvey

Electrocardiogram

Chest X-Ray

Cardiac Diagnostic Laboratory: Non-Invasive and Invasive Techniques

Part II
Normal and Abnormal Structure and Circulatory Function

VOLUME II

Part IV
Coronary Heart Disease

Part V
Valvular Heart Disease

xxi

CLINICAL EVALUATION OF THE CARDIAC PATIENT: THE "FIVE-FINGER APPROACH" OF DR. W. PROCTOR HARVEY

CHAPTER 1

Clinical Approach to the Patient with Heart Disease

Antonio C. de Leon, Jr., M.D.

Whether or not heart disease is present depends on symptoms such as chest pain, shortness of breath, leg swelling (edema), fatigue, palpitations, dizziness, or fainting spells. It may also occur because of a cardiac murmur, abnormal heart sounds, cyanosis, or a rhythm disturbance. On other occasions, an abnormality noted in an electrocardiogram or chest X-ray directs suspicion for the possibility of heart disease. The patient therefore expects from the physician an opinion on whether heart disease is present, what kind of disease is present, its severity and prognosis, and management options available.

Traditionally, we have approached this process by obtaining the clinical history and performing a physical examination. Our ability to obtain useful information from this process relies upon understanding the symptoms and physical signs as manifestations of anatomic or pathophysiologic changes. This understanding and/or insight serves as the basis for determining if and what additional diagnostic tests are needed.

In recent years, there has been a tendency to rely on the multitude of diagnostic and imaging modalities available to determine if heart disease is present and define its nature and severity. Traditional "bedside" skills do not receive as much emphasis and, as a result, are not learned. Many factors contribute to this trend. There is a tendency by some to want to achieve absolute diagnostic certainty - a goal which is unattainable. It is also easy to confuse the informational value of a test with useful or meaningful information in a specific case, forgetting that as one approaches diagnostic certainty, the useful information provided by a diagnostic test approaches zero. The higher levels of

sensitivity and specificity of technologically-based diagnostic tools make the apparent lower yield of various aspects of physical examination to appear not worth the effort. However, it should be remembered that the sensitivity and specificity arrived at applies to one physical finding viewed as an independent finding. In the context of a clinical evaluation, they are but a part of the total correlation made from the clinical history, the rest of the physical examination, and simpler, less expensive tests.

The "Five-Finger" Approach

It was to emphasize the importance of the various aspects of the clinical examination that Dr. W. Proctor Harvey proposed the "five-finger" approach (Figure 1). Using the analogy of the five fingers of the hand, he assigned the clinical history to the thumb to signify that it was of special singular value since the thumb is the most important, useful finger of the hand.

He then assigned the physical examination to the next most important finger - the index finger - and other sources of useful information to the rest of the fingers. He further underscores the need for correlation of information by pointing out that if the fingers of the hand were clenched into a fist, a powerful weapon, a fist, results.

CARDIAC PEARL

Never has the need been greater than it is today for the physician to learn and apply the art of bedside and office diagnosis of cardiovascular disease. In today's world, there is an unfortunate, as well as very expensive (for the patient) trend to obtain the "noninvasive" as

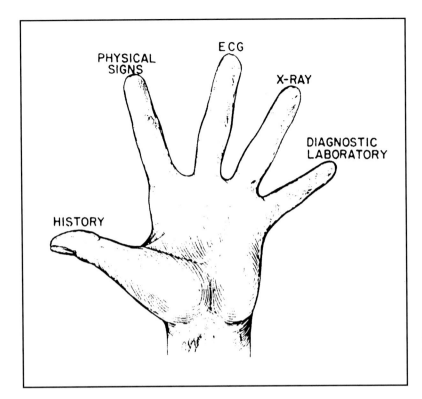

Figure 1. The Five-Finger approach to cardiac evaluation. (Courtesy of W.P. Harvey.)

well as "invasive" laboratory test for diagnosis before there is a careful clinical evaluation of what we term the "five-finger approach" to cardiovascular diagnosis. This includes: a complete detailed history, physical examination, electrocardiogram, x-ray and appropriate laboratory tests. We should make a "fist" of these fingers using all of them to make the correct diagnosis in the great majority of patients. However, if we were allowed only one of the five "fingers", we would, of course, choose the thumb, the history. By this method probably 90% of patients seen for some form of heart disease, can be evaluated at the bedside or in a physician's office. The remaining patients screened do, indeed, need hospital admission to make use of the excellent ingenious and sophisticated laboratory equipment and studies in our modern hospitals.

W. Proctor Harvey, M.D.

In an effort to assess the lasting value of clinical skills learned in training, Kern et al surveyed graduates of an internal medicine program with at least one year of practice experience after formal training. The top five categories of importance listed by those surveyed were the physical examination (90.6%), history taking (90.2%), diagnosis/problem definition competence (88.8%), interpersonal skills (88.4%), and selecting diagnostic studies (88.4%). This underscores the value of emphasis on basic clinical skills in training.

Fletcher and Fletcher emphasize that "bedside" skills be used to recognize when more powerful tests are needed and high technology diagnostic tests "should only supplement the clinician's physical diagnosis skills and not replace them". The strategy of continued emphasis in the clinical history and physical examination is strongly patient-oriented and thus invaluable in establishing patient-physician relationship. It is therefore well worth the effort for any clinician.

CARDIAC PEARL

When we meet our patients for the first time, we usually do not know what pertinent findings may be present which will provide clues to the diagnosis or, perhaps, make the diagnosis. Also, each day we often do not know what specific cardiovascular problems or findings they will present to us. It is still true that the great majority of our patients can be diagnosed in the physician's office and at the bedside. This is part of what we call the "fun of medicine."

W. Proctor Harvey, M.D.

Clinical History

Collecting historical clinical information is a basic goal, but the method of collection is equally important. It has been shown in patients with chest pain that when a physician interview is compared to patient questionnaire, disagreement in data collected can occur, and that this disagreement led to a significantly different diagnosis.

Dr. W. Proctor Harvey has always emphasized that the physician should always allow time for the patient to respond to the questions posed, and the questions posed should not be a leading question. It is more helpful to have the patient express his or her symptoms in their own words. The physician should have the ability to place himself or herself into the patient's situation and be able to impart by ones' demeanor sympathy, understanding, and a sense of caring.

Watching a patient's facial expression, tone of voice, and hand and body movements may impart more information than the actual words the patient speaks. It is important that the physician not give the patient a hurried impression since important details of the history may be unwittingly withheld by the patient. In arriving at a diagnosis of angina, an unhurried, painstaking interview has been emphasized as essential.

CARDIAC PEARL

The most important part of the total clinical evaluation of a patient is the history. A student of medicine should try as much as possible to observe a physician who has mastered this art in action with his patients. It will be noted that he/she rapidly establishes a rapport with his patients based on true and sincere empathy. He allows time for his patient to respond to his questions. The clinician should have a real ability to put himself into the patient's situation. It is important when taking a history not to give a rushed impression to the patient; this may make some feel they are taking too much of the doctor's valuable time and often results in inadequate descriptions of valuable signs and symptoms. The physician's demeanor should impart sympathy, understanding, and, probably most important, a sense of caring. At the same time, the patient should be given hope and encouragement that the problem can be diagnosed and treated. To allay unnecessary fears and anxieties, we often tell the patient at presentation, "You know, there are few patients that cannot be helped."

W. Proctor Harvey, M.D.

Ischemic Chest Pain

• Stable Angina

Recurrent chest pain is an important and common cardiovascular symptom. In a middle aged or older patient (with or without coronary risk factors) one could hurriedly conclude that the complaint of chest pain, especially if substernal, represents angina. This can lead to a cascade of increasingly expensive diagnostic tests. However, there are many other causes of chest pain, the majority of which are non-cardiac such as esophageal spasm, esophageal reflux, gall bladder disease, chest wall muscle or cartilage, parenchymal lung disease, and diseases of the cervical spine.

It is therefore important to secure added information such as the character of the pain, its location of onset, radiation, duration, factors which cause the pain and measures which relieve it. Visceral pain (of which angina is one) is a deep pain usually described by patients as "dull" or "pressure-like" and referred to cutaneous sites served by the same spinal cord level as the heart. Referred pain is a characteristic of visceral pain and is not specific for angina pectoris. True angina is rarely described as "sharp" or "knife-like". More often, it is described as a "pressure sensation", "tightness", "constricting feeling", "heaviness", "band-like" constriction, or a "burning" sensation like "indigestion". Less commonly, the patient complains of a "suffocating feeling" or breathlessness. The latter two may represent anginal equivalents and are more commonly encountered in older or diabetic patients. Breathlessness on exertion has also been observed to precede the onset of angina. Regardless of how the patient describes the discomfort, characteristically, it is similarly described with recurrent episodes.

Anginal pain usually is in the general substernal area or parasternally, or epigastric and is diffuse enough so that the patient is unable to point to a spot with a finger. It may radiate to one or both arms, usually the inner aspect and can extend all the way to the fingers. Less commonly, radiation can extend to the throat, mandible, or maxilla. The arm radiation may be described as "numb" or "heavy" rather than actual pain. The discomfort lasts one to five minutes (unless it is unstable angina or acute MI where it may last as long as 20 minutes to many hours).

The discomfort is precipitated by physical effort and/or mental or emotional stress. Reproduceability of discomfort with a consistent level of effort is also a helpful clue for angina.

Characteristically, the patient stops activity to obtain relief but is not relieved by lying down. Relief from sublingual nitroglycerin is prompt and usually complete within a minute or two. Remember that similar prompt relief occurs from the drug with pain from esophageal spasm. Thus, relief with

---

TABLE 1

Grading Effort Angina

GRADE I – Ordinary physical activity does not cause angina. (Angina occurs with strenuous, rapid, or prolonged exertion at work or recreation.)

GRADE II – Slight limitation of ordinary activity. (Angina occurs with walking or climbing stairs rapidly, walking uphill, walking or stair climbing after meals, in cold, in wind, under emotional stress, or only during the few hours after awakening; walking more than two blocks on the level, and climbing more than one flight of stairs at a normal pace and in normal conditions.)

GRADE III – Marked limitation of ordinary physical activity. (Angina occurs with walking one to two blocks on the level and climbing one flight of stairs in normal conditions and at normal pace.)

GRADE IV – Inability to carry on any physical activity without discomfort. (Angina occurs at rest.)

---

nitroglycerin should not be construed as diagnostic for angina.

It should also be remembered that physical activity, which a person is used to performing, and indoor activity are less likely to provoke angina. Additionally, the pace of activity can influence when angina occurs.

Cutaneous pain is sharp or burning and can be localized unlike true angina. Pain that is fleeting or lasts for a few seconds, or for days or weeks is not of cardiac origin.

Remember that a normal coronary arteriogram can be encountered in a patient with ischemic pain such as in those with hypertrophic cardiomyopathy, severe aortic stenosis, coronary spasms, and those with abnormality of the microvascular circulation. Conversely, patients with pain from non-cardiac causes may have demonstrable atherosclerotic coronary artery disease on coronary arteriography, so a good clinical history is still essential.

Grading effort angina as proposed by the Canadian Cardiovascular Society can be useful in categorizing and following patients (Table 1).

• Unstable Angina

An increase in severity, frequency and/or duration of angina from it's previously predictable and reproducible character is a feature readily obtained by careful history taking. This change should alert the clinician to possible progression of coronary atherosclerosis, the addition of coronary vasospasm, reduction in myocardial oxygen supply because of anemia, significant arrhythmia, or an increase in myocardial oxygen consumption caused by hyperthyroidism. New onset angina can present with the features of unstable rather than stable angina and influence the type and rapidity of diagnostic work-up and management.

• Variant Angina

Angina at rest, in the early morning after arising or with initial low level exertion (with no symptoms at subsequent higher effort levels) should suggest coronary artery spasm. Patients with fixed lesions (and stable angina) may also develop coronary spasm at or near the lesion site.

In some patients with exercise or effort induced angina, angina at rest also occurs. This is also referred to as "mixed angina" and represents a vasospastic component added to a fixed coronary artery stenotic lesion.

• Acute Myocardial Infarction

The ischemic chest pain of acute myocardial infarction characteristically lasts longer than angina. It usually is sustained, lasting 30 minutes or more. The discomfort may be reported by the patient as more severe than the angina they have previously experienced. Additional symptoms such as nausea, diaphoresis, light-headedness, or syncope may accompany the chest discomfort.

The lack of relief from nitrates, when previously prompt relief was obtained during anginal episodes, further raises suspicion for infarction. In the elderly, pain may not be a prominent symptom. Instead, shortness of breath or an altered sensorium may dominate the clinical presentation.

Chest Pain in Other Cardiovascular Disorders

• Mitral Valve Prolapse

Although chest pain in mitral valve prolapse may indeed mimic angina pectoris, more often there are atypical features which can be elicited by careful history taking. The location and radiation varies with different episodes in the same patient: there may be spontaneous variation in severity of symptoms which are unrelated to the level of activity; the pain may be brief or fleeting, but recurrent over a long time, occurring at rest or exercise without demonstrable consistency. Response to nitrates is unpredictable. Palpitations are a prominent feature and commonly co-exist with periods of chest pain. The association of light headedness, syncope, chronic fatigue, anxiety, and/or hyperventilation are more common features in mitral valve prolapse than angina pectoris of coronary artery disease. Confirmation of mitral valve prolapse on physical examination strengthens the historical information obtained above.

• Aortic Dissection

Onset of sudden chest pain commonly raises the possibility of acute myocardial infarction. However, aortic dissection should be an equally important consideration. Aortic dissection should be considered, especially when pain is severe, unrelieved, or only minimally relieved by opiates. Some patients describe the pain as "tearing".

Prominent radiation of pain to the back and localization in the interscapular area would increase suspicion for this possibility. Physical findings such as disparity in amplitude of the carotid pulses, disparity in upper extremity blood pressures, and new onset of the murmur of aortic insufficiency - especially one that is louder on the right compared to the left parasternal areas - are all helpful in directing the diagnostic consideration toward aortic dissection.

• Pericarditis

The character of chest pain in pericarditis has been described as sharp, dull, stabbing, or an ache. Pain may be brief but is recurrent, may wax and wane in intensity, usually over a period of hours; discomfort may be aggravated in the recumbent posture or by swallowing. Relief is obtained by assuming an upright posture or leaning forward. Finding a pericardial friction rub on physical examination helps establish diagnosis. Fever in association with pain onset is not a usual feature of acute myocardial infarction and its presence can help direct suspicion away from it.

• Pulmonary Hypertension

Chest pain can occur in patients with pulmonary hypertension and may be related to exertion. The mechanism for its genesis is unclear but is presumed to be secondary to right ventricular ischemia. The finding of a giant "A" wave in the jugular venous pulse, a loud pulmonary valve closure sound and a right ventricular lift on physical examination helps the clinician entertain this consideration.

• Pulmonary Embolism

Chest pain which occurs with this entity may be due to the resulting pulmonary hypertension or to development of pulmonary infarcts. In the case of the latter, the pain is pleuritic - (i.e. changes in severity with respiration), may be located in portions of the chest other than substernal, and also be associated with hemoptysis.

Chest Pain from Non-Cardiovascular Causes

• Esophageal Abnormalities

In esophageal abnormalities, esophageal spasm and esophageal reflux can cause visceral pain with the character, location, and radiation similar to that encountered in angina pectoris. Unless this possibility is included in the differential diagnosis, extensive work-up in the direction of coronary artery disease can result. It is further compounded by the possibility of finding coronary artery lesions on angiography in patients with symptomatic esophageal disease. It is easy to fall into the trap of ascribing the symptoms to the demonstrated coronary artery lesions, especially if one has no objective evidence of myocardial ischemia from other sources. Furthermore, true angina can occur with normal coronary arteries.

As previously pointed out, pain from esophageal spasm is promptly relieved by nitrates and can also be provoked by ergonovine. When one can obtain from clinical history that the discomfort is brought on by the recumbent position, large meals or spicy foods, when there is associated dysphagia, relief from antacids or bland food, or a history of previously demonstrated hiatus hernia, suspicion for an esophageal cause rises. It has been suggested that radiation of the pain through to the back occurs more frequently in esophageal disorders.

• Thoracic Wall

Chest wall pain can be localized, diffused, perceived as sharp or ache, or a tightness across the chest. Finding areas on the chest wall which upon palpation reproduce the symptoms is useful in their recognition. Pain which is sharp or stabbing, momentary or fleeting, and inframammary in location are of chest wall origin and do not represent angina. Costochondrodynia is readily recognized by palpation during the physical examination. Pain from lower cervical or upper thoracic nerve root compression may at times have an apparent relation to effort. Dorsal root compression usually produces a sharp, piercing pain, of lightning characteristics, and may have associated superficial paresthesias. Ventral root pain presents as a deep, boring or dull discomfort which thus mimics angina. However, root pain is also characterized by pain upon body movement, pain on coughing or sneezing, and pain after prolonged recumbency. Pain may be precipitated by bending or hyperextension of the spine, or by throwing back the shoulders; development of the pain after several hours in bed is a common feature, while original onset may have been noted after a vigorous sneeze. Repeated jarring may provoke pain, and paresthesias occur and may precede pain onset.

Tingling, numbness, and stiffness, especially of the fingers, are aggravated by the same maneuvers which provoke pain. On physical examination, provocative maneuvers such as stretching the arm across the chest while pulling the head toward the flexed shoulder and inhaling deeply, applying pressure to the top of the head as it is tilted to either side, and deep palpation over the spinous processes, can all help establish diagnosis. Thus, correlation of the clinical history and physical examination allows one to come to a diagnostic conclusion. Recognition of radicular features of pain during history taking ensures that the physician perform the provocative maneuvers.

• **Gastrointestinal and Other Entities**

Peptic ulcer, gallbladder disease, or irritable bowel may produce epigastric discomfort or pain with substernal or precordial radiation. Other features of the clinical history usually allow for their recognition.

Hyperventilation may be associated with chest pain or discomfort and mistakenly thought to be angina. This is further compounded by ST segment changes which can occur on exercise testing in some patients. Associated symptoms of air hunger, dizziness or light headiness, syncope in some, numbness, and tingling of the fingers and palpitation enable its recognition as a benign entity.

CARDIAC PEARL

Hyperventilation can sometimes cause symptoms similar to those of heart disease, including chest discomfort, dyspnea, dizziness, near syncope, or tachycardia.

Illustrating this point are two patients; the first was a middle aged man who had congenital ventricular septal defect. He had a moderate sized defect, and had been asymptomatic. However, he was admitted to the Emergency Room of a local hospital when he developed chest discomfort, shortness of breath, paresthesias of both arms and hands, dizziness, and near syncope while eating in a restaurant. On examination there was no change from previous examinations. Also there was no reason why an uncomplicated ventricular septal defect should produce his symptoms.

He was instructed to hyperventilate and, sure enough, started to have symptoms similar to those he had in the restaurant. He perspired, complained of substernal chest pain, appeared anxious and had dizziness and obvious respiratory distress. Carpal spasm appeared bilaterally. Subsequently a movie was made of him again showing the same symptoms and signs due to hyperventilation. To stop the hyperventilation syndrome, he was told to look at his watch and stop breathing for every 15 seconds before he took another breath. At first this was difficult, but he did so.

Then, on repeating the purposeful breath holding alternating with breathing, one could see the reversal of all of the symptoms and signs of his hyperventilation. Subsequently this film was used to show this patient and other patients how to manage, as well as prevent, these episodes. Fortunately, the patient learned to control as well as prevent subsequent attacks.

Another patient, a 32-year-old unmarried woman, was evaluated because of what had been called "symptoms related to her mitral valve prolapse." The patient had a history of what reportedly had been documented by echocardiography to be mitral valve prolapse. Her father, who accompanied her, stated that she had recently seen her physician who again described her heart as "still clicking away." However, a careful evaluation did not reveal a systolic click or any other auscultatory evidence of mitral valve prolapse. She then had an echocardiogram at our institution, searching carefully for any evidence of mitral valve prolapse, and none was found. A follow-up examination with a repeat echocardiography was performed; again no evidence of mitral valve prolapse. During her physical examination while sitting upright on the examining table, she was asked to hyperventilate (which had been demonstrated to her). Shortly thereafter she had chest discomfort, perspiration, paresthesias of the upper extremities, and subsequent carpal spasm. Her father was present at the time of the examination; both said these were the identical symptoms that the patient had been having and had been attributed to her "mitral valve prolapse." She had been misdiagnosed as having mitral valve prolapse.

W. Proctor Harvey, M.D.

Dyspnea, Orthopnea, and Paroxysmal Nocturnal Dyspnea

Dyspnea (shortness of breath) as an isolated symptom does not always indicate cardiac failure. Pulmonary, thoracic cage, and thoracic muscle abnormalities are equally important diagnostic considerations; more benign entities such as anxiety and panic disorders may also exhibit this symptom. In hospitalized patients, five diagnostic entities account for 66% of patients whose principal com-

TABLE 2
New York Heart Association Functional Status Classification

Class I	– Symptoms only with unusual exertion. No symptoms with ordinary activity.
Class II	– Symptoms with ordinary exertion.
Class III	– Symptoms with minimal exertion
Class IV	– Symptoms at rest.

plaint is dyspnea, left ventricular failure, asthma, chronic obstructive lung disease, cardiac tachyarrhythmias, and bacterial pneumonia. Unless there is associated orthopnea and/or paroxysmal nocturnal dyspnea, the clinical judgement on the cause of dyspnea requires correlation of physical examination and/or additional diagnostic tests.

Paroxysmal nocturnal dyspnea is a breathless sensation which awakens patients 2 to 4 hours after having fallen asleep. It is presumed that gradual resorption of interstitial fluid, resulting in increased intravascular volume causes elevation of pulmonary venous pressure, interstitial edema or even alveolar edema. The resulting increased work of breathing then awakens the patient. By its occurrence, it implies that mean left atrial pressure is elevated to start with and that the intravascular fluid shift occurring after a period of recumbency is sufficient to make the patient symptomatic.

Orthopnea represents breathlessness upon assuming the recumbent position. As such, it represents a more advanced state of left heart failure than the patient who only experiences paroxysmal nocturnal dyspnea. Increased venous return from the lower extremities and abdomen resulting from the recumbent position is sufficient to further increase pulmonary venous pressure and increase breathing to the point at which the patient is aware of it. While, typically, elevation of the head and upper trunk is needed for relief, in its milder form, the patient experiences cough on recumbency.

Presence of paroxysmal nocturnal dyspnea and/or orthopnea in association with effort dyspnea identifies left heart failure and directs attention to conditions which affect the left heart such as obstruction at mitral valve level, or left ventricular abnormalities associated with elevation of left ventricular end-diastolic pressure. Like the previous discussion on chest pain, it is valuable to obtain information from clinical history of the circumstances which brought on the symptoms.

For example, a history that these symptoms started only after development of palpitation perceived as a rapid irregular heart beat suggest that onset of rapid atrial fibrillation was the precipitating event. Loss of "atrial kick" and resulting symptoms would suggest conditions associated with a diminished left ventricular compliance, such as a hypertrophied left ventricle.

In a young female with rapid atrial fibrillation and resulting decrease in diastolic filling period, symptoms raise the possibility of mitral stenosis as the underlying cardiac pathology.

In patients with effort dyspnea, it is useful to categorize their functional state using the New York Heart Association's functional cardiac classifications (Table 2). It is of value in following a patient's clinical course and response to treatment, as well as for providing other physicians some objective measure of the patient's functional state.

Peripheral Edema

Leg edema does not always imply right heart failure. More commonly, it is due to local reasons rather than cardiac disease. When leg edema and/or ascites is a manifestation of right heart failure, it is valuable to note the associated elevated mean venous pressure (jugular venous pressure) and congestive hepatomegaly on physical examination.

Fatigue

This symptom is also not specific for cardiac disease and is more commonly due to non-cardiac causes; however, it can be a complaint of patients with cardiac disease. Often it occurs with other symptoms such as those of left ventricular failure and abnormalities demonstrated on physical examination. In cardiac disease, the symptom usually implies a low or inadequate cardiac output, especially when fatigue is constant and present even after a sound night's rest.

An example would be the patient with severe mitral regurgitation and chronic left ventricular failure. It can also be the result of vigorous diuresis in patients in congestive failure. It has been suggested that excess fatigue and feelings of general malaise may represent premonitory symptoms of future coronary events.

Syncope or Near-Syncope

There are many non-cardiac causes for dizziness or syncope. However, it is an important symptom of various forms of obstruction to left ventricular outflow. It should especially be considered if there is associated angina and/or symptoms of left ventricular failure. Intracardiac mass lesions such as right or left atrial myxoma can present with syncope.

Slow cardiac rates such as complete heart block, or rapid rates such as ventricular tachycardia or fibrillation, can also result in syncope; it is not a symptom usually associated with supraventricular tachycardias. Effort syncope, especially in a young female with no murmurs, should raise suspicion for primary pulmonary hypertension.

Physical examination will usually provide confirmatory evidence in the form of a giant "A" wave in the jugular venous pulse, a second left interspace lift over the pulmonary artery, a palpable, loud pulmonic valve closure sound (P_2), and the left parasternal lift of right ventricular hypertrophy. Syncope in a cyanotic patient should raise the possibility of Tetralogy of Fallot.

Palpitations

This symptom refers to a patient's awareness of their heartbeat. The careful history taker can usually discern whether the patient is simply aware of a forceful heartbeat as a result of excitement or apprehension, or whether the patient is aware of the more forceful, larger stroke volume of a post extra-systolic beat. The latter is usually described as a sensation of something "flopping" over in the chest or throat, a "flip-flop", "fluttering", "skipping", or "jumping". It may represent a sensation of a tachyarrhythmia.

For the latter instance, it is helpful to obtain the patient's perception of onset and offset of the rapid rhythm - i.e., sudden or gradual. Paroxysmal atrial tachycardia usually has a sudden onset and offset. Sometimes patients can relate maneuvers they have learned to terminate these episodes, such as inducing gagging, or briefly immersing their face in a bucket of cold water. It is also helpful to ascertain the patient's perception of the regular or chaotic nature of the tachycardia. Dr. W. Proctor Harvey usually would place a hand over the precordium and mimic the various arrhythmias by tapping the hand over the precordium and inquiring which resembles what the patient feels during those episodes.

In some, a history of marked diuresis during or shortly after the tachycardia can be obtained. In those instances, dysrhythmia is usually paroxysmal atrial tachycardia and, less commonly, paroxysmal atrial fibrillation.

Hemoptysis

Coughing up blood occurs from cardiac and non-cardiac causes. However, the character and circumstance of hemoptysis can be helpful in diagnostic considerations. The "pink, frothy" sputum resulting from the mix of air, alveolar edema fluid and red blood cells is characteristic of the hemoptysis in acute pulmonary edema.

The blood-streaked sputum from coughing spells in bronchitis, the rusty-colored or bloody sputum of pulmonary infarction, and the spontaneously welling up of bright red blood from rupture of bronchial submucosal veins in mitral stenosis are features obtainable by a careful clinical history.

Having obtained a detailed clinical history, it is useful to formulate diagnostic possibilities and, where possible, mentally list them in descending order of probability. For example, in a patient with palpitation, effort dyspnea, and orthopnea, one considers all possible clinical entities that can result in left ventricular failure.

However, the additional information that the palpitation suggests atrial fibrillation, that its onset preceded the dyspnea and orthopnea, that previous episodes of syncope and near syncope have occurred, or that a sibling died young of unexplained causes would all lead the physician to place hypertrophic cardiomyopathy high on the list of diagnostic possibilities.

In another patient with similar palpitation suggesting atrial fibrillation preceding the onset of effort dyspnea and orthopnea, and who has had spontaneous bright red hemoptysis in the past, mitral stenosis would be a more likely diagnostic consideration. Diagnostic inferences derived from the clinical history ensures a focused physical examination which then either strengthens the original hypothesis or directs the physician to one or more of the other diagnostic considerations. This approach also helps to determine what, if any, other diagnostic tests are needed to establish a diagnosis sufficient to enable appropriate determination of prognosis or therapeutic action. Generation of a hypothesis is an essential element of the diagnostic process and cannot be emphasized enough.

Physical Examination

Once the physician has formulated a working hypothesis based on a careful clinical history, the physical examination can then be conducted to either corroborate or deny this hypothesis. On occasion, the physical findings demand that a new hypothesis be considered. In an asymptomatic patient, the first hypothesis for diagnostic possibility occurs after the physical examination.

In the case where hypertrophic cardiomyopathy was the leading diagnostic possibility, physical examination can confirm presence of atrial fibrillation, brisk bifid arterial pulse, normal pulse pressure, a lower parasternal and apical systolic ejection murmur, as well as absence of the diastolic

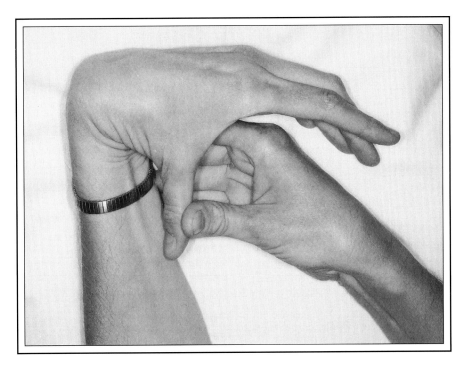

Figure 2. Joint hyperextensibility in a patient with Marfan's Syndrome.

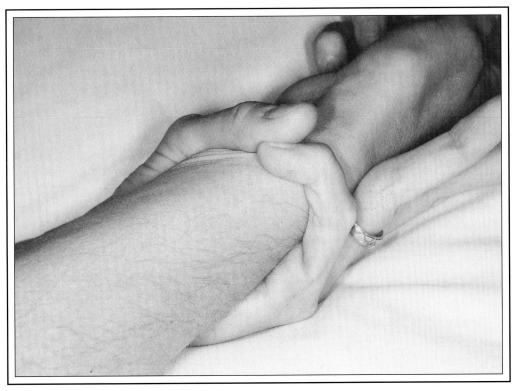

Figure 3. The "wrist sign" in a patient with Marfan's Syndrome; note how readily the wrist is encircled by the thumb and 5th digit.

decrescendo murmur of aortic regurgitation; all would tend to support the original hypothesis.

Furthermore, if the patient's clinical status permits, it would ensure that the physician takes time to observe the response of the systolic murmur to bedside maneuvers. Such corroboration of the initial hypothesis might then make the physician decide that the single most important therapeutic maneuver would be to restore normal sinus rhythm as promptly as possible. An echocardiogram would then be the definitive diagnostic test.

The physical examination provides objective clues for the physician and is valuable in that it is now dependent upon the physician's skills, and not subject to the patient's ability to communicate, or their reliability as a historian. Aspects of the physi-

11

cal examination most rewarding in helping a diagnosis are inspection, palpation, and auscultation.

Appearance and Habitus

Facial and general appearance, cutaneous lesions, body habitus, musculoskeletal abnormalities, cyanosis, and clubbing can provide clues to presence and type of heart disease.

Marfan's Syndrome is characterized by an abnormally wide arm span, arachnodactyly, and joint hyperextensibility (Figure 2). The "wrist" sign (Figure 3), grasping the wrist of the opposite hand proximal to the styloid process using the thumb and fifth finger and showing a 1 to 2 cm overlap, and the "thumb" sign (Figure 4), having the patient make a fist over the clenched thumb and demonstrating that the thumb extends significantly beyond the ulnar aspect of the hand, can all be useful in identifying patients with Marfan's Syndrome.

The cardiovascular abnormalities noted in this syndrome include aneurysmal dilatation of the ascending aorta, aortic dissection, aortic regurgitation, mitral and tricuspid regurgitation, mitral valve prolapse, and chordal rupture which may be spontaneous or secondary to bacterial endocarditis.

Down's Syndrome (Trisomy 21) can be recognized by the "mongoloid" appearance due to the widely set eyes, upward slanting palpebral fissures, epi-

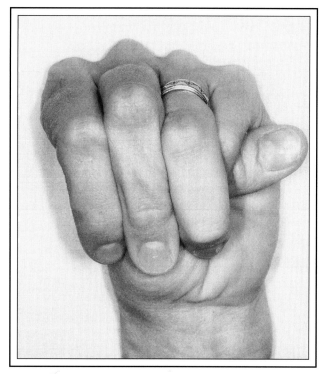

Figure 4. The "thumb sign" in a patient with Marfan's Syndrome. Note how much of the thumb extends beyond the ulnar aspect of the hand as it is grasped by the other fingers.

canthal folds, and large tongue. The cardiovascular abnormality associated with this syndrome is usually a persistent common atrioventricular canal.

Turners Syndrome (XO Chromosomal Anomaly) is recognized in a female with short stature, neck webbing, cubitus valgus, a shield-like chest, and facies characterized by a small mandible, prominent ears, ptosis, and epicanthal folds. The cardiovascular anomaly commonly noted is co-arctation of the aorta.

Ullrich-Noonan Syndrome represents patients with the physical characteristics of Turner's Syndrome but who have XX or XY Chromosomes. Pulmonary stenosis secondary to a dysplastic valve is the most common cardiac lesion.

There are many other entities with known associated cardiovascular lesions such as the Holt-Oram Syndrome, associated with secundum atrial septal defect and ventricular septal defect; the patient with ankylosing spondylitis who may have mitral or aortic regurgitation. Acromegaly, scleroderma, osteogenesis imperfecta, or muscular dystrophy are some additional entities recognizable from their physical appearance with known associated cardiovascular abnormalities.

Familiarity with these associations enable the physician to focus the search for confirmatory evidence of the expected abnormality during the rest of the physical examination.

Jugular Venous Pulse

Although examination of the jugular venous pulse is brief, it tends to be ignored or, if comment is made, limited to the observation of whether it is "distended" or not. Measurement of mean venous pressure and observation of the wave form can provide information about right heart pathophysiologic events which, when correlated with the other clinical symptoms and the rest of the physical examination, can lead to diagnostic conclusions.

Obvious elevation of mean jugular pressure (>7 cm of blood) would contribute supporting evidence if one is considering right heart failure, right ventricular infarction, tricuspid obstruction, constrictive pericarditis or cardiac tamponade. It can be useful in following the patient's clinical course during therapy and conversely, alert the physician about deteriorating hemodynamic status as mean venous pressure begins to rise.

It has been shown that a 4 cm to 5 cm (blood) rise in mean venous pressure, maintained for ten seconds, as a result of applying mid-abdominal pressure (20 mm Hg force) suggest an elevated pulmonary artery wedge pressure unless right ventricular infarction is present.

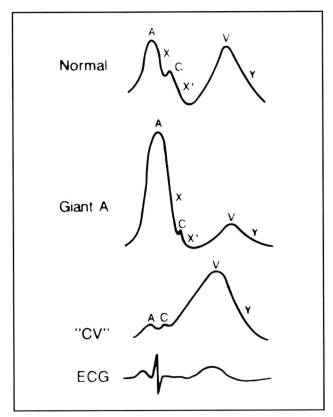

Figure 5. Diagrammatic representation of a giant "A" wave and abnormal "CV" wave compared to a normal jugular venous wave form. (From de Leon AC and Cheng TO with permission).

Inspiratory rise of mean venous pressure (Kussmaul's sign) is a sign of restriction to right ventricular filling and thus noted in constrictive pericarditis.

Recognition of a giant "A" wave (large, regularly occurring "A" waves) raises the possibility of tricuspid stenosis or atresia, significant pulmonic stenosis or pulmonary hypertension, or pathology resulting in significantly diminished diastolic compliance of the right ventricle (Figure 5). On occasion, this large "A" wave may be appreciated as pre-systolic pulsation of the liver.

Cannon "A" waves are large intermittent "A" waves of varying amplitude resulting from atrial contraction against a closed mitral valve. They therefore serve as a clue to forms of atrio-ventricular dissociation, and can be noted during ventricular extrasystoles, complete heart block, and with electronic right ventricular pacing.

Abnormal "V" waves are a hallmark of significant tricuspid regurgitation (Figure 5). It is systolic in time, and the large systolic expansion of the internal jugular vein (especially to the right) results in visible leftward head nodding ("no, no sign"). On occasion, in patients with severe tricuspid regurgitation and incompetent venous valves, systolic pulsation can be observed in visible varicose veins. In some with elevated mean venous pressure and severe regurgitation, systolic pulsation of the eyeballs may be observed.

Routine observation of the jugular venous waveforms develops expertise and a "sense" of normal amplitudes and rates of descent (X and Y). Such an observer may then recognize a slow rate of Y descent relative to the height of the "V" wave and be able to infer the presence of tricuspid stenosis. The practiced examiner can also better appreciate

A more recent study suggests that mean jugular venous pressure >7cm and/or a positive abdomino-jugular test as outlined above has an 81% sensitivity, 80% specificity, and 81% predictive accuracy for elevation of the pulmonary capillary wedge pressure to ≥18 mm Hg in patients with chronic left ventricular dysfunction.

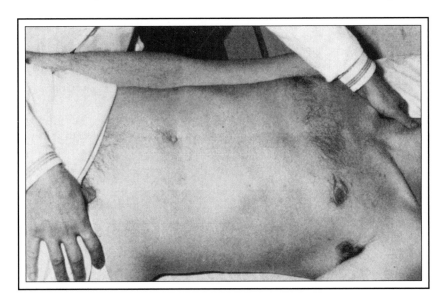

Figure 6. Simultaneous palpation of carotid and femoral arteries. (From de Leon AC and Harvey WP with permission).

the "M" or "W" shaped venous pulse created by the brisk X and Y descents in a patient with an elevated mean venous pressure and constrictive pericarditis or restricted cardiomyopathy.

Arterial Pulse

Palpation of the arterial pulse readily provides information about rate (regular and irregular) rhythms. Additionally, palpation of all major peripheral arteries, and especially simultaneous comparisons, can provide information on specific vessel stenosis or obstruction. One of the earliest clues to the presence of co-arctation of the aorta can come from comparison of the right carotid with the femoral artery (Figure 6). In adults, developed collateral circulation usually results in a femoral pulse, but simultaneous comparison with the right brachial allows the examiner to more readily appreciate the lower amplitude and/or late arrival of the femoral pulse.

By varying the degree of compression of a large peripheral artery (usually the brachial or carotids) information about the rate of rise, character of the

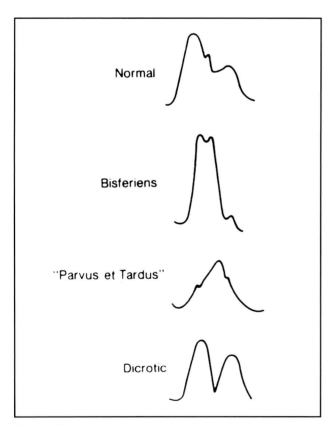

Figure 7. Diagrammatic representation of some arterial pulses.
Top: Normal
2nd: Bisferiens pulse
3rd: Slow-rising and late peaking (parvus et tardus)
4th: Dicrotic pulse
(From de Leon AC and Cheng TO with permission).

peak and/or presence of a dicrotic wave can be appreciated. Furthermore, the examiner also obtains an impression of the rigidity or elasticity of the arterial wall. The small amplitude and sometime discernible slow rate of rise can be consistent with left ventricular failure. Alternation of the rate of rise and/or peak (pulsus alternans) strongly suggest a left ventricle with diminished ejection fraction. When the small amplitude pulse has a "shudder" as it rises to a late peak (pulsus parvus et tardus – Figure 7), valvar aortic stenosis should be the first consideration.

On the other hand, a patient with a clinical history of effort syncope, angina, and/or symptoms of left heart failure (i.e. the history suggests aortic stenosis as a possibility), whose arterial pulse is brisk-rising and even twin-peaked, hypertrophic cardiomyopathy (IHSS) would be the more likely possibility. Usually, the bifid, rapid rising pulse (water hammer or Corrigan pulse) is a characteristic of significant aortic regurgitation or of a patent ductus arteriosus (Figure 7). In patients with a low cardiac output and high peripheral vascular resistance, as is often the case in dilated cardiomyopathy, a diastolic wave (dicrotic wave) is felt after the systolic peak (Figure 7). More recently, experimental data suggest that the dicrotic wave is not actually exaggerated. Rather, reduction of the systolic upstroke, together with a normal amplitude of the incisural down slope and rebound is responsible for the "double" pulse felt. The arterial pulse which substantially decreases or even disappears on inspiration is called a paradoxical pulse. A blood pressure inspiratory decrease of greater than 10 mm Hg systolic pressure is also usually present. Although it is most commonly noted in chronic obstructive lung disease, in the context of possible heart disease, constrictive pericarditis or pericardial effusion with tamponade should be considered.

Precordium

Palpation of the point of maximum impulse (PMI) is commonly construed to represent the left ventricular apex. However, this is not always so, since in right ventricular hypertrophy the point of maximum impulse is caused by the right ventricle. In 1908, McKenzie pointed out ". . . . . confusion in regard to the correct interpretation of the heart movements has arisen from associating the shock conveyed to the chest wall with the cardiac apex".

In the normal heart, this impulse is brief and although caused by the left ventricle as it contracts to initiate systole, does not necessarily represent the anatomic apex of the heart. However, by common usage, the point of maximum impulse is com-

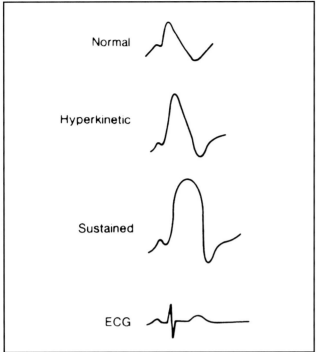

Figure 8. Diagrammatic representation of apical motion.
Top: Normal
2nd: Hyperkinetic apical impulse
3rd: Sustained (hypertrophied) apical thrust with pre-systolic motion from "atrial" kick
(From de Leon AC and Cheng TO with permission).

monly referred to as the apex beat. If one accepts that this point of maximum impulse which we refer to as the cardiac apex does not necessarily represent the anatomic apex, it is easier to understand the poor correlation of apex beat location relative to the mid-clavicular line or mid-sternal line cardio-thoracic ratio by chest x-ray, or volume measurement by echocardiography.

Observation and palpation of the point of maximum impulse (PMI) is still a useful clinical tool. In the supine position, patients with increased left ventricular volume have a laterally displaced PMI, although lateral displacement alone does not always mean increased left ventricular volume.

More importantly, in a volume loaded left ventricle, observing the activity in the region of the apex usually reveals rather diffuse motion instead of a small isolated thrust (Figure 8). By echocardiographic correlation, an apical diameter greater than 3 cm has been shown to be a good indicator of left ventricular enlargement. As emphasized previously, this as well as other physical examination findings must still be correlated before definitive conclusions are made.

The outward thrust of the PMI may also have duration and thus feel "sustained" (Figure 8). Pre-

systolic outward motion may be seen and felt and when present represents left atrial contraction and is a mechanical counterpart of the S_4. Presence of these findings usually suggests left ventricular hypertrophy, but they are also encountered in coronary artery disease.

In coronary artery disease, a sustained apical thrust represents abnormal left ventricular function. When a pre-systolic ("atrial kick") component is also present, moderate left ventricular dysfunction is usually present. Whether the "atrial kick" is felt and/or heard as an S_4, conditions associated with increased left ventricular diastolic stiffness should be considered. A double systolic outward thrust is often noted in IHSS, although by itself is not specific for the entity. The "atrial kick" commonly present in conjunction with the double outward systolic thrust results in a palpatory sensation that has been referred to as a "triple ripple" (Figure 9). For purposes of better appreciating these characteristics of the apical impulse, examination should also be carried out with the patient in the left lateral decubitus.

When the PMI is caused by the left ventricle, retraction medial to it may be observed. Systolic outward motion in the area just medial and above the PMI is abnormal and can represent a clue to left ventricular wall dyskinesia (Figure 10).

Motion in the immediate left parasternal area is

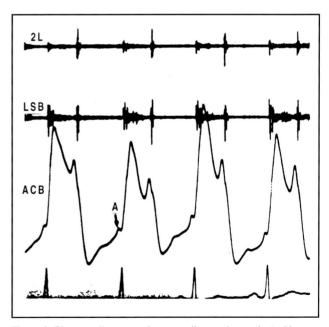

Figure 9. Phonocardiogram and apex cardiogram in a patient with obstructive hypertrophic cardiomyopathy (IHSS). Note the pre-systolic wave (A) and the double systolic peaks of the apex cardiogram. The systolic murmur associated with this condition is recorded best at the lower sternal border (LSB). (From de Leon AC and Cheng TO with permission).

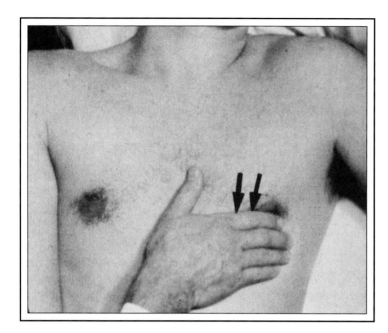

Figure 10. Outward impulse in systole made by the ventricular aneurysm (arrow). (From de Leon AC and Harvey WP with permission).

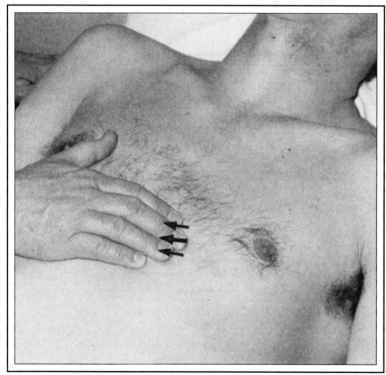

Figure 11. Location of parasternal lift caused by the right ventricle (arrows). (From de Leon AC and Harvey WP with permission).

usually ascribed to the right ventricle (Figure 11). When the systolic outward motion begins with the PMI, this usually represents right ventricular hypertrophy. Retraction lateral to the PMI would further suggest that the hypertrophied right ventricle occupies the PMI. When this left parasternal lift occurs in late rather than early systole, there is a "rocking" motion between the PMI and left parasternal area. Severe mitral regurgitation should be considered since the late parasternal lift is caused by left atrial expansion in systole.

It is also worthwhile to palpate throughout the precordium for additional clues. A systolic lift at the second left interspace, especially with a concurrently palpable second heart sound, should raise consideration for significant pulmonary hypertension. Thrills may also be appreciated. Location and direction of a thrill can reduce the diagnostic possibilities. For example, a left parasternal versus an apical systolic thrill may help distinguish between a ventricular septal defect and mitral regurgitation - both of which generate a holosystolic murmur.

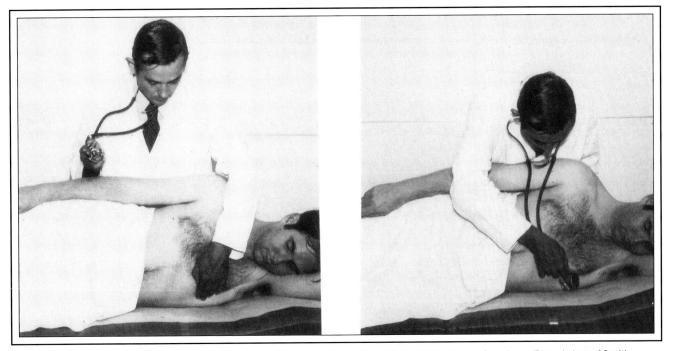

Figure 12. The left lateral decubitus position, finding the cardiac apex and ausculting with the bell for S_3 and S_4 gallops. (From de Leon AC with permission).

When a murmur is loud and widely transmitted, it can be difficult to decide where it is loudest; location of the thrill could then be helpful. Thrills are not always systolic although most of them are. An apical diastolic thrill, especially with a palpable first heart sound, is likely to represent rheumatic mitral stenosis.

Auscultation

The basic purpose of cardiac auscultation is to deduce or infer normal as well as pathophysiologic alterations of the heart based upon audible events after examining the thorax and precordium. Thus, to simply go through the motion of placing the stethoscope over various portions of the precordium and note sounds heard without further thought given to them, or correlation with other physical findings and the clinical history, defeats its purpose and represents a waste of the examiner's time. If the examiner is to obtain useful information, it is essential to identify cardiac systole from diastole.

Correctly identifying the first and second heart sound is therefore a paramount first step. With slow and normal heart rates, this task is usually easy, but with more rapid heart rates can be a more difficult task. Simultaneous palpation of the apex beat, or an arterial pulse to identify systole, and thus the first heart sound (S_1) which immediately precedes it, are methods used.

When heart rate is rapid, quick, and almost instantaneous, correlation between tactile sense and hearing, or eye and hearing can be difficult for some. The alternative is to utilize the same sense (hearing) to accomplish this task. Dr. W. Proctor Harvey has advocated "inching" as a means of recognizing the first (S_1) from the second heart sound (S_2). He has suggested using the stethoscope diaphragm, and starts at the second (right or left) interspace to note the loudest sound which is usually S_2. When S_2 splitting is present, this further aids in its identification.

Then, listening for a few cardiac cycles at a time, he listens sequentially at the 3rd left, 4th left, 5th left and lastly the cardiac apex, keeping in mind the sound representing S_2. From this, S_1 is deduced, since it gets louder as one approaches the apex and S_2 gets softer. From this point on, the interval between S_1 and S_2 defines systole, and the interval between S_2 and the following S_1 diastole.

The examiner should also develop the ability to concentrate ("tune in") to one sound event at a time while temporarily ignoring ("tune out") other sound events. In this manner, details such as intensity, character, and splitting can be more readily noted. Routinely drawing a diagram of the sounds and murmurs heard and represented in one cardiac cycle is one way to ensure that each event has been adequately assessed.

To obtain the greatest possible information from auscultation, the examiner should strive, when cir-

17

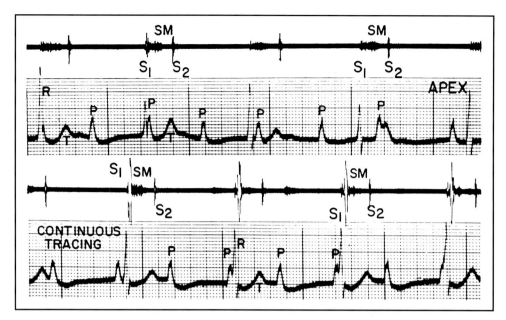

Figure 13. Continuous tracing: Phonocardiogram and electrocardiogram in a patient with complete heart block. Note the systolic murmur (SM), the changing intensity of the first heart sound (S$_1$) and the lack of conduction from atria (P) to ventricle (R) in the electrocardiogram. (From de Leon AC and Harvey WP with permission).

cumstances permit, to achieve a quiet room, a comfortable patient (and examiner), and eliminate sources of extraneous noise. Depending upon the auscultatory events sought for, the patient should be examined supine, in the left lateral decubitus (Figure 12; right if the patient has dextrocardia), sitting and standing, leaning forward, as well as utilizing various bedside maneuvers.

The examiner should be aware that the stethoscope bell, applied lightly, is best for low frequency events (such as gallops), and that the diaphragm piece applied firmly is best for higher frequency events (such as heart sounds and most murmurs). As previously mentioned, the diagnostic differential evolved from the clinical history and other aspects of the physical examination also directs the examiner to a concerted search for specific findings on auscultation.

• First Heart Sound (S$_1$)

The first heart sound is usually split — the splitting being best appreciated along the lower left sternal edge (4th and 5th interspaces). The first component is due to mitral valve closure (M$_1$) and is normally the louder component. The second component due to tricuspid valve closure (T$_1$) is softer and thus best heard over the right ventricle. The sound results from the abrupt deceleration of the valve structures at the point of maximal travel toward their respective atria.

Rate of acceleration of ventricular pressure rise at the moment of valve closure is an important determinant of the intensity of S$_1$. Since this rate of pressure development progressively increases in early systole, the later the A-V valve closes, the louder the valve closure sound produced. Position of the mitral valve leaflets at the onset of systole also influences intensity. A loud M$_1$ is a hallmark of mitral stenosis, and is also seen when the PR interval is short, as well as in conditions associated with increased left ventricular contractility.

A softer M$_1$ occurs when mitral leaflets are almost in a closed position, such as in 1st degree A-V heart block and when left ventricular contractility is impaired (acute myocardial infarction). It is absent when mitral valve closure occurs in diastole in some patients with acute severe aortic regurgitation.

The tricuspid component (T$_1$) is loud in atrial septal defect and in Ebstein's anomaly. Variation in

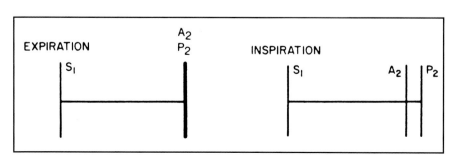

Figure 14. Diagrammatic representation of the first heart sound (S$_1$) and the second heart sounds (A$_2$ and P$_2$). Aortic valve closure (A$_2$) and pulmonic valve closure (P$_2$) are heard separately (split) on inspiration but occur simultaneously on expiration. This is normal physiologic splitting of the second heart sound. (From de Leon AC with permission).

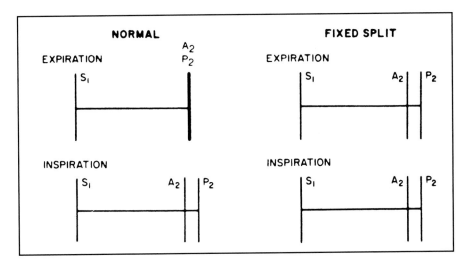

Figure 15. Diagrammatic representation of "fixed" splitting of the second heart sound (A_2, P_2) compared to physiologic splitting (normal). (From de Leon AC with permission).

intensity of the first heart sound occurs in complete heart block (Figure 13), A-V dissociation, and atrial flutter-fibrillation. Variation in position of the mitral leaflets at the time of ventricular systole is responsible for the changing intensity of S_1.

• **Second Heart Sound**

The sound produced by aortic semilunar valve closure (A_2) and pulmonary semilunar valve closure (P_2) constitute the two components of the second heart sound (S_2).

In the normal sound, A_2 precedes P_2 and this separation (splitting) increases with inspiration and decreases (or becomes single) on expiration. This sequence of splitting is also referred to as "physiologic" (Figure 14). When onset of right ventricular systole is delayed (e.g. RBBB), P_2 is also delayed and this normal splitting becomes exagger-

ated, such that the second sound does not become single on expiration. Other causes of delay in P_2 such as pulmonic stenosis, idiopathic dilatation of the pulmonary artery, and right ventricular failure can also result in exaggerated splitting of S_2.

Persistent delay of P_2 results in a "fixed" S_2 splitting - a hallmark of left to right shunts at atrial level - particularly atrial septal defect (Figure 15). The inspiratory delay in P_2 is caused by the delay in occurrence of the dicrotic notch in the pulmonary arterial pressure ("hang-out") occasioned by the inspiratory decrease in pulmonary vascular impedance. In atrial septal defect, this increased capacitance of the pulmonary vascular bed results in the persistent delay in P_2.

Exaggerated splitting is not always because P_2 is delayed. An earlier A_2 can also increase the degree of splitting. This may be encountered in patients

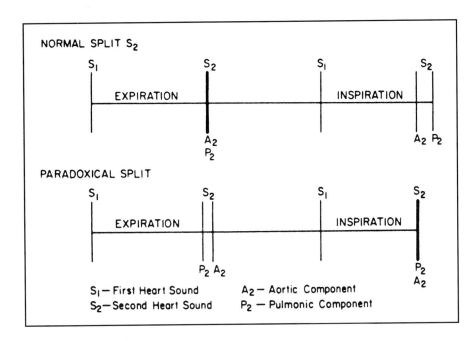

Figure 16. Diagrammatic representation of reversed or "paradoxical" splitting of the second heart sound compared to normal. Note the reversal in sequence of second heart sound components (P_2 and A_2) resulting in splitting on expiration. The reverse of normal (co-incident P_2 and A_2) occurs on inspiration. (From de Leon AC with permission).

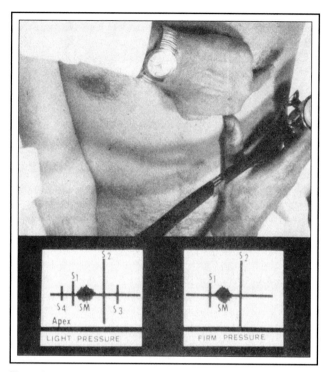

Figure 17. With the patient in the left lateral decubitus and the point of maximum impulse identified, the pressure with which the stethoscope bell is held against the chest wall may determine whether an S_3 or S_4 gallop is heard. Note that gallops may disappear with firm pressure. (From de Leon AC and Harvey WP with permission).

with severe mitral regurgitation or in a large left to right shunt ventricular septal defect. In these cases, the unloaded left ventricle has a shorter systolic ejection time. In any patient thought to have "fixed" or exaggerated splitting, the finding is not definitive until similarly demonstrated while auscultation is carried out in the sitting position. This is especially important in children and adolescents.

When the normal A_2 P_2 sequence is reversed such as encountered in complete left bundle branch block, the S_2 components are single or almost single on inspiration, and more widely split on expiration. This reversal from normal is referred to as a "paradoxic" split (Figure 16). In addition to complete left bundle branch block, conditions which prolong left ventricular ejection can result in paradoxic splitting. Thus it may be encountered in severe aortic stenosis and in myocardial ischemia.

It is also of value to pay attention to the intensity of A_2 or P_2. The sound is accentuated in systemic hypertension (A_2) and pulmonary hypertension (P_2). Intensity of semilunar valve closure sound relates to the rate of ventricular pressure decline and thus the rate of pressure gradient change across the valve.

In some patients, especially the elderly, A_2 may have a "tambour" quality in the absence of abnormal elevation in aortic diastolic pressure. A dilated

aortic root resulting in stretched and taut aortic cusp on closure is a possible explanation. A diminished intensity of P_2 is noted in association with a delay in severe pulmonic stenosis. In calcific aortic stenosis, the resulting diminished mobility of the aortic cusps results in a soft or even inaudible A_2. Thus in this entity (aortic stenosis), a single second heart sound (P_2) is most commonly encountered.

• Diastolic Gallops

The third heart sound (S_3) and fourth heart sound (S_4) are also referred to as ventricular diastolic gallop and atrial diastolic gallop respectively. Both are low-frequency events and of relatively lower intensity than the first and second heart sounds. Because of these characteristics, they are more difficult to hear and probably explain the inter-observer variability noted for S_3. Experience however improves yield as has been shown for S_4.

The experienced examiner learns to integrate precordial inspection and palpation with auscultation. Additionally, technique is also important. It has been shown that the amplitude of apical diastolic sounds and movements are greater in the left lateral compared to the supine position. This positioning plus the proper use of the stethoscope bell (i.e. lightly applied to just obtain a skin seal; Figure 17) will enhance yield in appreciating these low frequency events.

The third heart sound (S_3) occurs in early diastole, usually 0.14 to 0.16 second after the second heart sound. It is common in the young and in the absence of any cardiac abnormality, is referred to as a physiologic third heart sound. It tends to disappear with age as the left ventricle increases thickness in the process of growth from childhood to adulthood. This change in left ventricular compliance results in a decrease in early diastolic filling and rate of deceleration of inflow, resulting in diminution of the amplitude of S_3 and its audibility.

In the middle aged and older adult, its presence could be a clue to heart disease. Its appearance in this age group suggests increased left ventricular wall thickness, impaired relaxation and increased resistance to filling (Figure 18); it can thus be one of the early signs of heart failure. In patients with moderate to severe mitral regurgitation, the increased volume of flow into the left ventricle in early diastole also contributes to the generation of S_3 (Figure 19). A similar situation results from a large left to right shunt due to ventricular septal defect. Conversely, this auditory event cannot occur in the presence of tight mitral stenosis. Although the foregoing discussion relates to a left ventricular S_3, it should be remembered that right ventricular

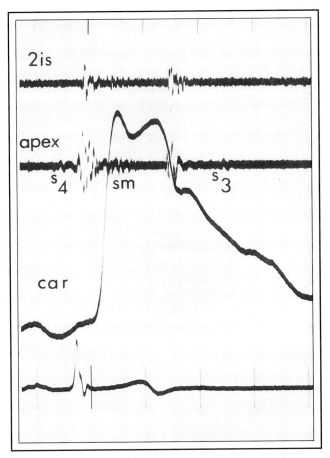

Figure 18. Note the S₄ (atrial gallop) and S₃ (ventricular diastolic gallop) at the apex recorded as a low-frequency event. (From de Leon AC with permission).

However, a normal intensity of S_1 and absence of a diastolic rumble should deny the possibility of rheumatic mitral stenosis. A possibility in the differential could be a tumor plop which would be an uncommon finding.

The fourth heart sound (S_4) is not a common finding in normal children and young adults. It is, however, a frequent finding in patients with a stiff, non-compliant ventricle and thus encountered in significant aortic stenosis, hypertrophic cardiomyopathy, systemic hypertension, acute myocardial infarction, ischemic heart disease, during episodes of angina, and in dilated cardiomyopathy (Figure 18). Right ventricular origin of S_4 can also occur in similar circumstances of a stiff, non-compliant right ventricle.

Occurrence of an S_4 in other conditions such as in first degree A-V block and its frequency in the older age group tends to detract from its usefulness as an isolated finding. Furthermore, the inexperienced observer can confuse a split S_1 with an S_4. However, when presystolic distension is visible and palpable, and correlation with the rest of the clinical history and physical findings are made, the S_4 is usually significant. Its absence in certain circumstances - such as a patient with chest pain and suspected of having an acute myocardial infarction or angina, should make one reconsider these diagnostic possibilities.

In patients seen in congestive failure with sinus tachycardia, the S_3 and S_4 may occur simultane-

S_3 occur and can be recognized by inspiratory augmentation of intensity and correlation with other physical findings.

Recent studies suggest that the S_3 results from the sudden limitation of longitudinal expansion of the left ventricle during early diastolic filling. It is likely that this abrupt deceleration sets up vibrations of the ventricular wall resulting in the sound. In patients with marked cardiomegaly, the ventricle may actually strike the chest wall in early diastole producing a loud sound of similar timing and has been called a ventricular knock sound.

Studies suggest that this could also be a mechanism for generation of S_3. A change in the intensity of S_3 can be helpful in following the patient's clinical course. It tends to decrease in intensity, or even disappear as heart failure improves. Its continued loud presence usually implies a poor prognosis. In constrictive pericarditis, the S_3 sound occurs earlier (0.10 to 0.12 second), tends to have a higher frequency than the usual gallop and is called a pericardial knock sound. Because of its early location in diastole, it can be mistaken for an opening snap.

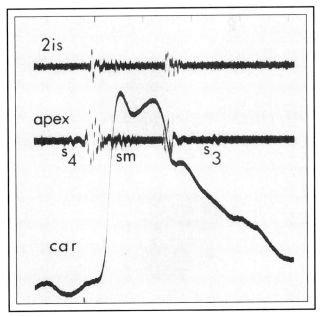

Figure 19. A patient with mitral regurgitation. Recorded at the apex are the first heart sound (S_1), the second heart sound (S_2), a third heart sound (S_3) and a holosystolic murmur (SM). (From de Leon AC with permission).

21

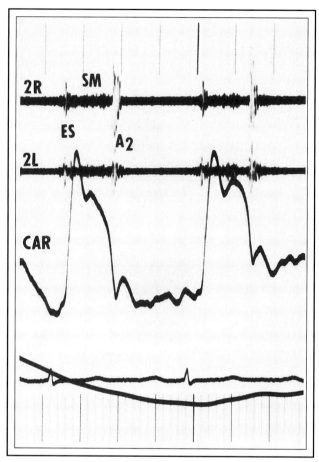

Figure 20. A patient with congenital bicuspid aortic valve and resulting mild aortic stenosis. Note the aortic ejection sound (ES) and the systolic ejection murmur (SM) following it. (From de Leon AC with permission).

ously or close together (summation gallop). The resulting sound may be louder than the first and second heart sound and result in mistiming systole and diastole. The issue is readily resolved by repeating the examination as failure improves and the heart rate decreases.

In patients presenting in congestive heart failure with no audible S_3 but with a loud S_4, one should suspect the possibility that the congestive failure results primarily from diastolic ventricular dysfunction.

The technique involved in eliciting an S_4 is similar to that utilized for an S_3. Listening at the cardiac point of maximum impulse in the left lateral decubitus maximizes yield (Figure 12). Also, using the stethoscope bell held lightly over the skin will emphasize the lower frequency events (Figure 17). Since a split S_1 or S_1-ejection sound represent the differential with S_4-S_1, one should take advantage of the higher frequency characteristics of the former two options.

One quick way is to alternately press firmly or

lightly with the bell. Pressing firmly stretches the skin and converts it to a "diaphragm". The S_4 gallop decreases in intensity or disappears on firm pressure (Figure 17) while S_1 split or S_1-ejection sound becomes sharper and distinct. An alternative would be to shift from stethoscope bell to stethoscope diaphragm.

Additionally, an S_4 is rarely loud enough to transmit to the left or right second interspace where ejection sounds tend to be loudest. A left ventricular S_4 is usually confined to the left ventricular PMI and should not be louder and better heard along the lower left sternal border where a split S_1 is best appreciated.

Of course, a right ventricular S_4 will be better heard along the lower left sternal border and xiphoid area but demonstrating inspiratory augmentation of the sound will identify it's right sided origin. When all else fails, correlation with the rest of the physical findings and the clinical history will often shed light on the correct option.

• **Sounds in Systole**

There are two important categories of sound most frequently encountered in systole: ejection sound and systolic clicks.

The ejection sound is a high-frequency sound noted at the onset of ventricular systole. Most frequently, they occur at the time of maximal opening travel of an abnormal semilunar valve (Figure 20) and less commonly when the great vessel (aorta or pulmonary artery) is dilated.

The pulmonic ejection sound is of right-sided origin and, when due to a stenotic pulmonary valve, is usually followed by an ejection systolic murmur (Figure 21). The ejection murmur may be of variable length, depending upon severity of stenosis. When the murmur is early and brief, it sounds like an innocent systolic ejection murmur. However, the presence of the preceding ejection sound identifies it's pathologic origin. Characteristically, this sound selectively decreases in intensity on inspiration and the converse occurs on expiration. It is best heard at the left second interspace and along the left 3rd and 4th sternal border.

The aortic ejection sound is of left heart origin and is common in patients with a bicuspid aortic valve. It is a high frequency sound following the first heart sound and often is louder than S_1. While it is well heard at the right second interspace, it may be equally heard at the cardiac apex. When what is thought to be "S_1" is louder at the second right interspace than at the apex, one should suspect that the sound is in reality an aortic ejection sound rather than S_1. Like it's right heart counter-

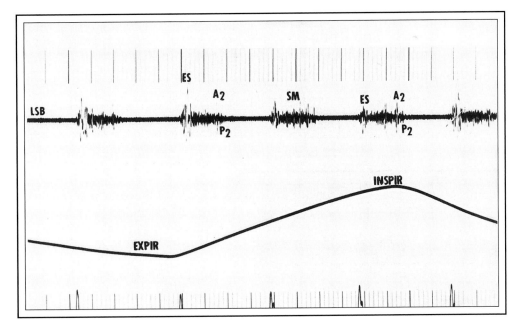

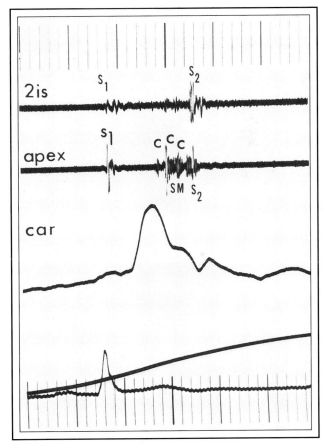

Figure 21. A patient with valvar pulmonic stenosis. The pulmonic ejection sound (ES) which introduces the ejection systolic murmur (SM), decreases in intensity on inspiration and conversely increases in intensity on expiration. (From de Leon AC with permission).

part, it is usually followed by a systolic ejection murmur of variable length depending on whether obstruction (and corresponding severity) is present.

A blowing, decrescendo early diastolic murmur of aortic regurgitation is also a useful clue toward identifying its presence. Recognition of the presence of an aortic ejection sound and therefore suspicion for the presence of a biscuspid aortic valve is important since the valve is susceptible to bacterial endocarditis. Appropriate endocarditis prophylaxis should be prescribed.

A normally functioning aortic mechanical prosthetic valve produces an opening sound with the timing of an aortic ejection sound. The character of the sound is usually readily recognizable as prosthetic in origin.

Systolic clicks may be of extracardiac or intracardiac origin. Clicks of extracardiac origin are of pleuro-pericardial or pericardial origin and are recognized by their relatively fixed location in systole. The more commonly encountered systolic click is of intracardiac origin and results from abrupt halting and tensing of the prolapsing mitral valve (or tricuspid valve) leaflets (Figure 22).

It may be a single click or a series of clicks and are readily recognized by demonstrating movement in their location in systole by simple bedside maneuvers designed to alter left ventricular volume (Figure 23). In some patients the click(s) is followed by a late systolic murmur which when present clearly identifies an intracardiac origin.

• **Murmurs**

Murmurs result from turbulent blood flow of sufficient magnitude to produce audible noise; it is therefore usually loudest at or near its site of genesis and radiates toward the direction of blood flow. Murmur intensity is usually expressed using the 6 level grading system of Levine and Harvey. A grade

Figure 22. A patient with mitral valve prolapse. Note at the apex, the multiple systolic clicks (C) and the late systolic murmur (SM). (From de Leon AC with permission).

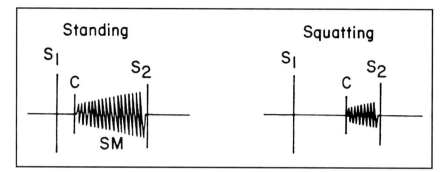

Figure 23. Diagrammatic representation of the movement within systole of the systolic click (C) and onset of the late systolic murmur (SM) in patients with mitral valve prolapse. Note that as left ventricular volume gets smaller (standing) the systolic click occurs earlier and the late systolic murmur starts sooner. Conversely, when left ventricular volume increases (squatting), the systolic click (C) occurs later and murmur onset is correspondingly later. (From de Leon AC with permission).

1/6 murmur is faint and heard only after a period of concentration; a grade 2/6 murmur is faint but heard immediately; a grade 3/6 murmur is of moderate intensity; a grade 4/6 murmur is loud and associated with a thrill on palpation; a grade 5/6 murmur can be heard with only a portion of the stethoscope piece touching the chest wall; a grade 6/6 murmur can be heard with the stethoscope piece off the chest wall.

Grade 5/6 and 6/6 murmurs usually represent pathology but faint murmurs also may be pathologic. It is thus not good practice to equate loudness of the murmur with pathology or benign origin nor does loudness necessarily define the severity of a pathologic lesion present. The configuration, length, location in the cardiac cycle, and other associated sounds such as second heart sound splitting, ejection sound, systolic clicks, and gallops are more

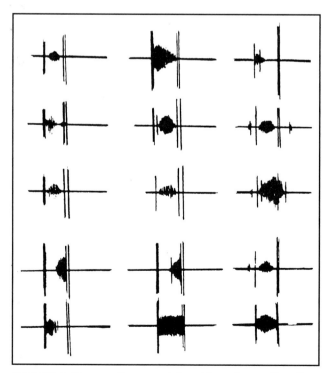

Figure 24. A diagrammatic representation of the various configurations and onset of systolic murmurs. (From de Leon AC and Harvey WP with permission).

useful in deciding whether a murmur is physiologic or represents cardiac pathology. In trying to arrive at a diagnostic conclusion, it is helpful first to determine if the murmur heard is systolic, diastolic, or continuous.

On occasion, a murmur will have a musical quality. This is because a structure, usually a valve leaflet, vibrates in a uniform and periodic fashion to produce a musical tone. Musical murmurs generally comprise the grade 6/6 murmurs. The most common cause of a musical systolic murmur in the young adult is mitral valve prolapse. Tricuspid insufficiency can be a less frequent cause. In the elderly, sclerosis and thickening of the aortic leaflets are most common. The musical diastolic murmur is usually noted in aortic insufficiency especially those of luetic etiology.

• Systolic Murmurs

Systolic murmurs are the most frequently encountered in clinical practice (Figure 24). The most common systolic murmur is a physiologic or "innocent" systolic murmur, especially in children and young adults. It is crescendo-decrescendo in configuration, starts in early systole and is usually short. Because it results from turbulence as the ventricle rapidly ejects blood into its corresponding great vessel, it is usually best heard at the left or right second interspace and is of grade 3/6 or less in intensity.

Conditions which increase the force of ventricular contraction such as tachycardia, excitement, thyrotoxicosis and fever all tend to increase murmur intensity. In the child or young adult, a physiologic third heart sound is also present. The benign nature of this murmur is best arrived at by demonstrating absence of abnormal findings such as a fixed S_2 split, or an ejection sound preceding the murmur onset. In some patients, one might encounter a vibratory left parasternal murmur (Still's murmur). It is a readily recognizable innocent murmur which currently is thought to result from vibration of left ventricular bands in the left ventricular outflow tract caused by increased ejection velocity from the left ventricle.

Short systolic ejection murmurs can also occur when pathology is present. Many elderly patients have such a murmur as a result of sclerosis or thickening of the aortic leaflets. In some elderly patients, the murmur may have a musical quality. Similar short systolic ejection murmurs can be noted with aortic or pulmonary dilatation, ascending aortic aneurysm, or because of unusually large stroke volume from aortic regurgitation or as a result of slow heart rate such as complete heart block. A short systolic ejection murmur is a frequent finding in patients with an aortic or mitral prosthetic valve.

Obstruction to right or left ventricular outflow is always a consideration when one encounters a systolic ejection murmur (Figure 25). With mild forms of obstruction the murmur may be brief and mimic a physiologic murmur; hearing a preceding ejection sound helps to identify its pathologic origin. With moderate to severe obstruction, the systolic ejection murmur occupies more or all of systole and late peaking of the crescendo-decrescendo murmur signifies significant obstruction (Figure 26). Usually there are other supporting findings from physical examination and corresponding symptoms obtained from clinical history.

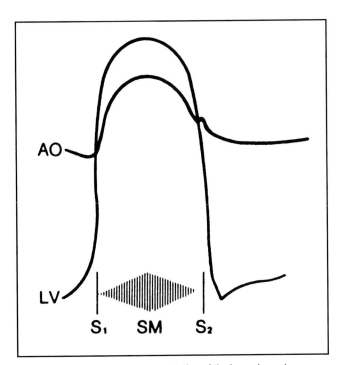

Figure 25. A diagrammatic representation of the hemodynamic correlates of the ejection systolic murmur in aortic stenosis. Note that murmur onset occurs after isometric ventricular contraction and the murmur must end upon closure of the aortic valve (S_2). The murmur (SM) has a crescendo-decrescendo configuration. (From de Leon AC and Cheng TO with permission).

Vascular bruits are usually systolic and often have the crescendo-decrescendo configuration of cardiac ejection systolic murmurs. Some are innocent, such as the supraclavicular bruit, which can be abolished by hyperextending the shoulders. Some result from vascular pathology such as carotid artery stenosis, coarctation of the aorta and pulmonary artery branch stenosis.

• Holosystolic Murmurs

Learning to recognize a holosystolic murmur is valuable and clinically useful. A holosystolic murmur always represents pathology (i.e., an innocent or physiologic murmur is not an option). Further, its presence limits the possible cause to either mitral regurgitation, tricuspid regurgitation, or ventricular septal defect.

The murmur starts with the first heart sound and is present during isovolumic contraction and extends to or just beyond the second heart sound (Figure 27). It is usually even frequency throughout, except in ventricular septal defects where some mid-systolic accentuation may be present.

The holosystolic murmur resulting from mitral regurgitation is usually loudest at the point of maximum impulse (apex) and can radiate to the mid-axilla or posteriorly, or radiate toward the left parasternal area or both. Feeling a thrill at the cardiac apex essentially establishes the mitral origin of the holosystolic murmur. Ventricular septal defect is usually loudest along the 3rd and 4th left parasternal areas, and radiates across the sternum to the right side and/or superiorly along the path of the right ventricular outflow toward the second left interspace. In the left parasternal area, a thrill which traverses the sternal body to the right side is additionally helpful in establishing the diagnosis.

Tricuspid regurgitation is also usually loudest along the lower left parasternal area, but can be distinguished from the holosystolic murmur of ventricular septal defect by being able to elicit inspiratory increase in murmur intensity. Other associated findings such as abnormal "CV" waves in the jugular venous pulse and systolic liver pulsation additionally help to establish the diagnosis.

Although finding a holosystolic murmur allows the examiner to consider the above three diagnostic possibilities, these entities may present with systolic murmurs which are not holosystolic.

Mitral regurgitation may present as a late systolic murmur and if so, mitral valve prolapse or papillary muscle dysfunction are the most likely cause. Presence of systolic clicks in addition to the late systolic murmur identifies mitral valve prolapse as the likely etiology. In acute severe mitral

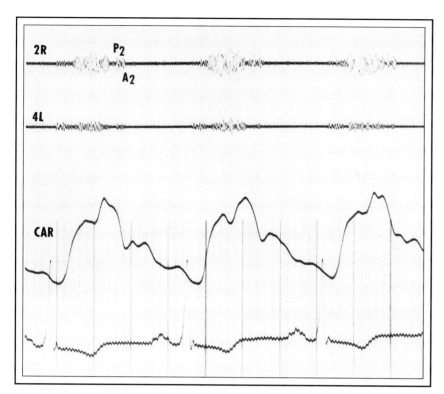

Figure 26. A patient with severe aortic stenosis illustrating the long, late peaking of the systolic ejection murmur and paradoxic splitting of the second heart sound (P$_2$ and A$_2$). (From de Leon AC with permission).

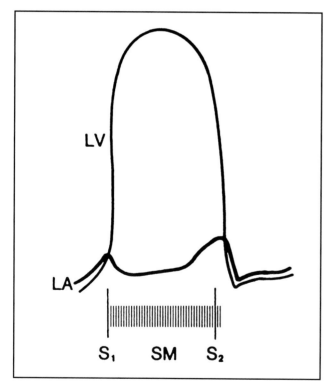

Figure 27. A diagrammatic representation of the hemodynamic correlates of the holosystolic murmur. Note that murmur (SM) onset occurs right after the first heart sound (S$_1$) and is therefore present during isovolumic ventricular contraction, and extends through semilunar valve closure (S$_2$) into part of isovolumic relaxation. This murmur tends to be even-frequency throughout systole. (From de Leon AC and Cheng TO with permission).

regurgitation, the murmur, if holosystolic, may have a late systolic decrease in intensity and, in some, a less than holosystolic murmur which ends before S$_2$ (Figure 28). Papillary muscle dysfunction also presents in a variable fashion, in that the systolic murmur encountered may be early, mid, late, or holosystolic.

A useful clinical feature of the murmur of mitral regurgitation that helps to separate it from a long systolic ejection murmur is its response to an extrasystole. The holosystolic murmur of mitral regurgitation usually does not appreciably change in intensity in the immediate post extrasystolic beat, and if the systolic murmur is due to papillary muscle dysfunction, may actually decrease in intensity (Figure 29).

The systolic murmur of aortic stenosis increases in intensity following the extra-systolic pause. Severe paravalvular mitral prosthetic leaks may be silent or produce a murmur that is less than holosystolic.

Tricuspid regurgitation similarly may be silent, or when a murmur is present, be early or mid-systolic, or late systolic rather than holosystolic. As previously alluded to, the murmur may be musical as well; demonstrating inspiratory increase of the lower parasternal murmur identifies its right heart origin.

Ventricular septal defect murmurs may be less than holosystolic when a small muscular defect becomes physiologically closed as the ventricular

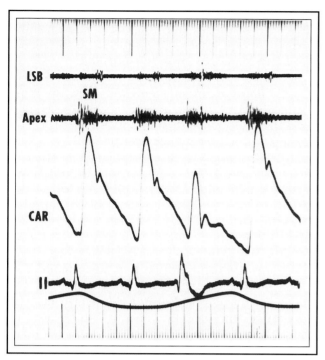

Figure 28. A patient with spontaneous chordal rupture resulting in acute severe mitral regurgitation. Note the crescendo configuration of the mitral regurgitant murmur (SM). Note as well the absence of post extra-systolic change in murmur intensity - a characteristic of mitral regurgitant murmur. (From de Leon AC with permission).

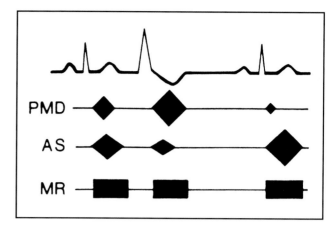

Figure 29. A diagrammatic representation of the effect of ventricular extra-systole on the murmur intensity of the post extra-systolic beat in papillary muscle dysfunction (PMD), aortic stenosis (AS) and mitral regurgitation (MR). (From de Leon AC and Cheng TO with permission).

septum contracts in systole. It may also be less than holosystolic because of development of pulmonary hypertension resulting in progressive decrease in left to right shunting. In this latter instance, other physical signs of pulmonary hypertension would be expected to be present.

• Diastolic Murmurs

Presence of a diastolic murmur is presumptive evidence that a cardiac abnormality is present. It can only occur when blood is flowing from atrium to ventricle (a normal direction of blood flow), or backwards from great vessel through the semilunar valve into its corresponding ventricle.

Large volume of blood flowing from atrium to ventricle during the period of passive rapid filling can create turbulence and hence murmur in the absence of AV valve stenosis. These mid-diastolic murmurs are usually brief, follow a third heart sound, are of low energy and low-frequency components and thus heard best the same way that gallops are listened for. This murmur is useful in inferring the severity of the cardiac abnormality present. Thus, a mid-diastolic flow murmur across the tricuspid valve and heard along the lower parasternal border, could be because of the moderate to large left to right shunt from an atrial septal defect, or because of moderate to severe tricuspid regurgitation (Figure 30).

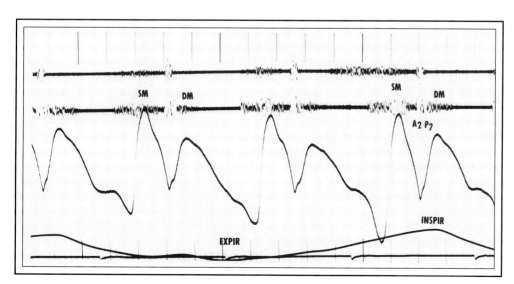

Figure 30. A patient with tricuspid regurgitation. Note the systolic murmur (SM) increase in intensity on inspiration, as well as the diastolic murmur (DM) resulting from increased diastolic flow through the tricuspid valve because of the severe degree of tricuspid regurgitation. (From de Leon AC with permission).

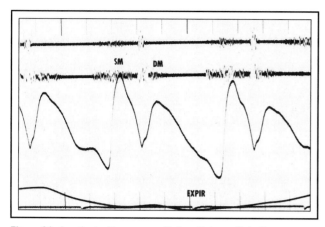

Figure 31. A patient with severe aortic insufficiency. Note the decrescendo, diastolic murmur (DM) and the short, early systolic ejection murmur (SM) resulting from a large left ventricular stroke volume. (From de Leon AC and Harvey WP with permission).

Actual obstruction at tricuspid valve level because of tricuspid valve stenosis, or presence of a right atrial intracardiac mass also would give rise to a similar, low-frequency mid-diastolic murmur. Severity of obstruction will tend to determine the length of the diastolic murmur — i.e., longer in more severe degrees of obstruction. Atrial systole can also cause pre-systolic crescendo-decrescendo configuration to the diastolic murmur; this murmur also increases with inspiration.

A mid-diastolic flow murmur across the mitral valve can occur in severe mitral regurgitation, or because of a large left to right shunt from a ventricular septal defect or patent ductus arteriosus. Like its right heart counterpart, the murmur is of low frequency, usually low energy and therefore soft, introduced by a left ventricular S_3, and best heard at the PMI using the stethoscope bell. As indicated above, its presence provides information regarding the severity of the lesion (MR, VSD, or PDA).

When mitral valve stenosis is present, the resulting diastolic murmur is usually introduced by an opening snap, and when normal sinus rhythm is present, has a presystolic crescendo to the first heart sound. When cycle length changes occur as in atrial fibrillation, the length of the diastolic murmur provides a clue to the severity of obstruction by the length of time it takes to achieve diastasis. Continued murmur presence implies gradient across the mitral valve and ends when left atrial and left ventricular diastolic pressure equalize (diastasis).

This mid-diastolic murmur of mitral stenosis can be mimicked by severe aortic regurgitation with an Austin-Flint murmur. The aortic regurgitant jet strikes the ventricular surface of the anterior mitral leaflet and moves it toward a closed position.

It has been postulated that the resulting rapid mitral inflow causes the "blubbery" mid-diastolic murmur. Recent studies suggest that aortic regurgitant flow alone can cause the murmur.

Semilunar valve insufficiency results in an early diastolic murmur; in aortic insufficiency, the murmur begins right after aortic valve closure (A_2) and has a decrescendo configuration (Figure 31). The murmur is high frequency and hence best heard with the diaphragm piece; as previously mentioned, it may be musical. When the murmur is faint, it my be heard only in full held expiration while the patient is seated and leaning forward. The murmur is usually best heard along the left sternal border. When the murmur is louder along the right 2nd, 3rd and 4th interspaces compared to the left, causes of aortic regurgitation from abnormalities of the ascending aorta (rather than aortic valve) should be considered. Neither the length nor the intensity of the diastolic murmur can be used to judge severity of the aortic regurgitation. The diastolic blood pressure, pulse pressure, evidence of left ventricular enlargement and when present, an Austin-Flint murmur are the clinical points used to judge severity.

Acute severe aortic regurgitation represents a dif-

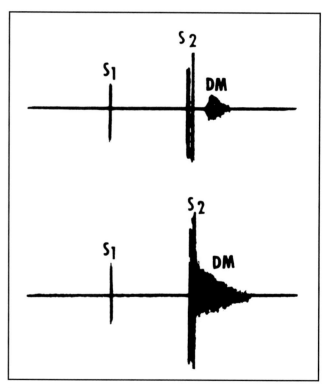

Figure 32. A diagrammatic illustration of the difference between the diastolic murmur (DM) of low (normal) pressure pulmonary valve insufficiency (top) and the diastolic murmur (DM) of pulmonary hypertensive pulmonary valve insufficiency (bottom). (From de Leon AC and Harvey WP with permission).

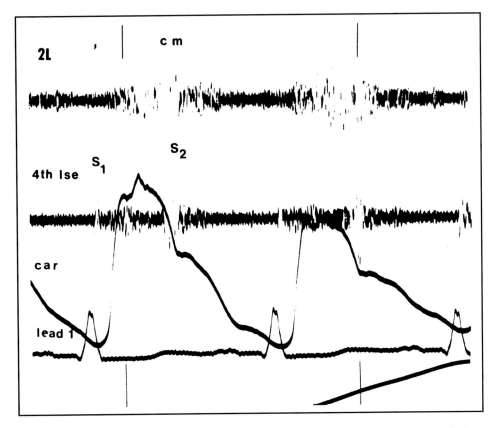

Figure 33. A patient with a patent ductus arteriosus. Note the continuous murmur (CM) at the 2nd left interspace. The murmur envelops the second sound (S$_2$). (From de Leon AC with permission).

ferent clinical presentation in that the aortic diastolic pressure may only be modestly low, pulse-pressure may be normal, and diastolic murmur short. The large volume of regurgitant blood into a normal left ventricular cavity results in marked elevation in left ventricular pressure and may even close the mitral valve in diastole. When this occurs, the loudest heart sound heard at the apex is S$_2$ but is miscalled S$_1$ resulting in mistiming of the murmur.

Pulmonary semilunar valve regurgitation presents differently depending upon whether pulmonary artery pressure is normal or elevated. When pulmonary artery pressure is normal, the murmur of pulmonary valve insufficiency is low to medium-frequency, does not start right with P$_2$, has a crescendo-decrescendo configuration, and is likely to demonstrate inspiratory increase in murmur intensity at the 2nd and 3rd left sternal border (Figure 32).

When pulmonary hypertension is present, the resulting murmur of pulmonary valve regurgitation is very similar in frequency and configuration to chronic aortic valve regurgitation (Graham Steell; Figure 32). Some may manifest inspiratory increase in murmur intensity but others do not. Other associated physical findings of pulmonary hypertension are needed to support the hypothesis of a Graham-Steell murmur as opposed to aortic regurgitation.

• Continuous Murmurs

Continuous murmurs extend from systole into diastole through the second heart sound. Some continuous murmurs are of benign origin, such as the venous hum encountered over the internal jugular vein especially in children and young adults. On occasion, such a venous hum transmits to the infraclavicular area and is mistaken for the murmur of a patent ductus arteriosus. This is recognized by demonstrating murmur disappearance by turning the patient's head forward or by transient finger compression of the internal jugular vein.

A typical example of a cardiac anomaly causing a continuous murmur is a patent ductus arteriosus. The murmur characteristically envelops the second heart sound. Eddy sounds present throughout the murmur can give it a "machinery-like" character (Figure 33). Sinus of Valsalva rupture into the right atrium or ventricle also gives rise to a continuous murmur. Surgical aorto-pulmonary communication such as a Blalock-Taussig or Waterston Shunt also produce a continuous murmur.

Because coronary artery bypass surgery is commonly performed, one should be alert to the possibility of finding a continuous murmur along the left upper sternal border in such patients. Although an uncommon occurrence, it is caused by the inadvertent attachment of the bypass graft to the great cardiac vein which is located adjacent to the left anterior descending artery. Arterio-venous fistulae are surgically created for hemodialysis and produces a continuous murmur. This murmur can be transmitted and most commonly is to the infra-clavicular area on the same side as the fistula. It may also radiate to the supraclavicular area and neck. It is rare for it to transmit to the sternal edge, but the systolic component of the continuous murmur may have sufficiently wide transmission to be mistaken for having cardiac origin.

Presence of combined lesions result in more than one murmur. Thus, aortic stenosis and insufficiency results in a systolic and diastolic murmur. Mitral regurgitation and aortic insufficiency or ventricular septal defect and aortic insufficiency produce a holosystolic murmur, followed by a decrescendo diastolic murmur. They are also referred to as a "to and fro" murmur. These murmurs can be mistaken for a continuous murmur.

However, the two murmurs involved are of different frequency and quality, the second heart sound separates the two murmurs, and one can usually identify two different locations where each murmur is loudest.

The three component pericardial friction rub (systolic, early diastolic, and pre-systolic) is pathognomonic of pericarditis. It is usually best heard along the lower left sternal border and xiphoid area and typically waxes and wanes with respiration. When the pre-systolic component is absent and only the systolic and early diastolic components are present, it can mimic a "to and fro" murmur.

Bedside Aids

The physician who is truly committed to obtaining the most information from the clinical examination has many options. Throughout the preceding discussion, we have referred to use of respiration and change of body position from supine to sitting or standing, and the usefulness of paying attention to the post extrasystolic beat. Many other bedside maneuvers may be utilized such as Valsalva, isometric hand grip, prompt squatting, transient arterial occlusion, and amyl nitrate inhalation.

The Valsalva maneuver is useful in assessment of various auscultatory events and also provides information about autonomic dysfunction, congestive heart failure and left ventricular end-diastolic pressure.

Technologic Aids

Electrocardiogram

The 12 lead electrocardiogram and chest x-ray are relatively less expensive tests and more widely

and quickly available to the physician. Thus they are still useful tools for the clinician.

Based upon the clinical suspicion for right or left ventricular hypertrophy because the clinical findings suggest pulmonary hypertension, tetralogy of Fallot, Eisenmenger, severe pulmonic stenosis, systemic hypertension, severe valvar aortic stenosis, hypertrophic cardiomyopathy, etc., the electrocardiographic finding of hypertrophy then corroborates the working hypothesis. Its absence does not always necessarily deny the working hypothesis but should alert the clinician to reconsider how the clinical data has been integrated; conduction abnormalities such as right or left bundle branch block can be correlated with the observations on the second heart sound. Certain cardiac abnormalities such as the Wolff-Parkinson-White syndrome can best be recognized in the electrocardiogram.

Finding electrocardiographic changes of myocardial infarction can serve as confirmatory evidence. However, absence of such changes should not detract from a clinical diagnosis of infarction since not all infarctions have diagnostic electrocardiographic changes. Documenting ST segment changes during an episode of pain is clinically helpful. On the other hand, global T wave changes do not necessarily imply coronary artery disease. Many noncardiac conditions can cause global T wave inversion and is thus non-specific. Thus even with this very useful tool, there continues to be a need for total correlation and integration of clinical findings.

Chest X-Ray

Chest x-ray is similarly useful and provides information about pulmonary arterial blood flow and pulmonary venous congestion. Enlargement of the main pulmonary artery, ascending aorta, right atrium, and left ventricle are readily provided. Early left atrial enlargement can best be appreciated in the appropriate oblique or lateral view with barium filled esophagus. An increase in tracheal carinal angle as noted in the PA view, is helpful only when the degree of left atrial enlargement is considerable.

One study suggests that a carinal angle of 100° or greater accurately predicts a left atrium that is 5 cm or greater in diameter when measured with echocardiography.

Since elevation of the left main bronchus is most likely to occur before the tracheobronchial cartilages become rigid and non-compliant, its presence suggests that left atrial enlargement occurred during childhood or adolescence.

Obvious enlargement of the left atrial appendage noted as a bulge along the left cardiac border suggests rheumatic mitral stenosis and/or insufficiency. Valvar, annular, cavitary mass, coronary, aortic and pericardial calcifications are also useful findings in the chest roentgenogram and represents information not available by clinical examination.

Diagnostic Laboratory

There are currently many non-invasive tests available such as echocardiography, pulsed and continuous doppler, as well as color doppler studies, stress echocardiography, ECG stress testing, ambulatory holter monitoring, heart rate variability measurements, signal averaged electrocardiogram, nuclear imaging tests, computed tomography and magnetic resonance imaging. Invasive studies such as cardiac catheterization, angiography and electrophysiologic studies are also available.

The clinician's task is to determine which additional tests, if any, are needed by a particular patient to provide information vital to arriving at a diagnosis or determining the appropriate direction of therapy. This judgement can only be made in an appropriate and cost effective manner after the information from the clinical history, physical examination, and simpler, less expensive tests have been properly integrated.

Further, the working hypothesis arrived at from this reasoning then determines the sequence of additional tests obtained.

Selected Reading

1. Allen SJ, Naylor D. Pulsation of the eyeballs in tricuspid regurgitation. *Can Med Assoc J.* 1985:133;119-120.
2. Appels A, Mulder P. Excess fatigue as a precursor of myocardial infarction. *European Heart J.* 1988:9;758-764.
3. Bethell HJN, Nixon PGF. Examination of the heart in supine and left lateral positions. *BHJ.* 1973:35;902-907.
4. Butman SM, Ewy GA, Standen JR, Kern KB, Hahn E. Bedside cardiovascular examination in patients with severe chronic heart failure: Importance of rest or inducible jugular venous distension. *JACC.* 1993:22;968-974.
5. Campeau L. Grading of angina pectoris. *Circulation.* 1975:54;522.
6. Cannon RO, Watson RM, Rosing DR. Angina caused by reduced vasodilator reserve of the small coronary arteries. *JACC.* 1983:1;1359.
7. Cha SD, Gooch A. Diagnosis of tricuspid regurgitation. Current status. *Arch Intern Med.* 1983:143;1763-1768.
8. Cheng TO. Esophageal function in patients with angina and normal coronary arteriogram. *Ann Surg.* 1984:199;123.
9. Cheng TO. Mechanism of Still's murmur. *AJC.* 1992:69;839.
10. Christie LG Jr, Conti RC. Systematic approach to evaluation of angina-like chest pain: Pathophysiology and clinical testing with emphasis on objective documentation of myocardial ischemia. *AHJ.* 1981:102;897-912.
11. Cook DG, Shaper AG. Breathlessness, angina pectoris and coronary artery disease. *Am J Cardiol.* 1989:63;921-924.
12. Darazs B, Hesdorfer CS, Butterworth AM, Ziady F. The possible etiology of the vibratory systolic murmur. *Clin Cardiol.* 1987:10;341-346.
13. Denef B, DeGeest H, Kesteloot H. The clinical value of the calibrated apical A wave and its relationship to the fourth heart sound. *Circ* 1979:60;1412-1421.
14. Eilen SD, Crawford MH, O'Rourke RA. Accuracy of precordial palpation for detecting increased left ventricular volume. *Ann Intern Med.* 1983:99;628-630.
15. Emi, Fukuda N, Oki T, Iuchi A, Tabata T, Kiyoshige K, Fujimoto T, Manabe K, Ito S. Genesis of the Austin Flint Murmur: Relation to mitral inflow and aortic regurgitant flow dynamics. *JACC.* 1993:21;1399-1405.
16. Ewy GA. The abdominojugular test: Technique and hemodynamic correlates. *Ann Intern Med.* 1988:109;456-460.
17. Ewy GA. Bedside evaluation of precordial pulsations. *Cardiol In Practice.* 1984:1;127-133.
18. Fletcher RH, Fletcher SW. Editorial: Has medicine outgrown physical diagnosis? *Ann Intern Med.* 1992:117;786-787.
19. George DS, Marsh C, Leier CV. "A-Wave" Liver. *Clin Cardiol.* 1988:11;349-350.
20. Gibson TC, Madry R, Grossman W, McLaurin LP, Craige E. The A wave of the apexcardiogram and left ventricular diastolic stiffness. *Circ.* 1974:49;441-446.
21. Glower DD, Murrah RL, Olsen CO, Davis JW, Rankin JS. Mechanical correlates of the third heart sound. *JACC.* 1992:19;450-457.
22. Hickman DH, Sox HC Jr, Sox CH. Systematic bias in recording the history in patients with chest pain. *J Chron Dis.* 1985:38;91-100.
23. Ishmail AA, Wing S, Ferguson J, Hutchinson TA, Magder S, Flegel KM. Interobserver agreement by auscultation in the presence of a third heart sound in patients with congestive heart failure. *Chest.* 1987:91;870-873.
24. Johnson HA. Diminishing returns on the road to diagnostic certainty. *JAMA.* 1991:265;2229-2231.
25. Jordan MD, Taylor CR, Nyhuis AW, Tavel ME. Audibility of the fourth heart sound: Relationship to presence of disease and examiner experience. *Arch Intern Med.* 1987:147;721-726.
26. Kassirer JP. Diagnostic Reasoning. *Ann Intern Med.* 1989:110;893-900.
27. Kassirer JP. Teaching clinical medicine by iterative hypothesis testing. *N Engl J Med.* 1983:309;921-923.
28. Kern DC, Parrino TA, Korst DR. The lasting value of clinical skills. *JAMA* 1985:254;70-76.
29. Kono T, Rosman H, Alam M, Stein P, Sabbah HN. Hemodynamic correlates of the third heart sound during the evolution of chronic heart failure. *J Am Coll Cardiol.* 1993:21;419-423.
30. Lembo NJ, Dell'Italia LJ, Crawford M, O'Rourke RA. Bedside diagnosis of systolic murmurs. *NEJM.* 1988:318;1572-1578.
31. Lembo NJ, Dell'Italia LJ, Crawford M, O'Rourke RA. Diagnosis of left-sided regurgitant murmurs by transient arterial occlusion: A new maneuver using blood pressure cuffs. *Ann Intern Med.* 1986:105;368-370.
32. Levine HJ. Difficult problems in the diagnosis of chest pain. *Am Heart J.* 1980:100;108-118.
33. Lown B, Graboys TB. The art of taking a history. *J Myocardial Ischemia.* 1992:4;14-24.
34. Mangione S, Neiman LZ, Gracely E, Kaye D. The teaching and practice of cardiac auscultation during internal medicine and cardiology training. *Ann Intern Med.* 1993:119;47-54.
35. Nishimura RA, Tajik AJ. Cardiovascular Clinics: The valsalva maneuver and response revisited. *Mayo Clin Proc.* 1986:61;211-217.
36. O'Neill TW, Barry M, Smith M, Graham IM. Diagnostic value of the apex beat. *Lancet.* 1989:1;410-411.

37. Ozawa Y, Smith D, Craige E. Origin of the third heart sound. II Studies in human subjects. *Circ.* 1984:67;399-404.

38. Pathy MS. Clinical presentation of myocardial infarction in the elderly. *BHJ.* 1967:29;190-199.

39. Quyyumi AA, Cannon RO, Panza JA, Diodati JG, Epstein SE. Endothelial dysfunction in patients with chest pain and normal coronary arteries. *Circulation.* 1992:86;1864-1871.

40. Ranganathan N, Juma Z, Sivaciyan V. The apical impulse in coronary heart disease. *Clin Cardiol.* 1985:8;20-33.

41. Rault R. Transmitted murmurs in patients undergoing hemodialysis. *Arch Intern Med.* 1989:149;1392-1393.

42. Reddy PS, Haidet K, Meno F. Relation of intensity of cardiac sounds to age. *Am J Cardiol.* 1985:55;1383-1388.

43. Reddy PS, Meno F, Curtiss EL, O'Toole JD. The genesis of gallop sounds: Investigation by quantitative phono and apex cardiography. *Circ.* 1981:63;922-933.

44. Ronan JA Jr. Cardiac Auscultation: The first and second heart sounds. *Heart Disease and Stroke.* 1992:1;113-116.

45. Ronan JA Jr. Cardiac Auscultation: The third and fourth heart sounds. *Heart Disease and Stroke.* 1994:1;267-270.

46. Schmitt BP, Kushner MS, Weiner SL. The diagnostic usefulness of the history of the patient with dyspnea. *J Gen Intern Med.* 1986:1;386-393.

47. Schofield PM, Whorwell PJ, Jones PE, Brooks NH, Bennett DH. Differentiation of "esophageal" and "cardiac" chest pain. *Am J. Card.* 1988:62;315-316.

48. Sheikh MU, Lee WR, Mills RJ, Dais K. Musical murmurs: Clinical implications, long term prognosis, and echo-phono-cardiographic features. *AHJ.* 1984:108;377-386.

49. Shuford WH. Detection of cardiac chamber enlargement with the chest roentgenogram. *Heart Disease and Stroke.* 1992:1;341-347.

50. Silber EN. Tracheal Carinal angle in evaluating left atrial size. *Arch Intern Med.* 1991:151;2096 and 2100.

51. Smith D, Craige E. Enhancement of tactile perception in palpation. *Circ.* 1980:62;1114-1118.

52. Smith D, Craige E. Mechanism of the dicrotic pulse. *BHJ.* 1986:56;531-534.

53. St. Clair EW, Oddone EZ, Waugh RA, Corey GR, Feussner Jr. Assessing housestaff diagnostic skills using a Cardiology Patient Simulator. *Ann Intern Med.* 1992:117;751-756.

54. Taskin V, Bates MC, Chillag SA. Tracheal carinal angle and left atrial size. *Arch Intern Med.* 1991:151;307-308.

55. Van De Werf F, Boel A, Geboers J, Minten J, Williams J, DeGeest H, Kesteloot H. Diastolic properties of the left ventricle in normal adults and in patients with third heart sounds. *Circ.* 1984:69;1070-1078.

56. Van De Werf F, Geboers J, Kesteloot H, DeGeest H, Barrios L. The mechanism of disappearance of the physiologic third heart sound with age. *Circ.* 1986:73;877-884.

57. Vieweg WVR. Continuous murmur following bypass surgery. *Chest.* 1981:79;4-5.

58. Walder LA, Spodick DH. Global T Wave inversion. *JACC.* 1991:17;1479-1485.

59. Wilken MK, Myers DG, Laski PA, Yi FP, Starke H. Mechanism of disappearance of S3 with maturation. *AJC.* 1989:64;1394-1396.

60. Zoneraich S, Spodick DH. Bedside Science Reduces Laboratory Art. Appropriate use of physical findings to reduce reliance on sophisticated and expensive methods. *Circ.* 1995: Vol. 91; No. 7. pp. 2089-2092.

Figure Sources

1. de Leon AC Jr, Cheng TO; Cheng TO, ed. *History and physical examination: The International Textbook of Cardiology.* New York, Macmillan Publishing Co., 1986

2. de Leon AC Jr, Harvey WP; Spittell, JA Jr, ed. *Clinical approach to the patient with suspected heart disease in Clinical Medicine.* Philadelphia, Harper and Row, 1981.

3. de Leon AC Jr. *A handbook on cardiac auscultation.* Newton, New Jersey, Laennec, 1989.

CHAPTER 2

The Doctor-Patient Relationship

Richard B. Perry, M.D.

"No one cares how much you know, until they know how much you care"

L.E. Fuller, M.D.

Throughout medical history, physicians have studied and written about the unique relationship between the doctor and the patient; it is universally considered as benevolent. Its goal is to improve the health related quality of life for each patient encountered. However, with today's rapid advances in medical technology, this traditional relationship is in danger of deteriorating due to lessened emphasis on the interpersonal and humanistic qualities of the physician. Yet, from the patient's standpoint, these qualities are considered to be equally as important as technical competence. Factors such as discontinuity of care caused by changing methods of patient reimbursement, poor communication and lessened compliance with treatment regimens, reduced time of physician-patient contact secondary to economic realities, and defensive medical practices due to malpractice threats make rededication to the ideals of the patient-centered doctor-patient relationship more important now than ever.

CARDIAC PEARL

The author has put his finger on a very important aspect of medical practice and patient care. Something has to be done about the national disgrace of the plethora of unjustified malpractice suits against physicians, medical institutions, and other medical personnel.

Some advocate a "medically qualified hearing officer, rather than a lay jury." This would be advantageous, but I believe that if a panel, composed of unquestionably well trained and qualified members, screened and evaluated these suits, that most of them could be eliminated, or settled fairly out of court. If on this panel there were several physicians, several attorneys, several religious leaders, plus two or three other selected individuals, that prompt and efficient justice could be better administered. By its strength in numbers, such a large authoritative panel would carry more weight and be better than the opinion of one or two persons.

Also, it is likely that a marked reduction in the numbers of legal suits would occur if attorney contingency fees (such as one third of the award) were banned. I also favor, as some have suggested, that if the suit is determined to be unjustified, that the cost incurred by the defendant physician or other party being sued, be paid by the person (or persons) initiating the law suit.

W. Proctor Harvey, M.D.

Let us consider, then, what the patient needs and the physician must provide. The eponym **P-A-T-I-E-N-T** lists characteristics that are highly valued by the patient and essential to this relationship.

P   Patience
A   Advocacy
T   Thoroughness
I   Information
E   Empathy
N   Nuances
T   Treatment

The physician must *listen*, with minimal interruptions, gather accurate *information* and record it precisely, be *thorough* in both data collection and data analysis, acknowledge and feel, if possible, the *emotions* of the patients, whether *expressed* directly or *indirectly;* determine the best *treatment* and enlist the patient's participation; and act as the patient's *advocate* in all matters determined on medical grounds to be in the patient's best interest.

This relationship requires physicians to focus their entire attention on the total patient. These qualities must be provided by the physician without conscious effort and will require a constant and life-long dedication to the principles involved.

P: Patience

Physicians are born interrupters. Observers have shown that on the average, they do not allow patients to complete their opening statements of concern 70% of the time, interrupting after a mean time of 18 seconds. This is done in order to take charge and to direct the interview. But investigators have shown that once the patient begins talking, if the doctor says nothing for the first 30 seconds and is content with any type of information, more data will be obtained than by the closed-end type of questioning. This non-interrupted interviewing is associated with increased patient satisfaction and compliance. It shows that the physician is listening and is considering the patient and not focusing on the disease. If too many problems are presented for the time scheduled, the physician then negotiates an agenda for further investigation.

The patient's history unfolds best if the interviewing techniques include silence, nonverbal responses to encourage talking, neutral utterances and echoing of the patient's own words, and short summaries or paraphrases. Practical measures for improving communication include making the office setting unintimidating; that is, moving out from behind the desk to a chair closer to the patient, slowing the physician's actions and rate of speech to match that of the patient, acknowledging all complaints even if they seem trivial, and encouraging patients to bring problem lists and helping them rank concerns.

Studies have shown that there is generally little significance in the order in which patients list their complaints. Physicians should also keep as much eye contact as possible by paying more attention to the patient than to the chart, ask patients what they think is the cause of their symptoms and how they think you, the physician, can help, use repetition in explanations, and give good results first if the condition is serious and bad news is delivered. Patients' retention rate of positive information has been found to be almost five times greater when

they are given the positive information first. With practice this does not take long. Allowing patients to tell their stories completely, with minimal interruptions, is a first therapeutic step in itself, as well as an opportunity to gather information. The end result will be more helpful to the patient and more meaningful to the physician in learning about the total experience of the patient's illness.

A: Advocacy

The physician must be the patient's advocate in all things determined on medical grounds to be in the patient's best interest. The physician must facilitate a chosen course of action as much as possible, whether arranging optimal medical care or enlisting the help of the patient's family, friends, employer, or others. Doctors are placed by their professions and by society right at the crossroads where needs of the individual and of society might conflict. Advocacy must include concern for the total patient. The physician must be available when needed and take personal responsibility for attention to detail. It is often necessary that the physician be able to convince the patient to undertake a course of action which he or she would rather avoid, which the physician knows is in the patient's best interest. Much of the trust the patient grants the physician is based on this quality and grows or shrinks in proportion to the attention the physician gives to this quality in a caring relationship.

Advocacy includes respecting the autonomy of the patient by involving him or her in the decision making process. When patients see doctors as their advocates, they permit the doctor's entrance into their most private selves, laying aside society's rules of behavior and expectation. Physicians must keep in mind at all times that they are the inhabitants of a respected role. They must be sensitive and flexible, practicing with integrity and a high sense of altruism. There is something special about being a doctor, so special that in virtually every culture, in good times or bad, people invariably treat doctors with singular respect and esteem. Patients dread sickness and death, and they know that physicians have learned to work without fear among the sick and dying.

In this era of managed care contracts and HMO's, the physician has added responsibilities as the patient's advocate. Third party payers, when they deny requests for medical services, do not determine standards of medical care. The physician has the obligation and the patient has the right to expect excellent standards of care regardless of the insurance contract. The courts have recognized that in insurance conflicts, the physician must be the advocate of the patients under his or her care.

T: Thoroughness

Thoroughness has been described as the most enduring and critical quality of the excellent physician. Thoroughness is the characteristic that makes the physician trustworthy. It includes attention to detail, maintenance of knowledge, self discipline and understanding of self. Doctors are believed to be always probing and searching for the mysteries of diseases. When a physician says "I do not know," the implications are that he or she has competence and that he or she will try to find out. Good physicians are perpetual students and the patient is the teacher.

Thoroughness applies both to data collection and to data analysis. Studies have shown that "thoroughness of data gathering is uncorrelated with obtaining the correct diagnosis unless there is equal thoroughness in hypothesis formation." While listening, diagnostic possibilities must be considered and tested and revised as information is gathered. This is the process of clinical problem solving. It is learned by trial and error from our teachers and peers, by examples and role modeling, and is not easily taught by any systematic educational approach. More mistakes result from lack of thoroughness than from lack of knowledge. Every patient-physician encounter should be a problem solving exercise which organizes information and experience into the doctor's long term memory for future applications. Complex interpersonal and social issues will play an important role and clinical decisions ultimately are influenced by the interactions of the doctor, the patient, and the sociocultural environment.

The principal maxims to be remembered are that "common diseases occur commonly" and "uncommon manifestations of common diseases are more common than common manifestations of uncommon diseases". An index of suspicion to consider less common is required only if the more common diseases do not fit the available data base. Clues often come in small clusters and are always worth remembering. Dr. W. Proctor Harvey uses the term "Cardiac Pearl" to define facts or findings that either make the diagnosis or lead one to it. They do not change with the passage of time and are gleaned by astute observers from the clinical manifestation of many patients over long periods of time. These clusters of clues lead, with experience, to the recognition of patterns. These patterns can be learned only by study of and working with patients. It is the physician's responsibility to

observe each patient as thoroughly and carefully as possible. This inquisitive, reflective, and thorough approach to clinical thinking is a required behavior throughout the career of any successful physician.

CARDIAC PEARL

A cardiac pearl is defined as a fact or a finding that either makes a diagnosis or is a clue that leads you to it. The cardiac pearl often has "stood the test of time" and is not changed with the passage of time. Fifty years from now, what we discuss as a cardiac pearl will still be apropos to that particular finding.
W. Proctor Harvey, M.D.

I: Information

One's professional life is spent gathering information, based on history taking, examination and diagnostic studies. It is vital to be mindful of the difference between information and conclusions. The physician must note the history and findings carefully, since they will always be open to possible reinterpretation due to subsequent data. Physicians who only record conclusions, such as "the murmur of mitral insufficiency was heard at the cardiac apex" gradually weaken their observational skills and tend to prematurely close off diagnostic options. Developing excellent observational skills requires discipline and practice. These skills give you confidence to stand by your findings. Dr. Harvey often has said when presented with a negative 2-D echo, that the echocardiographer had "missed" the mitral valve prolapse, since he had heard a typical systolic click and murmur; and the repeat echo proved him to be correct. The clinician's task is to always increase the accuracy of information to the highest possible degree. Each step in the diagnostic process is dependent on the information obtained in the preceding steps, and all are in pursuit of a basis for the action which will most benefit the individual patient. Medical education requires that physicians be precise in their record keeping. Studies have shown that House Officers model the record keeping practices of their preceptors, particularly in ambulatory care settings.

The information that the clinician needs however, includes not only the name of the disease, but just as importantly, those factors that modify the disease within the patient, plus the whole myriad of external nonmedical factors, such as where the patient lives, availability of medical services, presence or absence of family, the patient's occupation, or other environmental exposures, etc. All such information has a bearing on the most appropriate treatment for each patient. We must focus on the total threat to the patient and not merely diagnose what disease is present.

E: Empathy

Empathy is difficult to describe despite the fact that civilization could not exist well without it; basically it is feeling the feelings of others. In the physician, it is the capacity of the clinician to identify with the patient and to feel his or her pain. Many writers view this as the most fundamental quality of the physician. It is an essential and highly developed skill in master clinicians. It is part of the kindness and compassion that doctors must have, but it also serves practical diagnostic and therapeutic ends. We are much better able to appreciate the importance of a particular symptom if we are aware of the distress that the symptom causes. This requires attending to and concentrating on the patient rather than on the words alone. When a patient becomes aware that the physician understands their feelings, the patient overcomes inhibitions and embarrassments, and gives a deeper and clearer picture of their medical problems.

These empathetic connections with patients provide physicians with much of the pleasure in medicine. It is this quality that enables those who care for the sick to extend themselves to all levels of the human condition. Because of it, physicians expect from themselves a higher quality of behavior with patients than they use in their own personal interactions. This increased awareness, however, brings added responsibilities, and the physician must have adequate personal strength to cope with the worries and burdens encountered through patients. Care must be both compassionate and competent. Learning how to balance competent care and to manage these emotional strains, produced by caring for the sick and dying, will take virtually all of one's professional career. Medical training is a never-ending apprenticeship and the teachers are the patients. Most patients expect to be liked, and it is the physician's smile and pleasantries throughout the encounter that provides the setting in which the patient will relax and share their story and feelings. It is this quality of shared empathy that now allows the doctor-patient relationship to be benevolent.

CARDIAC PEARL

Don't be a prophet! It is better to tell the patient and/or members of the family that no one can usually accurately prognosticate and to think positively rather than negatively:

"Let's talk about living- not dying."

I have found it unwise to quote statistics when answering the question, "Doctor, what are my chances of surviving the operation?" This simple answer usually suffices: "The risk of having the surgery is less than not having it;" or when appropriate, to say: "There is always some risk of surgery, but in your case it is low."

The great majority of patients and their families are satisfied and often relieved with this answer.

I have found that when numbers concerning mortality are cited, undue fears and anxiety can result; helpful to counteract this" "You are not a number, a statistic. You are an individual and will be treated as such."

Putting ourselves in the place of patients and/or their families will remind us and insure that we talk, explain and reassure them; also letting them know we care. These simple things which we and the staff can provide should not be absent in any hospital.

"You have a problem with your heart, but you would be an unusual patient if you cannot be helped." This is certainly true of the great majority of patients we see with cardiovascular disease. Whether in the hospital or office, a patient being evaluated for the first time should have this encouragement as an initial and integral part of treatment. All we have to do is put ourselves in the patient's place to realize how important this is.

W. Proctor Harvey, M.D.

Physicians must also be understanding of their own feelings. While listening to the patient's problem, the physician should be thinking, "What am I feeling now about this patient?"; "In what way can I be more helpful and comforting to this patient?"; "Are my reactions to the patient interfering with my judgment?". Most of the behaviors we accept in patients are behaviors we would not permit in ourselves. We must remember that the patient is a collaborator in the doctor-patient relationship and any achievements or successes are due to this collaboration between the patient and the physician. Throughout their personal lives, physicians must develop a personal philosophy that allows them to understand suffering and to accept the limitations of their ability to control disease. Fortunately, the doctor-patient relationship allows the physician to share not only the pain and suffering, but also the patient's joys and successes. But the patients won't let us in until we let them know that it is okay for them to tell us all, that is, their symptoms, their reactions, their feelings, and their secrets. Beyond feeling understood, patients also need to feel accepted. As physicians we must be tolerant of our patients' inhibitions, embarrassments, fears, weaknesses and physical limitations. The patient must feel not only compassion, but unconditional acceptance; the rapport that is so essential to the doctor-patient relationship depends on this mutual respect expressed in words and behavior between the physician and the patient. The doctor should try not only to understand but to actually feel the feelings of the patient.

Doctors should be kind, courteous, and compassionate.

Make sure that a patient is never embarrassed, and give him every boost you can. When patients come into a hospital, they are discouraged and frightened. I often tell a patient, "It's a rare patient that we cannot help." And this is true. You need to impart the positive side. I hate for doctors to use scare tactics. When I make rounds with students, I use the time in a patient's room as an opportunity to lift his morale. When I go into the room, I shake the patient's hand and go to the pulse. While I'm talking to him – if I haven't met him before, asking him where he's from and so forth – I have my hand on his wrist, and I can get quick clues. I can tell if the pulse is alternating in intensity, and, if it is, I know there's an element of heart failure; it takes me ten seconds to get this information. I wish all doctors would do this; most don't.

Then, in front of the patient, as I'm feeling the pulse, I will say, "Strong . . . strong . . . strong." Later, when I'm outside of the room with the students, I'll say, "Why didn't I say, "Strong, weak, strong, weak?" It's because the patient would remember the word weak.

W. Proctor Harvey, M.D.

N: Nuances

The nuances of the patient's story are the emotions expressed indirectly. If these clues are not noted and interpreted, there will be a higher rate of diagnostic error. The physician's task is not only to discover what the patient's disease is, but to uncover who is this patient who has this disease, with all the worries, anxieties, and misconceptions that the disease is causing. Once an emotion is expressed, whether directly or indirectly, the physician must not let it pass, thinking to save embarrassment to the patient, but should acknowledge it to let them know that the physician understands. The time it takes is negligible, but the benefit can

be enormous. Clinical problem solving becomes more accurate as the physician gains skill in dealing with the emotions generated by the patient's disease. Do not ignore mixed messages. If the doctor asks the patient if he or she has any more concerns and the patient says no, but the body language indicates hesitation, probe for more information or worries. Sometimes switching to the third person, that is, saying "Many patients with your symptoms seem to worry that they..." is helpful. Let the patient know that you are not only comfortable with their asking questions and expressing concerns, but that you are encouraging it. Much information is to be gained by noting not only what is said, but also how it is said and what is left unsaid.

Some cardiovascular disease terms, or conversations should be avoided in the presence of patients.

I have learned to explain to my patients that when the ECG term "block" is used, it is an electrical description, and does not connote blockage of blood in the heart or circulation.

The term "bundle branch block", which may be either left or right, is an unfortunate one in many respects. Illustrating this was a nursing instructor about 55 years of age. I first examined her approximately six years before. At that time she had hypertension for which she was treated, with satisfactory control of her blood pressure. I was asked to now evaluate her again and when I took her history, I read a report from her physician stating that she now showed left bundle branch block on her electrocardiogram. I then said to her, "I think I may know what is bothering you, in that you now think that you have blockage of blood in your heart from circulation." She said, "Yes." When I explained to her that this was not the case she proclaimed, "Thank God! I have been worried sick for the past months thinking I might get a complete blockage of the heart and then I would die suddenly." Her treatment: Merely understanding bundle branch block does not mean blockage of blood. It does not necessarily mean that some dire event is bound to happen. In fact, there are many patients that have left bundle branch block for many, many years without any symptoms whatsoever. However, this can be evaluated and explained to the patient by a physician. As a rule, the outlook can be good as far as this specific finding is concerned. Right bundle branch block carries an even better outlook, if this is the only finding, and

can be present for many years without any symptoms whatsoever.

With patients having mitral valve prolapse, stress the good aspects and prognosis of this common cardiac lesion. Avoid bringing up the rare dire-complication of sudden death (unless the patient has been aware of this or, of course, if the patient is unnecessarily frightened by this possibility). Make a point to explain the excellent outlook and to emphasize that the patient can usually lead a normal life. Also, emphasize that about 90 percent of patients need no treatment except an explanation and reassurance.

W. Proctor Harvey, M.D.

T: Treatment

Thorough consideration of all the appropriate information, obtained by proper attention to the patient's story and emotions, reveals the sequence by which the patient changed from a healthy person to a sick person. All diseases are processes that involve a chain of events taking place over time. Treatment is the activity that interrupts the chain in order to change the outcome. Treatment may sometimes stop the disease, but any intervention that interferes with the disease process is equally acceptable. Patient education and promotion of preventative measures ultimately may be the more effective therapy than treating the immediate process. The determination of which treatment is best for the patient is based on medical judgment, but the therapeutic action depends on the physician's ability to elicit the participation of the patients in their own care. Treatment includes also the physician's skill and need to prognosticate for the patient's benefit. If the physician warns a patient going home after a significant surgery or illness, that a temporary period of depression may occur, it not only prepares the patient for this, but lets him or her know that it is alright.

Conclusion

The final goal, then, in the doctor-patient relationship is to improve the health related quality of life of each patient encountered. All the diagnostic methodologies from history to angiography are in pursuit of a basis for action that will most benefit this individual patient. The responsibility is burdensome and requires each physician to focus his entire attention on the patient's problem, to act in the patient's best interest, and to always seek help when in doubt. We tend to forget that most cardiovascular diagnosis can be made at the bedside or in the office by careful history and physical examination; electrocardiogram; chest X-ray; and simple laboratory tests.

CARDIAC PEARL

We tend to forget that most diagnoses of cardiovascular disease are made in the office or at the bedside. Also, we usually do not need the sophisticated, elegant laboratory diagnostic equipment that we all have in our modern hospitals. Most patients with cardiovascular disease can be diagnosed in the physician's office – or should be. This diagnosis can be accomplished by combining the findings of a complete clinical cardiovascular evaluation, which includes a careful, detailed history and physical examination, electrocardiogram, x-ray examination, and simple laboratory tests. This procedure is known as the "five–finger" method of diagnosis. The fingers make a fist, which is an excellent and efficient way to evaluate our patients.

W. Proctor Harvey, M.D.

Ultimately, however, the success of the doctor-patient relationship depends on one paramount quality in the physician. This is measured by Dr. Harvey's *Give-Take* ratio (G/T ratio) concept. It means that the best physicians *give* to their patients, to their families, and to medicine and society in general without thought of reward or gain. This ratio must be *positive* to be the "compleat" physician. We must *give* more than we *take*. This applies to our relationships with our patients and our fellow physicians, to our teachers and our students. The role model for this quality, for myself and all of the co-authors of this book is Dr. W. Proctor Harvey.

CARDIAC PEARL

The problems that we encounter in life generally relate to a *person* or *people*, in some way. If we meet with a person to try to solve a particular problem, and his or her G/T ratio is 1.0 or more, we have no problem. On the other hand, if it is below 1.0, then we often cannot arrive at a satisfactory solution.

It is gratifying that we still meet many people whose ratio well exceeds the 1.0 – What a pleasure to meet and work with such people! In today's society, alas, we still need many more people with high G/T ratios. The high ratio is infectious and good. Also, we know that those who are "givers" in life are the likely "receivers" of much more than is ever realized or anticipated. People young and old learn by example. Frequently this is the way high G/T ratios are transmitted and perpetuated. May they transcend to all aspects of our lives and society! Many of the world's serious ills would be solved if enough leaders of nations could increase their G/T ratios. Certainly the medical profession is the ideal one to set the example.

W. Proctor Harvey, M.D.

Selected Reading

1. Arnold RM, Forrow L: Rewarding medicine: Good doctors and good behavior. *Ann Intern Med* 113:10:794-798, 1990.
2. Delbanco TL: Enriching the doctor-patient relationship by inviting the patient's perspective. *Ann Intern Med* 116:5:414-418, 1992.
3. Duffy TP: Getting the story right. *NEJM* 328:18:133-136, 1993.
4. Fuller LE: Primary caring. *JAMA* 270:1033, 1993.
5. Harvey WP: *Cardiac Pearls.* Laennec Publishing Inc., 1993.
6. Judge RD, Zuidema GD, Fitzgerald FT: *Clinical Diagnosis.* Fifth Edition. Little Brown Co, 1989.
7. Matthews DA: The boundaries and frontiers of empathy. Presentation University of Texas, March, 1992.
8. Matthews DA, Feinstein AR: A review of systems for the personal aspects of patient care. *AJTMS* 31:3:159-171, 1988.
9. Matthews DA, Sledge WH, Lieberman PB: Evaluation of intern performance by medical inpatients. *Amer J Med* 83:938-944, 1987.
10. Matthews DA, Suchman AL, Branch WT: Making "connexions": Enhancing the therapeutic potential of patient-clinician relationships. *Ann Intern Med* 118:12:973-977, 1993.
11. Mirvis DM: Physicians autonomy - the relation between public and professional expectations. *NEJM* 238:18:1346-1349, 1993.
12. Parmley WW: The decline of the doctor-patient relationship. *JACC* 26:287-288, 1995.
13. Rowland-Moran PA, Carol JG: Verbal communication skills and patient satisfaction: A study of doctor-patient interviews. *Eval* and *Health Prof.* 13:165-185, 1990.
14. Smith RC, Hoppe RB: The patient's story: Integrating the patient and physician centered approaches to interviewing. *Ann Intern Med* 115:6:470-477, 1991.
15. Suchman AL, Matthews DA: What makes the patient-doctor relationship therapeutic? Exploring the connexional dimension of medical care. *Ann Int Med* 108:125-130, 1988.

CHAPTER 3

The History

Ron J. Vanden Belt, M.D.

Evaluation of the patient with known or suspected cardiac disease begins with a carefully obtained history. A thoughtful, sympathetically conducted interview sets the stage for the patient-physician relationship that will continue for days, months, or years to come. In addition, important facts that are not uncovered in a meticulous initial history have an uncanny way of eluding later detection as work-up progresses and the patient and physician become focussed on high technology studies and more aggressive therapeutic interventions. After the history is obtained, important observations may be made during the physical examination; sophisticated physiologic data and images of astonishing clarity may be acquired, yet a thorough and careful history is the foundation for a rational approach to diagnostic evaluation and ultimate therapeutic recommendations.

CARDIAC PEARL

Never has the need been greater than it is today for the physician to learn and apply the art of bedside and office diagnosis of cardiovascular disease. In today's world, there is an unfortunate, as well as very expensive (for the patient) trend to obtain the "non-invasive" as well as "invasive" laboratory test for diagnosis before there is a careful clinical evaluation of what we term the "five–finger approach." We should make a "fist" of these fingers using all of them to make the correct diagnosis in the great majority of patients. However, if we were allowed only one of the 5 "fingers," we would of course, choose the thumb, the history. By this method probably 90% of patients seen for some form of heart disease, can be evaluated at the bedside or in a physician's

office. The remaining patients screened do, indeed, need hospital admission to make use of the excellent ingenious and sophisticated laboratory equipment and studies in our modern hospitals.

The history (thumb) is generally the most important finger; next is the physical exam (index finger). Often, by the time these two have been completed, the diagnosis is already evident. Too often, today, these simple basic important components of evaluation of a patient are neglected or deemphasized. Specialized "invasive" or "non invasive" laboratory procedures are often top priority, which may be unnecessary, expensive and sometimes even risky.

W. Proctor Harvey, M.D.

One should always be sure that the findings of the diagnostic evaluation fit the patient's history, and that treatment recommendations seem appropriate for the level of symptoms and disability reported by the patient and are commensurate with severity of disease identified. It's important to gain a clearcut understanding of the patient's symptoms and their impact on his/her lifestyle. As diagnostic and therapeutic procedures that carry risks and costs are employed, one must be certain that the risk/cost/benefit ratio remains reasonable.

For example, proceeding with an especially high-risk intervention will be much more acceptable to all if the patient is highly symptomatic. Conversely, it is not uncommon to see an individual at very low risk for cardiac disease whose symptoms and resulting apprehension regarding heart disease are so great that they have greatly modified their lifestyle. In this situation, a more aggressive evaluation than usual may be needed. Symptoms should be explored in a context relevant to the patient being evaluated. Ranch house dwellers rarely climb stairs; running a vacuum cleaner, changing bed linen, pushing a lawn mower, or raking leaves are domestic chores with which most people can identify. But a host of conditions such as advanced age, marked obesity, generalized arthritis, peripheral vascular disease, decreased vision, to name only a few, may impose sufficient limitation of activity that effort-related symptoms are denied by the patient.

Obtaining a history from the patient with cardiac disease is similar to taking a history from any other patient, except that a different set of symptoms is explored in more detail as one reconstructs chronology of the illness, gleans clues to formulate a diagnosis, and identifies various problems to which attention must be directed. Although the focus of the initial history is appropriately the cardiovascular system, the past medical history, other intercurrent symptoms and diseases should be assessed. For example, not only does a history of long-standing diabetes identify a patient at increased risk for atherosclerosis, but may be the clue to impaired renal function that could be aggravated by the contrast medium given at the time of cardiac catheterization. An individual with multiple disorders involving other organ systems or limiting life expectancy may be approached more conservatively as the diagnostic and therapeutic program is developed. Specific symptoms associated with cardiovascular disease are discussed below.

CARDIAC PEARL

Unfortunately, the history is not adequately emphasized and utilized. Certainly, if the physician is allowed to use only one "finger", or one aspect, of the evaluation he/she should choose the history. Of course, the total cardiovascular examination is used and is necessary. Too often, mainly because a careful history is time consuming, a busy physician may try a "short cut", only to find that he has penalized himself. For example, a typical history of angina pectoris is often readily elicited by appropriate questions to the patient, whereas the other components of the cardiovascular evaluation may not indicate an abnormality; the ECG may be read as normal in about 50% of patients who have a typical history of angina pectoris, and the heart is also interpreted as being normal in size and contour. Key questions can often aid in the diagnosis.

Asking the Right Questions: To elicit a description of the typical pain caused by myocardial ischemia, ask the question, "What happens if you walk briskly up a hill, against the wind, in cold weather?"

The patient may pause and then state, "Nothing", or "I get some shortness of breath." Does anything else happen? "Yes, I get a pressure or tightness here" (and the patient may put his hand or fist over the midportion of his sternal area). The patient may not use the word pain, but rather "pressure" or "burning," or simply "discomfort," particularly if the symptom is not severe. Some patients may only note this typical discomfort of angina pectoris after they have eaten a large meal and then walk up a hill, against the wind, in cold weather.

Be careful not to suggest to the patient that pain or discomfort might occur with this situation. That's why the question is put, "What happens if...etc." rather than saying, "Do you get pain or discomfort...etc." If the patient answers in the affirmative, it is not as easy to interpret as it would be if they describe their symptoms in response to the former question.

W. Proctor Harvey, M.D.

Cardiovascular Symptoms

Chest Pain

Most people experience chest pains at some point in their life. While chest pain is a symptom of many cardiovascular, pulmonary, and gastrointestinal disorders, it frequently is encountered as well in the absence of any underlying organic disease. Careful analysis of the characteristics of chest pain (Table 1) frequently will lead one to the correct diagnosis. The chest pain history usually is more helpful than the physical examination in the patient with uncomplicated coronary disease. With the spontaneous recital of a history of typical angina characteristics, one often can be confident of diagnosis within a few minutes. Familiarity with the usual patterns of pain is helpful in reassuring the patient without cardiac disease. It is not uncommon for patients to have two or three distinct types of pain that may take some effort to sort out during the interview. Sometimes a presenting symptom of noncardiac pain may be masking the more subtle symptoms of angina pectoris. Although there is overlap, it is helpful to think of chest pain as being chronic, recurring as opposed to the single acute episode.

In general, the former is more likely to be evaluated electively in the outpatient setting and includes stable angina, musculoskeletal or gastrointestinal pain, anxiety, etc. The acute episode is more frequently seen in the hospital or Emergency

42

TABLE 1
Characteristics of Chest Pain

Location – Pain may be retrosternal, diffuse across precordium, in left inframammary area, left precordial ("over the heart"), mainly in the back, shoulder(s), or subscapular area. Some cardiac pain may be felt in the epigastrium only. The consistency of the location of the pain should be determined. Pinpoint or sharply localized should be distinguished from more diffuse or generalized pain.

Quality – Pain may be described as squeezing, burning, a fullness, pressure, dull ache, sharp, gas, heartburn, indigestion, a need to belch, numbing or prickly.

Frequency – Does the pain occur many times per day or only occasionally in response to specific precipitating factors? What has been the pattern of the episodes - more or less frequent/severe in recent days/weeks?

Duration – Does the pain last for seconds, minutes or hours? Are there quick jabs or stabs or does the pain last for hours at a time? Is there lingering pain after the worst of the episode has cleared?

Course of pain – Does the pain remain steady or wax and wane during an episode? Does the pain begin abruptly at full intensity or does it build up gradually? How rapidly does the pain subside?

Precipitating/relieving factors – Do activities such as walking uphill, hurrying, exposure to cold, emotional stress, sex, or the postprandial state bring on the pain? Is pain influenced by motion, position, respiration? Does the supine position influence the pain? Does pain come on without any precipitating factor or during sleep?

Radiation – Are any extrathoracic sites affected? Radiation of pain to shoulders, arm, back, neck, throat, jaw or the interscapular area is not uncommon. Sensation of numbness/tingling in upper extremities may be manifestation of referred pain.

Associated symptoms – Breathlessness, marked fatigue, diaphoresis, pre-syncope, syncope, apprehension and sense of impending doom may occur.

Department and includes the more pressing problems of myocardial infarct, unstable angina, aortic dissection, pulmonary embolus, etc. In the non-urgent setting, one should take advantage of the opportunity for a repeat interview to clarify the history. Once the patient has been interviewed regarding chest pain, he or she may have better answers and observations at a second visit. Diseases affecting most of the thoracic and some extrathoracic structures can cause chest pain.

CARDIAC PEARL

A history of chest discomfort or pain warrants careful, detailed analysis.

If there is a family history of coronary disease, this provides a caution flag. It is especially important if present in both the mater-nal and paternal sides of the family and/or if there is a family history of death from coronary artery disease occurring at a young age (premature coronary disease). Any patient with such a history and who complains of chest discomfort, should have a careful review of the electrocardiogram which may reveal some abnormalities. If there is any question as to the presence of coronary disease, additional screening studies such as an echocardiogram, exercise treadmill, thallium exercise treadmill, and even coronary angiography may be indicated.

Chest discomfort in an athlete also should alert the physician to the possibility of hypertrophic cardiomyopathy, the leading cause of sudden death in athletes less than 30 years of age. Many patients with hypertrophic cardiomyopathy have no symptoms. However, if symptoms are present, chest discomfort is the most common. It often simulates the type of pain seen in coronary ischemic disease. Some complain of dizziness, while others have both chest discomfort and dizziness.

W. Proctor Harvey, M.D.

• **Myocardium (Myocardial Ischemia):** The fear and concern aroused when an individual experiences chest pain in large part reflects concern regarding coronary heart disease and its well-known sequelae. Given the potential serious and rapid changes which can occur with myocardial ischemia, it is important to be able to make a good clinical judgement as to whether or not the patient has myocardial ischemia. In a typical clinical practice, myocardial ischemia is the most frequently encountered serious cause of chest pain and most commonly is the condition which needs to be "ruled out". While the vast majority of patients with symptoms of myocardial ischemia have coronary disease, aortic stenosis or hypertrophic cardiomyopathy can cause myocardial ischemia in the setting of normal coronary arteries. Severe pulmonary hypertension can cause anginal type chest pain, presumably due to right ventricular ischemia.

When blood flow to the myocardium is inadequate (increased demand and/or decreased supply) to meet its metabolic demands, ischemia of myocardial tissue results. Although not completely understood, the mechanism of chest discomfort due to myocardial ischemia is thought to be the accumulation of metabolites and/or vasoactive substances that result from ischemia. While the typical discomfort of myocardial ischemia is perceived in the substernal area, radiation of pain to other areas is common. This "referred" pain occurs in the C7-T4 distribution; the segments from which the cardiac nerves arise. With heavy afferent stimuli coming in from the heart, adjacent neurons supplying other sites may become activated, leading to the perception of pain in the arm(s), back, throat, or neck. Numbness or tingling, especially in the arms, is a common manifestation of referred pain.

The classic symptom of myocardial ischemia, angina pectoris, is an oppressive retrosternal sensation. Although generally perceived as painful, it is not uncommon for patients to describe an ache, pressure or fullness and to deny chest pain if that is the only symptom sought. It is well-recognized that myocardial ischemia and even infarction, can be "silent" without any evident symptoms. Diabetic patients have a high incidence of painless ischemic episodes. Some patients present with symptoms such as dyspnea or extreme weakness which represent "anginal equivalents".

Typical angina pectoris (AP) is usually described as a squeezing, pressing, constricting, full, aching, or burning. The discomfort frequently has a visceral quality. Characterizing chest discomfort with the sign of a clenched fist (Levine's sign) is highly suggestive of angina. Usually precordial in location, angina tends to be somewhat diffuse and does not localize to a small area such that a single finger can point to the pain. Occasionally, angina will be low enough to be described as epigastric in location. AP typically occurs during physical effort or with strong emotion, and is more readily precipitated in cold weather or wind and following meals.

The combination of physical and emotional stress, such as hurrying to catch a plane, is especially likely to cause angina. Many patients with severe angina can accomplish considerable activity as long as they pace themselves and do not hurry. Duration of typical angina is minutes, usually not more than 20, especially if the inciting activity is discontinued. AP is not a fleeting stab of pain, nor does it last hours or days, and does not begin at peak intensity but takes some period of time (several seconds to minutes) to build. Sublingual nitroglycerin usually will produce relief from pain within a minute or two of its dissolution or prevent an attack altogether if taken prophylactically.

Angina tends to be more readily provoked shortly after arising. Some patients will experience angina early in the day with light activity and much heavier activity later in the day without symptoms. Also, angina may occur early in the course of a given activity, then subside as the patient continues to "walk through".

The amount of activity required to bring on angina tends to be consistent, but some patients have a variable threshold for angina. Coronary vasospasm is believed to be operative in some of these patients; while typically precipitated by physical activity, angina can occur while the patient is inactive, or during sleep. During an anginal episode, most patients want to remain in the sitting or standing position and will resist the supine position. A single breath does not influence angina. Frequently there is radiation to the arm(s), throat, lower jaw, or back. On occasion, anginal distress will be perceived only in an extrathoracic site(s); dyspnea, diaphoresis, or weakness may accompany angina. The pattern of the anginal episodes needs to be explored with care. The recent onset of angina, increasing frequency, severity or duration of attacks, provocation with less activity, or occurrence of chest pain may be indicative of unstable angina that requires more aggressive management than longstanding stable effort angina.

In contrast to transient myocardial ischemia, which usually results from increased oxygen demand, myocardial infarction results from an interruption in myocardial blood flow (decreased supply), which is not restored. Most myocardial infarcts result from formation of a clot in one of the epicardial coronary arteries at site of an atherosclerotic plaque. The pain of an acute myocardial infarct (AMI) is similar to that of AP, but usually more severe and unremitting, although it can be deceptively mild. Other symptoms such as nausea, vomiting, diaphoresis, dyspnea, weakness, syncope, or an ashen color frequently occur in AMI. An episode of diaphoresis during the pain may be the symptom that distinguishes an infarct from an anginal episode. It is well recognized that +/- 25% of all infarcts are silent. Sometimes there are absolutely no symptoms, but some patients will be able to recall an episode that probably was the infarct. Some patients will present with predominant symptoms of congestive heart failure, atrial fibrillation or heart block with mild or no pain.

• **Pericardium:** Inflammation of the pericardial surfaces may cause anterior chest pain, sometimes of great severity. Radiation of pericardial pain to the cap of the left shoulder and the neck is common. Pain usually is accentuated by respiration, and may be relieved by sitting up and leaning forward. It's usually described as sharp by the patient, but may mimic the pain of myocardial infarction.

• **Aorta:** Dissection of the aorta typically results in severe anterior chest pain of abrupt onset at maximal intensity, often with a "tearing" quality and radiation to the back. Location of pain is related to the portion of the aorta involved by dissection. Involvement of the neck, upper extremity, or abdominal vessels by dissection may result in pain in those sites, and migration of pain may reflect extension of the dissection.

• **Pleura:** Inflammation or irritation of the pleura (often seen with pulmonary infarction) results in pain, usually related to site of involvement, that is sharp, of variable severity, and increased with inspiration. Patients frequently describe pleuritic pain as a "stitch" or "catch." Some patients with pulmonary embolus may experience an anginal type of pain, thought to be due to pulmonary hypertension. Massive pulmonary embolism is more likely to present with dyspnea, collapse, hypoxemia, etc than with chest pain.

• **Muscles and Skeleton:** Pain originating in the chest wall is a common complaint, especially in healthy young people. Individual episodes may be fleeting, with frequent recurrences, or may last several hours to days. This pain, which typically occurs at rest, can be severe, often is affected by change in position or respiration, and may be reproduced by palpation of the chest wall. Cervical osteoarthritis or intervertebral disc disease may cause pain in the upper extremities, shoulder, or neck and raise concern regarding myocardial ischemia. Examination of a patient with chest pain of uncertain cause always should include palpation of the ribs, spine, and costochondral junctions.

CARDIAC PEARL

Pain in the left arm can be misinterpreted as being of coronary origin. One such pain is similar to that caused when a blood pressure cuff is left inflated too long and the radial pulse is occluded.

One can occlude his own radial pulse by moving the arm backwards and rotating it in such a manner that there is interference of the arterial blood supply to the left arm. Occasionally a patient will sleep in such a position that his or her left arm is extended and partially occluding the arterial pulse. The pain from this condition can simulate the arm pain from coronary ischemic pain. One such patient is recalled who would have pain lasting for hours or days; it extended from the shoulders down his left arm to the hand. To further complicate the picture, the patient also had a hiatal hernia. At first, coronary artery disease was suspected, but an extensive cardiovascular workup was negative. A detailed history revealed that the patient often awoke with the pain, which led to questions about the positioning of his arms while sleeping. His answers indicated that he might be occluding the arterial blood supply to his arm in his sleep. The patient was advised to sleep in a position where his arms and shoulder were not in a position to occlude the pulse. This solved his problem.

W. Proctor Harvey, M.D.

• **Esophagus:** The pain of esophageal spasm can mimic angina, including radiation to the neck, arms or back, with associated diaphoresis and relief with nitroglycerin. Presence or absence of other gastrointestinal symptoms is not especially helpful in assigning a cardiac or gastrointestinal cause to the pain. Radiation of the pain to the back has been reported to support diagnosis of GI pain (Schofield). Since both coronary heart disease and esophageal reflux are common disorders, it is not unexpected that a patient may experience symptoms of reflux and angina.

• **Atypical Chest Pain:** Many patients are seen whose chest pain is not characteristic of any of the specific disorders discussed above. Although there are many variations, several patterns commonly are encountered. This sort of pain usually occurs at rest, is not aggravated by activity, and may be present for long periods. Sometimes the pain is in the left inframammary area, especially in women, and associated with a sense of constriction (desire to loosen clothing). Other patients report ill-defined diffuse anterior precordial pressure, present for hours or days at a time, and unrelated to exertion. Sharp stabs of pain, either single or repetitive, are almost never of cardiac origin. Sometimes stretching or deep breaths will decrease distress. Sighing respirations or a feeling of needing to take in a deep breath frequently accompany noncardiac chest pain. Numbness or paresthesias in the left upper extremity are a frequent source of concern in patients with no apparent organic disease; cause of these symptoms is unclear, believed by many to be related to stress or anxiety.

It has been suggested that a substantial number of patients with atypical chest pain actually have Panic Disorder or Generalized Anxiety Disorder (Beitman/Kane). Through the years, a variety of diagnoses such as DaCosta's Syndrome ("irritable heart syndrome"), neurocirculatory asthenia, cardiac neurosis, etc have been applied to these patients. Certainly, the hyperventilation syndrome with its symptom complex including dyspnea, chest pain, circumoral and acral paresthesias, and carpal pedal spasm, is generally accepted as being related to anxiety. Once the serious causes of chest pain have been excluded, further extensive diagnostic evaluation usually is not revealing.

Non-Coronary Chest Pains: It is worthwhile to explain to the patient the type of chest pain that generally is not related to heart disease:

• **A constant "aching" pain that might be in the substernal area and lasts all day is usually not caused by heart disease. Nor is pain that is present only in one position and not in others.**

• **Coronary pain is not accentuated by external pressure over the precordium.**

• **Pain over the apical region of the heart or over the right anterior chest region is not typical of coronary artery pain.**

• **The fleeting, momentary pain in the chest described as a needle jab or stick, lasting only a second or two, is not heart pain.**

The patient can be reassured that these types of pain are not significant and not signs of a new or recurrent coronary artery disease.

It is reassuring to tell patients who have had an acute myocardial infarction and are returning home- back to physical activities and their occupation- about these noncoronary chest pains. Point out that it will be natural for them to look for pain, and almost certainly some of the pains described will occur. If patients are aware of them and are reassured, unnecessary fears and anxieties can be prevented.

W. Proctor Harvey, M.D.

Dyspnea

Dyspnea is defined as difficult or labored respiration, or the unpleasant awareness of one's respiration. Dyspnea is a very common symptom experienced at one time or another by most healthy people, as well as occurring in many diseases. Heavy activity in a well-conditioned individual can cause dyspnea as can lesser degrees of activity in a deconditioned or obese individual without apparent cardiac or pulmonary disease. Dyspnea is a very common symptom in heart disease (usually left ventricular failure), ranging from mild dyspnea with heavy effort to the gasping and wheezing of pulmonary edema. A bronchospastic component of acute heart failure, apart from underlying airways disease, is well-recognized and accounts for appellation of cardiac asthma. As the ventricle fails, there is a compensatory increase in its diastolic pressure (Frank-Starling Mechanism). This elevation of pressure is transmitted to the left atrium, pulmonary veins, and capillary bed with a reduction in pulmonary compliance, the common denominator underlying the dyspnea of left heart failure.

Increased work of respiration due to the reduced pulmonary compliance is a major determinant of the sensation of dyspnea. The symptom of dyspnea may be the patient's major concern and presenting problem, or may require careful inquiry to elicit. It is helpful to get some quantitative sense as to how much the patient can do before dyspnea occurs, such as flights of stairs or distance walked. Pace of the activity needs to be ascertained since patients with chronic heart disease often accommodate by slowing their pace to avoid dyspnea.

Obviously, pulmonary disease is also a common cause of dyspnea. Generally, pulmonary disease of severity sufficient to cause dyspnea should be readily detectable by routine clinical methods (history, physical, x-ray, and pulmonary function tests). A long history of dyspnea, wheezing, cough and sputum production supports an element of pulmonary disease. Given a high rate of smoking (past or present) in patients with cardiac disease, some component of chronic obstructive pulmonary disease which often has not been a major symptomatic problem in the past, is common in this population. A recent or dramatic increase in the dyspnea in this setting is more likely to be due to the development of heart failure than to the lung disease. Attribution of increasing dyspnea or wheezing to pulmonary disease often leads to a missed diagnosis of heart failure. Determination of relative contributions of pulmonary and cardiac components of dyspnea at the bedside when heart and lung disease coexist can be very difficult.

Cheyne-Stokes respiration is a form of periodic breathing characterized by cycles beginning with shallow respirations that increase in rate and depth to significant hyperpnea, followed by decreasing rate and depth of respiration, then a period of apnea that may last 15 seconds to 30 seconds or longer. This pattern of respiration is encountered in advanced congestive heart failure and in some forms of CNS disease. Cheyne-Stokes respiration occurs during sleep without the patient's awareness, but may be reported by a companion. When Cheyne-Stokes respiration occurs in the awake patient, the patient will experience dyspnea during the hyperpneic phase; the patient cannot voluntarily slow his respiration during this phase of the cycle.

Cheyne-Stokes respiration as a manifestation of heart failure is generally missed, simply because it is not looked for.

Remember, while we find what we look for,

we also must know what we are looking for. If the patient is not under the influence of a sedative or a narcotic, and there is no significant cerebrovascular disease present, the presence of Cheyne-Stokes respiration usually indicates the patient has very advanced heart failure. I have observed a number of patients who had not been considered to have heart failure and Cheyne-Stokes respiration had not been noted. That finding alone should alert the physician to promptly institute all necessary measures and medications to alleviate the cardiac decompensation. Adequate auscultation may be accomplished during the apneic phases of Cheyne-Stokes respiration, but may be impossible during the dyspneic phase.

W. Proctor Harvey, M.D.

Dyspnea also occurs without any significant cardiopulmonary abnormality and is a frequent manifestation of anxiety or emotional disturbance. This sort of dyspnea may be part of the classic hyperventilation syndrome or simply is a vague sensation of breathlessness not associated with physical effort and punctuated by deep sighing respirations or feeling breathless during ordinary conversation.

• **Orthopnea:** Increase in hydrostatic pressure in the lungs that occurs with assumption of the supine position may cause cough and dyspnea in patients with left ventricular failure or mitral valve disease and necessitates the use of two or more pillows when they lie down. Patients with severe obstructive pulmonary disease, especially acute asthma, cannot lie flat comfortably.

• **Paroxysmal Nocturnal Dyspnea (PND):** PND is development of dyspnea during sleep, usually 2 hours to 3 hours after going to bed, relieved by assumption of the upright position. It usually does not recur after the patient goes back to sleep. These episodes may be fairly mild but can be severe, with wheezing, cough, gasping, and apprehension. Some of these episodes will progress to frank pulmonary edema requiring medical attention. The most likely explanation for this frequent symptom of left heart failure is redistribution of body water in the supine position, with increased intravascular volume.

Other Symptoms

• **Edema:** Edema is commonly reported by patients with right and/or left heart failure. Fluid retention in heart failure is believed to result from increased venous pressure and abnormal activity of salt-retaining hormones. In an average-sized individual, it takes about 6 lbs to 10 lbs of excess fluid for edema to become apparent; history of recent weight gain will often correlate with a deterioration in clinical status. Amount of weight loss in response to treatment for heart failure in the past will be a clue as to severity of the problem. Minor degrees of edema are apparent only after a period of dependency of the legs and decrease after rest. Edema fluid may be most evident over the sacrum when the patient has been at bed rest. Although edema of cardiac origin may progress to anasarca involving thighs, genitalia, flanks, and rib cage, cardiac edema rarely involves the face or upper extremities. Edema mainly affecting the face and arms is more likely to be due to venous or lymphatic obstruction by clot or neoplasm. Facial edema is a feature of the nephrotic syndrome, angioneurotic edema, glomerulonephritis, etc. Swelling or "puffiness" of hands and fingers is not ordinarily a symptom of cardiac disease. Persistent edema in the leg(s) from which veins were harvested at the time of bypass surgery is common. Other causes of edema, such as varicosities, obesity, tight girdle, renal insufficiency, or cirrhosis with hypoproteinemia, must be considered before congestive heart failure is invoked.

• **Ascites (Fluid in the Peritoneal Cavity):** Patients will be aware of ascites because of increased abdominal girth. Previously comfortable trousers or skirts may no longer fit. Bending at the waist is uncomfortable, and there often is ill-defined abdominal fullness. Patients with severe edema due to ordinary congestive heart failure may develop ascites, but ascites is especially frequent in patients with restrictive pericardial disease, sometimes occurring before peripheral edema becomes apparent. Ascitic fluid is formed when elevated venous pressure leads to exudation of fluid from the serosal surfaces. Other causes of ascites, such as cirrhosis, nephrosis, and tumor must be excluded.

• **Fatigue:** This very nonspecific symptom, which is seen in many illnesses, both organic and psychiatric, especially depression, is common in patients with cardiac disease. Although dyspnea and fatigue often coexist, patients usually can distinguish between the two. The hemodynamic correlate of fatigue in patients with cardiac disease is a reduction in cardiac output. As congestive heart failure worsens, the descending limb of the Frank-Starling curve is reached and fatigue may supervene, replacing dyspnea as the major symptom. Beta blockers used to treat angina or hypertension commonly will cause fatigue and lethargy. Hypotension or hypokalemia caused by diuretics or ACE inhibitors can cause fatigue and weakness.

Worthy of emphasis is the symptom of fatigue. This is a very common compliant occurring in many of us even without heart disease. Recalled to mind are some examples of women in their twenties or thirties who attributed their unusual fatigue to their role as mother and housewife. However, once a diagnosis was made of atrial septal defect and operation successfully performed, fatigue was no longer a complaint.

W. Proctor Harvey, M.D.

• **Nocturia/Oliguria:** Formation of greater-than-normal volumes of urine during sleep when the patient is recumbent is a common symptom in early heart failure. Diuretic administration late in the day is a usually avoidable cause of nocturia. Some patients will report a fall in their urinary output in the days prior to an exacerbation of heart failure.

• **Palpitation:** Most normal people intermittently are aware of their heart action, usually at the time of physical or emotional stress. When the heart action is more vigorous than usual or its perception is unpleasant the term palpitation is appropriate. The symptom of palpitation and the concern it evokes are a common reason for consultation. Palpitation is frequently a benign symptom without any serious cardiac disease present, but at the other extreme may signal a potentially life-threatening condition. Simple extrasystoles or premature beats may be perceived as a fluttering or flopping sensation in the chest or as if something "turned over." This symptom may be due to the more forceful beat that occurs after the pause rather than the premature beat itself. Sometimes a transient feeling of fullness in the neck (due to cannon waves) is perceived with premature beats. There is great variability in the degree to which patients are aware of arrhythmias when symptoms are correlated with electrocardiographic recordings. Some patients feel almost every premature beat they have, while others are totally unaware of even frequent or advanced arrhythmias, with all gradations between. A report of skips or irregularity during perfectly regular sinus rhythm is not uncommon. Generally, thin, tense individuals tend to be more aware of their cardiac activity than others. Awareness of one's heartbeat is most common during periods of inactivity and quiet. People with and without arrhythmias are often aware of their cardiac activity when they first lie down on their side to sleep, especially if they lie on their left side.

Rapid heart action of a paroxysmal tachycardia is usually of abrupt onset and offset and causes a pounding sensation in the chest. Patients will often know whether tachycardia is regular or irregular, and may be able to tap out the rate and rhythm of the spell. During such an episode, patients will often be aware of precordial movements or will report that it felt like their "heart would jump out of their chest". Chest pressure or pain suggesting angina may occur with an episode of tachycardia even in young healthy patients without coronary heart disease. On the other hand, patients with coronary disease may develop severe angina with a sustained arrhythmia because of the increased myocardial oxygen demand. Depending on the rate and mechanism of the rhythm disturbance, altered level of consciousness with faintness or syncope may occur and one should always inquire in this regard. A lack of altered consciousness cannot be taken as reassurance as to the benignity of the arrhythmia. It is well recognized that sustained ventricular tachycardia can occur in the setting of serious underlying cardiac disease without a significant compromise in hemodynamics. Syncope due to tachyarrhythmias may occur without the patient being aware of palpitations.

• **Syncope (Fainting):** Syncope is a common problem which accounts for many office and emergency department visits. A history of an isolated syncopal episode at some time in the past is not unusual in an otherwise healthy person. Most syncopal episodes of cardiac origin have as their final common pathway, a reduction in cardiac output or blood pressure with decreased cerebral perfusion and loss of consciousness. In assessing the patient with syncope, it is important to determine if there were precipitating factor(s), premonitory symptoms, whether injury occurred with the episode, whether seizure activity or incontinence were present, and what the status was immediately post-syncope. Injury incurred during an episode suggests sudden profound loss of body tone and raises concern regarding the more serious causes. Brief seizure activity can occur with syncope due to a cardiac arrhythmia but sustained activity does not occur.

A patient may be incontinent during cardiogenic syncope. Loss of consciousness due to seizure activity frequently is preceded by an aura; visual, auditory, olfactory, etc. Sustained tonic-clonic movements, incontinence, and tongue biting are features of a typical grand mal seizure. A period of confusion or drowsiness and muscle pain from seizure activity after the episode characterize syncope due to CNS disease. In contrast, return of consciousness and the alert state is prompt after reversal of the arrhythmia or hypotension which caused cardiogenic syncope. Frank syncope is an unlikely presentation of carotid artery stenosis. The common faint results from bradycardia and hypotension caused by excessive vagal discharge. This "vasovagal" syncope is often associated with some precipitating event, and has brief premonitory signs and symptoms such as nausea, yawning, diaphoresis and sometimes a feeling of decreasing hearing or vision. There frequently is sufficient warning that the patient does not abruptly fall. With the advent of head up tilt table testing, it has become clear that a vasovagal mechanism is operative in some patients with syncope who do not have classic premonitory symptoms. Following a vagal episode the patient will be described as pale and diaphoretic and have a slow heart rate. Syncope occurring in the setting of any GI symptoms, nausea, abdominal cramps, diarrhea etc. is likely to be vagal in origin. A history of similar episodes dating back over several years is common in patients with vagal syncope.

A hypersensitive carotid sinus can cause similar episodes. On occasion, a patient will relate a history of episodes occurring with an activity which would apply pressure to the carotid sinus, such as shaving, tight collar, or extreme turning of the head. Most of the time this history is not obtained, even though a sensitive carotid sinus is shown to be the cause of syncope. Syncope following urination (micturition syncope) is a well-recognized phenomenon in men at the time of rapid decompression of a distended bladder which typically occurs after a period of sleep. Paroxysms of cough, usually in patients with underlying pulmonary disease can result in syncope.

Excessively fast or slow arrhythmias may decrease the cardiac output enough to cause alteration in consciousness ranging from abrupt profound syncope to mild light headedness. Stokes-Adams syncope is the type of spell caused by intermittent complete heart block or sinus arrest (occasionally ventricular tachyarrhythmias) characterized by abrupt loss of consciousness without warning, a variable period of unconsciousness (seconds to minutes), followed by rapid return of normal mental status without amnesia or postictal state.

CARDIAC PEARL

I have long realized the importance of listening carefully and paying attention to what our patients tell us. This was duly impressed upon me when I started my Fellowship in cardiology. I was taking a history from an elderly lady I was evaluating in the outpatient cardiac clinic. When I asked her what was bothering her, she replied that she had been having a lot of "spells". As if to demonstrate to me, her body stiffened; her eyes became a stare and rolled upward. Her hands and arms not only stiffened but trembled to some degree. This episode lasted a matter of seconds, probably four or five. She did not fall over. She promptly started talking again. A few minutes later she said, "I'm having another one." The same sequence of events just described occurred again. By this time, I was ready to diagnose her as a neurotic. However, when I was listening to her heart, she had a couple of recurrent episodes, each characterized by a sudden cessation of the heart beat and accompanied by the signs I observed when she was relating her history; after a brief period, her heart beat returned to her former normal rhythm. The electrocardiogram showed sinus pauses which, of course, explained her clinical symptoms and signs. This was a good lesson to me, reinforcing the importance of taking time to listen to our patients. She was subsequently followed for four to five years until her death. Autopsy revealed scarring in the region of the sinoatrial node. Unfortunately the pacemaker was not available for treatment at that time.

W. Proctor Harvey, M.D.

In the presence of severe left ventricular outflow obstruction (aortic stenosis or hypertrophic cardiomyopathy), loss of consciousness with effort may occur. These syncopal episodes occur when the heart is unable to increase its output because of fixed obstruction to outflow in response to the peripheral vasodilatation that occurs during exercise. These spells frequently follow a sudden burst of activity such as a brief periods of running or walking fast. Intermittent obstruction of a cardiac valve by an intracavitary tumor or thrombus is a rare cause of syncope, which may be precipitated when the patient changes position.

Many normal individuals experience transient lightheadedness with rapid changes in position. This is more common in older patients since the ability of the peripheral vasculature to respond is blunted with aging. Postural hypotension is a well-documented cause of fainting or dizziness. These spells usually happen when the individual is in an upright position and often take place after arising from a sitting or standing position. Possible causes which need to be explored include peripheral neuropathy, autonomic dysfunction, volume depletion or drug side effects.

• **Embolization:** The entry of a blood clot, vegetation, or tumor fragment from the heart into the systemic circulation results in an arterial embolus. Clots may occur in the left atrium behind a stenotic mitral valve, within a ventricular aneurysm or in the ventricle of a patient with cardiomyopathy. While many emboli originate in the heart, since the advent of transesophageal echo it has been recognized that atherosclerotic material in the ascending and descending aorta can embolize to the periphery. Symptoms resulting from emboli are related to the vessel in which it has lodged. It is recognized that many emboli are asymptomatic. Symptoms of a stroke occur with emboli to the cerebral vessels. Myocardial infarction can result from an embolus to a coronary artery. Hematuria, flank pain and hypertension can result from embolization to a renal artery. The abrupt development of a cold, painful extremity follows embolic obstruction of an arm or leg artery. Emboli from the vegetations of acute endocarditis may produce characteristic areas of necrosis in the fingers or toes. Extensive atherosclerosis in the abdominal aorta and iliac vessels can be resposible for showers of peripheral emboli with multiple small reddish blue lesions on the lower extremities sometimes causing small areas of gangrene ("trash toes"). An embolic event may be the presenting manifestation of previously unrecognized cardiac disease so other clues to cardiac disease in the history should be sought when a patient's clinical presentation is consistent with an embolic event.

• **Cyanosis:** Although cyanosis is a sign rather than a symptom, patients or family members may describe cyanosis during the history. Cyanosis is a bluish color of the skin and/or mucous membranes caused by excess amounts of reduced hemoglobin. About 4 gm of reduced hemoglobin is required for cyanosis to be apparent. Severely anemic patients will not exhibit cyanosis. Central cyanosis refers to a distribution of cyanosis involving the mucous membranes as well as the periphery and is caused by the admixture of venous blood at the level of the heart or great vessels. Peripheral cyanosis does not involve the mucous membranes, the result of slow peripheral flow with accumulation of excess reduced hemoglobin in the setting of circulatory failure, shock or peripheral vasospasm.

• **Cough:** A chronic non-productive cough may be a prominent feature of mild-to-moderate heart failure, but can also be a side effect of the ACE inhibitors being used to treat the heart failure. Cough can be a major symptom during paroxysmal nocturnal dyspnea or acute pulmonary edema. A large left atrium or thoracic aortic aneurysm can stimulate an irritative cough by impingement on the recurrent laryngeal nerve. Obviously, a primary lung problem often will account for the cough.

• **Hemoptysis:** Coughing of blood occurs in many cardiac disorders. Bright red pulmonary venous blood from ruptured submucosal pulmonary venules may be expectorated by patients with pulmonary venous hypertension due to mitral stenosis or severe left ventricular failure. Darker blood and/or clots occur with some pulmonary emboli, but certainly are not a diagnostic requisite. Pink, frothy sputum may be produced during acute pulmonary edema. Blood-streaked sputum is a feature of the "winter bronchitis" of mitral stenosis. Rarely, hemoptysis due to mitral stenosis can be life threatening. Massive hemoptysis with exsanguination or death from asphyxiation can follow rupture of an aortic aneurysm or one of the cardiac chambers into the bronchial tree. Rupture of a pulmonary artery by the balloon of an indwelling pulmonary artery catheter can cause abrupt severe hemoptysis in the inpatient setting.

• **Fever, Chills, and Sweats:** These symptoms in any patient with a heart murmur should lead one to suspect infective endocarditis. A history of valvular heart disease is not a prerequisite for a diagnosis of endocarditis, since previously normal valves become infected. A history of recent dental work, genitourinary surgery, or illicit drug use (potential causes of bacteremia) strengthens suspicion of infective endocarditis. Rarely, an intracardiac tumor (myxoma) may produce systemic symptoms in the absence of infection. Low grade fever in a patient with heart failure may be a sign of pulmonary emboli.

• **Diaphoresis:** Profuse "cold sweat" mediated by sympathetic discharge often accompanies early stages of acute myocardial infarction. Excessive sweating may occur in patients with severe aortic regurgitation. Diaphoresis often is a sign of congestive heart failure in infants.

• **Gastrointestinal:** Anorexia, nausea, and vomiting may occur as a result of digitalis excess. Hepatomegaly associated with tricuspid valve disease or severe right heart failure may cause right upper quadrant and epigastric pain and fullness, as well as anorexia. Abdominal pain due to visceral ischemia/infarction may occur in a patient who has or has had a period of very low cardiac output. The pain of some gastrointestinal diseases may be referred or extend to the chest or back and lead to confusion with myocardial ischemia.

• **Neck Pulsations:** Patients with severe tricuspid or aortic regurgitation may be aware of pulsations (venous and arterial, respectively) in the neck.

• **Squatting:** Patients with Tetralogy of Fallot will squat during physical activity. The squatting position increases systemic resistance which reduces the amount of right to left shunting of nonoxygenated blood which increases as systemic resistance falls during exercise. Frequent occurrence of one or more of these symptoms in patients without any organic cardiovascular disease is well recognized. The constellation of chest pain, dyspnea, fatigue, lightheadedness and palpitations is familiar in most practices.

Special Features of the Cardiac History

In addition to carefully eliciting and chronologically ordering the patient's symptoms, inquiry directed to some other specific aspects of the history is important.

• **Prior Cardiac Events and Procedures:** Patients will frequently give the history of having had a "heart attack", which in reality may have been an episode of unstable angina, heart failure, or arrhythmia. The heart attack history is then transposed to myocardial infarction in the medical record by medical personnel and will confuse the examiner unless more detail about the episode is sought or source documentation is reviewed. It is common, especially in a referral practice, to encounter patients who have had several catheterizations, angioplasties and one or more bypass operations in addition to multiple noninvasive studies. A painstaking and often time-consuming review of records from other institutions, operative notes, catheterization films, and noninvasive studies will be required to develop an accurate picture of the patient's current status and to avoid unnecessary repetition of expensive and potentially risky procedures.

• **Treatment:** The patient's therapeutic program, both past and present, must be reviewed carefully. Unyielding heart failure may be significantly improved with the institution of a low-salt diet. A surprising number of patients with typical angina pectoris have never been given sublingual nitroglycerin. The drugs currently utilized for the treatment of various cardiovascular diseases have a large number of potential side effects (not true allergy) which can result in cardiovascular and non-cardiovascular symptoms with which the clinician needs to be familiar (Table 2).

• **Risk Factors:** Multiple risk factors for development of coronary heart disease have been identified and include age, male sex, hypertension, hypercholesterolemia, low HDL cholesterol, cigarette smoking, and diabetes. Presence or absence of the risk factors increases or decreases the statistical likelihood that an individual patient may or may not have coronary disease. However, risk factor status, especially their absence, generally

TABLE 2	
Symptoms Attributable to Cardiovascular Drugs	
SYMPTOM	CARDIOVASCULAR DRUG/MECHANISM
CNS	
Headache	Nitroglycerin
Syncope	IA antiarrhythmic (torsade de pointes)
	Beta blockers } bradycardia
	Calcium channel blocker } hypotension
	Warfarin - blood loss
Tremor/ataxia	Amiodarone
Gastrointestinal	
Xerostomia	Disopyramide
Anorexia	Digitalis
Nausea/vomiting	Quinidine, digitalis
Diarrhea	Quinidine
Constipation	Verapamil, cholestyramine
Peptic disease	Nicotinic acid
Pulmonary	
Cough	ACE inhibitors
Pulmonary fibrosis	Amiodarone
Genitourinary	
Nocturia	Diuretics
Hesitancy	Disopyramide
Impotence	Beta blockers
Renal insufficiency	ACE inhibitors, contrast medium
Endocrine	
Hyper/hypothyroid	Amiodarone
Diabetes aggravated	Nicotinic acid
Hypoglycemia masked	Beta blockers
Musculoskeletal	
Arthritis/lupus	Procainamide, hydralazine
Muscle weakness/cramps	Diuretics/electrolyte depletion
Cutaneous	
Sunlight sensitivity	Amiodarone
Flushing	Nicotinic acid
Fatigue/lethargy	Beta blockers

should not be used to make management decisions about an individual patient, especially in the emergent/urgent evaluation of chest pain. Risk factors such as hypertension, hypercholesterolemia, diabetes, and smoking should be explored in sufficient detail to determine the duration and severity of the condition, past and present therapy and the degree of control which has been achieved. The designation of male sex as one of the major risk factors for coronary heart disease and the observations in some studies that women with chest pain seem to have a fairly benign prognosis have led to a failure to appreciate the importance of chest pain in women. There is substantial recent literature regarding "gender bias" in diagnosis and treatment of heart disease in women. Although coronary disease does develop about ten years later in women than in men, coronary disease is highly prevalent in women and is the most common cause of mortality in women, accounting for twice as many deaths in women as all forms of cancer. It has been implied that there is a tendency for the significance of chest pain in women to be underestimated, especially by physicians. Additionally, Birdwell and colleagues suggest that the style (dramatic vs business-like) of the patient's presentation to the physician can significantly impact the physician's approach to diagnosis and treatment.

• **Family History:** Although most of the common cardiovascular disorders are sporadic, there are several examples in which genetic transmission can occur. These include mitral valve prolapse and the hypertrophic or dilated cardiomyopathies. Other disorders which are more frequently regarded as genetically determined include some of the inborn errors of metabolism, muscular dystrophies, the Ehler-Danlos syndrome, Marfan's Syndrome and the long QT syndrome with and without deafness. A family history of congenital heart disease confers a higher risk of a congenital cardiac lesion. A strong family history is common in patients with coronary disease which may reflect a familial predisposition to the development of atherosclerosis, presence of one or more major risk factors (diabetes, hypercholesterolemia, etc) in the family or a high-risk behavior such as smoking.

• **Congenital Heart Disease Suspected:** Symptoms of congestive heart failure in infancy include labored respirations, frequent respiratory infections, sweating, difficulty feeding and poor growth and development, and are common in patients with large VSDs or patent ductus. Maternal rubella is a cause of pulmonary artery stenosis and patent ductus arteriosus. A high incidence of prematurity is present in patients with patent ductus as is birth at higher altitude. Determining the time when a murmur was first detected will be helpful in the differential diagnosis (vide infra). A family history of the same or other congenital cardiac malformations may be obtained.

• **Rheumatic Fever:** Many patients with obvious rheumatic heart disease have no history of acute rheumatic fever, whereas other patients give histories of clear-cut, well-documented rheumatic fever, often multiple episodes. Inquiry about growing pains, St. Vitus' dance (chorea), frequent streptococcal throat infections, or prolonged febrile illnesses as a child with absence from school, may be helpful if the patient denies rheumatic fever. Questions about features of the illness are important even when a patient says he has had rheumatic fever, since many patients have been told that they "had rheumatic fever," based on pres-

ence of a heart murmur heard many years later, when, in fact, there never was a clinically apparent episode. Remember, rheumatic fever is unusual before the age of 4 years.

• **Heart Murmur:** Has a murmur been heard previously? Recent onset of a murmur may suggest endocarditis or a serious complication in a patient with coronary heart disease. Murmurs due to rheumatic heart disease rarely are heard before age 5 or 6. Murmurs heard in the newborn nursery usually are due to outflow obstruction, whereas murmurs of the common left-to-right central shunts are not heard until the child is older (shunt flow does not begin until the high pulmonary resistance of the newborn has fallen). Is the murmur heard by everyone who examines the patient? A faint murmur of aortic regurgitation often is missed, but the harsh murmur of pulmonic or aortic stenosis is unlikely to escape even the most casual examiner.

• **Previous Examinations:** In addition to being examined at the time of routine physicals or in association with other medical treatment, patients often have been examined for the armed forces, for athletics or insurance and may have been told of a heart murmur or hypertension on those occasions. Rejection by the military or an insurance company often is prompted by a cardiovascular abnormality. This line of questioning should also ascertain if the patient has, in fact, ever been examined. Many people have not seen a physician for some years or never had their heart adequately examined when they were seen.

• **Pregnancy:** Increased hemodynamic burden of pregnancy may cause an otherwise marginally compensated cardiac patient to become symptomatic. Inquiry should be made about heart failure, edema, dyspnea or requirement for prolonged periods of bed rest during pregnancy. Many normal women will have a murmur detected during pregnancy. Remember that dyspnea, edema, and episodes of light-headedness due to uterine compression of the inferior vena cava are common during pregnancy in the absence of cardiopulmonary abnormality. Patients with long standing paroxysmal supraventricular tachycardia may report either amelioration or aggravation of symptoms during pregnancy.

• **Drug and Alcohol Use:** A history of illicit parenteral drug use should raise the suspicion of infective endocarditis, especially in a febrile patient. Cocaine can cause coronary vasospasm and also raises myocardial oxygen demand by increasing heart rate and blood pressure. Angina, myocardial infarct, and sudden cardiac death have been well-documented after cocaine use. This possibility should be considered, especially in the young patient otherwise at low risk for coronary disease. Since continued use can lead to recurrence, it is imperative to identify this inciting factor.

Alcohol depresses myocardial function. Taken in sufficient quantity, not necessarily "skid row" levels, alcohol is a well recognized cause of cardiomyopathy in some patients and may be a contributing factor in patients with heart failure of other etiologies. Moderate alcohol consumption is associated with increases in HDL cholesterol and there is some evidence that the incidence of coronary disease is less at this level of alcohol use.

• **Cardiac Enlargement:** Often patients have been told about an enlarged heart on a routine chest x-ray sometime in the past.

• **Weight:** Recent rapid weight gain suggests fluid retention from heart failure. Weight loss may reflect cardiac cachexia (related to low cardiac output), digitalis toxicity, or hyperthyroidism.

• **Other Illnesses:** History of a prior malignancy, connective tissue disease, or renal failure may explain pericarditis or cardiac tamponade. Diabetes is a frequent concomitant of atherosclerotic heart disease. Treatment of malignancy with the anthracycline agents can cause myocardial dysfunction and heart failure.

• **Prior Diagnosis:** Often the questions "What have your doctors told you the problem is?" and "What do you think the problem is?" will result in very revealing answers. Sometimes you may learn the precise diagnosis; on other occasions, you may find that the patient is harboring totally unfounded fears about a diagnosis that you have not even considered.

CARDIAC PEARL

On Taking a History: When taking a history, ask your patient, "What have you been told about the diagnosis of your heart condition?"

Surprisingly, in some, an accurate diagnosis is made by the patient who knows specific details of his or her problem, including laboratory findings, results of diagnostic workup, and surgery if this had been performed. However, we should not cut short our own careful clinical evaluation because of this, because the facts related by the patient can be incorrect and misleading.

It is my impression that lawyers give the most accurately detailed account of their history. Sometimes when I do not know an occupation of a particular patient and he states, "On July 19, at 1:00 PM I was walking on the left side of Main Street, I noticed, etc." Then I ask, "By the way, are you an attorney"; and the answer is "Yes."

W. Proctor Harvey, M.D.

Goals for the History

At the conclusion of your initial interview, which ideally has included a complete medical history with emphasis on the cardiovascular system, the following should have been accomplished:

• You should have a very good idea as to what major type of heart disease, if any, the patient has (coronary, congenital, valvular, etc).

• You should be planning your physical examination and thinking of things for which you will carefully look and listen.

• Appropriate diagnostic studies should be coming to mind.

• Since changes in medical treatment and recommendations for intervention frequently are based on information derived from the patient's history, your plan of management should be beginning to take shape.

• You should have some feeling for your patient's reaction to his disease and how the disease or its treatment is affecting lifestyle. Therapeutic recommendations for a laborer with no vocational alternative may be very different from those given to a bank president. Perfect control of a symptom or risk factor at the price of intolerable side effects may be a Pyrrhic victory.

Classifications of Cardiac Disability

Several schema have been proposed and used over a number of years for systematic and reproducible grading of disability due to cardiac disease. Although the full New York Heart Association method of cardiac diagnosis originally proposed many years ago is not used widely now, the portion of the classification which addressed functional capacity (deleted in later versions) still receives some use. Despite the fact that the Canadian Cardiovascular Society's grading system for angina is more widely utilized, references to the NYHA class continue to appear in the literature and in clinical practice.

New York Heart Association Classification

Functional Class I: Patients who have heart disease without limitation of physical activity. Ordinary activity does not cause symptoms.

Functional Class II: Patients with heart disease with slight limitation of physical activity; ordinary physical activity causes fatigue, dyspnea, palpitation, or angina pectoris.

Functional Class III: Patients with heart disease who have marked limitation of activity and experience symptoms with less than ordinary activity; they do not have symptoms at rest.

Functional Class IV: Patients who cannot engage in any physical activity without symptoms and may have symptoms at rest.

Canadian Cardiovascular Society Grading System

The Canadian Cardiovascular Society's grading system for severity of effort angina is a modification of the NYHA classification. Believed to be more precise and reproducible than the NYHA classification, this system has been used in a large number of research studies and is widely applied in clinical practice. It has the limitation of being applicable to angina only.

Grading of Angina of Effort by the Canadian Cardiovascular Society:

I. Ordinary physical activity does not cause angina, such as walking and climbing stairs. Angina with strenuous or rapid or prolonged exertion at work or recreation.

II. Slight limitation of ordinary activity. Walking or climbing stairs rapidly, walking uphill, walking or stair climbing after meals, in the cold, in wind, or under emotional stress, or only during the few hours after awakening. Walking more than two blocks on the level and climbing more than one flight of ordinary stairs at a normal pace and in normal conditions.

III. Marked limitation of ordinary physical activity. Walking one to two blocks on the level and climbing one flight of stairs in normal conditions and at normal pace.

IV. Inability to carry on any physical activity without discomfort; anginal syndrome *may be* present at rest.

Goldman Scale

This system of grading cardiovascular disability is based on the metabolic cost of the activity in question. It has the advantage of being relatively quantitative and reproducible but has not been widely applied.

Selected Reading

1. Beitman BD, Basha I, Flaker G, et al: Atypical or nonanginal chest pain. *Arch Intern Med* 147:1548-1552, 1987.
2. Birdwell BG, Herbers JE, Kroenke K: Evaluating chest pain: patient's presentation style alters diagnostic approach. *Arch Int Med* 1991-1995, 1993.
3. Christie LG, Conti CR: Systematic approach to evaluation of angina-like chest pain: pathophysiology and clinical testing with emphasis on objective documentation of myocardial ischemia. *AHJ* 102:897-912, 1981.
4. Constant J: Clinical diagnosis of nonanginal chest pain: differentiation of angina from nonanginal chest pain by history. *Clin Card* 6:11-16, 1983.
5. The Criteria Committee of the New York Heart Association. *Nomenclature and criteria for diagnosis and diseases of the heart and great vessels.* 9th Ed. Boston: Little, Brown and Co., 1994.
6. DeMeester TR, O'Sullivan GC, et al: Esophageal function in patients with angina-type chest pain and normal coronary angiograms. *Ann Surg* 196:488-498, 1982.
7. Goldman L, Hashimoto B, Cook EF, Loscalzo A: Comparative reproducibility and validity of systems for assessing cardiovascular functional class: advantages of a new specific activity scale. *Circ* 64:1227-1234, 1981.
8. Hickam DH, Sox HC, Jr, Sox CH: Systematic bias in recording the history in patients with chest pain. *J Chron Dis* 38:91-100, 1985.
9. Kane FJ, Harper RG, Wittels E.: Angina as a symptom of psychiatric illness. *South Med J* 81:1412-1416, 1988.
10. Maserl A.: Pathogenetic mechanisms of angina pectoris: expanding views. *BHJ* 43:648-660, 1980.
11. Mellow MH: A gastroenterologist's view of chest pain. *Current Problems in Cardiology.* Year Book Medical Publishers 1983.
12. Schofield PM, Whorwell PJ, Jones PE, et al: Differentiation of "esophageal " and "cardiac" chest pain. *AJC* 62:315-316, 1988.
13. Singh S, Richter JE, et al: Contribution of gastroesophageal reflux to chest pain in patients with CHD. *Ann Int Med* 117:824-830, 1992.
14. Wasserman K: Dyspnea on exertion: is it the heart or the lungs? *JAMA* 248:2039-2043, 1982.
15. Wenger NK, Speroff L, Packard B: Cardiovascular health and disease in women. *NEJM* 329:247-256, 1993.
16. Wood P: *Diseases of the Heart and Circulation,* Ed 2. Philadelphia: JB Lippincott Co., 1956.

CHAPTER 4

The General Appearance
of the Patient

Donald F. Leon, M.D.

Observation of the general appearance of individual patients often provides the physician insight into the nature and severity of cardiac disability, and at least some information about duration of illness. The clues are many and varied, and are not always apparent to the hurried observer. Thus, in every encounter, a few moments should be dedicated to having a good and thoughtful look at the patient.

The general demeanor of the patient may provide considerable information. Heart disease is usually fatiguing, particularly over time, so the energy and gait of the patient may be signs of the adequacy of systemic blood flow (cardiac output relative to usual activity).

A particularly informative observation can be made while greeting the patient alongside the hospital bed, or on the examining table, by shaking hands and engaging the patient in brief conversation while maintaining physical contact. Holding the patient's hand or forearm is usually reassuring, and permits observation of the temperature of the extremity, some clues as to the adequacy of circulation, and an opportunity to evaluate volume and rate of the peripheral pulse. Information about skin texture and wall structure of the peripheral arteries may be available, and hyperkinetic circulatory states can usually be recognized. Systolic expansion of the forearm, when detected, suggests presence of advanced aortic regurgitation.

Body Conformation

There are numerous clues to be found in the general morphology and stature of cardiovascular patients. Wasting and cachexia are almost certain

indicators of curtailment of systemic blood flow, whereas substantial obesity should cause the observer to consider the congestive syndrome that marked obesity can cause. Severe obesity associated with intermittent somnolence and signs of congestive heart failure leads rapidly towards diagnosis of Pickwickian syndrome. Severe obesity itself can produce congestive heart failure in the absence of pulmonary hypoventilation; mechanisms are complex but treatable.

CARDIAC PEARL

Sleep – what an important and integral part of our lives, and where we spend approximately one-third of our time. Most of us usually take it for granted – but what a problem when we can't, or don't get our "night's sleep;" without it we have numerous complaints; fatigue; malaise; lassitude; feeling "dull," depressed, nervous, irritable, and crotchety. In other words, when we miss our sleep during each 24 hours we are definitely affected, both physically and emotionally.

I have always marveled at those individuals who are able to get by on little sleep each night, several hours instead of the usual eight. Edison, the great inventor, was such a person. I must confess I have often wondered if people like him make up for this by "napping" during the day. I suspect they do. Of course, there are those who give the appearance, at least, of being "sleepy" during much of the day. These individuals may well be free of any definite disease such as hypothyroidism. They just look and act that way. Along these lines, there is an interesting disease known as the "Pickwickian Syndrome," described so appropriately by that astute physician, the late Dr. Sydney Burwell. But first I will quote from The Pickwick Papers by Charles Dickens:

The object that presented itself to the eyes of the astonished clerk, was a boy – a wonderfully fat boy – habited as a serving lad, standing upright on the mat with his eyes closed as if in a sleep. He had never seen such a fat boy, in or out of a traveling caravan; and this, coupled with the calmness and repose of his appearance, so very different from what was reasonably to have been expected of the inflicter of such knocks, smote him with wonder.

"What's the matter?" inquired the clerk.

The extraordinary boy replied not a word; but he nodded once, and seemed, to the clerk's imagination, to snore feebly.

"Where do you come from?" inquired the clerk.

The boy made no sign. He breathed heavily, but in all other respects was motionless.

The clerk repeated the question thrice, and receiving no answer, prepared to shut the door, when the boy suddenly opened his eyes, winked several times, sneezed once and raised his hand as if to repeat the knocking. Finding the door open, he stared about him with astonishment, and at length fixed his eyes on Mr. Lowten's face.

"What the devil do you knock in that way for?" inquired the clerk angrily.

"Which way?" said the boy in a slow and sleepy voice.

"Why, like 40 hackney-coachmen," replied the clerk.

"Because master said I wasn't to leave off knocking till they opened the door, for fear I should go to sleep," said the boy.

The Pickwickian Syndrome is also known as the Obesity Hypoventilation Syndrome. When first presented by Dr. Burwell, he listed the following findings: "Extreme obesity (like Dickens' fat boy), somnolence, hypoventilation, twitching of muscles, cyanosis, periodic respiration, polycythemia, right ventricular hypertrophy, and heart failure."

There are a number of anecdotes concerning these sleepy fat people (Pickwickians). One was about a judge in one of our southern states who would at times fall asleep when presiding at court. This, of course, was a subject of much concern. I understand he was eventually retired, illustrating again that "justice will triumph."

Some Pickwickians may snore in a very loud, jerky, raucous manner, which may even wake them up. I remember once standing in the nurses' station and hearing loud snoring from a room down the hall. Because the snoring was so loud, I walked down to the end of the hall, thinking it was emanating from a patient with a cerebral vascular accident. Instead, to my surprise, it was a very fat man sitting in a large chair in the visitor's lounge – T.V. going full blast, other people in the room, but he was sound asleep. It turned out he was a typical Pickwickian and would often fall asleep while driving his car and waiting for the stop light to change.

W. Proctor Harvey, M.D.

Long-standing heart disease may produce gradual wasting of body mass due to suboptimal perfusion of a variety of body tissues. Cardiac cachexia, an unpleasant term, is a common manifestation of advanced heart disease. Patients with congestive heart failure who require a salt restricted diet also gradually lose body mass. The mechanism may not be related to inadequate tissue perfusion, but rather reduced caloric intake over the long term secondary to absence of flavor of unsalted food. The modern treatment of congestive heart failure calls for use of peripheral vasodilators, especially angiotensin-converting enzyme inhibitors, with smaller amounts of potent diuretics. As a result, there may be room for liberalizing salt intake and thereby maintaining body mass.

CARDIAC PEARL

Ear Lobes- At times you may see movement of the patient's ear lobes coincident with systole. This should immediately suggest two possible causes: severe aortic regurgitation or severe tricuspid regurgitation.

In each instance, the movement of the ears reflects transmitted impulse from the carotid artery (aortic regurgitation) or the jugular vein (tricuspid regurgitation).

A prominent V-wave as noted in the jugular venous pulse may increase with inspiration, also producing an increase in the tricuspid systolic murmur. The more advanced degrees of tricuspid regurgitation can even cause systolic movement of the ear lobes as well as rightward lateral movement of the head coincident with systole. (This has been called the "no-no" sign as compared with the "yes-yes" sign of advanced aortic regurgitation which produces the "up and down" bobbing of the head.)

W. Proctor Harvey, M.D.

Patients with Marfan's syndrome have a characteristic appearance not unlike that of Abraham Lincoln. They are usually tall and slender with sharp facial features, and their arms and legs may be somewhat long. There may be hyperextensibility of the small joints and subluxation of the ocular lens, the hard palate is often arched, and there may be some skeletal deformity of the anterior thorax. Marfan's syndrome is associated with cystic medial necrosis of the aorta predisposing to aneurysm of the ascending aorta, perhaps aortic regurgitation, and often mitral regurgitation due to connective tissue deficiency in the mitral leaflets themselves. Incomplete penetration of the Marfan genetic defect may result in patients who do not have the completely characteristic physiognomy, but have one or another physical manifestation.

CARDIAC PEARL

Marfan's Syndrome or Variant

A patient with typical Marfan's syndrome is likely to be identified by his or her physical appearance: tall, thin, long arm span, long supple fingers and joints, and a high arched palate (Figures A,B and C). Due to eye defects such as dislocation (subluxation) of the lens, thick glasses may be worn, thereby affording another clue to the presence of this condition. I remember one patient who told me, "People say I look like Abraham Lincoln." The patient did indeed resemble Lincoln and had the classical pathological finding of aortic root pathology with aneurysmal dilatation of the ascending aorta. Associated clinical findings were aortic diastolic murmur, systolic ejection sound, systolic murmur, and accentuation of the aortic component of the second sound — typical auscultatory findings. Rupture of an aneurysm can result in sudden death in these patients.

Not all patients with Marfan's syndrome have all of the typical features. Thus, the physician must be alert and use extra care to look for Marfan's variant where only some of the features are present.

Of course, Marfan's is most likely to be found in basketball or volleyball players rather than in football players or volleyball players. In screening athletes, the typical physical appearance, even in the absence of diagnostic physical and auscultatory findings, should prompt one to order additional laboratory tests.

Marfan's patients can have mitral rather than aortic valve involvement as the predominant lesion. They may have varying degrees of mitral valve regurgitation, the etiology of which may be related to mitral valve prolapse.

W. Proctor Harvey, M.D.

Of these, this writer has observed that the high arched palate may be the most frequent manifestation. Many additional conditions associated with major cardiovascular manifestations are readily diagnosable by observation of body conformation. Among these, acromegaly, Cushing's syndrome, hypothyroidism, kyphoscoliotic disorders, and numerous congenital syndromes will be mentioned elsewhere in this chapter.

Individuals whose thoracic spine is straight often have reduced thoracic antero-posterior dimensions and flattening of the heart: the straight back syndrome. This often goes undetected if the patient is inspected in the reclining position — the patient

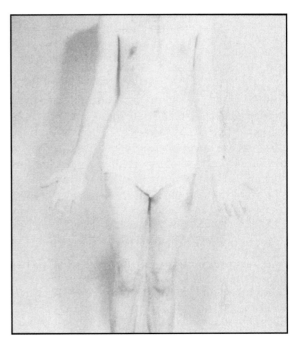

Fig A: Signs of Marfan's Syndrome - Typical body habitus of Marfan's Syndrome: tall, long legs, wide arm span.

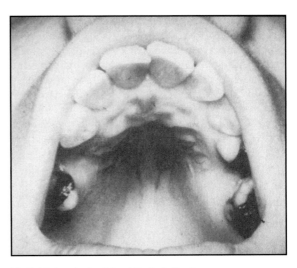

Fig B: High arched palate of Marfan's Syndrome.

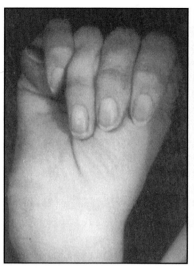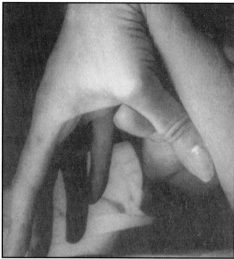

Fig C: More Signs of Marfan's - Note the supple joints and long fingers. Also, note the position of the patients thumb in both photos (compare to your own hand).

should be erect. The heart is usually normal in the straight back syndrome even though it may appear enlarged in a P-A radiograph of the thorax. Patients with marked pectus excavatum may also appear to have cardiomegaly in chest radiographs. However, a lateral view clarifies the picture that can be suspected on physical inspection (Figure 1).

CARDIAC PEARL

It is apparent that a number of patients have been misdiagnosed as having congenital heart disease, particularly atrial septal defect, pulmonary stenosis, and others, because of some similar features produced by the straight back syndrome. At times, there is a wide splitting of the second heart sound along with a systolic murmur, which may be confused with atrial septal defect. At other times, a systolic murmur, even with a palpable thrill, might be present over the pulmonary outflow tract. These findings along with the x-ray and electrocardiogram also add to the confusion, unless one carefully inspects the patient's body build and A-P diameter of the chest.

W. Proctor Harvey, M.D.

Cutaneous Manifestations

At the very least, the skin has texture, temperature, color, and thickness, and observations about each may be important.

CARDIAC PEARL

The Malar Flush of Mitral Stenosis- The malar flush of mitral stenosis generally occurs in patients who have more advanced degrees of stenosis. Today this sign is not found as frequently as in the past when mitral stenosis was so prevalent. It simulates the color of makeup such as "blush" or "rouge" over the cheeks.

W. Proctor Harvey, M.D.

Certainly patients with hypothyroidism, with or without accompanying coronary artery disease, and cardiac manifestations of the endocrinopathy, have dry, moderately coarse skin that is sometimes thickened, particularly over the extremities. Conversely, patients with hyperthyroidism have normal or even soft skin that is warm and radiates heat, most easily detected over the upper anterior thorax.

CARDIAC PEARL

Bird-like Movements- A clue to the presence of thyrotoxicosis.

A lady of about 70 years of age had no venous hum that could be elicited. She had cervical arthritis to the degree that it was difficult to listen over the right supraclavicular area in the neck with her head turned to the opposite direction, and on a stretch. However, she did have (what my mentor, the late Samuel A. Levine, taught me) quick bird-like movements that sometimes are apparent with thyrotoxicosis. When asked to sit up from a lying position, she did so very quickly. Most

70-year-old patients would do so slowly and gradually. She also had a quick wit.

Other subtle "pearls" of thyrotoxicosis: If we ask the patient to sit up and we feel where he or she has been lying it may be warmer than expected, due to the increased metabolism.

Husbands and wives may get into arguments because one wants a lot of bed covers and the other doesn't want any. Guess which one has the increased metabolism? Menopause, of course, could be a "red herring".

Another interesting patient: A young boy was referred for evaluation because his muscle and bone development was definitely impaired. He had had a congenital patent ductus repaired about one year before. The question was, could his problem be related to his congenital heart disease, now surgically corrected, or did he have some additional congenital problems? Neither of these possibilities proved to be present. He appeared to be about six years of age, but actually was nine years old. It was summer time and his hospital room was comfortable, although there was no air conditioning. It was noticed that he was sleeping with his socks on and under blankets. He stated he always did so. This was now a clue to his problem: He had primary hypothyroidism. With thyroid medication, "he grew like a weed", as was subsequently reported by his physician.

W. Proctor Harvey, M.D.

Central cyanosis, bluish discoloration of the skin, due to desaturation of five or more grams per 100ml of hemoglobin is of particular importance. Central cyanosis should first be distinguished from simple peripheral cyanosis. Usually, simple peripheral cyanosis is not indicative of disease, but rather relates to slowing of cutaneous blood flow due to environmental cold in the hands, feet, nose, and ears. The most likely mechanism is vasoconstriction with slowing of flow and excessive regional oxygen extraction from hemoglobin.

Central cyanosis may be caused by shunting of venous blood into the systemic circulation through a variety of possible intracardiac defects. These shunts are usually, but not always, associated with elevated right ventricular pressures due to pulmonary hypertension or right ventricular outflow tract obstruction. Eisenmenger's syndrome and tetralogy of Fallot are typical examples, but by no means the only mechanisms. Endocardial cushion defects, for instance, may result in arteriovenous mixing within the heart, and isolated severe pulmonary valvular stenosis may cause increases in right heart pressures to the extent that the foramen ovale may be opened and permit right-to-left intratrial shunting. Whatever the precise anatomical defect, central cyanosis due to a cardiac defect is a serious matter.

Central cyanosis may also be caused by advanced pulmonary disease with intrapulmonary right-to- left shunting. In both cardiac and pulmonary defects causing central cyanosis, clubbing of the nail beds occurs. However, hypertrophic osteoarthropathy of the bones of the forearms and calves is observed more commonly in association with pulmonary causes of cyanosis.

Differential cyanosis refers to cyanosis of some extremities but not others. The usual example is seen in association with pulmonary hypertensive

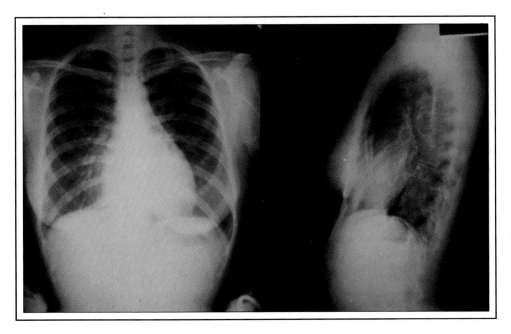

Figure 1. PA and lateral chest radiographs of a woman with pectus excavatum. Note the appearance of cardiomegaly on the frontal image, and anterior compression of the heart by the sternum and calcified cartilage in the lateral view.
(Courtesy James J. Leonard, MD)

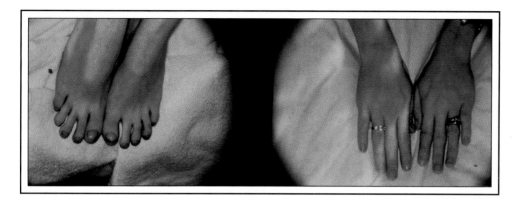

Figure 2. The feet and hands of a woman with pulmonary hypertensive patent ductus arteriosus. Note cyanosis and nail bed clubbing in the feet and the left hand with relatively normal right hand.
(Courtesy James J. Leonard, MD)

patent ductus arteriosus in which both feet are cyanotic and perhaps clubbed while the right hand is normal; the left hand may be less cyanotic (Figure 2). In pulmonary hypertensive patent ductus, unsaturated blood from the high pressure pulmonary artery flows through the patent ductus into the descending aorta; thus the lower extremities receive unsaturated blood. The right arm and hand are perfused by blood which has transversed the lungs and is pumped into the ascending aorta by the left ventricle. The left arm is perfused by the left subclavian artery which normally takes its origin from the aorta quite close to the insertion of the ductus arteriosus, thereby being perfused by a mixture of blood from the ductus and the ascending aorta.

Quite rarely, infants are observed with cyanotic upper extremities and normally colored lower extremities: reversed differential cyanosis. This physical finding indicates presence of pulmonary hypertensive patent ductus in association with transposition of the great arteries. Slate blue discoloration of the skin, in distinction from the violaceous color of cyanosis, is one of the many side effects of the long-term use of amiodarone and is due to chemical deposits in the skin. Methemoglobinemia may be caused by nitrates and is associated with a slate blue discoloration of the skin which should be distinguished from cyanosis.

CARDIAC PEARL

Carcinoid Syndrome- Another facial characteristic that is important is the violaceous hue over the cheeks and face of the patient with carcinoid syndrome.

I remember seeing the first patient ever diagnosed with the carcinoid syndrome in the United States (Figure A). The patient was first diagnosed by General Thomas Mattingly at Walter Reed Army Hospital; she had been examined at Johns Hopkins Hospital by Dr. Helen Taussig. I saw her at a conference at Walter Reed Army Hospital. Her face was a deep purplish color that I had never seen before and her only cardiac finding was a systolic murmur heard over the pulmonic area. This was subsequently documented to be a mild to moderate degree of pulmonic valve stenosis. There was no shunt to explain this particular coloration, which some had believed was cyanosis.

Dr. Mattingly had read an article in one of the cardiology journals describing a new "carcinoid syndrome" described by Dr. Bjork of Scandinavia. Dr. Mattingly thought this particular patient had the features described in this syndrome. By chance, Dr. Bjork was attending the World Congress of Cardiology being held in Washington at that time and the patient was presented to him on rounds at Walter Reed Army Hospital. He agreed that

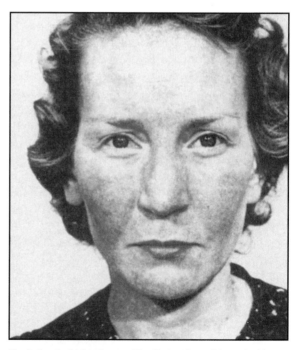

Fig A: Carcinoid Syndrome - The first patient with carcinoid syndrome diagnosed in the United States. She had a permanent violaceous hue over her face, as shown.

this patient had the carcinoid syndrome. She was therefore the first carcinoid patient diagnosed in the United States; she was then studied by Dr. Al Sjordsma and his colleagues at the National Institutes of Health. They demonstrated the relationship of serotonin in producing features of this syndrome.

Carcinoid Tumor- When flushing occurs or the patient has persistent violaceous or erythematous facial flushing, then the carcinoid tumor of the intestine has metastasized to the liver.

A patient was evaluated because of the finding of a systolic murmur over the pulmonic area. He described flushing of his face when he ate his breakfast and his noonday meal, but not with his evening meal. The next morning, however, he would again flush when eating. To explain the lack of flushing at the evening meal, it was postulated that his serotonin stores in the body had been depleted by the evening, but were replenished during the night.

The carcinoid syndrome can also cause a reddish-pink facial hue, as if a person were blushing. I recall examining a woman who had such a coloration constantly. Evaluation was requested because of the presence of a systolic murmur. The murmur was diagnosed as a mild degree of obstruction of the pulmonic valve. She was asked whether she had been out in the sun, because her facial appearance simulated a sunburn. She said no, she had not been out in the sun at all. She had a variant of the violaceous facial hue that can occur with a carcinoid.

The serotonin in the bloodstream of patients with the carcinoid syndrome can cause scarring of the pulmonic valve, producing the pulmonic systolic murmur.

W. Proctor Harvey, M.D.

Blue sclerae are frequently observed in persons with osteogenesis imperfecta. These patients are of small stature and sometimes have aortic regurgitation.

CARDIAC PEARL

Osteogenesis Imperfecta (blue sclera, brittle bones) belongs to the hereditary group of disorders of connective tissue which includes Marfan's syndrome, Ehlers-Danlos syndrome, pseudoxanthoma elasticum and Hurler's syndrome. Patients with osteogenesis imperfecta may present in the same way as with those seen more commonly with Marfan's syn-

drome. There may be aortic insufficiency associated with aortic root disease or there may be varying degrees of mitral valve involvement varying from systolic clicks with late apical systolic murmur to advanced severe mitral valve insufficiency with a holosystolic murmur. These patients often have a "right- sided" aortic diastolic murmur with the murmur heard best along the right sternal border as compared with its counterpart on the left. On the other hand, the murmur may well be heard best along the left sternal border, as with more common causes of aortic insufficiency. Also, osteogenesis imperfecta can affect the mitral valve in the same way as Marfan's syndrome with the variant spectrum of clicks to advanced mitral insufficiency with cardiac decompensation. When a patient has blue sclera and a history of fractures (brittle bones), one should always look carefully for an aortic diastolic murmur, including listening carefully along the right sternal border as well as the left, and also for the possibility of systolic clicks at the apex and systolic murmurs over that area.

W. Proctor Harvey, M.D.

Jaundice due to hepatic dysfunction secondary to heart failure is no longer commonly observed because of improved treatment modalities. With icterus, the patient is at end stage and may be too disabled to be a heart transplant candidate (unless the serum bilirubin can became normal with intensive heart failure treatment).

The oral mucosa should also be inspected. Vascular lesions on the oral mucosa are associated with pulmonary vascular malformations (Figures 3 to 6).

CARDIAC PEARL

The Osler-Weber-Rendu Syndrome (a pulmonary arteriovenous fistula)- Careful examination of the lips and buccal membranes may reveal small, reddish-purple telangiectasia which provide an immediate clue to the possible presence of this syndrome. If searched for carefully, a continuous murmur might be detected over an arteriovenous shunt in the lung.

Such a lesion can produce clubbing of the fingers and toes and cyanosis. The x-ray and angiography may document one or more lesions that might be amenable to surgical correction. This is another example of a curable type of heart disease.

W. Proctor Harvey, M.D.

61

Other Congenital Anomalies and Syndromes

In addition to Marfan's syndrome, there are a variety of defects probably related. Reference is made to Ehlers-Danlos and Hurler's syndromes, both of which are rare and are clinically severe defects producing aortic and mitral regurgitation. Down's syndrome is common and may be associated with cardiac defects, mild to severe, typically endocardial cushion defects.

Turner's syndrome, ovarian agenesis, is associated with coarctation of the aorta and bicuspid aortic valve. Holt-Oram syndrome is associated with ostium secundum atrial septal defect. Patients with broad frontal bones and therefore widely set eyes should be examined for right ventricular outflow tract obstruction, especially valvular pulmonic stenosis. The presence of an elf-like appearance, elfin facies, suggests the possibility of supravalvular

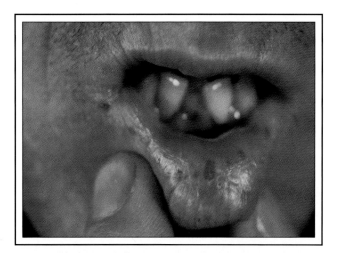

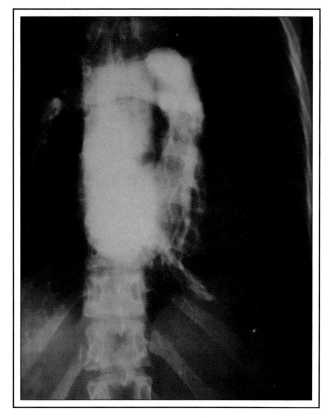

Figures 3 and 4. Vascular lesions detected on the mucous membranes may be associated with pulmonary arteriovenous communication, as seen in the left lower lobe of the same patient. *(Courtesy of James J. Leonard, MD)*

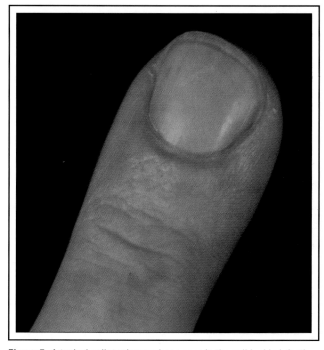

Figure 5. A typical splinter hemorrhage seen in the nail bed in infective endocarditis. *(Courtesy James J. Leonard, MD)*

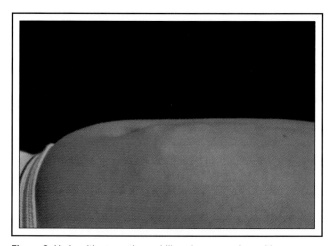

Figure 6. Varicosities near the umbilicus in a young boy with congenital cirrhosis. *(Courtesy James J. Leonard, MD)*

aortic stenosis. This may be manifest by a disparity between left and right arm blood pressure due to streamlining of flow by the supra aortic membrane.

CARDIAC PEARL

Physical Signs of Supravalvular Aortic Stenosis- Figure A shows characteristic facies of a boy with supravalvular aortic stenosis.

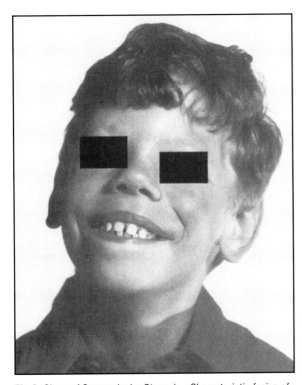

Fig A: Signs of Supravalvular Stenosis - Characteristic facies of boy with congenital supravalvular aortic stenosis.

It is interesting that a patient with this problem has enough look-alikes to think they might be members of the same family. Note the large mouth, large lips, prominent teeth in poor alignment, receding chin and eyes that are more widely set apart than usual. In many, the carotid artery pulsations are stronger on the right than the left. A typical harsh aortic systolic murmur is present, but the aortic ejection sound and aortic diastolic murmur are absent.

W. Proctor Harvey, M.D.

The list of congenital abnormalities associated with cardiac defects is long indeed and beyond the scope of this chapter. However, each defect has its characteristic appearance and, likewise, the associated cardiac defect is reasonably predictable based upon appearance of the patient. It is clear that there are innumerable clues as to the nature and extent of heart disease to be found on careful examination of the patient. Skill in this particular aspect of physical examination requires time and patience, but over time proves very rewarding.

Selected Reading

1. Harvey WP: *Cardiac Pearls.* Laennec Publishing, Inc., 1994.
2. Hurst JW: *Cardiovascular Diagnosis: The Initial Examination.* Mosby-Year Book Inc. St. Louis 1993.
3. Wood P: *Diseases of the Heart and Circulation;* Third Edition, J.B. Lippincott Co., Philadelphia 1968.
4. Zuberbuhler JR: *Clinical Diagnosis in Pediatric Cardiology.* Churchill Livingstone. New York, 1981.

CHAPTER 5

Venous and Arterial Pulsations: Bedside Insights Into Hemodynamics

Gordon A. Ewy, M.D.

The correct interpretation of the jugular venous and arterial pulsations are important aspects of the non-invasive assessment of the cardiovascular system, providing insights into the patient's hemodynamics. Their evaluation can be accomplished with ease and economy of time, but like all skills, optimal davelopment requires practice and, at times, tutelage.

Identification of the Jugular Venous Pulse

The jugular venous pulse is recognized by its location in the neck and by the characteristic pulsations. The internal jugular vein is a relatively deep structure lying lateral to the carotid artery. In the mid and lower neck, this large vein runs beneath the sternocleidomastoid muscle. The lower end of the sternocleidomastoid muscle splits into two heads that originate from the clavicle. The triangle formed by the two heads of the sternocleidomastoid muscle and the clavicle is the internal jugular triangle and marks the location of the internal jugular bulb. Normally, pulsations from the internal jugular vein are reflected in the lower portion of the neck by the motion of the skin over the internal jugular triangle and when relaxed, the sternocleidomastoid muscle. The external jugular vein is superficial and located more laterally. Because of its superficial location, the external jugular vein pulsations are often easier to appreciate and may be especially prominent in patients who have chronic elevation of venous pressure. Characteristically, the venous pulse is a series of subtle, wavy, nonpalpable impulses, contrasting to the stronger easily palpable carotid arterial pulse. An important exception to this generalization are the venous pulsations of the patient with severe tricuspid regurgitation. With severe incompetence of the tricuspid valve, the high right ventricular systolic pressure is transmitted to the right atrium and hence to the veins, resulting in a venous pulse that is large and sometimes palpable. These prominent systolic venous impulses might be mistaken for prominent arterial pulsations. However, the discrepancy between the forceful pulsation in the neck and a relatively weak radial arterial pulse should arrest one's attention and suggest that the prominent neck pulsations are venous.

The distinction is easy, however, as pressure at the base of the neck will obliterate venous pulsations but has little effect on arterial pulsations. Another differential diagnostic feature is the fact that venous pulsations are likely to be altered by changes in position. Arterial pulsations are little changed with varying positions. Venous pulsations are subject to a much greater respiratory variation than arterial pulsations. And finally, abdominal compression may result in changes in the height of venous pulsation and has no effect on arterial pulsations. With attention to these details, the recognition of venous pulsations can be reliably accomplished.

Evaluating Jugular Venous Pulsations

Evaluation of the jugular venous excursions requires the patient to be in an optimal position; this position varies depending upon the venous pressure. The patient's head and thorax are gradu-

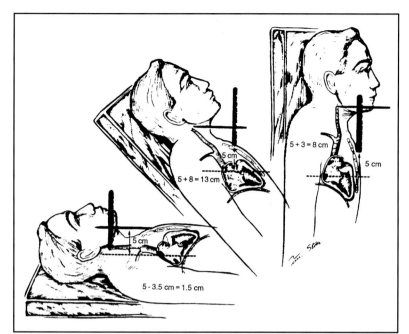

Figure 1. This figure illustrates the technique of estimation of venous pressure in *three different patients,* although they look alike. As shown, the sternal angle or the angle of Lewis is approximately 5 cm above the mid-right atrium with the patient in any position from supine to upright. The patient is positioned so that the jugular venous pulsations are best seen. A centimeter ruler is placed vertically on the sternal angle if the venous pressure is above the angle of Lewis. The distance above the sternal angle is then determined by forming a right angle to the ruler with a pencil or other straight edge as shown. The first supine patient has a normal venous pressure. Since the pulsations are below the sternal angle, the vertical distance is subtracted from the reference point. The second patient is in an intermediate position, as this is where his venous pulsations are best seen. The venous pressure is 3 cm above the sternal angle or about 8 cm of water. The third patient has a marked elevation of venous pressure. The venous pulsations at the top of the venous blood column are visible only in the upright position. Again measured vertically, the venous pulsations are 8 cm above the sternal angle, equivalent to a venous pressure of approximately 13 cm of water (with permission, 2).

ally raised or lowered until the maximum venous pulsations are visible. Evaluation of the jugular venous pulses can be divided into three general categories: estimating jugular venous pressure, assessing the response of the venous pressure to abdominal compression, and interpreting the jugular venous wave form.

Estimating Central Venous Pressure

Perhaps the greatest myth, and the greatest impediment to accurate interpretation of the jugular venous pressure is the misconception that venous pressure needs to be evaluated with the patient at a 45 degree angle. When estimating the venous pressure, one is estimating the hydrostatic filling pressure of the right heart. Hydrostatic fluid pressure is measured vertically regardless of the shape of the fluid container. This concept is applicable to the clinical estimation of venous pressure, since venous pressure is measured as the vertical distance between the mean venous pulsations at the top of the column of venous blood and mid right atrium. The reference point for the estimation of the height of venous pressure is the sternal angle or the angle of Lewis. Sir Thomas Lewis called attention to the fact that the angle between the manubrium and the body of the sternum bears a near constant relationship to the right atrium in the supine, the sitting, or any intermediate position (Figure 1).

The sternal angle then is the benchmark for the noninvasive determination of venous pressure. This angle can be felt as a transverse ridge formed by the connection between the manubrium and the

body of the sternum at the articulation of the second ribs. For practical purposes, if the venous pulsations are equal to or lower than the sternal angle, the venous pressure is normal. An elevation in pressure is said to be present when the height of the venous column in the neck is 2 cm to 3 cm above the sternal angle, indicating a mean right atrial pressure of 7 cm to 8 cm of water. As noted above, it is a common misconception that patients must be examined with the trunk at an angle of 45 degrees from horizontal. This is incorrect, as the patient should be placed in the position where the venous pulsations are best seen. In the normal individual, the patient must be near horizontal if the venous pulsations are to be seen. On the other hand, in a patient with markedly elevated venous pressure, the summit of the venous column may not be appreciated unless the patient is sitting bolt upright (Figure 1). The patient's head should be resting comfortably on the bed or examining table. Pillows usually need to be removed before one can accurately evaluate the venous pulse, as they tend to bend the neck, placing the patient's chin near the chest, and thus interfering with evaluation. Since the internal jugular pulse is often reflected by motion of the skin over the sternocleidomastoid, this muscle must be relaxed. The pulses of the veins of the neck are best seen when lighting is tangential so that shadows are cast, causing the pulses to stand out in relief. Use of a pocket flashlight is often helpful with the beam directed tangentially across the neck; shadow of the pulsations on the bed will magnify the venous pulsation and may help in their interpretation.

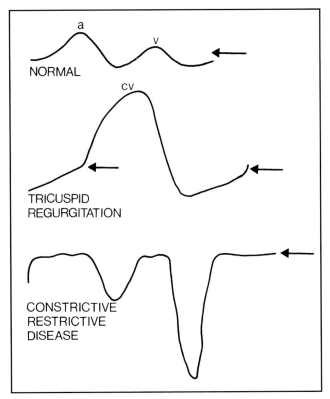

Figure 2. When estimating the right ventricular filling pressure, one normally uses the mid point of the excursions as illustrated by the arrow, top tracing. The two exceptions are illustrated. In patients with large CV waves of tricuspid regurgitation (middle tracing) the right ventricular end diastolic filling pressure correlates best with the pressure at the bottom of the pulse, or at the beginning of the CV wave (arrow, middle tracing). In contrast, in patients with constrictive or restrictive disease, the right ventricular end diastolic pressure correlates most closely with the top of the jugular venous pulse (arrow, bottom tracing).

The technique of estimating venous pressure has distinct limitations, and these deserve emphasis. Obstruction of the superior vena cava will result in bilateral venous engorgement. In this situation the veins fill from above and not from below. The lack of venous pulsation indicates a block between the right atrium and the jugular veins. Unilateral venous obstruction also occurs, at times from previous placement of catheters or pacing leads; estimation of the venous pressure is usually not possible in the patient in shock because of the marked venous constriction that accompanies the increased sympathetic tone. In pulmonary disease, there is often such marked fluctuation of intrathoracic pressures that accurate assessment is difficult. Finally, in the morbidly obese patient, estimation of the venous pressure is often impossible. The patient with extreme elevation of venous pressure may have such venous distention that the pulsations may not be appreciated even with the patient sitting upright. In this situation, the neck often

appears full (a bullneck appearance) and the fact that the venous pressure is elevated may be overlooked. If this question arises, palpation of the neck may be helpful. Distended venous veins have a characteristic soft feeling in contrast to the relatively non-compliant nature of the very muscular individual with a so-called "bullneck". In some patients with markedly elevated venous pressure, it is only after the venous pressure decreases with therapy that pulsations can be visualized. A marked increase of venous pressure can at times be suspected by the engorgement of the veins under the tongue or on the forehead of the patient in the sitting or upright position.

What point of the venous pulsation should be used to estimate the height of the venous pressure? It is usually not the peak of the waves; one wants to estimate the right ventricular end-diastolic pressure; thus, the height of the pulse just preceding the C wave is used. This point is difficult to see, but in normals is located near the midpoint of the venous excursion. The jugular venous pressure is then estimated by height of mean venous pulsations above the angle of Lewis. The two exceptions to this rule are patients with tricuspid regurgitation or constrictive pericarditis (Figure 2). In tricuspid regurgitation, the right ventricular filling pressure is the trough of the venous pulse as the peak of the wave occurs during systole (Figure 2). The height of the regurgitant wave reflects the degree of regurgitation rather than the filling pressure of the right ventricle. In constrictive pericarditis, the right ventricular filling pressure correlates with the peak of the venous pulse (Figure 2).

Abdominojugular Test

The abdominojugular test (AJT), previously referred to as either the hepatojugular reflux (HJR) or the abdominal jugular reflux (AJR), is an important bedside test that provides insights into the patient's hemodynamics. The ability to perform and accurately interpret AJT is essential to optimal management of patients with chronic heart failure. A positive hepatojugular reflux, according to cardiovascular textbooks of the 1980s, indicated right heart failure. Even though isolated right heart failure is rare and the most common cause of right heart failure is left heart failure, it was assumed that elevated jugular venous pressure and a positive hepatojugular or abdominojugular reflux indicated right heart failure.

Burch was the first to suggest that a positive hepatojugular test was a sign of left heart failure, as he noted a positive test in a number of hypertensive patients. He postulated that increased sympa-

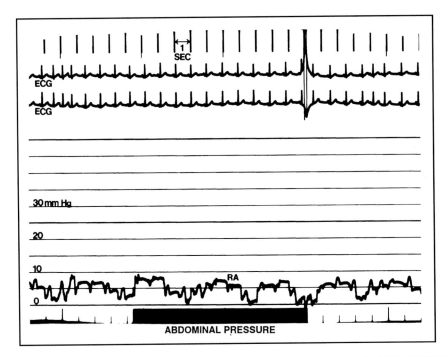

Figure 3. A negative abdominal jugular test. With 10 seconds of mid-abdominal pressure there is no change in the right atrial (RA) pressures. Time lines are one second. ECG = electrocardiogram.

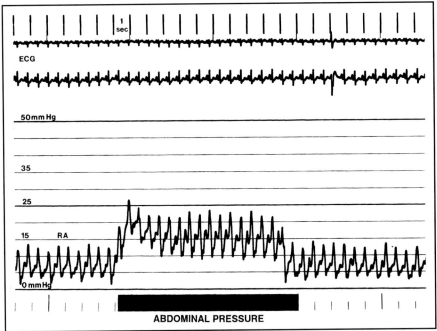

Figure 4. A positive abdominojugular test. With 10 seconds of mid-abdominal pressure in a patient with dilated cardiomyopathy the right atrial pressure rises abruptly, and remains elevated until abdominal pressure is released. This pressure pattern is called a square wave response. ECG = electrocardiogram; RA = right atrial (with permission, 4).

thetic tone of heart failure resulted in increased venoconstriction and decreased venous compliance. When the abdominal veins were compressed, there was generalized increase in venous pressure that was visible in the jugular veins. This concept was disregarded until Ewy studied the hemodynamic correlates of a positive abdominal jugular test. Studying 63 consecutive patients undergoing both right and left cardiac catheterization, Ewy recorded the right atrial pressure before, during, and after 10 seconds of mid-abdominal pressure and correlated the response with the hemodynamics

obtained during the cardiac catheterization (Figure 3, 4). This procedure was renamed to abdomino-jugular test (AJT) to not only emphasize the difference in technique (10 seconds of mid-abdominal pressure rather than one minute of pressure over the liver or over the mid-abdomen as described for the hepatojugular or abdominal jugular reflux), but also to emphasize the different interpretation that should be ascribed to a positive response.

Ewy found that while there was a correlation between left ventricular ejection fraction and other indices of left heart failure, these correlations were

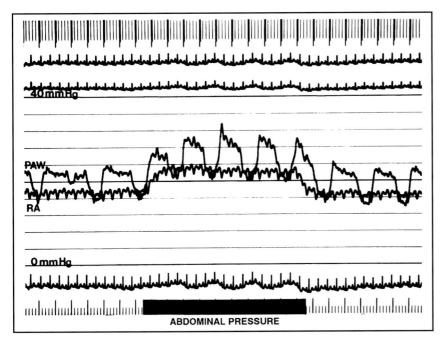

Figure 5. A positive abdominojugular test. While both the right atrial (RA) and pulmonary arterial wedge (PAW) pressures are elevated, they both increase further together with mid-abdominal pressure and both fall with release of mid-abdominal pressure. This patient had restrictive cardiomyopathy.

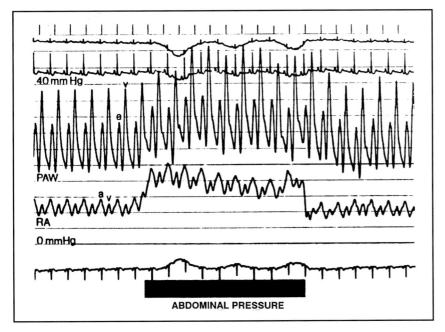

Figure 6. Simultaneously recorded right atrial (RA) and pulmonary artery wedge (PAW) pressure in a 60-year-old patient with mitral valve disease who had a positive abdominojugular test (with permission, 4).

not clinically significant. The best correlation was between the left ventricular filling pressure (as assessed by the pulmonary artery occluded pressure obtained by the Swan-Ganz catheter). The exact reason for this correlation is yet to be proven, but the hypothesis is closely related to that of Burch. When the venous or capacitance system of the cardiovascular circulation is filled (leaving little residual capacitance) or is less compliant due to increased sympathetic tone and increased plasma catecholamines present in heart failure, abdominal pressure increases the intravenous pressure that is in turn reflected in an elevated jugular venous

pressure. Support for this hypothesis is the observation that in patients with a positive AJT, ten seconds of mid-abdominal pressure cause a rise and fall in the pulmonary artery wedge pressure along with the rise and fall in right atrial pressure (Figures 5,6).

To perform the abdominojugular test, the technique is as follows: the patient's pillow is removed and the head of the bed is raised to the position where one can best estimate jugular venous pressure. The patient is told that you are about to apply abdominal pressure, but that for the test to be valid, he or she must continue to breathe normally

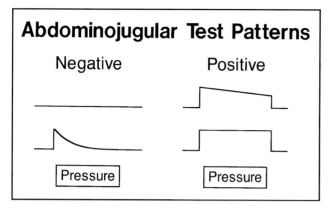

Figure 7. A schematic representation of the four patterns of jugular venous or right atrial responses to 10 seconds of mid-abdominal pressure.

and not strain. Mid-abdominal pressure is applied with the flat of the right hand for 10 seconds. The reason 10 seconds is used is because Ewy noted that in the occasional patient who has an initial rise in jugular venous pressure in response to abdominal pressure, the jugular venous pressure would return to normal before ten seconds. Ducas and colleagues noted that of patients with jugular venous pressures elevated at one minute of abdominal pressure, all had elevated jugular venous pressure at 12 seconds. Ten seconds of abdominal pressure is all that is necessary. Figure 7 illustrates negative and positive responses. A positive AJT is a fall in jugular venous pressure of 4 cm or more with the abrupt release of ten seconds of mid-abdominal pressure. The validity of the AJT was confirmed by a subsequent study by Butman and associates studying patients with chronic heart failure referred to our hospital for cardiac transplant evaluation.

In this study of 52 patients (mean age 53 years) with chronic heart failure (mean NYHA Class III, mean left ventricular ejection fraction 18± 6%) jugular venous distension or a positive abdominal jugular test provided the best sensitivity, specificity, and predictive accuracy for the non-invasive assessment of a pulmonary arterial wedge pressure over 18 mmHg (Table 1). While presence of pulmonary rales in this study was more specific, rales were much less sensitive (Table 1).

In fact, when patients with other diseases are considered along with patients with chronic heart failure, the adage that most patients with rales do not have heart failure and most patients with chronic heart failure do not have rales, appears to hold true. In patients with chronic heart failure, Ewy confirmed the findings of Stevensen and Perloff that the presence of rales, jugular venous distension, and edema always indicated a markedly

elevated wedge pressure (Table 2). However, clinical usefulness of the abdominal jugular test is greatest in those patients without jugular venous distention, that is, elevated jugular venous pressure (Table 3). In these patients, a negative AJT indicated that neither the left ventricular nor the right ventricular filling pressure is elevated; therefore, the patient with peripheral edema and a negative AJT has the edema due to conditions other than heart failure; drugs (such as calcium channel blockers), decreased albumin, orthostasis, or due to venous or lymphatic obstruction (Table 4). The AJT is equally helpful when the jugular venous pressure is normal and the AJT is positive. These patients have elevated wedge pressure and need to be assessed and treated according to the etiology of the elevated pulmonary artery wedge pressure (Table 3). As illustrated in Table 3, patients with chronic heart failure without jugular venous distention (JVD) and a negative abdominal jugular test (AJT) have the lowest left ventricular filling pressure. Those without JVD but with a positive AJT have intermediate wedge pressure. Finally, those with JVD and AJT will almost always have rales, or evidence of venous congestion on chest roentgenograms. These observations hold for acute exacerbations of chronic heart failure as well as in patients with stable chronic heart failure, but they do not hold for acute left heart failure seen in acute myocardial infarction. Early use of the Swan-Ganz catheter in patients with acute myocardial infarction showed no correlation between the central venous pressure (and therefore jugular venous pressure) and left ventricular filling pressure. Why is chronic heart failure so different?

In contrast to acute heart failure, in chronic heart failure there is increased lymphatic clearance

T A B L E   1
Non-Invasive Examination in Patients With Chronic Heart Failure: Detection of Pulmonary Artery Wedge Pressure Greater Than 18 mm Hg

	SENSITIVITY	SPECIFICITY	PREDICTIVE ACCURACY
Rales	24%	100%	46%
JVD	57%	93%	67%
AJT or JVD	81%	80%	80%
S₃	68%	73%	69%
X-ray	65%	80%	69%

JVD = jugular venous distention; AJT = positive abdominal jugular test; S_3 = third heart sound; X-ray = roentgenographic evidence of pulmonary venous congestion. (with Permission, 2)

TABLE 2

Non-Invasive Evaluation in Patients With Chronic Heart Failure

FINDING	MEAN PAo (mm Hg) ABSENT	MEAN PAo (mm Hg) PRESENT
Rales	20+9	29+5
JVD	17+8	27+6
AJT or JVD	15+9	27+6
S_3	17+8	25+7
X-ray	17+7	26+7

JVD = jugular venous distention; AJT = positive abdominal jugular test; S_3 = third heart sound; X-ray = roentgenographic evidence of pulmonary venous congestion. (with Permission, 2)

TABLE 3

Venous Pressure in Patients With Chronic Heart Failure

	−JVD −AJT	−JVD +AJT	+JVD +AJT
Number of Patients	19	11	22
RA mean (mm HG)	4+3	8+5	13+5
PAW mean (mm HG)	15+9	22+5	27+6

TABLE 4

Ankle Edema Without Jugular Venous Distention and a Negative Abdominal Jugular Test (AJT)

Drugs (such as calcium channel blockers)
Low Albumin (Age, Liver disease or dysfunction)
Prolonged Orthostasis
Venous Obstruction
Lymphatic Obstruction
Decreased Tissue Turgor

of fluid from the pulmonary circulation. Therefore, patients with chronic heart failure may have elevated left ventricular filling pressures, no rales, and no evidence of pulmonary venous congestion on chest roentgenograms. If the left ventricular filling or pulmonary arterial occluded or wedge pressure is markedly elevated, rales and pulmonary venous congestion on chest roentgenogram will be present. In such patients the jugular venous pressure will also be elevated. The abdominal jugular test is most useful in identifying those patients with chronic heart failure who do not have elevated jugular venous pressure, do not have rales, nor evidence of pulmonary venous congestion on chest roentgenogram, but who nevertheless have elevated left ventricular filling pressures and would benefit from more aggressive therapy of their congestive heart failure (Table 3).

Jugular Venous Pulsations

Jugular venous pulsations are normally the result of repeated interference with the relatively steady flow of venous return by the contractions and relaxations of the right atrium and ventricle. The normal venous pulse therefore, consists of intermittent increases of blood volume in the veins due to intermittent slowing or halting of blood flow to the right heart. Because they are low pressure impulses, the venous pulsations are interpreted by inspection rather than by palpation. The normal venous pulsation is classically taught to consist of two major waves and two major troughs. The A wave results from atrial contraction and is presystolic in timing, peaking near the time of the first heart sound. The second major wave, the V wave, is caused by continuous venous return to the right atrium during systole, a time when the tricuspid valve is closed. The X descent follows the A wave and the Y descent follows the V wave (Figure 8).

Relaxation of the atrium is the major factor that contributes to the normal X descent; the V wave is terminated and the Y descent initiated by the fall in right atrial pressure coincident with the opening of the tricuspid valve. Thus, the V wave peaks just after the second heart sound. The A wave is larger than the V wave and the X descent is more prominent than the Y descent.

On occasion, the X descent is interrupted by a third small wave, the C wave. The C wave in the neck is partly due to transmitted carotid artery pulsations and partly due to the upward bulging of the closing tricuspid valve early in ventricular systole. The normal C wave is difficult to recognize as a separate wave. However, this idealized description of the venous pulsation has confused many physicians. In many normal individuals, the A and V waves may not be prominent at all. The most clearly discernible venous motion is a rhythmic collapse or inward motion of the jugular venous pulse during systole. Instead of two distinct peaks and two distinct troughs, one sees low amplitude, undulant venous motion, and one dominant collapsing motion. Timing of this inward or collapsing motion shows it to be systolic and recordings reveal this motion to be the X descent. The reason for these findings is the presence of a third positive wave, the H wave (Figure 9). The H wave follows the Y descent and is the result of passive filling of the right atrium and ventricle during diastole. The H

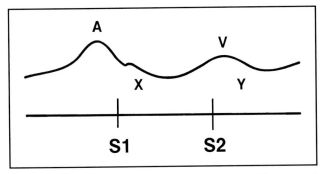

Figure 8. A normal jugular venous pulse illustrating A and V waves and X and Y descents.

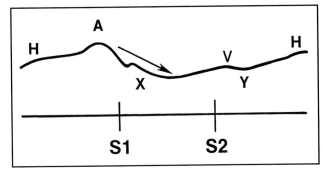

Figure 9. Normal venous pulse showing the H wave.

wave is present only at normal or slow heart rates, since at faster heart rates diastole is shortened. In the normal, the subtle changes in venous amplitude from the H to the A wave, and the low amplitude motion of the V wave makes these waves difficult to appreciate (Figure 9). Large changes in amplitude are easier to recognize than small undulations, and therefore, the most obvious event of the normal jugular venous pulse is the X descent. Fortunately, recognition of these subtle changes in the H, A, C, and V waves are usually unnecessary since one can conclude that there is no significant abnormality of the venous pulsation when the venous pressure is normal, the abdominal jugular test is negative and there is regular systolic collapse of the venous pulsation. The X descent can be timed by several techniques: one is by observing the jugular venous pulse on the right side of the neck while palpating the opposite carotid. The X descent occurs during systole, at the time of the carotid pulse. An alternative method of timing is by observing the jugular venous pulsations while auscultating over the precordium. As illustrated in Figures 8 and 9, the X descent occurs during systole. Absence of the X descent, the presence of prominent systolic waves, easily appreciated A or V waves, or prominent diastolic collapse of the venous pulse indicates the need for more detailed analysis.

The best way to detect the specific waves of the jugular venous pulse in the neck is to be able to see both the venous pulsation and the carotid arterial pulsation in the same localized area. If this can be done, remember that the venous pulsation is lateral and the arterial is medial (Figure A).

If we detect a pulsation of the jugular vein just before that of the carotid artery, then this has to be an A-wave. Sometimes this cannot be seen, but it is worth the time to concentrate using only one sense, the visual. If it is not possible to visualize this pulsation, then the carotid arterial pulsation (on the same side or opposite side) can be felt with the thumb or finger, noting that the venous impulse preceded the arterial; this would represent an A-wave.

When both the arterial and venous waves occur simultaneously, this would be a V-wave or C-wave.

Of course, timing can be accomplished by palpating the carotid artery pulsation, or listening to the first heart sound, and correlating it with the jugular pulse.

W. Proctor Harvey, M.D.

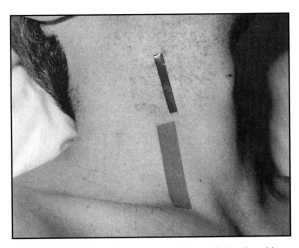

Fig A: Pulses - The carotid arterial pulse is medial to the midline of the neck. The jugular venous pulse (larger marker) is lateral. It is helpful to see both pulsations simultaneously. If the jugular pulse precedes the carotid, this is an A-wave; if they are occurring at the same times, this is a V-wave of the jugular pulse.

Abnormalities of the Venous Wave Form

• **The A Wave:** Abnormal increases in the A wave occurs when there is an increase in force of atrial contraction in response to increased resistance to atrial emptying. Examples are tricuspid stenosis, decreased compliance of the right ventricle, or, rarely, clots or tumors of the right heart.

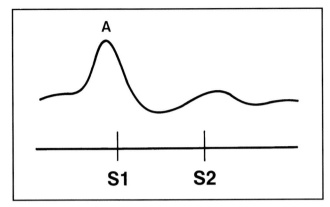

Figure 10. Illustration of a giant A wave in the jugular venous pulse.

Most causes of right ventricular hypertrophy result in an increase in the A wave of the venous pulse. Tetralogy of Fallot is said to be the exception to this rule. Right ventricular hypertrophy usually results from pulmonary hypertension. Right ventricular outflow obstruction and hypertrophic cardiomyopathy must be considered in patients with prominent A waves. As the A wave increases in height it becomes more conspicuous and easier to recognize. When very large, these waves are termed "Giant A Waves" (Figure 10).

CARDIAC PEARL

There are only a few conditions that cause a "giant" A-wave in the jugular venous pulse:

1. Obstruction between the right atrium and the right ventricle occurring with tricuspid stenosis or atresia, or right atrial myxoma, can cause a prominent A-wave with atrial systole.

2. Increased pressure in the right ventricle, as may occur from severe obstruction of the pulmonary outflow tract with pulmonic stenosis, will result in a significant A-wave on atrial contraction.

3. Pulmonary hypertension ("Eisenmenger syndrome" - pulmonary hypertension with atrial septal defect, ventricular septal defect, and patent ductus arteriosus) can cause pressure to be reflected back to the right ventricle, which produces an A-wave with atrial systole.

4. Primary pulmonary hypertension (unknown etiology).

5. Recurrent pulmonary emboli can produce a prominent A-wave of the jugular venous pulse.

W. Proctor Harvey, M.D.

Small A waves may occur because of a poorly contracting right atrium. In atrial flutter, the small rapid F waves may appear as shimmerings on the surface of the venous pulsations. The A wave completely disappears with atrial fibrillation or with atrial standstill.

• **Cannon A Waves:** When the right atrium contracts against the closed tricuspid valve, the full force of atrial contraction is transmitted into the venous system. The resultant impulses are called "Cannon A waves" or "Cannon waves". These waves differ from the giant A wave in two respects. First, the Cannon A wave is systolic in timing, whereas, the giant A wave is presystolic. Also, the Cannon A wave tends to have a more rapid rate of rise and therefore appears to have a more flicking motion. Intermittent cannon A waves may occur with premature ventricular or nodal contractions; they are classically seen in patients with complete heart block. Intermittent Cannon A waves may also occur in patients with ventricular pacemakers and dissociation between the independent atrial and the paced ventricular contractions. Regular occurring cannon A waves may accompany paroxysmal supraventricular or junctional tachycardias, or in patients with ventricular pacemakers and normal AV nodal retrograde conduction.

• **The X Descent:** The explanation for the X descent has been the subject of some controversy. Since the X descent is often decreased in patients without atrial contraction, such as atrial fibrillation, the X descent has been thought to be related to atrial relaxation. The trough of the X descent is usually the lowest point of the jugular venous pulsation, dropping well below the onset of the A wave. This observation does not preclude the explanation that the X descent is due to atrial relaxation since some atrial filling (inscribing the H wave) occurs before onset of active atrial contraction. Atrial fibrillation itself could decrease the X descent by interfering with atrial relaxation. Another factor contributing to the genesis of the X descent is the descent of the tricuspid valve or "floor of the right atrium" toward the right ventricular cavity during

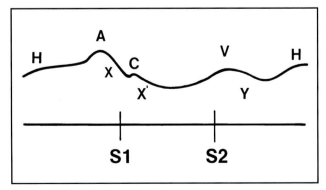

Figure 11. Normal jugular venous pulse with all components labeled. See text.

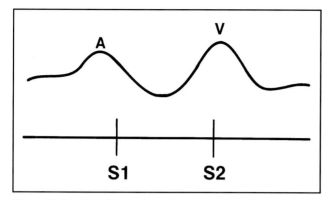

Figure 12. Prominent V wave in a patient with atrial septal defect.

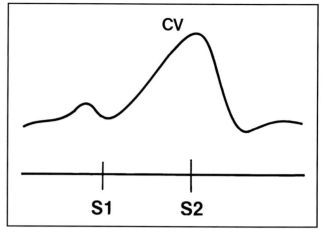

Figure 13. Regurgitant CV wave of tricuspid regurgitation. Because the patient is in sinus rhythm, there is a small A wave prior to the onset of the CV wave.

systole. Some authors divide the X descent in two components, referring to the initial descending limb of the A wave as the X descent and the continued descent following the C wave as the X prime descent (Figure 11). These authors ascribe the X descent to atrial relaxation and the X prime descent to tricuspid valve motion towards the right ventricle during systole (Figure 11). In cardiac tamponade the venous pressures may be so elevated that the specific wave form is difficult to determine; if recorded, the X descent may be prominent. In experimentally produced tamponade, the dominant right atrial wave is the X descent.

• **The C Wave:** The C wave of the jugular venous pulse was originally thought to be secondary to transmitted carotid pulsations. Dr. Paul Wood agreed with this opinion, as he could not find a wave of similar magnitude in right atrial tracings. Rich and Tavell demonstrated that the C wave of the jugular venous pulse occurred a similar distance from the QRS complex in both controls and in patients with left bundle branch block, whereas the onset of the carotid pulse was significantly delayed in the latter group. These investigators concluded that the C wave was not transmitted from the carotid. Tavell's method of recording jugular venous pulsations was by placing a funnel shaped pickup held with some pressure between the two heads of the sternocleidomastoid muscle over the internal jugular bulb, directed posteriorly and caudally. This type of tracing produces records that can resemble right atrial pressure tracing. In contrast, the jugular venous tracings that are recorded over the sternocleidomastoid by displacement techniques may record a transmitted carotid impulse.

As emphasized by Coleman, there are in all probability two mechanisms that produce the C wave in the jugular venous pulse. One, transmitted from the right atrium due to bulging of the tricuspid valve in early systole and the other due to transmission from carotid pulsations.

• **The V Wave:** Normally, the A wave is the dominant venous wave. In patients with an atrial septal defect, the V wave is increased in height so that it equals or is of slightly greater amplitude than the A wave (Figure 12). Normally, the left atrial V wave is larger than the left atrial A wave. In patients with large atrial septal defects, the venous pulse resembles the left atrial pressure tracing. The most common cause of an increase in the magnitude of V wave is incompetence of tricuspid valve. These waves are more than just augmented V waves, since when severe they begin with the C wave. Therefore, they are often referred to as "CV waves", "regurgitant CV waves", or systolic "S waves" (Figure 13). The appearance and height of the CV wave will depend not only upon the amount of blood that is regurgitated into the atrium during right ventricular systole, but also upon the compliance or the stiffness of the right atrium. Mild degrees of tricuspid regurgitation may be manifest only by an obliteration of the X descent. With increasing degrees of tricuspid insufficiency, the height of the V wave will usually increase. Patients with severe tricuspid regurgitation can have very prominent systolic venous pulsations. At times these waves are so forceful that they can be palpated and thus are the exception to the generalization that venous pulsations are visible but not palpable. On the other hand, patients with large right atriums may have significant tricuspid regurgitation with CV waves in the jugular venous pulse that are not impressive.

Patients with chronic tricuspid regurgitation usually have associated atrial fibrillation. In this rhythm the CV wave is not preceded by an A wave. In patients with severe aortic regurgitation, the forceful arterial pulse may produce a dominant

74

transmitted C wave. This wave might be confused with a regurgitant CV wave. In these patients the examining physician should apply pressure to the base of the neck. Venous pulsations will be abolished.

• **The Y Descent:** The most obvious abnormality of the venous wave form in patients with constrictive pericarditis or restrictive myocardial disease is the striking diastolic collapse of the venous pulse. The distended veins not only collapse suddenly, but redistend just as quickly (Figure 2). In cardiac constriction or restriction the veins are distended because of resistance to filling of the right ventricle. When the tricuspid valve opens, the column of blood falls into the right ventricle. Since in both restrictive and constrictive heart disease, the right ventricle has decreased compliance, it quickly fills and the Y ascent is nearly as rapid as the Y descent. The rapid drop and rise of the venous pulse of several mm Hg with each arterial pulse is readily apparent on inspection. It should be emphasized that it is not possible to differentiate between restrictive cardiomyopathy and constrictive pericardial disease by inspection of or recording the venous pulsations, since both conditions result in similar venous pulsations.

A rapid Y descent is not diagnostic of constrictive pericarditis or restrictive heart disease. Since the Y descent is caused by a fall in venous pressure with the opening of the tricuspid valve, whenever the venous pressure is elevated, the Y descent will be prominent and rapid, provided there is no obstruction in the atrium or the tricuspid valve. Thus, the Y descent is prominent in patients with large CV waves due to tricuspid regurgitation and in patients with right heart failure. However, the ascent following the Y descent is not rapid as it is in patients with restrictive or constrictive disease. When tricuspid stenosis is present, the Y descent is slowed and the Y trough may be absent.

Respiratory Variation and Kussmaul's Sign

The mean jugular venous pressure normally falls with inspiration, passively following the intrathoracic pressure. In some patients with decreased right ventricular compliance, relative height of the A wave will increase with inspiration even though the mean venous pressure falls. This is thought to be related to an increased force of atrial contraction with atrial distention that is caused by the ventilatory increase in the venous return.

In patients with a marked decrease in right ventricular compliance, such as those with constrictive pericarditis, there is a rise in the mean height of the jugular venous pulse during inspiration. This

phenomenon is known as Kussmaul's sign and is present in about 40% of the patients with constrictive pericarditis. Inspiratory increase in venous pressure is generally not seen in patients with pericardial tamponade.

Right Ventricular Infarction

Right ventricular myocardial infarction is not uncommon, and when present is virtually always associated with transmural infarction of the inferior or posterior wall of the left ventricle. This diagnosis should be suspected in any patient with inferior or posterior myocardial infarction who develops an elevated venous pressure without evidence of significant pulmonary congestion. Right ventricular infarction is usually well tolerated, but when extensive can lead to cardiogenic shock and serious cardiac dysrhythmia. It may mimic cardiac tamponade or pulmonary embolism. Therefore, it is essential to recognize. Hemodynamic alterations gradually appear within the first two days. An early hemodynamic sign is an otherwise unexplained elevation of the jugular venous or central venous pressure; in patients with right ventricular infarction, jugular venous pressure in the range of 12 cm to 15 cm of water are common. The venous pressure may fail to fall or even rise with inspiration (Kussmaul's sign). Associated pericarditis is occasionally present and pulsus paradoxus in excess of 10 mm Hg has been reported in 40% of patients in some series.

Thus, the clinical triad of pericardial rub, pulsus paradoxus, and hypotension strongly suggest cardiac tamponade. However, closer analysis reveals that the hemodynamics are those of cardiac constriction and not cardiac tamponade. Presence of an inspiratory increase in venous pressure is distinctly uncommon in tamponade. In addition, balloon-tipped catheter recordings will show that the morphology of the right heart pressure tracings more closely resembles that of constrictive pericarditis than tamponade. This morphology includes a prominent X and Y descent in the right atrial pressure recording and the early diastolic "dip and plateau" configuration of the right ventricular pressure tracing. In addition, there is loss of the normal inspiratory decrease of right atrial and ventricular pressures. In cardiac tamponade, Y descents are not ordinarily seen, the dip and plateau phenomenon in the right ventricle is usually absent, and an inspiratory increase in right atrial pressure (Kussmaul's sign) is distinctly uncommon.

It has been postulated that the constrictive hemodynamics of acute right ventricular infarction are due to the abrupt limitation of diastolic filling of the dilated infarcted right ventricle by the rela-

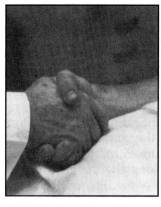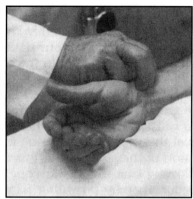

Fig B: Palpation of the radial pulse.

tively nondistensible pericardium. Because of this, intervascular volume depletion may mask the hemodynamic signs of right ventricular infarction. It is therefore important to insure that the patient's volume is adequately expanded before this diagnosis is excluded. Occasionally, regurgitant CV or systolic waves can be seen in right atrial tracing or the jugular venous pulse as the result of tricuspid insufficiency secondary to dysfunction of an infarcted right ventricular papillary muscle.

Right ventricular infarction is one condition that will produce a positive abdominal jugular test without elevation of the pulmonary artery wedge pressure.

Arterial Pulsations

Interest in arterial pulsations dates to antiquity. The common disorders of rate and rhythm were well described in the early part of this century by Sir James MacKenzie and Sir Thomas Lewis, who used recordings of the venous pulse to reflect atrial activity and simultaneous recordings of the apex beat or arterial pulse to reflect ventricular activity. Although a trained observer can on occasion diagnose a dysrhythmia by simultaneously observing the venous pulse and palpation of an artery, few would initiate therapy based on these observations without first confirming and documenting the abnormality with an electrocardiogram. Yet, symptoms and the routine examination of the arterial pulse for rate and rhythm as well as observation of the jugular venous pulse, frequently suggest when an electrocardiographic rhythm tracing is necessary. Careful evaluation of the character or contour of the carotid pulse and an evaluation of the peripheral pulse for volume alterations (pulsus alternans) and abnormal respiratory variations (pulsus paradoxus) as well as for rate and rhythm, will reward the examiner with invaluable diagnostic information.

In past decades, palpation of the arterial pulses, with the information derived by the physician, represented one of the important facets of the physical examination. It is indeed an ancient art of medicine that can be mastered by the student and practicing physician; however, today, for all practical purposes, it almost represents a lost art.

Worthy of continued reemphasis is the importance of palpating the radial pulse as one of the first steps in examining patients. It is a very natural and simple maneuver, after greeting a patient and shaking hands, then to move our fingers to palpate the radial pulse (Fig. B). A number of clues regarding the presence of cardiovascular disease may then become immediately evident, e.g., a paradoxical pulse, pulsus alternans, quick rise pulse of aortic insufficiency or idiopathic hypertrophic subaortic stenosis, pulsus bisferiens of aortic stenosis plus insufficiency or aortic insufficiency alone, slow rise pulse of aortic stenosis and dicrotic pulse. This often takes 15-30 seconds or less and can provide an important indication of heart disease.

The art of feeling the arterial pulse is an important part of the total cardiovascular evaluation. It is also part of what a good physician can do themselves. I call it part of "the fun of medicine."

W. Proctor Harvey, M.D.

Arterial Pulse Contour

Arterial rate and rhythm can be assessed from any palpable pulse. However, since the arterial pulse contour is altered as it travels to the peripheral arterial vessels, the arterial pulse closest to the heart, that is, carotid pulse is evaluated when assessing pulse contour. During peripheral transmission of the arterial pulse, pulse pressure increases and the rate of rise of the arterial pulse is accentuated. These phenomena make it easier to appreciate pulsus alternans and pulsus paradoxus from the peripheral pulses. But as stated above, when one is evaluating the central arterial pulse contour the carotid artery should be assessed.

CARDIAC PEARL

I routinely feel the radial pulse as one of my first steps in the physical examination of a patient. After greeting the patient and shaking hands, I move the palpating fingers (index and third) of my right hand to the patient's right radial pulse. This is a very "natural" thing to do and, at the same time, can be reassuring to the patient. Palpation should be performed gently and with light pressure. By paying strict attention to the character of the pulse, valuable information can be obtained. For example, pulsus alternans often can be detected even though it may be slight and easily overlooked. However, this finding generally provides an immediate clue as to the presence of myocardial weakness. It can represent one of the earlier subtle signs of cardiac decompensation. This simple procedure takes only a short time (15-30 seconds) and alerts the physician to concentrate carefully on auscultation of the heart. A ventricular (S₃) diastolic gallop may be heard as well as alternation of heart murmurs and sounds (particularly the second sound).

Another practical example of a clue provided by the radial pulse at the very start of the physical examination is to note a "quick rise" of the pulse. A common cause of this would be some degree of aortic insufficiency, and the physician is alerted to this possibility as he carefully listens with the flat diaphragm of his stethoscope exerting firm pressure along the left sternal border. Detection of an early, blowing, high-frequency diastolic murmur usually would be diagnostic. However, if no diastolic murmur of aortic insufficiency is heard, but instead a systolic murmur, one always should consider the possibility of hypertrophic cardiomyopathy.

The final step in diagnosis is to perform the squatting maneuver: on standing, the systolic murmur is heard but may diminish or disappear on squatting. Even more important is to have the patient quickly resume the standing position, at which time the systolic murmur may increase in intensity even louder than at the beginning of the maneuver. If this sequence of events occurs, the diagnosis of hypertrophic cardiomyopathy is quite likely.

In fact, of patients in whom I have made this diagnosis and not knowing their problem beforehand, this sequence of observations accounted for the diagnosis in the great majority. Many of these patients present to the physician with chest pain thought to be that of ischemic heart disease and a smaller number with symptoms of dizziness or syncope.

A pulse that is quick rising but promptly collapsing is typical of aortic insufficiency, whereas the pulse of aortic stenosis is slower to rise and is sustained. Pulsus paradoxus, with the pulse decreasing in amplitude on inspiration, may be the first clue as to the presence of pericardial effusion or constrictive pericarditis. This is best detected with the blood pressure cuff. Sounds decreasing in intensity or becoming absent with inspiration ≥ 10mm Hg range suggests paradoxus.

The term "paradoxical pulse" is really a misnomer because when it is clinically apparent, it is really only an exaggeration of the normal pulse. The decrease in amplitude of the pulse coincident with inspiration is an important sign of pericardial tamponade, and may be a sign of restrictive cardiomyopathy, or chronic pulmonary disease such as emphysema or asthma.

Pulsus paradoxus can be present with constrictive pericarditis, but it is more likely to occur with cardiac tamponade.

W. Proctor Harvey, M.D.

When assessing the carotid pulse, the examining finger is placed lightly over the artery just below the carotid sinus. Increasing pressure is applied until the pulse is readily appreciated. One should assess selectively the upstroke, the peak and the collapse of the carotid pulse.

• **Ascending Limb or Upstroke:** Rate of rise of the carotid pulse upstroke is altered by various disease states; rate of rise is increased in patients with

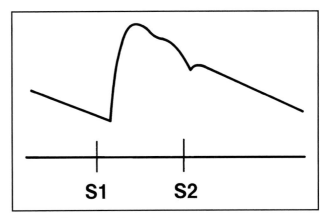

Figure 14. Normal carotid pulse tracing.

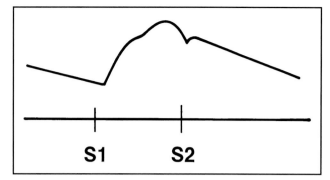

Figure 15. Slow rising carotid pulse with anacrotic shoulder of patients with aortic stenosis.

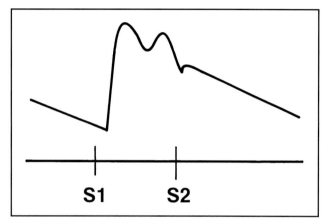

Figure 16. Bisferiens carotid pulse.

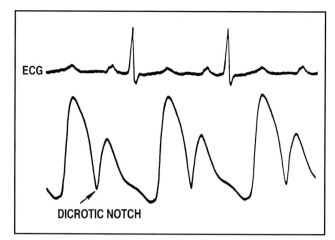

Figure 17. Dicrotic pulse.

hyperdynamic contractions such as in anxiety, hypertrophic cardiomyopathy, and with increased aortic run-off such as aortic regurgitation. The forceful arterial pulse of severe aortic regurgitation is referred to as a water-hammer pulse. The water-hammer is a toy consisting of water and vacuum in a small glass container. When inverted, the water falls abruptly to the bottom.

CARDIAC PEARL

Often careful analysis of the arterial pulse may provide an important clue as to whether we are dealing with aortic or pulmonary valve regurgitation. The aortic insufficiency produces a "quick rise" or a "flip" detected by the palpating fingers, which would not be present with pulmonic valve regurgitation. Also, if an early blowing diastolic murmur is heard over the aortic area, this would practically rule out that of pulmonary valve origin. The pulmonary valve insufficiency of a low pressure leak such as that occurring with a congenital valve insufficiency typically, although not always, has a pause between the pulmonic valve closure and the onset of the diastolic murmur, which may be of a low frequency

rumble rather than of a high frequency early blowing decrescendo murmur immediately following the second heart sound. The pulmonary regurgitant murmur of the low pressure type also characteristically increases with inspiration.

W. Proctor Harvey, M.D.

The pulse of mitral regurgitation associated with good ventricular function is sometimes referred to as a "small water-hammer" pulse. In acute mitral regurgitation the stroke volume and the pulse pressure is small, but rate of rise is quite brisk but non-sustained.

Rate of rise of the carotid pulse is decreased in patients with fixed obstruction to left ventricular outflow tract and severe heart failure. Slowly rising carotid pulsations may be found in patients with significant fixed obstruction of the left ventricular outflow, whether the obstruction be discreet, sub-valvular, valvular, or supravalvular aortic stenosis. Figure 14 illustrates the normal while Figure 15 shows the slow rising pulse of aortic stenosis; presence or absence of a palpable thrill does not correlate with severity of stenosis. Patients with significant aortic regurgitation may have a palpable carotid thrill in the absence of aortic stenosis. Since the carotid pulse contour changes with age, hypertension and atherosclerosis, the rate of rise of the carotid pulse loses some of its diagnostic qualities in the elderly patients. Elderly patients with significant aortic stenosis can have a normal rate of rise of the arterial pulse.

The aortic and carotid pulses of younger patients with severe aortic valve stenosis have an anacrotic notch in addition to the slow rate of rise. This anacrotic notch is appreciated as a shoulder on the ascending limb of the carotid pulse (Figure 15). The anacrotic notch is thought to relate to the decreased

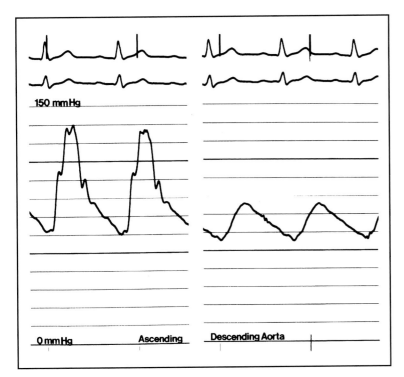

Figure 18. Pressure recordings from a patient with coarctation of the aorta.

velocity of flow. A slowly rising carotid pulse is not necessarily an indication of left ventricular outflow obstruction. A poorly functioning ventricle develops pressure more slowly and the rate of rise of the carotid pulse may be slow. However, a slow rising carotid pulse associated with an anacrotic notch or palpable thrill should suggest presence of aortic stenosis.

• **Peak of the Carotid Pulse:** The peak of the carotid pulse can be nonsustained, sustained, or bisferiens. Fries and associates have shown that the externally recorded carotid pulse has an early and a late systolic component. In youth, the first component is dominant. With age the second component increases relative to the first, producing a more sustained carotid impulse. Disease states such as systemic hypertension, atherosclerosis or both, also increase the relative height of the second peak. Thus, in these patients the peak of the carotid pulse is more sustained. On occasion, there are two distinctly palpable pulsations in systole. This type of pulse is said to be bisferiens or twice beating (Figure 16). Presence of a bisferious arterial pulse should immediately bring to the clinician's mind one of two diagnoses: aortic regurgitation, and hypertrophic obstructive cardiomyopathy. In its most florid form, the contour of the carotid pulse of hypotrophic obstructive cardiomyopathy has a "spike-dome" configuration. It should be emphasized however, that in the majority of patients with obstructive or nonobstructive hypertrophic cardiomyopathy, a bisferious pulse is not present. A bisferious pulse suggests that the obstruction is severe. Most patients with hypertrophic cardiomyopathy have only a rapidly rising carotid pulse.

CARDIAC PEARL

A double systolic impulse in the radial pulse is called a bisferiens pulse. When this is present, think of three possibilities: 1. A combination of aortic stenosis plus aortic regurgitation; 2. More severe aortic regurgitation; 3. Hypertrophic cardiomyopathy.

W. Proctor Harvey, M.D.

• **Descending Limb of the Carotid Arterial Pulse:** Normally, the carotid pulse collapses rather briskly. In a small subset of patients the dicrotic wave is very prominent and is palpable. This is the "dicrotic pulse". The dicrotic pulse is a twice-beating pulse in which the first peak is in systole and the second is in early diastole (Figure 17). The second peak is an exaggeration of the normal dicrotic wave that occurs following the closure of the aortic valve. Characteristics of the dicrotic pulse are a slow rate of rise, small pulse pressure, low dicrotic notch and large dicrotic wave. Measurement of systolic time intervals of the dicrotic pulse revealed a prolonged pre-ejection period and a shortened left ventricular ejection time.

Although the exact cause of the dicrotic pulse is unknown, the hemodynamic correlates are clear; a low stroke volume, low cardiac output, and high peripheral vascular resistance in a relatively young adult. This constellation is found most often in the young patient with congestive cardiomyopathy; many patients have a low stroke volume and a high peripheral vascular resistance, but presumably because of the less compliant or less resilient arterial vascular system, these middle aged or older patients do not have a dicrotic arterial pulse. The dicrotic pulse has also been recorded in young patients with advanced states of cardiac decompensation due to ischemic heart disease. A striking dicrotic pulse was recorded in a 42-year-old man who had aortic valve replacement with a Starr-Edwards ball-valve prosthesis six years earlier. Presence of clots resulted in malfunction of the valve, with severe compromise of his cardiac stroke volume. Following valve replacement, the striking dicrotic pulse was no longer present.

The importance of low stroke volume to the genesis of the dicrotic pulse has been confirmed by two other observations. The first is the fact that in patients with a dicrotic arterial pulse, the post premature beat, a beat with a larger stroke volume, is frequently normal. The other is the observation of a dicrotic arterial pulse in young patients with cardiac tamponade only during inspiration, the time when left ventricular filling is compromised and stroke volume is low. A dicrotic pulse is also seen in post operative patients operated for either aortic or mitral regurgitation. When observed it reflects poor ventricular function and when persistent, indicates a poor prognosis.

Peripheral Arterial Pulses

Peripheral arterial pulses should be routinely checked in all four extremities and in both carotid arteries in patients being evaluated for the first time, for hypertension, possible aortic dissection, cerebral ischemia, subclavian steal syndrome, claudication and in patients with suspected cardiac decompensation or cardiac tamponade. Figure 18 shows the arterial pressure tracings from the central aorta and lower aorta in a patient with severe coarctation of the aorta. Note that the onset of the femoral artery pressure is only slightly delayed, but the rate of rise of the femoral artery pressure is much slower, imparting a distinct impression to the palpating fingers that there is a radial-femoral delay. Simultaneous palpation of the radial and femoral pulses should be carried out in the initial evaluation of all patients with hypertension to rule out the presence of coarction of the aorta. Atherosclerotic lesions in the subclavian artery can result in a significant discrepancy in the blood pressure between the upper extremities.

CARDIAC PEARL

On first shaking hands with the patient and then palpating the radial pulse (Figure C), a quick rise to the arterial pulse may be noted. This finding can be a clue to the following:
- **Aortic regurgitation**
- **Mitral regurgitation**
- **Ventricular septal defect**
- **Hypertrophic cardiomyopathy**

All of the foregoing can cause a quick rise or "flip" of the arterial pulse.

The quick rise or "flip" of the radial pulse may be even better detected by having the patient raise his arms over his head (Figure D). This simple maneuver may make this type of pulse more evident.

W. Proctor Harvey, M.D.

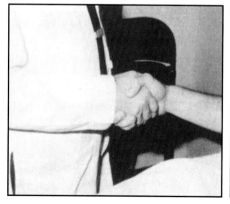
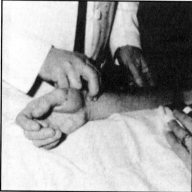

Fig C: Shaking hands and then palpating the radial pulse.

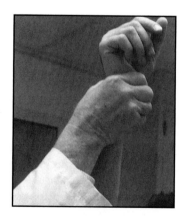

Fig D: Aortic regurgitation - the "quick rise" or "flip" of the radial pulse may be even better appreciated by palpation with the patient's arm elevated as shown.

Pulsus Alternans

Pulsus alternans is a peripheral manifestation of left ventricular decompensation. When simultaneous recording of arterial pressures and their first derivative are made, there is alternation not only at the height of the pressure pulse but also the rate of rise of the arterial pulse. Some have suggested that it is this latter phenomena that is appreciated during palpation rather than small alternations in systolic pressure.

Although a more central arterial pulse is used to evaluate pulse contour, pulsus alternans is best detected by palpation of the more distal radial or femoral artery pulsations. Rate of rise and the peak pressure developed are accentuated during peripheral transmission of the arterial pulse pressure. This phenomenon accentuates the degree of alternation, making it easier to appreciate the presence of pulsus alternans in the distal arteries. Light pressure, like blowing on your fingertips, is applied over the pulse. Mild degrees of pulsus alternans can be detected by using the blood pressure cuff and deflating it very slowly around systole. Rarely, the weak pulse is too small to feel, in which case total alternans is said to be present.

Pulsus alternans often represents one of the earliest and most subtle indications of myocardial weakness or decompensation. Of course, pulsus alternans can be detected by searching for it and can be easily detected by palpation of the peripheral pulses. A simple but very effective maneuver is to shake hands with the patient at the first meeting and then to move your palpating fingers of the middle and index fingers to the radial artery, which may reveal a finding such as pulsus alternans. This initial maneuver can thereby quickly indicate the presence of underlying heart disease. Of course, all arterial pulses, in addition to the radial, should be subsequently palpated to identify any abnormal findings. If pulsus alternans is noted, then one can expect to find alternation of the second heart sound and alternation of any murmur if present. However, they will not be detected unless they are specifically looked for. These findings represent one of the most constantly overlooked clinical clues that are present in patients that I examine today.

Most physicians do not do this, thereby missing a unique opportunity to know that the patient has heart disease. For example,

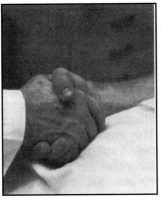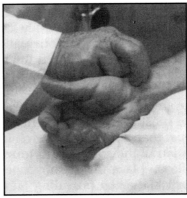

Fig E: Left: Greeting and shaking hands with patient. Right: Next, move hand to palpate radial pulse.

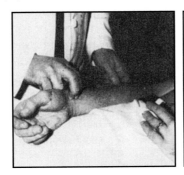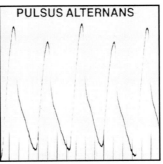

PULSUS ALTERNANS

Fig F: Pulsus alternans detected with "light" palpation of the radial pulse.

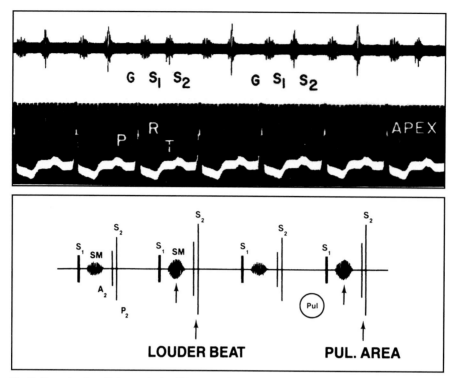

Fig G: Upper tracing: Note ventricular (S₃) gallop (G) and alternation of the second sound (S₂).
Lower tracing: Note alternation of the systolic murmur (SM) and second sound (S₂).

palpating the pulse may indicate that it alternates in amplitude with each beat- strong, weak, strong, weak. This is pulsus alternans. Every other beat is weaker than the preceding one, and after a premature beat, the alternation is more accentuated. We do not detect the pulsus alternans if we palpate with very firm pressure over the artery; instead, a very light pressure is needed, similar to what might be felt by a blow of breath on our fingers. It is rewarding how often pulsus alternans is found because it is such a common finding, but we have to look for it. As is true in life, especially in medicine, we find what we look for. However, there are two parts to the observation. Not only do we find what we are looking for, but we also have to know what we are looking for. Then we will find it. Here is a practical example, which represents a valuable cardiac pearl: if the alternating radial pulses are found, then alternation of the second heart sound will be heard on auscultation of the heart in most patients if we search carefully. If a murmur is present, it too will alternate in intensity. A ventricular (S₃) diastolic gallop should be heard, if the simple, basic techniques discussed here are used. Thus it can be readily known. It often takes less than several minutes to know that our patient has heart disease. These findings, which can be detected in the examiner's office or at the bedside, establish the clinical diag-

nosis of cardiac decompensation. As a rule, the more prominent these findings, and the easier they are found, the greater the degree of heart failure (Figures E, F and G).

W. Proctor Harvey, M.D.

Pulsus Paradoxus

Pulsus paradoxus was described by Kussmaul more than a century ago when he found an inspiratory increase in venous pressure, but a decrease in arterial pulse volume in patients with chronic constrictive pericarditis. It is now known that arterial pulsus paradoxus is distinctly rare in constrictive pericarditis, but is common in severe asthma and chronic obstructive lung disease, and is the *sine qua non* of pericardial tamponade. Tamponade can occur without pulsus paradoxus as will be discussed later. Pericardial effusion without tamponade does not produce pulsus paradoxus, for only when the pericardium is filled and tensed does hemodynamic embarrassment of the heart ensue. Recognition and appropriate therapy are life-saving. Pulsus paradoxus is generally ascribed to a fall in systolic blood pressure of at least 10 mmHg to 12 mmHg during normal inspiration. The technique for the bedside measurement of pulsus paradoxus is illustrated in Figure 19. Pulsus paradoxus is most commonly found in patients with obstructive lung disease. In this condition the marked

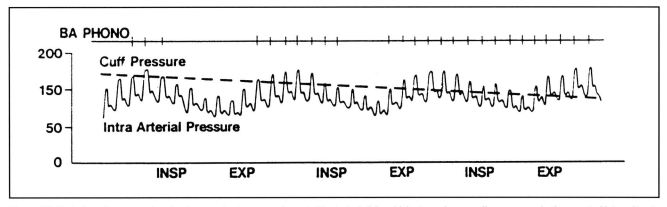

Figure 19. Technique for measuring the degree of pulsus paradoxus is illustrated. A brachial artery phonocardiogram reveals the onset of intermittent Korotkoff sounds on the left and continuous sounds on the right. The pressure difference between the onset of Korotkoff sounds and continuous Korotkoff sounds indicates the degree of pulsus paradoxus. The measurement should be taken while the patient is breathing normally.

decrease in intrathoracic pressure with forceful inspiration is transmitted to the intrathoracic arterial structures resulting in a fall in systolic pressure. The presence of pulsus alternans in patients with chronic obstructive lung disease correlates with the degree of pulmonary obstruction.

Etiology of pulsus paradoxus in patients with cardiac tamponade has been shown by the work of Shabetai, Fowler, and their co-workers to be related to the inspiratory increase in right ventricular filling that causes a decrease in left ventricular filling. Because the fluid filled pericardial sack has reached its limits of distensibility, further increase in right heart volume can only occur if there is compensatory decrease in the volume of the other intrapericardial structures. Echocardiograms have demonstrated a decrease in left ventricular diameter and a decrease in excursion of the mitral valve opening during inspiration in patients with pericardial tamponade. Decreased left ventricular filling with inspiration results in a smaller stroke volume and a lower arterial pressure. Tamponade can occur without pulsus paradoxus in patients with aortic regurgitation or atrial septal defects. These cardiac lesions compensate for inadequate left ventricular filling during inspiration inspite of tamponade. Tamponade can also occur without pulsus paradoxus in patients with marked elevation of left ventricular filling pressure prior to the onset of tamponade. Cardiac dysrhythmias can cause "pseudo" pulsus paradoxus. Some patients with atrial ventricular dissociation can have phasic swings in systolic blood pressure that mimic pulsus paradoxus.

CARDIAC PEARL

Another cardiac pearl related to the initial handshake with our patient and then palpating the radial pulse: the patient may have a quick-rise "flip" type of pulse which immediately suggests aortic regurgitation as one possible diagnosis. The examiner is immediately clued in to listen carefully for the detection of this condition, which on auscultation of the heart might show a typical aortic diastolic murmur, confirming the first observation obtained from palpation of the arterial pulse.

Another poorly recognized position where the aortic diastolic murmur can often be easily heard is with the patient turned to the left lateral position and the stethoscope over the mid left sternal border. Firm pressure with the diaphragm of the stethoscope should be exerted against the skin of the chest wall with the patient holding his or her breath in deep expiration.

W. Proctor Harvey, M.D.

Commentary

Over the years, some physicians have tended to place less emphasis on the physical diagnosis; this is unfortunate, since a detailed cardiovascular examination is invaluable, not only to determine when more sophisticated and expensive tests are needed, but when therapy or alteration in drug therapy is needed. Numerous examples are provided throughout this book, but in the area covered by this chapter, evaluation of the jugular venous pressure and the patient's response to the abdominal jugular test is critical to the optimal management of patients with chronic heart failure. One finds daily chest roentgenograms being ordered to follow the progress of a hospitalized patient with chronic severe heart failure, when a better and less costly approach is a careful daily bedside evaluation of the jugular venous pressure and the response to the abdominal jugular test.

Selected Reading

1. Burch GE, Ray CT: Mechanism of the hepatojugular reflux test in congestive heart failure. *AHJ* 48:373-382, 1954.
2. Butman SM, Ewy GA, Kern KB, Standen JR: Resting and/or provable jugular venous distention (abdominojugular test) are the best discriminators in bedside examination of patients with chronic heart failure. *Circ* 86:1-529, 1992.
3. Butman SM, Ewy GA, Standen JR, Kern KB, Hahn E: Bedside cardiovascular exam in patients with severe chronic heart failure: importance of resting or inducible jugular venous distention. *JACC* 22:968-74, 1993.
4. Coleman AL: *Clinical Examination of the Jugular Venous Pulse.* 11-68, Charles C Thomas, Springfield, Illinois, 1966.
5. Coleman AL: Jugular C wave. *NEJM* (letter) 285: 462, 1971.
6. Coma-Cannella I, Lopez-Sandon J, Gamallo C: Low output syndrome in right ventricular infarction. *AHJ* 98: 613-620, 1979.
7. Constant, J: *Bedside Cardiology.* Little, Brown; Boston 1969.
8. Ducas J, Magder S, McGregor M: Validity of the hepatojugular reflux as a clinical test for congestive heart failure. *AJC* 52:1291-1303, 1983.
9. Ewy GA: The abdominojugular test: Technique and hemodynamic correlates. *Ann Int Med* 109; 456-460, 1988.
10. Ewy GA, Marcus Fl: Bedside estimation of venous pressure. *The Heart Bulletin* 17:41-44, 1968.
11. Ewy GA, Rios JC, Marcus F: The dicrotic arterial pulse. *Circ* 39:655-661, 1969.
12. Ewy, GA: Venous and arterial pulsations (in) Horwitz LD, Groves BM. *Signs and Symptoms in Cardiology* 1985, Lippincott, Philadelphia.
13. Feigenbaum H: *Echocardiography,* Second Edition, p. 255-262 Philadelphia, 1976, Lea and Febiger.
14. Freis ED, Heath WC, Luchsinger PC et al: Changes in carotid pulse which occur with age and hypertension. *AHJ* 71:757-765, 1966.
15. Hancock EW: On the elastic and rigid forms of constrictive pericarditis. *AHJ* 100: 917-923, 1980.
16. Hirschfelder AD: Variations in the form of the venous pulse. A preliminary report. *Johns Hop Hos Bul* 18:265-267, 1987.
17. Isner JM, Roberts WC: Right ventricular infarction complicating left ventricular infarction secondary to coronary heart disease. *AJC* 42:885-894, 1978.
18. Lange RL, Botticelli JT, Tsagaris TJ, et al: Diagnostic signs in compressive cardiac disorder: constrictive pericarditis, pericardial effusion, and tamponade. *Circ* 33:763-777, 1966.
19. Lorell B, Leinbach RC, Pohost GM et al: Right ventricular infarction: clinical diagnosis and differentiation from cardiac tamponade and pericardial constriction. *AJC* 43:465-479, 1979.
20. Orchard RC, Craige E: Dicrotic pulse after open heart surgery. *Circ* 62:1107-1114, 1980.
21. Perloff JK: *Clinical Recognition of Congenital Heart Disease.* WB Saunders, Philadelphia 1970.
22. Rebuck AS, Pengelly LD: Development of pulsus paradoxus in the presence of airway obstruction. *NEJM* 288:66-69, 1973.
23. Reddy PS, Curtiss EJ, O'Toole JD and Shaver JA: Cardiac tamponade: hemodynamic observations in man. *Circ* 58:265-272, 1978.
24. Rich LL, Tavel ME: The origin of the jugular C wave. *NEJM* 284:1309-1311, 1971.
25. Roberts, WC, Perloff, JK, and Costantino, T: Severe valvular aortic stenosis in patients over 65 years of age. A clinico-pathologic study. *AJC* 27:497-506, 1971.
26. Shabetai R, Fowler NO, Fenton JC, Masangkay M: Pulsus paradoxus. *J Clin Invest* 44:1882-1898, 1965.
27. Shah PK, Shellock F, Berman D et al: Predominant right ventricular dysfunction in acute myocardial infarction: frequency, clinical, hemodynamic, and scintigraphic findings. *Circ* 62:111-313, 1980.
28. Sharpe, DN, Botvinick EH, Shames DM et al: The non-invasive diagnosis of right ventricular infarction. *Circ* 57:483-490, 1978.
29. Stevenson LW, Perloff JK: The limited reliability of physical signs for estimating hemodynamics in chronic heart failure. *JAMA* 261:884-888, 1989.
30. Tavell ME, Bard RA, Franks LC, Feigenbaum H, Fisch C: The jugular venous pulse in atrial septal defect. *Arc Int Med* 121:524-529, 1968.
31. Wade WG: Pathogenesis of infarction of the right ventricle. *BHJ* 21:545-554, 1959.
32. Wood P: *Disease of the Heart and Circulation.* 2nd edit. 42-57; JB Lippincott, Philadelphia 1956.

CHAPTER 6

Precordial Palpation: Let Your Fingers Do the Walking

Jonathan Abrams, M.D.

One of the oldest aspects of the cardiac physical examination is precordial palpation. Feeling for cardiac activity on the chest is as ancient as the use of the stethoscope, and a considerable amount of information can be intuited from a careful examination and description of precordial motion in normal and cardiac disease states. For much of the mid-portion of the 20th century, various means were employed to record this activity, and the role of apex cardiography was well established in the 1950s and 1960s. Since the advent of echocardiography and the widespread use of cardiac catheterization, graphic recordings of precordial motion have fallen by the wayside. Nevertheless, the knowledge and deductions generated several decades ago remain valid today and help us understand the physiology of the normal and abnormal cardiac impulse.

Information derived from astute palpation of the cardiac area on the chest wall can be very useful in the evaluation of patients with overt cardiac disease. While it is true that in the majority of patients with adult heart disease who suffer from acute and chronic coronary artery syndromes or arrhythmias, palpation of the apex is generally unrewarding, it is clearly a valuable component of the examination in patients with structural heart disease, cardiomegaly, systolic and diastolic overload states, major wall motion abnormalities secondary to coronary artery disease, and elevated pulmonary artery pressure from a variety of causes. It therefore behooves the clinician to be familiar with the normal and abnormal cardiac impulses. The examination is relatively straightforward and when abnormal, careful attention to apical and parasternal wall motion abnormalities can be useful in the assessment and quantification of the underlying cardiac disorder. While graphic recordings of precordial motion contain considerable information, these are rarely available, and in any case, require skilled technicians for acquisition of high quality recordings, as well as skilled phonocardiographers to interpret the apexcardiographic tracings.

The Normal Precordial Impulse

In normal adults the only palpable precordial movement is derived from the left ventricle, resulting in a detectable outward impulse at the "apex beat" or point of maximal impulse (PMI) on the left anterior chest wall. The left ventricle moves anteriorly during early systole, with rotation of the chamber in a counter-clockwise fashion in its long axis during isovolumic systole while intraventricular pressure rapidly rises. The apical area of the heart, including the left ventricular septum, lifts slightly and makes contact with the inner left anterior chest wall. After aortic valve opening and early ejection, the left ventricular chamber begins to decrease in volume and the LV epicardium moves away from chest wall, particularly during the second half of ejection. The left ventricle continues to decrease in size throughout systole until the second heart sound. Diastolic filling of the ventricle is not usually palpable unless it is abnormally augmented and/or the diastolic pressure is excessively high. Thus, the normal apex impulse is generated by an anterior and counter-clockwise motion of the interapical por-

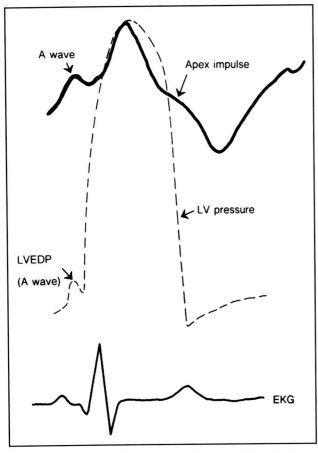

Figure 1. Relationships of the normal apex impulse to left ventricular pressure. LVEDP = left ventricular end-diastolic pressure. *(From Abrams J: Precordial motion. In Signs and Symptoms in Cardiology. Edited by LD Horwitz and BM Groves. Philadelphia, JB Lippincott Co, 1985).*

erally only found in patients with congestive heart failure and/or major mitral regurgitation.

Right Ventricular Activity

The right ventricle is located just beneath the sternum between the left third to fifth ribs, in the so-called parasternal area. Normally, right ventricular activity is not detectable, presumably because right ventricular systolic pressure is low and the right ventricular free wall is rather thin. Furthermore, the right ventricle pulls away from the anterior chest as the heart rotates in a counter clockwise fashion during presystole. However, in children, young adults, or particularly thin individuals with a narrow chest, some degree of parasternal or right ventricular activity may be palpable in the right ventricular area. This is typically a gentle lifting motion. In patients who have large chests, COPD, or obesity, careful subxiphoid palpation during deep and/or held inspiration may bring out right ventricular activity.

Palpable Diastolic Events

Diastole is typically quiet with respect to precordial motion; a palpable diastolic impulse is distinctly abnormal except in very young individuals with vigorous cardiac output. Altered ventricular diastolic volume or compliance can result in prominent third and fourth heart sounds which may become palpable at the apex or over the right ventricle.

tion of the left ventricle, which impinges on the inner chest wall to produce a palpable lifting motion under the examiner's fingers (Figures 1 and 2). It should be obvious that the normal physiologic left ventricular impulse in systole is of relatively brief duration. It is palpable only over a relatively small area of the chest and should not be particularly forceful. Table 1 outlines the classic criteria for the normal apical impulse. Figure 2 shows a normal apex recording with several components, as initially described during the era of apex cardiography.

While the atrial deflection, O-point and rapid filling wave are readily detectable with high quality recording equipment, these are not usually palpable under normal circumstances. An augmented A-wave or pre-systolic movement may be felt when there is increased left ventricular end diastolic pressure and enhanced left atrial booster function producing an S_4. Similarly during the rapid filling phase into a dilated ventricle with an increased end diastolic volume and pressure, a left ventricular filling transient or S_3 may be palpable. This is gen-

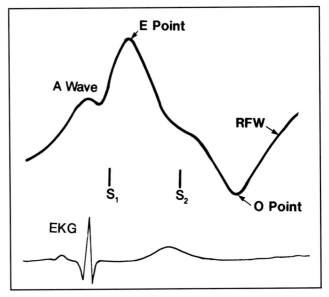

Figure 2. Normal precordial impulse. Note that the outward motion occurs entirely within the first half of systole. The left ventricle retracts from the chest wall as it becomes smaller during late systole. The palpable apex impulse is brief. Normally, the A wave and diastolic events are not palpable. RFW = rapid filling wave. *(From Abrams J: Cardiac Physical Diagnosis. Philadelphia, Lea & Febiger, 1987).*

TABLE 1
The Normal Apical Impulse

- A gentle, nonsustained tap
- An early systolic anterior motion that ends before the last third of systole
- Location within 10 cm of the midsternal line in the fourth or fifth left intercostal space
- A palpable area less than 2 cm^2 to 2.5 cm^2 and detectable in only 1 intercostal space
- RV motion that is not normally palpable
- Diastolic events that are not normally palpable
- Complete absence in some older individuals

Genesis of Precordial Activity: The Normal Apex Impulse

The supine apex impulse is normally formed by the left ventricle. Right ventricular activity is not palpable in healthy subjects as a rule. Table 1 lists the characteristics of the normal apex impulse in the supine position. Note that Figure 1 diagrams the outward and inward components of left ventricular apical activity. Only the early outward motion is normally felt, which is typically not forceful nor sustained. As previously mentioned, the apex impulse should not be felt over a large area. In many individuals, the apex beat will not be palpable in the supine position. This is particularly true in subjects with large chests and an increased A-P diameter, women with large breasts, obese subjects and very muscular men. Furthermore, for uncertain reasons (perhaps because of an increasing thoracic dimension over time) older individuals may not have a palpable apex beat in the supine position. This is not an abnormality, and it is common in people in their 50's and 60's or older.

When the supine apical impulse is not detectable, the examiner should always ask the patient to turn on the left side to achieve the so-called left lateral decubitus position (Figure 3). This maneuver should also be accompanied by requesting the subject to bring his or her left arm above the head. This tends to pull the skin taut over the left precordium; breast tissue as well as the normal chest wall moves away from the apex area. In the majority of instances, precordial left ventricular activity can be detected in the left lateral position, but this is not always the case. The same factors that tend to decrease the likelihood of detecting the apex impulse in the supine position are also likely to decrease the likelihood of feeling left ventricular activity in the 45 degree left decubitus position. In spite of difficult-to-feel apex impulses, careful examination and exploration of

the precordial area usually is rewarding. Often, with the finger on the apex in the left lateral decubitus position, when the patient is asked to return to the supine position, the apex impulse is then readily found. One must also pay attention to the respiratory cycle; apical activity is sometimes masked during inspiration and is only felt during expiration, and occasionally vice versa. Thus, the apex impulse itself may wax and wane in strength and detectability. When an abnormal precordial motion is found or suspected, careful attention to detail is important with the examiner noting the general size of apex beat, its forcefulness, and most importantly whether the impulse is brief and outward only during the first half of systole, or whether it is sustained. When an apical impulse is sustained or prolonged in quality it is called a lift or heave. This non-scientific expression implies protracted systolic outward motion, and in the supine position it indicates a definite cardiac abnormality.

Right Ventricle

As previously indicated, the thin walled and low pressure right ventricle, while directly under the left parasternal region, does not typically generate palpable precordial activity. In very thin or young individuals, such as children, gentle parasternal

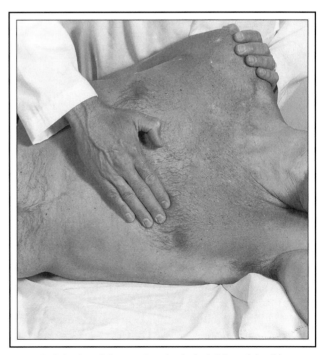

Figure 3. Palpation of the apex impulse in the left lateral decubitus position. This maneuver should be used in any patient with suspected left ventricular disease. The patient should be turned 45 to 60 degrees onto the left side with the left arm extended above the head. *(From Abrams J: Precordial palpation. In Signs and Symptoms of Cardiology. Edited by LD Horwitz and BM Groves. Philadelphia, JB Lippincott Co, 1985).*

87

TABLE 2 Major Types of Precordial Impulses			
IMPULSE	**HYPERDYNAMIC**	**SUSTAINED**	**LATE SYSTOLIC**
Left ventricular impulse (apical beat)	Hyperkinetic circulatory states Thin chest wall Pectus excavatum Volume overload Aortic regurgitation Mitral regurgitation Ventricular septal defect	Pressure overload Hypertension Aortic stenosis Chronic or severe volume overload states LV dilatation, especially with decreased ejection fraction LV dysfunction LV aneurysm Cardiomyopathy	LV dyssynergy Hypertrophic cardiomyopathy Mitral valve prolapse (rare)
Right ventricular impulse (parasternal area)	Hyperkinetic circulatory state in young subjects Volume overload Atrial septal defect Tricuspid regurgitation	Pressure overload Pulmonary stenosis Pulmonary hypertension Cor pulmonale Mitral stenosis Pulmonary emboli Cardiomyopathy	Severe mitral regurgitation

(Abrams J: Modified from Precordial motion in health and disease. Mod Concepts Cardiovasc Dis 49:55-60, 1980. By permission of the American Heart Association, Inc.)

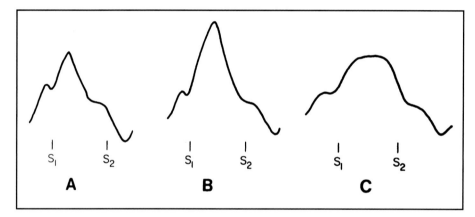

Figure 4. Major types of left ventricular precordial motion. **A.** Normal. **B.** Hyperdynamic. **C.** Sustained. With a patient in the supine position, the presence of sustained left ventricular activity detectable in the latter half of systole is distinctly abnormal. Some experts believe that palpation of a sustained impulse when patients are in the left lateral decubitus position may have less specificity for underlying left ventricular enlargement. *(From Abrams J: Precordial palpation. In Signs and Symptoms of Cardiology. Edited by LD Horwitz and BM Groves. Philadelphia, JB Lippincott Co, 1985).*

right ventricular anterior motion may be detectable, particularly at the end of expiration. Only experience and clinical judgement can resolve the question as to whether this is or is not abnormal in a particular subject.

Abnormal Precordial Motion

There are three basic aspects of abnormal left ventricular activity (Table 2, Figure 4). In essence, the normal left ventricular impulse may be increased in amplitude but maintain its contour (hyperkinetic); the impulse may be prolonged or sustained; and occasionally the impulse may be more prominent in late systole than early systole. Furthermore, ectopic impulses are clearly abnormal; this term or phrase refers to precordial activity that is outside of the normal LV apical area or right ventricular parasternal

region. Ectopic impulses typically occur following myocardial infarction when there is an akinetic or dyskinetic anterior wall motion abnormality or perhaps a left ventricular aneurysm. Rarely, dilated great vessels may be palpable. In the presence of severe pulmonary hypertension a palpable pulmonary artery tap in the second-third left interspace area of the sternum is often found. Table 3 lists the common causes of palpable precordial abnormalities, which include transmitted sound transients or murmurs.

Responses of Left and Right Ventricles to Various Stresses

Left Ventricle

• **Pressure Overload:** Response of the LV to increased outflow resistance (such as aortic steno-

TABLE 3

Causes of Palpable
Precordial Abnormalities

- LV hypertrophy and/or dilatation
- LV wall motion abnormalities (fixed or transient)
- Increased force of left atrial contraction (palpable S_4)
- Accentuated diastolic rapid filling (palpable S_3)
- Anterior thrust of the heart from severe mitral regurgitation
- RV hypertrophy and/or dilatation
- Loud murmurs (thrills)
- Loud heart sounds (normal and abnormal)
- Dilated or hyperkinetic pulmonary artery
- Dilated aorta

sis, hypertension) is concentric hypertrophy with minimal change in LV cavity size and preservation of LV contractile or systolic function. If pressure overload results in a myocardial hypertrophic response, or there is marked increase in resistance to ejection, the LV impulse may become abnormal, and in such instances, usually becomes prolonged in duration, reflecting increased left ventricular ejection time. This results in sustained or protracted left ventricular motion, usually called a heave or a thrust. Such patients typically have a normal to increased ejection fraction and little chamber dilatation. An increased force of the apex impulse is not uncommon, not necessarily with any accompanying leftward and/or downward displacement of the apex impulse. With longstanding disease and/or depression of cardiac systolic function, the LV enlarges and often becomes more spherical, with the apex impulse moving more leftward or lateral on the chest wall. The apex impulse in pressure loaded hearts is not usually palpable over as large an area of the precordium as is found in chronic volume overload states.

• **Volume Overload:** Increases in left ventricular volume, such as in mitral or aortic regurgitation, result in an increase in amplitude of the apex impulse but not necessarily a change in contour. The resulting apex motion is known as a hyperkinetic impulse; early systolic motion and late systolic retraction are preserved (Figure 4B). In mild to moderate degrees of mitral or aortic regurgitation, there may be no change in either the amplitude or the contour of the LV impulse. As the volume overload increases one is more likely to detect an apex impulse of increased amplitude. With major, and particularly chronic, overload conditions the left ventricle changes from an elliptical to more of a spherical shape, and as left ventricular dilata-

tion ensues the apex impulse is likely to become sustained as well as increased in amplitude (Figure 4C). The PMI in the patients with chronic severe aortic regurgitation typically is felt over a very large area, palpable in two or more interspaces, is displaced leftward, and has increased force as well as a sustained characteristic. When left ventricular contractile function decreases and ejection fraction falls, it is even more likely that a sustained impulse will be palpable (Figure 4C).

• **Abnormalities in LV Contractile Function:** In cardiomyopathy or coronary artery disease with impaired ejection fraction, the apex impulse is often abnormal, and occasionally strikingly so. The apex motion may become sustained into the second half of systole. Mid or late systolic bulges may be palpated, reflecting dyskinetic contractile patterns during systole. Ectopic precordial impulses may be detected, located at sites away from normal apical impulse, usually superior and medial. This may be seen with anterior wall dyskinesis with or without the presence of an overt left ventricular aneurysm. Garden variety left ventricular dilatation with a depressed ejection fraction, as is found in many coronary patients, individuals with heart failure due to systolic dysfunction, or volume overload states, usually results in an apical impulse that's displaced laterally and downward. It's felt over a larger than normal area, has increased forcefulness and has a sustained lift or heaving quality. In addition, palpable third or fourth heart sounds may be associated with such apex impulses. In these circumstances, careful precordial palpation by an experienced physician may be very rewarding in predicting left ventricular size and function, as subsequently determined by echocardiography or cardiac catheterization.

Right Ventricle

The normal RV impulse is impalpable, but in the presence of volume and/or pressure overload palpable right ventricular activity may be detected in the parasternal region.

• **Pressure Overload:** Pulmonary hypertension from any cause usually results in sustained systolic right ventricular activity manifested as a palpable and often visible anterior motion at the left lower parasternal region. The RV inflow area is located at the fourth to fifth intercostal spaces just beneath and to the left of the sternum; the RV infundibulum is located more superiorly at the third to fourth left intercostal spaces. Care is needed to detect the usually low amplitude and easily missed right ventricular activity. Firm pressure with the heel of the hand (Figure 5) is advised.

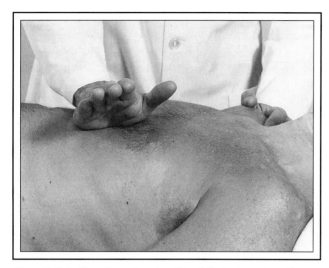

Figure 5. Detection of parasternal or RV activity. Instruct the subject to hold his or her breath in end-expiration. Use firm downward pressure with the heel of the hand. *(From Abrams J. Cardiac Physical Diagnosis. Philadelphia, Lea & Febiger, 1987.)*

• **Volume Overload:** A volume overload of the right ventricle is likely to produce a hyperdynamic, high amplitude impulse that isn't sustained, and is dominantly felt in early systole. The motion felt may be a brief anterior thrust. As right ventricular end diastolic volume increases or right ventricular contractile function decreases, or both, the parasternal RV impulse may become sustained.

• **Mitral Regurgitation:** In the unusual circumstance where mitral regurgitation is moderate to severe but pulmonary hypertension does not co-exist, the large regurgitant jet going from the left ventricle posteriorly into the left atrium may result in anterior displacement of the precordium in the parasternal area that can mimic right ventricular hypertrophy. In this case, this motion is produced by a dilated left atrium that expands in late diastole as a result of a major degree of mitral reflux into the left atrial chamber (Figure 6). It is difficult to dissociate the parasternal impulse of secondary pulmonary hypertension in the presence of severe mitral regurgitation from the cardiac motion related to the regurgitation itself; however, careful studies have indicated that severe mitral regurgitation can produce a late anterior systolic motion in the parasternal area in the absence of severe pulmonary hypertension (Figure 7B).

Clinical Examination of the Precordium

It is useful to approach the precordial examination with a knowledge base as to what forms the left and right ventricular impulses in normal and diseased states, and to literally seek out the abnormalities that are likely to be found in specific car-

diac conditions. Thus, having some indication as to what is the existing cardiovascular problem is desirable, as it will enable the examiner to extract the largest amount of useful information from the precordial exam.

Patient Preparation

Accurate examination of the precordium cannot be done in a hurried fashion. Both the patient and physician should be as relaxed as possible under the circumstances. The room should be warm, the patient's chest should be completely bare with appropriate gowns or sheets to prevent unnecessary exposure, and the patient should be lying in supine or with the head elevated no more than thirty degrees. Normally, the precordial palpation will follow the examination of the carotid arterial and jugular venous pulses, and precede the use of the stethoscope. The examiner must be prepared to count intercostal spaces, measure the distance of the precordial impulse from the sternum or axillary line, etc. As previously suggested, patients with known or suspected cardiovascular disease should be examined in both the supine and left lateral decubitus positions.

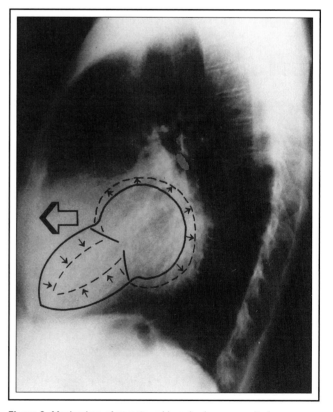

Figure 6. Mechanism of parasternal impulse in severe mitral regurgitation. Systolic expansion of an enlarged left atrium thrusts the right ventricle anteriorly, producing a late systolic impulse at the lower left sternal border. *(From Abrams J: Cardiac Physical Diagnosis. Philadelphia, Lea & Febiger, 1987).*

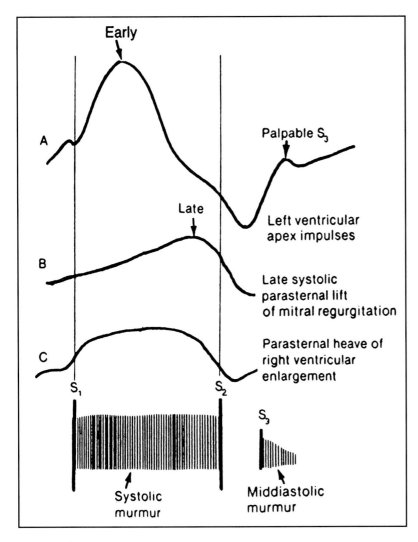

Figure 7. Precordial motion patterns in mitral regurgitation. **A.** The left ventricular impulse is hyperdynamic with a normal contour and increased amplitude of the early systolic outward motion. A palpable third heart sound may be felt in the left decubitus position. In severe chronic mitral regurgitation the left ventricular impulse may be sustained and heaving in quality (not diagrammed). B and C represent parasternal (right heart) activity. **B.** A late systolic parasternal lift. This reflects an anterior thrusting motion of the heart that occurs in late systole. It is produced by regurgitation of a large volume of blood into an enlarged left atrium (see Fig. 6). *(From Abrams J. Cardiac Physical Diagnosis. Philadelphia, Lea & Febiger, 1987).*

Inspection

Careful visual observation of the chest is useful, particularly after the apex beat has already been identified and other impulses have been detected. Retraction may occasionally be more prominent than the outward motion of the PMI, and such motion may be better seen with an examining lamp or penlight providing tangential lighting to the chest wall to accentuate visible movements. When the precordial impulse is visible, it should be measured as to which interspace and the distance from the left sternal border.

Palpation

The examiner should be positioned to the patient's right side. Initially the palm of the hand and the ventral surface of the proximal metacarpals and fingers should be used for exploratory palpation. Individuals should know which aspect of their hand has the best sense of touch (Figure 8). Once the PMI has been localized, it is advisable to use the fingertips for precise local-ization and assessment of LV activity (Figure 9). The palm and proximal metacarpals are often best to detect palpable precordial motion and precordial thrills. Applying pressure with the hand is suggested once a precordial impulse is identified. High frequency sounds such as an increased S_1, an opening snap or ejection click, or a transmitted thrill, are best detected with the hand firmly applied to the chest wall. Low frequency sounds, such as an S_3 and S_4 may be palpable and will be detected only with light pressure of the pads of the fingers. A palpable S_4, imparts a double systolic apical impulse with a "shelf" on the upstroke of the apex beat (Figure 10). Precise timing of precordial events is occasionally necessary, and is best done with simultaneous palpation of the carotid pulse with the left hand while the right hand is on the apex impulse. Auscultation may also be used for timing and identification of S_1 and S_2 by visual inspection of the stethoscope head while it is placed directly on the apex beat.

If the apex impulse is only felt in the left decubi-

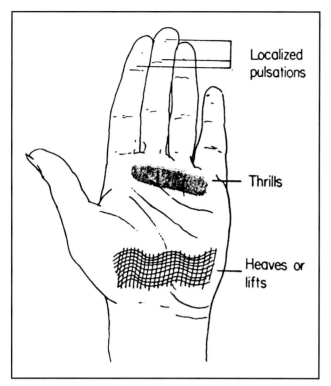

Figure 8. Optimal areas on the examiner's hand for detecting precordial events. *(From Constant J: Bedside Cardiology, 2nd ed. Boston, Little, Brown and Co. 1976).*

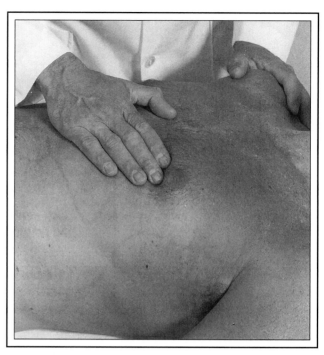

Figure 9. Palpation of the apex impulse, supine position. The patient may also be examined with the thorax and head elevated 20°-30°. *(From Abrams J: Cardiac Physical Diagnosis. Philadelphia, Lea & Febiger, 1987).*

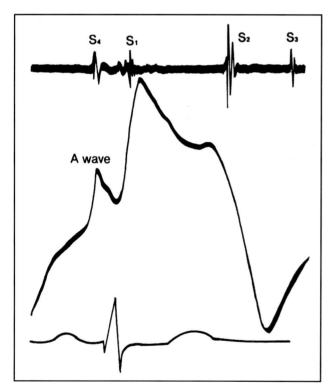

Figure 10. Palpable atrial or fourth heart sound. Light pressure with the fingertips will often detect presystolic distention of the left ventricle when the patient is turned to the left lateral decubitus position. *(From Abrams J. Cardiac Physical Diagnosis. Philadelphia, Lea & Febiger, 1987).*

tus position, the patient should return to the supine position to see if the precordial motion can then be felt in this position. It is more reliable to measure the distance of the PMI from the left sternal border or the midsternal line in the supine rather than in the left lateral position. While turning the subject 45° onto his or her left side will enhance the ability of the examiner to detect left ventricular precordial motion, it often will result in an impulse that is somewhat leftward or lateral of its position when the patient is supine; in addition, the impulse may become sustained in the left lateral position.

Right Ventricular Examination

The right ventricular examination is carried out with the breath held at end expiration. Firm pressure, often with the heel of hand with the wrist cocked upwards, is advisable (Figure 5). The lower sternum and adjacent areas from the third to fifth ribs and interspace should be carefully examined. Low amplitude RV activity is often more readily seen than felt, with the examiner's hand gently moving anteriorly from the chest wall. Subxiphoid or epigastric palpation may be used on individuals where the RV impulse cannot be felt but is suspected to be enlarged, such as individuals with cor pulmonale (Figure 11). This technique is particularly useful when there is obesity, a large chest, or chronic obstructive lung disease.

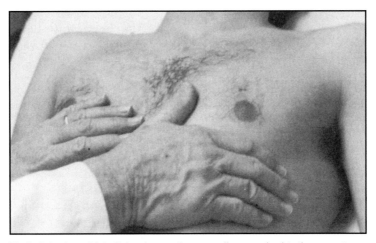

Fig A: Palpation with both hands over the precordium may lead to the prompt detecting of dextrocardia.

On physical examination, when starting to palpate the precordium, the examiner should use both hands as shown in Figure A, which enables the observer to feel both the left side and the right-side counterpart. Cardiac pearl: In this way the examiner should not overlook dextrocardia (provided the patient is of normal build, not greatly obese, and does not have an increase in anteroposterior diameter of the chest, as with obstructive emphysema).

At a teaching conference some years ago at Walter Reed Army Hospital, I was presented several "unknowns" for me to examine, diagnose and discuss. Examining the next to last patient, I placed both hands over the precordium and said:

"This is a cardiac pearl: if there is dextrocardia present (in a patient with a normal sized chest and not obese) we should not miss diagnosing this immediately, since we would feel the cardiac impulse on the right side instead of the left."

This patient, however, did not have dextrocardia. As I said this, I noticed two physicians in the front row turn to each other and grin (I wondered if they were smiling about a private joke or something and not paying attention to the patient's examination).

The next-and last-patient had to be examined quickly, since the conference was just about to end. The patient was obese. She had symptoms consistent with mitral stenosis: shortness of breath on exertion and effort, such as making beds, vacuuming and/or scrubbing the floor, climbing stairs, etc. She even had what appeared to be a malar flush of mitral stenosis (a reddish coloration over the malar eminences of the face as if she used rouge or "blush").

On physical examination, I forgot to use both hands on palpating the chest, and I had difficulty palpating the left ventricle, which I attributed to her significant obesity and very large breasts. On auscultation, I had difficulty in hearing the sounds. I was then told by the moderator of the conference to hurry up and conclude. It then dawned on me that they were playing a trick on me, and had presented a patient that had a history and physical appearance of mitral stenosis, but did not have it.

I was then asked, "Show us the diastolic rumble of mitral stenosis." I replied, "I don't hear it." Then, I was asked, "Why don't you use both hands on palpation of this patient?" I did so and you have guessed it – the cardiac impulse was on the right side, not the left and a classic diastolic rumble of mitral stenosis was present and heard by all (by means of multiple stethoscopes)- in the midst of continuing chuckles and laughter. No one attending that conference will ever forget this cardiac pearl, especially me. I don't think I have overlooked dextrocardia since that time.

W. Proctor Harvey, M.D.

Other Precordial Abnormalities

Palpable thrills are often detectable at the aortic or pulmonic area, and on occasion at the apex in the presence of severe mitral regurgitation or hypertrophic cardiomyopathy. Sound transients, such as ejection clicks, a loud S_1 or opening snap, are often palpable with the palm of the hand.

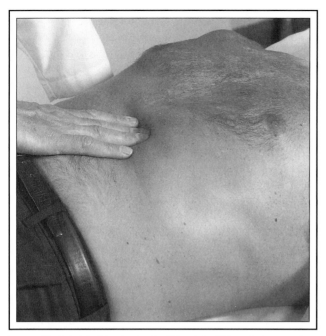

Figure 11. Subxiphoid palpation for RV activity. This technique can be useful for subjects with large chests, obesity, or COPD. Instruct the patient to hold breath in end-inspiration. Do not mistake abdominal aortic pulsations for cardiac motion. *(From Abrams J: Cardiac Physical Diagnosis. Philadelphia, Lea & Febiger, 1987).*

CARDIAC PEARL

It is important to palpate over the base of the heart, as shown in Figure A.

The palpating hand can feel:
- A loud pulmonic valve closure of P_2.
- A systolic ejection sound.
- A systolic thrill of pulmonic valve stenosis.
- A right ventricular lift with the bottom (heel) of the palm.

- A loud aortic valve closure of A_2.
- An aortic systolic ejection sound.
- A systolic thrill of aortic stenosis.
- A diastolic thrill of aortic regurgitation.
  W. Proctor Harvey, M.D.

Absent Apical (LV) Impulse

As already mentioned, many individuals over the age of 50 do not have palpable cardiac activity in the supine position. When this is the case, the left heart border may be percussed to see whether there is dullness that extends to the left beyond the normal range. In most adults, if the subject is turned on the left side, left ventricular activity can usually be detected, particularly during expiration.

Lateral Displacement of PMI Without Cardiomegaly

Individuals with skeletal muscle deformities, such as scoliosis or the straight back syndrome, or who have intrathoracic pathologies, may have an apical impulse that is displaced leftward and laterally in the absence of cardiomegaly. Thus, pseudo-cardiomegaly may be detected on examination as well as on x-ray in individuals with characteristics of the straight back syndrome (narrow A-P diameter of the thorax, loss of normal thoracic kyphosis).

Precordial Motion in Specific Cardiac Disorders

Pressure Overloaded Ventricles

- **Valvular Aortic Stenosis:** There may be no abnormality of the PMI in mild aortic stenosis, but once hemodynamically significant obstruction to left ventricular outflow is present, the character-

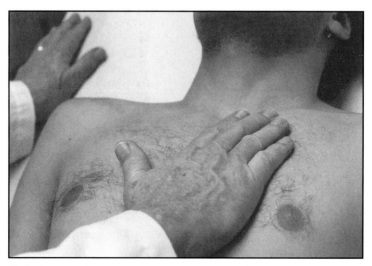

Fig A: Precordial Palpation - The palpating hand, as shown above, gathers valuable information from the base of the heart and the right and left sternal borders.

istic apical impulse becomes sustained and forceful (Figure 4C). The continuing outward motion is felt throughout much of systole. As a rule, the LV impulse is not displaced very much, as the typical left ventricle in aortic stenosis has concentric left ventricular hypertrophy without dilatation. Presystolic distention of the left ventricle or a palpable A wave is common in this condition, particularly when the patient is turned to the left lateral position (Figure 10). In a young individual, presence of a palpable S_4 indicates a major left ventricular-aortic pressure gradient and is indicative of at least moderately severe aortic stenosis. In older individuals, when hypertensive or coronary artery disease may also contribute to the formation of an augmented fourth heart sound, presystolic distention is less specific. In moderate to severe aortic stenosis, a systolic thrill is usually found most commonly in the second right interspace and right clavicular area. Some individuals may have a thrill that is present over the manubrium or second left interspace. In older patients or those with an increased thoracic A-P diameter, a systolic thrill may be detected at the apex and not at the base, concordant with the occasional radiation pattern of the systolic murmur of aortic stenosis which may be best heard at apex and not at the base in such subjects (Gallivardin phenomenon). Having the patient lean forward with the breath held in end expiration will increase likelihood of detecting the basal precordial thrill of aortic stenosis. A palpable aortic ejection sound is often felt in patients with congenital bicuspid aortic valves, with or without significant stenosis. This palpable sound transient will only be felt at the apex and must be differentiated from the PMI itself, which is a more rounded and sustained impulse. Note that presence of a thrill indicates that the systolic murmur is quite loud (grade 4 or greater intensity) but does not necessary mean that the degree of obstruction is severe, particularly in young individuals, or those with co-existing aortic regurgitation, when a large stroke volume is ejected across a deformed valve. On the other hand, presence of a sustained forceful apex impulse, especially if felt over two interspaces and/or presence of a palpable atrial sound in the left decubitus position, is suggestive of severe aortic stenosis.

CARDIAC PEARL

Using both hands, the observer places the right hand over the apex of the left ventricle and the other over the aortic area. A left ventricular pulse, indicating hypertrophy of the left ventricle, can be felt, and a palpable systolic thrill may be noted over the aortic area (Fig. A), the direction of which is toward the right neck and right shoulder. Cardiac pearl relating to the palpable thrill: the direction of the thrill with aortic stenosis is toward the right neck or clavicle. The palpable thrill of pulmonary valve stenosis is in a direction toward the left neck and left clavicle. The detection of a palpable thrill, which is easily identified if searched for, means that an aortic systolic murmur of at least grade 4 intensity will be heard. Therefore the patient has aortic stenosis, which is diagnosed by palpation. If the physician finds, when he or she initially greets the patient and pays attention to the radial pulse (also the brachial and carotid), that the pulse has a slow rise and also a slow descent, aortic stenosis is indicated. If no quick rise or "flip" of the pulse was associated, the physician could be sure that no significant aortic degree of aortic regurgitation existed. Therefore the diagnosis from palpation is that of a significant aortic stenosis, with no or minimal aortic regurgitation. Many times after a complete workup, this initial diagnosis obtained from palpation is confirmed.

The finding of a palpable thrill is very helpful in diagnosis. The thrill generally is best felt by placing the palm of the hand lightly over the precordium. The vibrations of a thrill are best detected by one's palmar surface of the hand rather than the tips of the fingers, which generally are best to detect impulses, localized precordial movements or arterial pulses. As

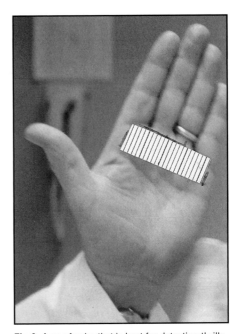

Fig A: Area of palm that is best for detecting thrills.

95

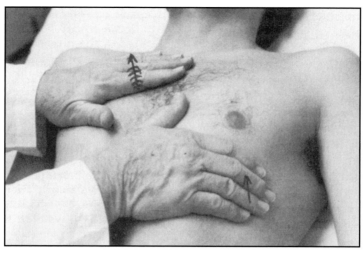

Fig B: The diagnosis of aortic stenosis by palpating the precordium with both hands. A left ventricular impulse is felt with the physician's right hand, a palpable systolic thrill with the left hand, the direction of which is toward the right shoulder and neck. The thrill indicates the murmur is grade 4 or above.

shown in Figure A, the area of the palm adjacent to the fingers is generally best for detecting thrills. Probably the reason why some physicians are able to detect thrills better than others is because they use this part of the hand. One can easily convince himself as to which area is most sensitive by gently stroking with the tips of the fingers, the palmar surface of the opposite hand, from the tips of the fingers down to the wrist, noting which area is most sensitive. Also do this with the opposite hand; one may note that one hand is more sensitive than the other (Figure B).

W. Proctor Harvey, M.D.

• **Hypertrophic Cardiomyopathy or IHSS:** In obstructive hypertrophic cardiomyopathy, an unusual condition, precordial palpation can be very revealing. In such individuals, the left ventricle has moderately decreased diastolic compliance and the A wave is typically prominent and usually palpable. Furthermore, the LV impulse itself is forceful and vigorous, and may be sustained. As with valvular aortic stenosis, the apex impulse is not usually displaced laterally, unless there is massive hypertrophy with a marked increase in the total muscle mass. IHSS may also be associated with a mid- or late systolic wave or bulge, resulting in a double or bifid impulse. If the A wave is palpable in the left decubitus position, the precordium action will be trifid in nature ("triple ripple") (Figure 12). As opposed to valvular aortic stenosis, the presence of a palpable A wave in IHSS or hypertrophic cardiomyopathy does not correlate with the magnitude of the gradient across the left ventricular outflow tract.

With the patient turned to the left lateral position and palpating over the maximum impulse of the left ventricle, three impulses may be felt: The presystolic movement and a double systolic impulse. This is called the "triple ripple" impulse associated with hypertrophic cardiomyopathy.

W. Proctor Harvey, M.D.

A thrill commonly accompanies a loud murmur in this condition, and is usually detected somewhat superior and medial to the cardiac apex. The murmur does not radiate well to the base or neck.

• **Hypertension:** Long-standing hypertension will result in a left ventricular impulse that is more forceful. A sustained left apical impulse (LV heave) and/or a palpable A wave in the left decubitus position is indicative of increased left ventricular mass, as is the presence of the apex beat in two interspaces. Leftward displacement in the hypertensive patient without obvious valve disease suggests cardiac dilatation. Once a patient has developed congestive heart failure as a result of hypertension, it is likely that most of the above mentioned abnormalities will be present.

Volume Overload Conditions

• **Mitral Regurgitation:** As with all other valve lesions, the apex impulse in mitral regurgitation may be normal when the hemodynamic burden is mild to moderate. The typical LV response to moderate to severe mitral regurgitation is a precordial impulse that is hyperdynamic with an increased amplitude but maintained normal contour. As the LV dilates and becomes more spherical, the apex impulse becomes sustained. If this is the case, one can anticipate that the degree of mitral regurgitation is severe and that the hemodynamic burden has been chronic. On the other hand, a sustained PMI in the setting of severe mitral regurgitation may indicate that left ventricular systolic function has decreased and that the ejection fraction is subnormal. In chronic mitral regurgitation, the apex impulse may be quite large, felt in two or more interspaces. A systolic apical thrill will often accompany the abnormal PMI in the presence of a severely incompetent valve. As previously emphasized, mitral regurgitation is a cause of the unusual late systolic impulse at the parasternal or right

ventricular area (Figure 7). In the presence of sustained pulmonary hypertension, secondary to a large mitral regurgitant volume, an RV impulse would be expected, along with a palpable P_2. Remember that left atrial expansion alone can produce a parasternal lift; careful simultaneous palpation of the parasternal and left ventricular areas is important in order to determine whether the parasternal or right ventricular lift is due to pulmonary hypertension (sustained systolic lift) or to the mitral regurgitation, when it will be felt in the second half of systole after the earlier LV apex pulse has been felt.

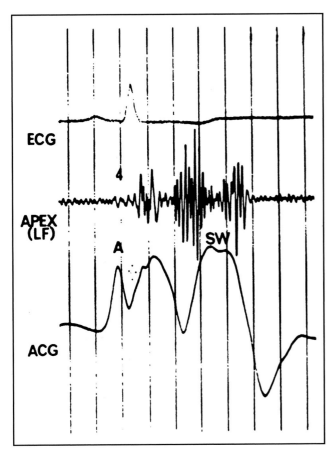

Figure 12. Apical impulse in hypertrophic cardiomyopathy. In this apex recording the huge presystolic A-wave is followed by a normal systolic impulse and subsequently by a late systolic wave or bulge (SW). These events produce the characteristic "triple ripple"; all three waves may be palpable on careful examination. *(From Tavel NE: Clinical Phonocardiography and External Pulse Recording, Year Book Medical Publishers, Chicago, 1972).*

CARDIAC PEARL

Use of two hands is also helpful in detecting the presence of significant chronic mitral regurgitation (Fig. A). If the right hand is placed over the left ventricle and the left hand is placed over the lower left sternal border, the examiner may feel an impulse in systole indicating left ventricular hypertrophy. The left hand feels a delayed impulse along the lower left sternal border. This situation usually indicates an advanced degree of mitral regurgitation into an enlarged left atrium that can impinge on the spine. With systole, which produces the left ventricular impulse, left ventricular contents are emptied into the large left atrium, which then impinges on the spine, and a "bank shot" results, with the heart being moved forward, producing the delayed impulse along the right sternal border. This is an excellent cardiac pearl, poorly appreciated and seldom investigated. It is readily appreciated that if only the area along the lower left sternal border was palpated, a misdiagnosis of right ventricular hypertrophy would be made. By using both hands and getting a delayed impulse, this erroneous "trap" would not occur. It is true, of course, that right ventricular hypertrophy develops in some patients with mitral regurgitation. This situation is caused by the regurgitant mitral leak extended up into the pulmonary veins, eventually resulting in increased pressure on the pulmonary circuit and, in turn, right ventricular hypertrophy. When hypertrophy of the right ventricle is also present, palpation with both hands reveals that the impulse is not delayed but is occurring simultaneously with the left ventricular impulse.

W. Proctor Harvey, M.D.

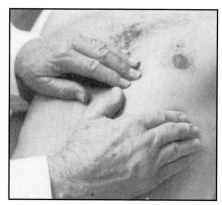

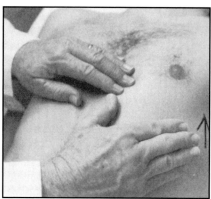
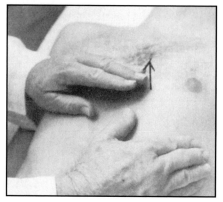

Fig A: Severe chronic regurgitation. Diagnosis by palpation. Use both hands simultaneously. Top panel, Right hand detects left ventricular impulse; the left hand feels the right ventricular impulse. Lower left panel, A left impulse is first detected (↑). Lower right panel, A delayed impulse (↑) is noted over lower left sternal border. This is a basketball "bank shot," not right ventricular hypertrophy.

Visible and palpable third heart sounds are common in severe mitral regurgitation, particularly in the left lateral position (Figure 13). In acute mitral regurgitation, the left ventricular impulse may not be particularly remarkable, although perhaps of high amplitude. However, a palpable fourth heart sound is quite common in recent onset mitral regurgitation of moderate to severe nature. Thus, the finding of pre-systolic distension of the LV is a very important finding in the patient with mitral regurgitation, as pre-systolic distension is rarely found in chronic rheumatic or myxomatous mitral regurgitation. When left ventricular failure and marked systolic dysfunction ensues, the physical findings of mitral regurgitation may be altered, particularly with a decreased intensity of the systolic murmur and thrill. In such cases, a large, displaced, and sustained apical impulse would be the rule.

• **Aortic Regurgitation:** As with mitral insufficiency, a mild to moderate volume overload due to aortic regurgitation may not produce an abnormality of the PMI but a moderate degree of insufficiency usually produces some detectable abnormal precordial motion. The early response is of a hyperdynamic impulse, which moves laterally and downward as the LV cavity dilates over time. Aortic regurgitation usually results in eccentric hypertrophy of the left ventricle with chamber dilatation out of proportion to hypertrophy. The left ventricle can be enormous in chronic severe aortic regurgitation, producing a large apical heaving motion that is felt over two interspaces, as well as a palpable third heart sound; the precordial impulse is usually forceful in such cases and medial retraction is commonly seen. Acute or recent onset aortic regurgitation of moderate to severe magnitude is usually superimposed upon a normal left ventricle or one that is not markedly dilated. Thus, a sudden major volume overload results in a marked increase in left ventricular wall stress, altered compliance of the left ventricle and/or an elevation of left ventricular filling pressure and left atrial pressure, typically causing left ventricular failure or pulmonary edema.

This is comparable to the situation in acute mitral regurgitation (see above). In such instances, a very prominent and often palpable fourth sound

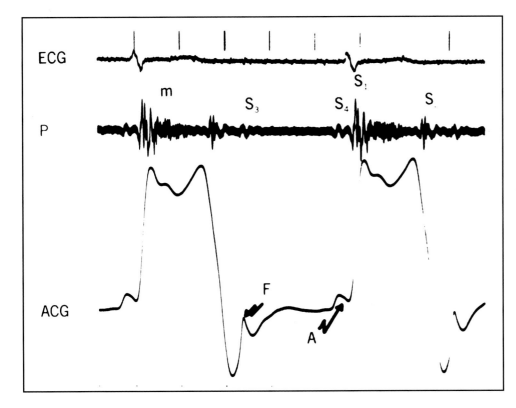

Figure 13. Palpable and audible third heart sound in mitral regurgitation. A loud S₃ may be transmitted as a palpable diastolic event and indicates moderate to severe mitral regurgitation. The third sound is simultaneous with the peak of the rapid filling phase of the recorded apexcardiogram (F-wave). Note the holosystolic murmur (m) at the apex. *(From Stefadorous MA and Little RC: The cause and clinical significance of diastolic heart sounds. Arch Intern Med 140: 537, 1980).*

appears resulting in pre-systolic distension of the ventricle (Figure 13). If the LV chamber was completely normal prior to the onset of the aortic regurgitation (for example, acute infective endocarditis or trauma to the aortic valve and root, or dissection) the LV impulse will not be displaced but may be somewhat forceful and increased in amplitude. In such instances, one can exclude mitral stenosis as a cause for a mid-to late-diastolic frequency murmur at the apex, often found in severe aortic regurgitation. This murmur, the Austin Flint murmur, is related to a severe regurgitant volume impinging on the anterior leaflet of the mitral valve which forms a considerable portion of the left ventricular outflow tract; the regurgitant volume literally pushes the leaflet into the path of diastolic flow of blood entering the left ventricle from the left atrium. The increased turbulence in the volume overloaded ventricle may produce a diastolic murmur that is acoustically identical to the mitral rumble of mitral stenosis.

Occasionally, a palpable diastolic thrill along the left sternal border can be felt, particularly when there is a perforation, eversion, or prolapse of an aortic cusp which results in a particularly loud diastolic murmur. A diastolic thrill from a loud regurgitant murmur will more likely be detected with the patient sitting up, leaning forward with the breath held in end expiration.

Other Conditions

• **Mitral Stenosis:** While the left ventricle in pure mitral stenosis is usually normal and even underfilled because of limitation to inflow of blood from the obstructed mitral valve, the precordial examination in this condition may be quite rewarding. For instance, the loud first heart sound and opening snap are frequently palpable. One should explore the precordium with the palm of the hand to detect the sound transients. A parasternal lift is the rule rather than the exception in mitral stenosis, and this can be quite prominent in presence of significant pulmonary hypertension. In the left decubitus position, a diastolic apical thrill may be detected, the palpable counterpart of a loud mitral diastolic murmur.

CARDIAC PEARL

A patient who has a tight mitral stenosis with a loud first sound, prominent second sound, opening snap, and a diastolic rumble with presystolic accentuation can have palpatory counterparts that can be detected by placing the palm of the hand over the point of maximum impulse of the left ventricle (Figure A).

The loud first heart sound is easily felt, as are the vibrations of the accentuated second sound, opening snap, and then the palpable

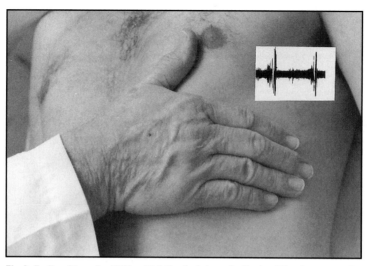

Fig A: Feeling Stenosis - With a "tight" mitral stenosis, the loud first heart sound, second sound, and opening snap can be palpated, as can the diastolic rumble occupying all of diastole with presystolic accentuation, which produces a palpable diastolic thrill.

diastolic thrill of the rumble. There is practically no other condition that simulates these specific findings of mitral stenosis.

W. Proctor Harvey, M.D.

Left ventricular activity in pure mitral stenosis is unimpressive. As many individuals with mitral stenosis have concomitant mitral regurgitation, mild to moderate, there may be some increased left ventricular prominence (amplitude or duration) if the chronic mitral regurgitation exerts a significant hemodynamic burden on the ventricle.

CARDIAC PEARL

The diagnosis of mitral stenosis is an example of how palpation is of such benefit in enabling the physician better to listen. One may "zero in" on the spot where the rumble is best detected by carefully palpating the point of maximal impulse in the apical area. When this is located, the bell of the stethoscope, as shown in Figure B, is placed lightly over this area (barely making an air seal) and the physician listens specifically for a diastolic rumble. Unless this point of maximal impulse in the apical area is carefully searched for, the diastolic rumble of mitral stenosis may easily be overlooked. In addition, auscultation may be required at the time the patient is actually turning to the left lateral position, provided care is taken that the stethoscope still remains over the point of maximal impulse; the diastolic rumble, if present, will be heard over this area. Various other maneuvers may be used to "bring out" this rumble: having the patient breathe deeply five or six times, take several coughs, or exert slight effort such as several "sit ups" on the bed or examining table. Auscultation after any one of these maneuvers sometimes enables detection

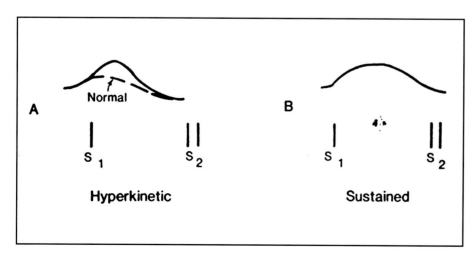

Figure 14. Parasternal or right ventricular activity in atrial septal defects. **A.** A hyperkinetic right ventricular impulse is the initial response to volume overload of the right ventricle. The low amplitude parasternal pulse contour is accentuated and becomes palpable; there is systolic retraction in the second half of systole. **B.** Sustained right ventricular lift or parasternal heave. This contour is present when there is a large right ventricular volume overload. When a sustained impulse is present, it indicates a very large right ventricular chamber and/or the presence of pulmonary hypertension. *(From Abrams J; Cardiac Physical Diagnosis. Philadelphia, Lea & Febiger, 1987).*

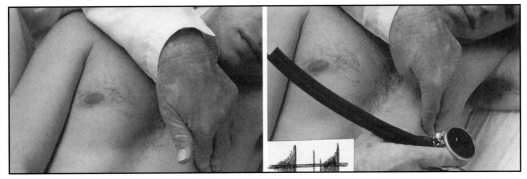

Fig B: Finding the diastolic rumble of mitral stenosis. Left: Point of maximal impulse (P.M.I.) in the apical area is located and "held" by palpating finger. Right: Bell of stethoscope is being placed over this point. Bell chest piece held lightly (but making an air seal) to hear typical rumble of mitral stenosis, as shown by phonocardiogram.

of an otherwise previously unrecognized diastolic rumble.

The cardiac pearl of "one sense at a time."

If difficulty is experienced in locating the point of maximal impulse of the left ventricle with the patient turned to the left lateral position, remember to remove the ear pieces of the stethoscope from the ear canals. The impulse, often the size of a quarter, may then be promptly found. We need to concentrate on one sense at a time; removing the ear tips enables specific single concentration on the sense of touch over the chest wall.

W. Proctor Harvey, M.D.

• **Cardiomyopathy:** Typical precordial abnormalities in a dilated or congestive cardiomyopathy include a large or diffuse anterior precordial heave; a palpable third heart sound; and occasionally presystolic distension of the left ventricle (palpable A-wave). Parasternal activity is often prominent, as myopathies tend to involve both left and right ventricles. The precordium may be diffusely heaving or rocking, with minimal systolic retraction between the RV and LV impulses. On occasion, a mid- or late-systolic bulge at or near the apex may be detected. A completely normal precordial exam in a patient not overweight or who has a large A-P diameter is indirect evidence against a significant cardiomyopathic process.

• **Coronary Artery Disease:** The most common adult cardiac condition is coronary heart disease. Patients with angina pectoris who have not had a previous myocardial infarction in general have no detectable abnormality on palpation other than the occasional finding of a palpable atrial sound or presystolic distention of the ventricle. Thus, patients with angina should be routinely examined in the left decubitus position to see if a fourth sound can be

felt. On the other hand, in patients with prior myocardial infarction, particularly when anterior or extensive, left ventricular apical impulse abnormalities are common. These may consist of an increased size of the impulse, a heaving or sustained duration of the PMI, an ectopic bulge, as well as a palpable fourth heart sound. In a severe ischemic cardiomyopathy, with chronic heart failure and a markedly depressed ejection fraction, palpable third heart sounds may be present. Occasionally, right parasternal activity can be felt that reflects either right ventricular hypertrophy or anteroseptal dyskinesis. A sustained left ventricular impulse suggests marked left ventricular hypertrophy or an anteroapical wall motion abnormality. Left ventricular aneurysms produce large, often hyperdynamic or sustained impulses usually felt over two precordial impulses.

CARDIAC PEARL

When palpating the precordium over the apex (Fig. A), the examiner might find an abnormal systolic impulse, which indicates left ventricular hypertrophy. Along the lower left sternal border, the tricuspid area, a systolic impulse is consistent with right ventricular hypertrophy. In between the lower left sternal border and apex, systolic impulses are most likely related to coronary artery ischemic heart disease. This finding might be indicative of a ventricular aneurysm. In systole, it is seen as an outward paradoxical bulge that is felt and is an immediate clue to the presence of a ventricular aneurysm. Other impulses can be felt over this area that indicate coronary artery disease caused by akinesia or dyskinesia types of contractions, which may occur with coronary artery disease.

W. Proctor Harvey, M.D.

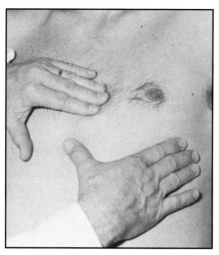 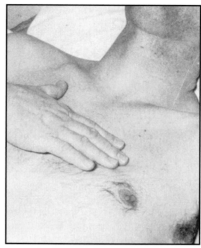

Fig A: Left panel, Left ventricular impulse is palpated at the apex. Right ventricular impulse is felt along the lower left sternal border. Right panel, A systolic outward impulse palpated in the middle (between the right and left impulses) is most likely the result of coronary ischemic heart disease such as ventricular aneurysm.

Right-Sided Lesions

• **Atrial Septal Defect:** In an uncomplicated atrial septal defect (ASD), there is considerable volume overload of the right ventricle, resulting in an increased amplitude non-sustained left lower sternal pulsation (hyperdynamic RV, Figure 14). A pulmonary artery lift is commonly felt in the second to third interspace, secondary to a dilated pulmonary artery. When there is co-existing pulmonary hypertension, the parasternal or RV impulse is sustained and heaving in quality. This may be present even when there is not substantial pulmonary hypertension. A palpable P_2 may be felt over the pulmonary artery area in this condition.

• **Tricuspid Regurgitation:** In adults, tricuspid regurgitation usually means there is secondary pulmonary hypertension with subsequent right ventricular hypertrophy and dilatation. The most common cause of this is left heart disease with sustained pulmonary hypertension. Thus, mitral valve disease, chronic left ventricular failure, or coronary artery disease with multiple wall motion abnormalities and depressed ejection fraction may be associated with pulmonary hypertension. The right ventricle does not tolerate pressure overload very well and the RV cavity dilates as well as the tricuspid annulus. Thus, tricuspid regurgitation is dynamic in nature, changing in magnitude according to the volume and contractile state of the right heart. Tricuspid regurgitation is actually quite common in patients with underlying heart disease and congestive heart failure. In addition to the characteristic jugular venous pulse with large systolic V waves, the right ventricle has both a volume and often a pressure load which result in an abnormal parasternal impulse. In cases with chronic obstructive pulmonary disease or obesity, subxyphoid palpation may be useful in detecting abnormal right ventricular activity. In such cases, a downward and forceful displacement of the right ventricular apex will be palpated. Rarely, severe tricuspid regurgitation can result in right anterior lower chest pulsations which are palpable and visible, reflecting right atrial expansion during systole. Careful examination of the liver is critical in patients suspected of having tricuspid regurgitation. Exploration of the right upper quadrant from below with the patient's breath held in end inspiration is the ideal way to feel for hepatic pulsations. These are usually undulant and low pressure in nature, and visual observation of the examining hand and fingers is more helpful than palpation itself.

Selected Reading

1. Abrams J: The precordial impulse. In: *Essentials of Cardiac Physical Diagnosis.* Philadelphia. Lea and Febiger, 1987.
2. Abrams J: Precordial motion. In: Horowitz LD, Groves BM (eds.); *Signs and Symptoms in Cardiology.* Philadelphia. JB Lippincott, 1985.
3. Abrams J: Precordial motion in health and disease. *Mod Concepts Cardiovasc Dis* 49:55, 1980.
4. Basta LL, Bettinger JJ: The cardiac impulse: A new look at an old art. *AHJ* 97:96, 1979.
5. Basta LL, Wolfson P, Eckberg D, et al: The value of left parasternal impulse recordings in the assessment of mitral regurgitation. *Circ* 48:1055, 1973.
6. Bethell HJN, Nixon PCF: Examination of the heart in supine and left lateral positions. *BHJ* 9:902, 1973.
7. Chizner MA: Bedside diagnosis of acute myocardial infarction and its complications. *Curr Prob Card* 7:14, 1982.
8. Conn RD, Cole JS: The cardiac apex impulse: Clinical and angiographic correlations. *Ann Intern Med* 75:185, 1971.
9. Constant J: Inspection and palpation of the chest. *In Bedside*

102

Cardiology, 2nd ed; Boston, Little, Brown, 1976.

10 deLeon A, Perloff JK, Twigg H, et al: The straight back syndrome: Clinical cardiovascular manifestations. *Circ* 32:193, 1965.

11. Eddleman EEJ, Langley JO: Paradoxical pulsation of the precordium in myocardial infarction and angina pectoris. *AHJ* 63:579, 1962.

12. Ellen SD, Crawford MH, O' Rourke RA: How accurate is precordial palpation for detecting increased left ventricular size? *Circ* 66:11-266, 1982.

13. McGinn FX, Gould L: The phonocardiogram and apexcardiogram in patients with ventricular aneurysm. *AJC* 21:567, 1968.

14. Mounsey JPD: Inspection and palpation of the cardiac impulse. *Prog Card Dis* 10:187, 1967.

15. Perloff JK: The movements of the heart—observation, palpation, and percussion. In *Physical Examination of the Heart and Circulation,* pp 130-170. Philadelphia, WB Saunders, 1982.

16. Reddy PS, Meno F, Curtiss EF, et al: The genesis of gallop sounds: Investigation by quantitative phono- and apexcardiography. *Circ* 63:922, 1981.

17. Ronan JA, Steelman RB, DeLeon AC, et al: The clinical diagnosis of acute severe mitral insufficiency. *AJC* 27:284, 1971.

18. Shah PM: Newer concepts in hypertrophic obstructive cardiomyopathy, II. *JAMA* 242:1771, 1979.

CHAPTER 7

The Art of Cardiac Auscultation: Normal and Abnormal Heart Sounds

Michael A. Chizner, M.D.

The great majority of patients seen in clinical practice for evaluation of the possibility of heart disease can be diagnosed in the physician's office, or at the bedside, by employing the "five-finger approach" to cardiovascular diagnosis espoused by Dr. W. Proctor Harvey. The "five fingers" include the patient's history, physical examination, electrocardiogram, chest x-ray and appropriate laboratory tests. In this orderly and systematic method of evaluation, the physical examination ranks second in importance only to the clinical history.

When one considers the physical examination of the cardiac patient, the thought of auscultation most often comes to mind. The experienced clinician, however, is often greatly aided by the diagnostic clues derived from inspection and palpation, even before careful attentive listening with the stethoscope. Auscultation of heart sounds and murmurs, therefore, although of vital importance, is only one part of the complete clinical cardiovascular examination, and is most informative and rewarding when combined with the information derived from a thorough clinical history, coupled with a careful, detailed assessment of the jugular venous pulse, arterial pressure and pulse, precordial movements and pulsations, and the general physical appearance of the patient.

Today, the need for the talents of the well-trained clinician, who can make sophisticated diagnoses at the patient's bedside, is becoming increasingly more apparent. In this era of cost containment, the practicing physician must learn to develop his or her clinical skills and rely on them with confidence in daily clinical decision-making to help direct the patient to further non-invasive and invasive "high-tech" diagnostic evaluation on a more selective basis when necessary.

This chapter will review the fundamental aspects of the art and technique of cardiac auscultation, emphasizing the clinical significance of the normal and abnormal heart sounds that may be encountered in the routine everyday practice of medicine. Since these sounds provide many valuable diagnostic and prognostic clues and draw attention to the presence, type and severity of an underlying cardiovascular abnormality, their accurate identification and characterization is of paramount importance.

The Art of Auscultation

Auscultation of the heart is one of the most challenging and rewarding diagnostic skills that can be learned and mastered by the astute clinician who aspires to it. Proficiency in this time-honored art requires experience, repeated practice and a great deal of patience. The most important prerequisite for effective auscultation is the proper state of mind. The ability to detect faint, often subtle acoustic findings, is not merely a reflection of more sensitive ears, but of a mind trained to be aware of, and alert to, their occurrence. As so aptly emphasized by Dr. Harvey, "We find what we look for, but we must know what to look for."

During auscultation, the well-trained clinician should have a mental image of the dynamics of the cardiac cycle, integrating and correlating each heart sound and murmur heard with the corresponding hemodynamic event. Although the most

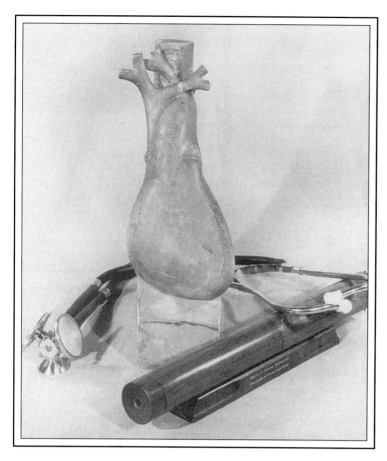

Figure 1. The Stethoscope. Front, Replica of Laennec's original monaural stethoscope. Back, The Harvey Triple-Head Stethoscope. *(From Harvey WP, 18.)*

important component of the auscultatory apparatus lies between the ear pieces, the importance of a well-designed and efficient stethoscope can not be overemphasized; and in the hands of the person properly trained in its use, it is an instrument of precision.

The Stethoscope

The era of modern cardiac auscultation began with the introduction of the stethoscope in 1816 by the French physician, Dr. Rene Theophile Hyacinthe Laennec. Inspired by a children's game of scratching and listening to sounds at the end of a wooden beam, coupled with the modesty of his female patients and the extreme obesity of one in particular, Laennec rolled a "quire" of paper into a cylinder, placed one end of it on the patient's precordium and the other to his ear, and was able to hear the heart more clearly and distinctly than if he had applied his ear directly to the chest, the customary practice at the time. After considerable experimentation, the rolled paper was replaced by a wooden cylinder, the monaural stethoscope. This primitive instrument was further improved upon years later, becoming the flexible binaural device in use today (Figure 1).

Since its introduction, the stethoscope has endured as a most valuable and reliable medical tool, enabling many diagnoses to be made without recourse to more complicated, expensive, potentially hazardous and burdensome methods of examination. Despite this, many contemporary physicians have not taken full advantage of cardiac auscultation, nor have they developed the art to that level of competence where the instrument proves its true worth. Now, more than ever before, the practice of medicine should apply the scientific lessons learned in the laboratory to the clinical art of auscultation at the bedside.

The modern technologic advances that initially may have seemed to supersede the use of the stethoscope have, on the contrary, provided new insights that have clarified the meaning and increased the importance of the myriad acoustic findings heard in clinical practice. They have contributed greatly to our knowledge and understanding of the pathophysiologic mechanisms of cardiovascular disease, thereby helping the practicing physician apply his or her clinical acumen and cardiac auscultatory skills more accurately to the simple solution of problems at the bedside.

The choice of a stethoscope is a very personal one. Since many physicians purchase only one stethoscope in a lifetime, great care should be taken in its selection. The physician can be reassured that a stethoscope is of high quality when he or she is able to clearly identify the lowest and highest frequencies that the human ear can detect. The stethoscope should be equipped with both bell and diaphragm chest pieces. Proper use of these chest pieces will enhance the quality of heart sounds and murmurs heard, and maximize the effectiveness of auscultation.

The bell, when applied gently to the skin, is designed primarily to "bring out" low frequency sounds and murmurs, e.g., the atrial "S_4" and ventricular "S_3" diastolic gallops, and diastolic rumbles across the mitral and tricuspid valves. If the examiner exerts too much pressure on the bell chest piece, the stretched skin beneath it will serve as a diaphragm and filter out these low-pitched sounds and murmurs.

The diaphragm chest piece, when pressed firmly against the skin, applying sufficient pressure so that an indentation remains after its removal, will selectively reinforce and accentuate the higher-pitched sounds and murmurs, e.g., first (S_1) and second (S_2) heart sounds, aortic and pulmonic ejection sounds, systolic clicks, the opening snaps of mitral and tricuspid stenosis, most systolic ejection and regurgitant murmurs, the diastolic murmurs of aortic and pulmonic insufficiency, and pericardial friction rubs.

CARDIAC PEARL

How do you tell a good stethoscope from an inferior one? The answer is simple: a good stethoscope can pick up the faintest high frequency murmur (such as an early, blowing, aortic diastolic murmur) and the faintest low frequency sound, such as a diastolic rumble or gallop (S_3, S_4).

If your stethoscope can't do this, discard it. You are penalizing yourself as well as the patient.

Use all chest pieces on each patient. The flat diaphragm chest piece is best for detecting a faint, early blowing aortic diastolic murmur; also for analysis of systolic clicks, ejection sounds, and most systolic murmurs. The flat diaphragm chest piece is the "work horse." As a rule, the bell is best for the detection of low frequencies, such as diastolic rumbles and faint gallop sounds. Low frequency sounds are better heard with the bell-type chest piece touching the skin very lightly and barely making an air seal. The length of the stethoscope tubing is important. Actually, the closer one gets to the heart, and thus the shorter the tubing, the better. However, the

physician must also be comfortable and a tall physician would be uncomfortable using short tubing. From experience with postgraduate courses where one has to use the stethoscope for long periods, it has become evident to me that the eartips should be large enough to fit snugly in the ear canals, and be made of firm, smooth plastic. Stethoscopes with soft rubber tips or even hard rubber tips have resulted in more discomfort and irritation for me, although some people prefer them. The small size ear tips, often of a hard material, may not fit snugly and can, in fact, cause discomfort, which I refer to as "somewhat like having a myringotomy in one's ear."

W. Proctor Harvey, M.D.

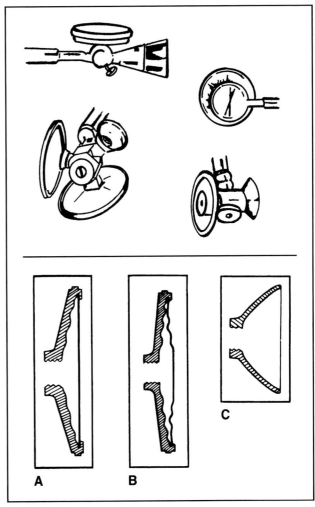

Figure 2. Top, Composite of many types of double head and triple head (Harvey) stethoscopes. Bottom, Stethoscope chest pieces. **A. Flat diaphragm:** Excellent for all sounds and murmurs. Best for higher frequencies, e.g., faint diastolic murmur of aortic regurgitation, splitting of heart sounds, systolic clicks, and ejection sounds. **B. Corrugated diaphragm:** Amplifying quality. Excellent for an "overview" of heart sounds, especially low frequency gallop sounds and murmurs. **C. Bell:** Particularly useful in detecting faint, low frequency heart sounds and murmurs, e.g., gallop sounds or diastolic rumble. *(Modified from Harvey WP 18.)*

107

Although many different types of stethoscopes have been developed over the years and remain in widespread use today, none has surpassed the quality, acoustical excellence and effectiveness of the unique triple-headed model designed by Dr. Harvey (Figure 2). In addition to the standard flat diaphragm and bell, the Harvey triple-head has a third chest piece, the corrugated diaphragm, which is designed to amplify sound and provide an "overview" of the acoustic events.

Regardless of the type of stethoscope chosen, the ear pieces should fit the examiner snugly, yet comfortably, and the binaurals should be directed so that proper alignment with the external auditory canal is ensured. The stethoscope system must be air-tight. Air leaks, by destroying the integrity of the acoustical seal, will admit extraneous noise and diminish the quality of sound transmission. The length and diameter of the stethoscope tubing make considerable difference on how well the auscultatory findings are perceived. In general, the tubing should have an internal diameter of 1/8" and should be thick-walled and as short as possible for efficiency, (12" to 15"), yet compatible with a convenient listening posture. Double tubing is preferable, as it results in less sound distortion than single tubing. Care should be taken, however, to ensure that the tubes are not touching each other, or the patient, since such contact may create extraneous friction noise and interfere with one's ability to listen effectively.

CARDIAC PEARL

Emphasizing the importance of a good stethoscope is the following anecdote: When I first became Director of the Division of Cardiology at Georgetown, I was working on a teaching project in which we were recording heart sounds and murmurs on high fidelity tape. We produced a collection of 4-1/2 hours of these teaching tapes and donated copies to any medical school or medical institution that requested them. We also set up a small room in our hospital with high fidelity equipment for self teaching.

Dr. Carl Wiggers, one of the most eminent physiologists ever produced in the United States, somehow heard of our teaching efforts, and paid us a visit personally to observe the setup.

He appeared quite interested in this teaching project and listened to a number of the recordings. After a while he said, with a twinkle in his eye- "You know, when I was a medical student, I never seemed to hear with my stethoscope what my instructors and others seemed to hear." He said he was puzzled and wondered about his ability to hear- or whether his difficulty could be explained on individual differences in aptitude of auscultation. (Probably because of this difficulty, he was not attracted to this aspect of medicine, and subsequently pursued his brilliant career in Physiology.) He then related an incident that occurred when he was at the Rockefeller Institute in New York City. He was driving home after a day's work. It was dark and he was crossing one of the major bridges in New York City when the lights of his automobile suddenly went out. The lights worked from an acetylene source. As he examined the connections from the source to the lights of his car, he found that a "Y tube" type of connection had broken. Fortunately, he remembered that his stethoscope tubing also connected to a T tube and guessed that it might serve as a temporary substitute. Sure enough, on removing the Y tube from his stethoscope it proved to be a good replacement and the light reappeared! However, there was one puzzling aspect- only one light went on. This was sufficient for him to continue home, but having the inquisitive mind that made him such an outstanding scientist, the next day in his laboratory he examined his stethoscope's "Y" connection. To his surprise, he found only one arm of the "Y" had been bored- the other was solid and obstructed! No wonder Dr. Wiggers had difficulty with auscultation! This twist of fate may have prevented us from having a master of auscultation in medicine, but perhaps it was actually a blessing, giving him an even greater stimulus to pursue his career in Physiology, one of the greatest in the history of medicine.

W. Proctor Harvey, M.D.

Fundamentals of Auscultatory Technique

For maximum auscultatory yield, the examination should be conducted in a warm, adequately lit, quiet room, free of background noise and distractions. Both the patient and the examiner should be relaxed and comfortable. The patient should be properly gowned and draped in order to avoid embarrassment, yet allowing for sufficient exposure of the precordium to enable adequate inspection, palpation and auscultation. The height of the bed should be adjusted to permit the physician to listen and concentrate at ease, and without strain. An orthopneic patient may not tolerate the supine position, and will require elevation of the head of the bed or examining table, to maximize comfort and facilitate auscultation.

As a rule, most physicians conduct the examination from the right side of the patient, and begin

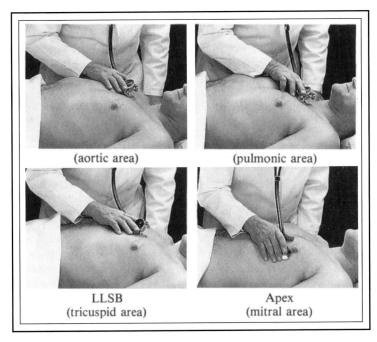

Figure 3. Systematic method of cardiac auscultation over the traditional "valve" areas. In the aortic area (second right intercostal space) the second heart sound (S_2) is louder than the first heart sound (S_1). By keeping S_2 in mind as the stethoscope is moved down along the left sternal border to the apex, extra sounds or murmurs can be accurately timed as systolic if occurring before S_2 or diastolic if after S_2 ("inching" technique). *(From Harvey WP, 18.)*

(aortic area)   (pulmonic area)

LLSB
(tricuspid area)   Apex
(mitral area)

with the patient reclining in the supine position. A systematic and organized method of examination is essential. As suggested by Dr. Harvey, one may listen with the corrugated diaphragm chest piece applied lightly along the lower left sternal border to obtain an "overview" of the auscultatory events. The examiner then proceeds to listen over the second right intercostal space (aortic area) and slowly moves ("inches") the stethoscope across to the second left intercostal space (pulmonic area), progresses downward along the left sternal edge to the lower left sternal border (tricuspid area), and then laterally to the cardiac apex (mitral area), using both the diaphragm and bell chest pieces. Some physicians prefer to reverse this examining sequence. Although it makes little difference whether one starts at the aortic area and progresses to the mitral area, or vice versa, it is important to adopt a routine procedure for auscultation which becomes automatic, beginning in one area, and then carefully exploring all areas, in an orderly and unhurried fashion so that nothing is overlooked (Figure 3).

Every patient should be listened to lying flat, turned to the left lateral position, sitting upright with the legs dangling over the edge of the bed or examining table, standing and squatting. These positions are quite valuable and often enable clues to be heard in one position, which might not be appreciated in another. After the initial evaluation is conducted in the supine position, the patient should be turned to the left lateral decubitus position, which brings the cardiac apex closer to the chest wall. The physician then "tunes in" to faint,

low-frequency sounds and murmurs, e.g., atrial (fourth heart sound) and ventricular (third heart sound) gallops, and the diastolic rumble of mitral stenosis, using the bell of the stethoscope applied lightly to the chest wall at the cardiac apex, barely making an air seal. The apex should be auscultated not only after the patient has turned, but also while the patient is actually turning. Diagnostic rumbles and other low-frequency sounds are frequently best heard in this manner. Then, using the diaphragm chest piece pressed firmly enough against the chest wall to leave a temporary imprint (after-ring) on the skin, the patient is examined over the base or left sternal border, while sitting upright and leaning forward with the breath held in deep expiration, to detect high-pitched sounds and murmurs, e.g., the blowing diastolic murmur of semilunar valve insufficiency, and the pericardial friction rub of pericarditis. Firm pressure with the diaphragm chest piece further enhances the high-frequency response of the stethoscope, so that a faint Grade I or II aortic or pulmonic diastolic murmur might not be overlooked, thus allowing the patient to be instructed in the appropriate use of antibiotic prophylaxis to cover bacteremic procedures, such as dental work (Figure 4).

CARDIAC PEARL

An illustration of the importance of combining palpation with auscultation is the simple but practical point that if one palpates at the point of maximum impulse at the apical area, places the bell or low frequency diaphragm piece over this area and listens specifically for a diastolic rumble, he may quickly detect here the low frequency rumble of mitral stenosis. However, auscultation may be required at the time when the patient is actually turning to the left lateral position if care is taken that the stethoscope is then placed over the point of maximal impulse; the diastolic rumble, if present, will be heard over this area. Various other maneuvers to bring out this rumble can be used, such as having the patient breathe deeply five or six times, take several healthy coughs, or make slight effort such as several "sit-ups" in the bed. Thus an otherwise previously unrecognized diastolic rumble may be brought out. The patient is then asked to sit upright, and again the same areas are explored by the physician using all chest pieces and listening in different phases of respiration. With the patient in the sitting position, one listens with particular care to the aortic and pulmonary areas and along the left and right sternal borders, remembering to have the patient stop breathing, lean forward, exhale, and hold his breath in deep expiration. Forceful pressure should

be applied with the diaphragm chest piece to make sure that a faint blowing diastolic murmur is not present. A good practical rule is not only to listen specifically for the high frequency blowing murmur of aortic or pulmonary valve insufficiency along the sternal borders, but also to exert pressure on the flat diaphragm of the stethoscope; if an imprint of the diaphragm chest piece of the stethoscope is not left on the skin of the patient, then the faintest diastolic blow may possibly have been overlooked. This firm pressure does not cause any particular discomfort to the patient. In case of emphysema, one should always listen particularly carefully with the patient in the upright position, as sounds are frequently very distant and in some cases even absent when the patient is in the supine position. When the patient sits up and leans forward, his heart is closer to the chest.

W. Proctor Harvey, M.D.

In the presence of chronic obstructive pulmonary disease, heart sounds over the precordium are usually faint. The examiner should listen over the xiphoid or upper epigastric region with the patient

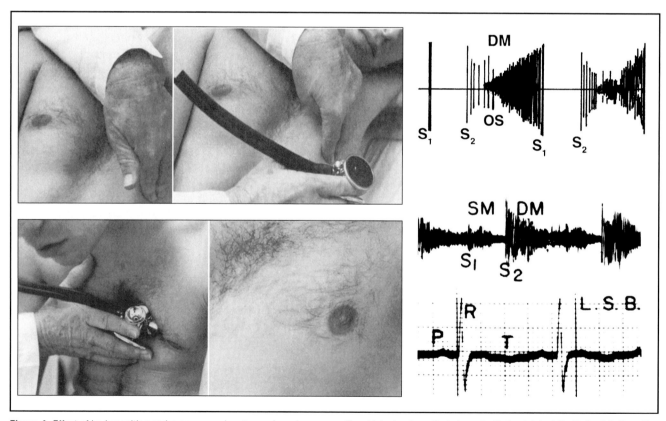

Figure 4. Effect of body position and pressure on heart sounds and murmurs. Top, Listening for mitral stenosis. To best detect the "tell-tale" diastolic rumble, turn the patient to the left lateral position. The index and middle fingers of the left hand palpate the point of maximal impulse of the left ventricle; holding that spot, the bell of the stethoscope is placed lightly over it, barely making an air seal with the chest wall. Bottom, Listening for aortic insufficiency. To detect the faintest diastolic blow, sit the patient upright, leaning forward with the breath held in deep expiration. Listen with the flat diaphragm exerting enough pressure against the chest wall to leave a momentary imprint on the chest wall. *(From Harvey WP, 18.)*

110

in the upright position, to avoid interference from emphysematous lung tissue.

Another cardiac pearl- a faint gallop, ventricular (S_3) or atrial (S_4), might be overlooked in a patient who has an emphysematous chest with an increase in anteroposterior diameter as a result of chronic obstructive pulmonary disease. This oversight might occur if the examiner listens over the usual areas of the precordium, the lower left sternal border, and apex; however, by listening over the xiphoid area or epigastric area, the examiner might easily detect the gallop (Fig. A).

W. Proctor Harvey, M.D.

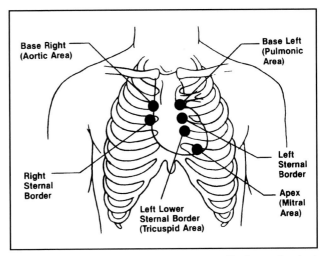

Figure 5. Sites of auscultation. These are the specific sites on the chest wall most principally used for cardiac auscultation. See text for details. *(From Harvey WP, 18.)*

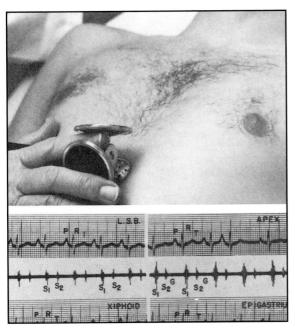

Fig A: If a patient has an emphysematous chest, a faint ventricular (S_3) diastolic gallop might not be heard over the lower left sternal border or apex; it may be detected over the xiphoid or upper epigastric area. Note heart sounds (S_1 and S_2) are also louder.

In routine practice, it is customary to listen for specific heart sounds and murmurs over the traditional so-called "valve" areas. These classic sites of auscultation on the chest wall correspond to points over the precordium where events originating in each heart valve are best transmitted and heard (Figure 5). It should be realized, however, that these auscultatory "valve" areas do not correspond to the anatomic location of the valves themselves. Sounds and murmurs of the aortic valve and aorta are well heard at the second right intercostal space, close to the sternal border (aortic area). Sounds and mur-

murs from the pulmonic valve and pulmonary artery are usually heard best at the second left intercostal space (pulmonic area), or third (mid) left sternal border. The mid-left sternal border is usually the best site to detect the high-frequency diastolic murmur of aortic insufficiency. The lower left sternal border (tricuspid area) is the customary location for evaluation of the first heart sound, systolic clicks, right-sided gallop sounds, and tricuspid valve sounds and murmurs. The characteristic increase in the intensity of the holosystolic murmur of tricuspid regurgitation with inspiration (Carvallo's sign) is best appreciated at this site. The holosystolic murmur of ventricular septal defect, often accompanied by a palpable thrill, is also located over this area. It tends to radiate out, like the spokes of a wheel, about its loudest point. The apex (mitral area) is usually best for identification of left-sided gallop sounds and murmurs of mitral valve origin. Aortic ejection sounds, however, are often well heard in this location as well.

Although these favored acoustic sites on the chest wall enable identification and analysis of most heart sounds and murmurs, auscultation should not be limited to these principal areas alone. Important findings may be present in additional locations, e.g., the neck (transmitted systolic murmur of aortic stenosis, bruit of carotid arterial occlusive disease), clavicles (bone transmission of the systolic murmur of aortic stenosis), supraclavicular fossa (continuous murmur of a jugular venous hum), left axillary region and posterior lung base ("band-like" radiation of the holosystolic murmur of chronic mitral regurgitation), interscapular region (systolic murmur of coarctation of the aorta), lung areas (pulmonary arteriovenous fistula, pulmonary artery branch stenosis), right sternal border, third

111

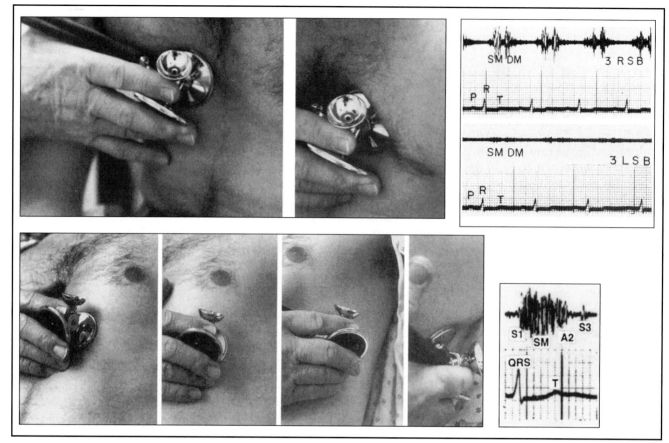

Figure 6. Transmission of heart sounds and murmurs. Top, "Right-sided" murmur of aortic insufficiency. Note that the diastolic murmur (DM) is louder over the third right sternal border (3RSB) (upper panel) as compared with the third left sternal border (3LSB) (lower panel). Bottom, "Band-like" radiation of the holosystolic murmur (SM) of mitral regurgitation from the lower left sternal border (left) to the left axillary region and posterior lung base (right). *(from Harvey WP, 18.)*

and fourth "key" interspaces (the so-called "right-sided" murmurs of aortic insufficiency due to rightward displacement and pathology of the aortic root, as seen in aortic dissection, aneurysm and Marfan's syndrome), and over scars (continuous murmur of peripheral arteriovenous fistula). Thus, the site of maximal intensity and direction of transmission of certain heart sounds and murmurs may prove to be of diagnostic value in the evaluation of their origin and clinical significance (Figure 6).

CARDIAC PEARL

Listen to Areas Other than the Precordium-We should not limit our auscultation to the heart, but in every patient examined we should listen over the neck, back, and anterior chest, abdomen and groin. One can listen over these areas quickly and efficiently. Make it a routine of the physical examination and it will be rewarding.

A short systolic murmur heard over multiple areas of the back of the chest and often over the right and left anterior chest may afford the first clue as to the diagnosis of pulmonary branch arterial stenosis.

With very large shunts (3:1 or greater) of atrial septal defect, a systolic murmur similar to the pulmonary arterial branch stenosis may be found over the back, if searched for. An arteriovenous fistula might be detected by the presence of a continuous murmur.

A systolic murmur of coarctation may be heard of almost equal intensity in the upper back as well as the front. Larger intercostal arteries of coarctation and Tetralogy of Fallot may at times be felt and have a systolic murmur. (In Tetralogy patients, a continuous murmur may also be detected over the intercostal arteries.)

The transmitted holosystolic murmur of severe mitral regurgitation can be detected at the left posterior lung base. (The murmur has radiated- "band-like"- from the lower left sternal border, apex, and axillary lines to the posterior lung base.)

Some very musical systolic murmurs are heard at the apex. Listen to the abdomen of every patient being examined. The bell of the

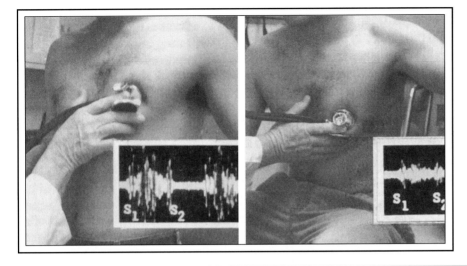

Figure 7. Squatting maneuver. Note that the systolic murmur of hypertrophic cardiomyopathy is louder on standing (left) and becomes softer on squatting (right). *(From Harvey WP, 18.)*

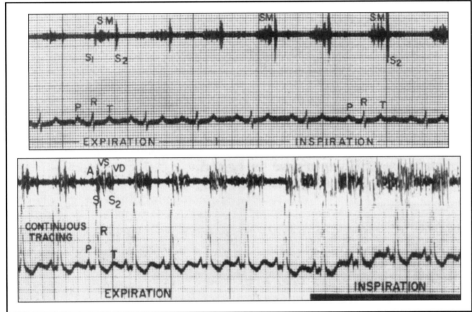

Figure 8. Effect of respiration on heart sounds and murmurs. Top, Note the striking increase in intensity of the systolic murmur (SM) of tricuspid regurgitation with inspiration. Bottom, Typical three-component pericardial friction rub which generally gets louder with inspiration. A = Atrial component. VS = Ventricular systolic component. VD = Ventricular diastolic component. *(From Harvey WP, 18.)*

stethoscope is best, using firm pressure to indent the abdomen.

A faint, short, midsystolic murmur, grade 1 to 3, may be a normal finding over the mid-abdomen and over the aortic pulsation. Systolic murmur (bruits) no longer in duration may be a clue to arterial obstruction, as is the case with carotid bruits in the neck. A continuous murmur may indicate an arteriovenous fistula.

Also listen with the bell of the stethoscope over each femoral artery. If you hear a "pistol shot" ejection sound, suspect aortic regurgitation. Pressure over the femoral artery with the bell of the stethoscope may also detect a systolic murmur and a higher frequency diastolic murmur (Duroziez's Sign).

W. Proctor Harvey, M.D.

Changes in body position and bedside physical maneuvers that increase or decrease blood flow through the heart, e.g., Valsalva maneuver, isometric hand grip, squatting and standing, may also be helpful adjuncts in enhancing the evaluation of specific sounds or murmurs heard in such conditions as mitral valve prolapse and hypertrophic cardiomyopathy (idiopathic hypertrophic subaortic stenosis) (Figure 7). As a practical clinical point, the physician need not squat and stand with the patient while the patient performs the squatting maneuver. Instead, the physician should remain comfortably seated in order to concentrate and focus attention with ease on any subtle and evanescent auscultatory changes. Paying careful attention to the effect of respiration on the splitting and variation in intensity of heart sounds and murmurs, especially those generated within the right side of the heart, can also be very useful during auscultation, and should be specifically listened for (Figure 8). If respiration is shallow, the depth of breathing may be controlled by

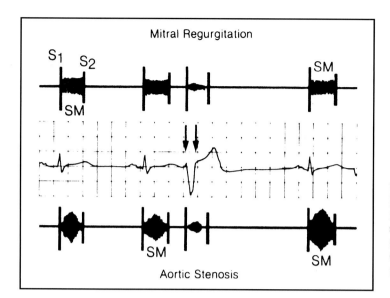

Figure 9. Effect of cycle length on heart sounds and murmurs. Note that the systolic murmur (SM) of mitral regurgitation (top) remains unchanged after the compensatory pause following the spontaneously occurring premature ventricular contraction (PVC). In contrast, the systolic murmur (SM) of aortic stenosis (bottom) is louder after the pause following the PVC. *(From Harvey WP, 18.)*

instructing the patient to inhale and exhale, as the examiner slowly raises and lowers his hand.

CARDIAC PEARL

At times, proper and efficient auscultation over the chest and neck is accomplished by having the patient stop breathing. In this way breath sounds are not interfering. When we ask the patient to do so, we too, should also stop breathing. This reminds us when to tell the patient to resume breathing; if we don't remember, we may find our patient struggling to keep from taking a breath.

When listening over the supraclavicular area and neck, it is absolutely necessary to have the patient stop breathing because of the distraction of the loud breath sounds.

Sometimes a particularly garrulous patient continues to talk while we try to listen; several things are helpful: (a) politely ask to please stop talking, (b) say: "Let me see your tongue," (c) "Hold your breath." Along these lines and pertaining to some of our fellow men and women: one of the most common of the tachycardias and often the hardest to treat, is "mandibular tachycardia;" some even have "mandibular fibrillation." Sometimes I, too, am guilty of this when giving a lecture.

W. Proctor Harvey, M.D.

Alterations in diastolic filling period caused by changing cycle lengths as in atrial fibrillation, or the long diastolic period created by the compensatory pause following a premature ventricular contraction, are also helpful, when present, in the differentiation of murmurs at the bedside. The systolic ejection murmur of aortic stenosis, for example, increases in intensity after the pause following shorter cycle lengths in atrial fibrillation or a pre-

mature ventricular beat. By contrast, the holosystolic murmur of mitral regurgitation remains essentially unchanged (Figure 9).

Since the entire "key" to successful auscultation is the proper timing of heart sounds and murmurs in the cardiac cycle, the first (S_1) and second (S_2) heart sounds, which divide the cardiac cycle into systole and diastole, must be identified in each auscultatory area on the precordium. Both heart sounds are usually well heard over all traditional "valve" areas, and in most cases can be readily differentiated from each other when the heart beats regularly, or at normal or slow rates. Since systole is shorter in duration than diastole, the recognition of a longer pause between S_2 and S_1 (diastole) than between S_1 and S_2 (systole), will enable immediate identification of these corresponding heart sounds. In the presence of tachycardia, however, diastole shortens more than systole and may be approximately equal in duration, making it difficult at times to distinguish between the two. Under these circumstances, it has been suggested that one may properly time the first and second heart sounds by palpation of the carotid or apical impulse. The first heart sound is approximately synchronous with the onset of the apical impulse and immediately precedes the carotid upstroke. The second heart sound occurs after the carotid pulse and apical impulses are felt. In clinical practice, however, it is often difficult to apply two senses simultaneously, e.g., palpation and auscultation, as this may dull the perception of either sense.

CARDIAC PEARL

There is no question in my mind that the simultaneous use of two senses, such as seeing and feeling (palpating) or listening and seeing or listening and palpating, often dulls the perceptiveness of either sense. A couple of examples: (1) Searching for the point of maximal impulse (PMI) of mitral stenosis with the patient turned to the left lateral position (LLP). If one does so with the tips of the stethoscope still in place in the ear canals, difficulty may be experienced in finding the point of maximal impulse. However, on removing the stethoscope from the ears, the impulse often is promptly found. (2) Timing of the jugular venous pulse. To do so, I find that always is easier if I can concentrate solely on the visual. If the carotid arterial pulsation is identified, and within a small area of vision the jugular venous pulse is also seen, timing is not difficult. For example, a venous wave preceding the carotid pulse is an "a" wave, a venous wave occurring at the same time as the arterial pulse is a "v" or "cv" wave.

W. Proctor Harvey, M.D.

The accurate timing of heart sounds and murmurs, even at faster rates, may be achieved by concentrating on auscultation alone, if one employs the simple, but important, technique referred to as "inching." This classic auscultatory technique is based on the fact that the second heart sound is usually the louder of the two heart sounds heard at the base of the heart (aortic and pulmonic areas). By focusing attention and keeping the second heart sound in mind, as the stethoscope is moved or "inched" from the aortic area across to the pulmonic area and down along the left sternal border to the apex, any extra sound or murmur occurring before S_2 can be recognized as systolic in timing, and after S_2 as diastolic (Figure 10). This valuable "inching" technique, therefore, helps make the timing of heart sounds and murmurs relatively easy. As a practical point, it is often easier to keep the first heart sound in mind as a reference at the lower left sternal border or apex, where it is loudest, and "inch" the stethoscope up to the aortic area for proper identification of the atrial "S_4" gallop.

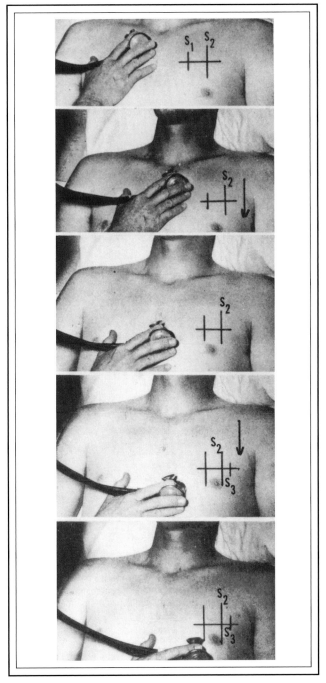

Figure 10. Inching Technique. A sound in diastole, e.g., the ventricular (S_3) gallop or physiologic third heart sound can be detected by moving or "inching" the stethoscope down from the aortic area (top) to the apex (bottom). By keeping the second heart sound (S_2) in mind as a reference, the S_3 is heard shortly after S_2 at the lower left sternal border and apex. *(From Harvey WP, 18.)*

CARDIAC PEARL

The "Inching" Technique: For the most accurate timing of heart sounds and murmurs, the simple technique called "inching" is the best (Fig. A). The physician uses the clinical fact that in most patients, the second heart sound is the louder of the two over the aortic area. It may not be loud, but it is louder than the first heart sound over this area. Therefore we have the second sound (S_2) as a reference point as we "inch" our stethoscope from the aortic area down to the apex. By keeping our second sound in mind as the stethoscope is inched, the physician can hear the extra sound that occurs in systole before the second sound, thereby diagnosing a systolic click. If the sound occurs after the second sound, then it is a diastolic sound such as a ventricular (S_3) or diastolic gallop. If a murmur appears before the second sound, then it is obviously a systolic murmur. If it occurs after the second sound, then it is a diastolic murmur.

The examiner can be practically 100% accurate in timing by using this technique. Although the ventricular rate may be rapid, the inching technique can correctly place the sound or murmur in systole. If this technique is not used, these sounds might be placed erroneously in diastole. A ventricular diastolic gallop (S_3) is generally absent at the base, so that as inching downward to the apex occurs, the S_3 appears after the second heart sound and is easily detected.

On the other hand, if an S_4, a presystolic atrial gallop, is present, it is best to inch from the apex and lower left sternal border upward to the base. In this instance, the first heart sound is used as the reference point because the extra heart sound is occurring in presystole before the first heart sound. Then, as the stethoscope is inched up the precordium, the S_4 disappears. This sound is also easily detected and identified as being a sound in presystole rather than in early diastole.

Another cardiac pearl: at times, both S_3 and S_4 occur in the same patient. This situation is often present with advanced heart failure such as can occur in patients with coronary artery disease or dilated cardiomyopathy. At times, when the examiner first listens, a gallop rhythm is heard, and it is not clear that two gallop sounds instead of only one might exist. By using the inching technique, moving the stethoscope from the aortic area to the apex, the physician will discover that the extra sound coming shortly after the second sound is that of an S_3 gallop. In the same patient, with the examiner starting from the lower left sternal border and apex and inching upward, a presystole sound in diastole disappears; therefore this sound is an S_4 diastolic gallop.

W. Proctor Harvey, M.D.

The examiner should allow sufficient time to become oriented to the various heart sounds and murmurs, and listen through several cardiac cycles in order to determine the underlying heart rate and rhythm (e.g., fast or slow, regular or irregular). If necessary, having the patient take a deep breath, or gently massaging the carotid sinus, may slow excessively rapid heart rates and permit more reliable appraisal of the auscultatory findings.

Expertise in clinical auscultation requires the ability to train one's ear to detect the details of the various auscultatory events occurring in the cardiac cycle at each area. In order to recognize and interpret acoustic events correctly, one must

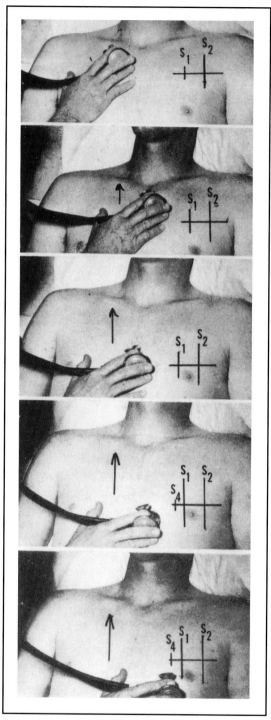

Fig A: "Inching" technique. As previously demonstrated in Figure 10, start at the aortic area (top panel), keep the second sound (S_2) in mind as a reference, and move (inch) the stethoscope downward to the apex (bottom panel). The extra sound (S_3) appears in diastole and continues to the apex. This is the ventricular (S_3) gallop. Starting at the lower left sternal border or apex, an extra sound is heard in presystole. Keep the first sound in mind as a reference and move (inch) the stethoscope upward to the aorta area (top panel). The extra sound disappears (middle panel) and remains absent at the base. This is an atrial (S_4) diastolic gallop.

116

develop the ability to "tune in," i.e., listen selectively to one specific aspect of the cardiac cycle at a time. While mentally "tuning in" and concentrating on S_1 first, and simultaneously blocking out all other sounds and events, the physician should pay special attention to intensity (e.g., faint, average, loud or varying), and listen for any splitting. After S_1 has been carefully appraised, S_2 is likewise concentrated on and analyzed with respect to the intensity and the type (physiologic, "fixed," paradoxical), degree (narrow, normal, wide) and effect of respiration on splitting. After the physician has listened to the first and second heart sounds, extra sounds in systole (e.g., ejection sounds and systolic clicks), and extra sounds in diastole, (e.g., atrial {S_4} and/or ventricular {S_3} gallops, normal physiological third heart sound, opening snap of mitral stenosis, pericardial knock sound of constrictive pericarditis) are then appraised. Following this, the examiner concentrates and listens for murmurs in systole, and then for murmurs in diastole. Continuous murmurs begin in systole and spill over into diastole without interruption. In patent ductus arteriosus, for example, blood flows from a high pressure system to a low pressure system throughout systole and diastole. The typical continuous "machinery" murmur peaks around ("envelops") the second heart sound. Cardiac conditions that result in combinations of systolic and diastolic murmurs, e.g., aortic stenosis and insufficiency, ventricular septal defect and aortic insufficiency, may occasionally be mistaken for a continuous murmur. Careful, attentive listening to S_2, however, will reveal that the systolic murmur in these conditions ends before or with S_2, and the diastolic murmur begins after S_2.

CARDIAC PEARL

We should practice and train our ears to detect the details of the various auscultatory events occurring in the heart cycle. By concentrating on the first sound, and at the same time mentally blocking out other events, we can detect the loudness (faint, average intensity or loud), the degree of splitting and variability of the first heart sound, etc. Then the second heart sound is analyzed. Only the second heart sound is concentrated on, noting the degree of splitting and the effect of respiration on splitting; then sounds in systole (systolic clicks, ejection sounds), sounds in diastole, atrial (S_4) and/or ventricular (S_3) gallops or a normal physiologic third sound (S_3). Next, concentrate specifically on murmurs in systole and then murmurs in diastole. Careful analysis of a systolic murmur will enable the

listener to determine its duration, intensity and what part of systole it occupies (holosystolic, early to middle, middle or late systole). Does the crescendo-decrescendo murmur peak in a specific portion of systole? Does it decrease in intensity in the latter part of systole? the same type of careful analysis is necessary for diastolic and continuous murmurs.

For those who have not been in the habit of making this careful detailed dissection of the heart sounds and murmurs occurring in the heart cycle, this may at first appear difficult. However, it is not, and with concentration and practice it can be accomplished readily. In fact, we do this all the time in our daily lives. A clock, for example, may be ticking in a room and we may not be aware of it until, for some reason, we hear it or listen specifically for it. We have, at times, had a clock ticking in the auditorium during a postgraduate course of 250 participants. At the end of the day's session, the question is asked, "How many heard the clock ticking?" None had. Then it was related that the clock had been ticking all day. Now, all listen specifically for it- and 100% hear it. Another example: if we stop whatever activities we are engaged in to listen for any noises in a room, we immediately hear various events, such as the motor of an air conditioner, a fan, voices in another room, a typewriter down the hall or other noises that previously we were unaware of.

W. Proctor Harvey, M.D.

This meticulous, detailed auscultation of the heart sounds and murmurs occurring in the cardiac cycle may, at first, appear difficult. With continued practice and concentration, however, it can be accomplished readily and with a gratifyingly high degree of accuracy. To emphasize this point, when teaching auscultation of the heart, Dr. Harvey often uses the analogy of listening to music, e.g., one of Beethoven's symphonies, concentrating on the sounds and selectively identifying the various instruments playing in the orchestra, one at a time. The difference in the auscultatory ability among physicians, he demonstrates, lies not in the difference in ability to hear the various heart sounds and murmurs, but a difference in the ability to listen specifically to each individual component of the heart cycle, concentrate ("tune in") and then carefully interpret what can be heard.

CARDIAC PEARL

On first thought it would appear that this process of "dissection" might take considerable time, but actually only a few moments of

concentration are required for each component analyzed. Probably the best analogy of this method of study of heart sounds and murmurs is that of listening to music. When discussing auscultation of the heart before an audience we have often purposely had a tape recording of symphonic music, such as one of Beethoven's symphonies, played as the audience files into the room. The audience is immediately curious as to why the music is being played at this time. The music is then stopped, and before starting the discussion the question is asked, "How many heard a violin, French horn, or kettle drum?" Very few would say that an individual instrument was specifically heard. However, if the music is replayed, and the audience is asked to listen specifically for a violin, then everyone immediately hears this instrument. The sounds of other instruments may be quickly searched for and detected. Following this, the analogy of listening to the heart and that of listening to music is easily understood. Proper emphasis can then be made that for adequate auscultation one must listen specifically to the various components of the heart cycle and not attempt to listen to everything at once, which would be equivalent to hearing only the melody of the music.

I am convinced that the difference in ability to practice adequate auscultation of the heart, which varies with students and physicians, is in general not a difference in ability to hear heart sounds and murmurs, but a difference in ability to "tune in" and at the same time to dissect the various specific events of the heart cycle. True, some individuals with impaired hearing may be handicapped, but the great majority of students and physicians are shown by tests with audiograms to have the ability to hear within the range covered by all the important heart sounds and murmurs.

W. Proctor Harvey, M.D.

The appropriate identification and characterization of the myriad heart sounds heard in clinical practice, in terms of their intensity, pitch, duration, timing, intervals, etc., is of great help in the bedside interpretation of heart murmurs. Unfortunately, too many physicians become so intent on and unduly preoccupied with the detection of murmurs that they fail to recognize the clinical significance of the heart sounds themselves. The recognition that a systolic murmur is "significant" or "pathologic," rather than "innocent," often rests on the "company it keeps," rather than the characteristics of the murmur itself. Thus certain abnormal heart sounds that reflect cardiac pathology, e.g., the wide,

so-called "fixed" splitting of the second heart sound in atrial septal defect, the ejection sound in valvular aortic or pulmonic stenosis, and the systolic click in mitral valve prolapse, all serve as immediate clues to the presence of a "significant" murmur. In contrast, the "innocent" systolic murmur is characteristically accompanied by normal physiologic splitting of the second heart sound, the absence of these abnormal heart sounds and the frequent presence of a physiologic third heart sound. An effective way to improve one's auscultatory ability is to draw a diagram or "sketch" of the acoustic findings heard on every patient examined.

CARDIAC PEARL

If not already being done, we should develop the habit of drawing or sketching the various heart sounds and murmurs that we hear when examining our patients (Fig. A). Include it as part of the patient's record on both the office and hospital charts. If done, this invariably increases the accuracy of our auscultation because if we have to sketch what we are hearing, we obviously have to pay strict attention to the various components of the heart cycle. Note should be made of the intensity and splitting of the first heart sound and whether or not it varies in intensity; also, the features of the second sound- its intensity and type of splitting, normal or abnormally widely split ("fixed"). Sketch the murmur as to what part of systole and/or diastole it occurs, as well as any ejection sounds, systolic clicks, gallops, pericardial knocks and normal physiologic third sounds that are heard. If a continuous murmur is present, where in systole or diastole is it loudest? Does it "envelop" the second sound, as is typical of patent ductus arteriosus? I have yet to find a physician or student who sketches what he is hearing who does not greatly improve his expertise in clinical auscultation of the cardiovascular system. Making this a continuing lifelong habit will also result in continued progressive improvement over the years.

W. Proctor Harvey, M.D.

Heart Sounds

Heart sounds are brief, discrete, auditory vibrations of varying intensity (loud, normal or soft), frequency (high, medium, low-pitched), tonal quality (muffled, snapping, tambour, sharp, dull), and timing (location within the cardiac cycle), generated within the heart and great vessels, that travel through the surrounding tissues to the surface of the chest wall, where they may be detected by the

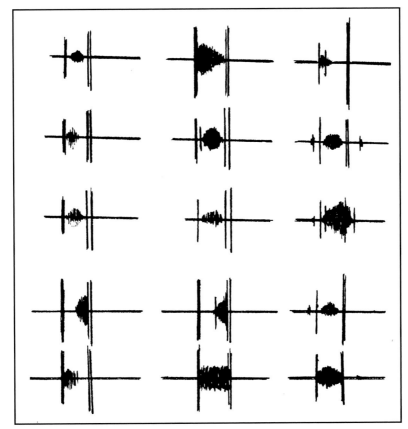

Fig A: Sketches of various murmurs and heart sounds. Top 3, left to right: (1) Note that systolic murmur is short in midsystole with normal aortic and pulmonic components of second heart sound, consistent with innocent murmur. (2) Note holosystolic murmur decreasing in the latter part of systole. This configuration of murmur is seen in acute mitral valve insufficiency, such as with ruptured chorda tendineae. (3) Note ejection sound and short systolic murmur in early systole, plus accentuated, closely split second heart sound, consistent with pulmonary hypertension as with Eisenmenger's ventricular septal defect. Line 2: (1) Early to mid systolic murmur with vibratory component, consistent with innocent murmur (Still's). (2) Note ejection sound following first sound with diamond-shaped murmur and wide splinting of second heart sound that may be present with milder degrees of pulmonic stenosis or atrial septal defect. Ejection sound more likely with valvular pulmonic stenosis. (3) Crescendo-decrescendo systolic murmur, not holosystolic; however, atrial (S_4) and ventricular (S_3) diastolic gallops present, consistent with mitral systolic murmur heard with congestive cardiomyopathy or coronary artery disease with papillary muscle dysfunction and cardiac decompensation. Line 3: (1) Longer, somewhat vibratory crescendo-decrescendo systolic murmur with wider splitting of second heart sound. If second heart sound became single with expiration, atrial septal defect less likely and if remainder of cardiovascular evaluation normal, then consistent with innocent murmur. (2) Midsystolic murmur, wide splitting of second heart sound that was "fixed"; atrial septal defect. (3) Prolonged diamond-shaped or "kite-shaped" systolic murmur masking the aortic component of second sound with delayed pulmonic component, atrial sound present in presystole, ejection sound present. Typical of valvular pulmonic stenosis of increasing severity. Line 4: (1) Late apical systolic murmur. Prolapsing mitral valve leaflet (systolic click-murmur syndrome, Barlow's syndrome). (2) Systolic click-late apical systolic murmur. Prolapsing mitral leaflet syndrome. (3) Midsystolic murmur, not holosystolic, atrial sound in presystole, consistent with mitral systolic murmur of cardiomyopathy or ischemic heart disease. Bottom line: Early crescendo-decrescendo systolic murmur ending at midsystole, consistent with innocent murmur; or can be seen with small ventricular septal defect, often closing. (2) Holosystolic murmur consistent with mitral insufficiency, ventricular septal defect. (3) Holosystolic murmur peaking in midsystole, also consistent with mitral insufficiency, tricuspid insufficiency, ventricular septal defect. An acute mitral insufficiency may take this configuration where there is a decrease in the murmur in the latter part of systole (in this latter case, atrial and ventricular diastolic gallops are frequent, and the second heart sound may be accentuated).

chest piece of the stethoscope and carried via the tubing to the listening ear.

First Heart Sound

The first heart sound (S_1) clinically signals the onset of ventricular systole. It is normally composed of two audible high-frequency components. The first component (M_1) is considered to correspond to mitral valve closure, and the second component (T_1) to tricuspid valve closure. The first heart sound is best heard with the diaphragm of the stethoscope at the cardiac apex and lower left sternal border. Both valves close at the beginning of ventricular systole, but mitral closure usually precedes tricuspid closure by 0.02 - 0.03 seconds, so that audible splitting of the first heart sound is a common and normal occurrence. Splitting of S_1 into the loud early mitral component and the softer tricuspid component is best appreciated along the lower left sternal border (tricuspid area). Since the tricuspid component is much softer and radiates poorly, S_1 is usually perceived as a single sound at the cardiac apex (mitral area), where it is loudest.

Most of the abnormalities of the first heart sound that are of clinical significance are those of intensity rather than of splitting (Table 1). Clinical variations in S_1 intensity are usually due to alterations in the mitral (M_1) component. The intensity of the normal first heart sound will usually be different in each of the auscultatory areas examined. The clinician judges the sound to be loud, average or faint according to his or her perception of normal, based on experience listening to heart sounds. Since S_1 is characteristically louder than S_2 at the cardiac apex, if S_1 is softer than S_2 over this site, then one is dealing with a reduced intensity of S_1. However, it may be difficult to detect by listening there alone whether the intensity of S_1 is increased. On the other hand, since S_2 is normally louder than S_1 at the aortic area, one may identify an accentuated S_1 with a high level of confidence if S_1 is equal to or louder than S_2 over this site.

• Loud S_1

The intensity of the first heart sound is augmented by any condition which increases the force of ventricular contraction and the rate of pressure development in the ventricle, or brings the heart closer to the chest wall. Thus, S_1 is physiologically more intense in children and young adults, in patients with a thin chest wall, and in hyperkinetic states (e.g., exercise, tachycardia, anemia, hyperthyroidism, fever, pregnancy, excitement). In the presence of a normal ventricular rate, however, a loud S_1 should alert the physician to the possibility

---

T A B L E 1

Abnormalities of the First Heart Sound

Increased intensity of S_1

Mitral stenosis.
Short PR interval.
Hyperkinetic states (e.g., hyperthyroidism, fever, anemia, exercise, tachycardia, pregnancy).
Physiologically normal in children, young adults, patients with a thin chest wall and narrow A-P diameter.
Holosystolic mitral valve prolapse.

Decreased intensity of S1

Long PR interval (first-degree AV block).
Diminished LV contractility (e.g., congestive heart failure, acute myocardial infarction, cardiomyopathy).
Premature mitral valve closure with high LV end-diastolic pressure (e.g., acute severe aortic insufficiency).
Ineffective valve closure due to loss of leaflet substance or thickening, fibrosis, calcification, or shortening of mitral valve apparatus.
Increased tissue, air, or fluid between the heart and the stethoscope (e.g., emphysema, obesity, large breasts, thick chest wall, increased A-P diameter, pericardial effusion).

Changing intensity of S_1

AV dissociation (varying PR intervals, e.g., complete heart block, ventricular tachycardia).
Atrial fibrillation.

Wide splitting of S_1

RBBB
PVCs, ventricular tachycardia
Atrial septal defect
Ebstein's anomaly

S_1 = first heart sound; AV = atrioventricular; LV = left ventricular; RBBB = right bundle branch block; PVC = premature ventricular contraction; A-P = anterior-posterior. *(From Chizner MA, 5.)*

---

of a short PR interval on the electrocardiogram and mitral stenosis (Figure 11). Unless the mitral valve is immobilized by calcific deposits, this increase in intensity of S_1 in mitral stenosis is so well established, that it can be considered an auscultatory hallmark of this condition, and may be the first indication of its presence.

According to the classic valvular theory, the chief factor in determining the intensity of S_1 is the position of the atrioventricular (AV) valves at the onset of ventricular contraction. If the valve leaflets are wide open as systole begins, the excursion is large and the vibrations amplified, thus producing a loud first heart sound. In mitral stenosis with mobile cusps, the loud first heart sound relates to the high left atrial pressure, which causes the supple and not severely calcified valve to remain open more widely until a very sharp high-velocity closing movement is produced by ventricular systole.

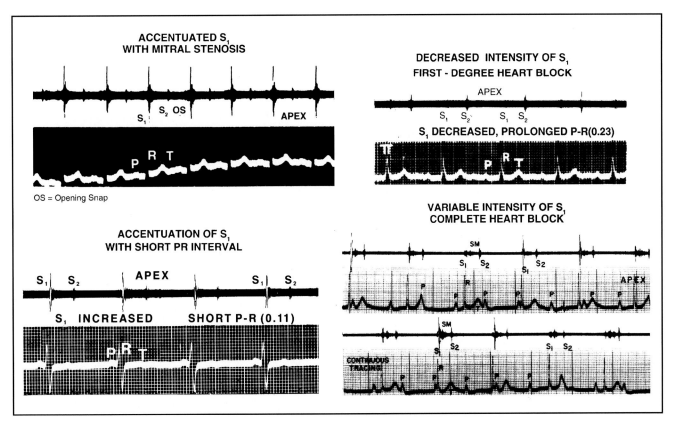

Figure 11. Composite of four patients with variation in intensity of S_1. Left, S_1 is loud in mitral stenosis (top) with a short PR interval (bottom). Right, Faint S_1 with long PR interval in first degree atrioventricular block (top). Varying intensity of S_1, in complete heart block (bottom). Note the loud S_1 with short PR interval and faint S_1 with prolonged PR interval. A short systolic murmur (SM) is present, due to the slow rate and exaggerated stroke volume. *(From Harvey WP, 18.)*

A loud S_1 is also heard in association with a short PR interval (0.10 - 0.14 seconds), since the valve leaflets are also in a wide open position at the onset of ventricular contraction. When a loud S_1 is heard in the presence of a holosystolic murmur of mitral regurgitation, one should also consider the diagnosis of mitral valve prolapse. The loud first heart sound may be due to an increased amplitude of leaflet excursion beyond the line of closure and/or the summation of the first heart sound and systolic click as they move into each other and merge together.

CARDIAC PEARL

Loud First Heart Sound- If a patient who has a normal heart rate has a loud first sound, always think of two conditions: mitral stenosis and a short P-R interval on the electrocardiogram.

The length of a P-R interval can affect the first heart sound. The increase in intensity of the sound is most likely due to the position of the atrioventricular (A-V) valves at the time systole occurs. If the valves are deeper in the ventricles and systole occurs promptly after the atrial systole, the valves close, making a louder sound. If the P-R interval is prolonged and the A-V valves have had time to move upward in the ventricles, systolic contraction produces a faint first sound.

A loud first heart sound due to a short P-R interval can simulate the sound of mitral stenosis. The presence of a normal physiologic third heart sound can be misinterpreted as an opening snap.

A young college track star, a long distance runner, had been diagnosed as having mitral stenosis, which, of course, was devastating news to this young person. He was referred to us for consultation; examination showed that he had a short P-R interval, which caused the accentuated first sound, and a normal physiologic third heart sound- misinterpreted as an opening snap. These were normal findings, which made one happy athlete!

In the case of mitral stenosis, an opening snap should be heart and by turning the patient to the left lateral position and listening over the point of maximum impulse of the left ventricle, the telltale diastolic rumble should be present.

If the ventricular heart rate is normal and the first heart sound is loud, a short P-R interval or mitral stenosis should be considered. The increased intensity of the first heart sound of mitral stenosis may be the first indication of the presence of this condition. Also, if the second sound is accentuated and closely split, and if in addition there is an opening snap, the physician may be alerted to the importance of listening specifically over the point of maximum impulse in the apical area. It is helpful if the patient turns to the left lateral position, or performs other maneuvers such as breathing rapidly five or six times, coughing, or exercising, to bring out the typical, diagnostic diastolic rumble to be heart over this area. Worthy of emphasis is the occasional misdiagnosis of mitral stenosis because of a loud first heart sound due to a short P-R interval, especially when in combination with a prominent third heart sound. The differentiation can be accomplished by the total cardiovascular evaluation, but this still remains a recurring source of confusion. An aid in differentiation is the usual variability of the normal physiological third heart sound waxing and waning coincident with respiration, and occurring later in timing after the second sound than the typical opening snap. Also, the absence of a diastolic rumble, as well as additional normal findings on the x-ray film and electrocardiogram can further aid in this differentiation.

W. Proctor Harvey, M.D.

• **Soft S_1**

When the valve leaflets are in close apposition at the onset of ventricular contraction, the excursion is minimal, the vibrations are small and the ensuing sound is soft and often faint. Therefore, a soft, or faint, S_1 may accompany a prolonged PR interval (0.20 - 0.24 seconds), as occurs in first degree AV block and may, in fact, be the first clinical indication of its presence. Here the atrioventricular valves have had more time to "float" to a partially closed position after atrial contraction and before the delayed onset of ventricular contraction. As a general rule, S_1 will be normal in intensity when the PR interval is in the range of 0.16 seconds. With some practice, the physician can become quite adept in estimating the PR interval on the electrocardiogram by attentive auscultation.

The intensity of S_1 may also be modified by the rate and force of valve closure. Depressed left ventricular contractility and a diminished rate of pressure development within the left ventricle will tend to soften S_1 (Table 1). Thus, S_1 may be soft in con-

gestive heart failure, acute myocardial infarction and cardiomyopathy with diminished left ventricular contractility. In acute, severe aortic insufficiency, a sudden volume overload in a nondilated left ventricle results in a markedly elevated end-diastolic pressure, which may lead to premature closure of the mitral valve at the onset of systole and therefore reduce the intensity of the first heart sound. The faint S_1 is an important clue to this urgent diagnosis, where early surgical replacement can be life-saving.

The first heart sound may also be softened by loss of leaflet substance or thickening, fibrosis, calcification and shortening of the valve apparatus, resulting in ineffective valve closure and loss of valve mobility and elasticity, which leads to mitral regurgitation. Body build, chest configuration and other extracardiac factors that influence how far away the stethoscope is to the heart may also play a role in diminishing the intensity of S_1, e.g., pulmonary emphysema with an increased anteroposterior diameter of the chest, obesity, large breasts, increased chest wall thickness, and pericardial effusion. These conditions, however, will diminish the intensity of the second heart sound and the ability to detect all other sounds and murmurs present as well.

In applying the above principles, an auscultatory maneuver that is useful in detecting the presence of pericardial fluid is to listen for heart sounds and murmurs with the patient first lying in the supine position, and then on the stomach, propped up on the elbows, with the stethoscope in the same spot over the precordium. Heart sounds and murmurs in the normal heart usually become louder in this position, but may decrease in the patient with pericardial effusion, because the fluid tends to gravitate anteriorly, interposing itself between the heart and the chest wall.

• **Variable Intensity of S_1**

A variation in the intensity of the first heart sound may be detected during the presence of atrioventricular dissociation, e.g., complete heart block and ventricular tachycardia, and with changes in cycle lengths during atrial fibrillation (Table 1). A variation in the position of the AV valve leaflets (varying PR intervals) and changes in the rate of pressure development in the ventricle resulting from the change in left ventricular end-diastolic volume (varying RR intervals) respectively explain the variation in intensity of S_1. Alternation in S_1 intensity (auscultatory alternans) may also be heard in patients with cardiomyopathic conditions where regular alternation in the rate of intraventricular pressure development is responsible. The clinical finding of a slow heart rate of approximately forty beats per minute, accompanied by a varying intensity of S_1, at times very loud (bruit de canon), when atrial systole happens to occur immediately before ventricular systole (short PR interval), and at other times faint (long PR interval), is an auscultatory hallmark that often leads to the bedside diagnosis of complete heart block.

Ventricular tachycardia, another condition characterized by varying temporal relationships in atrial and ventricular contraction, is also marked by a changing intensity of S_1. Further auscultatory clues to the diagnosis may be afforded by the detection of multiple sounds which are best heard along the lower left sternal border and are created by a wide splitting of S_1 and S_2 due to asynchronous ventricular contraction and the presence of atrial and ventricular diastolic gallops. The presence of intermittent cannon A waves, and the lack of response of the arrhythmia to carotid sinus pressure, lend confirmatory evidence to the diagnosis.

Auscultation during atrial fibrillation also reveals a varying intensity of S_1 that is dependent on the length of the previous diastole. At the end of short cycles, a loud S_1 is produced since the AV valves close from a wide open position. A faint S_1 occurs at the end of longer cycles, as the valve leaflets are in close apposition at the onset of ventricular contraction.

• Split S_1

Splitting of the first heart sound is a frequent normal occurrence. In the normal person, when S_1 is split into its mitral (M_1) and tricuspid (T_1) components, the time interval between them is very short (0.02 - 0.03 seconds). Wide splitting of S_1 is almost always abnormal. It can be heard in pathologic conditions which delay electrical activation and contraction of the right ventricle, and thus delay tricuspid valve closure. Wide splitting of S_1, therefore, can be heard in complete right bundle branch block, during premature left ventricular contractions, or ventricular tachycardia. In atrial septal defect, wide splitting of S_1, in addition to a loud T_1, is present because the valve is held open by the increased flow of blood from the right atrium to the right ventricle. This results in valve closure from a more open position, and at a greater velocity than normal. Occasionally, this finding can serve as a valuable, subtle clue to the diagnosis of atrial septal defect. Wide splitting of S_1 with an accentuated, delayed T_1 ("sail sound") caused by the abnormally large size and increased excursion of the anterior

tricuspid valve leaflet, can also be heard in Ebstein's anomaly of the tricuspid valve.

Second Heart Sound

The second heart sound clinically signifies the end of systole and identifies the onset of diastole. It is higher in pitch, shorter and sharper than S_1, and has two audible components. The first is the aortic component (A_2), and the second is the pulmonic component (P_2), resulting from closure of the aortic and pulmonic valves, respectively. The normal second heart sound is usually single (fused) during expiration. Auscultation using the diaphragm of the stethoscope in the second left intercostal space (pulmonic area), or mid-left sternal border during the inspiratory phase of respiration, usually reveals splitting of S_2 into two distinct high-pitched components (A_2 and P_2). Since the closing pressure is higher in the aorta than in the pulmonary artery, the aortic component (A_2) is normally louder and earlier than the pulmonic component (P_2), and is also louder than S_1 in the second right and left intercostal spaces (aortic and pulmonic areas). It can be heard well over the entire precordium. The pulmonic component is normally heard only at the second left intercostal space and along the mid-left sternal border, and does not usually radiate to the apex as a separate detectable sound, except in young, thin individuals with a delicate build and narrow anteroposterior chest diameter, or when pulmonary hypertension is present. It should be noted that the abbreviations A_2 and P_2 refer to the aortic and pulmonic components of S_2 respectively, and not to the intensity of S_2 over the aortic or pulmonic areas.

A great deal of diagnostic information can be obtained from a careful clinical analysis of S_2. The second heart sound should be judged with regard to the intensity of its components (A_2 and P_2) and the presence, degree and type of S_2 splitting. As Dr. Harvey so aptly demonstrates, the physician can simulate the degree of splitting by striking one's knuckles or fingertips against a hard surface, varying the degree of asynchrony. Paying close attention to the splitting of the two components of S_2 and their behavior during the respiratory cycle may provide important clues to the presence and severity of underlying cardiovascular disease, and is one of the most rewarding observations during cardiac auscultation.

CARDIAC PEARL

Most physicians report difficulty in detecting the various degrees of splitting. It is

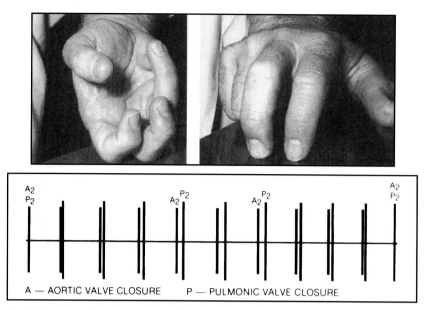

A — AORTIC VALVE CLOSURE   P — PULMONIC VALVE CLOSURE

Fig A: Simulation of heart sounds by striking knuckles or fingertips on a hard surface.

merely a matter of practicing concentration on the second heart sound and hearing successive degrees of synchrony of sounds. Any physician can become expert in the bedside detection of the spectrum of splitting of sounds. This can be simulated by striking two knuckles or fingertips on a hard surface (Figure A); one can easily vary the degree of synchrony. Striking only one knuckle produces a single sound. Striking both knuckles not quite simultaneously imitates a close split, and a wide split is simulated by delaying the second knuckle before striking it. The tips of the fingers on one hand can also be used in place of the knuckles as just described.

It is also possible, using this technique, to simulate the first sound, second sound, opening snap- all in proper sequence. Many physicians have been able to apply what they have learned from this technique to the accurate auscultation of actual patients.

W. Proctor Harvey, M.D.

• Normal Splitting of S_2

Normally, A_2 and P_2 separate with inspiration and fuse with expiration. Normal physiologic inspiratory splitting of S_2 varies from 0.02 to 0.06 seconds and is due chiefly to a delay in P_2 and less to earlier closure of the aortic valve. During inspiration, intrathoracic pressure decreases, favoring greater venous return of blood to the right side of the heart. This results in an increase in right ventricular stroke volume, which prolongs right ventricular ejection time and delays pulmonic valve closure. In addition, inspiratory expansion of the lung allows the resistance (impedance) of flow in the pulmonary vascular bed to decrease, causing the blood leaving the right ventricle to be carried forward through inertia, continuing after the right ventricular force has been dissipated, thereby delaying P_2 (prolonged "hang-out" interval).

The net effect of inspiration, therefore, is the delay of the pulmonic component of S_2 by increasing pulmonary vascular compliance and right ventricular volume and ejection time. Inspiration will also favor earlier aortic valve closure, since pooling of blood in the pulmonary bed will decrease flow to the left side of the heart, thereby shortening ventricular systole, with left ventricular ejection ending earlier than right ventricular ejection. A_2 is heard earlier, therefore, than P_2. The above mechanisms account for the normal physiologic respiratory splitting of S_2.

• Wide Splitting of S_2

Abnormally wide splitting of the second heart sound occurs in a variety of pathologic conditions that cause delayed pulmonary closure or early aortic closure (Table 2, Figure 12). Conditions that delay the transmission of right ventricular systole electrically (complete right bundle branch block, left ventricular ectopic beats) or mechanically (valvular pulmonic stenosis) delay pulmonic valve closure and, therefore, widen the splitting of S_2. This results in audible wide splitting of S_2 over the pulmonic area and mid-left sternal border, even on expiration, which widens further coincident with inspiration. Increased splitting of S_2 may also occur in severe mitral regurgitation and ventricular septal defects with large left-to-right shunts. In these conditions there is a second lower resistance route of exit for

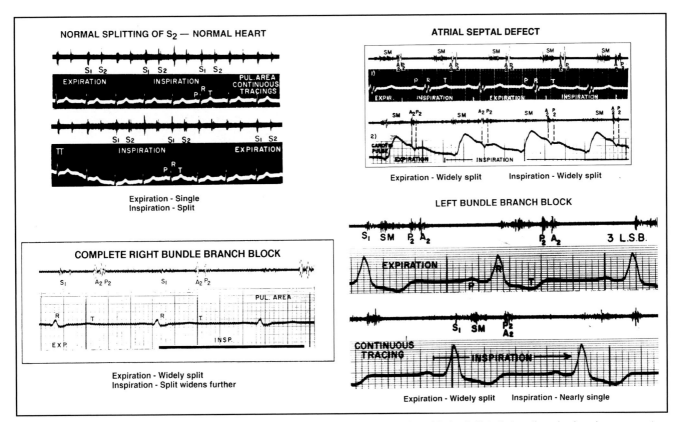

Figure 12. Variations in splitting of the second heart sound. Left, Normal physiologic splitting of S_2 (top). Note that aortic and pulmonic components of S_2 are synchronous (fused) during expiration and split (A_2-P_2) during inspiration. Note the persistent splitting of S_2 in right bundle branch block (bottom). During expiration, S_2 is split with wide physiologic increase in split, coincident with inspiration. Right, Two patients with atrial septal defect (top). Note the wide, relatively "fixed" splitting of S_2 (A_2-P_2) without significant respiratory variation of the interval between aortic closure and pulmonic closure. A faint systolic murmur (SM) is present. Although the term "fixed" splitting is used, there may be some movement of the components of S_2. Left bundle branch block (bottom). Note that the wide reversed "paradoxical" splitting of S_2 (P_2-A_2) during expiration becomes more closely split or a single sound (fused) during inspiration. *(From Harvey WP, 18.)*

blood flow from the left ventricle to the right ventricle in ventricular septal defect and to the left atrium in mitral regurgitation. This unloading of the left ventricle results in a shorter left ventricular ejection time and earlier closure of the aortic valve.

Wide physiologic splitting may also occur in idiopathic dilatation of the pulmonary artery, due to the decrease in impedance (increased capacitance and ability to receive blood volume) in the pulmonary bed and the prolonged "hang-out" time. In all of these instances there is an appropriate inspiratory and expiratory directional change in splitting, i.e., wide splitting on expiration and further widening during inspiration (wide physiologic splitting of S_2).

• "Fixed" Splitting of S_2

One of the acoustic hallmarks of atrial septal defect is the respiratory behavior of the second heart sound. In "classic" atrial septal defect, A_2 and P_2 are not only widely split, but also remain relatively "fixed" throughout the respiratory cycle. So-called "fixed" splitting of S_2 (i.e., little or no respiratory variation) is thus a valuable bedside diagnostic sign of a left-to-right shunt at the atrial level, and when present in association with a systolic murmur, may afford an immediate clue to the diagnosis of atrial septal defect. The proposed mechanism for "fixed" splitting of the second heart sound is twofold. The increase in pulmonary vascular compliance resulting from longstanding pulmonary shunt flow creates an inertial delay in closure of the pulmonic valve ("hang-out"). In addition, the increase in flow to the right ventricle from both shunted blood and the periphery during inspiration and expiration prolongs right ventricular ejection, thereby negating the usual influences of respiratory variation on venous return to the right side of the heart. Although the term "fixed" is appropriate, it should be mentioned that there may be some movement of A_2 and P_2 in approximately one fourth to one third of patients.

For practical purposes, auscultation should be performed with the patient in the sitting position before one can conclude that there is truly abnormal splitting of the second heart sound. Normal

125

TABLE 2

Abnormal Splitting of the Second Heart Sound

Wide "physiologic" splitting (increases with inspiration)

RBBB	
LV ectopic beats	Due to delay of pulmonic valve closure
Pulmonic stenosis	
Mitral regurgitation	Due to shortening of LV ejection time
Large VSD	and early aortic valve closure
Idiopathic dilatation of pulmonary artery	Due to decreased impedance in the pulmonary bed

Wide "fixed" splitting (no change with inspiration)

Atrial septal defect	Due to prolonged RV ejection time and decreased impedance in the pulmonary bed

Paradoxical or reversed splitting (decreases with inspiration)

LBBB	
RV ectopic beats, RV pacing	
Severe AS or Hypertrophic cardiomyopathy	Due to delay
Severe LV dysfunction, e.g., Acute MI	of aortic
Transient LV dysfunction during angina (rare)	valve closure
Large PDA	

RBBB = right bundle branch block; LV = left ventricular; VSD = ventricular septal defect; LBBB = left bundle branch block; RV = right ventricular; AS = aortic stenosis; PDA = patent ductus arteriosus. *(From Chizner MA, 5.)*

---

children, young adults and trained athletes may have persistent expiratory splitting of S_2 when examined supine, which disappears when they sit or stand owing to decreased venous return. By contrast, S_2 remains audibly split during expiration in pathologic conditions, even when the patient is examined sitting or standing and is, therefore, a valuable clue to an underlying cardiovascular abnormality.

Wide, relatively "fixed" splitting of S_2 may also be heard in severe right ventricular failure, since the compromised right ventricle is unable to accommodate the additional amount of blood coincident with inspiration, and no change in the position of pulmonary valve closure occurs. In patients with pulmonary hypertension, therefore, wide, relatively "fixed" splitting of S_2 instead of single (fused) or close splitting, becomes a useful sign of abnormal right ventricular performance.

• Paradoxical Splitting of S_2

Paradoxical, or reversed, splitting of S_2 occurs when the order of semilunar valve closure is reversed (P_2 preceding A_2) and is noted in a variety of conditions which interfere with ejection on the left side of the heart (Table 2). This may be due to electrical delay as in complete left bundle branch block, right ventricular ectopic beats and right ventricular pacing. It may also be due to mechanical delay as in left ventricular outflow obstruction (severe valvular aortic stenosis, hypertrophic cardiomyopathy {idiopathic hypertrophic subaortic stenosis}, and significant left ventricular dysfunction). Paradoxical splitting of S_2, however, is more likely to occur in hypertrophic cardiomyopathy than in valvular aortic stenosis. In hypertrophic cardiomyopathy A_2 is well preserved, but in severe calcific aortic stenosis the aortic component may not be heard due to impaired mobility and compliance of the valve leaflets.

Paradoxical S_2 splitting is also a helpful clue in distinguishing hypertrophic cardiomyopathy from acute mitral regurgitation, where many of the auscultatory features may be similar. If reverse splitting of S_2 is present, the diagnosis of hypertrophic cardiomyopathy is favored. Physiologic splitting of S_2, on the other hand, favors mitral regurgitation. Reversed splitting of S_2 in valvular aortic stenosis, in the absence of a conduction defect, i.e., left bundle branch block, implies hemodynamically significant outflow tract obstruction (Figure 13). When the mobility of the aortic valve is markedly reduced, however, as in severe calcific aortic stenosis, S_2 may have a single component because the aortic contribution is no longer audible.

Other infrequent causes of paradoxical splitting of S_2 include coronary artery disease, e.g., during an attack of angina pectoris or acute myocardial infarction, large patent ductus arteriosus, and rarely systemic arterial hypertension. At the bedside, paradoxical splitting may be recognized when there is audible splitting of S_2 on expiration (P_2-A_2) that becomes narrower or single during inspiration, as pulmonic valve closure occurs later as anticipated, and the two components merge, or fuse, into a single sound.

In many normal older patients (greater than fifty years of age), splitting of S_2 is less discernible to the listening ear, with a single audible S_2 on inspiration and expiration. This results from a delayed A_2 and earlier P_2 secondary to decreased pulmonary "hangout" time. An inaudible pulmonic component of S_2 may also exist in older adults with increased anteroposterior chest diameter. This may result in a single second heart sound (A_2) heard during both expiration and inspiration, or during inspiration alone, leading to the false impression of paradoxical splitting of S_2.

• Loud S_2

Elevation of pressure in either of the great vessels will result in a forceful valve closure sound.

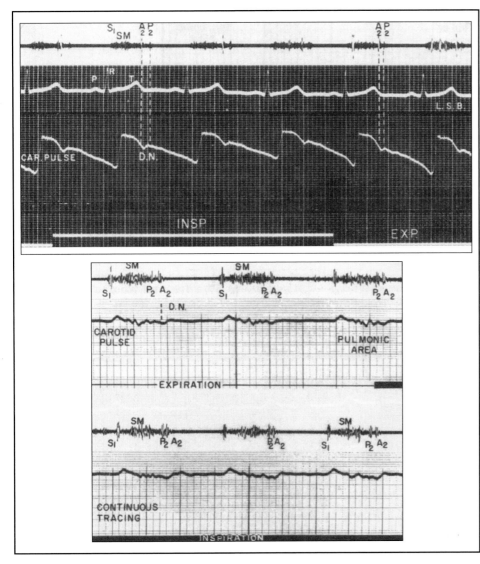

Figure 13. Top, Mitral insufficiency. Note persistent splitting of S_2 (A_2-P_2). During expiration, S_2 is split with wide "physiologic" increase in split coincident with inspiration. Bottom, Aortic stenosis. Note reversed ("paradoxical") splitting of S_2 (P_2-A_2) during expiration, which becomes more closely split during inspiration. *(From Harvey WP, 18.)*

The intensity of aortic or pulmonic valve closure, therefore, provides a crude indicator to the pressure levels in their respective great arteries. During auscultation, both components of S_2 must be heard for accurate evaluation of the loudness of A_2 and P_2. In systemic arterial hypertension, a loud "tambour" (ringing or musical) quality of A_2 is audible (Figure 14). In "olden days," a tambour second sound was said to occur in luetic aortitis. Today, the most common cause of a tambour S_2, heard in clinical practice is systemic arterial hypertension.

In pulmonary hypertension, a loud, often palpable, single (fused) or closely split second heart sound with an accentuation of P_2 is present, widening slightly coincident with inspiration. This loud P_2 transmits from the pulmonic area along the left sternal border as far as the apex. Thus, with inspiration, S_2 splits normally, but with less than usual inspiratory separation of A_2 and P_2. This results from the increase in impedance and decrease in

hang-out time of the pulmonary bed, in the presence of advancing degrees of pulmonary hypertension. With severe pulmonary hypertension, the S_2 components may be virtually fused. It should be emphasized that P_2 is usually inaudible at the apex, except in young, thin individuals, where P_2 may be accentuated as a normal variant. The occurrence of two audible components of S_2 at the apex, therefore, should alert the physician to the presence of pulmonary hypertension. P_2 may be louder in such conditions as congestive heart failure, mitral stenosis, Eisenmenger's syndrome or other congenital heart diseases (Figure 15). Splitting of S_2 is more pronounced in patients with Eisenmenger's syndrome due to atrial septal defect than with ventricular septal defect or patent ductus arteriosus. In addition, the increased size and relative proximity of the aorta, or pulmonary artery, and the enhancement of sound transmission to the chest wall, as may occur with dilatation of the aorta

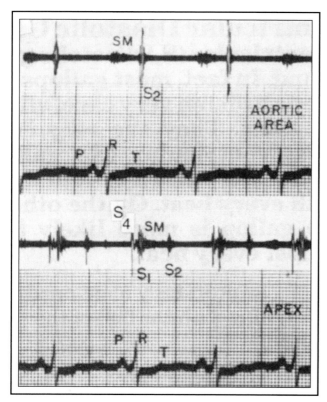

Figure 14. Note the loud "tambour" second heart sound (S₂) due to accentuation of the aortic component in a patient with systemic hypertension. Also note the atrial (S₄) gallop sound in presystole heard at the apex, not over the aortic area, and the short early midsystolic murmur (SM). *(From Harvey WP, 18.)*

(in hypertension, thoracic aneurysm, coarctation of the aorta) or pulmonary artery (in hypertension, idiopathic dilatation of the pulmonary artery) is often associated with accentuation of A_2 or P_2, respectively.

• Soft S_2

Impaired mobility of the aortic or pulmonic valve will result in the diminished intensity of their respective closure sounds. In severe calcific aortic stenosis with a completely immobile valve, A_2 may be faint, or even absent. This is in contrast to congenital aortic stenosis in a young adult, where the valve is still mobile and the aortic closure sound remains well-preserved. A_2 intensity may also be diminished when ventricular decompensation is present, e.g., after an acute myocardial infarction and in the setting of hypotension and shock with decreased pressure beyond the semilunar valve. A decreased intensity of the pulmonic component is most common in the patient with pulmonic stenosis. In this case, P_2 is often markedly delayed (wide splitting of S_2), faint or absent. In a cyanotic patient with classic Tetralogy of Fallot, P_2 may also be faint or absent. It should be realized that one of the most

common causes of a soft S_2, especially the pulmonic component, is the inability to hear this fainter sound in the presence of emphysema, obesity, respiratory noise or an abnormal chest configuration.

Sounds in Systole

Ejection Sounds

Normally, the opening of the aortic or pulmonic valves and the onset of ventricular ejection is acoustically silent. In certain cardiac conditions, extra sounds in early systole occurring shortly after S_1 may be heard and are referred to as aortic or pulmonic ejection sounds, since they occur at the onset of ventricular ejection and systolic flow into the great vessels (Table 3). Heard best with the diaphragm chest piece, these sounds are brief, sharp and high-pitched, and frequently occur close enough to S_1 to simulate splitting. They are usually the result of "doming" of the maximal opening motion of a congenitally stenotic, but mobile and compliant, aortic or pulmonic valve (valvular origin). The presence of an ejection sound, when heard in association with evidence of LV or RV outflow tract obstruction, helps to identify the site of obstruction at the valvular level. In other cases they are due to abrupt "checking" of the rapid initial systolic distention of a dilated ascending aorta, or main pulmonary artery with resultant vibrations of the cardiohemic system (vascular origin). It is important that the physician become adept in the detection of ejection sounds, as they often serve as one of the first clues to the diagnosis of these conditions.

• Aortic Ejection Sounds

Aortic ejection sounds are widely transmitted over the precordium, but are best heard in the aor-

---

TABLE 3

Ejection Sounds

Aortic ejection sounds

Aortic valve abnormality (e.g., congenital bicuspid aortic valve, AS, AI)

Dilatation of the aortic root (aneurysm, hypertension)

Forceful LV ejection (e.g., thyrotoxicosis, anemia, pregnancy, exercise, high cardiac output states)

Prosthetic (mechanical) aortic valve opening

Pulmonic ejection sounds

Pulmonic valve abnormality (e.g., PS)

Dilatation of the pulmonary artery

AS = aortic stenosis; AI = aortic insufficiency; LV = left ventricular; PS = pulmonic stenosis. *(From Chizner MA, 5.)*

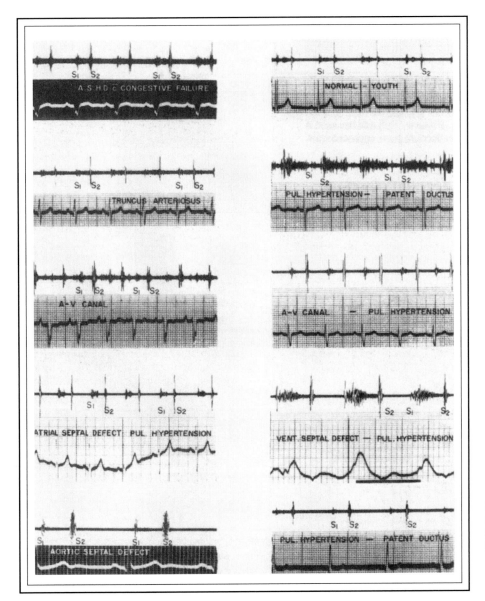

Figure 15. Composite tracings of various causes of a loud second heart sound (S₂) due to an accentuated pulmonic valve closure. *(From Harvey WP, 18.)*

tic area (second right intercostal space) and at the cardiac apex, where they may even be loudest. They are commonly heard in conditions in which an abnormality of the aortic valve is present, e.g., congenital bicuspid aortic valve, valvular aortic stenosis, or aortic regurgitation, or when dilatation of the aortic root exists, e.g., hypertension or aneurysm of the ascending aorta (Figure 16). They may also be heard in clinical conditions associated with forceful left ventricular ejection, e.g., thyrotoxicosis, anemia, pregnancy, exercise, high cardiac output states.

An ejection sound in a patient with coarctation of the aorta is a practical auscultatory finding that may afford the physician an immediate clue to the presence of a bicuspid aortic valve, which is the most common congenital defect associated with this condition. In persons between ages fifteen and sixty-

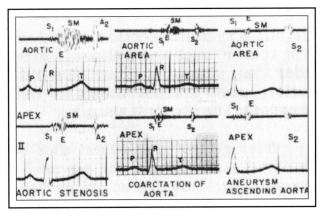

Figure 16. Composite of aortic ejection sounds (E) in patients with bicuspid aortic valve (aortic stenosis, coarctation of aorta) and dilated aorta (aneurysm of ascending aorta). The aortic ejection sound is well heard at the apex and the base (aortic area) and is not influenced by respiration. *(From Harvey WP, 18.)*

129

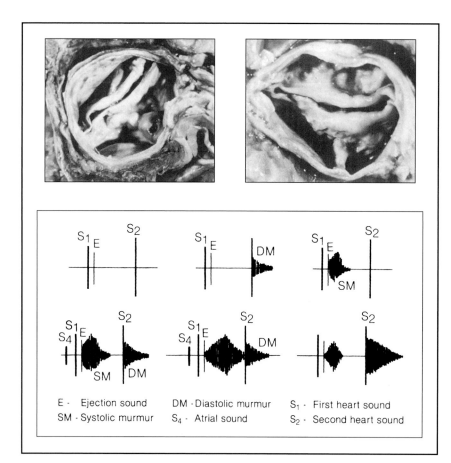

Figure 17. Top, Pathologic specimen of bicuspid aortic valve. Bottom, Schematic diagram of the auscultatory findings present with a bicuspid aortic valve. The spectrum may vary from only an ejection sound (E) and no murmur, to a systolic murmur (SM), diastolic murmur (DM) or both. An atrial (S_4) gallop is present with the more severe degrees of stenosis. *(Courtesy of WC Roberts; from Harvey WP and Canfield D, 19.)*

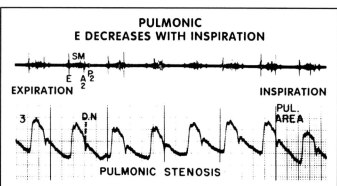

Figure 18. Patient with congenital pulmonic stenosis. Note the pulmonic ejection sound (E) that characteristically decreases during inspiration. This is in contrast to the aortic ejection sound which does not change with respiration. Note also the crescendo-decrescendo systolic murmur (SM) extending up to and including aortic component of S_2, and widely split S_2 with faint, delayed P_2. *(From Levine SA, Harvey WP, 30.)*

five (particularly male), it is highly probable that aortic stenosis, unassociated with a mitral valve lesion, is caused by a congenital bicuspid valve rather than rheumatic fever. In a number of patients with a congenital bicuspid aortic valve, an ejection sound is an early (and may be the only) auscultatory finding signaling its presence. The spectrum of findings, however, is variable (Figure 17).

Worthy of emphasis, when an early to midsystolic murmur is present, even if brief and with all of the characteristics resembling an "innocent" murmur, an audible ejection sound should provide an immediate clue that the murmur is one of significance, and serves to pinpoint the presence of underlying aortic valve pathology. The clinical recogni-

tion of this sound, therefore, enables these patients to receive antibiotic prophylaxis to protect against infective endocarditis.

Unlike pulmonic ejection sounds, the aortic ejection sound does not fluctuate in intensity with respiration. It is of much value in identifying the level, but not the severity, of left ventricular outflow tract obstruction. The presence of a crisp ejection sound in aortic stenosis, often accompanied by a well-preserved A_2, implies that the valve is supple, noncalcified, and still capable of movement, and is commonly heard in mild or severe congenital aortic stenosis in children and young adults. By contrast in older adult patients with severe calcific aortic stenosis and frozen immobile valves, the ejection

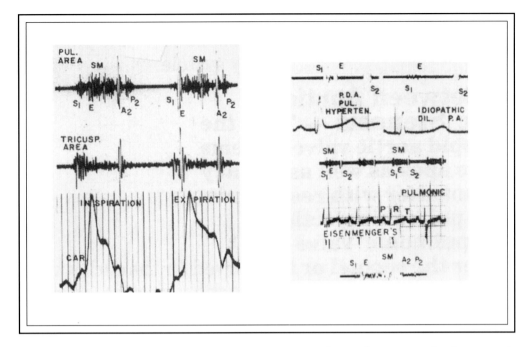

Figure 19. Composite of various pulmonic ejection sounds in pulmonic valvular stenosis, pulmonary hypertension, and idiopathic dilatation of the pulmonary artery. *(From Harvey WP, 18.)*

sound is no longer heard, and the aortic second sound diminishes or is absent as well.

• Pulmonic Ejection Sounds

Pulmonic ejection sounds, e.g., those caused by pulmonic valve stenosis are best heard in the pulmonic area and along the left sternal border. The timing, intensity and presence of the pulmonic ejection sound is related to the severity of the stenosis and to the respiratory cycle. These brief, high pitched, sharp sounds, unlike those of aortic stenosis, radiate poorly and characteristically and selectively diminish in intensity or disappear with inspiration, becoming louder again during expiration (Figure 18). In fact, pulmonic ejection sounds, in contrast to other right heart events, are the only sounds originating from the right side that decrease in intensity on inspiration. During expiration the valve leaflets are in the closed position and have a greater forward excursion before being abruptly checked in systole, thereby creating a loud systolic ejection sound. However, during inspiration, the inflow of blood to the right ventricle may move the stenotic pulmonary valve leaflets to a more open position, resulting in little additional systolic excursion and thereby diminishing the intensity of the ejection sound.

The interval between the first heart sound and the pulmonic ejection sound varies inversely with the degree of obstruction. The milder the obstruction, the later and louder the ejection sound. As the severity of stenosis increases, the pulmonic ejection sound moves closer to S_1, and in severe pulmonic stenosis when there is very little valve motion at the time of valve opening, the ejection sound is absent. The presence of an ejection sound identifies the obstruction at the valvular level and helps differentiate pulmonic valve stenosis from infundibular stenosis.

Pulmonic ejection sounds, however, are also heard in patients with dilatation of the pulmonary artery due to pulmonary hypertension, primary or secondary to a variety of causes, e.g., ventricular septal defect, atrial septal defect, patent ductus arteriosus, or to a large pulmonary blood flow in the absence of pulmonary hypertension (Figure 19). Under these conditions, the origin of the sound is probably vascular rather than valvular, and the selective respiratory variation in intensity may be absent or less prominent, in contrast to the valvular pulmonic ejection sound. Timing of the pulmonary artery ejection sound varies with the distensibility or compliance of the vessel. The greater the distensibility, the greater the delay and the later the timing of the ejection sound.

Ejection sounds may also accompany the opening movement of a mechanical prosthetic aortic valve, e.g., the Starr-Edwards ball-in-cage valve, Bjork-Shiley tilting-disk, and St. Jude bi-leaflet prosthesis. The relative intensity of these sounds varies according to the type and design of the prosthetic valve. The ball-in-cage valve produces the loudest sounds, simulating the rolling of dice as the ball "jiggles" at the top of the cage during systole. They are normally absent, however, with a porcine heterograft (tissue) valve, e.g., Hancock-Carpentier-Edwards bioprosthesis. Alteration in intensity, presence, and timing of these distinctive sounds

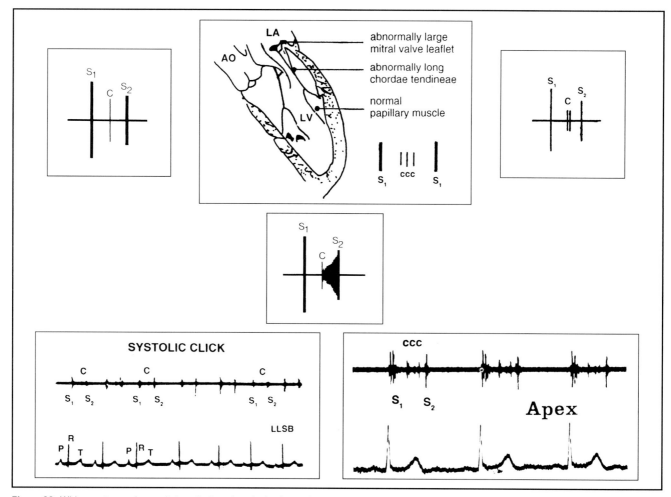

Figure 20. Wide spectrum of auscultatory findings in mitral valve prolapse: single click, multiple clicks, and/or systolic murmur. The number of clicks may vary, even in the same patient. Note the schematic diagram of the left ventricle and mitral valve; clicks occur when the mitral leaflet is checked at the farthest extent of its valve motion. *(Courtesy of WP Harvey)*

and the characteristic features of associated murmurs, provide clues to the state of prosthetic valve function. The disappearance or absence of previously heard opening or closing sounds with a mechanical prosthesis and the development of a new murmur usually indicates significant prosthetic valve dysfunction, e.g., due to thrombus, tissue ingrowth or ball variance.

Systolic Clicks

Systolic clicks are discrete high-frequency sounds caused by prolapse of the mitral valve leaflets into the left atrium during systole. Either or both of the anterior and posterior leaflets may be involved. Prolapse may also occur in the tricuspid valve. Isolated tricuspid valve prolapse, however, occurs only rarely, and in most instances accompanies mitral valve prolapse. Systolic clicks may be single or multiple, heard best at the cardiac apex or lower left sternal border, and are usually mid to late systolic in timing, although occasionally they occur suf-

ficiently early to simulate an ejection sound. They are thought to be generated by the sudden tensing of the redundant mitral valve leaflets and elongated chordae tendineae, and they coincide in timing with the maximal excursion of the prolapsed leaflets of the mitral valve into the atrium (Figure 20).

The auscultatory findings in these patients, and even in the same patient at different times on serial examinations, are notoriously variable and represent a wide spectrum. Occasionally, no click or murmur is present. One negative examination, therefore, does not exclude the diagnosis. At other times, an isolated systolic click (or clicks) with or without a mid to late systolic (crescendo-decrescendo or crescendo to the second heart sound), or holosystolic murmur, or musical "whoop" or "honk" of mitral regurgitation may be audible (Figure 21). The presence of a click or clicks without a murmur, is often associated with anterior mitral leaflet prolapse, whereas murmurs of mitral regurgitation occur frequently when the posterior leaflet alone prolapses.

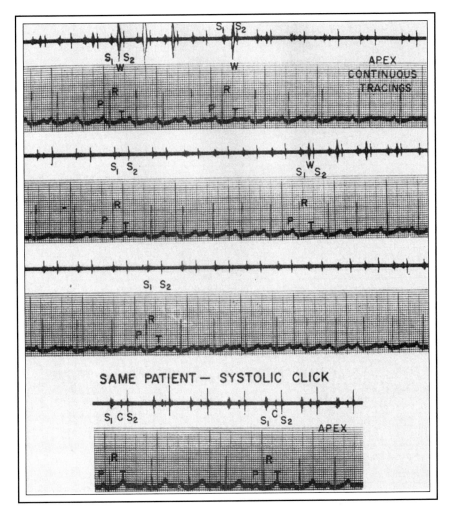

SAME PATIENT — SYSTOLIC CLICK

Figure 21. Variable auscultatory spectrum in mitral valve prolapse. At times no click (C) or murmur is present (panel three). At other times an isolated systolic click (or clicks), systolic murmur or musical systolic "whoop" (W) of mitral regurgitation is heard.
(From Harvey WP, 18.)

Careful auscultation in multiple positions (supine, left lateral decubitus position, sitting, standing, squatting) or after bedside maneuvers, e.g., Valsalva, may be required to "bring out" or enhance these auscultatory features. Sometimes the typical findings are heard only in one phase of respiration, e.g., some in the early part of inspiration, others during expiration. Another variant present on occasion, is a succession of systolic clicks simulating the flipping of a deck of cards, heard only in the early part of systole along the mid to lower left sternal border rather than at the apex. When these multiple clicks occur in such close succession, they may be misinterpreted as a "scratchy" systolic murmur.

CARDIAC PEARL

Seldom Recognized Variant of Mitral Valve Prolapse- Systolic clicks generally occur in mid to late systole. However, a seldom recognized variant of mitral valve prolapse is that they can occur in early to mid systole; they can be multiple and rapid and can simulate the flipping of a deck of cards or the creaking of new leather. Once one has heard this variant of mitral valve prolapse, it should be accurately diagnosed in others.

This variant is also different in that these clicks are usually better heard over the third left sternal border and pulmonic area rather than the lower left sternal border and apex. Although I have seen about 100 patients having this variant (also documented on echocardiography) I have not seen it reported in the medical literature.

It can simulate and be misdiagnosed as a pericardial friction rub because of these multiple rapid sounds in systole. However, if we remember the cardiac pearl of friction rubs, this confusion should not occur.

A pericardial friction rub has 2 or 3 components rather than only one is systole: (1) the atrial systolic, (2) the ventricular systolic, and (3) the ventricular diastolic.

W. Proctor Harvey, M.D.

Although there is no strict correlation between murmur intensity and severity of mitral regurgita-

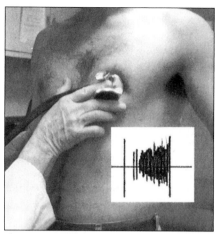
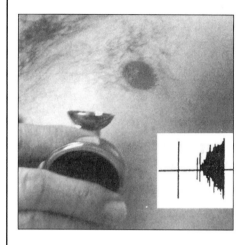
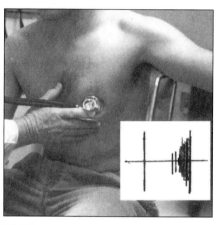

Figure 22. Movement of systolic click(s) and murmur of mitral valve prolapse with change of position. Left: Supine, note two systolic clicks in midsystole followed by late apical systolic murmur (SM). Top right: Standing, the systolic clicks and murmur move toward the first heart sound (S_1) and the murmur becomes longer and often louder. Bottom right: Squatting, the clicks and murmur move toward the second heart sound. *(From Harvey WP, 18.)*

tion, as a rule, the combination of a midsystolic click (or clicks) and a murmur confined to late systole is associated with a mild degree of mitral regurgitation rather than with the more severe degrees of regurgitation. When the leak is severe, the prolapse occurs early in systole, and the click fuses with the first heart sound, resulting in a loud S_1 followed by a holosystolic murmur, accompanied by a rapid ventricular (S_3) filling sound. The presence, intensity, and timing of the clicks heard at the bedside may vary dramatically depending upon the degree of left ventricular volume. Any physiologic maneuver or manipulation that decreases left ventricular cavity size and volume, e.g., sitting, standing, Valsalva maneuver or inspiration, will increase the amount of redundancy, causing the valve leaflets to prolapse into the left atrium earlier in systole, thereby accentuating and moving the onset of the click and murmur toward the first heart sound (Figure 22). Conversely, maneuvers that augment venous return and increase ventricular volume or increase systemic vascular resistance and raise afterload, e.g., squatting, leg raising, hand grip, cause the mitral valve leaflets to prolapse at a

later time in systole, and the click to move toward the second heart sound, and the murmur to become shorter and softer. The click and murmur may be masked or disappear altogether with the increased blood volume and ventricular dimensions during pregnancy, returning after delivery in the postpartum state. Likewise, beta blocking agents, frequently used in these patients, decrease heart rate and contractility and increase ventricular volume, and may attenuate or abolish the classic auscultatory findings of mitral valve prolapse. These auscultatory phenomena, therefore, may help explain why patients with mitral valve prolapse may have no acoustic findings on one occasion yet prominent findings on another.

Today, careful examination with a stethoscope is still the most valuable and cost-effective means of diagnosing the prolapsing mitral valve leaflet syndrome. The diagnostic acoustic hallmark, the systolic click, may even be heard in patients with no evidence of mitral valve prolapse on echocardiography. Although it does not require special skill to hear these clicks, they have often been overlooked when the physician does not properly time them or

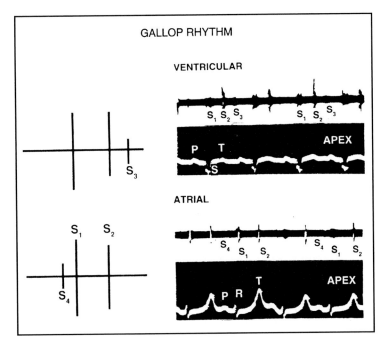

GALLOP RHYTHM

VENTRICULAR

S_1 S_2 S_3 S_1 S_2 S_3

P   T   APEX

S

S_3

ATRIAL

S_4 S_1 S_2 S_4 S_1 S_2

P   R   T   APEX

S_1 S_2

S_4

Figure 23. Gallops are diastolic filling sounds. Top, The ventricular gallop (S_3) is a low-frequency sound occurring after S_2 in early diastole, at the end of rapid ventricular filling. Bottom, The atrial gallop (S_4) is a low-frequency sound in late diastole that is generated in the ventricle but is secondary to atrial contraction and is heard before S_1. *(From Levine SA, Harvey WP, 30.)*

listen specifically for these high pitched sounds in systole. As a rule, the findings are best detected using the flat diaphragm chest piece of the stethoscope. The auscultatory phenomena described usually occur in otherwise healthy asymptomatic individuals, often young women. However, a variety of symptoms and associated complications may occur. These include: atypical chest pain, dyspnea, palpitations (attributed to arrhythmias), chronic anxiety, panic reactions, fatigue, autonomic nervous system dysfunction, high adrenergic tone, orthostatic hypotension, dizziness, syncope, transient cerebral ischemic attacks, musculoskeletal abnormalities of the rib cage and thoracic vertebrae (e.g., pectus excavatum, straight back, narrow anterior-posterior diameter, kyphoscoliosis), hypermobility of the joints, hypomastia, asthenic body habitus, progressive mitral regurgitation, ruptured chordae tendineae, mitral anular calcification, and rarely sudden death. Infective endocarditis may occur on the mitral valve in these cases, even when only click (or clicks) and no murmur is detected. Accurate diagnosis is therefore essential in this syndrome to ensure that these patients receive antibiotic prophylaxis before dental cleaning and manipulation as well as other surgical and diagnostic bacteremic procedures.

Idiopathic mitral valve prolapse (myxomatous degeneration) has proved to be the most common basis for systolic clicks. Other heart diseases, however, have been associated with systolic clicks including Marfan's syndrome, ostium secundum atrial septal defect, papillary muscle dysfunction secondary to coronary artery disease, and car-

diomyopathy. Systolic clicks have also been noted after trauma and following mitral commissurotomy.

Sounds in Diastole

Third Heart Sound

Filling sounds are referred to as third (S_3), or ventricular and fourth (S_4), or atrial gallop sounds and are produced by papillary-chordal apparatus tensing and blood deceleration during early diastolic rapid filling (S_3) and following atrial contraction (S_4) in late diastole (pre-systole) (Figure 23). The third heart sound is a low frequency, often soft and faint sound, which is closely associated with the rapid influx of blood into the ventricles in early diastole. It follows the second heart sound by an average of 0.15 seconds and may originate in either the left or right ventricle (Table 4).

These heart sounds may be normal or physiologic, or they may be pathologic. They are a common and physiologic finding when heard in a healthy child and young adult with rapid filling rates and large flow volumes without any other stigmata of heart disease. A physiologic S_3 is often accentuated and more easily heard in normal pregnant women during the third trimester of pregnancy because of increased cardiac output and more active filling of the ventricles during diastole. This sound waxes and wanes during respiration and is best heard at the beginning of expiration. The physiologic S_3 is common in children and young adults, since the left ventricle is normally compliant, thus permitting rapid filling. The occurrence of a physiologic S_3 diminishes with advancing age,

---

T A B L E   4

Third Heart Sound

- Physiologic S₃: normal sound heard in healthy child or young adult, athlete, hyperkinetic states, or third trimester of pregnancy.

- Pathologic S₃: abnormal sound heard in ventricular failure (LV and RV) and mitral or aortic regurgitation, VSD or PDA (due to large volume of ventricular flow).

LV = left ventricular; RV = right ventricular; VSD = ventricular septal defect; PDA = patent ductus arteriosus. *(From Chizner MA, 5.)*

---

however, as the left ventricle becomes less compliant, disappearing in most men by the age of twenty to thirty years, and in most women by the age of thirty to forty years. Occasionally, however, both men and women retain their normal third heart sounds beyond these age limits, especially those who have continued to engage in athletic endeavors, e.g., jogging, swimming, and squash. Ironically, in later life, age fifty and above, the presence of the third heart sound which was a perfectly normal finding heard in youth, may now afford one of the earliest and most subtle clinical clues to the presence of circulatory overload or cardiac decompensation in adults, and thus has a great diagnostic and prognostic value.

The determination of whether an S₃ is a normal "physiologic" sound or a "pathologic" ventricular diastolic gallop often rests on the clinical context in which it occurs, i.e., the presence or absence of other evidence of heart disease, rather than on any distinctive auscultatory properties of the sounds themselves. "Gallop rhythm" describes a sequence of tripling or quadrupling of heart sounds, a characteristic auscultatory cadence which resembles the canter of a horse. Since gallops are low in frequency and faint, they may be difficult to detect by auscultation. One must be careful, therefore, to search specifically for these sounds in a quiet room using special stethoscopic techniques. Maximal audibility of left-sided S₄ and S₃ gallops can be facilitated by turning the patient to the left lateral decubitus position, locating the point of maximum impulse of the left ventricle with the palpating hand, and then placing the bell of the stethoscope lightly over this localized area, barely making an air seal. Worthy of re-emphasis, care must be taken not to press the bell too firmly on the skin, since tension makes the skin act as a diaphragm which will tend to filter out low frequency sounds. This simple, but fundamental, bedside maneuver may detect gallops when they are not heard or are overlooked in any other location. Because S₃ is associated with blood volume and velocity, listening intently and specifically

after extrasystoles, exercise, leg-raising, and cough, may augment stroke volume and rapid ventricular filling, and accentuate or "bring out" this faint gallop sound.

Gallops can originate in either the left or right ventricle. Right-sided gallops usually exhibit inspiratory increase and are heard best along the lower left sternal border or over the xiphoid region. On the other hand, left-sided gallops do not vary with respiration and are more easily audible during expiration, (less interposed lung space). They are heard best over the apex. Right ventricular gallops become louder during inspiration because of the increase in venous return and blood flow to the right ventricle. In patients with an increase in the anterior-posterior diameter of the chest, e.g., in pulmonary emphysema, right-sided gallops are often best heard over the xiphoid area or just below the xiphoid in the epigastric region. Right-sided S₃ gallops are present in patients with dilated right ventricles and elevated right heart pressures. These sounds, therefore, may even be heard over the cardiac apex when the dilated right ventricle occupies it. They are commonly heard in those patients with right ventricular failure, tricuspid insufficiency, pulmonary hypertension, cor pulmonale due to pulmonary emboli or pulmonary parenchymal or vascular disease, etc.

Ventricular diastolic gallops may be present when ventricular dilatation and failure occur, and they provide valuable bedside information regarding myocardial function. These gallops are frequent in patients with acute myocardial infarction and are associated with an abnormally elevated left ventricular filling pressure. In these circumstances, the appearance of a ventricular gallop denotes more severe changes in left ventricular compliance and usually implies more extensive and advanced left ventricular damage and dysfunction. The intensity of an S₃ gallop tends to diminish spontaneously during the healing phase of the infarction. If louder and more persistent, however, particularly when associated with sinus tachycardia, the S₃ gallop reflects a greater loss of LV function and carries a poor prognosis. Prompt subsidence of the S₃ gallop suggests that cardiac compensation is restored with recovery of function of "stunned" or "hibernating" myocardium, a favorable response to therapy, and thus a brighter outlook.

Gallop rhythm is the hallmark of cardiomyopathy. The detection of pulsus alternans on careful palpation of the radial arterial pulse is often associated with this ventricular filling sound, and may also be one of the earliest and most subtle signs of heart failure and cardiac decompensation. The bedside recognition of pulsus alternans, ventricular

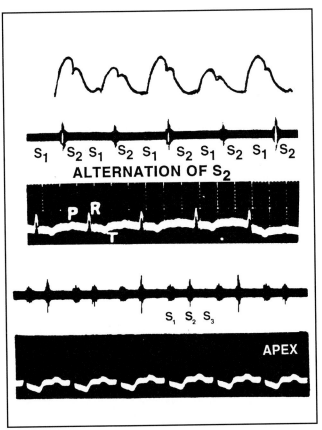

Figure 24. Pulsus alternans on palpation of the radial pulse (top) has a high correlation with alternations of the second heart sounds (middle) and with ventricular diastolic gallops (S_3) (bottom).
(From Harvey WP, 18.)

diastolic gallop, and alternation of the intensity or quality of heart sounds, especially the second heart sound and heart murmurs, are all clues to the presence of myocardial weakness (Figure 24).

The physician can usually palpate these filling sounds over the point of maximal impulse with the patient in the left lateral decubitus position. They may even be seen or felt better than they can be heard, a fact that supports the concept that these sounds may be caused by the impact of the heart on the chest wall. However, if one listens carefully and specifically, and "tunes in" for these faint low-frequency sounds using the special stethoscopic techniques previously mentioned, they will generally be heard in the majority of cases.

CARDIAC PEARL

The ventricular (S_3) diastolic gallop has clinical connotations different from those of the atrial (S_4) gallop. It is frequently one of the first signs that one can detect indicating serious heart disease and/or cardiac decompensation. This gallop appears in the early part of diastole, later than the opening snap of mitral stenosis but at the same time as the normal physiological third heart sound heard in the young. If searched for, the ventricular diastolic gallop is a common finding and can appear in a great variety of diseased states of the heart, including those due to coronary heart disease; cardiomyopathy; and others. A ventricular diastolic gallop may be one of the earliest clinical findings of cardiac dysfunction. The majority of these gallop sounds are faint, and because of this they are frequently overlooked.

Since most gallop sounds are faint, a special technique must be employed to detect them. The patient should be recumbent and examined in a quiet room. Closing the door that leads to the corridor of the hospital, closing windows, or turning off fans or the air conditioner may make the difference as to whether a gallop is heard or not. If one exerts normal pressure with the flat diaphragm of the stethoscope, the gallop, though present, may not be heard, or may be greatly diminished (Fig. A). Very light pressure with the bell of the stethoscope is necessary to hear the low-frequency vibrations. Gallop sounds from the left ventricle are often best heard by having the patient turn to the left lateral position; the physician then listens at the point of maximum impulse in the apical area (this is similar to the maneuver that one uses when listening for the localized rumble of mitral stenosis) (Fig. B). It is of great importance to use palpation first to detect this point of maximum impulse of the left ventricle after the patient has turned to the left lateral position.

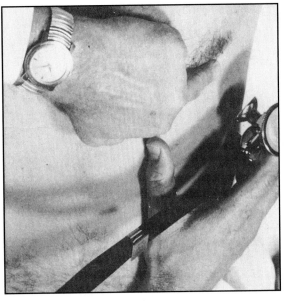

Fig A: Note disappearance of S_3 with firm pressure of stethoscope.

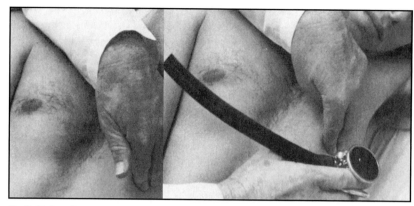

Fig B: To Best Detect an S₃ Gallop - The patient is turned to the left lateral position. The index and middle fingers of the left hand palpate the point of maximal impulse of the left ventricle; holding that spot, the bell of the stethoscope is placed lightly over it, barely making an air seal with the skin of the chest wall.

The stethoscope is then placed over this localized area, and the gallop sound is either heard for the first time or is accentuated in intensity. At times, however, a ventricular gallop sound is well heard along the lower left sternal border and apex and with the patient recumbent. This usually indicates the gallop sound originates in the right ventricle. Right ventricular (S₃) gallop sounds usually become louder with inspiration. Both atrial and ventricular gallops generally become fainter when the patient sits or stands. At times the gallop sounds are better heard after slight physical effort, and when the blood flow and heart rate are somewhat accelerated. Having the patient cough five or six times may bring out the faint gallop. Occasionally, a gallop sound is detected when one listens after the patient has had brief exertion, such as walking, climbing a flight of stairs, or performing a number of sit-ups on the examining table. The quality of sounds simulating a horse galloping is more likely to be noticed when the heart rate is increased. It should be emphasized, however, that a gallop occurring at a slow rate still has the same significance that it would have when heard at a faster rate.

W. Proctor Harvey, M.D.

Sometimes, especially in the presence of sinus tachycardia, both atrial and ventricular diastolic gallops can occur in close proximity to one another, producing a short, low-pitched, rumbling diastolic murmur which may at times simulate the murmur of mitral stenosis. If these gallops occur at the same time and fuse in diastole, a prominent sound referred to as a "summation" gallop may result, which may be louder than both the first and second heart sounds.

Pathologic third heart sounds do not always connote heart failure and may result not only when blood entering the ventricle decelerates rapidly in the presence of a stiff noncompliant failing left ventricle, but also if blood rapidly accelerates into the ventricle because of an increased volume of flow. A rapid left ventricular filling sound may occur, therefore, in the setting of hemodynamically significant mitral or aortic regurgitation, and a large left-to-right shunt, e.g., ventricular septal defect or patent ductus arteriosus. In the more severe cases, a mid- diastolic flow rumble and an enlarged, inferolaterally displaced left ventricular apical impulse, in addition to the S₃, may also be present. Likewise, a right-sided S₃ and a parasternal mid-diastolic flow rumble of right-sided origin that increases in intensity with inspiration are heard with large left-to-right shunts at the atrial level (atrial septal defect) and the more severe cases of tricuspid regurgitation. These findings are often accompanied by abnormal CV waves of the jugular venous pulse and palpable systolic pulsations of the liver. In contrast, a ventricular third heart sound would not be the expected finding in tight mitral or tricuspid stenosis. In fact, an audible third heart sound in isolated mitral or tricuspid valve disease virtually excludes the diagnosis of severe mitral or tricuspid stenosis.

Fourth Heart Sound

The fourth heart sound or atrial (S₄) gallop is related to atrial contraction and may occur with or without clinical evidence of cardiac decompensation (Table 5). The atrial gallop sound usually just precedes the first heart sound in presystole and may be heard with ventricular failure, but unlike the S₃ gallop, it is not by itself a sign of ventricular decompensation. Instead, an S₄ gallop implies the presence of decreased ventricular compliance which necessitates a more forceful atrial contraction for

138

TABLE 5

Fourth Heart Sound

- Due to forceful atrial contractions necessitated by decreased ventricular compliance ("stiffer ventricle"), e.g., AS, hypertension, coronary artery disease (AMI, angina), cardiomyopathy (dilated, hypertrophic, restrictive), PS, pulmonary hypertension.
- Acute severe mitral regurgitation (not chronic where the LA is dilated and unable to generate a forceful atrial contraction).
- Long PR interval (first-degree AV block).
- Normal in some apparently healthy older persons.

AS = aortic stenosis; AMI = acute myocardial infarction;
PS = pulmonic stenosis; LA = left atrium. *(From Chizner MA, 5.)*

completion of ventricular filling. This change in compliance may be related to ventricular hypertrophy, ischemia, infarction, fibrosis or an increased afterload, e.g., elevated aortic or pulmonary artery pressure (systemic or pulmonary arterial hypertension) (Figure 25).

An S_4 gallop may be detected, if carefully searched for, in almost all patients with an acute myocardial infarction due to the presence of a stiff, noncompliant, ischemic recipient left ventricle, and may become louder during the early phase of infarction or during an episode of angina pectoris. The S_4 gallop may therefore provide a useful clue if it appears intermittently during attacks of chest

pain suspected of being ischemic in etiology. Likewise, since the atrial (S_4) gallop appears almost universally in patients with acute myocardial infarction, its absence should raise serious doubts as to the diagnosis. It is most unusual not to hear an S_4 gallop in those patients who are in normal sinus rhythm and have had a prior myocardial infarction.

CARDIAC PEARL

An atrial (S_4) gallop sound is related to atrial contraction and may occur with or without any clinical evidence of cardiac decompensation. A left ventricular gallop sound is heard at the apex and a right ventricular atrial gallop sound is heard over the right ventricle. The latter may be louder during inspiration. An atrial gallop sound (S_4) is a frequent finding in patients with cardiomyopathy (primary myocardial disease), coronary artery disease, hypertension (systemic and pulmonary), and with the more severe degrees of aortic and pulmonic stenosis. It can also occur when there is a delay in atrioventricular conduction (prolongation of the PR interval on the electrocardiogram) and, in addition, may be heard in some normal hearts. If one searches carefully for an atrial sound or gallop, it is most commonly heard in

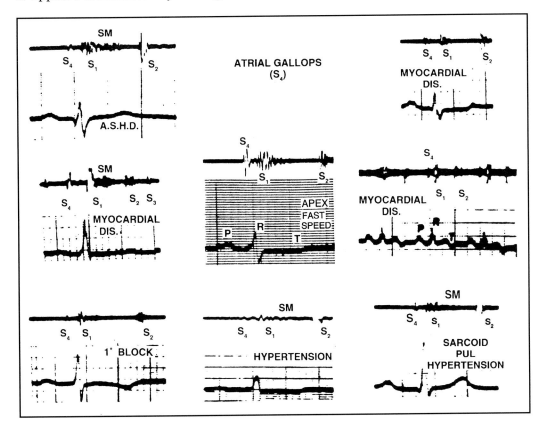

Figure 25. Composite of various atrial gallops (S_4) in coronary artery disease, hypertensive cardiovascular disease, cardiomyopathy, and first degree atrioventricular block. *(From Levine SA, Harvey WP, 30.)*

139

patients with coronary artery disease, and at times this may be one of the first clues from the physical examination as to the presence of underlying heart disease. It would be unusual not to hear a faint atrial gallop sound in a patient who has had a previous myocardial infarction.

The atrial gallop sound associated with myocardial infarction may be easily heard, or it may be faint- more commonly, it is faint. The sound is often louder during an episode of acute myocardial ischemia and pain, or during the initial phases of myocardial infarction. Subsequently, usually with improvement of the patient, the gallop sound becomes fainter but, if carefully searched for, can generally be heard.

W. Proctor Harvey, M.D.

Various myocardial diseases, e.g., cardiomyopathy (congestive-dilated, hypertrophic, restrictive-obliterative), increase resistance to ventricular filling by reducing myocardial compliance, thereby causing atrial sounds. An atrial gallop may also be heard in significant valvular aortic stenosis and systemic hypertension, associated with concentric left ventricular hypertrophy and stiffening of the ventricular wall, leading to a more vigorous atrial contraction. The detection of an atrial (S_4) gallop and a loud "tambour" second heart sound (A_2) are the earliest auscultatory findings detected in hypertensive cardiovascular disease, often preceding electrocardiographic and other signs of left ventricular hypertrophy.

It has been stated that an audible S_4 gallop in a patient under the age of forty, with valvular aortic stenosis, correlates with higher degrees of severity of outflow tract obstruction (peak systolic gradient of 70 mmHg). Since older patients may have an atrial sound for additional reasons (e.g., the coexistence of coronary artery disease, hypertension and the aging effects on the myocardium), its diagnostic specificity is markedly reduced. The presence of an atrial (S_4) gallop, therefore, may be difficult to interpret as an index of severity of obstruction in these patients.

Atrial gallops are also commonly heard in patients with acute severe mitral regurgitation (e.g., ruptured chordae tendineae, papillary muscle rupture following an acute myocardial infarction), reflecting the persistence of vigorous left atrial contraction resulting in acceleration of blood flow into the left ventricle. This contrasts sharply with the absence of an S_4 gallop in chronic mitral regurgitation, since the left atrium is large, dilated and unable to generate much contractile force. The presence of an atrial (S_4) gallop sound in conjunction with the murmur of mitral regurgitation is, therefore, an important clue alerting the physician that the valve insufficiency is acute or of recent onset.

An audible S_4 is an unusual finding in the normal heart in patients under fifty years of age, except in the presence of AV heart block. When there is a delay in AV conduction, as occurs with first degree AV block (prolonged PR interval), the resulting separation of atrial contraction from ventricular contraction creates an audible prominent S_4. The presence of an atrial gallop, in association with a faint S_1, lends confirmation to the bedside suspicion of first degree AV block. Likewise, severe pulmonic stenosis, pulmonary hypertension from various causes (e.g., massive pulmonary embolism, chronic cor pulmonale) and right ventricular compliance changes, as may occur when a right ventricular infarction complicates an inferior-posterior wall myocardial infarction, are all associated with right-sided atrial (S_4) gallops. These gallops are best heard over the tricuspid area, becoming louder during inspiration as venous return to the right side of the heart is increased.

Atrial sounds may also be heard in apparently healthy individuals, particularly in young athletes with physiologic left ventricular hypertrophy and in the older population, owing to decreased ventricular compliance with increasing age, even in the absence of clinically detectable heart disease. The atrial (S_4) gallop is absent, however, in atrial fibrillation, because of the loss of effective coordinated atrial contraction. By contrast, the ventricular (S_3) diastolic gallop does not disappear with atrial fibrillation, but may require more concentration and attentive auscultation for its detection.

The fourth heart sound must be differentiated from other sounds which occur closely around the first heart sound. When the physician hears the double first sound complex, the differential includes a split S_1, S_4-S_1, S_1-ejection sound and, less frequently, an S_1-systolic click (See Table 6). This common auscultatory problem provides an important diagnostic challenge to the clinician. In general, the two components of a split S_1 (M_1 and T_1) are similar in frequency and are heard best with the diaphragm of the stethoscope at the left sternal border. The S_4 gallop, however, is of lower frequency than S_1 and is heard best at the cardiac apex with the bell of the stethoscope lightly applied to the point of maximal impulse of the left ventricle, and with the patient turned to the left lateral decubitus position. If firm pressure is exerted on the stethoscope, the bell functions as a diaphragm and filters out low frequency sounds. An S_4 gallop, therefore, should decrease in intensity, or even disappear when pressure on the bell of the stethoscope is increased, and it should reappear when light pressure is resumed. This would not occur with a split S_1, or an S_1 ejection sound. The two components around S_1 are higher in frequency and would tend to either persist unchanged, or become accentuated by this maneuver. In addition, the S_4 gallop may be associated with a palpable presystolic distention of the left ventricle, an additional diagnostic clue confirming its presence. The intensity of S_4 may also be increased by certain bedside maneuvers that increase venous return to the heart, e.g., exercise, leg raising, coughing, etc.

CARDIAC PEARL

When listening along the lower left sternal border, a faint sound, possibly atrial (S_4), is noted in presystole. Pearl: turn the patient to the left lateral position and listen over the point of maximum impulse of the left ventricle, with the bell of the stethoscope barely touching the skin of the chest wall to make a seal; the sound (S_4) becomes louder. Now press on the bell chest piece- this sound disappears or becomes fainter. This sound definitely is the S_4. Both atrial (S_4) and ventricular (S_3) diastolic gallops may be present in a patient. This occurrence is common in patients with cardiac decompensation associated with coronary heart disease, hypertensive heart disease, and dilated cardiomyopathy. When these diastolic filling sounds occur in close proximity, a short rumbling murmur may be heard. In fact, in the past a patient on two occasions was referred to me for mitral commissurotomy because of the presence of a diastolic rumble. This erroneous diagnosis of mitral stenosis occurred because two gallop sounds were heard, each with low frequency after-vibrations. Occurring close together, these sounds produced a low-frequency diastolic rumble. Surgery was, of course, avoided. Gallops occurring in close proximity should not be called a summation gallop. However, when diastole is shortened with an increase in heart rate in patients having both S_3 and S_4 gallops, these two gallops can occur exactly at the same time, producing a single loud sound in diastole, often louder than either S_1 or S_2. This is the true summation gallop.

W. Proctor Harvey, M.D.

Ejection sounds may be more difficult to differentiate from a split S_1, however, separation of S_1 and an ejection sound, or S_1 and an early systolic click, is generally wider. These sounds have a high pitch and

T A B L E 6	
Auscultatory Features of Double First Sound Complex	
DOUBLE FIRST SOUND COMPLEX	**AUSCULTATORY FEATURES**
A. Split S_1	Both components of S_1 (M_1 and T_1) are similar in frequency, and heard best with diaphragm chest piece at lower left sternal border and occasionally at apex, not at base.
B. S_4-S_1	S_4 is lower in frequency than S_1 and heard best at cardiac apex using light pressure of bell chest piece with patient in left lateral position. S_4 decreases or disappears with firm pressure on bell. Palpable presystolic distention of LV frequently present.
C. S_1/Ejection Sound (ES)	Separation of S_1 and ES is usually wider than split S_1.
	ES is high pitched, heard best with diaphragm chest piece.
	Aortic ES is loudest at aortic area and cardiac apex with no respiratory variation.
	Pulmonic ES is loudest at pulmonic area and decreases coincident with inspiration.
	Firm pressure on bell or diaphragm chest piece enhances audibility.
D. S_1/Systolic click (SC)	SC usually mid to late systolic in timing, varies in position with bedside maneuvers (standing - earlier in systole, squatting - later in systole).
	Late systolic murmur of mitral regurgitation frequently present.

are best heard with the diaphragm chest piece. By paying careful attention to location (aortic ejection sounds are loudest at the aortic area and apex, pulmonic ejection sounds are loudest at the pulmonic area) and selective respiratory variation in intensity (pulmonic ejection sounds decrease in intensity with inspiration, aortic ejection sounds do not vary with respiration), one should be able to differentiate the ejection sound from a split S_1. A split first heart sound is heard best at the lower left sternal border (tricuspid area) and occasionally at the apex, but not over the base (the right or left second interspace).

CARDIAC PEARL

In some patients having congenital heart disease, the first heart sound over the pulmonic area and third left sternal border may at first seem to be split. Often, however, this is

141

not splitting, but rather a pulmonary ejection sound occurring in early systole and related to: Congenital valvular pulmonic stenosis, idiopathic dilation of the pulmonary artery or pulmonary hypertension due to ventricular defect, atrial defect, patent ductus, and primary pulmonary hypertension. The pulmonary ejection sound may be well heard in expiration and decrease in intensity with inspiration.

The aortic ejection sound, however, is usually well heard at the apex and also at the aortic area. It does not diminish in intensity with inspiration.

The aortic ejection sound occurs when there is "doming" of the bicuspid valve in early systole. The same holds true for congenital stenosis of the pulmonary valve- the ejection sound occurs with it"doming" in early systole.

The ejection sound of a bicuspid aortic valve is generally well heard at the apex as well as over the aortic area. It does not alter with respiration. On the other hand, a pulmonic ejection sound from a congenital pulmonic valve stenosis usually localized over the second or third left sternal border, characteristically has an ejection sound that may decrease or even disappear coincident with inspiration. It is generally not heard at the apex as is the rule with a bicuspid aortic stenosis.

W. Proctor Harvey, M.D.

If the practitioner hears what appears to be a loud first sound in the pulmonic area, while remembering that S_2 is normally louder than S_1 in this location, it should be an immediate clue that this represents an ejection sound, unless the patient has an unusually loud S_1 at the apex, as may occur with mitral stenosis or short PR interval. One should not confuse the tricuspid closure sound (T_1) with the pulmonic ejection sound, since the intensity of T_1 tends to increase rather than decrease during inspiration.

TABLE 7
Early Diastolic Sounds

- Opening snap of mitral stenosis
- Pericardial knock sound of constrictive pericarditis
- Physiologic third heart sound
- Ventricular (S_3) diastolic gallop
- "Tumor plop" of atrial myxoma
- Opening sound of mechanical prosthetic mitral valve

S_3 = third heart sound. *(From Chizner MA, 5.)*

CARDIAC PEARL

Rule out a systolic ejection sound when the "first sound" over the pulmonic area seems louder than usual. This may be a pulmonary ejection sound masquerading (or being misinterpreted) as the first sound.

W. Proctor Harvey, M.D.

The timing of a systolic click is usually later (midsystole to late systole), and if early, will vary in position with various bedside maneuvers that alter ventricular volume (sitting or standing will cause the click to occur earlier in systole and closer to S_1, squatting will cause the click to occur later in systole and closer to S_2). These physical maneuvers, therefore, are helpful in distinguishing the systolic click of the mitral valve prolapse syndrome from aortic and pulmonic ejection sounds, because the ejection sound is relatively fixed in timing in early systole, compared with the first heart sound, despite maneuvers that alter the ventricular volume.

The fourth heart sounds emanating from the right side of the heart are heard best over the lower left sternal border and xiphoid region, and are enhanced by inspiration. They may be accompanied by other features of right ventricular involvement, including sustained parasternal lifts, palpable pulmonary artery systolic impulse, accentuated pulmonic component of S_2, and elevated jugular venous pressure and pulse with large A or V waves. Left-sided fourth heart sounds usually either decrease, or do not change in intensity, during inspiration. Right-sided S_4 gallops may be prominent in those patients with significant pulmonic stenosis, pulmonary hypertension, cor pulmonale, etc.

Opening Snap of Mitral Stenosis

The mitral opening snap (OS) is another important valve opening sound heard in clinical practice (Table 7). The opening of a normal mitral valve does not produce a clinically audible sound. When the valve becomes thickened and stenotic, however, a "classic" high-pitched, sharp snapping sound is heard as the opening movement of the mitral valve apparatus reaches its fullest extent and is suddenly arrested in early diastole. In the asymptomatic patient, or the symptomatic patient with unexplained dyspnea, atrial fibrillation or system embolism, the presence of an opening snap often affords the first clue to the diagnosis of mitral stenosis. It also provides useful information which strongly suggests that the valve is still capable of movement, an important surgical consideration. The intensity of the opening snap may be influ-

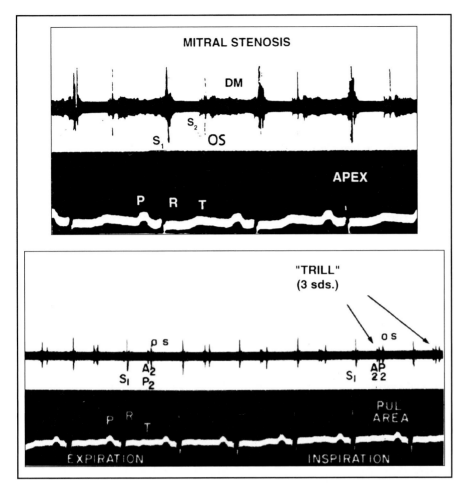

enced by the condition of the mitral valve itself, the level of left atrial pressure and cardiac output, and the presence of concomitant mitral insufficiency or aortic valve disease. A loud mitral opening snap suggests a supple, significantly stenosed valve with at least moderate cardiac output and significant left atrial pressure elevation.

In the most severe cases of mitral stenosis, however, heavily calcified or rigid, immobile valve cusps will diminish or abolish the opening snap and decrease the intensity of S_1 at the apex as well. A soft to absent opening snap may also be present with dominant mitral insufficiency, concomitant aortic valve disease, a low cardiac output, or very mild mitral stenosis.

The opening snap is usually heard best with the diaphragm of the stethoscope at the lower left sternal border and apex, but can transmit widely, radiating well to the base of the heart. At the base of the heart the opening snap is often mistakenly confused with the pulmonic component of the second heart sound, which may appear to be a wide, fixed split of S_2 (A_2-P_2), as occurs in atrial septal defect. Careful auscultation over the pulmonic area and mid-left sternal border, however, will reveal physio-

logic splitting of S_2 into its aortic and pulmonic components during inspiration, followed by the opening snap (producing a "trill" effect of three sounds: A_2, P_2 and OS) (Figure 26). This often subtle auscultatory finding, therefore, may be the important diagnostic clue in the differential diagnosis of an atrial septal defect and mitral stenosis.

When an opening snap is suspected, the physician should listen for a loud first heart sound and search carefully for the characteristic diastolic rumble of mitral stenosis. This is accomplished by turning the patient to the left lateral decubitus position, finding the point of maximal impulse of the left ventricle with the palpating index and third fingers, and placing the bell of the stethoscope lightly over this localized area, barely touching the skin. As emphasized by Dr. Harvey, the "tell-tale" rumble, if present, will always be heard over this localized spot. Although "silent" mitral stenosis can exist, it is not common, and is more often related to the highly localized nature of these auscultatory findings, rather than true silence. With practice, the timing of an opening snap relative to aortic closure (A2-OS interval) can be approximated with a high degree of accuracy by careful auscultation, and is valuable in

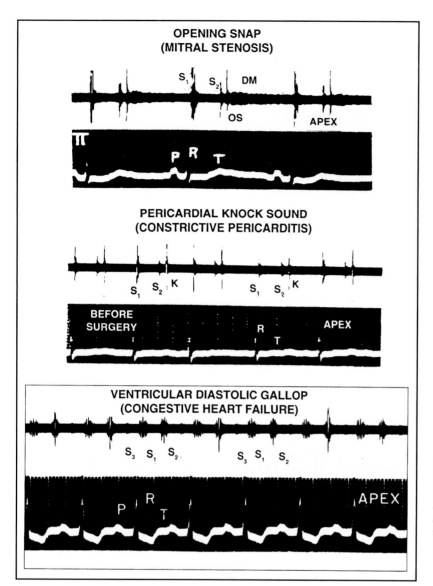

**OPENING SNAP
(MITRAL STENOSIS)**

**PERICARDIAL KNOCK SOUND
(CONSTRICTIVE PERICARDITIS)**

**VENTRICULAR DIASTOLIC GALLOP
(CONGESTIVE HEART FAILURE)**

Figure 27. Note the timing of the extra diastolic sound in each of the examples. The pericardial knock (K) (0.10 seconds after S_2) occurs earlier than a ventricular (S_3) diastolic gallop (0.14-0.16 seconds after S_2) and later than the opening snap (OS) of severe mitral stenosis ($\leq$0.08 seconds after S_2). *(From Levine SA, Harvey WP, 30.)*

the bedside assessment of the severity of the stenosis. The opening snap generally follows A_2 by an interval of 0.04 to 0.12 seconds. In normotensive patients with pure or dominant mitral stenosis, and a normal heart rate and cardiac output, the duration of the A_2-OS interval is inversely related to the severity of mitral stenosis. The more severe the mitral stenosis, the higher the left atrial pressure, the earlier the opening snap and the shorter the A_2-OS interval. In general, an A_2-OS interval of less than 0.08 seconds indicates severe mitral stenosis, and an interval of greater than 0.10 seconds indicates mild mitral stenosis. It should be realized, however, that this interval is influenced by several factors. In older patients with systolic hypertension, for example, significant mitral stenosis may be present despite a relatively long A_2-OS interval since the elevated left ventricular systolic pressure takes longer to fall below left atrial pressure.

Pericardial Knock Sound

The early diastolic filling sound of constrictive pericarditis is termed the pericardial knock. This special variation of the early diastolic sound is generated by the sudden, early arrest of blood flow by the restricting envelope of rigid pericardium during rapid ventricular filling, resulting in sudden checking of myocardial expansion. The sound generally occurs approximately 0.10 to 0.12 seconds after S_2, slightly later than the usual opening snap of a tight mitral stenosis (less than 0.08 seconds), but earlier than the normal physiologic third heart sound, or ventricular diastolic gallop (0.14 - 0.16 seconds from A_2) (Table 7, Figure 27).

In general, it is of a higher pitch and intensity than the gallop, is widely transmitted over the entire precordium, and usually becomes louder with inspiration. On occasion, pericardial knock sounds can be multiple rather than single. In those

144

patients who have milder degrees of constriction, the pericardial knock sound may only be heard with inspiration coincident with the increase in venous return, and is absent or diminished on expiration. It can occur with or without pericardial calcification. The more severe the constrictive process, the earlier and louder the knock sound. Following successful surgery, the sound becomes later and softer. Because of its higher frequency characteristic, the pericardial knock sound may be mistaken for an opening snap. The presence of this early diastolic heart sound, however, in association with an elevated jugular venous pressure increasing during inspiration (Kussmaul's sign) and in the absence of a loud S_1 and diastolic rumble of mitral stenosis, should provide the physician with an immediate clue to the diagnosis of constrictive pericarditis. Nowadays, one should specifically search for these findings in the patient who presents with unexplained congestive heart failure, especially right-sided, following open heart surgery.

Additional Early Diastolic Sounds

The presence of an early diastolic sound may also be caused by left or right-sided atrial myxomas and is referred to as a "tumor plop." The sound is created when the mobile pedunculated tumor, attached by a long stalk to the interatrial septum, has moved and come to an abrupt halt at the full extent of its excursion and descent into the ventricle during early diastole. Although the auscultatory findings may simulate rheumatic mitral stenosis, this sound is usually lower in pitch than an opening snap and may vary in intensity and timing, after the second sound, accompanied by changing systolic and diastolic murmurs as the tumor is altered in position with various postural changes. An early diastolic click may, on rare occasion, also be heard in mitral valve prolapse, thus creating a potential cause for confusion.

Early diastolic sounds may also be caused by the opening movement of a mechanical mitral valve prosthesis, e.g., Starr-Edwards ball-in-cage, Bjork-Shiley tilting-disk, and St. Jude bi-leaflet valve. The sounds vary in intensity and quality, depending upon the design of the prosthesis. A change in the intensity or timing of the prosthetic valve sound, on serial auscultation, may serve as the first clue to the presence of a malfunction of the artificial valve.

In the presence of a cardiac pacemaker, iatrogenic sounds may occur at any time during the cardiac cycle. They are frequently brief, high-pitched and "clicking" but occasionally may be low-pitched. These sounds are heard best at the apex, or lower left sternal border, and may be loud or faint.

Intercostal muscle contraction may cause pacemaker sounds, and these are usually presystolic in timing, occurring immediately after the onset of the pacing stimulus just preceding the first heart sound. A midsystolic click, or late systolic murmur, whoop or honk have also been observed, and suggest pacemaker-induced tricuspid regurgitation.

CARDIAC PEARL

Extracardiac Sounds Produced by Cardiac Pacemakers: It is now well established that the pacemaker can produce a sound in presystole that is related to skeletal muscle contraction rather than being of cardiac origin. At times one can see precordial muscle contraction coincident with the sound, and the patient may be aware of it, occasionally feeling some discomfort. Also, uncommonly, the pacemaker can produce unusual auscultatory findings. This may result in peculiar musical murmurs such as a whoop or honk. These are often loud and occur in late systole. In one patient personally observed, a murmur having a musical quality resembling a "grunt" or "groan" (also described as sounding like "the croaking of a frog") was heard in systole, and at times in diastole. Apparently this was related to the position of the pacing catheter across the tricuspid valve, since repositioning it resulted in disappearance of the murmurs.

W. Proctor Harvey, M.D.

The proper identification of two heart sounds occurring around S_2 also provides a diagnostic challenge to the clinician (Figure 28). The physician should distinguish the wide splitting of the second heart sound due to aortic and pulmonic valve closures from an extra sound, such as the mitral opening snap, pericardial knock sound, or ventricular diastolic gallop. A split second heart sound is high-pitched. Its splitting interval usually lasts 0.02 to 0.06 seconds, displays characteristic respiratory variation, and is usually heard best along the pulmonic area and mid-left sternal border, with little radiation to the apex. The opening snap (OS) is also higher in pitch with a snapping quality, and in severe mitral stenosis usually follows the second heart sound by less than 0.08 seconds. However, this sound radiates more widely, generally over the entire precordium. When an opening snap is suspected, one should listen for the other features in the auscultatory spectrum of mitral stenosis, i.e., a loud S_1, a loud P_2 if pulmonary hypertension is present, and the characteristic acoustic hallmark, the diastolic rumble, using the appropriate auscultatory techniques previously described. The pericar-

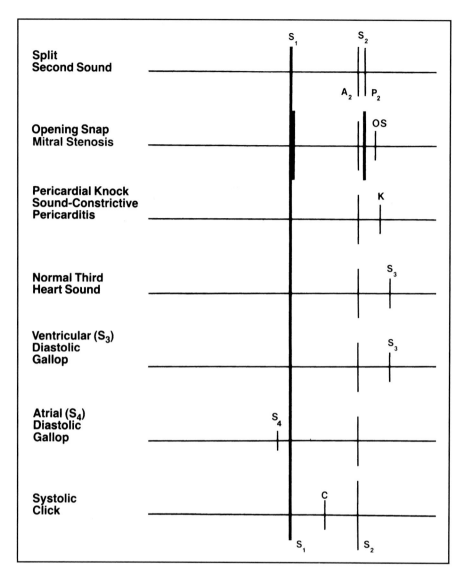

Figure 28. Comparison of the timing of extra sounds and events. Note that S_1 and P_2 are accentuated with mitral stenosis. With constrictive pericarditis a pericardial knock sound (K) occurs later than the opening snap (OS) and S_1 is not accentuated. *(From Harvey WP, 18.)*

dial knock sound is generally later in timing (0.10 - 0.12 seconds after S_2) than the opening snap of severe mitral stenosis, and is accompanied by significant jugular venous distention that increases during inspiration (Kussmaul's sign) with a rapid X and Y descent noted. This sound occurs earlier than the usual ventricular diastolic gallop or normal physiologic third heart sound (0.14 - 0.16 seconds after A_2), radiates widely, increases in intensity during inspiration, and is of value in confirming a clinical diagnosis of pericardial constriction.

CARDIAC PEARL

How to differentiate the opening snap of mitral stenosis from the pericardial knock sound of constrictive pericarditis.

These two sounds can be similar and cause confusion. Here are clues to differentiate them.

1. The first sound in mitral stenosis is usually loud when the opening snap is heard. The first sound associated with the pericardial knock is often not accentuated, although it can be.

2. P_2 is associated with mitral stenosis, but not with constrictive pericarditis.

3. The diastolic murmur of mitral stenosis is usually heard over the point of maximum impulse of the left ventricle. A diastolic murmur is hardly ever present with constrictive pericarditis. An exception: Very, very rarely, constriction between the left atrium and left ventricle has occurred, resulting in a diastolic murmur.

4. Neck vein distention is characteristic of constrictive pericarditis, but does not usually occur with mitral stenosis.

5. Rheumatic heart disease usually has two valves involved, the aortic and the mitral. This is not so with constrictive pericarditis.

W. Proctor Harvey, M.D.

146

Conclusion

This chapter is a timely reminder of the primary importance of cardiac auscultation in the modern practice of clinical cardiology. As discussed, the astute clinician derives a great deal of useful clinical information from careful, attentive auscultation of heart sounds. When used properly, the time-honored stethoscope remains a powerful and indispensable tool in the clinical evaluation of the cardiac patient, often allowing the expert examiner, skilled in the art of auscultation, to arrive at a definitive and accurate physiologic and anatomic diagnosis. It also enables the physician to derive intellectual satisfaction and personal fulfillment in the use of his or her own senses and clinical skills in the making of sophisticated diagnoses at the bedside (the "fun of medicine"). Furthermore, in this era of high technology and managed care as the practice of medicine becomes increasingly more instrumental and dehumanizing in its approach, the sense of care and comfort the patient receives from the "laying on of hands" fosters the close rapport, trust and confidence so important to the doctor-patient relationship.

Selected Reading

1. Abrams J. *Essentials of Cardiac Physical Diagnosis.* Philadelphia: Lea & Febiger. 1987.

2. Barlow JR, Bosman CK, Pocock WA, et al. Late systolic murmurs and non-ejection ("mid-late") systolic click. *BHJ* 1968; 30:203.

3. Bedford E. Cardiology in the days of Laennec: the story of auscultation of the heart. *BHJ* 1972;34:1193.

4. Braunwald E. The physical examination. In: Braunwald E, ed. *Heart Disease: A Textbook of Cardiovascular Medicine.* 4th ed. Philadelphia: WB Saunders. 1992:13.

5. Chizner MA. Cardiac auscultation: heart sounds. *Cardiology in Practice.* Sept/Oct 1984:141-156.

6. Chizner MA. Bedside diagnosis of the acute myocardial infarction and its complications. *Curr Prob Cardiol.* 1982;7:1-86.

7. Chizner MA. Valvular aortic stenosis in adults. *Primary Cardiology.* 1981:7.

8. Chizner MA, Pearle DL, deLeon AC Jr. The natural history of aortic stenosis in adults. *AHJ* 1980;99:419.

9. Constant J. *Bedside Cardiology.* 2nd ed. Boston: Little, Brown & Co. 1976.

10. Craige E. On the genesis of heart sounds: contributions made by echocardiographic studies. *Circ.* 1976; 53:207.

11. Craige E. Should auscultation be rehabilitated? *NEJM.* 1988;318:1611.

12. Crawford MH, O'Rourke RA. A systematic approach to the bedside differentiation of cardiac murmurs and abnormal sounds. *Curr Prob Cardiol.* 1977; 2:1.

13. Fontana ME, Wooley CF, Leighton RF, et al. Postural changes in left ventricular and mitral valvular dynamics in the systolic click-late systolic murmur syndrome. *Circ* 1975;51:165.

14. Hancock EW. The ejection sound in aortic stenosis. *AJM* 1966; 40:561.

15. Harvey WP. Technique and art of auscultation. In: Segal BL, ed. *Theory and Practice of Auscultation.* Philadelphia: FA Davis Co. 1964.

16. Harvey WP. Heart sounds and murmurs. *Circ* 1964;30:262.

17. Harvey WP. Auscultatory findings in diseases of the pericardium. *AJC.* 1961;7:15.

18. Harvey WP. *Cardiac Pearls.* Laennec Publishing Co. 1993.

19. Harvey WP, Canfield D. *Clinical Auscultation of the Cardiovascular System..* Laennec Publishing Co. 1989.

20. Harvey WP, deLeon AC Jr. The normal third heart sound and gallops, ejection sounds, systolic clicks, systolic whoops, opening snaps and other sounds. In: Hurst JW, ed. *The Heart.* 5th ed. New York: McGraw-Hill. 1982.

21. Harvey WP, Perloff JK. The auscultatory findings in primary myocardial disease. *AHJ* 1961;61:199.

22. Harvey WP, Ronan JA. Bedside diagnosis of arrhythmias. *Prog Cardiovasc Dis.* 1966;8:429.

23. Harvey WP, Stapleton J. Clinical aspect of gallop rhythm with particular reference to diastolic gallops. *Circ* 1958; 17:1007.

24. Hultgren HN, Reeve R, Cohn K, et al. The ejection click of valvular pulmonic stenosis. *Circ* 1969;40:631.

25. Laennec RTH. *Traite de L'Auscultation Mediate.* 2nd ed. Paris: Brosson et Chaude. 1826.

26. Leatham A. *Auscultation of the Heart and Phonocardiography.* Edinburgh: Churchill Livingstone. 1975:181.

27. Leatham A, Gray I. Auscultatory and phonocardiographic signs of atrial septal defect. *BHJ* 1956;18:193.

28. Leatham A, Leech GJ. The first and second heart sounds. In: Hurst JW, ed. *The Heart.* 5th ed. New York: McGraw-Hill. 1982.

29. Leon DF, Shaver JA, eds. *Physiologic Principles of Heart Sounds and Murmurs.* AHA monograph, No. 46. 1975.

30. Levine SA, Harvey WP. *Clinical Auscultation of the Heart.* 2nd ed. Philadelphia: WB Saunders Co. 1959.

31. Mangione S, Nieman LZ, Gracely E, Kaye D. The teaching and practice of cardiac auscultation during internal medicine and cardiology training. *Ann Intern Med.* 1993;119:47-54.

32. Mounsey P. The opening snap of mitral stenosis. *BHJ* 1952;15:135.

33. Mounsey P. The early diastolic sound of constrictive pericarditis. *BHJ* 1955;17:143.

34. O'Rourke RA, Crawford MH. The systolic click-murmur syndrome: clinical recognition and management. *Curr Prob Cardiol.* 1976;1:1-60.

35. Perloff JK. *Physical Examination of the Heart and Circulation.* 2nd ed. Philadelphia: WB Saunders Co. 1990.

36. Ronan JA Jr. Cardiac sound and ultrasound: echocardiographic and phonocardiographic correlations. *Curr Prob Cardiol.* 1981;6.

37. Ronan JA Jr. Cardiac auscultation: the first and second heart sounds. *Heart Disease and Stroke.* 1992;1:113.

38. Ronan JA Jr. Cardiac auscultation: the third and fourth heart sounds. *Heart Disease and Stroke.* 1992;1:267.

39. Ronan JA Jr. Cardiac auscultation: opening snaps, systolic clicks, and ejection sounds. *Heart Disease and Stroke.* 1993;2:188.

40. Ronan JA Jr, Perloff JD, Harvey WP. Systolic clicks and the late systolic murmur: intracardiac phonocardiographic evidence of their mitral valve origin. *AHJ* 1965;70:319.

41. Shaver JA: Cardiac Auscultation: A cost-effective diagnostic skill. *Curr Prob Cardiol*, 1995; 20:441-532.

42. Shaver JA, Leonard JJ, Leon DF. *Examination of the Heart, Part 4: Auscultation of the Heart.* Dallas, Tx: American Heart Association. 1990.

43. Shaver JA, Salerni R. Auscultation of the heart. In: Schlant RC, Alexander RW, O'Rourke RA, et al, eds. *Hurst's The*

Heart. 8th ed. New York: McGraw Hill. 1994:253-314.

44. Shaver JA, Salerni R, Reddy PS. Normal and abnormal heart sounds in cardiac diagnosis, Parts I and II. *Curr Prob Cardiol.* 1985; 10:No.3,No.4.

45. Smith ND, Raizada V, Abrams J. Auscultation of the normally functioning prosthetic valve. *Ann Intern Med.* 1981; 95:594, 1981.

46. Stapleton JF. Third and fourth heart sounds. In: Horwitz LD, Groves BM, eds. *Signs and Symptoms in Cardiology.* Philadelphia: JB Lippincott Co. 1985:chap 9.

47. Stapleton JF, Harvey WP. Systolic sounds. *AHJ* 1976;91:383.

48. Stapleton JF, Harvey WP. Heart sounds, murmurs and precordial movements. In: Sodemen WA, Sodeman TM, eds. *Pathologic Physiology: Mechanisms of Disease.* 6th ed. Philadelphia: WB Saunders Co. 1979; chap 11.

49. Tavel ME. *Clinical Phonocardiography and External Pulse Recording.* Chicago: Yearbook Medical Publishers. 1985.

50. Wood P. An appreciation of mitral stenosis. *Br Med J.* 1952;15:135.

51. Wood P. Chronic constrictive pericarditis. *AJC* 1961;7:48.

52. Wood P. *Diseases of the Heart and Circulation.* 2nd ed. Philadelphia: JB Lippincott Co. 1957.

CHAPTER 8

Physiologic Mechanisms of Heart Sounds and Murmurs

Donald F. Leon, M.D.
James J. Leonard, M.D.

The mechanisms responsible for the generation of heart sounds and cardiac murmurs are well-established. However, they are somewhat complex and not particularly intuitive. As a result, much that is taught is incomplete and, after multiple repetitions, may become misrepresented. The advent of diagnostic and interventional methods for patients with coronary heart disease has opened a floodgate for those who can now be treated effectively. Much of the clinical activity of the average cardiologist has become more technical, thus diverting attention away from the physiologic considerations that have been the hallmark of the discipline since its founding. There is some risk that these important principles will be forgotten.

In this chapter, we will summarize a large body of physiologic information so as to provide the reader with a working understanding of the important mechanisms responsible for the production of heart sounds and murmurs.

Heart Sounds as Transient Events

The sounds of mitral and tricuspid valve closure, the various early systolic ejection sounds, mid- and late systolic clicks, the sounds of aortic and pulmonic valve closure, and mitral and tricuspid opening snaps are considered in this category. Their mechanisms are similar in many respects.

The heart and its contents are suspended from the great vessels in the pericardial space in the thorax. Within this mass structure, blood is propelled forcefully by contracting myocardium, and closure of atrioventricular valves prevents reflux.

Thereafter, blood is reflected back toward the heart as the functional capacities of the systemic and pulmonary vascular beds are reached, thus closing the aortic and pulmonic valves. As the flow of blood is abruptly checked by closure of individual heart valves, the cardiohemic mass generates sharp pressure transients that are audible and palpable. This mechanism is responsible for mitral, tricuspid, aortic, and pulmonic valve closure sounds.

Similar transients occur when stenotic valves reach their maximum excursion and stop abruptly prior to the onset of flow through the stenotic orifice. These transients are responsible for mitral and tricuspid opening snaps and ejection sounds associated with aortic and pulmonic stenosis.

Transients may occur when the proximal great arteries become distended and sharply reach their elastic limits during early systolic ejection. This mechanism is enhanced by high stroke volume and also by presence of abnormal distensibility characteristics in walls of the great vessels in the absence of semilunar valve stenosis. Transients produced in this way account for a different type of aortic or pulmonic ejection sound, those of vascular origin.

The non-ejection systolic sounds of mitral leaflet prolapse deserve a special comment. This particular valve deformity is characterized by presence of several billowing segments, particularly in the posterior leaflet. These large redundant billows reach their elastic limits at varying times in mid and late systole and, when abruptly halted, produce one or more transients. Thus, mid- and late-systolic clicks of mitral leaflet prolapse may be single or multiple.

The First Heart Sound Complex

High resolution acoustic analysis of the first heart sound reveals that it is made up of four components which occur sequentially. The first component is composed of small, low frequency vibrations, usually inaudible, and which coincide with the beginning of left ventricular contraction. The second component is a large high frequency vibration, usually audible and related to closure of the mitral valve. The third component is an additional high frequency component related to closure of the tricuspid valve. This component occurs in close proximity to the mitral component. A fourth component is of variable frequency, coinciding with acceleration of blood into the great vessels. The second and third components of this complex, M_1 and T_1, are separated by only 20 to 30msec and therefore are usually heard as a single sound in normal subjects. M_1 and T_1 are not due to the clapping together of the delicate leaflets but rather are the cardiohemic vibration transients that occur when the mitral and tricuspid valves reach their elastic limits of closure, 20msec-40msec following atrioventricular pressure crossover.

Splitting of the mitral and tricuspid components of the first heart sound is rarely audible in the normal subject but, if so, it is often heard at the lower sternal edge. If a duplicated first heart sound is heard at the apex, it usually represents either a preceding atrial sound or a subsequent ejection sound. The principal cause for obvious splitting of the mitral and tricuspid components is delayed activation of the right ventricle due to right bundle branch block. The tricuspid component is enhanced in pulmonary hypertension. In mitral stenosis, M_1 is delayed and therefore may unmask T_1. In some instances of left bundle branch block, the sound of mitral valve closure is delayed, thus reversing the sequence of the first heart sound components.

CARDIAC PEARL

A question frequently asked: "I hear splitting of the first sound; why is this?" Splitting of the first sound usually is a normal occurrence in a healthy heart. We find it if we look for it. However, when it is more widely split than usual it may still be normal, but also can be a clue to an abnormality. Wide splitting of the first heart sound can occur with complete left bundle branch block, complete right bundle branch block, Ebstein's anomaly, and at times with premature ventricular beats.

Splitting of the first sound can be confused with an atrial sound (S_4) plus a first sound, or a first sound plus an ejection sound. How to tell the difference is a question frequently asked.

Press firmly with your stethoscope against the skin of the chest wall at the lower left sternal border and/or apex.

The S_4 will disappear. The two components of the split first sound are not eliminated with pressure; they sound alike and at the aortic area only one component of the split S_1 is heard. The aortic ejection sound is also usually well heard at the apex as well as over the aortic area; pressure with the stethoscope does not eliminate it and it is not affected by respiration. The pulmonic ejection sound is usually not heard at the apex and it may decrease in intensity coincident with inspiration.

As a rule the first component of splitting of the first heart sound is the mitral component and is louder than the second (tricuspid). However, in atrial septal defect the second (tricuspid) component is often the louder. At times this finding can serve as a valuable subtle clue to suspect atrial septal defect. Ebstein's anomaly is another condition in which this finding may be present.

W. Proctor Harvey, M.D.

The intensity of the first heart sound is of great clinical importance. It is related primarily to three factors: position of the atrioventricular valves at the onset of ventricular systole, texture of the leaflets themselves, and rate of pressure development in the ventricle (Figure 1).

During and immediately following atrial contraction, the mitral and tricuspid valves open fully. If the PR interval is relatively short, 0.11 to 0.13 seconds, the first heart sound is augmented because

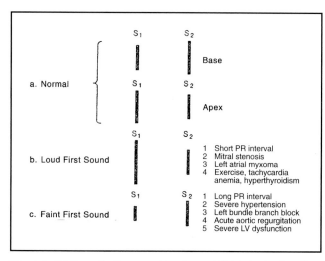

Figure 1. (A) Normally, the second heart sound (S_2) is louder than the first heart sound (S_1) at the base, while S_1 is usually more prominent at the apex. Causes of loud and faint first heart sounds are listed *(permission American Heart Association).*

the leaflets must traverse a full excursion before closure. If the PR interval is greater than 0.13 seconds the mitral and tricuspid valves start to float back towards the atrium and the first heart sound intensity starts to decline through a normal range. When the PR interval exceeds 0.20 to 0.26 seconds the first heart sound becomes faint because the leaflets have floated farther towards their closed position. This mechanism accounts for the changing intensity of the first heart sound in atrioventricular dissociation characterized by P-R interval variation from complex to complex.

CARDIAC PEARL

With practice, one can become expert in predicting the PR interval of the electrocardiogram by merely paying attention to the intensity of the first heart sound.

For example, a short PR interval such as 0.10 to 0.14 second, is generally associated with a loud first heart sound. On the other hand, a PR interval that is on the longer side, such as 0.21 to 0.24 second, is associated with a faint first heart sound. A person with a normal intensity of the first heart sound is more likely to have the PR interval in the normal range of around 0.16 second.

The detection of a faint first heart sound may be the first indication of a first degree heart block and this is often the first information furnished by auscultation that this condition might be present and can, in fact, be verified on the electrocardiogram. An atrial sound in presystole is not an uncommon association with a first degree block and is further support of the clinical impression of a first degree heart block.

W. Proctor Harvey, M.D.

Thickening and reduced mobility of the mitral leaflets due to rheumatic heart disease may cause the mitral valve to reach its elastic limit very abruptly during closure. In addition, the presence of a presystole pressure gradient places the leaflets as fully open as possible when left ventricular contraction begins, and the presence of elevated left atrial pressure results in the mitral valve closing at a much higher left ventricular rate of pressure rise. All of these factors result in an augmented first heart sound. However, rheumatic structural mitral changes resulting in total immobility lead to a marked reduction in intensity of the mitral first sound.

Hyperthyroidism, exercise, and anemia are associated with an augmented first heart sound related to increased stroke volume and enhanced contractile performance; similar changes are seen in tachy-

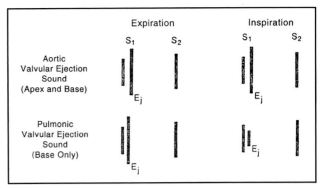

Figure 2. Aortic valvular ejection sounds are heard at the apex and at the base with little respiratory variation. They are found in nonstenotic congenital bicuspid valves and in the entire spectrum of mild-to-severe valvular aortic stenosis. Intensity of valvular ejection sounds correlates directly with the valve's mobility and becomes faint or disappears with calcific fixation of aortic valve, while intensity of aortic valve closure sound parallels intensity of aortic valvular ejection sound. There is little correlation between intensity and severity of obstruction, as long as stenotic valves are mobile. Pulmonary valvular ejection sounds are usually heard best at the base, with little radiation to apex. In contrast to valvular aortic ejection sounds, there is marked attenuation or disappearance of pulmonary valvular ejection sounds during inspiration. Such sounds are particularly well heard in mild-to-moderate pulmonic stenosis (S_1, first heart sound; S_2, second heart sound, E_j; ejection sound) *(permission American Heart Association).*

cardia. Conversely, a soft first heart sound may be observed in severe hypertension, left bundle branch block, acute aortic regurgitation and severe left ventricular dysfunction in addition to occurring with a prolonged PR interval.

Systolic Ejection Sounds

Early systolic ejection sounds may be vascular or valvular in origin and may be generated in either the left- or right-sided outflow tracts. Vascular ejection sounds occur a few milliseconds prior to valvular ejection sounds and so will be considered first. Vascular ejection sounds are transients resulting from an interplay of several variables. Among these variables are the velocity of ventricular ejection, the volume capacity of the proximal great arteries and the distensibility characteristics of these vessels. Dilated and atherosclerotic vessel walls are less compliant when subjected to a normal or increased early ejection velocity. Augmented ejection velocity in and of itself may produce an ejection sound transient.

The vascular ejection sound, whether of left- or right-sided origin, is synchronous with and probably identical to the fourth component of the first heart sound complex. Vascular ejection sounds are observed in many normal individuals, and those with fibrotic or atherosclerotic vessel wall changes, systemic or pulmonary hypertension, and dilated proximal great arteries.

Ejection sounds occur in the absence of valvular lesions of stenosis of either the aortic or pulmonary valve. Cardiac pearl: a pulmonic ejection sound can occur with a patient having pulmonary hypertension, which in some (similar to pulmonary valve stenosis) may also decrease in intensity coincident with inspiration. An aortic ejection sound may be present with aneurysm of the ascending aorta and in more advanced degrees of aortic regurgitation.

W. Proctor Harvey, M.D.

Valvular systolic ejection sounds occur in the presence of deformed and stenotic aortic and pulmonic valves (Figure 2). As the ventricle generates pressure in early systole, the stenotic valve with reduced mobility is thrust to its elastic limit, then suddenly checks at onset of ejection through the orifice. Ejection sounds are characteristic of valvular aortic and pulmonary stenosis and bicuspid semilunar valves. The valvular ejection sound disappears only after the semilunar valve has become totally immobile as a result of dense calcification or progressive fibrotic scarring.

The aortic ejection sound is heard in patients with valvular aortic stenosis. Such a sound is heard in patients with congenital bicuspid aortic valve stenosis. The ejection sound is not heard in patients with severely calcified valve leaflets.

The congenital bicuspid aortic valve is one of the most common congenital heart lesions. It presents with a spectrum of findings. An ejection sound may be heard in a patient with bicuspid valve when no murmur is audible. The ejection sound may be heard at the apex as well as at the base. More commonly, a short midsystolic murmur of grade 2 or 3 intensity is heard, together with the ejection sound and a prominent aortic valve closure sound. An early blowing aortic diastolic murmur plus an ejection sound and easily heard aortic valve closure may be present. Bicuspid aortic valve stenosis may progress over the years. The valve may become heavily calcified in the fifth to seventh decades of life, producing symptoms of congestive failure, syncope, dizziness, and myocardial ischemia, and aortic valve replacement may then be necessary.

An ejection sound can also be heard with aortic regurgitation, coarctation of the aorta, aneurysm of the ascending aorta. If a systolic ejection sound is heard at the apex and/or over the aortic area in a patient who has coarctation of the aorta, an associated bicuspid aortic valve is likely to be present. The ejection sound is usually produced by the bicuspid valve and not by the coarctation; however, an ejection sound can occur with coarctation and appears related to dilatation of the ascending aorta. An aortic ejection sound with aortic stenosis provides clinical support of the likelihood that the stenosis is of valvular type rather than infundibular, supravalvular, or idiopathic hypertrophic subaortic stenosis. Aortic ejection sounds, in contrast to the pulmonary ejection sounds, are usually well heard at the apex and have no respiratory variation. The aortic ejection sound occurs at the time of the abrupt stopping of the forward motion of the valve in early systole. With a stenotic bicuspid valve, it coincides with the "doming" of the valve in systole as seen on cineangiograms. The aortic ejection sound is often better heard at the apex than at the base of the heart. A harsh midsystolic ejection murmur of aortic stenosis over the aortic area may compete with detection of the ejection sound, or even mask it in some patients.

W. Proctor Harvey, M.D.

Ejection sounds are well heard at the base of the heart and are reflected into their corresponding ventricles of origin. Thus aortic ejection sounds are reasonably well heard at the apex and pulmonary ejection sounds are usually well heard at the lower left sternal edge. The aortic valvular ejection sounds are usually not affected by respiration whereas pulmonic valvular ejection sounds commonly decrease with inspiration and increase with expiration. This is particularly true in valvular pulmonic stenosis. In this setting, as venous return is augmented during inspiration, right ventricular end diastolic pressure increases to a level at which the domed pulmonic valve is displaced upward and actually reaches its elastic limit in late diastole. With onset of right ventricular systole, no further excursion occurs and the ejection sound becomes faint or absent only to reappear on expiration.

A pulmonary ejection sound is usually heard in patients with valvular pulmonic stenosis. It occurs in early systole when forward motion of the stenotic valve abruptly halts. The pulmonary ejection sound is best heard over the pulmonary area or third left intercostal space near the sternal border and is often misinterpreted as the first heart sound. To avoid this confusion one should always keep this possibility in mind and remember that the first heart sound is not well heard in this area. The pulmonary ejection sound, however, is usually poorly heard or absent at the apex. It is characteristic for the pulmonary ejection sound to diminish in intensity or disappear with inspiration and become louder with expiration. During inspiration, the right ventricular end-diastolic pressure exceeds the pressure in the main pulmonary artery, and no ejection sound can be heard or recorded. With expiration, the right ventricular end-diastolic pressure is lower and an ejection sound can be heard. These findings support a previous suggestion that during inspiration the inflow of blood to the right ventricle may move the stenotic pulmonary valve leaflets to the forward, more "open" position, thereby resulting in less movement with systole. During expiration, the valve leaflets are in a "closed" position, and with systole the stenosed valve is forced forward until it abruptly stops, producing the systolic ejection sound. An ejection sound is a common finding in pulmonary valve stenosis, particularly of the mild to moderate degrees. It may not be detected in the more severe forms of stenosis, or it may occur close to the first heart sound, thereby making specific identification difficult. An ejection sound is not heard with isolated infundibular stenosis.

W. Proctor Harvey, M.D.

Non-ejection Systolic Sounds

Non-ejection systolic sounds, formally referred to as systolic clicks, have had an interesting history in themselves. It was originally thought that they were extracardiac in origin because of their apparent association with a history of respiratory tract infection or pleuritis. However, several elegant intracardiac sound studies and correlations with echocardiographic and angiographic findings have documented the mitral and occasional tricuspid origin of non-ejection systolic sounds.

Mucoid degeneration of the mitral valve occurs in three to eight percent of otherwise healthy young adults; the tricuspid valve is involved less frequently. In this condition, the fibrous substrate of the valve leaflets is poorly structured and replaced with a mucoid material. Systolic ventricular pressure gradually stretches the leaflet tissue into redundant billowing scallops. The chordae tendineae are also involved and valvular regurgitation may be present.

During systolic pressure development the indi-vidual scallops are filled and protrude into the atrium. It is thought that the transients occur when the individual scallops reach their elastic limits; thus, non ejection systolic sounds may be single or multiple and often introduce the murmur of valvular regurgitation.

The timing of individual mid- and late-systolic clicks is related to ventricular volume (Figure 3). When the patient stands from a recumbent position venous return decreases and the heart becomes smaller. The systolic click occurs earlier than it had in the recumbent position. Squatting abruptly increases venous return and enlarges the heart. The click then moves towards the latter half of systole. These postural changes as well as volume changes related to the use of vasoactive agents are reliable identifiers of non-ejection systolic sounds as opposed to ejection sounds and widely split second heart sounds.

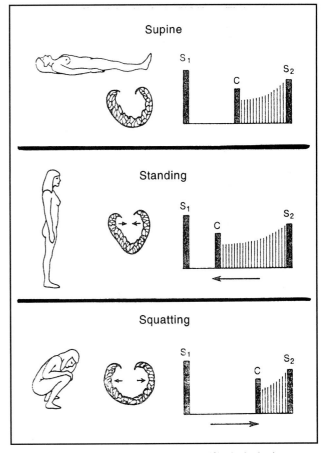

Figure 3. The midsystolic non ejection sound (C) of mitral valve prolapse is frequently followed by a late systolic murmur. Standing reduces venous return, heart size decreases, and C moves towards S₁. With prompt squatting, venous return increases and C moves toward S₂ *(permission American Heart Association).*

153

Terminology: It is suggested that the term "systolic click" be reserved for and identified with mitral valve prolapse. In other circumstances, rather than the term "systolic ejection click", use ejection sound. This terminology is clearer and more precise.

W. Proctor Harvey, M.D.

The Second Heart Sound

The aortic and pulmonic components of the second heart sound are related to closure of the respective semi lunar valves. At end systole forward flow into the great arteries has ceased and the previously ejected volume moves retrograde toward the heart, forcefully closing the semi-lunar valves and producing an audible transient. The reflux towards the heart is related to the capacitance of the arterial bed and rebound of distended elastic vessels.

The duration of left and right ventricular mechanical systole are nearly equal and occur almost synchronously in the absence of ventricle conduction defects. The forward flow from the right ventricle continues beyond forward flow from the left ventricle because of increased capacitance and decreased impedance in the pulmonary vascular bed.

The relatively higher level of impedance in the systemic vascular bed results in aortic closure concurrent with left ventricular pressure decline. Quite differently, the increased capacitance and decreased impedance of the pulmonary vascular bed permits the pulmonary artery pressure to decline less rapidly than the decline in the right ventricular pressure. The two pressure pulses become separated from each other by a readily detectable interval. This results in pulmonary valve closure occurring after aortic valve closure, P_2 occurs after A_2, and normal splitting of the second heart sound is established (Figure 4).

With inspiration, pulmonary vascular capacitance increases and the decline in pulmonary artery pressure is further delayed, thus delaying P_2. Simultaneously, there is a reduction in venous return to the left side of the heart during inspiration, causing aortic valve closure and A_2 to occur earlier. As a result, splitting of the second heart sound is increased with inspiration. A_2 and P_2 move closer together and sometimes become synchronous with expiration (Figure 5).

Right bundle branch block results in delayed activation of the right ventricle and in wide splitting of the second heart sound. Under these circum-stances, inspiration continues to increase the second heart sound splitting, but it is more difficult to detect because the splitting is wide even on expiration. Atrial septal defect is usually characterized by substantial increases in pulmonary vascular capacitance and substantial increases in pulmonary as opposed to systemic blood flow. As a result of this increased capacitance in atrial septal defect, P_2 is delayed and splitting is wide. Respiration does not significantly influence pulmonary vascular volume, so changes in duration of splitting are difficult to recognize.

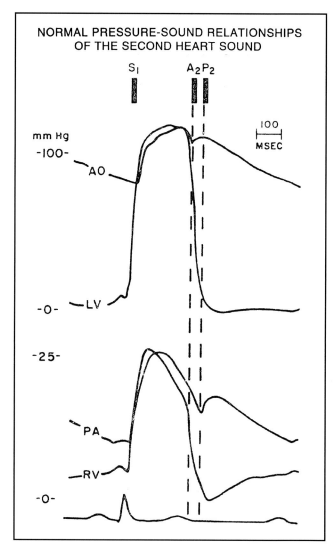

Figure 4. Left ventricular (LV) and proximal aortic (AO), right ventricular (RV) and proximal pulmonary artery (PA) pressures recorded with catheter-tipped micromanometers, thus eliminating delay. LV and RV systole are of nearly equal duration. A_2 and P_2 occur coincident with their respective incisurae. Note that the aortic incisura lies close to LV pressure, whereas the pulmonic incisura occurs later than RV pressure decline, causing S_2 splitting *(permission American Heart Association)*.

The importance of careful analysis of splitting heart sounds, particularly that of the second heart sound, is well established and is on a firm physiologic basis. Accurate clinical diagnosis of certain types of heart disease (such as atrial septal defect) cannot be made without paying detailed attention to splitting. To be noted are the intensity (loudness) and the degree of splitting of the second sound, which varies from a single or closely split sound to that of a wide split. Also to be noted is the effect of inspiration and expiration on the splitting of the second sound.

Splitting of the second heart sound is usually best appreciated over the pulmonic area or the third left sternal border. Most normal hearts have a split sound over these areas. With expiration, the splitting becomes closer or may even become single, and coincident with inspiration there is an increase in the degree of splitting.

When some patients are lying in the supine position, their second heart sound is distinctly split, thereby raising the possibility of atrial septal defect or bundle branch block. If on sitting or standing the sound becomes single or closely split, it tells you that the heart is normal.

This is more common in children, but also can occur in adults, especially athletes.

It is important to select the best spot over the pulmonic area or left sternal border where the two components of the second heart sound can be readily and clearly heard. The flat diaphragm of the stethoscope is usually the best chest piece to detect splitting of heart sounds.

The patient's respiration should be normal and quiet, and mouth slightly opened. It is important that the patient not force deep respirations. A helpful technique is to have the patient follow your free hand and to inspire when the hand moves upward, and exhale when it moves downward.

The splitting of the second heart sound has a significant relationship to various pathologic cardiac conditions. As might be expected, these disorders that delay contraction of the right side of the heart also result in delayed closure of the pulmonary valve. Therefore, even in expiration an increased degree of splitting might be present, and with inspiration there is an additional widening of the components of the second heart sound.

Complete right bundle branch block is a good illustration of this. Since there is an electrical delay of activation of the right side of the heart, the left ventricle contracts on schedule while there is some delay in right ventricular contraction. Therefore, with expiration there is a wider than normal splitting of the second heart sound, and with inspiration there is an additional increase in the normal degree of splitting.

Wider splitting of the second heart sound may also be heard in patients with right ventricular outflow obstruction. This occurs, for example, in patients with valvular or subvalvular pulmonic stenosis. Obstruction of outflow from the right ventricle results. Thus, pulmonic valve closure is delayed, because it takes longer for the right ventricle to empty its contents.

The wider the degree of splitting in pulmonic stenosis, the more severe the obstruction.

As the severity of stenosis increases, the second heart sound becomes prolonged and progressively fainter. Also, with increases in the degree of stenosis, the harsh "diamond-shaped" or "kite shaped" murmur of pulmonic stenosis becomes more prolonged, extending to, or even subsequently masking, the aortic valve closure sound so that one hears only the faint, delayed pulmonic valve closure.

W. Proctor Harvey, M.D.

Following successful surgical closure of the defect, splitting increases with inspiration but remains wide because of the large, dilated pulmonary artery and pulmonary vascular bed. A tabulation of the causes of wide physiologic splitting of the second heart sound can be found in Table 1 and Figure 6. There are a variety of causes of reversed splitting of the second heart sound other than true left bundle branch block (Table 2).

Narrow physiologic splitting of the second heart sound is commonly found in severe pulmonary hypertension in which pulmonary vascular capacitance is reduced and the pulmonic valve is closed almost synchronously with aortic valve closure. Occasionally in this setting, the right ventricle fails, its ejection time becomes prolonged, and P_2 is again split from A_2 (Figure 7).

Opening Snaps

Following closure of the semilunar valves, left and right ventricular pressures fall rapidly to the level of atrial pressure, which has begun to decline from the V wave peak. The ventricular and atrial pressures approximate and then decline together for a few milliseconds as the atrioventricular valve apparatus moves down into the ventricular cavity. The valves open and, under normal circumstances, the pressures continue to track each other as flow begins. When either atrioventricular valve (usually the mitral or, less commonly, the tricuspid) are deformed and thickened by the rheumatic process, the apparatus stops descending abruptly and the opening snap occurs; flow through the stenotic orifice then begins. It is the abrupt cessation of mitral or tricuspid descent that produces the opening snap transient; the opening snap sound is crisp and sharp, best heard from the apex to the left sternal border, and sometimes at the base, between 40 and 120 msec after aortic closure.

Shorter A_2-opening snap intervals are thought to represent more severe mitral stenosis. However, several factors actually influence the A_2-opening snap interval. In addition to the level of left atrial pressure, these include level of left ventricular pressure at time of aortic valve closure and rate of decline of left ventricular pressure after aortic valve closure. Intensity of the tricuspid opening snap is best heard at the lower left sternal border and is influenced by respiration.

Early diastolic opening snaps, then, are analogous to the valvular ejection sound heard in aortic

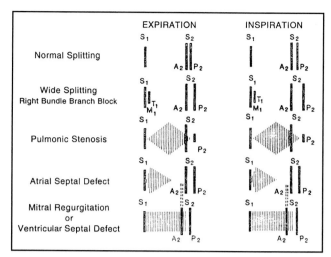

Figure 6. Causes of wide splitting of S_2. Although often difficult to appreciate S_2 splitting increases somewhat with inspiration in right bundle branch block and pulmonic stenosis, mitral regurgitation, and ventricular septal defect. In atrial septal defect, splitting is wide and usually not influenced by respiration (permission American Heart Association).

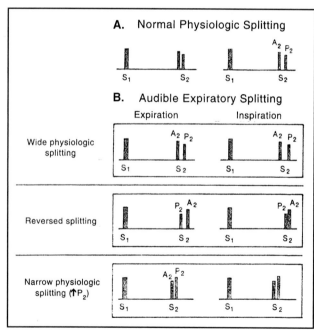

Figure 5. (A) Normal physiologic splitting. During expiration, aortic valve closure sound (A_2) and pulmonary valve closure sound (P_2) are separated by less than 30 msec and are heard as one sound. During inspiration, the splitting interval widens, and A_2 and P_2 are clearly separated into two distinctly audible sounds. (B) Audible expiratory splitting. In contrast to normal physiologic splitting, two distinct sounds are easily heard during expiration. Wide physiologic splitting is due to delay in P_2. Reversed splitting is due to delayed A_2, resulting in paradoxical movement; that is, with inspiration, P_2 moves toward A_2 and the splitting interval narrows. Narrow physiologic splitting is seen in pulmonary hypertension, and both A_2 and P_2 are heard during expiration at a narrow splitting interval due to increased intensity and high-frequency composition of P_2. S_1, first heart sound; S_2, second heart sound (permission American Heart Association).

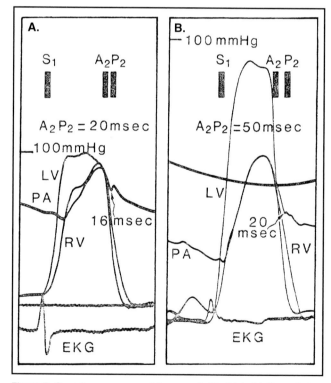

Figure 7. Sound-pressure correlates recorded by high-fidelity, catheter-tipped micromanometers in two patients with severe pulmonary hypertension. (A) Narrow physiologic splitting (less than 30 msec) is present. (B) Wide splitting is shown. There is marked reduction in hangout interval in both patients. In (A) duration of left and right ventricular (LV and RV) systole is nearly equal, and narrow splitting of second heart sound results. In (B) significant prolongation of RV mechanical systole beyond LV systole delays pulmonic valve closure sound (P_2) resulting in wide splitting of second heart sound. S_1, first heart sound; A_2 aortic valve closure sound; PA, pulmonary artery (permission American Heart Association).

TABLE 1
Wide Physiologic Splitting of the Second Heart Sound
DELAYED PULMONIC CLOSURE
Delayed electrical activation of the right ventricle   • Complete right bundle branch block (proximal type)   • Left ventricular paced beats   • Left ventricular ectopic beats
Prolonged right ventricular mechanical systole   • Acute massive pulmonary embolus   • Pulmonary hypertension with right heart failure   • Pulmonic stenosis with intact septum (moderate to severe)
Decreased impedance of the pulmonary vascular bed (increased hangout)   • Normotensive atrial septal defect   • Idiopathic dilation of the pulmonary artery   • Pulmonic stenosis (mild)   • Atrial septal defect, postoperative (70%)   • Unexplained audible expiratory splitting in normal subject
EARLY AORTIC CLOSURE
Shortened left ventricular mechanical systole (left ventricular ejection time)   • Mitral regurgitation   • Ventricular septal defect

TABLE 2
Reversed Splitting of the Second Heart Sound
DELAYED AORTIC CLOSURE
Delayed electrical activation of the left ventricle   • Complete left bundle branch block (proximal type)   • Right ventricular paced beats   • Right ventricular ectopic beats

Prolonged left ventricular mechanical systole
 • Complete left bundle branch block (peripheral type)
 • Left ventricular outflow tract obstruction
 • Hypertensive cardiovascular disease
 • Arteriosclerotic heart disease
   – Chronic ischemic heart disease
   – Angina pectoris

Decreased impedance of the systemic vascular bed (increased hangout)   • Poststenotic dilation of the aorta secondary to aortic stenosis or regurgitation   • Patent ductus arteriosus
EARLY PULMONIC CLOSURE
Early electrical activation of the right ventricle   • Wolff-Parkinson-White syndrome, type B

and pulmonic stenosis. The mechanisms are almost identical, with abrupt cessation of movement of a deformed valve producing an audible transient due to vibration of the cardiohemic mass (Figure 8).

Diastolic Gallops

The term "gallops" continues to be used for diastolic filling sounds. The term takes its origin from the cadence observed when filling sounds occur during a rapid heart rate. Diastolic filling sounds, including the third and fourth heart sounds, are ordinarily lower in frequency than the first and second heart sounds. Both filling sounds result from an interplay of three variables: compliance of the ventricle, the volume being delivered from atrium

to ventricle, and velocity of diastolic flow. With the proper interplay of these three factors, the cardiohemic mass may vibrate at low frequency, producing gallop sounds. Abrupt transients are not observed, but rather, lower frequency wave forms occur. Reduced compliance, increased volume and increased velocity all favor production of third and fourth heart sounds (Figure 9).

CARDIAC PEARL

An old teaching is that gallops disappear with atrial fibrillation. This is true of the atrial (S_4) gallop (since there is no atrial contraction), but not of the ventricular (S_3) gallop, which persists.

Occasionally, a physician will talk about a "Tennessee" gallop or a "Kentucky" gallop with the Ten-nes-see being an S_4 gallop and the Ken-tuck-y gallop an S_3 gallop. It is best to discontinue such descriptions because they can cause confusion. By use of the inching technique, the correct identification of the type of gallop can be readily determined.

W. Proctor Harvey, M.D.

The Third Heart Sound

The third heart sound is heard in early diastole at the end of the rapid filling phase of the ventricle.

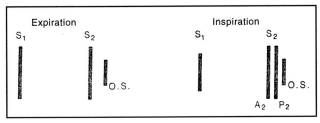

Figure 8. The mitral valve opening snap is best heard with the patient in a partial left lateral decubitus position and the bell of the stethoscope held lightly to the point of maximum impulse. OS is best differentiated from P_2 by listening for A_2 and P_2 and OS on inspiration *(permission American Heart Association).*

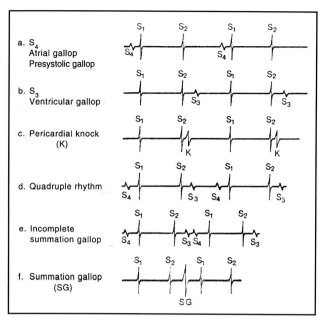

Figure 9. Various presentations of diastolic filling sounds. Note that a pericardial knock occurs earlier than S_3. In quadruple rhythm with increased heart rate, incomplete summation occurs. This may be mistaken for a mild diastolic rumble *(permission, American Heart Association)*.

Atrial contraction is not present or required. Third heart sounds may be physiologic or pathologic and may occur in the left and right ventricles. Physiologic third heart sounds are frequently observed in children and adolescents, and in adult males up to the end of the third decade. They are rarely observed after the age of 40, even in adult females. The sound is very low pitched and best heard at the apex.

CARDIAC PEARL

The Normal Third Heart Sound

A third heart sound is an expected finding in youth. Some years ago, the Division of Cardiology at Georgetown examined a large number of school children, the average age being approximately 10 to 12 years. A normal physiological third heart sound was detected in almost all of them. A normal venous hum was also heard in 100% of these children; an innocent systolic murmur in approximately 65%; a carotid bruit (short systolic murmur) in approximately one third, and a supraclavicular murmur in approximately one third.

The normal physiologic third heart sound in youth is usually best heard with the patient turned to the left lateral position, listening with the bell of the stethoscope held lightly, barely making an air seal over the point of maximal impulse over the left ventricle. The

normal third heart sound usually disappears in men in their 20's and women in their 30's, although those continuing in athletic endeavors in later years may retain their normal third sounds. It may be brought out by turning the patient to the left lateral position and listening over the point of maximal impulse. A prominent third sound may then be easily detected. It may, however, become faint or disappear after a few beats. Other maneuvers, such as having the patient cough several times or take a series of rapid deep breaths several times, might also bring out the third sound. (This same technique can be used to uncover the telltale diagnostic rumble of mitral stenosis: Turn the patient to the left lateral position, use the bell of the stethoscope barely making an air seal with the skin of the chest wall, and listen over the point of maximum impulse of the left ventricle.)

Elevation of the legs also may bring out the third heart sound in some patients, though this maneuver is usually not necessary. Speeding up the ventricular rate by a brief exercise of sit-ups or a short run-in-place also has been helpful in bringing out the third sound.

At times, low frequency vibrations producing a rumble murmur of short duration can follow the normal third heart sound. Occasionally, these normal findings have been mistaken for the opening snap and short rumble of mitral stenosis. This is more likely to happen if the first heart sound is accentuated due to a short PR interval on the electrocardiogram.

The normal third sound is not a surprising finding in swimmers, runners, basketball and baseball players, serious tennis players, and other athletes.

A ventricular diastolic gallop occurs with the same timing as the normal physiological third sound, approximately 0.14 to 0.16 s after the second heart sound. The technique employed to discover the normal third sound is the same as the technique used to find a ventricular gallop sound.

The normal third sound waxes and wanes in intensity with respiration. It is therefore preferable to listen while the patient continues to breathe in a normal fashion, since this aids left ventricular blood flow and production of the third sound. It is not heard as well when the patient is sitting or standing. As a rule, a low-pitched sound with this timing in a person in the forties, fifties, or older represents a ventricular diastolic gallop. It is ironic that a sound which in youth represents a normal, healthy condition should in later years be an unhealthy sign denoting a failing heart.

Since this diagnostic sound occurs at the time of the normal physiological third sound, it is frequently asked how one can tell the difference between a normal physiological third sound and a ventricular diastolic gallop. Practically, this differentiation is not difficult: after putting together all aspects of the cardiovascular evaluation, and considering the patient's age, one can generally make a correct identification. For example, a patient at age of 23 having a third heart sound occurring 0.15 seconds after the aortic component of the second sound, no history or symptoms of heart disease, a normal electrocardiogram and roentgenogram, and no other laboratory evidence indicating a heart problem, is assumed to have a normal physiological third heart sound. On the other hand, a faint heart sound occurring with the identical timing in a man aged 55 would immediately alert the physician to the presence of underlying heart disease. A total cardiovascular evaluation of such a patient will generally afford confirmatory evidence of heart disease in the history, electrocardiogram, x-ray, etc.

W. Proctor Harvey, M.D.

Third heart sounds heard in more mature adults and in association with myocardial dysfunction are likely to be pathologic, reflecting abnormal myocardial performance characteristics. In addition, in congestive heart failure increased volume and elevated left atrial pressure may result in enhanced flow during the rapid filling phase. Pathologic third heart sounds are reliable indicators of ventricular myocardial dysfunction or substantial volume overload as seen in mitral regurgitation, arteriovenous fistula, hyperthyroid state and others. Both physiologic and pathologic third heart sounds are influenced somewhat by postural changes, which affect venous return and sometimes by respiration. Third heart sounds may be made up of several components such that it may have detectable brief duration.

Elaborate studies concerning the genesis of the physiologic third heart sound have been reported by Shaver and colleagues. Their analysis of simultaneously recorded left ventricular intracavitary pressure and sound together with chest wall motion and sound at the cardiac apex demonstrates that the physiologic third heart sound, when present, occurs just after the end of the rapid filling wave, at the onset of a slower filling period and may be due to the heart striking the chest wall. The mechanism of production of the pathologic third heart appears to be similar.

The Fourth Heart Sound

The fourth heart sound occurs in late diastole and presystole during the period of active atrial contraction. The sound is generated in the ventricle and is substantially influenced by ventricular compliance and force of atrial contraction. Shorter PR intervals cause the mechanical event to merge with the onset of ventricular contraction and therefore are inaudible, whereas excessively long PR intervals may result in the presence of a fourth heart sound when compliance, volume, and velocity are not greatly different from normal. The fourth heart sound is a low frequency sound best heard at the apex; it is frequently associated with a palpable event that may be more easily detected than the sound itself. Fourth heart sounds can be detected in many myopathic conditions but are most prominent in severe ventricular hypertrophy.

During tachycardia or very prolonged PR intervals, timing of rapid ventricular filling and atrial contraction may approximate and the third and fourth hearts sounds occur almost synchronously. The acoustic events thus generated are known as summation gallops (Figure 9). Summation may be complete or incomplete. With incomplete summation the filling sounds of brief duration occur quite closely to each other and the perception of a short diastolic rumble may result. Third and fourth heart sounds occurring in the right ventricle wax and wane with respiration, unless the right heart is severely volume overloaded, in which case intensity varies little if any.

Sounds of Uncertain Origin

There is considerable conjecture about the mechanism responsible for the early diastolic knock frequently observed in constrictive pericardial disease. The presence of this sound is an important diagnostic clue to this diagnosis. The sound is crisp, sometimes excessively loud, and it occurs early in diastole, earlier than the usual third heart sound (Figure 9). The pericardial knock occurs at the end of rapid ventricular filling, when further expansion of the ventricles is limited by the thick adherent pericardium. The timing, intensity, and wide distribution of a pericardial knock suggest that the sound may be mechanical in origin, having been produced by the expanding ventricles striking the pericardium. However, in many instances, after surgical removal of the pericardium, the sound remains but occurs somewhat later in diastole, more typical of a third heart sound. Thus, the mechanisms for production of the pericardial knock and the third heart sound are similar.

159

CARDIAC PEARL

The filling sound of constrictive pericarditis, designated the "pericardial knock sound," is heard in the great majority of patients with constrictive pericarditis (if carefully searched for). It can be confused with an opening snap of mitral stenosis. Differential points are: the pericardial knock recurring about 0.10 second after S_2 is often later (after S_2) than the mitral opening snap, and no diastolic rumble is detected, which is the hallmark of mitral stenosis.

The third sound of significant mitral regurgitation generally occurs earlier after S_2 than the normal third sound. In addition, of course, a holosystolic murmur is indicative of mitral regurgitation.

W. Proctor Harvey, M.D.

Mechanical Third Heart Sounds

When cardiomegaly is excessive or when the chest wall is deformed, the ventricles may strike the chest wall during early rapid filling. This mechanism has been postulated as causing some third sounds. Certainly if the mechanism occurs at all, the phenomenon is quite rare.

Cardiac Murmurs

A classification and description of the various cardiac murmurs is beyond the scope of this chapter. Rather, the purpose is to shed some light on the mechanisms by which cardiac murmurs are produced. Rushmer has reported that murmurs are the result of turbulence in rapidly flowing blood. Flow through most vascular channels in humans produces no audible sound, unless there is a narrowing distortion or sharp angle, which would produce excessive turbulence.

In channels of constant caliber, conditions producing turbulence may be expressed mathematically as a relationship among velocity, viscosity, density, and the radius of the channel. The critical constant for turbulence is expressed as the Reynold's number: RVD divided by v. In this formula, R equals radius, V equals velocity, D equals density, and v equals viscosity. In this construct, fluids of low viscosity flowing at high velocity through tubes of large radius may produce turbulence; therefore, murmurs may be audible.

Rushmer further asserts that a specific Reynold's number for blood exists, 970+/-80, and this is frequently exceeded in the proximal aorta and pulmonary artery in early systole, thus perhaps explaining the common innocent murmur. Elegant intracardiac sound studies have shown that murmurs are most often produced across an obstruction in a large chamber or channel, or as the result of backward flow due to valvular or septal defects. Several mechanisms exist: eddy formation, vortex shedding, periodic wave formation, flittering, cavitation and turbulence due to flow striking an opposing surface.

Certainly, murmurs of stenosis of the semilunar valves, stenotic and regurgitant atrioventricular valves, and ventricular septal defects are due to eddy formation. Other mechanisms may be entailed in producing the murmurs of semilunar valve regurgitation, patent ductus arteriosus, and some of the less common congenital defects. One interesting phenomenon, not often considered, is the effect of the Doppler mechanism on murmurs. In a mechanical system when the source of sound is moving towards the listener, the sound has a higher frequency than when the source is moving away. In the same way the pitch of the same murmurs may differ when ausculted in two different areas. This is evident when one auscults over the carotid artery and then the cardiac apex in a patient with aortic stenosis. An appreciation of this mechanism will help avoid the impression of presence of two different murmurs. From a diagnostic standpoint, murmurs and their multiple characteristics are extraordinarily important, with skill in ausculting and interpreting cardiac murmurs achieved only via extensive study.

Selected Reading

1. Adolph RJ: *Second heart sound: The role of altered electromechanical events,* in: Leon DF, Shaver JA (eds): Principles of Heart Sounds and Murmurs. AHA Monograph no 46. New York, American Heart Association, 1975, pp 45-57.
2. Craige E: Gallop rhythm. Prog Cardiovasc Dis 1967; 10:246-261.
3. Curtiss EI. Mathews RG, Shaver JA: Mechanism of normal splitting of the second heart sound. *Circ* 1975; 51:157-164.
4. DiBartolo G, Nunez-Dey D, Muiesan G, MacCanon DM, Luisada AA: Hemodynamic correlates of the first heart sound. *Am J Physiol* 1961; 201:888-892.
5. Fontana ME, Kissel GL, Criley JM: *Functional anatomy of mitral valve prolapse,* in Leon DF, Shaver JA (eds): Physiologic Principles of Heart Sounds and Murmurs. AHA Monograph no 46. New York, American Heart Association, 1975.
6. Hultgren HN, Craige E, Fujii J, Nakamura T, Bilisoly J: Left bundle branch block and mechanical events of the cardiac cycle. *AJC* 1983; 52:755-762.
7. Hultgren HN, Leo TF: The tricuspid component of the first heart sound in mitral stenosis. *Circulation* 1958; 18:1012-1016.
8. Hultgren HN, Reeve R, Cohn K, McLeod R: The ejection click of valvular pulmonic stenosis. *Circulation* 1969; 40:631-640.
9. Hume L, Reuben SR: The effects of exercise or the amplitude of the first heart sound in normal subjects. *AHJ* 1978: 95: 4-11.

10. Leech G, Brooks N, Green-Wilkinson A, Leatham A: Mechanism of influence of PR interval on loudness of first heart sound. *BHJ* 1980; 43:138-142.

11. Leon, DF, Leonard JJ, Kroetz FW, Page WL, Shaver JA, Lancaster JF: Late systolic murmurs, clicks, and whoops arising from the mitral valve. *AHJ* 1966; 72:325-336.

12. Leonard JJ, Weissler AM, Warren JV: Observations on the mechanism of atrial gallop rhythm. *Circ* 1958; 17:1007-1012.

13. Leonard JJ, Weissler AM, Warren JV: Modification of ventricular gallop rhythm induced by pooling of blood in the extremities. *BHJ* 1958; 20:502-506.

14. Luisada AA, Slodki SJ, Krol B: Double (mitral and tricuspid) opening snap in patients with valvular lesions. *AJC* 1965; 16:800-806.

15. Martin CE, Reddy PS, Leon DF, Shaver JA: Genesis, frequency and diagnostic significance of ejection sound in adults with tetralogy of Fallot. *BHJ* 1973; 35:402-412.

16. Myers JD: *The mechanisms and significances of continuous murmurs,* in Leon DF, Shaver JA (eds): Physiologic Principles of Heart Sounds and Murmurs. AHA Monograph no 46. New York, American Heart Association, 1975, pp 201-208.

17. Myers, JD, Murdaugh HV, McIntosh HD, Blaisdell RK: Observations on continuous murmurs over partially obstructed arteries. An explanation for the continuous murmur found in the aortic arch syndrome. *Arc Intern Med* 1956; 97:726-737.

18. O'Toole JD, Reddy PS, Curtiss EL, Shaver JA: The mechanism of splitting of the second heart sound in atrial septal defect. *Circ* 1977, 56:107-1053.

19. Salerni R, Reddy PS, Sherman ME, O'Toole JD, Leon DF, Shaver JA: Pressure and sound correlates of the mitral valve echocardiogram in mitral stenosis. *Circ* 1978; 58:199-125.

20. Sakamoto T, Ichiyasu H, Hayashi T, Kawaratani H, Amano K: Genesis of the third heart sound. Phonoechocardiographic studies. *Jpn Heart J* 1976: 17:150-162.

21. Sakamoto T, Kusukawa R, MacCanon DM, Luisada AA: Hemodynamic determinants of the amplitude of the first heart sound. *Cir Res* 1965; 16:45-57.

22. Shah PM: *Hemodynamic determinants of the first heart sound,* in Leon DF, Shaver JA (eds): Physiologic Principles of Heart Sounds and Murmurs. AHA Monograph no 46. New York, American Heart Association, 1975.

23. Shah PM, Gramiak R, Kramer DH, Yu PN: Determinants of atrial (S4) and ventricular (S3) gallop sounds in primary myocardial disease. *NEJM* 1968; 278:753-758.

24. Shaver JA, Griff FW, Leonard JJ: *Ejection sounds of left-sided origin,* in Leon DF, Shaver JA (Eds): Physiologic Principles of Heart Sounds and Murmurs AHA Monograph no 46 New York, American Heart Association 1975.

25. Shaver JA, Nadolny RA, O'Toole JD, Thompson ME, Reddy PS, Leon, DR, Curtiss EI: Sound pressure correlates of the second heart sound. An intracardiac sound study. *Circ* 1974; 49:316-325.

26. Shaver JA, O'Toole, JD: The second heart sound: Newer concepts. Part I: Normal and wide physiological splitting. *Mod Concepts Cardiovasc Dis* 1977, 46:7-12.

27. Shaver, JA, O'Toole JD: The second heart sound: Newer concepts. Part II: Paradoxical splitting and narrow physiological splitting. *Mod Concepts Cardiovasc Dis* 1977; 46:13-16.

28. Shaver JA, O'Toole JD, Curtiss EI, Thompson, ME, Reddy PS, Leon DF: *Second heart sound: The role of altered greater and lesser circulation,* in Leon DF, Shaver JA (eds): Physiologic Principles of Heart Sounds and Murmurs. AHA Monograph no. 46 New York, American Heart Association, 1975.

29. Shaver JA, Rahko PS, Grines CL, Boudoulas H, Wooley CF: Effects of left bundle Branch Block on the events of the cardiac cycle. *Acta Cardiol* 1988; 43:459-467.

30. Shaver JA, Reddy PS, Alvares RF: Early diastolic events associated with the physiologic and pathologic S3. *J Car* 1984,14 (supp V) 30-46.

31. Shaver JA, Reddy PS, Alvares RF, Salerni R: Genesis of the Third Heart Sound. *Am J Noninvas Cardiol* 1987; 1:39-55.

32. Stapleton JF: *Third and fourth heart sounds,* in Horwitz LD, Groves BM (eds): *Signs and Symptoms in Cardiology.* Philadelphia, JB Lippincott Co, 1985, chap 9, pp 214-226.

33. Stept ME, Heid CE, Shaver JA, Leon DF, Leonard JJ: Effect of altering P-R interval on the amplitude of the first heart sound in the anesthetized dog. *Circ Res* 1969; 25:255-263.

34. Reddy PS, Memo F, Curtiss EI, O'Toole JD: The genesis of gallop sounds: Investigation by quantitative phono - and apexcardiography. *Circ* 1981; 63:922-933.

35. Ronan JA, Perloff JK, Harvey WP: Systolic clicks and the late systolic murmur: Intracardiac phonocardiographic evidence of their mitral valve origin. *AHJ* 1965; 70:319-325.

36. Rushmer RF: *Cardiovascular Dynamics,* 3rd ed. Philadelphia, WB Sanders Co, 1970, pp 313-317.

37. Tavel ME: *Opening snaps: Mitral and tricuspid,* in Leon DF, Shaver JA (eds); Physiologic Principles of Heart Sounds and Murmurs. AHA Monograph no 46. New York, American Heart Association, 1975, pp 85-91.

38. Thompson ME, Shaver JA, Heidenreich DP, Leon DF, Leonard JJ: Sound, pressure and motion correlates in mitral stenosis. *Am J Med* 1970; 49:436-450.

39. Thompson ME, Shaver JA, Leon, DF, Reddy PS, Leonard JJ: *Pathodynamics of the first heart sound,* in Leon DF, Shaver JA (eds): Physiologic Principles of Heart Sounds and Murmurs. AHA Monograph no 46. New York, American Heart Association, 1975.

40. Wooley CF, Klassen KP, Leighton RF, Goodwin RS, Ryan JM: Left atrial and left ventricular sound and pressure in mitral stenosis. *Circ* 1968,; 38:295-307.

161

CHAPTER 9

Heart Murmurs: Systolic, Diastolic, and Continuous

James J. Leonard, M.D.
Donald F. Leon, M.D.

As described in the previous chapter, the exact mechanism of murmur production is still the topic of some debate. Regardless of the exact mechanism of the sound formation responsible for them, murmurs can be attributed to basically three main factors. These have been described by Leatham: A. High rates of flow through normal valves; B. Forward flow through a constricted or irregular valve or into a dilated vessel; and C. Backward flow through a regurgitant valve, septal defect, or patent ductus arteriosus. Frequently a combination of these factors is operative.

The purpose of this chapter is to describe murmurs in terms of their essential characteristics. This is possible since phonocardiography, cardiac catheterization, angiocardiography, and echocardiography have correlated sound, pressure, and motion observations in a manner to place auscultation on a firm pathophysiological basis, rather than resorting to a purely descriptive one. This enhances understanding of the causes of heart murmurs, but in the final analysis, auscultation is a skill mastered only from experience at the bedside.

Classification of Murmurs

To facilitate verbal description, communication, and comparison of heart murmurs, they should be classified as to their timing (systolic or diastolic), loudness (intensity), location, and radiation. In addition, observation should be made concerning effects of respiration on a given murmur as well as its constancy over repeated examinations.

Observation of the behavior of murmurs in response to physiological maneuvers or pharmacologic agents which change preload and afterload heart rate or contractility may be helpful as diagnostic aids in assessing a given murmur.

- **Intensity:** The ear appreciates a murmur as having a given loudness related to amplitude and frequency of the vibrations. More than 50 years ago, Freeman and Levine graded the "loudness" of systolic murmurs based on a classification they themselves devised. The purpose of the grading system was to determine whether the loudness of a murmur correlated with its hemodynamic significance or with patient prognosis. Systolic murmurs under this classification were graded I to VI. A Grade I murmur is audible only after the listener has "tuned in". A Grade II systolic murmur is the faintest murmur which is audible immediately upon placing the stethoscope on the chest. A Grade V systolic murmur is a loud murmur which cannot be heard with a stethoscope removed from the chest wall but can be heard with just the rim or edge of the stethoscope touching the skin. A Grade VI murmur is one which is audible with the stethoscope removed from the chest wall. As stated by Harvey, grades III and IV are intermediate. Freeman, Levine, and others have shown that systolic murmurs of Grade III or more in intensity are usually hemodynamically significant. Although the "louder" murmurs (Grade IV or more) are likely to be accompanied by a palpable thrill, there is not a perfect correlation. For example, the blowing systolic murmur of mitral insufficiency may be perceived as equally as loud as a similar murmur caused by a ventricular septal defect and yet the latter murmur may be accompanied by a prominent thrill when the former is not.

In addition, although Freeman and Levine's classification of the loudness of a murmur has proved most helpful, it is important to note exceptions. Leatham, for example, has pointed out that a small VSD results in a high velocity jet which may give rise to a loud systolic murmur and thrill yet the lesion may be hemodynamically insignificant. On the other hand, a large atrial septal defect may result in shunting of a large quantity of blood in a low pressure, low velocity system without a signifi-

cant pressure gradient and, as a result, no murmur is heard.

The finding of a systolic murmur is a very common reason for our being asked to evaluate a patient. When we examine patients with significant systolic murmurs we find that the various murmurs have a special configuration or shape. They may occupy all of systole or only a part of it. A composite of the shapes of these murmurs is shown in Figure B.

If the murmur is holosystolic (pansystolic, that is, fills all of systole) we think of three

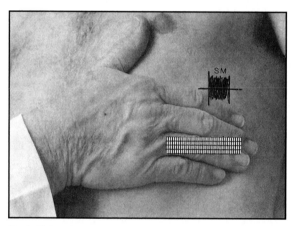

Fig A: Thrill - The detection of a palpable systolic thrill indicates the presence of a systolic murmur (SM) grade 4 or above.

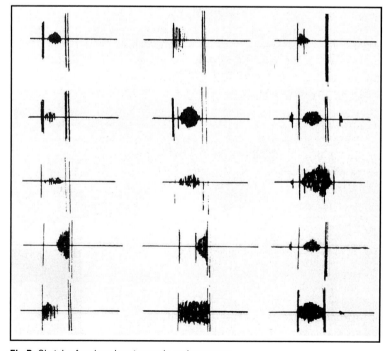

Fig B: Sketch of various heart sounds and murmurs.

lesions of the heart:
- **Mitral regurgitation**
- **Tricuspid regurgitation**
- **Ventricular septal defect**

Innocent murmurs (murmurs of no significance) are usually short in duration and occupy the early to mid-part of systole, or the middle of systole.

Murmurs vary in intensity and we grade them from one to six. (We are indebted to the late Samuel A. Levine of Boston for this practical classification).

A grade 1 murmur is the faintest murmur detected. After initially listening and not hearing a murmur, one adjusts the stethoscope in one's ears and concentrates more closely; then a faint systolic murmur is heard. Grade 2 is the faintest murmur heard, but it is detected immediately on auscultating the heart. At the opposite end, a grade 6 murmur is heard with the stethoscope off the chest. It is classified a grade 6 as long as the stethoscope does not touch the chest and one can "see daylight" between the chest wall and the stethoscope. At times, a grade 6 murmur can be heard even at a distance of several feet from the chest; this, of course, is very rare, but one does not go higher than a grade 6. Grade 5 is the loudest murmur heard, but it is not heard with the stethoscope not touching the chest. Grades 3 and 4 are in between, and it is obvious that the greatest jump in grading of the murmur with this system is between a 3 and 4. Grade 3 is a fairly faint murmur,. However, grade 4 is significantly loud and often accompanied by a palpable thrill. In fact, the finding of a palpable thrill on a physical examination generally means that the patient will have at least a grade 4 murmur (or louder) detected on auscultation (Fig. A).

This grading system is a cardiac pearl that has stood the test of time and is used throughout the world.

Remember, sketch the heart sounds and murmurs you hear. Sketch (draw) your findings on auscultation (Figure B) and include the drawings in your own patient records and also in the hospital record or medical report. If you do, you will get better and better with your auscultation expertise. We have never seen an exception.

W. Proctor Harvey, M.D.

Systolic Murmurs

Systolic murmurs are usually classified as midsystolic ejection or pansystolic regurgitant in nature. This classification has certain shortcomings as do all such classifications; nevertheless, this classification by Leatham is based on physiological principles, and the variation and exceptions can also be so explained. We favor this approach to murmurs rather than a purely descriptive one.

Midsystolic Ejection Murmurs

These murmurs are caused by the forward flow of blood through the aorta or pulmonary valves or outflow tract. The murmur begins when the systolic pressure in the respective ventricle exceeds the pressure in the aorta or pulmonary artery (Figure 1). There is a delay between the first heart sound and the beginning of the murmur; that is, the so-called isovolumic contraction time. These murmurs then wax and wane in a crescendo-decrescendo manner frequently described as diamond-shaped in configuration. Since forward blood flow ceases in the aorta and the pulmonary root in late systole and the second heart sound occurs as the result of incipient retrograde flow, it becomes obvious that the midsystolic ejection murmur always stops well before the closure sound of the respective ventricle.

In addition to obstruction, these murmurs may result from increased rate of ejection through a normal or nearly normal valve, flow across a damaged

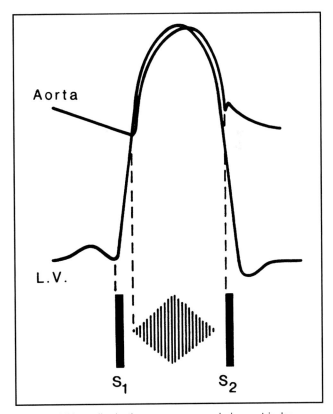

Figure 1. Midsystolic ejection murmurs occur during ventricular ejection. As a result, onset of murmur is separated from first heart sound (S_1) by a period of isometric contraction, and the murmur, which is crescendo-decrescendo in nature, stops before the respective semilunar valve closure. LV, left ventricle; S_2, second heart sound. (Permission AHA)

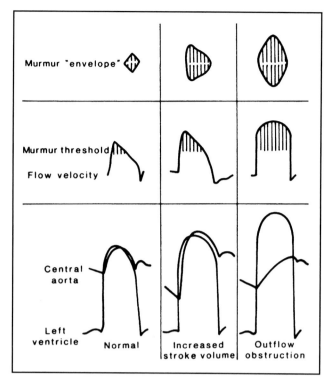

Figure 2. Left ventricular ejection dynamics are illustrated by simultaneous recording of left ventricular and aortic pressure, aortic flow velocity, and time intensity envelope of murmur. During normal left ventricular ejection (left panel), peak flow velocity is early, with two thirds of ventricular volume ejected during first half of systole. Murmur threshold may be exceeded during early peak flow and corresponding murmur envelope is inscribed. Center panel shows exaggeration of normal left ventricular ejection pattern, with large stroke volume as seen in high-output states. With critical left ventricular outflow obstruction (right panel), rapid early ejection is no longer possible; flow velocity is increased and contour becomes rounded and prolonged, producing typical diamond-shaped murmur of aortic obstruction. (Permission AHA)

but nonstenotic valve or flow across a normal valve into a dilated aortic root, or a combination of the above factors. The murmur envelope or time intensity pattern corresponds in general to contour of the flow velocity. A murmur is heard when the sound produced during peak turbulence exceeds the audible threshold. Not only is the intensity of the murmur proportional to the rate of ventricular ejection, but also its shape depends on the instantaneous flow velocity during ejection (Figure 2). High rate of flow across normal semilunar valves results in the murmur threshold being crossed but the ejection pattern is maintained giving rise to a murmur which peaks early and fades out in midsystole. Such murmurs have been described as "kite shaped" and are seen when forward flow velocity is high as in high output states, aortic regurgitation, and large stroke volume of heart block. Right ventricular systolic ejection time is longer than the equivalent period on the left. Maximal rate of ejec-

tion is less than in the aorta and the flow curve peaks later. This is probably the reason why right sided ejection murmurs related to flow are longer than those in the left. This is seen in atrial septal defects and straight back syndrome. In right-sided obstructive lesions, the murmur patterns follow the instantaneous gradient and flow pattern with the murmur waxing and waning in a symmetrical fashion which results in a diamond shaped murmur. Since intensity of an ejection murmur is closely related to stroke flow, any condition which increases flow velocity will increase the murmur. The mean and maximum rate of flow is increased in conditions which increase stroke volume, shorten systole or augment contractility. Exercise, anxiety, or fever will have such an effect. Physicians frequently exercise patients and note changes in intensity of a given murmur. All ejection murmurs will increase on exercise regardless of whether the turbulence is the result of high output or valvular obstruction.

• Aortic Valvular Murmurs (Figures 1, 2)

The murmur of valvular aortic stenosis is heard best at the second right and third left intercostal spaces just off the sternal edge. This murmur radiates widely into the neck and along the great vessels. Since murmurs are transmitted along bone, the murmur at times may be heard over the cervical vertebrae, the base of the skull or even the olecranon process. With radiation of the murmur to the apex the high frequency components predominate. The murmur heard at the apex has a higher pitch and frequently a musical quality (Gallavardin phenomena). This change in the pitch, although characteristic, is frequently the cause of some confusion. There is a tendency to assume that this murmur when heard at the apex represents a separate lesion such as mitral valve insufficiency. Observations confirmed by phonocardiograms repeatedly confirm that such a murmur regardless of its timber or harmonics still retains its diamond shaped configuration at various radiation sites. The differential diagnosis of a murmur heard at the apex in the presence of aortic stenosis may still be quite difficult. At times, the ejection murmur of AS is heard predominantly or exclusively at the apex. In this location neither semilunar valve closure may be audible. It is the fact that the aortic ejection murmur stops well before the second heart sound which defines the murmur as ejection in nature. If this sound is missing, the differentiation between aortic stenosis and mitral insufficiency becomes more difficult.

Acute Mitral Regurgitation: The murmur of severe acute mitral regurgitation is loud (grade 4 or above), occupies all of systole, peaks in mid-systole and decreases in the latter part of systole.

This is typical of chordal rupture, a serious complication of mitral valve prolapse. This murmur often radiates up the anterior chest to the aortic area and at times even into the neck. It may even be accompanied by a systolic thrill over the aortic area. It is easy to appreciate why this condition might be confused with aortic stenosis.

At times differentiation between this complication of mitral valve prolapse and hypertrophic cardiomyopathy has to be considered. Both of these conditions can be remarkably similar. A subtle but very important cardiac pearl:

Be sure to pay close attention to the splitting of the second heart sound. Paradoxical splitting immediately diagnoses hypertrophic cardiomyopathy (in the absence of left bundle branch block, of course, which would be rare).

Although women have a higher incidence of mitral valve prolapse, men are more likely to have rupture of chordae tendineae, producing mitral regurgitation. Mitral regurgitation is also a cause of wide splitting of the second sound. With systole, blood is ejected through the usual aortic outflow tract and simultaneously through the incompetent mitral valve into the left atrium. The left ventricular contents thereby empty earlier than usual, and the aortic valve closure (A_2) is earlier, which results in a wider split of both expiration and inspiration.

Another "cardiac pearl" is that paradoxical splitting of the second heart sound is more likely to occur in IHSS than with valvular aortic stenosis.

W. Proctor Harvey, M.D.

This is an important differential point since aortic stenosis and mitral insufficiency frequently occur together.

As has been stated, ejection murmurs vary greatly with changing cycle length. This does not occur with regurgitant murmurs. Forward flow against a high resistance in the aorta is more dependent on peak systolic pressure while regurgitant flow into the low pressure atrial system is not. With frequent extrasystoles or in the presence of atrial fibrillation, this contrasting response to cycle length may prove most helpful. With changing heart rates, regurgitant murmurs change only slightly while the change in intensity of the ejection murmur is dramatic. As a result, a murmur at the apex may be identified as a radiation of an ejection murmur or the presence of an additional regurgitant murmur of mitral insufficiency (Figures 3, 4). The same effect may be obtained pharmacologically by the inhalation of amyl nitrite, which increases the mean rate of ventricular ejection and hence augments the ejection murmur while the regurgitant murmur is unchanged. As aortic outflow obstruction becomes more severe, left ventricular systolic ejection is prolonged and splitting of S_2 becomes narrow. With progressive prolongation valve closure sounds are reversed, giving rise to paradoxical splitting. In the face of such a murmur with paradoxical splitting in the absence of a murmur of aortic insufficiency, a quick-rising pulse indicates the likely cause of obstruction to be hypertrophic subaortic stenosis.

At times, the differentiation between the systolic murmur of hypertrophic cardiomyopathy and that of rupture of the chordae tendineae can be quite difficult indeed. The ruptured chordae murmur may radiate upward to the base and may even be accompanied by a palpable thrill over the base Also at times the examiner hears this murmur, which originates from the mitral valve, even up into the neck. Cardiac pearl: to differentiate between these two similar murmurs, if paradoxical splitting of the second heart sound is present, the diagnosis of hypertrophic cardiomyopathy should be made immediately. Also, after a pause with a premature beat or with atrial fibrillation, a cardiac pearl: if the systolic murmur increases in intensity, this is of aortic origin, whereas if it remains about the same, it indicates mitral regurgitation of ruptured chordae.

W. Proctor Harvey, M.D.

In severe AI, there may be a loud systolic murmur secondary to the increased systolic flow compensating for the regurgitant volume. Such a murmur may become quite loud and even be accompanied by a thrill. If the classical peripheral signs of severe aortic insufficiency are present including low diastolic pressure and extremely wide pulse pressure, one can be certain that the murmur is secondary to increased forward flow and that no true aortic stenosis exists.

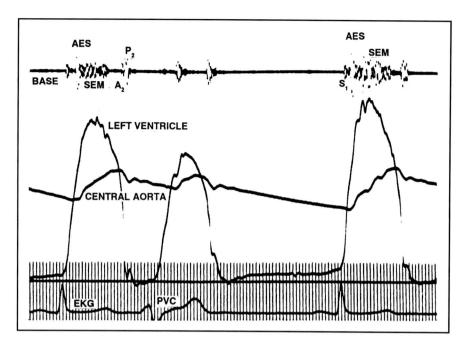

Figure 3. Simultaneous phonocardiogram, left ventricular and central aortic pressures in 23-yr-old patient with congenital valvular aortic stenosis. After premature ventricular contraction, note marked increase in peak left ventricular pressure and peak gradient across stenotic aortic valve. Note marked increase in intensity and duration of systolic ejection murmur accompanying this cycle, with a configuration of the systolic ejection murmur corresponding to instantaneous pressure difference between left ventricle and central aorta. Also note marked decrease in intensity of murmur during premature systole and its correlation with markedly decreased pressure gradient. (Permission, 33)

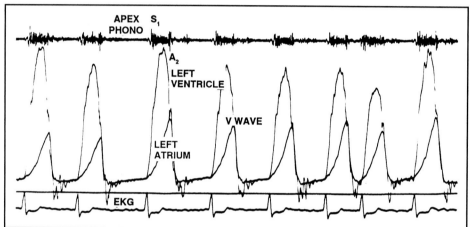

Figure 4. Mitral insufficiency with atrial fibrillation. Note the small variation of the amplitude of the systolic murmur in the presence of beat-to-beat intervals which vary markedly in length. (Permission, 29)

• Pulmonic Valvular Murmurs

Obstruction of the pulmonary outflow tract may be at the level of the valve or may be infundibular in nature. In valvular pulmonic stenosis (PS) with intact ventricular septum, the right ventricular ejection phase lengthens with increasing severity of the obstruction. As a result, the pulmonary closure sound is progressively delayed. The splitting widens and as the pulmonic murmur progressively lengthens, it encroaches, then masks, and finally completely envelopes the aortic closure sound. Under these circumstances, a pulmonary closure sound which is usually normal or increased in intensity in mild PS becomes increasingly faint and in most severe cases becomes inaudible (yet it can usually be recorded on the phonocardiogram). With progressive right ventricular hypertrophy secondary to severe pulmonary valve obstruction, the rising right ventricular end diastolic pressure

approximates or may exceed the end diastolic pressure in the pulmonary artery and cause the dome shaped stenotic valve to move upward, approaching or reaching its elastic limits before the onset of systole. As a result, with the onset of ventricular contraction the valve has a shorter distance of excursion or may have already reached its elastic limits. As a result, the ejection sound may occur sooner, blending with the first heart sound or disappear completely, especially if right ventricular end diastolic volume and pressure are further augmented by inspiration. The right ventricular hypertrophy also results in diminished compliance and a right sided atrial sound may appear together with a prominent A wave in the neck (Figure 5). Both of these are augmented on inspiration. Although the murmur of isolated infundibular stenosis is similar in nature, there is no pulmonary ejection sound and a pulmonary closure sound is absent. This helps

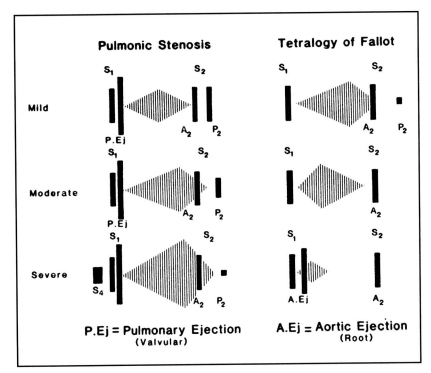

Figure 5. In valvular pulmonic stenosis with intact ventricular septum, right ventricular systolic ejection becomes progressively longer, with increasing obstruction to flow. As a result, murmur becomes louder and longer, enveloping aortic valve closure sound (A_2). Pulmonic valve closure sound (P_2) occurs later and splitting becomes wider but is more difficult to hear, because A_2 is lost in murmur and P_2 becomes progressively fainter and lower pitched. As pulmonic diastolic pressure progressively decreases, isometric contraction shortens until pulmonary valvular ejection sound fuses with first heart sound (S_1). In severe pulmonic stenosis with concentric hypertrophy and decreasing right ventricular compliance, fourth heart sound (S_4) appears. In tetralogy of Fallot with increasing obstruction at pulmonic infundibular area, more and more right ventricular blood is shunted across silent ventricular septal defect, and flow across obstructed outflow tract decreases. Therefore, with increasing obstruction, murmur becomes shorter, earlier, and fainter. P_2 is absent in severe tetralogy of Fallot, large aortic root receives almost all cardiac output from both ventricular chambers, and aorta dilates and is accompanied by root ejection sound, which does not vary with respiration. S_2, second heart sound.

differentiate the two levels of obstruction.

Pathophysiology of Tetralogy of Fallot on the other hand is quite different. In this setting, obstruction to the right ventricular outflow tract is usually primarily infundibular and the pulmonary closure sound is absent except in the mildest cases. As the obstruction becomes progressively severe, pulmonary blood flow diminishes and an increasing volume of blood is shunted right to left across the large septal defect which is a silent avenue of escape (Figure 5). With increasing severity of infundibular obstruction the murmur becomes shorter and cyanosis more severe. In fact, children with severe Tetralogy of Fallot may have hypercyanotic episodes with loss of consciousness. During such attacks the murmur may actually disappear. This is strong evidence that such spells are due to infundibular spasm with complete obstruction of the pulmonary outflow tract, all right ventricular blood shunting across the VSD into the arterial system.

In the most severe form of Tetralogy of Fallot there is pulmonary atresia (frequently called "pseudotruncus arteriosus") with no flow across the pulmonary outflow tract. As a result, no systolic ejection murmur is present. One hears instead a continuous murmur of increased flow through the enlarged bronchial vessels. In Tetralogy of Fallot the aorta is enlarged and somewhat transposed. A clear closure sound is heard in the pulmonic area, but this sound is single and due to aortic valve closure; an ejection sound is frequently heard in the same area. In children it arises from the dilated

aortic root. In adults, an ejection sound may indicate some element of pulmonary valvular stenosis in addition to the infundibular obstruction.

Dilation of the pulmonary artery as a result of pulmonary hypertension gives rise to an ejection murmur heard best at the base of the heart. The murmur is more likely to be prominent if pulmonary valve incompetence is also present, resulting in increased systolic ejection volume.

Such pulmonary hypertension may be primary in nature or secondary to mitral stenosis, intracardiac shunt, or chronic lung disease. Idiopathic dilatation of the pulmonary artery may result in a pulmonary ejection murmur which is delayed in onset accompanied by a late pulmonary ejection sound as well as wide physiological splitting of S_2. Delay in onset, late peaking of the murmur, late appearance of the click, as well as the late pulmonary valve closure, are all the result of the fact that the elastic limits of the large pulmonary artery and its branches are reached late in this abnormally high compliance, low impedance system.

Pulmonary ejection murmurs may result from increased rate of flow across the pulmonary valve. The increased flow can be selective to the pulmonary circulation as in atrial septal defect or anomalous venous return or as part of an overall increase in cardiac output. In the latter conditions, the murmur peaks in the first part of systolic ejection, and fades away during the latter third of systole. Wide splitting implies that the murmur is due to significant obstruction such as valvular pulmonic stenosis or selective increase in stroke volume on the right side as seen in atrial septal defect or anomalous venous return. When the splitting is normal, both sides of the circulation are involved in the hyperkinetic state. The increase in the mean and maximum rate of right ventricular ejection results in a kite shaped murmur. Such pulmonic murmurs are characteristic of exercise, excitement, fever, tachycardia, anemia, hyperthyroidism, pregnancy and peripheral AV fistula. This same type of murmur can be heard in children and young adults, especially those of asthenic habitus. The murmurs are short, ejection in nature, have a vibratory quality evoking the terms grunting, groaning or zipping. These murmurs have been recorded by intracardiac phonocardiography in the pulmonary artery root and also at times in the aorta. Unfortunately, these murmurs must be evaluated on the basis of history and physical findings including other auscultatory findings, since the murmur itself may overlap with systolic ejection murmurs due to cardiac or circulatory abnormalities.

CARDIAC PEARL

Some innocent murmurs have a vibratory, somewhat musical buzzing quality. They may sound like a tuning fork that is set in vibration. This vibratory type of innocent murmur is called Still's murmur, named after George Frederick Still (Common Disorders and Diseases of Childhood, London: Frode, Hodder and Stroughton, 1909).

When, in a young person, you hear a grade 1 to 3 vibratory, somewhat musical systolic murmur occupying the first to middle part of systole, you should be immediately reassured that this is probably an innocent murmur of Still's type.

The following is excerpted from Dr. Still's description of the murmur that bears his name:

"And here I should like to draw attention to a particular bruit which has somewhat of a musical character, but neither of sinister omen nor does it indicate endocarditis of any sort. In my own notebooks I am in the habit of labeling it physiologic bruit, but only for want of some better name. It is heard usually just below the level of the nipple and about halfway between the left margin of the sternum and the vertical nipple line; it is not heard in the axilla nor behind; it is systolic and is often so small that only a careful observer would detect it; moreover, it is sometimes very variable in audibility, being scarcely noticeable with some beats and easily heard with others; its characteristic fea-

ture is a twanging sound, very like that made by twanging a piece of tense string. This bruit is found mostly in children between the ages of 2 and 6 years; as a rule...the bruit is discovered only in the course of routine examination. It persists sometimes for many months. Have noted it as present in one case for two years. Whatever may be its origin, I think it is not due to any organic disease of the heart, either congenital or acquired; and I mention it in connection with endocarditis because I have seen several cases in which it has given rise not only to groundless alarm, but to uncertain restriction, so that the child has been treated as an invalid and not allowed to walk about."

Dr. Still's observations are of historical interest and value. His advice concerning "unnecessary restriction" still applies, eight decades later. One wishes it were possible to ask Dr. Still if any of the musical vibratory murmurs were in late systole, particularly those that were "sometimes very variable in audibility, being scarcely noticeable with some beats and easily heard with others." Of course today this would suggest mitral valve prolapse in which variability of the "systolic whoop" or "honk" is common. Almost certainly this is what Dr. Still was referring to, since an innocent murmur, while it can become louder with exercise, excitement, or fever, does not vary from beat to beat. Such variability is sometimes characteristic of mitral valve prolapse.

W. Proctor Harvey, M.D.

It is agreed that these are all ejection murmurs, therefore, they will become louder if the rate of ventricular ejection is increased by exercise, excitement or tachycardia. This response of ejection murmurs including innocent murmurs is of no value in establishing their cause. It is for this reason that innocent murmurs first come to the attention of physicians during intercurrent illness, fever and tachycardia or during the second or third trimester of pregnancy.

CARDIAC PEARL

The innocent systolic murmur is early to mid systolic. It is generally grade 1 to 3 on a basis of 6 (Samuel A. Levine's classification); splitting of the second heart sound is normal, becoming wider with inspiration and with expiration, single or closely split. The electrocardiogram and cardiac silhouette of the heart are normal. The findings of the history are negative, except for the discovery of a murmur. This diagnosis of the innocent murmur can be made accurately in the physician's office or at the bedside. Murmurs of other pathologic conditions can be similar, except they have other findings. For example, the atrial septal defect has the wide, so-called fixed splitting of the second heart sound. In particular, the electrocardiogram has changes that may be found in lead V_1 right ventricular conduction delay (RSR'), right bundle branch block, or right ventricular hypertrophy. The x-ray film shows increased blood flow in the lungs and enlarged pulmonary arteries. On auscultation, the innocent systolic murmur is similar, except that a wide, so-called fixed splitting of the second sound with atrial defect exists. The murmur of a congenital bicuspid aortic valve can in itself be similar to the innocent murmur, but an ejection sound is present with the aortic stenosis, which is well heard over the precordium from the aortic area to the apex. This illustrates another cardiac pearl: aortic events are often well heard at the apex. A mild pulmonic stenosis may also have a similar systolic murmur, but an ejection sound also exists, which may diminish in intensity on inspiration as compared with expiration. It may even become absent on inspiration. Significant murmurs of aortic stenosis and pulmonic stenosis are longer in duration, harsh in quality, and have other features of hypertrophy of the ventricles affected, which can be shown on electrocardiogram, chest x-ray film, or both. The differentiation of these lesions is not difficult. The

term "innocent murmur" is an excellent one and currently is accepted as the preferred description of this murmur. Innocent murmurs are better heard in young people who have thin chests, rather than in those who are obese or muscular. In the past a common term was "functional" heart murmur, which might still leave the patient or parent somewhat confused as to what the word "functional" means. By saying "innocent", everyone understands. Recently a mother said, "If I have an 'innocent' murmur, then are the other murmurs 'guilty'?" I said we call them "significant" murmurs, but when we think about it, the term "guilty" is a very good one (Fig. A).

W. Proctor Harvey, M.D.

Pansystolic Regurgitant Murmurs

These murmurs result from backward flow from a chamber of higher pressure to a chamber of lower pressure. Pressure differential persists throughout all of systole, hence, the term pansystolic or holosystolic. The classical examples of these murmurs are those of mitral insufficiency, tricuspid insufficiency and ventricular septal defect. In all three, the murmur starts with first heart sound at the onset of systole and continues up to and through the closure sound. In mitral insufficiency, the murmur continues up to and through the aortic closure sound since the left ventricular pressure continues to exceed the left atrial pressure at that time (Figure 6). In ventricular septal defect the same pressure differential occurs after aortic closure, since left ventricular pressure exceeds right ventricular pressure at the time of the aortic valve closure and the murmur continues. In tricuspid insufficiency the murmur continues through the aortic closure sound up to and enveloping the pulmonary closure sound. All of these murmurs are blowing in quality, of medium pitch, and basically are plateau in configuration with certain differentiating variations.

• Mitral Insufficiency

This murmur is heard best at the apex radiating well to the midaxillary line. The murmur may actually replace the first heart sound. Only the loudest murmurs give rise to a thrill. The murmur frequently demonstrates a late systolic accentuation and little change with respiration. In severe mitral insufficiency the murmur is frequently followed by a loud early diastolic filling sound which introduces a short diastolic rumble. When the filling sound becomes loud, the ear perceives it as higher pitched and it may be mistaken for or confused with the second heart sound, which is in turn enveloped by the

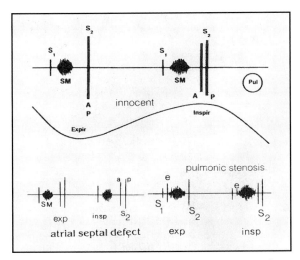

Fig A: Comparisons: (Top) A patient with an innocent systolic murmur (SM). The second sound (S_2) is single with expiration (expir) and widens with inspiration (inspir). Lower left: Atrial septal defect. The systolic murmur (SM) is similar to the innocent, but there is wide splitting of the second sound with both expiration and inspiration. Lower right: Congenital valvular pulmonic stenosis. The systolic murmur is similar to the innocent, but there is an ejection sound (e) which gets fainter with inspiration.

murmur at the apex and therefore inaudible. As a result of this confusion, the murmur will be thought to have stopped long before the aortic closure and may then be mistaken for an ejection murmur.

The holosystolic murmur of mitral regurgitation characteristically decreases coincident with inspiration (in contrast to that of tricuspid regurgitation, which increases).

It is sometimes said that the systolic murmur of mitral regurgitation "obscures" or "masks" the first heart sound. This is not so, as the first sound can be detected if carefully searched for; the murmur begins with that first sound.

A palpable thrill over the apex indicates mitral regurgitation as well as a grade 4, or above, systolic murmur.

A third heart sound (S3) is an expected finding in the more advanced, more severe leaks of the mitral valve. A short diastolic rumble may also be heard in such patients. These auscultatory findings are caused by the large volume of blood in the enlarged left atrium filling the ventricle and producing, in the rapid filling phase, the third sound plus low-frequency vibrations. This rumble is usually not the result of stenosis of the mitral valve.

A giant left atrium (large enough to hold a grapefruit or small bowling ball) can be identified on x-ray of the heart and by echo. Cardiac Pearl: if a diastolic rumble murmur is present in addition to the typical systolic murmur of mitral regurgitation, the significant and predominant lesion is that of mitral regurgitation.

W. Proctor Harvey, M.D.

• Tricuspid Insufficiency

This murmur is characteristically heard best at the lower left sternal border. In the presence of a large right ventricle it may be heard best laterally to the midclavicular line. Such a finding means that the right ventricle is occupying the region of the cardiac apex where one usually expects the murmur of mitral insufficiency to be maximal. Even under these conditions, the murmur of tricuspid insufficiency does not radiate well into the axilla region. When the murmur of tricuspid insufficiency is heard best at the apex, it can still be properly identified by the fact that it is strikingly influenced by respiration.

When listened for during continuous accentuated respiration, the murmur is found to increase at the

beginning of inspiration and to fade in early expiration. Intracardiac phonocardiography has documented the validity of these observations, as well as the fact that tricuspid valve gradient increases with inspiration while the mitral valve gradient and murmur are unchanged or somewhat diminished. Listening during held respiration results in the patient performing a Valsalva maneuver and confuses the issue.

Differentiation of these two murmurs is extremely important. For example, in a patient with rheumatic mitral stenosis, presence of complicating mitral insufficiency will alter the surgical strategy either as a possible contraindication to surgery or evidence for the need of valve replacement. On the other hand, tricuspid insufficiency complicating mitral stenosis is usually a manifestation of right ventricular hypertension with a dilated tricuspid ring. This latter set of findings indicates severe mitral stenosis, implying the need for surgery and the possibility of a mitral valve repair whether open or closed.

Pure tricuspid insufficiency, when severe, whether organic or relative, may give rise to a short diastolic rumble introduced by a right ventricular filling sound in much the same manner as seen in pure mitral insufficiency. In tricuspid insufficiency, both this rumble and the filling sound increase on

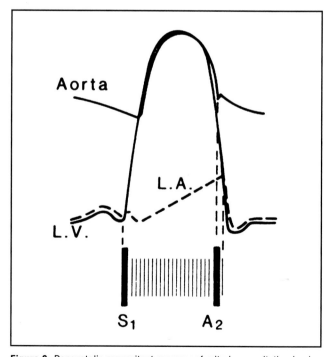

Figure 6. Pansystolic regurgitant murmur of mitral regurgitation begins with and may replace first heart sound (S₁) and continues up to and through aortic valve closure sound (A₂), as ventricular pressure continues to exceed left atrial (LA) pressure. Murmur has plateau configuration and varies little with respiration. LV: left ventricle. (Permission AHA)

inspiration. In acute severe tricuspid insufficiency right ventricular pressure elevates the right atrial pressure rapidly and the two pressures equalize early. As a result, there is severe regurgitation but no murmur. This diagnosis may be suspected by the huge A wave in the neck with inspiratory augmentation of its size.

Tricuspid insufficiency may be silent, particularly if one does not listen carefully to the changes that may occur with inspiration. In some patients, no murmur is audible over the lower left sternal border with expiration, but with inspiration a definite systolic murmur can be heard. Unless one specifically listens during both inspiration and expiration no murmur may be detected, and this would represent a "silent" lesion. This is particularly true with heroin addicts who have bacterial endocarditis on the tricuspid valve, and the early recognition of this lesion can be life-saving to the patient. Cases have been personally observed where no murmur was present except with the selective appearance coincident with inspiration. Coincidentally, the jugular venous pulse may demonstrate both an "A" wave and a "V" wave which increases with inspiration. Of additional aid is the detection along the lower left sternal border of an atrial sound that also increases in intensity with inspiration. Sometimes these findings suggest to the physician the possibility of tricuspid valve endocarditis in a patient whom he does not initially suspect of taking any drugs. This problem is becoming much more frequent today, and it is likely to be on the increase in the future. The presence of fever in a patient often being treated for isolated pneumonia or pneumonitis (multiple septic pulmonary emboli) together with the aforementioned findings may then lead to more careful questioning to see if the patient has been using narcotics. Also, a more careful search may reveal telltale scars along the veins of the extremities made by the previous intravenous injections of dope.

At times, in patients with mitral stenosis, the murmur of tricuspid insufficiency is erroneously diagnosed as that of mitral insufficiency. Sometimes these patients are not considered for commissurotomy because it is felt clinically that too much mitral insufficiency is present to warrant intervention. However, if the systolic murmur increases with inspiration, rather than decreases, and if at the same time there is an increase in the "V" wave in the jugular venous pulse, it should be recog-

nized that tricuspid insufficiency might be masquerading as mitral insufficiency. Echocardiography would be of great help in this instance in confirming the dominant and significant lesion to be that of mitral stenosis.
W. Proctor Harvey, M.D.

• Ventricular Septal Defect

The regurgitant murmur of the small ventricular septal defect is best heard at the left sternal edge in the fourth, fifth and sixth intercostal spaces (Roger's murmur). The murmur is accompanied by a prominent thrill. This murmur does not radiate well into the axilla as does the mitral insufficiency murmur, and it does not have the characteristic inspiratory augmentation seen in tricuspid insufficiency. The murmur of ventricular septal defect is an example of the lack of correlation between intensity of a regurgitant murmur and the seriousness of the lesion. The Roger's murmur is loud because of a high velocity, small volume shunt; defect is small and systolic gradient is large, therefore, velocity of flow through the shunt is great but the shunt volume itself is small.

With a large defect, there is no gradient. Shunt velocity is low, yet shunt volume may be great and the murmur less intense. As resistance rises in the pulmonary vascular bed the left to right shunt further diminishes and the classical Eisenmenger's complex regurgitant murmur disappears to be replaced by the short early ejection murmur of pulmonary hypertension.

Variations of the Pansystolic Regurgitant Murmur

• Early Systolic Murmurs (Figure 7)

Occasionally, in the presence of a small ventricular septal defect, a regurgitant murmur may be limited to early systole. This murmur begins in the usual manner with the onset of systole, but the murmur suddenly stops in early to mid systole (Figures 7, 8). Sudden cessation of the murmur is due to the fact that as ejection continues, ventricular size decreases, septum thickens, and the small defect is sealed shut with resultant cessation of the murmur. This type of murmur seen in infancy, childhood and young adulthood, is characteristic of small VSD's, many of which disappear with age.

Acute Severe Mitral Insufficiency: The prototype of mitral insufficiency is the chronic severe longstanding regurgitation seen in rheumatic heart disease. In acute mitral insufficiency secondary to papillary muscle or chordae tendineae rupture the left ventricle and the left atrium are normal in size

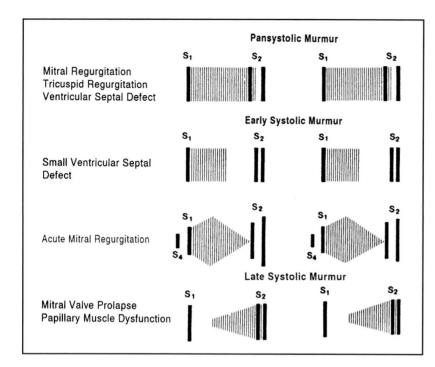

Figure 7. In addition to classic pansystolic regurgitant murmur seen in mitral regurgitation, tricuspid regurgitation, and ventricular septal defect, variations exist. In patients with small ventricular septal defects, murmur that starts with first heart sound (S$_1$) may suddenly stop during early or midsystole, purportedly because ventricular volume becomes smaller after maximal ejection, defect seals shut, and murmur ceases. In acute mitral regurgitation, regurgitant murmur may end well before aortic valve closure sound as a result of extremely high left atrial V wave, which abolishes left ventricular-left atrial pressure gradient during late systole. S$_1$ may be soft if flail mitral leaflet is present and is preceded by prominent fourth heart sound (S$_4$). Audible expiratory splitting with accentuated pulmonic valve closure sound is present. Midsystolic to late systolic regurgitant murmurs may be due to papillary muscle dysfunction and prolapse of mitral or tricuspid valve. In later conditions, valve is competent in early systole, but as ventricular volume decreases, leaflets become incompetent and murmur begins, building in late systole and becoming maximal at time of second heart sound (S$_2$).

and compliance and the rhythm is usually normal sinus in nature. With the sudden burden of severe mitral insufficiency, left atrial pressure rises rapidly in response to the large systolic regurgitant flow. The left atrial V wave peaks to or approaches the level of the left ventricular pressure towards the end of systole and the gradient from the left ventricle to the left atrium is small or absent during this part of the cardiac cycle. The murmur which signals the regurgitant flow and gradient wanes and may cease in late systole (Figure 9). This variant of the pansystolic regurgitant murmur

of mitral insufficiency coupled with the loud S$_4$ and a relatively normal sized heart, points to severe acute mitral insufficiency.

CARDIAC PEARL

Characteristically, the murmur of mitral valve insufficiency of the chronic type is holosystolic. When one hears a holosystolic (pansystolic) murmur one thinks of three conditions: mitral insufficiency, tricuspid insufficiency, and ventricular septal defect. If this murmur is maximal at the apex, then mitral insufficiency is the most likely cause. This is particularly likely if on moving the stethoscope in "band-like" fashion around to the back, one continues to hear the holosystolic murmur- not only at the apex, but also in the anterior axillary line, posterior axillary line, and posterior lung base (Fig. A). This "band-like" zone of radiation is characteristically of mitral valve insufficiency, especially of the chronic type. A filling sound (third sound or ventricular diastolic gallop) is a common finding. Also, following or coincident with the third heart sound, one often hears low-frequency vibrations which can produce a rumbling murmur although they do not reflect the lesion of mitral stenosis. The murmur of the acute form of mitral valve insufficiency is more likely to taper off in the latter part of systole. This is due to the fact that in the acute form the left atrium has not yet become distended (not having a large left atrium as in the case with the chronic mitral insufficiency)

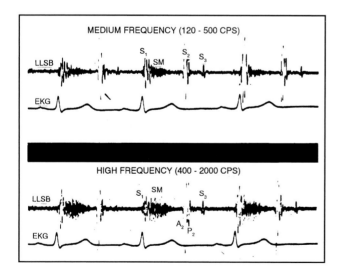

Figure 8. Typical murmur of small muscular septal defect in 19-yr-old asymptomatic girl. Early systolic murmur of high frequency starting with first heart sound and suddenly stopping about two-thirds through systole. *(With permission, 33).*

and when the acute significant leak of the mitral valve occurs as with a ruptured chorda tendineae, the pressure rises rapidly within the non-distensible left atrium during early systole. But the pressure builds up even higher in the latter part of systole, thereby concomitantly diminishing the rate of leakage and the intensity of the murmur. It is logical, therefore, that this murmur should be louder in the first or mid-portion of systole, and should decrease in the latter part.

In general, the murmur of acute mitral valve insufficiency tends to radiate anteriorly up the chest. A palpable thrill may be noted over the anterior precordium even at the base of the heart. At times the murmur radiates to the neck bilaterally. As a rule, if the murmur radiates anteriorly in this fashion it is more likely to reflect predominant involvement of the posterior leaflet of the mitral valve. If it radiates posteriorly and in the previously described "band-like" fashion to the back it is more likely to be the anterior leaflet of the mitral valve that is producing the major part of the regurgitant leak.

The differential diagnosis of acute mitral valve insufficiency versus the chronic has significant practical importance, and there are certain other differentiating features. It is important to make this distinction since corrective surgery can be performed for the acute problem to halt the progressive downhill course of congestive heart failure which often accompanies this complication. In the acute form the history of onset of symptoms is generally short whereas, in the chronic it occurs only after many years (after the appearance of the murmur). Men are more likely to have the acute as opposed to women who tend to have the chronic type. The acute form takes place in middle age or older, whereas the chronic form will have been noted for many years, often beginning in the second or third decade. Heart failure begins promptly with the onset of the murmur in the acute type. The patient may have had a period of temporary cardiac decompensation for several weeks or months, and then may become compensated. Occasionally, with the acute form there is a progressive downhill course without a period of improvement. This is in contrast with the chronic type where there is a more insidious, gradual onset of chronic cardiac decompensation coming on many years after the detection of the systolic murmur. Normal sinus rhythm is the rule

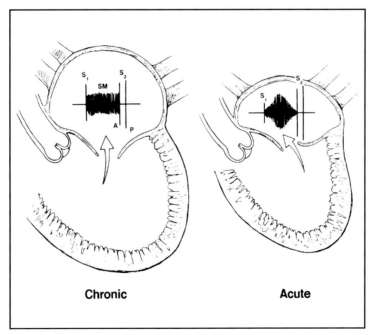

Fig A: During left ventricular systole, blood flows into the left atrium as well as the aorta, thereby emptying the left ventricle earlier. Therefore, the aortic valve (A_2) closes earlier, causing a wider split of the second sound (AP). Chronic regurgitation causes more left ventricular hypertrophy and left atrial enlargement, as well as more progressive regurgitation. Holosystolic murmur with chronic regurgitation extends up to A_2 and sometimes beyond. With acute regurgitation, the holosystolic murmur decreases in the latter part of systole because left atrial pressure significantly increases in a normal sized (or slightly enlarged) left atrium to about mid-systole and then decreases in late systole.

with the acute, whereas atrial fibrillation is very common in the chronic type. With the acute form the murmur is often rough or harsh, and it tends to decrease in the latter part of systole. Frequently it radiates anteriorly to the base of the heart, and even into the neck; it, therefore, can be confused with the murmur of aortic stenosis. On the other hand, the murmur of chronic mitral insufficiency is more likely to radiate laterally to the left posterior axillary line and the left posterior lung base. An atrial gallop is frequent in the acute problem, whereas it is unusual in the chronic. Cardiomegaly would be common in the chronic form, whereas in the acute the heart size might be normal or only slightly enlarged. Left atrial size tends to be moderately or greatly enlarged with chronic mitral valve insufficiency, whereas with the acute type it may be only slightly enlarged or not at all. Pulmonary hypertension is more likely to be a feature of the acute. By putting these various features together one can generally differentiate the acute versus the chronic type of mitral valve insufficiency.

W. Proctor Harvey, M.D.

• Mid- and Late-Systolic Regurgitant Murmurs

Papillary Muscle Dysfunction: These murmurs are recognized as regurgitant since they continue up to and through the aortic closure sound even though they do not start with the first heart sound but at a later time in mid or late systole. These murmurs are the result of papillary muscle dysfunction or mitral valve prolapse. Burch described the appearance of a late systolic murmur in patients with anterolateral subendocardial infarction. The murmur has been said to be due to anterior papillary muscle dysfunction secondary to ischemia or infarction of the structure. Appearance of late systolic murmur in a patient with chest pain and T wave inversion in V_4, V_5, and V_6, is said to be diagnostic of this syndrome.

Mitral Valve Prolapse: Mitral valve prolapse, a common condition, is the most frequent cause of late systolic murmurs. These murmurs are heard best at the apex and may crescendo at their termination with S_2 or may peak prior to this point in systole. Multiple studies have demonstrated that the scallops of the mitral leaflets (primarily those of the posterior leaflet) are large and redundant. During ventricular systole, as cavity size diminishes, the redundant leaflets prolapse or herniate into the left atrium. Their retrograde excursion is halted as the valve scallops reach their elastic limits due to the checking action of the chordae. At this point of deceleration, one or more clicks are heard and the

balloon leaflets are now incompetent. The multiple clicks introduce the murmur which continues through the remainder of systole (Figure 7).

The timing of the clicks as well as intensity, onset, and duration of the murmur may be altered by physiological and pharmacological maneuvers. Identification of these murmurs of mitral valve prolapse are of some importance because of increased incidence of embolic stroke and subacute bacterial endocarditis. It seems likely that in some patients, valvular dysfunction may progress so that the mitral valve is incompetent throughout all of systole with an unfavorable prognosis.

Systolic Whoop or Honk: A subset of the spectrum of late systolic murmurs with or without clicks is the systolic whoop or honk. This is a loud, high-pitched, musical or sonorous vibratory murmur usually heard at the apex and present in patients with known mitral valve dysfunction or occasionally in patients considered to have an otherwise normal

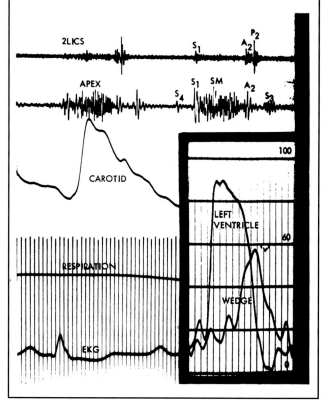

Figure 9. Forty-five-year-old male 12 weeks after myocardial infarction presents with severe congestive heart failure. Loud apical systolic murmur with atrial (S_4) and ventricular (S_3) gallop sounds. Note murmur starts with first heart sound (S_1) but fades and stops at aortic closure sound (A_2). Insert shows simultaneous left ventricular and pulmonary artery wedge pressure in the same patient. Note tall V wave of wedge pressure (reaching height of 60 mmHg) characteristic of acute mitral regurgitation. Murmur corresponds in timing and configuration to left ventricular-left atrial pressure gradient. *(With permission, 33).*

cardiovascular system. Such sounds are usually late systolic in nature, have a striking respiratory variation and may disappear and reappear on repeated examinations.

A very loud, musical systolic murmur- a "whoop"- occurring in the last half of systole is most likely due to mitral valve prolapse (Figure A).

Many years ago, a 23-year-old woman from another state was sitting outside of my office. On questioning her, she said, "I've come for the operation." I had no correspondence concerning her, but on examining her, she had no symptoms referable to her heart or cardiovascular system. On physical examination, the only positive finding was an intermittent, loud musical murmur occurring in the latter part of systole. It reminded me of the sound that occurs with a child who has whooping cough.

Thus, we gave it the name "systolic whoop" and believed it was a benign finding, even though at that time we could not explain its origin. Sometimes she would have no whoop sound, but would have a midsystolic click or clicks, and at still other times she had a late apical systolic murmur that did not have the musical "whoop" character. Subsequently, with the passage of years, this was documented as being part of the spectrum of auscultatory findings of mitral valve prolapse. Obviously no surgery was required.

Once this peculiar new sound had been described, others recognized and identified it in their own patients. Since then, we have seen many patients who have these musical "whoop" murmurs.

Subsequently, physicians at Duke University described a sound of similar nature and they termed it "systolic honk". Obviously more goose hunting is done in North Carolina than in the Washington, D.C. area. A "systolic whoop" can also be caused by a prolapse of the tricuspid valve. However, today the term "whoop" may not be a truly descriptive term, since most medical students have never seen and heard a patient with whooping cough and therefore would not

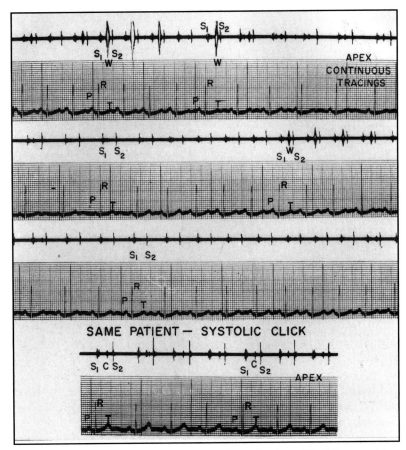

Fig A: Systolic Whoop - Note intermittent musical systolic whoop (W). At times, systole is clear of sounds or clicks (panel third from top). At other times only a click (C) is heard.

know what the whoop of that disease is like. Neither, I suspect, have most heard the "honk" of a goose.

Sometimes a late musical systolic "whoop" or "honk" may be a constant finding, or, more commonly, intermittently heard. Only very recently I saw a patient with mitral valve prolapse who had an intermittent "scraping" sound (like a metal blade scraping another metal) in late systole. These are variants of mitral valve prolapse and might only be heard in different positions.

The systolic "whoop" can be very loud; in fact, loud enough that others can hear it even several feet away. Several anecdotes: A woman "panicked" when she first heard loud noises emitting from her husband's chest (while in bed).

A young lady who was kind enough to be a patient we presented in some of our teaching conferences (group auscultation) would amuse the physicians in attendance by stating that the intermittent chest noise of her tricuspid valve might give a boyfriend the wrong impression that she cared for him more than she really did.

Another patient had such a loud late systolic whoop that she stopped coming to the cardiac clinic because of her embarrassing chest noise, which occurred with exertion; on climbing the stairs and boarding the subway people were aghast. However, she remarked, "I always got a seat."

Only recently, several residents told me about a peculiar sound that they were hearing in a patient; they had never heard anything like it before. The patient had an intermittent faint, but definite, "squeak" (like a mouse), in the latter part of systole. This was one of the many variants of mitral valve prolapse. Once hearing it, it will be readily identified when hearing it in another patient.

W. Proctor Harvey, M.D.

Traditionally, such sounds were thought to be extracardiac in nature but intracardiac phonocardiographic studies demonstrate that they originate from the mitral valve and together with the click and late systolic murmurs are part of a continuum representing mild mitral insufficiency. Such whooping murmurs may also be shown to emanate from the tricuspid valve. In addition, there are reports of such startling whooping sounds occurring in patients with transvenous right ventricular pacing electrode catheters in place. It is presumed that these catheters traversing the tricuspid valve have altered its normal function.

CARDIAC PEARL

Loud Murmurs That Can Be Heard Without a Stethoscope- Some very loud murmurs can be heard without a stethoscope, sometimes even several feet away from the patient. Conditions most likely to cause such a murmur are mitral valve prolapse, tricuspid valve prolapse, tricuspid regurgitation, or malfunction of a prosthetic valve.

Less likely causes are the loudest murmurs of aortic stenosis and pulmonic stenosis, traumatic arteriovenous fistula from shrapnel or bullet wounds or from automobile or airplane accidents, or traumatic rupture of a heart valve.

I recall one soldier who had an arteriovenous fistula due to a shrapnel wound. It produced a loud continuous murmur over his posterior chest. When he recovered consciousness after the injury, he thought the enemy tanks were coming because of the vibration due to his fistula while he was lying on the ground.

Another patient I remember was kicked in the chest by a horse. On recovery, he likened the sound emanating from his chest to that of a water pump on the farm where he grew up. He had traumatic rupture of his aortic valve, producing severe aortic regurgitation.

The presence of a transvenous pacemaker across a tricuspid valve can occasionally produce peculiar, bizarre musical murmurs.

I recall hearing such a murmur in a patient who had just had a pacemaker inserted. The sounds, heard in both systole and diastole, sounded like the "croaking of a frog." On repositioning of the catheter, the sounds disappeared.

In other patients, the catheter across any valve may cause a sound that simulates the systolic "whoop" of mitral valve prolapse. Again, it is related to the catheter position, and the sound disappears on removal or repositioning of the catheter.

W. Proctor Harvey, M.D.

Diastolic Murmurs

There are two types of diastolic murmurs: Diastolic rumbles, which are low pitched (hence, rumbling), created during flow across the mitral and tricuspid valve, and diastolic regurgitant murmurs caused by retrograde flow across an incompetent aortic or pulmonic valve.

Diastolic Rumbles

These murmurs are the result of an increased flow across normal atrioventricular valves or flow across diseased valves which are distorted, stiffened or stenotic.

Ventricular filling involves two rapid phases: the first is in protodiastole and is called the early rapid filling phase. The second occurs as the result of atrial systolic booster pump effect which is the presystolic or active ventricular filling period. Diastolic rumbles are most prominent during one or both of these filling phases. Since right-sided rumbles increase with inspiration, this finding aids in the differentiation of tricuspid from mitral rumbles. The latter vary little with respiration.

CARDIAC PEARL

A diastolic murmur almost always indicates the presence of underlying heart disease. Exceptions can occur. This is related to the after-vibrations of a normal physiologic third heart sound that is present. I have personally observed the normal physiologic third heart sound in all of more than 100 children approximately 10-11 years of age. It is a frequent finding in young people, including women in the childbearing age. Most women retain their third sound up to, and sometimes through the third and fourth decades, which are the childbearing ages. Indeed, a normal third heart sound is often accentuated and thereby more easily heard during pregnancy.

The normal third heart sound characteristically waxes and wanes with respiration, and at times, on careful auscultation, a short low-frequency rumble may be heard coincident with and shortly after its occurrence. This is sometimes described as "the third heart sound with duration" and can be interpreted as organic heart disease. One can readily understand why in a patient having a systolic

murmur of the innocent type, the finding of a third heart sound with low-frequency vibrations concurrently and just afterward could lead to the diagnosis of heart disease, such as rheumatic heart disease with mitral insufficiency and mitral stenosis. Patients with this combination of findings have been completely evaluated, and it has been shown that these are innocent murmurs.

W. Proctor Harvey, M.D.

• Mitral Stenosis

The rumbling murmur of mitral stenosis is heard best at the cardiac apex or slightly medial to this point. The murmur consists of low frequency vibrations which are close to the threshold of audibility. To listen for the murmur, one must place the patient in the supine position, then have the patient roll slightly on to the left side and listen with the bell of the stethoscope pressed lightly against the skin with just enough pressure to make a seal. The examiner should listen as the patient is rolling or immediately afterward. The murmur is introduced by an opening snap and, in severe mitral stenosis, continues up to the next first heart sound with a presystolic accentuation. The murmur of increased flow across a relatively normal valve is of higher frequency and higher amplitude than the murmur of severe MS, meaning that a loud rumble does not necessarily correlate with severity of the stenosis. Rather, it is the length of the murmur reflecting the duration of the mitral valve gradient which in turn indicates the severity of the valvular obstruction (Figure 10).

In the face of tachycardia, diastolic filling time is shortened and the potential length of the murmur is not challenged. Carotid sinus pressure, if it is successful in temporarily slowing the heart rate,

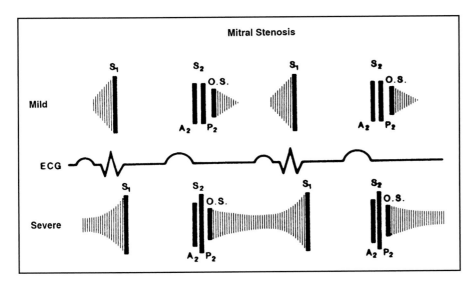

Figure 10. In mild mitral stenosis, diastolic gradient across the valve is limited to two phases of rapid ventricular filling in early diastole and presystole. Rumble occurs during either or both periods. As the stenotic process becomes severe, large gradient exists across mitral valve during entire diastolic filling period and rumble persists throughout diastolic filling period. As left atrial pressure becomes higher, time from aortic valve closure sound (A_2) to opening snap (OS) shortens. In severe mitral stenosis, secondary pulmonary hypertension results in louder pulmonic valve closure sound (P_2) and splitting interval usually narrows. S_1, first heart sound; S_2, second heart sound. (Perm. AHA)

will uncover the potential length of the murmur and severity of obstruction. In the face of atrial fibrillation, a common complication of mitral stenosis, one should listen patiently in an effort to hear the length of the diastolic rumble during a series of slow beats with long diastolic filling times. This will unmask the potential duration of the gradient and the murmur. The presystolic murmur of mitral stenosis is in fact an atrial systolic ejection murmur. In the presence of mitral stenosis complicated by heart block, one might hear a murmur or series of such murmurs occurring with each atrial contraction. When observed in this fashion, it becomes obvious that the usual presystolic murmur is the crescendo portion of an atrial systolic ejection murmur. At normal PR intervals, the first heart sound interrupts this murmur before the decrescendo half of the murmur occurs. The presystolic augmentation of the mitral diastolic rumble is not only the result of increased flow during atrial contraction, but also due to progressive narrowing of the mitral orifice during early ventricular systole as the left ventricular pressure rises but is still lower than the left atrial pressure and the first sound has not yet occurred. This early systolic closing of the mitral leaflets prior to the first sound is the explanation of the fact that a presystolic augmentation of the mitral rumble may sometimes occur in the face of atrial fibrillation. A mitral diastolic rumble may be heard in the presence of a left atrial myxoma, dynamically obstructing the mitral orifice. The tumor may protrude into the left ventricle during early left ventricular filling. When the tumor reaches the end of its excursion and is decelerated, a sound called a "tumor plop" may occur. Its mechanism and timing is similar to the opening snap. This murmur as well as the murmur of mitral regurgitation occurring in the presence of a left atrial myxoma varies from examination to examination and with changes in posture.

• Tricuspid Stenosis

The murmur of tricuspid stenosis is best heard just off the left sternal border in the xyphoid area. Right atrial systole occurs earlier than the equivalent event on the left side of the heart. Therefore, the presystolic murmur which is an atrial systolic ejection murmur occurs earlier and may have the classic diamond-shaped configuration with the murmur beginning to wane before the loud tricuspid closure sound. This early presystolic diamond-shaped murmur and a large A wave in the neck, both of which show inspiratory augmentation, is a useful sign in uncovering tricuspid stenosis in the presence of mitral stenosis. This is an important differential point since tricuspid stenosis occurs almost exclusively in the presence of mitral stenosis which in turn partially masks the signs of the tricuspid valve obstruction.

With onset of atrial fibrillation, total tricuspid diastolic flow may remain relatively unchanged, but hemodynamic observations show that the flow pattern is altered with the resultant predominant flow occurring in mid-early diastole. The bedside diagnosis of tricuspid stenosis in the presence of atrial fibrillation is quite difficult. It requires high index of suspicion and a careful search for the mid-diastolic rumble heard best off the left sternal border displaying inspiratory augmentation. The rumble of mitral stenosis does not demonstrate such inspiratory augmentation.

• Austin Flint Murmur

In cases of severe aortic regurgitation, early diastolic ventricular filling occurs simultaneously from both the left atrium and the aorta. The anterior leaflet of the mitral valve forms a curtain which separates the inflow and outflow tract of the left ventricle. The ventricle fills rapidly from both pathways. This causes the mitral leaflet, drawn partially closed, to be thrown into vibration and the diastolic rumble ensues. This rumble is introduced by a ventricular filling sound (S_3) rather than the usual opening snap which introduces the murmur of true mitral stenosis. The murmur as originally described by Flint was a presystolic murmur. This occurs, but less commonly than the mid-diastolic rumble. Use of amyl nitrite inhalation may help differentiate the two murmurs. The drug causes peripheral vasodilatation, unloading the ventricle, diminishing the aortic regurgitant flow, hence diminishing the Flint murmur. On the contrary, the resultant reflex tachycardia increases the mitral obstruction gradient and the murmur of true mitral stenosis is accentuated.

In acute severe aortic insufficiency, the pressure gradient between the aortic root and the left ventricle begins to equalize in mid-diastole and the mitral valve is closed in late diastole. In this setting there is no presystolic Austin Flint murmur and an absent or faint first heart sound.

Diastolic Regurgitant Murmurs

These murmurs, as with all diastolic murmurs, are usually highly significant and yet are frequently missed. At first this seems surprising since the murmurs are high pitched and in the frequency range where the ear is very sensitive, but they are frequently overlooked for a number of reasons. The murmurs frequently go unnoticed because the attention of the examiner is directed toward the medium frequency of the heart sounds and systolic murmurs. In addition, the examiner does not specifically listen for these murmurs in the high frequency range. Lastly, the examiner fails to listen for the murmur with the patient sitting up, leaning forward in deep fixed expiration with the diaphragm of the stethoscope pressed firmly against the chest wall. Such murmurs are specifically listened for in the second and third interspaces to the right and left of the sternal border. The character of the regurgitant murmur of itself will usually not define which set of semilunar valves is involved, nor is the location or radiation of the murmur sufficiently specific to be clinically helpful. One exception to this general rule is that murmurs which radiate more prominently down the right sternal border than the left alert the examiner to the fact that the murmur is aortic in origin and may be a manifestation of a dilated or aneurysmal aortic root. Such aneurysmal dilatation in turn may be the result of arteriosclerotic disease, syphilis, or Marfan's syndrome, etc. The contrary is not true since many patients with the above lesions still have a normal radiation of the murmur. The normal radiation of the diastolic regurgitant murmur of semilunar valve is down the left side of the sternum spreading out toward the apex.

• Aortic Regurgitant Murmur

The prototype of the regurgitant diastolic murmur is that of chronic aortic valve insufficiency. At the time of valve closure, a rapid gradient builds up between the aorta and the left ventricular cavity. This gradient is almost instantaneously maximal and thereafter the aortic pressure decreases and the left ventricular pressure begins to rise with the resultant gradient narrowing. In moderate to severe chronic aortic insufficiency, sufficient gradient exists so that the murmur continues through all of the diastolic cycle until the next first heart sound. In minimal aortic insufficiency, the valve may be incompetent only when it is supporting the highest gradient immediately after the second heart sound. The regurgitant flow disappears in early diastole.

A good example of this dynamic equilibrium was demonstrated by Partnope and Harvey, who administered a small dose of Hexamethonium to a small group of young patients with severe diastolic hypertension. This resulted in postural hypotension. When these patients were tilted upright, their diastolic pressures dropped and they lost their short regurgitant murmur. When the patients were returned to the horizontal position and the diastolic

pressure returned to control levels (120mmHg to 140mmHg) the murmur returned. The concept of the aortic left ventricular pressure gradient establishing the basis of the murmur when the valve is incompetent explains why the duration of the regurgitant murmur is a marker of the severity of insufficiency. As mild aortic insufficiency becomes increasingly severe, the murmur becomes longer and longer. The diastolic pressure volume curve of the left ventricle in chronic severe aortic insufficiency is flat enough so that there is usually a continuing gradient up until the next systole. This is not the case in acute severe aortic insufficiency. The previously normal or near-normal sized left ventricle has not had time to adapt to the large diastolic regurgitant flow and left ventricular diastolic pressure rises rapidly. The aortic left ventricular pressure gradient equalizes early and the murmur is short, rough and usually loud stopping in mid diastole. The finding of severe aortic insufficiency coupled with an absent first heart sound and a relatively normal sized heart confirms the fact that the condition is acute. The differential diagnosis of the etiological cause should include endocarditis, dissection, trauma, or dehiscence of an aortic valve graft or prosthesis.

As has been stated, etiology of aortic insufficiency is not readily determined by the quality of the murmur. Nevertheless, the presence of a "cooing dove" or "musical" diastolic murmur usually signals rupture or retroversion of one of the aortic cusps. Such a rupture may be a complication of bacterial endocarditis or trauma or may be an unusual complication of atherosclerosis involving the aortic valve. In the past, retroversion of the right anterior aortic cusp giving rise to a "cooing dove" murmur was a known complication of syphilitic aortitis. The syphilitic process resulted in dilation and widening of the aorta root with resultant spreading of the commissures. Therefore, the keystone support of the cusps approximating each other was lost and the valve edges began to roll and the cusps could be caught in the regurgitant stream and retroverted.

• Pulmonary Regurgitant Murmur

Graham Steele first described the pulmonary regurgitant murmur secondary to pulmonary hypertension, and the murmur bears his name. This murmur, secondary to pulmonary hypertension, has the same timing and quality as the aortic regurgitant murmur (Figure 11). Location of maximum intensity, as well as the radiation of the two murmurs overlap. Both are frequently heard best in the third left interspace just off the sternal border radiating down the left sternal edge to the

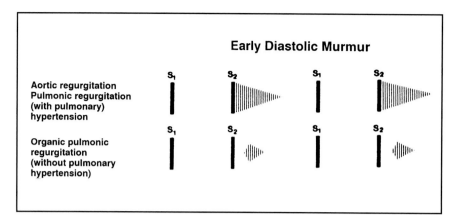

Figure 11. In aortic regurgitation or pulmonic regurgitation secondary to pulmonary hypertension, murmur begins almost simultaneously with second heart sound (S_2). Since gradient between aorta and left ventricle is maximal almost instantaneously and then slowly decreases, murmur is also high-pitched, slow decrescendo. In contrast, organic pulmonary regurgitation without pulmonary hypertension is manifested by murmur that starts later and has rapid crescendo with longer decrescendo. This murmur is lower pitched than usual early diastolic blowing murmur because regurgitant flow is across lower pressure system with small gradient. S_1, first heart sound. (Permission AHA)

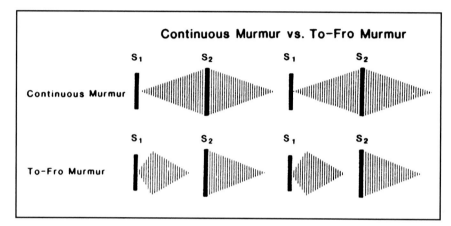

Figure 12. During abnormal communication between high-pressure and low-pressure systems, large pressure gradient exists throughout cardiac cycle, producing continuous murmur. A classic example is patent ductus arteriosus. At times, this type of murmur is confused with to-fro murmur, which is a combination of systolic ejection murmur and murmur of semilunar valve incompetence. A classic example of to-fro murmur is aortic stenosis and regurgitation. Continuous murmur builds to crescendo around second heart sound (S_2), whereas to-fro murmur has two components. Midsystolic ejection component decrescendos and disappears as it approaches S_2. S_1, first heart sound. (Perm. AHA)

apex. This regurgitant murmur of pulmonary valve incompetence when graphically displaced on high speed phonocardiograms is shown to occur immediately after the pulmonary closure sound. Since the pulmonary closure sound is delayed relative to the aortic closure, one might expect that the listener observing this delay could distinguish between the two murmurs at the bedside. In practice, this is not possible. The murmur is commonly seen in primary pulmonary hypertension or pulmonary hypertension secondary to intracardiac shunts such as Eisenmenger's complex. The combination of increased pressure coupled with pulmonary dilatation secondary to increased flow further favors the presence of such a murmur.

At one time, it was generally accepted that patients with severe rheumatic mitral stenosis and a diastolic regurgitant murmur were displaying the Graham Steele murmur since it was recognized that such patients frequently had pulmonary hypertension and the murmur was seen in absence of peripheral signs of aortic insufficiency. We now know that in such a setting these murmurs are almost all aortic, even in the absence of peripheral signs of aortic insufficiency. Rarely, pulmonic valve insufficiency may be organic in nature. The valve may be incompetent as a result of a congenital

defect, absence of the valve, as a complication of endocarditis or surgical correction of pulmonic stenosis, either valvular or infundibular in nature.

Pulmonary valve insufficiency without pulmonary hypertension gives rise to a murmur with characteristic timing and configuration. The murmur is separated from the pulmonary valve closure sound by the short interval necessary for the presence of a gradient between the pulmonary artery and the right ventricle to reach a threshold for turbulence to occur. The murmur builds up in a crescendo-decrescendo fashion as shown in Figure 11. This murmur is heard only during a short part of diastole where the gradient is maximal. The murmur is lower pitched than the usual early diastolic murmur of semilunar valvular insufficiency because the regurgitant flow is across a low pressure system with only a small gradient. The low frequency content of the murmur occurring in protodiastole may give rise to confusion in differentiating this murmur from that of the rumble of mitral or tricuspid stenosis.

Continuous Murmurs

High Pressure Shunts

A continuous murmur may be heard when there is an abnormal communication from a high pressure system to a lower pressure system resulting in a large pressure gradient throughout the cardiac cycle. The prototype of such a murmur is that of patent ductus arteriosus. This murmur is heard best in the pulmonic area. In coronary A-V fistula, in aortic pulmonary fenestration, in rupture of the sinus of Valsalva into the right side of the heart, or in the presence of an abnormal left coronary arising from the pulmonary artery, a continuous murmur may be heard at the right sternal edge (Figure 12).

CARDIAC PEARL

The most important auscultatory finding in the diagnosis of patent ductus arteriosus is a continuous murmur that envelops the second heart sound. When the second heart sound is not enveloped, always consider the possibility of another lesion simulating patent ductus arteriosus or of an associated defect. "All that is continuous is not patent ductus." In fact, there are about 30 causes of so-called continuous murmurs. When an associated congenital defect is present with patent ductus arteriosus, the classic machinery-like murmur may be changed when combined with the auscultatory features of the associated lesions.

It is important to listen carefully with both the bell and diaphragm of the stethoscope. Sometimes the continuous murmur is best heard with the diaphragm; at other times it is better heard with the bell (applying light pressure). A small ductus is more likely to have higher frequencies that are best heard with the diaphragm (applying firm pressure). The lower frequencies, associated with "eddy" sounds and louder murmurs, are more common with a larger ductus and are heard best with the bell. However, there appears to be no absolute correlation between the size of the ductus and the intensity of the murmur.

Sometimes the continuous murmur of patent ductus is heard louder over the third left sternal border rather than the pulmonic area. However, carefully check out such a patient to make sure there isn't another cause for the continuous murmur, such as coronary arteriovenous fistula, which can produce a murmur over the third or fourth sternal border.

Murmurs from medium sized ducti may have both high and low frequencies, averaging grade 3 or 4, and usually are easily heard on auscultation. These murmurs are loudest over the pulmonic area. We have used the analogy of a pipe organ in the church- the larger pipes have such low frequencies that the room seems to vibrate, while the small pipes produce the melodic high frequency sounds.

W. Proctor Harvey, M.D.

• Localized Arterial Obstruction

In coarctation of the aorta when the lumen is so small that a gradient exists across constriction at all times, a continuous murmur may be heard over the back. In pulmonary artery atresia (pseudo-truncus arteriosus) or in other conditions of obstruction to pulmonary flow, continuous murmurs may be heard over the chest which are the result of rapid flow through the large bronchial arteries. Similar murmurs may be heard in patients with pulmonary A-V fistulas.

Continuous Murmurs Due to Rapid Blood Flow

The prototype of the continuous murmur due to rapid blood flow is the cervical venous hum. This cervical venous hum is a continuous or almost continuous murmur with a diastolic accentuation. The murmur configuration reflects the flow pattern in the jugular system with diastolic accentuation and fading in presystole.

CARDIAC PEARL

A continuous innocent venous hum murmur in the neck is a common finding in children.

Such a murmur was personally observed in every one of approximately 100 school children 10 to 12 years old when it was carefully searched for using the following technique: The patient should be in the sitting position (the hum's origin is venous blood flow in the jugular vein which empties into the right atrium). On auscultation, the right hand places the bell of the stethoscope over the

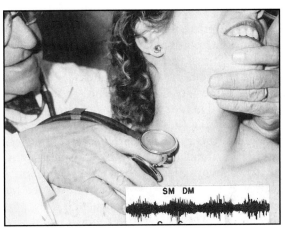

Fig A: Techniques to Detect a Venous Hum, (SM-DM) - The patient sits. The physician listens with the bell of the stethoscope over the right supraclavicular fossa, while his left hand holds the chin and moves it in the opposite direction and "on a stretch."

right supraclavicular fossa; the left hand holds the patient's chin from behind and tilts it upward and to the left. When an optimal position of the neck "on a stretch" is reached, the hum, if present, will be heard (Figure A).

W. Proctor Harvey, M.D.

Such vascular murmurs are most frequently seen in children and young adults. The hum is also frequent in high output states such as pregnancy, anemia and hyperthyroidism.

CARDIAC PEARL

Hyperthyroidism: the absence of a venous hum practically rules out hyperthyroidism.

Recently, as a coincidence, two patients, each nervous and very hyperactive types, were evaluated within a period of ten days. Each brought up the possibility of hyperthyroidism, but no venous hum was heard. Thyroid studies were normal in both.

The so-called "thyroid bruit" of hyperthyroidism is usually a venous hum.

Some patients with hyperthyroidism do have a "thyroid bruit" in addition to the venous hum. It is apparently due to the increased blood flow through the vascular thyroid gland. A few patients with hyperthyroids may have a true faint, high frequency, continuous murmur that can be clearly heard after the venous hum is temporarily eliminated by pressure over the jugular vein.

Furthermore, some venous hums not related to thyrotoxicosis can also have a residual high frequency continuous hum when pressure on the jugular vein has eliminated the louder low frequency components.

W. Proctor Harvey, M.D.

Venous hum is best elicited by placing the patient in the upright position with the head turned sharply to one side (preferably the left). The bell of the stethoscope is placed slightly over the supraclavicular fossa at the lateral edge of the sternocleidomastoid muscle. The venous nature of the murmur is confirmed by the fact that gentle compression over the jugular system higher in the neck obliterates the hum. If the hum obviously persists in the supine position, it favors the diagnosis of hyperdynamic circulation. Such continuous murmurs are also heard over the hyperactive thyroid, although they are not as common as the thyroid bruit which usually stops at the time of the second heart sound. Increased vascular flow is responsible for the mammary souffle as well as continuous murmurs associated with neoplasms such as renal cell carcinoma and hepatoma.

CARDIAC PEARL

A venous hum frequently has the character of a continuous loud, low frequency roaring murmur, and it usually can be made to disappear by moving the head to the forward position. Light pressure with the finger over the upper part of the jugular vein will cause the murmur to cease, although uncommonly a high frequency, faint, "whining" continuous murmur remains.

A venous hum is present in conditions associated with a rapid circulation and an increased cardiac output. It is an expected finding in pregnancy, anemia, and hyperthyroidism.

On careful examination of approximately 90 National Football League players, a venous hum was detected in all. The frequency of occurrence of a venous hum in these players (ages in their 20's or early 30's) was similar to that of children. Why is this? Remember that the venous hum is probably the result of a degree of normal mild obstruction of venous blood flow in the jugular vein to the right side of the heart, heard with the bell of the stethoscope placed over the supraclavicular fossa, especially when the patient's head is turned to the opposite direction and the neck is on a stretch. Many professional football players are large, muscular men weighing 250 to 300 pounds. They work out with weights and a common result is the development of large neck muscles.

It is interesting to theorize from the armchair that this muscular enlargement produces some degree of pressure on the jugular vein, which in turn results in some insignificant obstruction to blood flow, similar to what occurs when one listens with the bell of the stethoscope over the supraclavicular fossa with the neck "on a stretch" and turned in the opposite direction. The venous hum in the football players, however, could often be heard with the head in the forward position and became much more easily heard and often quite loud when the neck was put on a stretch.

A venous hum can be misdiagnosed as patent ductus arteriosus. This continuous murmur may be so prominent that it is heard transmitted over the pulmonic area, thereby being mistaken for patent ductus. This is uncommon, but does occur. In fact, in the past, once or twice a year we would have a young patient referred for surgical correction of a ductus. With tongue in cheek we would say these patients could be *medically cured* of a patent ductus by simple pressure with one's index finger or thumb over the jugular vein, thereby eliminating the murmur.

If routine auscultation in every patient examined includes the neck regions, a venous hum is often readily identified.

Even though a venous hum can be loud, the patient usually does not hear it, although one might expect them to. "Never say never." Personally observed was a woman who heard and was bothered by the noise of her loud venous hum. It was definitely proven that she could hear it. She represents the rare example "against the rule."

W. Proctor Harvey, M.D.

Continuous Murmurs Versus To-Fro Murmurs

Differentiation of continuous murmurs from to-fro murmurs is shown in Figure 12.

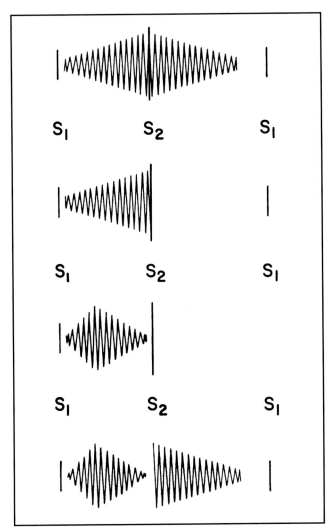

Figure 13. Upper panel shows a continuous murmur clustering around the second heart sound (S$_2$). The second panel shows that the diastolic component has dropped out. The third panel shows that the systolic murmur has become a midsystolic ejection murmur. The lower panel shows the addition of a diastolic component resulting in a to-fro murmur. For details, see text. *(With permission, 23).*

• Combination of Continuous and To-Fro Murmurs

While there is little difficulty differentiating a continuous murmur from a to-fro murmur, it should be remembered that such murmurs may occur together in the same patient. Figure 13 demonstrates a continuous murmur clustering around the second heart sound. The prototype would be a patent ductus arteriosus. With increasing pressures in the pulmonary circulation, the diastolic murmur may shorten and disappear, leaving only the systolic murmur which in turn with increasing pressure becomes an ejection murmur over the pulmonary artery. Finally, with severe pulmonary hypertension, a pulmonic insufficiency murmur appears, which together with the pulmonary ejection murmur results in a to-fro quality. Actually, in some patients with patent ductus arteriosus, a continuous murmur and a to-fro murmur may exist at the same time in the same patient. The presence of one may be masked by the other.

Figure 14 is an angiocardiogram taken from a patient with classical findings of aortic valve insufficiency. Because ECG demonstrated the appearance of a right bundle branch block and the chest x-ray showed a large pulmonary artery, the patient was carefully re-examined and found to have a continuous murmur as well as a to-fro murmur. In light of this combination of findings, the diagnosis of ruptured sinus of Valsalva was made in addition to that of aortic valve incompetence. The aortic arteriogram shows very clearly the fistulous track from the aortic root to the right ventricle but it also shows that the aortic valve as such is competent. The patient had two murmurs; the to-fro murmur dominated but the aortic valve was competent with the regurgitant flow going into the right ventricle. In patients with congenital aortic stenosis who demonstrate an early diastolic murmur, look carefully for an additional continuous murmur of patent ductus arteriosus, especially if the patient also has coarctation of the aorta.

CARDIAC PEARL

Murmurs (bruits) are not an uncommon finding over other portions of the body, such as the abdomen. The finding of a systolic murmur (bruit) over the abdomen in the absence of symptoms is not diagnostic of any pathology and is more frequent than generally appreciated. However, at times, the presence of a systolic or continuous murmur heard over the abdomen may be the clue as to changes in the caliber of one of the arteries of

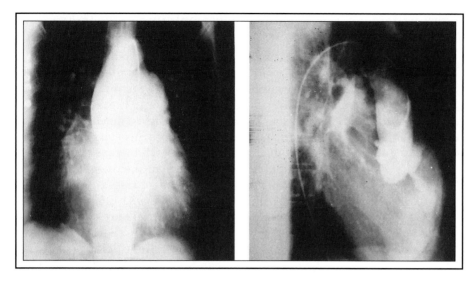

Figure 14. Retrograde aortogram with injection into the root of the aorta. Note fistula from the sinus of Valsalva to the right ventricle. Note also that there is no aortic regurgitation into the left ventricle. *(With permission, 23).*

the abdomen and may be of aid in the diagnosis. For example, appearance of a murmur over the abdomen may be the clue to the presence of renovascular hypertension.

We have seen several examples of an abdominal murmur formerly not present but subsequently associated with a new complaint of abdominal discomfort. This was illustrated by a woman in her 50s who had a new complaint and a new physical finding. (Previously, all of her symptoms were predominantly psychoneurotic in origin and had been above the diaphragm and had been present for many years.) Then, for the first time, she complained of abdominal pain, and a systolic bruit not present before was heard over the midepigastric area. The results of a complete work-up, including gastrointestinal series, gallbladder series, urinary tract studies, and liver and pancreatic scans, were negative. However, because of her persistent complaints and the presence of this new auscultatory finding, she had surgical exploration. Carcinoma of the pancreas was found that encroached on one of the arteries in the vicinity of the pancreas, reducing its caliber and producing the bruit. We have had several such examples. More attention, therefore, should be paid to detecting the presence of murmurs (bruits) in areas other than the heart.

W. Proctor Harvey, M.D.

Selected Reading

1. Barlow JB, Pocock WA, Marchand P et al: The significance of late systolic murmurs. *AHJ* 66: 443-452, 1963.
2. Burch GE, DePasquale NP, Phillips JH: Clinical manifestations of papillary muscle dysfunction. *Arch Int Med* 112: 112-117, 1963.
3. Burch GE, DePasquale NP, Phillips JH: The syndrome of papillary muscle dysfunction. *AHJ* 75:399, 1968.
4. Craige E: Phonocardiography in interventricular septal defect. *AHJ* 60: 51-60, 1960.
5. Criley JM, Hermer AJ: The crescendo presystolic murmur of mitral stenosis with atrial fibrillation. *NEJM* 285: 1284-1287, 1971.
6. Criley JM, Lewis XB, Humphries JO, et al: Prolapse of the mitral valve. Clinical and cine-angiocardiographic findings. *BHJ* 28: 488-496, 1966.
7. DePace NL, Nestico PF, Morganroth J: Acute severe mitral regurgitation: pathophysiology, clinical recognition and management. *AJM* 78:293-306, 1985.
8. Flint A: On cardiac murmurs. *AJMS* 44:29-54, 1862.
9. Fortuin NJ, Craige E: On the Austin Flint murmur. *Circ* 45:558- 570, 1972.
10. Fowler NO, Gause R: The cervical venous hum. *AHJ* 67:135-136, 1964.
11. Freeman AR, Levine SA: Clinical significance of systolic murmur: A study of 1000 consecutive "non-cardiac" cases. *Ann Int Med* 6:1371, 1933.
12. Gallavardin L, Pauper-Ravault: Le souffle du retrecissement aortique peot changer du timbre et devenir musical dans sa propagation apexienne. *Lyon Med* 523, 1925.
13. Harvey WP, Corrado MA, Perloff J: "Right-sided" murmurs of aortic insufficiency (diastolic murmurs better heard to the right side of the sternum rather than to the left). *AJMS* 245:533-543, 1963.
14. Henke RP, March HW, Hultgren HN: An aid to identification of the murmur of aortic stenosis with atypical localization. *AHJ* 60:354-363, 1960.
15. Hultgren HN, Reeve R, Cohn K, et al: The ejection click of valvular pulmonic stenosis. *Circ* 40:631-640, 1969.
16. Killip T III, Lucas DS: Tricuspid stenosis: Clinical features in twelve cases. *AJM* 24:836-852, 1958.
17. Leatham A: Systolic murmurs. *Circ* 17:601-611, 1958.
18. Leatham A: The spectrum of ventricular septal defect. In Leon DF, Shaver JA (eds): Physiologic Principles of Heart Sounds and Murmurs. *AHA* Monograph No. 46, pp 135-138. New York; AHA 1975.
19. Leatham A, Segal BL: Auscultatory and phonocardiographic signs of ventricular septal defect with left-to-right shunt. *Circ* 25:318-327, 1962.
20. Leatham A, Vogelpoel L: The early systolic sound in dilation of the pulmonary artery. *BHJ* 16:21-33, 1954.
21. Leon DF, Leonard JJ, Kroetz FW, et al: Late systolic murmurs, clicks, and whoops arising from the mitral valve. *AHJ*

72:325-336, 1966.

22. Leon DF, Leonard JJ, Lancaster JF, et al: Effect of respiration on pansystolic regurgitant murmurs as studied by biatrial intracardiac phonocardiography. *AJM* 39:429-441, 1965.

23. Leonard JJ, Allensworth D: Differential diagnosis of the early diastolic murmur. In Segal BL (ed): *Theory and Practice of Auscultation,* pp 487-499. Philadelphia: FA Davis Co, 1964.

24. Leonard JJ, Shaver JA: Acute mitral insufficiency. *Hospital Practice* 20:75-80, 84-89, 92-93, 1985.

25. Levine SA, Harvey WP: *Clinical Auscultation of the Heart.* Philadelphia: WB Saunders Co, 1959.

26. Martin CE, Reddy PS, Leon DF, et al: Genesis, frequency and diagnostic significance of ejection sound in adults with Tetralogy of Fallot. *BHJ* 35:402-412, 1973.

27. Murgo JP, Altobell SA, Dorethy JF, et al: Normal ventricular ejection dynamics in man during rest and exercise. In Leon DF, Shaver JA (eds): Physiologic Principles of Heart Sounds and Murmurs. AHA Monograph No. 46, pp 35-44. New York: AHA 1975.

28. Nasser WK, Davis RH, Dillon JC, et al: Atrial myxoma. II. Phonocardiographic, echocardiographic, hemodynamic and angiographic features in nine cases. *AHJ* 83:810-823.

29. Paley HW: Left ventricular outflow tract obstruction: heart sounds and murmurs. In Leon DF, Shaver JA (eds): Physiologic Principles of Heart Sounds and Murmurs. AHA Monograph No. 46, pp 107-117. New York: AHA, 1975.

30. Popp RL, Brown OR, Silverman JF, et al: Echocardiographic abnormalities in the mitral valve prolapse syndrome. *Circ* 49:428-433, 1974.

31. Reddy PS, Curtis EL, Salerni R, et al: Sound pressure correlates of the Austin Flint murmur: An intracardiac sound study. *Circ* 53:210-217, 1976.

32. Reddy PS, Leon DF, Krishnaswami V, et al: Syndrome of acute aortic regurgitation. In Leon DE, Shaver JA (eds): Physiologic Principles of Heart Sounds and Murmurs. AHA Monograph No. 46, pp 166-174. New York: American Heart Association, 1975.

33. Reddy PS, Shaver JA, Leonard JJ: Cardiac systolic murmurs: pathophysiology and differential diagnosis. *Prog Card Dis* XIV:1-37, 1971.

34. Rivero Carvallo JM: Signo para el diagnostic de las insuficiencias tricuspideas. *Arch Inst Cardiol Mexico* 16:531-539, 1946.

35. Roger H: Recherches cliniques sur la communication congenitale des deux coeurs par inocclusion du septum interventriculaire. *Bull Acad Med (Paris)* 8:1074-1094, 1879.

36. Ronan JA Jr, Steelman RB, deLeon AC Jr et al: The clinical diagnosis of acute mitral insufficiency. *AJC* 27:284-290, 1971.

37. Runco V, Levin HS: The spectrum of pulmonic regurgitation. In Leon DF, Shaver JA (eds): Physiologic Principles of Heart Sounds and Murmurs. AHA Monoraph No.46, pp 175-182. New York: AHA, 1975.

38. Runco V, Molnar W, Meckstrotl CV, et al: The Graham Steele murmur versus aortic regurgitation in rheumatic heart diseases. Results of aortic valvulography. *AJM* 31:71-80, 1961.

39. Sanders CA, Harthorne JW, DeSanctis RW, et al: Tricuspid stenosis, a difficult diagnosis in presence of atrial fibrillatlon. *Circ* 33:26-33, 1966.

40. Schilder DP, Harvey WP: Confusion of tricuspid incompetency with mitral insufficiency – a pitfall in the selection of patients for mitral surgery. *AHJ* 54:352-367, 1957.

41. Shaver JA: Innocent murmurs: innocent or pathologic? (Parts I and II). *Hospital Medicine,* June/July 1982.

42. Shaver JA, Leonard JJ, Leon DF: *Auscultation of the Heart.* AHA, 1990.

43. Steele G: The murmur of high pressure in the pulmonary artery. *Med Chron* 9:182-189, 1888.

44. Stembridge VA, Hejtmancik MR, Herrman GR: Unusual musical murmurs of anterior cusp aortic regurgitation: Report of 10 cases. *AHJ* 48:163-172, 1954.

45. Still SF Sir: Common Disorders and Diseases of Childhood (Ed 1). New York: Oxford University Press, 1909.

46. Sutton GC, Craige E: Signs of severe mitral regurgitation. *AJC* 20:141-144, 1967.

47. Tavel MD: Innocent murmurs, in Leon DF, Shaver JA (eds): Physiologic Principles of Heart Sounds and Murmurs. AHA Monograph 46, 102-106. New York: AHA, 1975.

48. Vogelpoel L, Schrire V: Auscultatory and phonocardiographic assessment of pulmonary stenosis with intact ventricular septum. *Circ* 22:55, 1960.

49. Vogelpoel L, Schrire V: Auscultatory and phonocardiographic assessment of Fallots Tetralogy. *Circ* 22:73-89, 1960.

50. Wood P: The Eisenmenger syndrome or pulmonary hypertension with reversed central shunt. *BMJ* 2:701-709 and 755-762, 1958.

51. Wooley CF: The spectrum of tricuspid regurgitation. In Leon DF, Shaver JA (eds): Physiologic Principles of Heart Sounds and Murmurs. AHA Monograph No. 46,139-148. New York: AHA 1975.

52. Wooley CF, Fontana ME, Kilman JW, et al: Tricuspid stenosis. Atrial systolic murmur, tricuspid opening snap and right atrial pressure pulse. *AJM* 78:375-384, 1985.

53. Zuberbuhler JR, Lenox CC, Neches WH, et al: Auscultatory spectrum of Tetralogy of Fallot. In Leon DF and Shaver JA teds): Physiologic Principles of Heart Sounds and Murmurs. AHA Monograph 46, 187-192. New York: AHA 1975.

CHAPTER 10

Dynamic Cardiac Auscultation: Bedside Interventions Useful in the Differential Diagnosis of Heart Sounds and Murmurs

Modestino G. Criscitiello, M.D.

Careful auscultation of the heart is a keystone of the general cardiovascular examination, but many present-day clinicians rely heavily on imaging techniques to aid in differential diagnosis and in assessing severity of heart disorders. At the bedside, they make note of any murmurs or abnormal heart sounds they detect, but tend to leave it entirely to the echocardiographic or catheterization laboratory to provide definitive information. Many overlook the usefulness of some simple interventions that can easily be performed at initial examination, including mild exercise, changes in position, squatting and standing, hand grip exercise, and the Valsalva maneuver. Resulting changes in heart rate, heart size, stroke volume, contractile state, venous return, and arterial pressure can alter heart sounds and murmurs in a way that helps differentiate between lesions with similar findings, or to detect subtle abnormalities that might otherwise be overlooked. There are also transient hemodynamic changes occurring spontaneously during normal respiration, after premature beats, or during episodes of ischemia, that can modify sounds or murmurs noted during preliminary examination.

Auscultation during these moments of spontaneous or induced hemodynamic change can provide important clues to heart disease and allow wiser selection of further laboratory testing.

Effects of Respiration

During a routine examination, it should be standard procedure to listen to the heart during a moment of respiratory silence following full expiration. By this means, as much air as possible is removed from the space between the heart and the chest wall, allowing for detection of very faint heart sounds and murmurs. For example, it may be only during the period of full expiration (with the patient sitting up and leaning forward) that one can detect the faint, blowing diastolic murmur of aortic insufficiency.

Normal respiration causes cyclical hemodynamic effects, influencing venous return, end-diastolic volume, stroke volume, and pulmonary arterial compliance. In this way, it influences behavior of the second heart sound, intensity (loudness) of some murmurs, and presence and timing of extra heart sounds.

Respiratory Variation in Splitting of the Second Sound

The second heart sound has two components: one produced by aortic valve closure (S_2-A), the other by pulmonic valve closure (S_2- P). Because pressure in the aorta at the end of ventricular systole exceeds that in the pulmonary artery, S_2-A normally precedes S_2-P. The degree of separation of these two components may be enough to result in audible splitting of the second heart sound. The degree of splitting is influenced by respiration with the interval between the two events increasing during inspiration. Normal inspiration expands the thorax and depresses the diaphragm, resulting in negative pressure in the chest and positive pressure in the abdomen. This pressure gradient augments venous return to the right ventricle, causing a transient increase in right ventricular stroke volume; duration of right ventricular systole is prolonged slightly. The negative intrathoracic pressure results in a reduction of pressure within the pulmonary vasculature, causing a decrease in impedance of the pulmonary arterial bed. Enhanced stroke volume and the reduced pulmonary arterial impedance result in a delay in pulmonic valve closure.

Negative intrathoracic pressure has less effect on the left side of the heart, but increased capacity of pulmonary veins may lead to a slight reduction of left ventricular filling, a decrease in left ventricular stroke volume, and shortening of left ventricular systole. Aortic closure occurs slightly earlier during inspiration, and the two components of the second sound become more widely separated. In most normal subjects, the second heart sound is single or narrowly split by an interval of 0.02 seconds or less during expiration. This interval may increase to as much as 0.06 seconds during inspiration. The greater part of the change in the S_2 A-P interval is due to delay in pulmonic valve closure.

During expiration, systemic venous return falls, pulmonary arterial impedance rises, and pulmonic closure returns to its earlier position with narrowing of the S_2 A-P interval. Unless pulmonary hypertension is present, the pulmonic component of S_2 is usually audible only in the second or third left interspace, and splitting is not easily heard at any point on the chest wall distant from this area. It is important to note that significant separation of S_2 A-P may be heard during expiration in many normal subjects while they are lying flat, and observations on splitting of the second sound are best made with the patient in a semi-upright or sitting position.

In some subjects, separation of the two components is not easily detected. Splitting may be brought out by a somewhat deeper inspiration, but unfortunately, a voluntary increase in the depth of respiration may add enough noise to obscure the heart sounds. The negative intrapleural pressure produces its maximum effect during the first beat or two at the end of normal inspiration, and venous return is not augmented further by breath-holding. On some occasions, splitting of the second sound is not readily apparent; when it is important to be certain of the presence of both semilunar valves, separation of S_2 A-P may be heard during inspiration immediately following release of the Valsalva maneuver. The markedly positive intrathoracic pressure caused by expiratory effort against a closed glottis results in marked reduction of venous return. There is a surge of blood flow to the right heart during inspiration following release of this pressure, and disparity between right and left ventricular stroke volumes may become sufficient to produce audible separation of closure of the two semilunar valves.

Deviations from the normal splitting pattern of the second heart sound during respiration provide major clues to a number of abnormalities. If right ventricular systole is prolonged because of right bundle branch block, right ventricular failure, pulmonic stenosis, or pulmonary hypertension, there may be unusually wide separation of S_2 A-P without fusion during expiration. Splitting can be heard during both phases of respiration, although there may be some narrowing during expiration. Some lesions such as atrial septal defect or anomalous pulmonary venous drainage cause maximal diastolic filling of the right ventricle to the extent that inspiration cannot further increase venous return to the right heart. Also, in some patients with right heart failure, the right ventricle cannot accommodate any further filling in diastole. In these circumstances, splitting of two components of the second sound is fixed with minimal or no respiratory variation. Left ventricular systole may be delayed or prolonged by abnormalities such as left bundle branch block, transient ischemia, left ventricular outflow obstruction, or volume overload. In these lesions aortic valve closure may be late enough to follow pulmonic closure. Splitting of the second sound will be heard during expiration, and inspiration will bring the two components closer together. This paradoxical pattern may also be present in patients being paced from the right ventricle (Figure 1).

Effect of Respiration on Heart Murmurs

There are several valvular lesions, usually right-sided, whose murmurs can be amplified by the transient increase in systemic venous return induced by inspiration. Since inspiration tends to reduce all heart sounds and murmurs by increasing volume of air between the heart and the chest piece of the stethoscope, one's attention may be arrested by detecting a selective increase instead. Rivero Carvallo noted almost 50 years ago that both the mid-diastolic rumble of tricuspid stenosis and the pansystolic murmur of tricuspid regurgitation are increased during inspiration; his name has become an eponym for the latter observation. In tricuspid stenosis the gradient across the valve increases measurably because right ventricular diastolic pressure falls during inspiration while right atrial pressure fails to do so. If there is a presystolic component of the tricuspid murmur (with sinus rhythm) this also may be enhanced by inspiration.

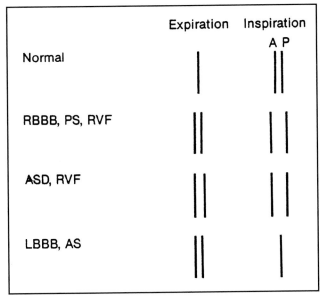

	Expiration	Inspiration
		A P
Normal		
RBBB, PS, RVF		
ASD, RVF		
LBBB, AS		

Figure 1. Behavior of the Second Heart Sound During Respiration – Aortic (A) and pulmonic (P) valve closure sounds occur simultaneously during expiration, but separate by 0.02-0.06 sec during quiet inspiration in normal persons. Delay in right ventricular ejection that occurs in right bundle branch block (RBBB), pulmonic stenosis (PS), or in right ventricular failure (RVF) results in wider than usual splitting on inspiration and causes failure of fusion of S_2 on expiration. Persistent fixed splitting with loss of respiratory variations occurs when right ventricular stroke volume exceeds left ventricular stroke volume, as in atrial septal defect (ASD) or in some instances of severe RVF. Prolongation of left ventricular ejection may result in reversal of the order of semilunar valve closure, causing inspiratory narrowing of the P-A interval, with "paradoxical splitting" during expiration. This may occur in left bundle branch block (LBBB), aortic stenosis (AS), or during left ventricular ischemia. *(From Quick Reference Guides To Cardiovascular Medicine, Primary Cardiology. PW Communications International, Secaucus, New Jersey, 1986.)*

The changes in these murmurs may be detected only at a selected site over the lower sternum, and careful listening during several respiratory cycles is necessary. If there is a tricuspid opening snap present, it also tends to become louder with inspiration. During the past three decades, the incidence of rheumatic fever has decreased in the United States and along with it occurrence of tricuspid stenosis. There are areas in the Third World where rheumatic heart disease remains a serious problem, however, and subjects from those regions may present with this lesion.

A pansystolic murmur may be heard along the lower left sternal border or just medial to the apical area in patients with hypertrophic subaortic stenosis, ventricular septal defect, or mitral insufficiency. Inspiration usually has no effect on these murmurs except for some dampening by the insulating effect of inspired air. If a murmur at the left sternal edge increases during quiet inspiration, it is almost certainly due to tricuspid insufficiency.

When tricuspid disease is caused by fibrous changes in the valve tissue as in rheumatic disease, the Carvallo sign is usually evident. If tricuspid regurgitation is the result of right ventricular dilatation due to failure, there may be no respiratory effect on the systolic murmur, since the failing ventricle is unable to accommodate an inspiratory rise in venous return. In fact, a systolic murmur may be inaudible altogether and the presence of regurgitation verified only by systolic expansion of the jugular veins or by Doppler ultrasound techniques. Under these circumstances, passive elevation of the patient's legs or compression of the right costal margin overlying the liver may augment venous return enough to increase flow into the right ventricle, thereby provoking or enhancing a systolic murmur of tricuspid insufficiency. On the other hand, the murmur may be heard best by having the patient suddenly stand upright. This will result in a temporary decrease in right-sided filling pressure, and respiratory fluctuations in venous return may then become apparent while the patient remains standing with restoration of the inspiratory increase in the tricuspid insufficiency murmur.

CARDIAC PEARL

Characteristically, the murmur of mitral valve insufficiency decreases with inspiration, becoming louder with expiration. This is in contrast to the murmur of tricuspid valve insufficiency which is best heard along the lower left sternal border or right sternal border rather than at the apex. This tends to increase in intensity with inspiration rather than decrease, as in the case of mitral insufficiency. A patient observed had cardiomegaly and a holosystolic murmur best heard at the cardiac apex. On inspiration the murmur definitely became increased rather than decreased, which seemed paradoxical since the initial impression was that this patient had mitral valve insufficiency. At that point, one could rightly wonder if this was a valid bedside sign of mitral insufficiency where the murmur is supposed to decrease with inspiration. Therefore, this paradoxical response with respiration afforded the first clue as to the presence of tricuspid insufficiency even though the systolic murmur was heard best at the cardiac apex. Eventually this patient was determined to have Ebstein's anomaly and, as correlated by the angiograms, the tricuspid valve was at the left anterior axillary line! Thus, this was the murmur of tricuspid insufficiency behaving in typical fashion.

W. Proctor Harvey, M.D.

Systolic ejection murmurs produced in most forms of right-sided outflow obstruction fail to change predictably with respiration. In some patients with valvular pulmonic stenosis, the systolic murmur will increase during inspiration, presumably from an increase in the transvalvular gradient resulting from a drop in pulmonary arterial pressure. In general, the response to inspiration does not help differentiate the murmurs of pulmonic stenosis and atrial septal defect from innocent or functional murmurs.

Aside from tricuspid stenosis, there are some unusual right-sided lesions causing diastolic murmurs, and these also may be amplified by inspiration. The low-frequency diastolic murmur of congenital pulmonic valve insufficiency is increased during inspiration. It is usually an early-to-mid-diastolic murmur heard best in the second and third left intercostal spaces. It is probably generated by turbulence resulting from the convergence of two streams, one flowing forward through the tricuspid valve, the other flowing backward through the incompetent pulmonic valve. This turbulence is enhanced by the increased venous return during inspiration. This type of pulmonic insufficiency may result from congenitally defective cusps, from idiopathic dilatation of the pulmonary artery, from cusp damage due to bacterial endocarditis, or from surgical correction of pulmonary stenosis. When pulmonary insufficiency is due to pulmonary hypertension, the murmur resembles that of aortic insufficiency and has a high frequency, blowing character. This murmur is generally not influenced by inspiration due to reduced diastolic compliance of the hypertrophied ventricle and high pulmonary arterial impedance.

In some patients with Ebstein's anomaly, there is a late diastolic or presystolic murmur; this has been noted to increase during inspiration. In some patients with atrial septal defect, the marked increase in pulmonary blood flow results in turbulence in some of the primary or secondary branches of the pulmonary arteries. This turbulence may generate murmurs, usually in systole, best heard in the axilla or over the upper back, and these may be strikingly increased during inspiration. There are also occasional instances of bruits occurring in pulmonary vessels resulting from arteriovenous fistulae, congenital branch stenosis or other lesions producing deformities of the vessels within the lung parenchyma. These bruits may vary with respiratory movement, presumably due to a shift in the location of the lesion in reference to the chest piece of the stethoscope or perhaps to torsion of the involved vessels.

Effects of Respiration on Extra Heart Sounds

A sound early in systole may be detected in some patients with congenital pulmonic or aortic stenosis. This event occurs as the deformed valve opens and is separated from the first heart sound by a very short interval, averaging 0.04 to 0.06 seconds. These sharp, discrete sounds are referred to as "ejection clicks" and usually occur at the onset of a systolic ejection murmur. The ejection click of aortic stenosis is not influenced by respiration, but that associated with pulmonic stenosis may undergo some tell-tale changes. The pulmonic click occurs at the end of isovolumetric contraction when the diaphragm-like pulmonic valve with its fused commissures reaches the limit of its excursion at ejection. This click typically decreases in intensity during inspiration and moves closer to the first sound, often fusing with it. In pulmonic stenosis, pulmonary arterial pressure is abnormally low. The right ventricle is hypertrophied with poor diastolic compliance resulting in elevation of the end-diastolic pressure. The increased venous return during inspiration may lead to a right ventricular end-diastolic pressure which actually exceeds that in the pulmonary artery just prior to the onset of ventricular systole. This forces the pulmonic valve upward to its open position prior to systole, and any vibrations produced in this structure by ventricular contraction are soft and merge with those of the first heart sound. During expiration, the pulmonic ejection click is later and louder.

An ejection sound may also be heard in circumstances where the pulmonic valve is normal but the proximal pulmonary artery is dilated as in atrial septal defect, idiopathic dilatation of the pulmonary

---

TABLE 1

Effects of Inspiration

Increased venous return to right ventricle leads to:

↑ Diastolic and presystolic murmur of tricuspid stenosis (TS)
↑ Intensity of tricuspid opening snap
↑ Intensity of right-sided third (S_3) and fourth (S_4) heart sounds
↑ Presystolic murmur of Ebstein's anomaly
↓ Intensity of pulmonic ejection sound, which fuses with S_1

Increased right ventricular stroke volume leads to:

↑ Pansystolic murmur of tricuspid regurgitation (TR)
↑ Systolic ejection murmur of mild to moderate pulmonic stenosis (PS)
↑ Early diastolic murmur of congenital pulmonic regurgitation (PR)

Decrease in pulmonary venous return and left ventricular stroke volume leads to:

↓ Diastolic murmur of mitral stenosis (MS)
↓ Intensity of left-sided S_3 and S_4

artery or pulmonary hypertension. A different mechanism is presumably involved in the production of this type of ejection sound. It is recorded as blood is ejected into the proximal portion of the pulmonary artery after the valve has opened and therefore may result from sudden distention of the enlarged vessel. Ejection sounds of this sort are not generally affected by respiration.

The interval between the second heart sound and the opening snap (OS) of mitral stenosis is not altered by inspiration, but when it is quite short (0.08 sec to 0.10 sec) the combination may simulate fixed splitting of S_2. During inspiration one can detect three events, S_2-A, S_2-P, and opening snap, in sequence, confirming mitral disease.

Early diastolic filling sounds in the right ventricle, either an atrial sound (S_4) or a ventricular gallop (S_3), may become louder during inspiration, whereas left-sided filling sounds tend to fade. Right ventricular filling sounds are usually best heard along the lower left sternal border or in the xiphoid area; those occurring in the left ventricle are better heard at apex, with the patient turned to the left lateral position. These filling sounds are often quite soft and are best heard using the bell piece of the stethoscope. A quiet environment is necessary. It is best to listen for these sounds with the patient in the horizontal position, since the sounds may disappear when the patient sits up (Table 1).

Changes in Position

Change in position may alter heart sounds and murmurs on a purely mechanical basis. A pericardial friction rub is heard best with the patient sitting up and leaning forward or with the chest entirely dependent while he is on his hands and knees. Assumption of this chest-down posture may cause a shift in the pericardial effusion, leading to a closer approximation of the roughened surfaces generating the rub. In the left lateral position, the left ventricle swings closer to the chest wall, and soft sounds or murmurs generated in that chamber become easier to hear, such as a left ventricular S_3 or a diastolic rumble of mitral stenosis. Murmurs generated by an atrial myxoma can be altered by mechanical displacement of the tumor mass induced by rotation of the torso. However, rapid changes in position such as standing or squatting, may also cause changes in heart sounds and murmurs by influencing venous return, stroke volume, heart size, and heart rate.

Recumbency and Passive Leg-Raising

Venous return can be augmented by having the patient suddenly lie flat from a sitting position, and the effect can be enhanced by passive leg-raising at the same time. Ventricular filling sounds, both S_3 and S_4, can be exaggerated with this technique. The Carvallo sign of inspiratory augmentation of the tricuspid insufficiency murmur may be detected only during passive leg-raising, especially in the patient with right heart failure. The systolic ejection murmurs of valvular pulmonic and aortic stenosis often increase and become longer during passive leg-raising. The effect is noticeable within two or three beats in the case of pulmonic stenosis, whereas several beats may elapse before the murmur of aortic stenosis is affected since the increased systemic venous return may take several beats to reach the left heart. Recumbency and passive leg-raising tend to decrease the murmur of hypertrophic subaortic stenosis. The left ventricle fills more completely during diastole and the subvalvular outflow channel is less severely obstructed.

Prompt Squatting

Prompt squatting provides an additional means of increasing venous return as a result of compression of capacitance veins in the legs and abdomen. In addition, squatting causes a rise in mean arterial pressure from the combined effect of increased cardiac output and increased arterial resistance. Diastolic murmur of aortic regurgitation is increased in intensity due to the rise in diastolic pressure and the impairment of arterial runoff during squatting. A barely audible diastolic blow can be readily amplified by this means.

Systolic murmurs of mitral regurgitation and ventricular septal defect increase during squatting since the greater arterial impedance leads to a rise in left ventricular systolic pressure. The ejection murmurs of aortic and pulmonic valvular stenosis are generally unchanged, or at most become slightly louder during the first few beats after squatting, but the murmur of hypertrophic subaortic stenosis decreases. The increase in venous return leads to greater filling of the left ventricle, which in turn leads to reduced obstruction during systole. In performing this, the examiner should be seated facing the patient with the stethoscope positioned while the patient is still standing. If the chest piece is held in place while the patient squats, any changes occurring within the first few beats can be readily detected. In those patients unable to perform squatting readily, similar circulatory changes can be induced by bending the patient's knees on his abdomen while he is in the supine position.

CARDIAC PEARL

Various bedside maneuvers affecting heart sounds and murmurs prove helpful in the diagnosis of heart disease.

In our experience, the squatting maneuver is usually the most efficient and reliable to test for hypertrophic cardiomyopathy. First, listen to the patient while he or she is standing; then have the patient squat down. If the systolic murmur becomes fainter or disappears when the patient squats and then becomes louder again when the patient resumes standing this is a definite positive response for hypertrophic cardiomyopathy. On standing, sometimes the systolic murmur doubles in intensity. Remember to repeat this maneuver several times, since the most striking change may not take place until the second or third sequence of standing.

Another condition where the squatting maneuver is helpful is mitral valve prolapse. At times, the squatting maneuver can "bring out" the auscultatory findings of this condition and can cause movement of clicks, murmurs, or both, in systole as a result of this change in position. A maneuver that increases volume to the left side of the heart, such as squatting, may delay these auscultatory findings, and therefore the click or murmur may move closer to the second heart sound. On prompt standing by the patient and with a decrease in volume, they may move in the opposite direction in systole- closer to the first heart sound. The fact that a change of the click or the murmur occurs strengthens further the bedside or office diagnosis of mitral valve prolapse. Squatting is an excellent procedure and is not used as often as it should be.

Most physicians squat as the patient squats and at the same time attempt to listen with the stethoscope. I too used to do this; however, not uncommonly, one of us might become unsteady and we would almost fall into each other. One cannot listen accurately if this awkward situation occurs. After a number of years, it finally dawned on me that there was a simple and effective way to remedy this situation: the physician sits comfortably in a chair (Fig. A), and the patient stands facing the physician, steadying himself or herself with the left hand on the examining table. The physician listens with the stethoscope over the patient's left sternal border or apex, thereby obtaining a baseline of the auscultatory findings. The patient is then told to squat, and the physician continuously listens as the patient squats and then returns to the standing position. This procedure is repeated

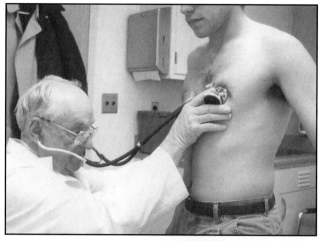

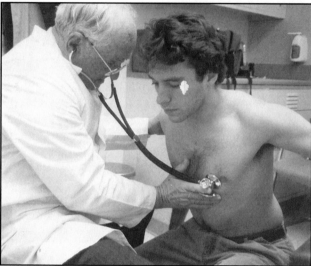

Fig A: Easiest and most efficient way to perform the squatting maneuver. The physician sits comfortably and listens to the standing patient (top panel). The patient (not the physician) does the squatting (lower panel).

several times. Once you use this method of performing the squatting maneuver, I must confess you feel somewhat foolish that you did not think of it sooner. We term this the cardiac pearl of the squatting maneuver.

W. Proctor Harvey, M.D.

Standing

When the lying or squatting patient stands upright, venous pooling takes place with a sharp reduction in venous return. This produces a momentary decrease in heart size, stroke volume and blood pressure followed by a reflex increase in heart rate and systemic resistance. Decreased left ventricular volume in the standing position results in an increase in the murmur of hypertrophic subaortic stenosis, whereas murmurs of pulmonic and aortic stenosis tend to soften a bit. Changes in position are helpful in evaluating patients with mitral prolapse who have a systolic click with or without a late systolic murmur; prolapse may result from attenuation of mitral leaflets or lengthening of the chordae tendineae. Systolic click occurs at the point of sudden checking of the mitral leaflet as it prolapses into the left atrium during ventricular systole. If the prolapse permits regurgitation, a murmur is generated in the latter half of systole. Changes in left ventricular end-diastolic volume influence the extent of leaflet prolapse during systole and therefore timing of the systolic click and loudness and duration of the murmur. During standing, the reduced left ventricular volume results in an earlier onset of the click and the murmurs since the mitral leaflet is somewhat closer to the position where prolapse begins. The murmur becomes longer and may in some cases fill all of systole. In some patients, the quality of the murmur may change, assuming a somewhat musical or "honking" character. Sudden squatting or lying flat increases end-diastolic volume, causing the click to mover toward the second sound and the murmur to become shorter or disappear altogether.

A mid or late systolic murmur may be heard in some individuals following myocardial infarction, presumably due to papillary muscle dysfunction. In this case, rise in ventricular systolic pressure following squatting may actually lead to a greater degree of stretching of the papillary muscle with a resultant increase in the extent of mitral regurgitation. In this respect, this group of patients differs strikingly from the usual mitral valve prolapse pattern.

In listening for the continuous murmur of patent ductus arteriosus it is important to examine the subject in the supine position since this murmur may decrease in duration or even disappear altogether in the upright posture. This is especially true in the case of a ductus of small diameter. Continuous murmur of a venous hum grows louder in the standing position. In some youngsters, this murmur, best heard over the internal jugular vein, may actually be loud enough to be detected below the level of the clavicle. Such a murmur can be confused with that of a patent ductus, but compression of the neck veins or institution of the Valsalva maneuver will suppress the murmur of a venous hum and eliminate any confusion. Ventricular filling sounds are influenced by change in posture. They may fade markedly when the patient is standing upright. The search for an S_3 or an S_4 is best made with the patient in the horizontal position. An atrial sound, easily audible with the patient lying down, may become quite soft and also merge with the first heart sound within a few seconds after standing. Physiologic third sounds also disappear in standing subjects whereas the pathologic third sound of congestive failure or severe mitral regurgitation tends to persist. It is therefore reasonable to conclude that diastolic filling sounds which persist when the patient stands upright are unlikely to be physiologic. Extra heart sounds such as the opening snap or ejection sounds are not much influenced by position changes (Table 2).

Effects of Exercise

In the patient not limited by dyspnea, a short period of mild exercise can be useful in augmenting some murmurs and filling sounds. Performance of a few step-ups or jogging in place will result in an

---

TABLE 2
Effects of Changes in Posture
(Listen for effect during first few beats in new position.)

RECUMBENCY AND PASSIVE LEG RAISING	PROMPT SQUATTING	STANDING AFTER SQUATTING
Augmentation of venous return leads to: ↑ Systolic murmur of PS (in first few beats) ↑ Systolic murmur of valvular AS (after 4-6 beats) ↑ Systolic murmur of TR ↑ Intensity of S_3 and S_4 (both right and left-sided) Increase in left ventricular volume leads to: ↓ Systolic murmur of hypertrophic obstructive cardiomyopathy (HOCM)	Increase in arterial pressure and peripheral resistance leads to: ↑ Diastolic murmur of aortic regurgitation (AR) Increase in left ventricular systolic pressure lead to: ↑ Systolic murmur of MR ↑ Systolic murmur of ventricular septal defect (VSD) Increase in left ventricular volume leads to: ↓ Systolic murmur of HOCM	Decrease in venous return leads to: ↓ Physiologic S_3 (pathologic S_3 usually unchanged) ↓ S_4 Decrease in left ventricular volume leads to: ↑ Systolic murmur of HOCM Earlier onset of systolic click (SC) and late systolic murmur (LSM) in mitral valve prolapse Decrease in stroke volume leads to: ↓ Systolic murmur of valvular AS and PS

increase in heart rate, cardiac output, systolic blood pressure, and augmentation of the contractile state. Increased velocity of ejection of blood from both ventricles leads to augmentation of murmurs generated by outflow obstruction including valvular and subvalvular stenosis. The so-called innocent or functional murmur also tends to increase with exertion, hence exercise is not useful in separating this murmur from those of organic valvular disease. Hemodynamic changes of exercise lead to significant increases in the diastolic murmurs of mitral or tricuspid stenosis. Third and fourth heart sounds are also more easily heard following exertion. Unfortunately the deep breathing following exercise often makes auscultation difficult. In checking for mitral stenosis, it is often easier to augment cardiac output by having the patient cough several times while lying in the left lateral position. Although the hemodynamic effect of this is quite transient, it may be enough to bring out the rumble of mitral stenosis quite readily. The exercise response in mitral regurgitation and mitral prolapse is unpredictable.

The Valsalva Maneuver

The Valsalva maneuver, a useful bedside intervention, has instantaneous effects on venous return and arterial pressure. After a few words of instruction or a demonstration, most patients can perform this maneuver which consists of forced expiration against a closed glottis. Some patients do best by inserting a finger in the mouth and attempting to blow out with lips sealed. The patient who does not understand such instructions may be induced to perform the equivalent of a Valsalva maneuver by pushing back against the examiner's hand, which is pressed downward on the mid-abdomen. In doing this most subjects close the glottis and strain effectively. The "bearing down" effort, no matter how initiated, should be sustained for 10 to 15 seconds to bring about the required hemodynamic changes. With onset of straining there is a sharp rise in arterial pressure resulting from direct transmission of the increased intrathoracic pressure to the walls of the large arteries (Phase 1). Continued straining impairs venous return, causing a decrease in output of both ventricles and a reduction in heart size. Mean arterial pressure drops (Phase 2), and this initiates a reflex increase in sympathetic activity with a rise in heart rate and vasoconstriction. After release of the straining effort, there is an immediate further decrease in arterial pressure as intrathoracic pressure drops acutely (Phase 3). Following this there is a surge of venous return to the heart producing an increase in cardiac output

---

TABLE 3
Effects of Valsalva Maneuver

The rise in intrathoracic pressure produced by forced expiration against a closed glottis causes, in sequence:

1. A momentary rise in blood pressure.
2. A decrease in venous return, and a decrease in cardiac output, reduction in heart size, and a decrease in arterial pressure that triggers a reflex rise in heart rate.
3. On release of the expiratory effort, blood pressure drops further for a few beats, but venous return is restored.
4. Blood pressure rises above control level, inducing reflex slowing of heart rate.

During phase 2 the diagnostic changes in murmurs occur. The patient should be instructed to maintain the Valsalva effort for at least 10 to 15 seconds and to avoid grunting.

During strain of Valsalva maneuver (phase 2)

Reduced stroke volume leads to:

↓ Systolic murmur of AS and PS

Reduced left ventricular volume leads to:

↑ Systolic murmur of HOCM

Earlier onset of SC and LSM of mitral prolapse

After Release

Increase in venous return to right ventricle before left ventricle leads to:

Wider splitting of S_2 for the first 3 to 4 beats

Earlier augmentation of right-sided (PS, TR, TS) than of left-sided murmurs (AS, MS)

---

and a rise in arterial pressure (Phase 4). In the non-failing heart there is an "overshoot" in the blood pressure which in turn triggers a short period of reflex bradycardia before return to control levels.

During Phase 2, innocent murmurs and those of pulmonic and aortic valve stenosis fade as stroke volume falls. The murmur of hypertrophic subaortic stenosis frequently increases strikingly as the reduction in left ventricular volume leads to more severe outflow obstruction. This murmur is often best heard at the lower left sternal border, where it may be mistaken for an innocent murmur. If it is heard well near the apical area it may be thought to represent mitral insufficiency, often present in patients with hypertrophic cardiomyopathy. Because the murmur of mitral regurgitation fades during the Valsalva strain, a definite increase in a systolic murmur in these areas should raise consideration of subaortic stenosis.

CARDIAC PEARL

The Valsalva maneuver, too, can be helpful in diagnosing hypertrophic cardiomyopathy. While listening along the left sternal border

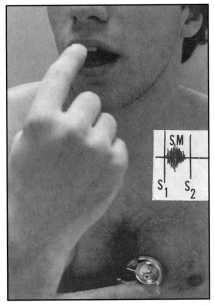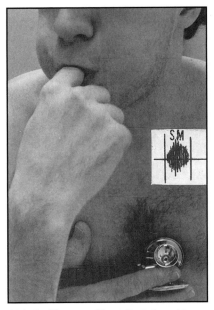

Fig A: Valsalva Maneuver - A different and efficient Valsalva Maneuver. The patient places his index finger in his mouth (left). He seals his lips around the finger (right) and is instructed to "blow hard." Note the increase in the systolic murmur.

or apex, have the patient take a deep breath, **blow the breath out and then strain as if having a bowel movement. The murmur may increase in intensity, indicating a positive response.**

However, some patients, such as the elderly, may have difficulty in performing this maneuver. A simple and efficient way is to have the patient place his index finger in his mouth, seal it with his lips, exhale and at the point of deep expiration, "blow hard" on the finger (Fig. A). This usually works.
W. Proctor Harvey, M.D.

In patients with mitral prolapse, the mid-systolic click moves toward the first heart sound and the murmur starts earlier as left ventricular dimensions diminish during the Valsalva effort. The intensity of the murmur does not change in a predictable way. During Phase 2, closure of the semilunar valves tends to become simultaneous and the second sound is single. In patients with atrial septal defect or right bundle branch block, however, discrepancy in duration of systole in the two ventricles persists and splitting of S_2 can still be heard. During Phase 4, the right heart receives the augmented venous return first, and right-sided murmurs and filling sounds become accentuated during the first two or three beats after release. Left-sided murmurs usually regain their baseline intensity after five to ten beats. In some normal subjects, splitting of the second heart sound cannot be detected during quiet inspiration. During Phase 4

the discrepancy between right and left ventricular stroke volumes may be great enough to bring about audible separation of aortic and pulmonic closure sounds in the first few beats (Table 3).

Hand Grip Exercise

Sustained isometric hand grip exercise provides a means of rapidly inducing an increase in heart rate and blood pressure. This procedure can be performed at bedside by having the patient clench his fist forcefully or squeeze a rolled-up facecloth. When sustained for 35 to 40 seconds, maximal effort of this sort results in a prompt rise in heart rate and blood pressure, leading to alterations in some heart sounds and murmurs. Moderate degrees of isometric effort produce tachycardia via a release of vagal tone, and the rise in blood pressure results from the increase in heart rate and cardiac output. More vigorous and sustained hand grip exercise will trigger sympathetic stimulation resulting in a further increase in heart rate and an additional rise in blood pressure due to vasoconstriction.

Increased left ventricular systolic pressure leads to enhancement of the murmurs of mitral regurgitation or ventricular septal defect, and increase in diastolic blood pressure helps to bring out the murmur of aortic regurgitation. The murmur of mitral stenosis may also become more easily audible as left atrial pressure rises secondary to the increased heart rate and blood flow. In many patients with impaired ventricular function, gallop sounds can be

TABLE 4

Effects of Handgrip Exercise

The patient performs isometric handgrip exercise by squeezing a rolled-up hand towel or clenching the fist forcefully for 40 to 50 seconds. Sinus tachycardia develops promptly, and arterial pressure rises as much as 15 to 30 mm Hg, due to increased cardiac output and generalized vasoconstriction. Left ventricular filling pressure and volume also increase.

Precautions:

Advise patient not to hold breath during isometric effort.

Avoid isometric handgrip in unstable angina or recent infarction.

Rise in arterial pressure leads to:

↑ Diastolic murmur of aortic regurgitation (AR)

Rise in left ventricular systolic pressure leads to:

↑ Systolic murmur of MR and VSD

Increase in left ventricular volume leads to:

↓ Systolic murmur of HOCM

Delayed onset of SC and LSM in mitral prolapse

Increase in heart rate and cardiac output leads to:

↑ Diastolic rumble of MS

Increase in left ventricular filling pressure leads to:

↑ Left-sided S_3 and S_4

---

evoked or accentuated by sustained hand grip. Patients with ischemic heart disease may even experience angina during isometric exercise of this type, and it should be avoided in patients with unstable angina or recent myocardial infarction. When ischemia involves the papillary muscle, a transient mid or late systolic murmur of mitral regurgitation may be produced (Table 4).

Effects of Pregnancy

In any discussion of circulatory changes that alter heart sounds and murmurs, it is appropriate to review the effects of pregnancy. The functional changes in the cardiovascular system that occur during normal pregnancy can produce symptoms and findings on physical examination that sometimes simulate organic heart disease where there is none present. These same changes can also modify the evidence of existing valvular heart disease, in some instances enhancing tell-tale murmurs, but in other circumstances obscuring them. Hyperkinetic circulation during pregnancy leads to accentuation of the intensity of the first heart sound, starting by the twelfth week. There also may be exaggerated splitting of the first sound heard along the lower left sternal border. A third heart sound is often audible at the cardiac apex during pregnancy, usually first detected at 15 to 20 weeks of gestation and disappearing during the first postpartum week.

A systolic ejection murmur, occasionally as loud as grade 3, is heard in a majority of women during the latter part of pregnancy, related to increased velocity of flow from the right ventricle into the pulmonary artery) and from the left ventricle into the aorta and its brachiocephalic branches. This murmur is best heard along the left sternal border either over the pulmonary area or in the third and fourth left interspaces. Occasionally, such murmurs lead to over-diagnosis of valvular heart disease; it is reassuring to note their disappearance in the postpartum weeks. Murmur of mitral stenosis is amplified during pregnancy as cardiac output increases; in the past, when rheumatic heart disease was more commonly encountered in the childbearing population, the disease was often first detected during pregnancy. Conversely, murmurs of aortic and mitral regurgitation may be reduced in intensity or become inaudible during pregnancy. This is most likely related to the drop in peripheral vascular resistance that occurs in pregnancy. Decrease in arterial impedance favors forward flow from the left ventricle and less regurgitation across an incompetent mitral valve. During diastole, the same phenomenon leads to greater forward run-off and less regurgitation across an incompetent aortic valve. There have been several reports of patients with mitral valve prolapse whose systolic clicks and late systolic murmurs have diminished or disappeared altogether during pregnancy. It is likely that increases in blood volume and left ventricular end-diastolic volume occurring during pregnancy realign the mitral valve complex so that there is less prolapse and less separation of leaflets during systole. If a woman has been known to have aortic or mitral regurgitation, she should receive the benefit of prophylactic antibiotics during delivery, even if corresponding murmurs are not audible during pregnancy.

Two bruits commonly detected during pregnancy, the cervical venous hum and the mammary souffle, may lead the unwary examiner to misdiagnosis of patent ductus arteriosus or arterial-venous fistula. The venous hum is best heard over the supraclavicular fossa, just lateral to the clavicular insertion of the sternocleidomastoid muscle. It can be detected at one time or another in almost all pregnant women, and is more readily heard on the right side of the neck. It consists of a continuous roaring noise which varies little during the cardiac cycle and can be obliterated by light compression over the internal jugular vein or by turning the neck. It rarely radiates below the level of the clavicle, but when it does, it may give the false impression of a patent ductus or some other communication between high-

and-low-pressure systems. The Valsalva maneuver will stop a venous hum but will have no effect on the abnormal circulatory shunts producing continuous murmurs.

A mammary souffle is heard chiefly in the early postpartum period, especially in lactating women, but it is sometimes heard in late pregnancy as well. It is usually systolic but may spill over into diastole, and it is generally heard best at the level of the second left or right interspaces. It may be louder in the third or fourth intercostal spaces, and is usually unilateral, although occasionally heard on both sides. It is frequently loudest near the sternal borders, but can also be heard in some women over the breast substance. It is heard best with the patient lying flat, and can be modified or obliterated by having the patient sit or stand or by compressing the chest piece of the stethoscope against the skin and subcutaneous tissue. There is still some controversy about the origin of the mammary souffle, some observers suggesting that it arises in the internal mammary artery or in junctions between this artery and the intercostal arterial system. Other investigators believe that it is of venous origin. In any event, it may be misinterpreted as evidence of a patent ductus arteriosus or of some form of arterial-venous fistula in the chest wall or mediastinum. Its day-to-day variation, alteration by change in position or local pressure, and eventual disappearance at the end of lactation distinguish it from these lesions.

A pregnant woman with mild aortic insufficiency may have her murmur undetected, particularly during her last trimester of pregnancy. This has been observed personally and was illustrated by a nurse who had a known faint aortic diastolic murmur which was absent on numerous examinations during her last trimester of pregnancy. After delivery of her child the murmur was again heard. The importance of this phenomenon is evident especially in patients who are first examined by their physician when they are pregnant. A careful examination on a subsequent date after pregnancy is therefore in order. It is easy to see how patients such as this might get bacterial endocarditis on a valvular lesion that was silent during pregnancy but could have been detected when she was not pregnant.

It is therefore wise to make sure that the faint aortic diastolic murmur has not been overlooked, and before the possibility of a significant murmur is dismissed at least one

careful cardiac examination should be made subsequent to delivery. The murmur of mitral regurgitation might also decrease in intensity during pregnancy, and a few of the fainter murmurs disappear.

Remember, also, that almost all pregnant women have an innocent grade 2 or 3, early to mid systolic murmur, which may not be heard before or after pregnancy.

An innocent versus hum over the neck is also an expected finding, particularly in the last trimester. Uncommonly, a continuous murmur can be heard over an engorged breast(s) of pregnancy- usually a nursing breast, but not always. It can be often eliminated by pressure with a finger over the area; if this mammary hum is over the left breast, it can be misinterpreted as patent ductus or an arteriovenous fistula over either breast. Of course, it disappears after pregnancy or cessation of nursing.

A maternal souffle is a continuous murmur that is usually high pitched and of musical quality. It is a constant finding in pregnant women and should present no problems in differential diagnosis. In addition, a systolic murmur of the type commonly heard over large vessels is frequently found over the lower abdomen of the pregnant patient, particularly during the latter trimesters. It often has a high-frequency musical quality that readily identifies it from the systolic murmur of lower frequency more commonly noted over large vessels in the nonpregnant patient.

W. Proctor Harvey, M.D.

Miscellaneous Diagnostic Maneuvers

The supraclavicular bruit, an innocent murmur heard over the subclavian artery in many children and young adults, may occasionally radiate downward toward the base of the heart and raise consideration of aortic or pulmonic stenosis. This innocent murmur may rise in an artery that undergoes sharp angulation as it passes from the superior mediastinum to the supraclavicular fossa. The bruit can be muffled entirely by compression of the artery. Also, having the subject extend the ipsolateral shoulder and reach backward can cause the bruit to disappear by straightening the course of the artery and reducing turbulence generated there.

Slowing heart rate with carotid sinus massage may be helpful in timing ventricular filling sounds. If heart rate is rapid, it is difficult to distinguish a gallop rhythm generated by a third sound vs a fourth heart sound. During temporary slowing heart rate, closer proximity to the first or second sound can be used to identify the event. If the mid-diastolic event is a summation gallop, it may divide into its separate components, producing a typical quadruple rhythm.

Muller's maneuver has not found a niche in the catalog of useful diagnostic techniques, but it is sometimes useful in studying hypertrophic cardiomyopathy. The patient is asked to inspire forcefully against a closed glottis, creating a markedly negative intrathoracic pressure. If this effort can be sustained for five seconds or more, the resultant increase in venous return may enlarge the left ventricle sufficiently to reduce any subvalvular obstruction causing the murmur to soften or disappear. Many subjects find it difficult to sustain the inspiratory effort for a long enough interval, and there is usually some noise generated by the trembling of muscles in the neck and upper thorax during the exertion involved.

Premature Beats

During examination, one should be attentive to the response of murmurs and heart sounds to spontaneously occurring premature beats. A premature beat may eject a smaller than usual stroke volume, resulting in sudden diminution of outflow murmurs across deformed semilunar valves. If the beat is premature enough, there may be no ejection at all, and therefore no murmur or second heart sound will be heard. There is usually a delay following a premature beat, lengthening the period of diastolic filling bringing about increase in stroke volume in the next beat. In addition, the beat which ends the pause demonstrates an increase in contractile force and in stroke volume. In the presence of aortic or pulmonic stenosis, this leads to a marked increase in intensity of the ejection murmur. However, the systolic murmurs of mitral or tricuspid regurgitation do not change after the pause.

In some patients, particularly those with an increase in chest diameter due to chronic pulmonary disease, the systolic murmur of aortic stenosis may be louder at the apex than at the base leading the examiner to think it due to mitral regurgitation. A striking increase in this systolic murmur in the first cycle following a premature beat provides an important clue to its aortic origin. Changes in the loudness and duration of ejection murmurs are often quite striking in patients with atrial fibrillation, whereas the pansystolic murmurs of mitral regurgitation show little beat-to-beat variation. The systolic murmur of hypertrophic subaortic stenosis usually becomes louder following a longer cycle length, presumably because of the increased force of contraction. In mitral valve prolapse, the behavior of the systolic murmur fol-

---

TABLE 5
Effects of Premature Beats

A premature beat of any type is usually followed by a short pause before regular rhythm resumes. The beat terminating the pause has enhanced contractile force and generates an increase in stroke volume and in velocity of ejection. This response is useful in differentiating lesions that may produce similar systolic murmurs.

Enhanced contractility after a pause induced by a premature beat leads to:

↑ Ejection murmur of valvular aortic (AS) or pulmonic stenosis (PS)

↑ Systolic murmur of hypertrophic obstructive cardiomyopathy (HOCM)

There is no change in pansystolic murmur of mitral regurgitation (MR) or tricuspid regurgitation (TR)

---

lowing a premature beat is somewhat variable, but most often the murmur starts later in systole and decreases in intensity.

The phenomenon of murmur alternans may be most readily detected for several cycles following a premature beat. In some patients with aortic stenosis and left ventricular failure, alternation of intensity and pitch of the systolic ejection murmur may be heard only during a short series of cardiac cycles following a single premature beat (Table 5).

CARDIAC PEARL

At times it is difficult to differentiate between the murmur of aortic stenosis and that of mitral regurgitation. A valuable cardiac pearl is to listen superficially to the murmur after a pause with a premature beat or listen to the beat after a pause with atrial fibrillation. The murmur of aortic stenosis increases in intensity, whereas the murmur of mitral regurgitation shows little change (Fig. A). Use of this pearl can make this diagnosis in patients where the differentiation can be extremely difficult. It can even be lifesaving, as it was in the following patient. A woman in her 60's was incapacitated because of advanced congestive heart failure. She could not climb even one flight of stairs because of her shortness of breath, and at night she had to sleep upright in a chair because of nocturnal dyspnea. She had all of the symptoms and signs of advanced cardiac decompensation. None of the medications she was taking were effective in affording relief, and she was considered at the end stage of her heart disease.

She stated that she had mitral stenosis and regurgitation and atrial fibrillation. On auscultation of her heart, she had atrial fibrilla-

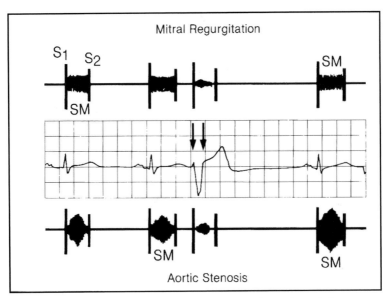

Fig A: Systolic murmur (SM) of mitral regurgitation remains unchanged after pause; in contrast, systolic murmur (SM) of aortic stenosis is louder after pause following premature beat.

tion, and by concentrating on the beat after a pause, the examiner could hear a definite increase in intensity of the systolic murmur over the lower left sternal border and apex. The murmur was not of a harsh quality but had frequencies that are often heard with mitral regurgitation. There was no opening snap of mitral stenosis; instead, there was an S3 diastolic gallop. The increase in the systolic murmur after the pause was the clue that this situation was consistent with aortic stenosis rather than with mitral regurgitation. The patient had cardiac catheterization after this observation, and she had a gradient over 100 mm across her aortic valve. She then had aortic valve replacement surgery, with a remarkable improvement in her condition to the extent that she was able to return to practically normal physical activities and a comfortable life. Approximately 10 years have passed since the cardiac surgery. In her case, paying attention to the cardiac pearl concerning the increase in the systolic murmur after a pause in atrial fibrillation (or a premature beat) proved to be lifesaving. She had a reversible type of heart disease. Such cases are gratifying to the patient, the family, and also to the physician.

W. Proctor Harvey, M.D.

Transient Myocardial Ischemia

During spontaneous or exercise-induced angina pectoris there are several changes in both systolic and diastolic performance of the ventricular myocardium. Heart muscle that has become transiently ischemic may fail to contract effectively or even undergo paradoxical expansion, leading to reduction of contractile force and of stroke volume. Diastolic compliance of ischemic areas is also abnormal with impaired relaxation in parts of the ventricular wall leading to elevation of the end-diastolic pressure. During spontaneous angina there is often an increase in mean arterial pressure, these various changes may be accompanied by alterations in heart sounds and murmurs and can provide clues to the presence of myocardial ischemia. For example, development of an easily audible fourth heart sound during an episode of chest pain strongly suggests that the pain is ischemic in origin; this is particularly true when the chest pain is spontaneous. Fourth heart sounds may develop following exercise in many normal adults without clinical evidence of heart disease, so the occurrence of a fourth heart sound during an exercise test is a less specific finding. A third heart sound is a less common accompaniment of angina.

Ischemia of a papillary muscle, leading to interference with its contraction, results in a temporary mid-systolic or late systolic murmur of mitral regurgitation. This form of papillary muscle dysfunction may lead at times to fairly marked mitral regurgitation, enough to raise left atrial pressure to pulmonary edema levels if ischemia is prolonged.

Pharmacologic Agents

Phenylephrine

There are a few drugs, chiefly potent vasocon-

TABLE 6

Responses to Amyl Nitrite

Fall in arterial pressure leads to:
- ↓ Early diastolic murmur of AR
- ↓ Austin Flint (middiastolic) murmur of AR
- ↓ Continuous murmur of patent ductus arteriosus (PDA)
- ↓ Systolic murmur of tetralogy of Fallot

Fall in left ventricular pressure leads to:
- ↓ Systolic murmur of VSD
- ↓ Systolic murmur of MR

Increase in cardiac output leads to:
- ↑ Diastolic murmurs of MS and TS
- ↑ Diastolic murmur of congenital PR
- ↑ Systolic murmur of TR

Increase in contractility and ejection rate leads to:
- ↑ Systolic murmurs of AS, PS, and HOCM
- ↑ Functional murmurs

Reduction in left ventricular volume leads to:
- Earlier onset of SC and LSM in mitral prolapse

---

strictor or vasodilator agents, that have been used to bring about rapid changes in vascular resistance, mean arterial pressure, and myocardial preload and afterload influence murmurs and heart sounds. Some of these agents have a sufficiently rapid onset of action and brief duration that contribute to easily-detected auscultatory changes. Of the pressor agents, phenylephrine has undergone the most extensive use, but the need for intravenous administration and careful titration of the dose has led most cardiologists to shy away from its routine use in the clinical setting. It is not surprising that a 15mm Hg to 20mm Hg rise in blood pressure produced by infusion of the drug can lead to enhancement of the diastolic murmur of aortic regurgitation or the systolic murmur of mitral insufficiency. Phenylephrine acts primarily on the systemic arterial network and has minimal effect on the pulmonary vasculature. This results in an increase in the systolic murmur of ventricular septal defect or in the volume of shunt flow through a patent ductus arteriosus.

Response to phenylephrine differs from that of isometric hand grip exercise in that it causes a reflex bradycardia and a drop in cardiac output. Therefore, the murmurs of valvular aortic stenosis and pulmonic stenosis change very little in response to this drug. A rise in left ventricular diastolic volume leads to a reduction in the outflow obstruction of hypertrophic subaortic stenosis causing a marked diminution of its murmur. Methoxamine and angiotensin, both potent vasoconstrictor agents, produce responses similar to those of

phenylephrine, but use of any of these pressor agents has not been looked upon with much enthusiasm in bedside diagnosis. Likewise, isoproterenol, a drug with a markedly positive inotropic effect, has gained little use at the bedside, although in the catheterization laboratory it may be used to increase left ventricular outflow gradient in hypertrophic cardiomyopathy.

Amyl Nitrite

Amyl nitrite is the pharmacologic agent most widely used in the bedside study of heart murmurs because of its ease of administration and its very transient effect. As a potent vasodilator, it causes a sharp drop in systemic arterial pressure, followed by a reflex increase in heart rate and myocardial contractility. Venous return is enhanced and cardiac output is increased. Circulation time is shortened. The faster heart rate leads to a shorter diastolic filling period. Pulmonary vasculature is less influenced by the vasodilating effect of inhaled amyl nitrite, since little of the drug reaches the pulmonary arteries and there is minimal reduction of pulmonary vascular resistance. The pulmonary arterial pressure, however, may rise slightly in response to the increased right ventricular output.

Although drop in systemic blood pressure is transient, the patient should be lying flat when administered amyl nitrite in order to avoid light headedness or syncope. He should also be warned of the peculiar odor of the drug and the transient feeling of flushing or fullness in the head. This is somewhat similar to the effect of sublingual nitroglycerin, but its duration is briefer. It is best to ask an assistant to administer the drug while the examiner listens to the heart. The standard perle is wrapped in a thin towel or gauze and crushed with a sharp squeezing motion. If the perle has maintained its proper charge, a sharp "popping" sound is produced when it is snapped open. After it is open it should be held within a few inches of the subject's nose. Three to five deep inhalations are usually sufficient to deliver an effective dose. The index of responsiveness is a reflex tachycardia, and the perle should be removed as soon as the heart rate increases by 20 to 30 beats/min. Dousing the perle in water will limit further drug release.

Within 30 seconds of inhalation, amyl nitrite has its maximal effect on the blood pressure, but the pressure returns to control levels within 90 seconds. Auscultation should be carried out during the control period and while the drug is being inhaled. As the heart rate rises, the first heart sound becomes louder in response to the more rapid rise of left ventricular pressure during reflex sympa-

TABLE 7

Response of Murmurs and Heart Sounds to Physiologic and Pharmacologic Interventions

This table provides a list of common cardiovascular disorders producing various types of murmurs and added heart sounds with an indication in each instance of the typical response to physiologic or pharmacologic interventions.

MURMURS AND CLINICAL DISORDER	INTERVENTION AND RESPONSE
Systolic murmurs	
Aortic outflow obstruction	
Valvular aortic stenosis	Louder with passive leg raising, sudden squatting, Valsalva release (after 5 to 6 beats), following a pause induced by a premature beat, after amyl nitrite; fades during Valsalva strain and with isometric handgrip
Hypertrophic subaortic stenosis	Louder on standing, during Valsalva strain, or with amyl nitrite; fades with sudden squatting, recumbency, or isometric handgrip
Pulmonic stenosis	Midsystolic murmur increases with amyl nitrite except with marked right ventricular hypertrophy; also increases during first few beats after Valsalva release.
Mitral regurgitation	
Rheumatic	Murmur louder on sudden squatting, with isometric handgrip, or phenylephrine; softens with amyl nitrite
Mitral prolapse	Midsystolic click moves toward S_1 and late systolic murmur starts earlier on standing, during Valsalva strain, and with amyl nitrite; click may occur earlier on inspiration; murmur starts later and click moves toward S_2 during squatting, with recumbency, and often after pause induced by a premature beat
Tricuspid regurgitation	Murmur increases during inspiration, with passive leg raising, and with amyl nitrite
Ventricular septal defect	
Small defect without pulmonary hypertension	Fades with amyl nitrite; increases with isometric handgrip or phenylephrine; if louder with amyl nitrite, suspect aneurysm of membranous septum.
Tetralogy of Fallot	Murmur softens with amyl nitrite
Supraclavicular bruit	Altered by compression of subclavian artery; may be eliminated by extension of ipsilateral shoulder
Diastolic murmurs	
Aortic regurgitation	
Blowing diastolic murmur	Increases with sudden squatting, isometric handgrip, or phenylephrine
Austin Flint murmur	Fades with amyl nitrite
Pulmonary regurgitation	
Congenital	Early or mid-diastolic rumble increases on inspiration and with amyl nitrite
Pulmonary hypertension	High-frequency blowing murmur increases with amyl nitrite
Mitral stenosis	Mid-diastolic and presystolic murmurs louder with exercise, left lateral position, coughing, isometric handgrip, amyl nitrite; phenylephrine widens A_2-OS interval; inspiration produces sequence of A_2-P_2-OS
Tricuspid stenosis	Mid-diastolic and presystolic murmurs increase during inspiration, with passive leg raising, and with amyl nitrite
Continuous murmurs	
Patent ductus arteriosus	Diastolic phase amplified with isometric handgrip, phenylephrine; diastolic phase fades with amyl nitrite
Cervical venous hum	Obliterated by direct compression of jugular veins or by Valsalva strain; louder with amyl nitrite
Added heart sounds	
Gallop rhythm	
Ventricular gallop (S_3) and atrial gallop (S_4)	Accentuated by lying flat with passive leg raising; decreased by standing or during Valsalva; right-sided gallop sounds usually increase during inspiration, left-sided during expiration
Summation gallop	Separates into ventricular gallop (S_3) and atrial gallop (S_4) sounds when heart rate is slowed by carotid sinus massage
Ejection Sounds	Ejection sound in pulmonary stenosis fades and occurs closer to the first sound during inspiration

thetic stimulation. As systemic diastolic pressure falls, murmur of aortic regurgitation fades. The Graham Steell murmur of pulmonic regurgitation in patients with pulmonary hypertension increases in response to the greater venous return induced by amyl nitrite. This quite opposite response makes this a useful drug in differentiating the diastolic murmur of pulmonary hypertension from that of

TABLE 8

Physiologic and Pharmacologic Maneuvers Useful in Differentiation of Similar Auscultatory Findings

This table lists those maneuvers which are particularly useful in differentiating lesions with similar auscultatory findings.

AUSCULTATORY PROBLEMS	HELPFUL MANEUVERS
Systolic murmur of valvular aortic stenosis or hypertrophic subaortic stenosis	Sudden squatting, Valsalva maneuver
Systolic murmur of valvular aortic stenosis or mitral prolapse	Sudden standing, amyl nitrite
Systolic murmur of valvular aortic stenosis or mitral regurgitation	Amyl nitrite, phenylephrine, variation in cycle length
Diastolic blow of aortic regurgitation or Graham Steell murmur of pulmonary regurgitation	Amyl nitrite
Diastolic rumble of mitral stenosis or Austin Flint murmur	Amyl nitrite
Diastolic murmur of mitral stenosis or tricuspid stenosis	Respiration
Systolic murmur of mitral regurgitation or tricuspid regurgitation	Respiration
Supraclavicular bruit or aortic stenosis	Extension of shoulder, compression of subclavian artery
Ejection sound in pulmonic stenosis or aortic stenosis	Respiration
Small ventricular septal defect or pulmonic stenosis	Amyl nitrite, phenylephrine
Systolic murmur of pulmonic stenosis or tetralogy of Fallot	Amyl nitrite
Continuous murmur of patent ductus arteriosus or cervical venous hum	Compression of neck veins
Fourth sound plus first sound or separation of two components of first heart sound	Respiration, sudden standing, lying with passive leg raising
Second heart sound plus opening snap or wide separation of S_2 components	Respiration, phenylephrine, sudden standing

From Criscitiello MG: 6.

aortic insufficiency. The low-frequency short diastolic murmur of congenital pulmonary valve insufficiency also grows louder. Amyl nitrite has also been used in separating the diastolic rumbling murmur of Austin Flint heard in aortic insufficiency from that of mitral stenosis. The Austin Flint murmur fades as aortic regurgitation is diminished. The mid-diastolic and pre-systolic murmurs of mitral stenosis are definitely accentuated as mitral flow increases. Morrison's 1918 report of the use of amyl nitrite to make this distinction represents the earliest record of employment of a pharmacologic agent to alter heart murmurs.

The amyl nitrite effect does not permit distinction between valvular and hypertrophic sub-valvular stenosis since both murmurs become louder in response to the increase in contractility and velocity of ejection. However, the murmur of mitral regurgitation is noted to fade markedly in response to the drop in left ventricular systolic pressure. In mitral valve prolapse amyl nitrite causes the click to occur earlier in systole and the murmur of mitral regurgitation to increase in duration, sometimes starting early enough to sound pansystolic. The intensity of the murmur may actually decrease, however. Because amyl nitrite lowers systemic pressure more than pulmonary pressure, the left to right shunt of a ventricular septal defect is reduced and its murmur diminishes. The diastolic component of the continuous murmur of patent ductus arteriosus also tends to decrease.

In the patient with pulmonic stenosis who has an intact ventricular septum, the systolic murmur grows much louder with amyl nitrite. When pulmonic stenosis is accompanied by a ventricular septal defect (Tetralogy of Fallot) the drop in systemic resistance produced by amyl nitrite permits a greater right to left shunt, with a resultant diminution in flow across the stenotic right ventricular outflow tract and a decrease in the systolic murmur. This difference in response in pulmonary stenotic patients with and without a septal defect is particularly useful in detecting acyanotic tetralogy (Table 6).

Selected Reading

1. Aronow WS, Uyeyama RP, Cassidy J, et al: Resting and post exercise phonocardiogram in patients with angina pectoris and in normal subjects. *Circ* 43:273,1971.
2. Beck W, Schrire V, Vogelpoel L, et al: Hemodynamic effects of amyl nitrite and phenylephrine on the normal human circulation and their relation to changes in cardiac murmurs. *AJC* 8:341,1961.
3. Brody W, Crilley JM: Intermittent severe mitral regurgitation. *NEJM* 283:673,1970.
4. Cochran PT: Auscultatory clues elicited by physical maneuvers and pharmacologic agents, in Abrams J (ed): *Essentials of Cardiac Physical Diagnosis;* pp 177-183 Philadelphia: Lea & Febiger 1987.
5. Crawford MH, O'Rourke RA: A systematic approach to the bedside differentiation of cardiac murmurs and abnormal sounds. *Curr Prob Card* -1, 1977.
6. Criscitiello MG: Physiologic and pharmacologic aids in cardiac auscultation, in Fowler NO (ed): *Cardiac Diagnosis and*

204

Treatment, Ed 3. pp 77-90. Hagerstown, MD, Harper & Row 1980.

7. Criscitiello MG, Harvey WP: Clinical recognition of congenital pulmonary valve insufficiency. *AJC* 20:765,1967.

8. Curtiss El, Matthews RG, Shaver JA: Mechanism of normal splitting of the second heart sound: *Circ* 51:157, 1975.

9. de Leon AC, Harvey WP: Pharmacological agents and auscultation. *Mod Concepts Cardio Dis* 44:23,1975.

10. Elkayam U, Gleicher N: *Cardiac problems in pregnancy,* pp 19-20 New York: Alan R. Liss, Inc. 1982.

11. Hultgren HW, Reeves R, Cohn K, et al: Ejection click of valvular pulmonic stenosis. *Circ* 40:631,1969.

12. Karliner JS, O'Rourke RA, Kerney DJ, et al: Hemodynamic explanation of why the murmur of mitral regurgitation is independent of cycle length. *BHJ* 35:397,1973.

13. Lauson HD, Bloomfield RA, Cournand A: The influence of the respiration on the circulation of man. *AJM* 1:315,1946.

14. Lembo NJ, Dell'ltalia LJ, Crawford MH, et al. Bedside diagnosis of systolic murmurs. *NEJM* 318:1572-78,1988.

15. McCraw DB, Siegel W, Stonecipher HK, et al: Response of heart murmur intensity to isometric (hand grip) exercise. *BHJ* 34: 605,1972.

16. Morrison A: The value of amyl nitrite inhalation in the diagnosis of mitral stenosis. *BMJ* 1:452,1918.

17. Nelson WP, Hall RJ: The innocent supraclavicular arterial bruit: utility of shoulder maneuvers in its recognition. *NEJM* 278:778,1968.

18. Perloff JK, Caulfield WH, de Leon AC: Peripheral pulmonary artery murmur of atrial septal defect. *BHJ* 29:411,1967.

19. Sharpey-Shafer EP: Effects of squatting on the normal and failing circulation. *BMJ* 1:1072,1976.

20. Thapar MK, Rao PS, Rogers JH, et al: Changing murmurs of patent ductus arteriosus. *J Ped* 92:939,1978.

21. Vitums VC, Gooch AS, Evans JM: Bedside maneuvers to augment the murmur of tricuspid regurgitation. *Med Ann DC* 38:533,1969.

22. Vogelpoel L, Mellen M, Beck W, et al: The value of squatting in the diagnosis of mild aortic regurgitation. *AHJ* 77:709,1969.

CHAPTER 11

The Electrocardiogram: Diagnostic Clues and Clinical Correlations

William P. Nelson, M.D. and Frank I. Marcus, M.D.

The electrocardiograph, over the past 80 years, has contributed substantially to diagnosis and treatment of cardiac patients, and remains an important and informative component of total cardiac assessment, as well as providing a better grip as part of the "five finger approach". Some abnormalities can be determined *only* by ECG (e.g. arrhythmias), some can be diagnosed or clarified (e.g. myocardial infarction), and others can be suggested when a specific pattern is observed (e.g. pericarditis). The accuracy of ECG interpretation is greatly improved when appropriate clinical information such as the patient's age, gender, presenting symptoms and list of pertinent medications is provided. Judgment regarding an abnormal tracing often cannot be made without such information.

Approach to ECG Interpretation

In an approach to ECG interpretation, there are a number of "commandments" that should be emphasized:

• **Commandment 1:** "Thou shalt not overinterpret the ECG". It is important to realize that the range of normal is broad and that clinical circumstances must dictate the importance of a particular ECG observation. Dr. H.J.L. Marriott has phrased it nicely — "Many an unfortunate individual is limping his apprehensive way through life maimed by the unkind cut of ECG misinterpretation."

• **Commandment 2:** "Beware the mischievous machine". The current three-channel electrocardiograph is an excellent electronic device and much of the problems of yesteryear have been removed. In the past, the frequency response of machines was often inadequate and careful adjustment of stylus pressure and heat was critical to avoid artifacts. The potential mischief today is the ECG analysis provided by computer. Those who have worked with computer interpreted ECGs will attest to problems with both overdiagnosis and underdiagnosis. The computer analysis must be carefully reviewed and edited before a final interpretation is provided by the clinician.

• **Commandment 3:** "Beware of technician errors". Even the most conscientious and dedicated ECG technician will have a "bad day" and provide tracings with rearranged or misplaced electrodes.

CARDIAC PEARL

Practically everyone who has taken a large number of electrocardiograms on patients had inadvertently reversed the limb leads in lead 1. Immediate recognition of this mistake can be seen in the tracing, as shown in Figure A with inversion of the P-wave and QRS complex- a mirror image of the complex when the electrodes are correctly placed. Always double check for correct attachment of the electrodes when first attaching them and also when removing them.

W. Proctor Harvey, M.D.

One must be particularly alert to tracings performed in the dead of night by house staff or nurses. The current practice of using disposable electrodes without any skin preparation can result in considerable baseline artifact and make the tracing difficult to interpret.

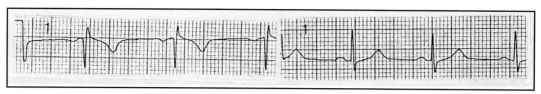

Fig A: Reversed Leads -Lead 1, right and left arm leads of ECG inadvertently reversed (left tracing). Note negative P wave and mirror image of complex when the limb leads are correct (right tracing). Always double check the lead wires when removing them. In this way the error is promptly detected.

CARDIAC PEARL

Do you have trouble with chest electrodes falling off? Not uncommonly, precordial electrodes may not stick to the hairy chest of a patient. Often all that is needed to correct this is to put extra paste or gel on the chest and with one's index and/or middle finger, mat down the chest hairs- the electrodes may now hold. Remember the smooth the hairs down on the skin with the fingers. Shaving the chest hair, I learned, has been used, at times, but usually is not necessary. Of course, some modern adhesive electrodes stick to the chest skin quite well.

W. Proctor Harvey, M.D.

• **Commandment 4:** "Thou shalt not interpret an ECG without reference to prior tracings". This is perhaps the most important and most often ignored commandment. A given tracing, even when correctly interpreted, may have an entirely different meaning when contrasted to prior tracings. On occasion, a new ECG abnormality can "erase" a previously existing abnormality.

CARDIAC PEARL

Very recently I evaluated a patient who had been previously examined in another medical facility. She had a photocopy of her electrocardiogram which was normal; however, it was a technically poor tracing as evidenced by the irregular artifact present in each of the 12 leads. This type of tracing can be prevented, or corrected, by paying attention to the following:

a. Make sure there is plenty of electrode paste.

b. Check the connections to insure that they are not loose.

c. Make sure the electrodes are clean.

d. Is the patient relaxed? If the muscles are tense, artifact can result. The patient can be told how to relax his or her muscles.

e. Are the patient's ankles pressing against the end of the examining table with the feet hanging over? If so, have the patient move upward on the table.

f. Make sure the electrode is positioned over the brachial artery where its pulsation moves the electrode.

g. Repeat the electrocardiogram, if necessary, to get a "good technical tracing."

W. Proctor Harvey, M.D.

Because there are numerous excellent ECG texts, we will limit ourselves to presenting a variety of interesting, instructive, or unusual tracings. The format selected is presentation of tracings as "unknowns", without clinical information (as is too often the case in practice!). It is suggested that the reader analyze the ECG and answer the questions before proceeding to the discussion and clinical correlation.

Abnormalities of Ventricular Depolarization

The ECG provides an inexpensive, non-invasive, and reproducible assessment of the electrical activity of the ventricles. A single tracing may not permit a decisive judgment, but serial tracings can often do so, and ECG conclusions always profit from clinical correlation. Common abnormalities that can be determined include changes in intraventricular conduction, alterations of QRS voltage, and identification of myocardial infarction. The ECG remains the best single diagnostic test for myocardial infarction. The ECG patterns of acute infarction are familiar to all clinicians. Typical examples are shown below (Figures 1 to 3).

ECG Example 1 (Figure 4)

• **Questions:** How would you interpret this tracing? (Note that the precordial leads are *right chest leads*). What might be present on an examination? What is "Kussmaul's venous sign"? What problems would you anticipate in this patient?

• **ECG Analysis:** The rhythm is sinus at 80 beats per minute with a PR interval of 0.20 seconds and a QRS axis of +30 degrees. There are Q waves in leads II, III, and aVF with ST segment elevation in these leads and reciprocal depression in leads I and aVL indicating an acute inferior myocardial infarction. The right precordial leads show ST elevation and a QS pattern in V3r through V6r —

changes consistent with right ventricular MI. The combination of abnormalities indicates that the left ventricular inferior wall MI is accompanied by infarction of the right ventricular free wall.

• **Clinical Correlation:** This 67-year-old woman presented with severe and protracted chest pain and the ECG shown above. On examination, there was prominent jugular venous distention with Kussmaul's venous sign (increase in jugular venous distention with inspiration). This occurs because the infarcted RV cannot accommodate normal venous return and the inspiratory increase in volume engorges the right atrium and distends the jugular veins. Such patients may be hypotensive owing to decreased pulmonary blood flow secondary to RV dysfunction. A high filling venous pressure is required and if the jugular venous engorgement is misconstrued to represent CHF and diuretics given, there may be further compromise in the patient's clinical condition.

ECG Example 2 (Figure 5)

• **Questions:** Two electrocardiograms are shown. The first tracing in each lead set was obtained one year before the second ECG. How many zones of myocardial infarction do you identify? What is the "cancellation phenomenon"?

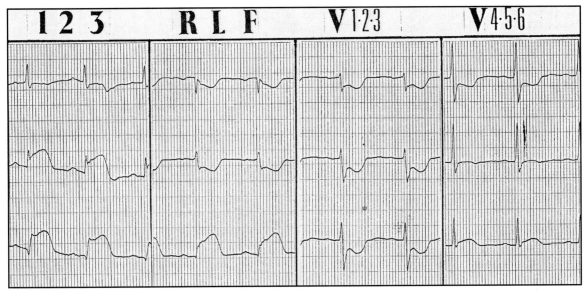

Figure 1. Acute Inferolateral MI

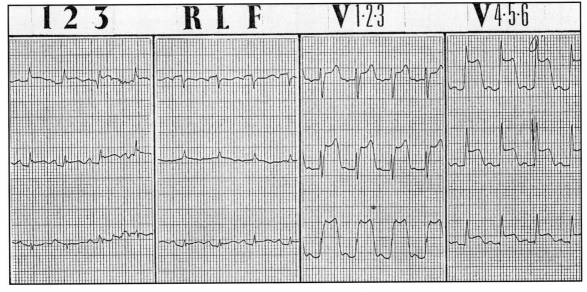

Figure 2. Acute Anterolateral MI

209

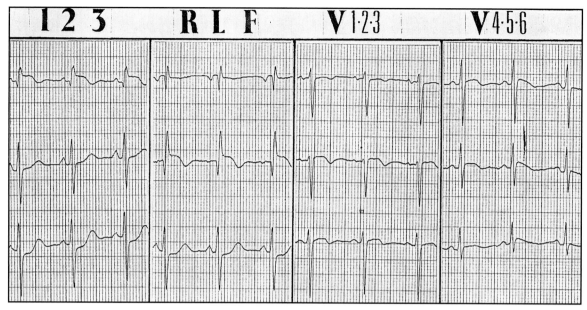

Figure 3. Acute Lateral MI

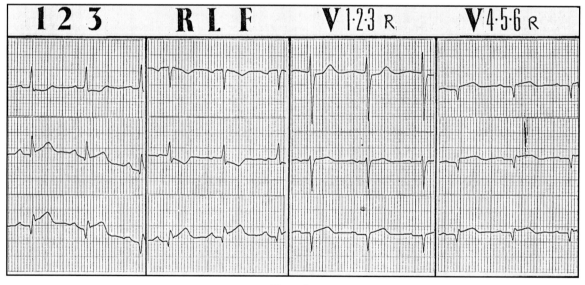

Figure 4

• **ECG Analysis:** In the first tracing, Q waves are present in leads II, III, and aVF with slight ST segment elevation in these leads. There are broad, tall R waves in leads V2-3 with ST segment depression. The tracing is consistent with an inferior-posterior MI of undetermined age. The second tracing is markedly different. The Q waves in the "inferior leads" have been replaced by positive deflections and the initial R waves in leads V2-3 are now Q waves. The second tracing is consistent with anterolateral myocardial infarction. The reorientation of initial forces in both frontal and horizontal planes has effectively erased the evidence of prior inferior-posterior MI.

• **Clinical Correlation:** This 53-year-old man sustained repeated myocardial infarctions. Without the sequence of tracings, the "cancellation phenomenon" would not be known.

ECG Example 3 (Figure 6)

• **Question:** This patient was hospitalized with chest pain. His ECG has been stable for three days. How would you interpret this tracing?

• **ECG Analysis:** There is sinus rhythm of 90 per minute with a normal QRS axis of 0 degrees and normal PR and QRS intervals. The QT interval is prolonged and the T waves negative in leads I and aVL and deeply inverted in leads V1-3. The

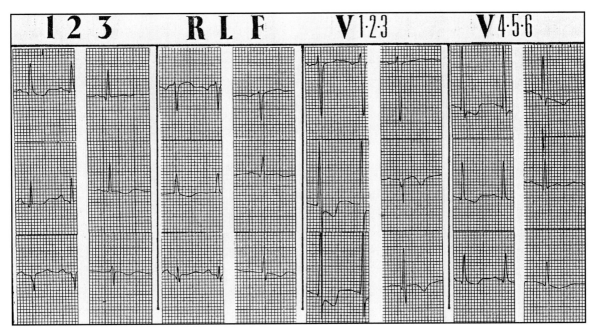

Figure 5

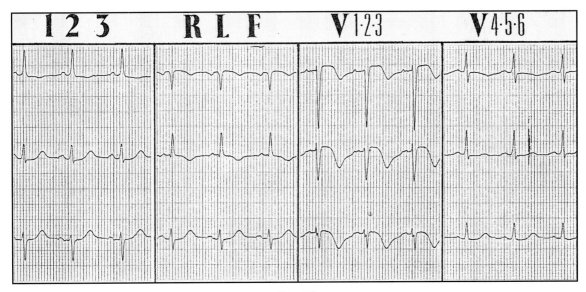

Figure 6

overall pattern is consistent with significant anteroseptal "ischemia" and probably represents non-Q infarction. In bygone days, this pattern was called "subendocardial MI" or "nontransmural MI", but pathologic studies have shown that the implications of these anatomic terms are often incorrect. These patients are often at risk of additional myocardial damage and the short-term prognosis is frequently poor.

• **Clinical Correlation:** This 78-year-old man presented with severe chest pain. Although his CPK enzyme levels were diagnostic of myocardial infarction, his ECG did not show the anticipated evolutionary features. Pain recurred on his fourth

hospital day and coronary arteriography was recommended. He declined the study and insisted on being discharged. His obituary appeared in the newspaper within a week.

ECG Example 4 (Figure 7)

• **Questions:** What do the wide QRS complexes represent? What additional abnormality is present?

• **ECG Analysis:** The QRS is wide with the morphology of complete LBBB. When there is normal ventricular activation, the general direction of the QRS and T forces (vectors) is the same and if the QRS is positive, the T wave is usually also positive. When LBBB is present, the sequence of ventricular

211

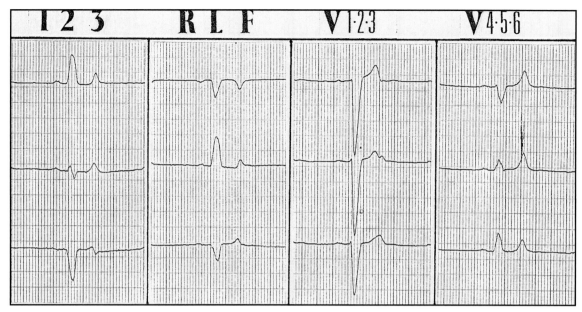

Figure 7

activation is altered and repolarization will also change. The anticipated morphology with LBBB is that the ST-T will be in opposite direction to the QRS, a "secondary repolarization abnormality". In this tracing, the T waves are inappropriately positive in leads in which the QRS is positive, and thus represent a "primary" disturbance of repolarization.

• **Clinical Correlation:** This 81-year-old woman has had typical complete LBBB for seven years. She presented with increase in severity of her usual angina pectoris and with the T waves shown. Subsequent evidence indicated myocardial infarction. This subtle change in T wave may be the only indication when LBBB is present that there is an acute myocardial process.

ECG Example 5 (Figure 8)

• **Questions:** In the middle QRS complex of each lead set, the last 0.04-0.06 seconds has been masked to emphasize the initial "pre-blocked" forces. What zone(s) of myocardium have been infarcted? What is the "pre-block axis"?

• **ECG Analysis:** The rhythm is sinus at 85 beats per minute. P waves are notched in leads II and aVF with a prominent terminal trough in lead V1 consistent with left atrial enlargement. The QRS is wide and the pattern in V1 is typical of RBBB. In RBBB the major alteration is in the late forces, i.e., the terminal vector. In order to determine the frontal plane axis, the late contribution due to RBBB should not be included. The "pre-block axis" is oriented inferiorly at approximately +90°. There are Q waves in leads I and aVL and in all the precordial leads. The QRS changes are due to recent

extensive anterolateral myocardial infarction.

• **Clinical Correlation:** This 75-year-old man presented with chest pain and features of congestive heart failure. Prior tracings showed normal QRS duration and no evidence of MI. The damage due to acute anterolateral infarction has resulted in right bundle branch block. The P wave abnormality anticipated the bedside findings of congestive heart failure.

ECG Example 6 (Figure 9)

• **Questions:** This tracing is from a 58-year-old normotensive man and all precordial leads except V4 are recorded at one-half standard. What ECG abnormality suggests a cause for this patient's symptoms of chest pain, dyspnea, and dizziness? What valvular lesion might be present and what abnormalities on physical examination would you anticipate?

• **ECG Interpretation:** There is sinus rhythm at 70 per minute with an increased P-R interval (0.32 seconds). The frontal plane QRS axis is normal at minus 15 degrees. Considering the half standard recording, there is striking precordial voltage diagnostic of left ventricular hypertrophy with ST-T changes consistent with a pressure loaded left ventricle, or "LVH with strain".

• **Clinical Correlation:** This man had known of a "slight heart murmur" since he was 25 years old. He presented with angina pectoris, postural dizziness, and marked dyspnea provoked by slight exertion. On examination, his pulse volume was small with a slow upstroke. The apical impact was sustained and forceful. A grade 4 late peaking systolic

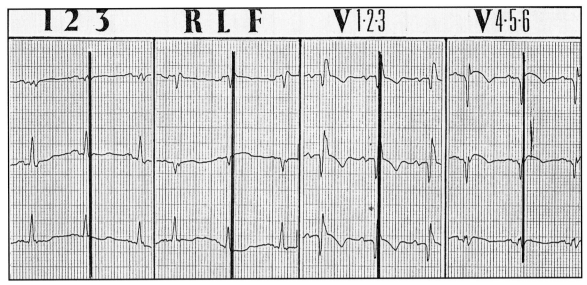

Figure 8

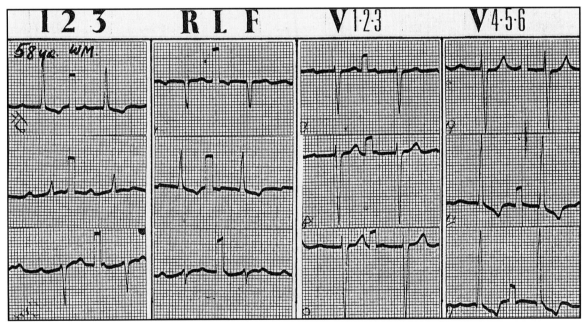

Figure 9

murmur was present in the second right interspace with radiation to the suprasternal notch and carotids. The impression of serious aortic obstruction was confirmed with a 100 mm Hg gradient recorded across the aortic valve.

ECG Example 7 (Figure 10)

• **Questions:** What is the pattern of "diastolic loading" of the left ventricle? What valve lesions might be present in this patient?

• **ECG Analysis:** There is sinus rhythm at 70 beats per minute with a normal frontal plane axis of +40 degrees. There is excessive precordial QRS voltage with delayed ventricular activation; both

support a diagnosis of LVH. Although there is ST segment sagging in leads V5-6, the T waves are upright. This finding suggests that the hypertrophy is secondary to a volume burden, LVH with "diastolic loading" pattern.

• **Clinical Correlation:** This active, energetic 52-year-old woman had known of a "leaky heart valve" for many years. On examination, blood pressure was 170/50. Peripheral pulses were quick rising and collapsing ("Waterhammer pulse"). The apical impulse was in the sixth intercostal space in the anterior axillary line and was forceful with a broad impact area. On auscultation, there was a harsh but brief grade 3 aortic ejection murmur and a loud

213

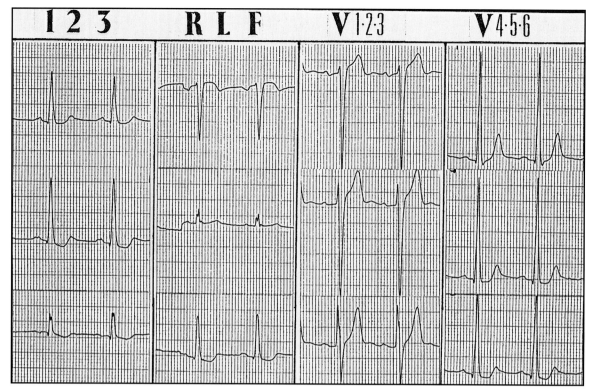

Figure 10

pan-diastolic murmur of aortic regurgitation. At the apex the first heart sound was faint and there was a prominent mid-diastolic rumble ("Austin-Flint murmur").

Both aortic and mitral regurgitation, when long standing, can result in left ventricular hypertrophy and dilatation due to the imposed volume burdens. Both of these valve lesions may result in the ECG pattern seen above.

ECG Example 8 (Figure 11)

• **Question:** A 35-year-old man has known of a "heart murmur" since age 15. He now complains of exertional chest pain and increasing effort dyspnea. Does his ECG suggest a cause for both his complaints and his murmur? (Single channel recording, leads V2-3-4 are recorded at one-half standard).

• **ECG Analysis:** There is sinus bradycardia at 55 per minute with normal intervals and an indeterminate frontal plane axis. (The initial forces in the limb leads are directed right and inferior and the terminal forces left and superior). Since the measured S wave in lead V2 is 27 millimeters and is one-half standard, there is ample voltage to indicate LVH. The prominent Q waves in leads I, aVL, and V4-6 are consistent with prior lateral wall MI. There are significant ST-T abnormalities in both frontal and horizontal planes.

• **Clinical Correlation:** This young man has echocardiographic features diagnostic of hypertrophic obstructive cardiomyopathy. On examination, he has quick rising pulses, paradoxical splitting of the second heart sound, and a grade 3 harsh, pansystolic murmur, audible over the entire precordium but loudest at mid precordium. The murmur decreases with a prompt squat and markedly increases on standing.

In IHSS, the ECG not only shows left ventricular hypertrophy but often "pseudo-infarct" Q waves. These are thought to be due to abnormal architecture of the ventricular myocardium with an altered sequence of depolarization.

CARDIAC PEARL

In the absence of any history, symptoms, or signs of coronary artery disease, the presence of significant Q-waves and ST and T-wave changes should alert one to the possibility of hypertrophic cardiomyopathy- particularly in a teenager or young adult.

A normal electrocardiogram practically rules out the diagnosis of hypertrophic cardiomyopathy. Dilated cardiomyopathy, too, often has some abnormality of the electrocardiogram.

W. Proctor Harvey, M.D.

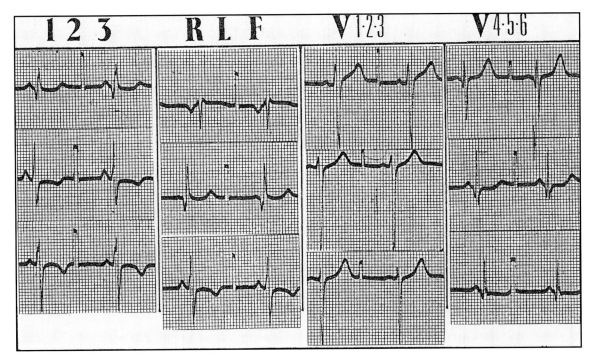

Figure 11

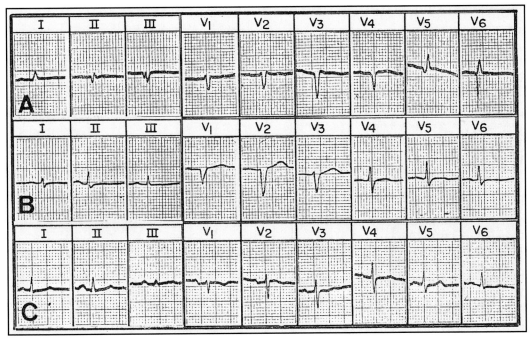

Figure 12

ECG Example 9 (Figure 12)

• **Questions:** What are the ECG criteria for "low voltage"? In what circumstances does low voltage occur and what would you guess are the causes in these three patients?

• **ECG Analysis:** Low voltage can be diagnosed when the total amplitude of the QRS complex is 5 mm or less in the limb leads and 10 mm or less in

the precordial leads. The causes can be grouped into two general categories: problems with the "electrical generator" and problems surfacing the electrical signal. "Generator problems" includes circumstances in which the myocardium has been replaced by non-electrical tissue (fibrous tissue, tumor, amyloid deposition, or sarcoid infiltrate). "Transmission problems" include situations in

215

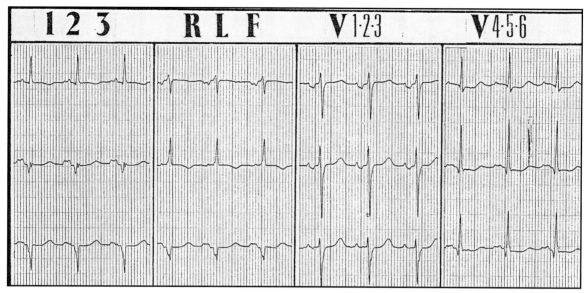

Figure 13

which the electrical event is insulated from the surface (air, fat, fluid). These causes are combined in the individual with myxedema. The heart's electrical activity is diminished in the hypothyroid state and there is frequently an accompanying pericardial effusion.

• **Clinical Correlation:** Patient "A" was a 58-year-old man who had repeated myocardial infarctions, including inferior, anterior, and lateral walls. The cumulative effect of the extensive myocardial destruction resulted in low voltage QRS complexes. Patient "B" was a 51-year-old man profoundly myxedematous. In such patients a clue that the low voltage is due to hypothyroidism is often significant bradycardia and generalized T wave flattening accompanying the depolarization abnormality. Patient "C" is a 55-year-old man who is 5 feet 2 inches with eyes of blue and weighs 330 pounds. His heart is insulated by surface fat.

CARDIAC PEARL

When low voltage is present on the electrocardiogram in a patient with an enlarged heart, not only conditions such as a pericardial effusion, emphysema, and diffuse myocardial fibrosis should be considered, but also amyloid cardiomyopathy. However, although this finding may be a clue to the present of amyloid, it is not specific.

W. Proctor Harvey, M.D.

Left Axis Deviation

Although there is some disagreement regarding the limits of normal of the frontal plane axis, a rea-

sonable range for the adult is +90 degrees to minus 30 degrees. An electrical axis greater than minus 30 degrees is a common ECG abnormality. Several causes will be reviewed with examples.

ECG Example 10 (Figure 13)

• **Questions:** What is the cause of left axis deviation in this patient? What might be the cause of the QT prolongation and the ST segment abnormality?

• **ECG Analysis:** There is normal sinus rhythm of 95/min with normal PR and QRS intervals. The frontal plane QRS axis is minus 45 degrees. There are broad, deep Q waves in leads II, III, and aVF diagnostic of inferior wall myocardial infarction. These initial forces are the cause of the LAD. Notched P waves in the limb leads and the broad, terminally negative P waves in leads V1-2 identify left atrial abnormality. The prominent Q waves present in leads V5-6 suggest an associated lateral wall MI. The QT interval is prolonged and is accompanied by sagging ST segments and T wave inversion in leads I and aVL. The combination suggests drug effect rather than "ischemia".

• **Clinical Correlation:** This 41-year-old man had an acute inferolateral myocardial infarction one year ago accompanied by atrial fibrillation and congestive heart failure. Digoxin and quinidine were administered and continued to the present. He developed mitral regurgitation thought to be due to papillary muscle dysfunction and regarded as the cause for left atrial enlargement. He is currently stable without evidence of angina pectoris.

ECG Example 11 (Figure 14)

• **Questions:** In each lead set, the first ECG was

216

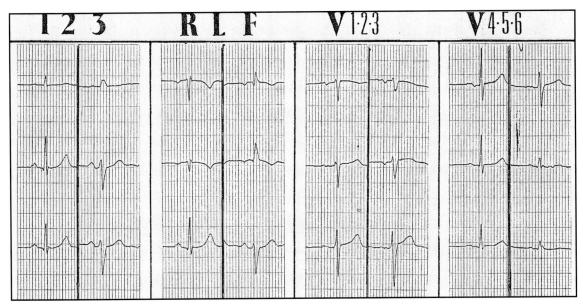

Figure 14

obtained five days before the tracing in the second column. What is the cause of the change in electrical axis due to?

• **ECG Analysis:** The QRS complexes in the first column have a frontal plane axis of +75 degrees and a duration of 0.08 sec. Insignificant Q waves are present in leads II, III, and aVF and the precordial progression is normal. In the second tracing, the mean QRS axis has shifted to minus 70 degrees and the QRS duration has increased to 0.10 sec. The left-superior shift in axis is due to directional change of the mid and terminal parts of the QRS. Another noteworthy observation is the change in direction of the initial forces of ventricular depolarization. They are now oriented inferiorly and recorded as + deflections in the same leads that were previously negative. This is an example of the change from normal activation to left anterior fascicular block. LAFB alters both initial and terminal portions of the QRS complex with the major change being the left axis shift. Without prior tracings, the slight increase in QRS duration may not be appreciated.

• **Clinical Correlation:** Although left axis deviation secondary to left anterior fascicular block is common and can occur without significant heart disease, in this 71-year-old man it represented progression of his coronary artery disease. Because of accelerating angina pectoris, coronary arteriography was performed showing a seriously obstructive proximal lesion in his left anterior descending coronary artery.

ECG Example 12 (Figure 15)

• **Questions:** What is the cause of left axis deviation in this patient? Is there evidence of intraven-

tricular conduction disturbance? Is there evidence of myocardial infarction?

• **ECG Analysis:** There is sinus rhythm at 70 beats per minute with a frontal plane QRS axis of minus 45 degrees. The PR segment is short and there are prominent slurs (delta waves) on the upstroke of the R waves in many leads. These are diagnostic of preexcitation. The location of the zone of preexcited myocardium results in early forces directed left and superior. The resultant broad, negative initial deflections in leads II, III, and aVF are really "inverted delta waves". Because ventricular activation is abnormal in WPW preexcitation, criteria for the diagnosis of myocardial infarction are not valid. In WPW, ventricular activation represents a blend of wave fronts — portions arriving over the normal AV junction and the accessory pathway. The amount of myocardium "preexcited" determines the increase in QRS duration.

• **Clinical Correlation:** This asymptomatic 64-year-old woman had a routine preoperative ECG. She had no history of cardiac arrhythmias and cardiac exam was normal. The projected surgery was accomplished without problems.

Right Axis Deviation

In children, the frontal plane QRS axis is usually directed to the right of +90 degrees, reflecting the electrical dominance of the right ventricle, present at birth. "Young adults" may also normally have an axis greater than +90 degrees with a reasonable limit of +105 degrees. Although there is no sharp dividing line of age, after 30 years an axis greater than +90 degrees should raise a question. Right axis deviation in the frontal plane is most often due

217

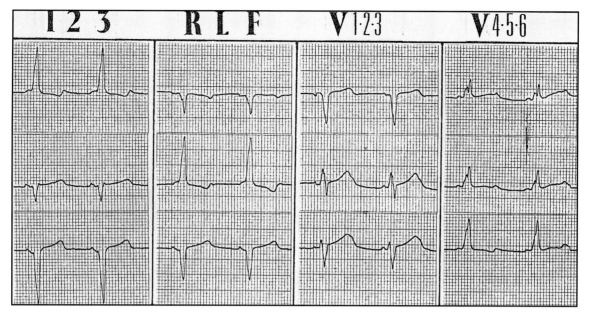

Figure 15

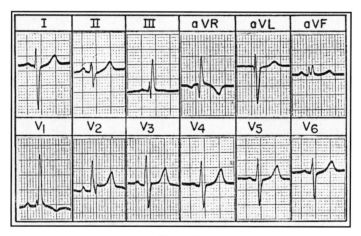

Figure 16

to right ventricular hypertrophy and less frequently to conduction disturbance, myocardial infarction, or abnormality of ventricular activation. Obviously, clinical correlation is essential to determine the cause and importance of this observation. Here are some examples:

ECG Example 13 (Figure 16)

• **Questions:** What is the most common cause of right axis deviation in the adult? What might be the cause in this 28-year-old woman?

• **ECG Analysis:** The QRS axis is +150 degrees, representing marked right axis deviation. Precordial leads show tall R waves in leads V1-2 with deep S waves in V4-6. The tracing is diagnostic of marked right ventricular hypertrophy and predicts a right ventricular pressure near systemic levels. Right ventricular hypertrophy remains the most

common cause of right axis deviation in the frontal plane.

• **Clinical Correlation:** This young woman presented after a syncopal episode. Bedside features of striking pulmonary hypertension were present and cardiac catheterization showed a pulmonary artery pressure of 100 mm Hg. No causes were evident and it was concluded that she had "primary pulmonary hypertension".

ECG Example 14 (Figure 17)

• **Questions:** Three months separate the two tracings on this 61-year-old man. In the upper tracing (Figure 17A), what is an important observation that identifies the cause of right axis deviation? Is there evidence of myocardial infarction in this ECG? In the lower tracing (Figure 17B), another cause for right axis has appeared, what is it?

218

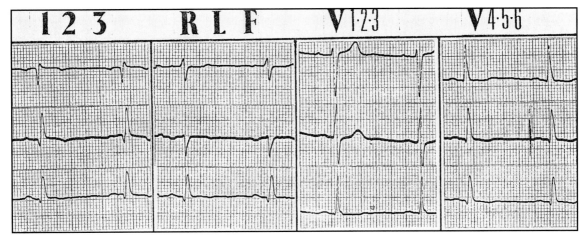

Figure 17A

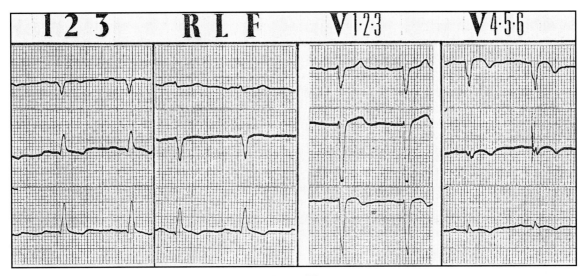

Figure 17B

• **ECG Analysis:** There is sinus bradycardia at 55 beats per minute with a normal PR interval and QRS duration. The frontal plane axis is +110 degrees. Q waves in leads I, II, III, aVF with the tall broad R waves in leads V2-3 identify a previous inferior-posterior-lateral myocardial infarction. An important observation is that the P wave is negative in lead I. Unless the patient has dextrocardia or unless there is a markedly abnormal site of impulse formation, a negative P wave in lead I always indicates misplaced right and left arm electrodes. This not only inverts the polarity of the P and QRS in lead I, but "switches" lead II for lead III, and aVR for aVL. Despite the technician error, the inferior-posterior MI can still be correctly interpreted, but when the QRS in lead I is inverted to compensate for the interchanged leads, the "diagnostic Q waves" of lateral wall MI are no longer present.

• **ECG Analysis:** (Figure 17B) The rhythm is sinus at 70 beats per minute. The PR interval is prolonged to 0.22 seconds and the QRS duration is

at the upper limit of normal (0.10 seconds). There is right axis deviation of +120 degrees. Marked changes have occurred in the precordial leads with evidence of anterolateral myocardial infarction. The frontal plane QRS forces have been redirected away from the "dead zone" of the lateral wall, resulting in right axis deviation.

ECG Example 15 (Figure 18)

• **Question:** What ventricular conduction abnormality results in right axis deviation?

• **ECG Analysis:** A sinus bradycardia of 55 beats per minute is present. The PR interval is prolonged at 0.22 seconds and the QRS is at the upper limits of normal minus 0.10 seconds. The frontal plane QRS axis is directed at +115 degrees. Small Q waves are present in leads III and aVF. Precordial R wave progression is normal with prominent S waves in the lateral precordial leads.

Although right axis deviation is usually due to right ventricular hypertrophy, in this instance, its

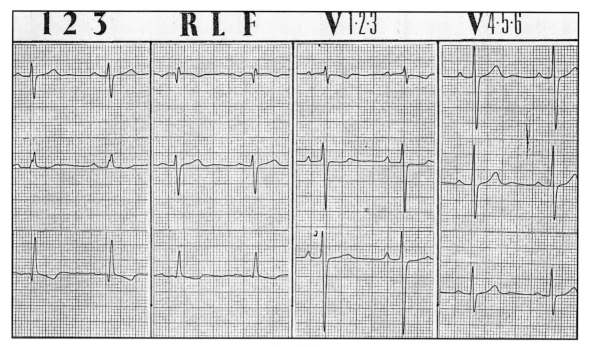

Figure 18

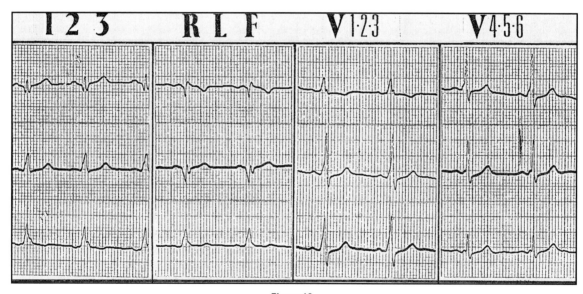

Figure 19

cause was a conduction disturbance, left posterior fascicular block. This abnormality results in reorientation of both initial and terminal forces. Early forces become directed to the left resulting in small Q waves in leads III and aVF; late forces are directed to the right and inferiorly, resulting in right axis deviation.

• **Clinical Correlation:** The patient was a healthy, active 70-year-old man with mild hypertension. A routine ECG the year before this tracing was within normal limits. On history and physical examination, there was no reason for right ventricular hypertrophy. No additional studies were per-

formed and he remained well during the subsequent four years.

ECG Example 16 (Figure 19)

• **Questions:** What is the reason for right axis deviation in this 53-year-old man? What was his recurring complaint?

• **ECG Analysis:** There is sinus rhythm of 80 beats per minute. The electrical axis in the frontal plane is +100 degrees. The QRS is wide (0.12 seconds) with abnormalities of both the early and late forces. Prominent "slurs" (delta waves) are present in the upstroke of the R wave. These are best seen

220

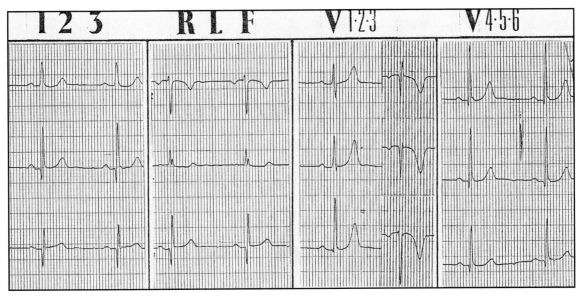

Figure 20

in the precordial leads and the PR segments are short in these leads. The pattern is WPW with the "preexcited" myocardium depolarizing to the right and anterior. The prominent Q waves in leads I and aVL are in reality "upside down" delta waves and do not represent lateral wall myocardial infarction. The delay in the terminal part of the QRS is due to associated incomplete RBBB. The combination of early and late forces results in right axis deviation.

• **Clinical Correlation:** This patient had no clinical features to suggest ischemic heart disease and his major complaint was "spells of heart racing". Holter monitoring showed recurrent brief bursts of paroxysmal supraventricular tachycardia regarded as reentrant tachycardia utilizing the accessory pathway.

Early R Wave Progression

In the normal individual, septal and right ventricular activation is oriented to the right and anterior, but these forces are quickly negated by the electrically dominant left ventricle. Thus, small R waves and large S waves are recorded in leads V1-2. When the initial R wave exceeds the terminal S wave in these leads, the term "early R wave progression" has been used. This pattern is normal in infancy and childhood. Causes for this in the adult include excessive right ventricular forces, loss of posterior LV forces, or changes in ventricular activation. Examples of these follow.

ECG Example 17 (Figure 20)

• **Questions:** What does this ECG example of "early R wave progression" represent? What is the difference between the first and second complexes in leads V1-2-3?

• **ECG Analysis:** Sinus bradycardia of 50/min is present with normal PR interval and QRS duration. The frontal plane axis is +30 degrees. There are deep narrow Q waves in leads II, III, and aVF and prominent initial R waves in lead V1-2-3. The combination indicates inferior wall myocardial infarction with posterior wall involvement. The complexes in the first set of V1-2-3 have been photographically altered in the second set to invert the images and make the QRS-T morphology more a "typical pattern" of infarction. Posterior wall MI frequently accompanies inferior infarction and is one of the very common causes of "early R wave progression".

• **Clinical Correlation:** This 64-year-old man sustained an acute inferior-posterior MI four years ago and has been stable since - taking daily aspirin and a small-dose beta blocker.

ECG Example 18 (Figure 21)

• **Questions:** Does the frontal plane axis help to determine the cause of the early R wave progression in this patient? What is a "right ventricular strain" pattern?

• **ECG Analysis:** P waves are present with a PR interval prolonged to 0.22 seconds. There is marked right axis deviation of +150 degrees. Impressive Q waves are present in leads II, III, and aVF. The R wave amplitude in V1 exceeds the S wave depth and there is an RS pattern across the precordium with a prominent S wave in leads V5-6. The composite is diagnostic of right ventricular hypertrophy and the associated T wave inversion in leads V1-5 constitutes the "RV strain" pattern. Right ventricular pressure at our near systemic levels would be anticipated in this patient.

221

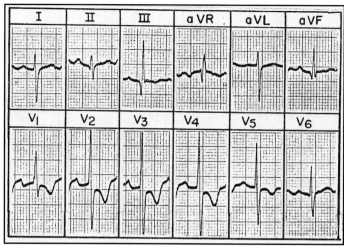

Figure 21

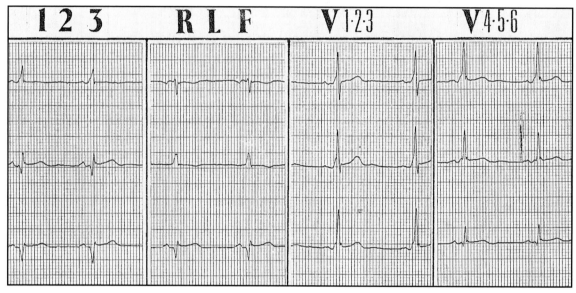

Figure 22

• **Clinical Correlation:** This 34-year-old man sustained a sports injury to his right leg one year ago. He did not seek medical attention but his description of subsequent events was consistent with deep venous thrombosis and repetitive pulmonary emboli. Exertional dyspnea gradually increased and when he presented for examination, there were striking bedside features of pulmonary hypertension. Pulmonary arteriography showed multiple filling defects and pulmonary artery pressure was 110/60. Anticoagulant therapy was initiated and in follow-up over two years there was gradual regression of the clinical evidence of pulmonary hypertension accompanied by marked symptomatic improvement. Serial ECG's showed a gradual shift in frontal plane axis to +90 degrees with virtual disappearance of the Q waves in leads II, III, and aVF.

ECG Example 19 (Figure 22)

• **Questions:** What is the cause of the prominent R wave in V1-2? Is there evidence of myocardial infarction?

• **ECG Analysis:** The rhythm is sinus at 64 beats per minute with normal PR interval and a QRS axis of minus 30 degrees. Prominent Q waves are present in leads II, III, and aVF and are associated with broad R waves in V1-3. The ECG could easily be misinterpreted as inferior-posterior MI, but it is an example of WPW conduction. The short PR segment and delta waves are evident in most leads. The direction of the delta waves creates the "Q waves" in the inferior leads and the prominent R waves in the precordial leads V1-2. Conduction over an accessory pathway results in preexcitation of a given area of ventricular myocardium. The abnormal ventricular activation in WPW therefore alters the initial forces and removes the ability to diagnose myocardial infarction.

• **Clinical Correlation:** This asymptomatic 34-year-old man had a "routine" ECG and was startled when told that he had "evidence of a heart attack". Happily he sought a second opinion and the situation was correctly identified. Have you seen a patient with WPW incorrectly diagnosed as myocardial infarction? (If not, you will!)

CARDIAC PEARL

A misdiagnosis of old anterior myocardial infarction can be made in a patient having a long asthenic chest build and a "tear drop" heart (Figure A). Electrode placement, even though in correct interspace, is the culprit. Place the chest electrodes one or one and one

half interspaces lower and the normal progression of R wave (rather than slow) may result.
W. Proctor Harvey, M.D.

Pattern of RSR' in Leads V1-2

This pattern can be seen in several circumstances and clinical information is essential for clarification. In the normal, healthy, young individual this morphology is often seen, reflecting persistence of the right ventricular forces that were dominant in childhood. In adults with either a volume or pressure load imposed on the right ventricle, the delayed terminal vector represents right ventricular hypertrophy. The pattern is most often seen in delayed activation of the right ventricle due to incomplete or complete right bundle branch block. The amplitude and duration of the terminal R' parallels the amount of RBBB delay.

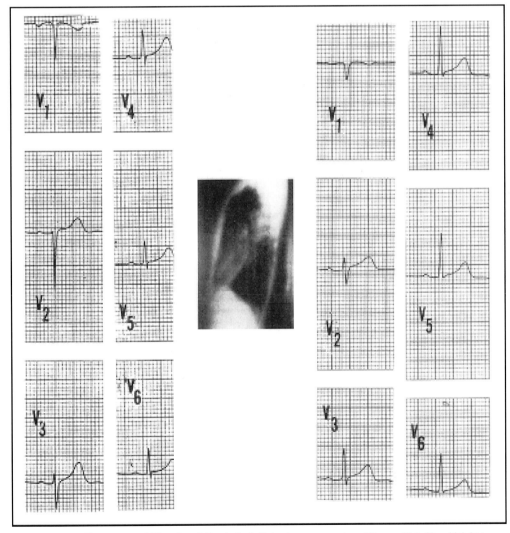

Fig A: Electrode Placement and "Tear Drop" Heart - Left: Note slow progression of R wave V₁ to V₄, which has been read as consistent with old myocardial infarction. Right: Electrodes placed 1 or 1-1/2 interspaces lower show normal progression of R wave. A "tear drop" heart may cause this misdiagnosis. Middle: Note long narrow silhouette of heart on lateral x-ray.

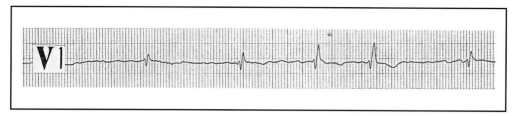

Figure 23

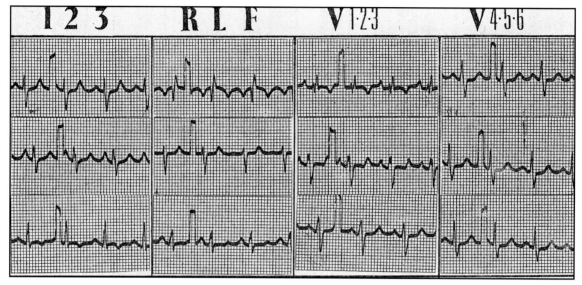

Figure 24

ECG Example 20 (Figure 23)

• **Question:** What explains the changing QRS morphology in this ECG strip?

• **ECG Analysis:** Atrial fibrillation is easily identified in this rhythm strip of lead V1. The conducted impulses are transmitted with RSR pattern. The initial portion of each complex is the same, but the height and breadth of the terminal part varies as the R-R interval changes. This example shows gradations of right bundle branch block, with minimal terminal force prolongation following long cycles and increasing duration with shorter cycles. The pattern is due to changing "degrees" of RBBB.

• **Clinical Correlation:** This 88-year-old man has had atrial fibrillation for fifteen years with rate control achieved with digoxin. When his rate was faster, all impulses were conducted with a pattern of complete RBBB.

ECG Example 21 (Figure 24)

• **Question:** This young woman has known of a heart murmur since grade school. What abnormalities would you anticipate finding on physical examination?

• **ECG Analysis:** There is sinus tachycardia of 120/min with normal PR interval and QRS dura-

tion. There is right axis deviation of +120 degrees and tall P waves in lead II consistent with right atrial enlargement. In lead V1 there is an RSR pattern and later precordial leads showed delayed progression with prominent S waves in leads V5-6. The pattern in lead V1 could represent right ventricular conduction delay (incomplete RBBB), but the electrical axis and the P wave abnormality is more consistent with right ventricular hypertrophy. This ECG is typical of atrial septal defect with significant left to right atrial shunt. The late vector in lead V1 (R') is characteristic of a volume burden of the right ventricle, the pattern of "diastolic loading".

• **Clinical Correlation:** This 24-year-old woman was not allowed to participate in school sports because of her "leaky heart". She recently completed a pregnancy and noted marked exertional dyspnea in its late stages. Noteworthy findings on cardiac exam included a palpable pulmonary artery thrust in the second left ICS, accompanied by a grade 3 ejection systolic murmur and persistent wide splitting of the second heart sound with an increased pulmonary component. A mid-diastolic flow rumble was heard at the lower left sternal border. The findings were regarded as characteristic of atrial septal defect and this was confirmed at cardiac catheterization. Surgical correction was accomplished.

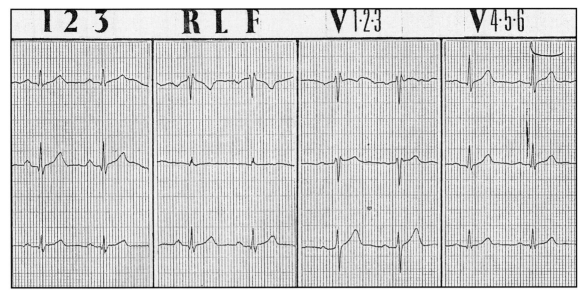

Figure 25

ECG Example 22 (Figure 25)

• **Question:** What would you advise this medical student regarding his ECG?

• **ECG Analysis:** There is sinus rhythm at 74/min with a normal PR interval and a frontal plane axis of +50 degrees. Small Q waves are present in leads I, II, III, and aVF. There is normal precordial QRS progression with an RSR pattern in leads V1-2.

• **Clinical Correlation:** A 24-year-old man volunteered for a research project. His ECG was interpreted as "probably normal but consider atrial septal defect". His cardiac examination was normal and he was reassured and told that his precordial pattern was normal for his age.

ECG Example 23 (Figure 26)

• **Question:** How would you interpret this ECG and what diagnosis does it suggest?

• **ECG Analysis:** There is sinus tachycardia of 120/min and the frontal plane QRS axis is +110 degrees. The P wave is isoelectric in lead I [+90°] and prominent in V1 consistent with right atrial enlargement. Although the precordial QRS transition is normal, there is an RSR pattern in lead V1. The V1 pattern accompanied by right axis deviation indicates some cause of right ventricular hypertrophy.

• **Clinical Correlation:** This 66-year-old man had smoked two packs per day since age 16. On examination, he showed features of advanced COPD. He declined to accept advice to stop smoking.

Repolarization Abnormalities

The clinician is frequently disappointed when a tracing is returned with an interpretation of "non-specific ST-T changes" and yet, without clinical data, a conclusive judgment is usually impossible. To suggest that such changes always represent "ischemia" seriously overstates the accuracy of the test. There are, however, repolarization abnormalities that are highly suggestive or at times virtually diagnostic of specific problems. These will be presented and, when appropriate, contrasted with similar ECG patterns.

ECG Example 24 (Figure 27)

• **Questions:** How would you interpret the negative T waves in leads V1-3 in this 18-year-old woman? Do you agree with the computer, "anterior ischemia"?

• **ECG Analysis:** There is sinus tachycardia of 120 bpm with normal axis of +60 degrees. There is normal QRS duration and voltage and appropriate precordial QRS transition. The T waves are inverted in leads V1-3. In young individuals, this may represent a normal variant and is of no clinical consequence.

• **Clinical Correlation:** For some reason, an ECG was requested on this young, pregnant woman. The patient was asymptomatic and no abnormalities were present on cardiovascular examination. She was reassured that her heart was normal. In childhood, the precordial T waves are commonly inverted in precordial leads V1-3 and their continued presence in young adults has been termed "persistent juvenile pattern", a common normal variant.

ECG Example 25 (Figure 28)

• **Questions:** What is the most noteworthy abnormality in this tracing? What is the differen-

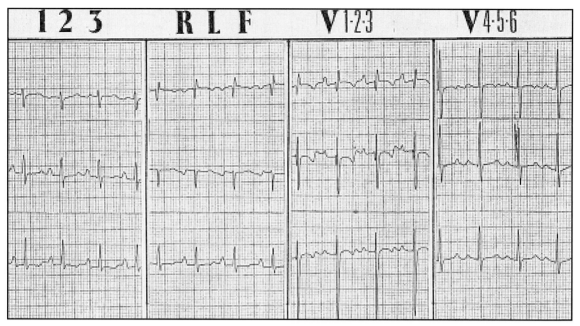

Figure 26

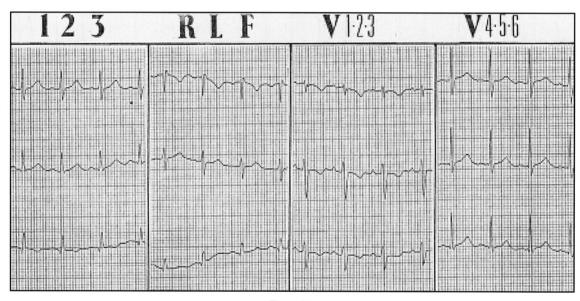

Figure 27

tial diagnosis of this condition?

• **ECG Analysis:** The rhythm is sinus at 95 beats per minute with a normal PR interval and QRS duration, and a frontal plane axis of +90 degrees. The ST segments are "sagging" in most leads and the QT interval is markedly prolonged. QT prolongation may be due to drug effect, myocardial ischemia, or electrolyte derangement. Common offending drugs are antiarrhythmic agents, tricyclic antidepressants, and phenothiazine drugs. Hypokalemia is a frequent cause.

• **Clinical Correlation:** This 24-year-old woman had the self image that she was "too fat" and began

a protracted fast, supplemented with the use of cathartics and emetics. When hospitalized she weighed 78 pounds and her serum potassium was 1.9 mEq/L.

ECG Example 26 (Figure 29)

• **Question:** What conditions come to mind as you look at this ECG?

• **ECG Analysis:** The sinus rate is markedly variable with periods of sinus arrest and junctional escape. The frontal plane axis is normal at +30 degrees and the QRS duration and morphology is normal. Strikingly deep and broad T waves and a

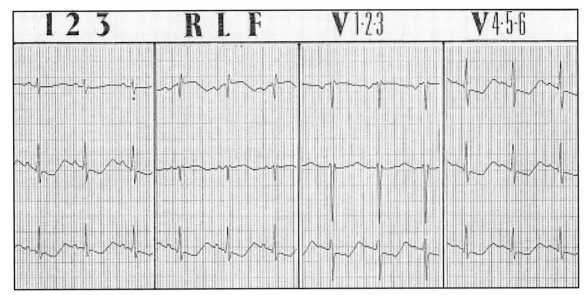

Figure 28

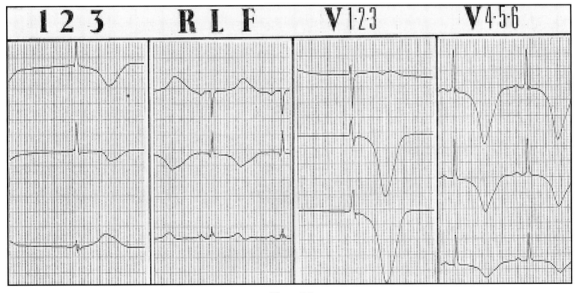

Figure 29

prolonged QT interval are present. This repolarization abnormality can be seen in patients with marked myocardial ischemia, but may also be seen with central nervous system abnormalities.

• **Clinical Correlation:** A 63-year-old woman presented to the Emergency Room complaining of severe headaches. CT scan of the head showed evidence of a large hematoma thought to be due to a subarachnoid hemorrhage.

ECG Example 27 (Figure 30)

• **Question:** What is the significance of "Wellens pattern"?

• **ECG Analysis:** The rhythm is of sinus origin at 62 beats per minute with normal PR and QRS intervals. There is left axis deviation of minus 40 degrees. P waves are bifid in lead II and in the precordial leads consistent with left atrial enlargement. There is striking ST-T change in leads V2-4. The ST segment is slightly elevated in these leads and rises in a concave fashion to the apex of a T wave and then drops sharply into a deep trough. This morphology has been termed "Wellens pattern". Dr. Wellens and his colleagues found that when patients presented with chest pain and this ECG pattern, coronary arteriography revealed a proximal and high grade lesion in the left anterior descending coronary artery. When untreated, they had significant incidence of extensive myocardial infarction within a few weeks to months.

• **Clinical Correlation:** This 43-year-old man presented with increasingly frequent and lasting

227

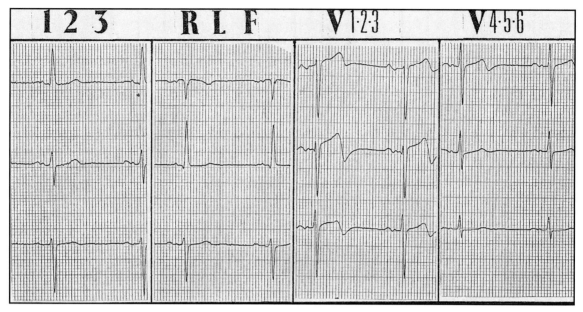

Figure 30

angina pectoris. After myocardial infarction was excluded, coronary arteriography was performed revealing a highly obstructive lesion in the LAD proximal to the first septal perforating branch. The other coronary vessels were normal. Angioplasty was performed with good results.

CARDIAC PEARL

When one sees straightening of the ST segment producing a right degree angle (as one might see particularly in the left precordial leads and the limb leads), some might refer to this finding as a "nonspecific" change. Actually, a common etiology is coronary artery disease (Figure A).

I learned this pearl from the late George Burch of Tulane.

W. Proctor Harvey, M.D.

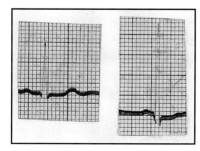

Fig A: Non-Specific Changes - Two patients having non-specific S-T and T wave change in Lead V_6. Note S-T segment is straightened coming off the R wave at approximately a 90° angle.

ECG Example 28 (Figure 31)

• **Questions:** This is a single channel recording from a 27-year-old black male. What is the differential diagnosis of this ECG? What is the "fish-hook sign"?

• **ECG Analysis:** Sinus rhythm of 60 beats per minute is present with a normal QRS axis of +75 degrees. Initial forces are directed right-superior and result in narrow Q waves in leads I, II, III, and aVF. ST segment elevation is present in the bipolar limb leads and particularly in precordial leads V4 and V5. Note the morphology of the ST-T in lead V4 and you can appreciate why Dr. Marriott suggested its similarity to a fish-hook. In addition, observe that the measured ST segment elevation is less than 25% of the T wave height. These features are identifying characteristics of the "early repolarization pattern". The cause of this repolarization variant is unknown but it may be a source of confusion regarding pericarditis or current injury.

• **Clinical Correlation:** A healthy 27-year-old black man had a routine ECG for flight status. He was athletically active and examination was normal. Review of prior tracings obtained during flight exams showed no changes over the past five years.

CARDIAC PEARL

Normal Variants: the absence of an S4 or S3 gallop may be helpful in evaluation of a patient who has findings on the ECG suspicious for coronary disease, myocarditis, or cardiomyopathy (dilated or hypertrophic).

I recall a young patient, a talented rookie

of one of the major baseball teams. Because of an electrocardiogram, he had been diagnosed as having either coronary artery disease, myocarditis, or cardiomyopathy. He had some elevation of ST segments and nonspecific ST and T-wave changes, including inversion of the T-waves in the left precordial leads. The patient was referred to me for evaluation.

On questioning this young, healthy-appearing athlete of about 22 years of age, no history could be elicited of any symptoms of or signs of heart disease other than the findings on the electrocardiogram, which the patient had with him and presented for review. The physical examination revealed no abnormality whatsoever. It was reasoned that if the patient had either coronary artery disease, myocarditis, or cardiomyopathy producing these findings on electrocardiogram, he should at least have an S4 and possibly and S3 gallop, detected on auscultation of the heart. However, with careful search no extra sound was present. Using this finding of absent gallop, together with a completely negative cardiovascular evaluation, it was suggested to the management of his baseball team that these findings were a variant of normal, particularly since the ST segment elevation and the ST and T-wave changes noted on his ECG are known to occur in healthy people (Figure

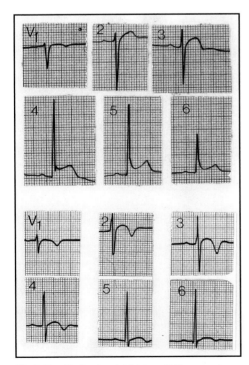

Fig A: Two Professional Athletes - S-T segment elevation and T wave inversions in both. These changes of early repolarization represent a normal variant but can be misdiagnosed as coronary heart disease, myocarditis, or cardiomyopathy.

A). We recommended that he be allowed to play baseball. The patient did so and I closely followed his performance as reported in the sports pages. He played on his team and had no problem.

About 15 years later, I received a telephone call from him and he asked if I remembered him. I told him that indeed I did. He said that he was in an Emergency Room in a midwestern town and had been diagnosed as having an acute heart attack. His electrocardiogram was described to me via telephone and it was the same as that when I originally saw him. On careful questioning, he had no symptoms consistent with coronary disease. He was therefore sent home.

On another occasion, he telephoned me about an insurance exam he had undergone. The company was reluctant to issue a policy because of the ECG findings. It was related to the officials of the company that these were normal variants and that the patient had no evidence of coronary disease at the time of my evaluation, and showed the same identical electrocardiographic changes.

In the case of this young baseball player, it was the absence of the finding of an atrial (S4) gallop and/or ventricular (S3) gallop that supported the clinical impression that his ECG changes were those of early repolarization, a normal variant, and not those of heart disease. Therefore he was able to play and was not deprived of the lucrative salary paid to professional baseball players.

W. Proctor Harvey, M.D.

ECG Example 29 (Figure 32)

• **Question:** A 33-year-old soldier presents with chest pain and fever. This ECG indicates that cardiac exam should include (Figure 32A)?

• **ECG Analysis:** There is sinus tachycardia at 130/min. The frontal plan QRS axis is normal at +45 degrees. There is diffuse ST segment change characteristic of acute pericarditis. It is evident that the *parietal* pericardium has no electrical activity and that ECG changes of "pericarditis" reflect *myocarditis*. The earliest ECG changes represent diffuse repolarization abnormality with a myriad of "injury vectors" to the left and inferior. The result is diffuse ST segment elevation in both frontal and horizontal planes. Importantly, the ST segment elevation occurs without reciprocal ST segment depression (except in lead aVR). Later, the ST segments return to the baseline and diffuse T wave inversion occurs. The process also involves the atria and an alteration in the *PR segment* occurs. This injury current is oriented toward the atria; that is,

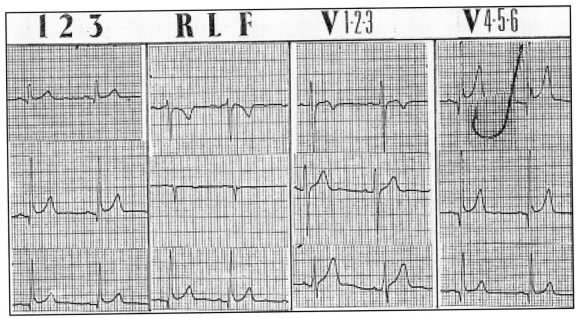

Figure 31

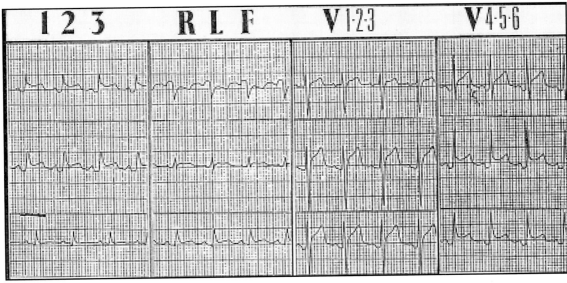

Figure 32A

to the right and superior, resulting in PR segment depression in leads II, III, aVF, and PR segment elevation in lead aVR. The PR segment changes help to confirm that the process is due to "pericarditis".

• **Clinical Correlation:** This young man presented one week after a respiratory infection with chest pain consistent with pericarditis. On examination, a loud three-part friction rub was present over the entire precordium. He was treated symptomatically and within two weeks was well and returned to his military duty (Figure 32B).

The contrasting morphology of the ST segment in pericarditis (upper tracing) compared to early

repolarization is shown. Note that the PR segment changes seen in acute pericarditis are absent in early repolarization.

ECG Example 30 (Figure 33)

• **Question:** What ECG finding suggests significant ongoing myocardial ischemia in this patient?

• **ECG Analysis:** There is sinus rhythm of 90 beats per minute with a frontal plane axis of +70 degrees. Q waves are present in leads II, III, and aVF and reflect a previous inferior MI. QRS complexes in precordial leads V1-2 and V4 exceed the limit of stylus excursion and their true amplitude is unknown, but there is probably excess precordial

230

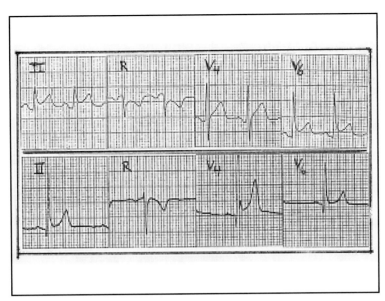

Figure 32B

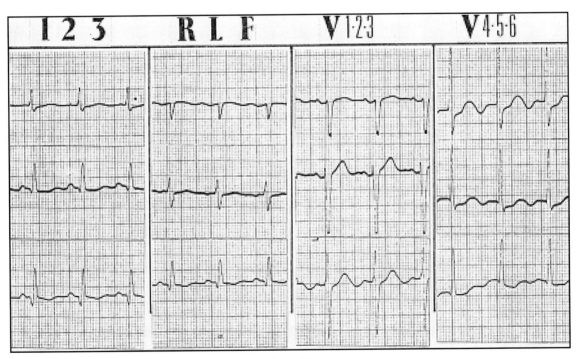

Figure 33

voltage (LVH). A noteworthy abnormality is prolongation of the QT-U interval with negative U waves well seen in leads V4-5. Although small U waves are normal, they are always positive in leads in which the T waves are upright. Negative U waves can be an indicator of significant myocardial ischemia, but also can occur with electrolyte imbalance (hypokalemia).

• **Clinical Correlation:** This 70-year-old man sustained an inferior MI five years ago and since has had stable angina pectoris. He presented to the Emergency Room with increasing chest pain and his ECG showed new inverted U waves. Coronary arteriography showed extensive but operable three vessel coronary artery disease and coronary artery bypass was performed.

CARDIAC PEARL

If possible, try to obtain an electrocardiogram while the patient still has the chest pain or discomfort.

If a patient has coronary artery disease, this may show ischemic changes that other-

231

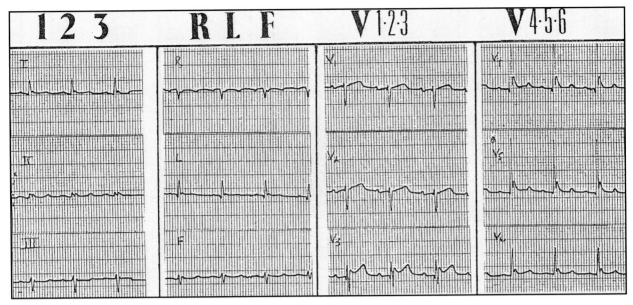

Figure 34

wise are not present on the electrocardiogram. Therefore, when a patient first comes in to the office or Emergency Room, if the complaint is chest pain and the patient states that he or she is still having it, be sure to do the ECG as one of the initial steps because the pain may be transient; if one waits until after a more detailed history, the opportune time might be missed.

Also helpful is to have the patient have an electrocardiogram during any arrhythmia or palpation or other symptoms of which he complains. This may be of great help in identifying the problem. Also, instruct the patient that, with the onset of any arrhythmia, he or she should promptly come to the office or Emergency Room to have an electrocardiogram.

W. Proctor Harvey, M.D.

ECG Example 31 (Figure 34)

• **Questions:** What would the first "diagnostic procedure" be on this patient? What is the significance of an "Osborne wave"?

• **ECG Analysis:** The most noteworthy observation regarding this tracing is the peculiar elevation of the "J point" best seen in leads V3-6. This morphology is seen in patients with hypothermia and its magnitude parallels the decrease in body temperature. It has been referred to as the "Osborne wave" and also with the picturesque term of "hypothermic hump".

• **Clinical Correlation:** A 76-year-old "street person" was found unconscious. When seen in the Emergency Room, his rectal temperature was 93 degrees. Using a warming blanket, body tempera-

ture gradually rose, accompanied by return of consciousness and normalization of his ECG.

ECG Example 32 (Figure 35)

• **Question:** The ECG segments shown demonstrate repolarization changes seen in patients with electrolyte abnormalities. Can you identify the derangements and guess the cause?

• **ECG Analysis and Clinical Correlation:**

Patient A: In these precordial lead strips, the arrows indicate large U waves and a markedly long QTU interval. Note the sagging ST segment and the prominent TU complex, features of hypokalemia. This 39-year-old woman had an aldosterone secreting tumor and presented with a serum potassium of 1.8 mEq/L.

Patients B - C - D: Gradations of hyperkalemia are shown. The earliest ECG change is increase in amplitude and symmetry of the T wave with minimal change in the QRS complex ("mild hyperkalemia"). As potassium levels rise, the QRS complex begins to broaden and the T wave remains large and pointed ("moderate hyperkalemia"). In advanced potassium excess, the QRS complex widens further and the T wave becomes smaller ("severe hyperkalemia"). Ultimately, the depolarization and repolarization wave forms merge into a "sine wave pattern". The most common cause of hyperkalemia is acute or chronic renal insufficiency.

Patient B is a 31-year-old woman with polycystic kidney disease: [K+] = 5.9 mEq/L.

Patient C is a 50-year-old man with acute alcoholic hepatitis: [K+] = 6.7 mEq/L.

232

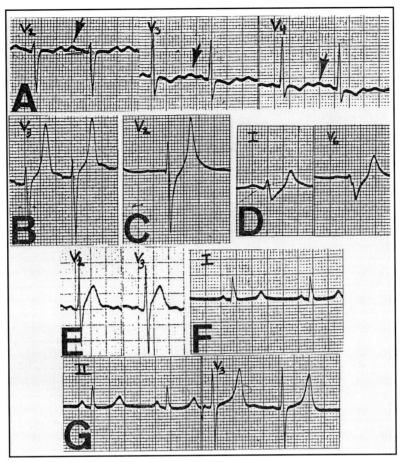

Figure 35

Patient D is a 58-year-old man with chronic renal failure: [K+] = 9.2 mEq/L.

Patients E and F: The level of extracellular calcium in great part determines the duration of repolarization phase II of the cellular action potential. Increases in calcium shorten the interval between the QRS and the beginning of the T wave (QoT = Q to the onset of the T wave) and its summit (QaT = Q to the apex of the T wave). Decreases in calcium prolong these intervals.

Patient E: A 29-year-old man with hematologic malignancy: [Ca++] = 13.6 mEq/L.

Patient F: A 50-year-old man undergoing chronic dialysis for renal failure: [Ca++] = 6 mEq/L.

Patient G: A combination of abnormalities is shown. The prolonged Q wave to the onset and apex of the T wave suggests hypocalcemia and the large symmetrical T waves suggest hyperkalemia. These strips were from a 50-year-old man with chronic renal failure — [K+] = 6; [Ca++] = 6 mEq/L.

Miscellaneous ECG Patterns

ECG Example 33 (Figure 36)

• **Questions:** What condition comes to mind when

you glance at this tracing? What would you expect on chest examination? What is "Schamroth's sign"?

• **ECG Analysis:** There is sinus tachycardia at 130 beats per minute with a QRS axis of +90 degrees. The P waves in the limb leads are tall - rivaling the QRS amplitude and indicating right atrial enlargement. Precordial leads show delayed R wave progression with prominent S waves in the lateral leads. The QRS voltage is borderline low. The overall pattern is that seen in chronic obstructive pulmonary disease.

• **Clinical Correlation:** The late Dr. Leo Schamroth described a distinctive pattern in which the P-QRS-T complexes are all isoelectric in lead I. He found that such patients had advanced COPD. This chronically ill 73-year-old man had accumulated 100 pack/years of cigarette smoking and at the bedside was markedly hyperinflated with a low-lying diaphragm and distant breath and heart sounds.

ECG Example 34 (Figure 37)

• **Question:** This tracing was obtained on a patient admitted because of dyspnea and hemoptysis. What does it suggest will be found on physical examination?

233

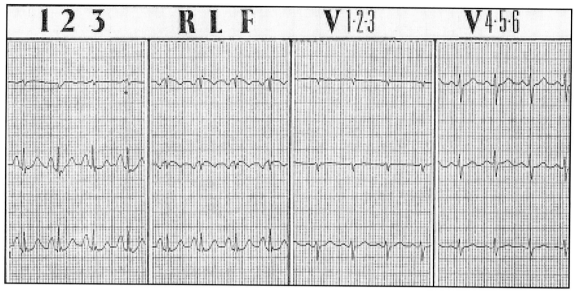

Figure 36

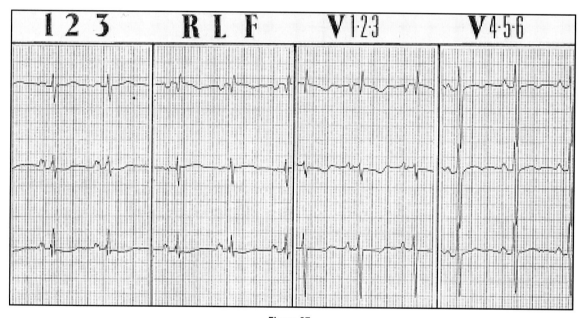

Figure 37

• **ECG Analysis:** There is sinus rhythm at 80 beats per minute. The QRS duration and PR interval are normal. Right axis deviation of +120 degrees is present. Notching of the P waves is evident in the limb leads and both early and late portions are prominent, consistent with bi-atrial enlargement. The breadth and depth of the P wave trough in V1 ("P-terminal force") confirm left atrial abnormality. There is a QR pattern in V1, delayed precordial progression, and the S waves exceed the R waves in leads V5-6. The composite of findings indicates combined atrial enlargement and right ventricular hypertrophy.

• **Clinical Correlation:** This 42-year-old woman had been told of a "heart murmur" during preg-nancy twenty years before. She had developed exertional dyspnea over the years and had gradually decreased her activity to prevent breathlessness. A recent house move necessitated increased exertion and she had recurrence of dyspnea on slight activity and had "coughed up blood".

On cardiovascular examination, the jugular venous column was normal, but the A wave pulsations were markedly increased in amplitude. Pulmonary artery pulsation and pulmonary valve closure were palpable in the second left interspace and there was excessive RV activity over the lower sternum. Second heart sound splitting was physiologic but the pulmonary component was markedly accentuated. At the apex, a loud and early opening

234

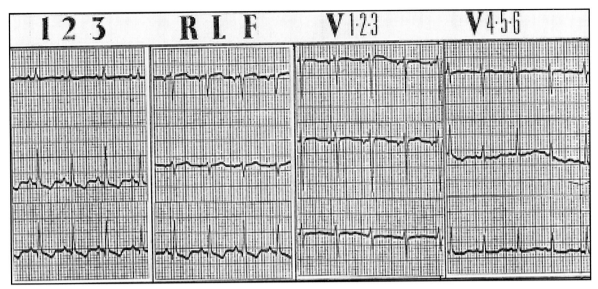

Figure 38

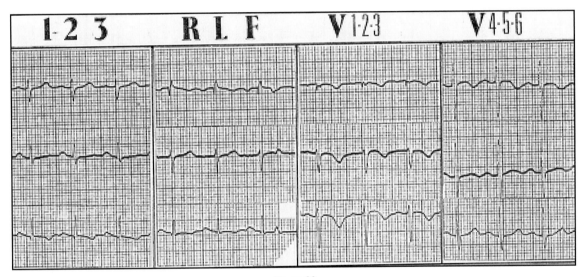

Figure 39

snap introduced a pan-diastolic rumble of mitral stenosis. Cardiac diagnostic studies confirmed the bedside impression of serious mitral obstruction with resultant pulmonary hypertension. Mitral valvotomy was successful.

ECG Example 35 (Figure 38)

• **Questions:** Other than the conspicuous repolarization abnormalities, what is the most important observation regarding this ECG? What bedside findings would you anticipate?

• **ECG Analysis:** Sinus tachycardia of 140/min is present. The intervals are normal and the QRS axis is +75 degrees. There are diffuse ST-T changes. The most noteworthy abnormality is the alternation in the amplitude of the QRS complexes — most evident in the precordial leads. This is an example of "electrical alternans".

• **Clinical Correlation:** This 42-year-old woman was seen two weeks after a febrile illness because of increasing dyspnea. Her blood pressure was 100/80 with a measured paradoxical pulse of 12 mm Hg. There was cervical venous engorgement with minimal pulsations in the jugular venous column. The precordium was dull to percussion and there was no palpable apical impact. A faint three-part friction rub was heard. There was moderate hepatomegaly and peripheral edema. With these characteristic physical findings and the ECG abnormality, a diagnosis of pericardial effusion with cardiac compression was made and echo-guided pericardiocentesis performed. Although electrical alternans is an uncommon ECG pattern, it is virtually diagnostic of pericardial effusion with tamponade. Usually, only the QRS complexes alternate ("QRS alternans"), but rarely the entire P-

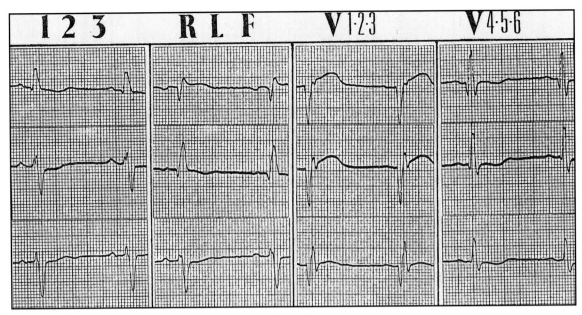

Figure 40

QRS-T wave pattern may change ("total electrical alternans"). The phenomenon is thought to be due to a pendular movement of the heart ("swinging heart"), so that its position changes as it beats.

ECG Example 36 (Figure 39)

• **Question:** A 64-year-old man is seen in the Emergency Room complaining of oppressive chest pain and shortness of breath. What is the "pattern of acute cor pulmonale"?

• **ECG Analysis:** Sinus rhythm of 100/min is present with right axis deviation of +120 degrees. T waves are inverted in leads III and aVF and there are negative T waves in leads V1 to 4. Right axis deviation in the frontal plane (S_I, Q_{III}, T_{III} pattern) accompanied by inverted T waves in V1 to 3 is very suggestive of an acute pulmonary process (pulmonary emboli, multilobar pneumonia, pneumothorax, etc).

• **Clinical Correlation:** This patient presented one week after abdominal surgery. The suspicion of pulmonary embolization suggested by his ECG and physical examination was confirmed by pulmonary perfusion scan.

ECG Example 37 (Figure 40)

• **Question:** This patient sustained a myocardial infarction six months ago. Does his ECG allow you to anticipate what might be found on physical examination?

• **ECG Analysis:** The rhythm is sinus bradycardia at 50/min. PR interval is 0.20 seconds and the QRS shows non-specific intraventricular conduction delay of 0.14 seconds. There is left axis deviation of

minus 60 degrees. Prominent Q waves are present in leads I and aVL with loss of expected initial R waves in V1-4. These depolarization abnormalities are consistent with anterolateral myocardial infarction accompanied by left anterior fascicular block. The elevated ST segments persisting six months after the acute MI suggest that a ventricular aneurysm has developed.

• **Clinical Correlation:** This 69-year-old man had protracted congestive heart failure during an anterolateral myocardial infarction six months earlier. After a lengthy convalescence, he stabilized at a low functional level. On cardiac exam, there was a prominent mid precordial systolic bulge consistent with dyskinetic motion of a ventricular aneurysm. A prominent third heart sound accompanied a murmur of mitral regurgitation - the latter regarded as due to "papillary muscle dysfunction".

ECG Example 38 (Figure 41)

• **Questions:** Contrast the two tracings shown on page 237 recorded three days apart. What is the electrical axis in the top ECG? Does it reveal evidence of myocardial infarction? In the bottom tracing, what change in axis has occurred? What is the result of this shift (Figure 41A)?

• **ECG Analysis:** The top tracing shows sinus bradycardia at 55/min with a prolonged PR interval. The frontal plane QRS axis is +60 degrees and the QRS duration is slightly prolonged. Prominent Q waves are present in leads II, III, and aVF and are an indication of a prior inferior MI. In the precordial leads, the ST segments are elevated in V1 to 4 consistent with acute anterior MI.

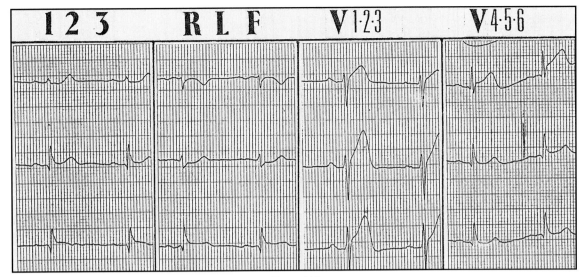

Figure 41A

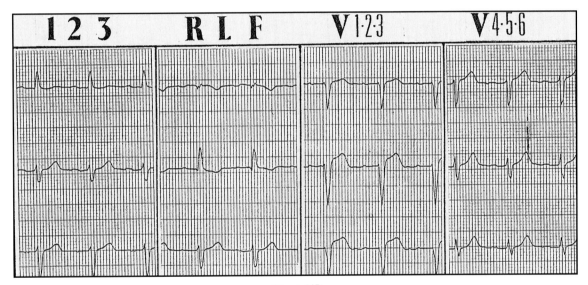

Figure 41B

In the bottom ECG (Figure 41B), the noteworthy change in the limb leads is an axis shift from +60 degrees to minus 60 degrees and in the precordial leads there has been loss of R waves in V1 to 4, representing the anticipated evolution of acute anterior MI. Of particular interest, the Q waves in limb leads II, III, aVF have disappeared. The development of left anterior fascicular block, with resultant change in direction of *initial* forces, effectively erases the evidence of previous inferior MI. This is an example of one abnormality cancelling another.

• **Clinical Correlation:** This 60-year-old man sustained an inferior wall MI in the remote past. He presented with severe chest pain and the ECG sequence seen above. In the lower tracing the acute anterior MI is obvious, but without the upper tracing existence of the prior infarction would be unknown.

ECG Example 39 (Figure 42)

• **Question:** What is "Bix's Rule"?

• **ECG Analysis:** There is a regular narrow QRS tachycardia at 140 per minute with a normal frontal plane QRS axis of +70 degrees. P waves are uncertain in the limb leads but are evident in lead V1. This could represent sinus tachycardia with prolonged PR interval or supraventricular tachycardia with 2:1 AV block. R waves are absent in V1 and V2 consistent with prior septal infarction. There are "sagging" ST segments in the limb leads of uncertain significance.

The late Dr. Harold Bix indicated that when evident P waves are *halfway between* QRS complexes that there is probably another P wave hiding in or near the QRS complex and that the rhythm represents some variety of supraventricular tachycardia with 2:1 transmission.

237

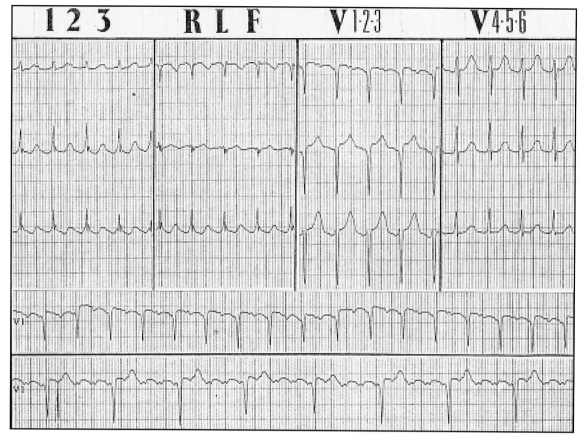

Figure 42

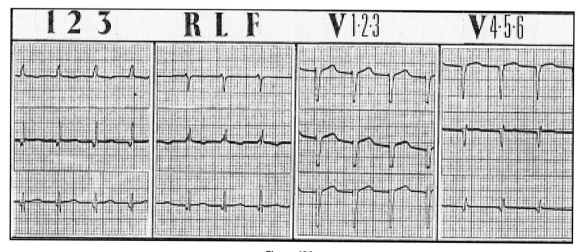

Figure 43A

• **Clinical Correlation:** This 60-year-old man sustained a septal infarction two years ago and for two days has been aware of "heart racing", fatigue, dyspnea on minimal exertion, and angina with slight provocation. Carotid sinus massage clarified his rhythm to be atrial flutter with 2:1 conduction (bottom strip of lead V1). All his symptoms disappeared after he was cardioverted.

ECG Example 40 (Figure 43)

• **Questions:** This 73-year-old man, with known ischemic heart disease, presented with increasing dyspnea. How many myocardial infarctions has he sustained? Is there an observation in tracing Figure 43A that would explain his breathlessness?

• **ECG Analysis:** The rhythm is regular at 130 per minute but P waves are inapparent. The elec-

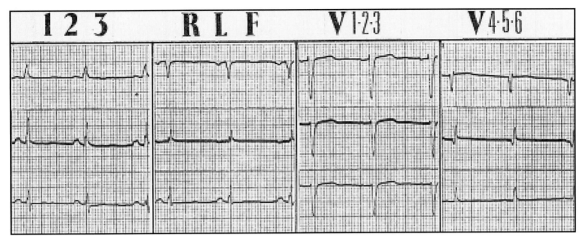

Figure 43B

trical axis and QRS duration are normal. There are broad Q waves in leads II, III, and aVF consistent with inferior wall myocardial infarction. Although the stylus excursion is limited in precordial leads V1 to 3, and the depth of the S waves is uncertain, the precordial pattern is typical of anterolateral myocardial infarction.

• **ECG Analysis:** A tracing three days later (Figure 43B) shows return of sinus rhythm with the P waves obvious and the "diagnostic" Q waves in the limb leads have disappeared. In reality, the initial forces in the first tracing are not the result of ventricular depolarization but are retrograde P waves inscribed before the QRS. In retrospect, his rhythm on the previous tracing was accelerated junctional rhythm with retrograde atrial activation — the negative P wave inscribed in front of the QRS complex. The inappropriate relationship of atrial and ventricular mechanical events can diminish his already compromised left ventricular function and explain his dyspnea. It was felt arrhythmia was due to digitalis excess and it disappeared on withholding the drug.

Selected Reading

1. ACP/ACC/AHA Task Force Statement. Clinical Competence in Electrocardiography. *JACC* 1995; 25:1465-1469.
2. Benhorin J, Moss A, Oakes D, et al: The Prognostic Significance of First Myocardial Infarction Type (Q Wave Versus Non-Q Wave) and Q Wave Location. *JACC* 1990; 15: 1201-7.
3. Flowers N: Left Bundle Branch Block: A Continuously Evolving Concept. *JACC* 1987; 9: 684-97.
4. Hands M, Cook EF, Stone PH, et al: Electrocardiographic Diagnosis of Myocardial Infarction in the Presence of Complete Left Bundle Branch Block. *AHJ* 1988; 116:23-30.
5. Karlson, BW, Herlitz, J, et al: Prognosis in Acute Myocardial Infarction in Relation to Development of Q waves. *Clin Cardiol* 1991; 14: 875-80.
6. Klein RC, Zakauddin V, DeMaria AN, et al: Electrocardiographic Diagnosis of Left Ventricular Hypertrophy in the Presence of Left Bundle Branch Block. *AHJ* 1984; 108:502-506.
7. Schweitzer P: The Electrocardiographic Diagnosis of Acute Myocardial Infarction in the Thrombolytic Era. *AHJ* 1990; 119:642-54.
8. Shah N, Sriharsa V, et al: Electrocardiographic Features of Restrictive Pulmonary Disease, and Comparison with Those of Obstructive Pulmonary Disease. *AJC* 1992; 70: 394.
9. Sreeram N, Cheriex EC, et al: Value of the 12-Lead Electrocardiogram at Hospital Admission in the Diagnosis of Pulmonary Embolism. *AJC* 1994; 73: 298-304.
10. Wong CK, Freedman SB, et al: Mechanism and Significance of Precordial ST-Segment Depression During Inferior Wall Acute Myocardial Infarction Associated with Severe Narrowing of the Dominant Right Coronary Artery. *AJC* 1993; 71: 25-30.

CHAPTER 12

The Chest X-Ray in Heart Disease

W. Bruce Dunkman, M.D. and Ron J. Vanden Belt, M.D.

The chest x-ray is an easily obtained, relatively inexpensive examination that provides considerable information in the evaluation of a patient with suspected or known heart disease. Overall cardiac size is readily assessed, as is pulmonary vascularity including both abnormal pulmonary arterial flow and pulmonary venous congestion. Sometimes specific diagnoses can be made from the chest film, but frequently radiologic findings must be correlated with the results of other examinations to reach a diagnosis. The chest x-ray can provide information regarding severity and progression of the disease process when diagnosis is known.

The routine radiographic chest examination includes a posteroanterior (PA) projection taken with the x-ray tube six feet from the film and a left lateral projection (left side of the chest adjacent to the film). Films may also be taken at the bedside with a portable x-ray machine, but interpretation of films taken in this manner is significantly limited as indicated below. In the past, it was common to obtain a "cardiac series" which, in addition to the PA and lateral views, included right and left anterior oblique projections with the esophagus filled with barium (Figure 1). This provided additional information regarding specific cardiac chamber enlargement, especially left atrial size. A number of x-rays using this technique are reproduced in this chapter, but technical advancements over the past decade allow the echocardiogram to provide more accurate information regarding specific chamber enlargement than was possible from the roentgenographic cardiac series.

Inspection of the Chest X-Ray

Interpretation of the PA chest film should proceed in a systematic fashion so that obscure findings are detected and technical variations do not lead to incorrect conclusions.

Technique

On a correctly exposed film, the vertebral bodies should be just visible behind the cardiac silhouette. The medial aspects of the clavicles should be equidistant from the midline (or vertebral bodies) to ensure that rotation of the patient's body has not produced a spurious abnormality of the cardiac silhouette. The degree of inspiration should also be assessed. On a film taken in deep inspiration the costophrenic angle should approach the level of the tenth rib posteriorly. If deep inspiration is not achieved, the costophrenic angle may be at the level of the eighth rib and the heart may appear falsely to be enlarged. Another cause of false cardiac enlargement may occur with pectus excavatum *(vide infra)*; therefore, inspection of the lateral chest film for this deformity is mandatory.

Although it is possible to obtain a nearly correctly positioned portable chest film (with the patient upright, the film cassette held anteriorly and the x-ray tube four to six feet away), portable chest films are commonly taken anteroposteriorly (AP), with the patient supine or with varying degrees of recumbency, with the film cassette posteriorly, and with the x-ray tube approximately 40 inches from the patient. In addition, the seriously ill patient may not be able to cooperate with a full

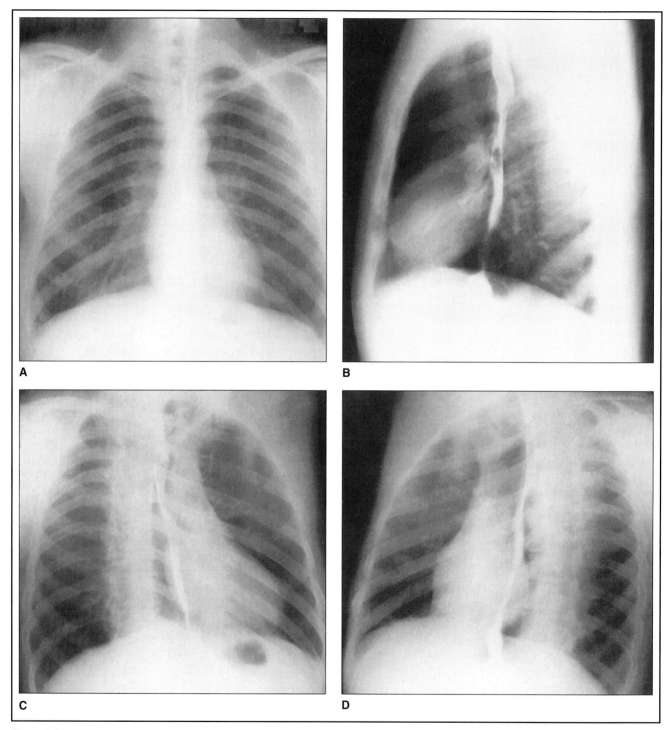

Figure 1. Cardiac series from a 39-year-old patient without cardiac disease. **A:** Posteroanterior (PA) projection. **B:** Left lateral projection. **C:** Right anterior oblique (RAO) projection. **D:** Left anterior oblique (LAO) projection. Note absence of posterior displacement of barium-filled esophagus by the left atrium, which is normal in size.

inspiratory effort. All of these factors result in a magnification of cardiac size. Thus, cardiac size should rarely be interpreted on a portable film and portable films should be compared with each other only if it is known that the technique used to obtain them is nearly identical. Portable chest films should always be so labeled. Likewise, all chest

films should be labeled to indicate the patient's right or left side so that dextroversion or situs inversus is not missed.

Approach to Interpretation

After assessing a chest film for these technical factors, it is then wise to inspect each film system-

242

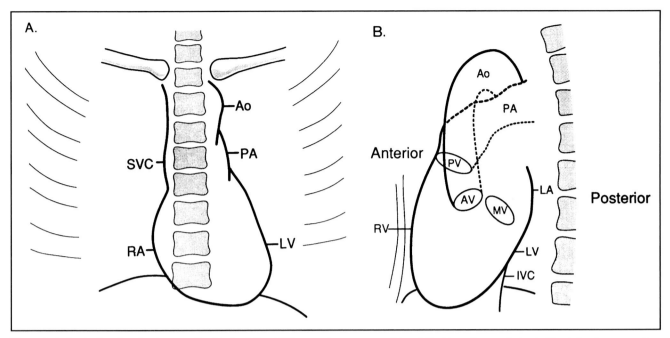

Figure 2. A: Border forming structures on the PA chest film. SVC = superior vena cava, RA = right atrium, Ao = aortic knob, PA = left pulmonary artery segment, LV = left ventricle. Compare to Figure 1A. **B:** Border forming structures and location of cardiac valves on the lateral chest film. RV = right ventricle, LA = left atrium, LV = left ventricle, IVC = inferior vena cava, Ao = aorta, PA = main pulmonary artery, PV = pulmonic valve ring, AV = aortic valve ring, MV = mitral valve ring. Compare to Figure 1B. *(Adapted from Vanden Belt RJ, Ronan JA: Cardiology: A Clinical Approach. 2nd Edition. Chicago: Yearbook Medical Publishers Inc, 1987; used with permission of Mosby-Yearbook, Inc.)*

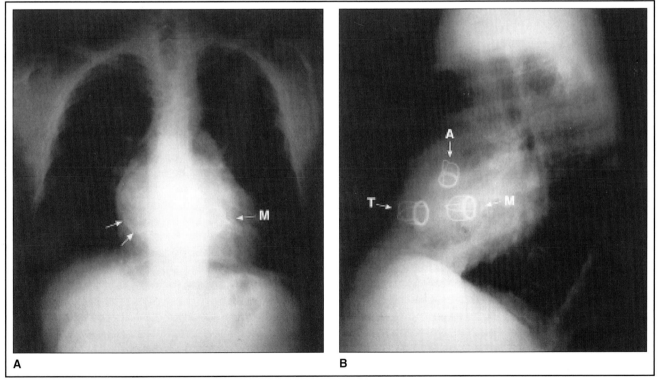

Figure 3. Location of cardiac valves illustrated by a patient with three prostheses. **A:** Frontal projection. Only the mitral valve prosthesis (M) is visible due to x-ray technique. Arrows at left indicate double density of left atrial enlargement. **B:** Lateral projection. T = tricuspid valve, A = aortic valve, M = mitral valve.

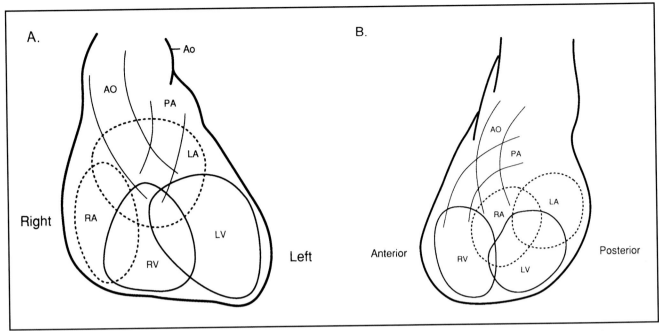

Figure 4. The location of cardiac chambers within cardiac silhouette. **A:** Posteroanterior projection. AO = aorta, Ao = aortic knob, PA = pulmonary artery, RA = right atrium, LA = left atrium, RV = right ventricle, LV = left ventricle. **B:** Lateral projection. Abbreviations as in panel A. (*Adapted from Miller WT: Introduction to Clinical Radiology. New York, NY: McGraw-Hill, 1982; used with permission*).

atically so that findings that do not relate to major abnormalities of the heart and lungs are not overlooked. It may be best to begin with bony structures, looking for such features as osteoarthritis of the spine, compression fractures of the spine (lateral view), recent or remote rib fractures, rib notching, metastatic bone disease, and pectus excavatum. Stainless steel sternal sutures, metal clips or loops marking saphenous vein coronary bypass grafts, and prosthetic valves or rings give evidence of prior cardiac surgery. Permanent pacemakers may be identified as to manufacturer and model number. Attention may then be turned to careful inspection of the costophrenic angles, the pleura, pulmonary parenchyma, pulmonary arteries and veins and, finally, the heart.

The Cardiovascular Silhouette

Figure 2 illustrates the border forming structures of the cardiac silhouette in frontal and lateral projections. In the frontal projection (Figure 2A), the right atrium forms the right heart border from the diaphragm to the lower aspect of the right hilus, where a small indentation marks the lower portion of the superior vena cava. The ascending aorta may also form a portion of the upper right heart border. The left side of the silhouette is marked by three rounded prominences. Superiorly is the aortic knob, comprised of the distal arch and proximal descending aorta. Below this is the main pulmonary artery segment from which the left pulmonary artery extends. Inferiorly, the left heart border is formed by the left ventricle. When left atrial enlargement is present, a fourth bulge may appear, located between the pulmonary artery segment and the left ventricular prominence, due to enlargement of the left atrial appendage.

In the lateral projection (Figure 2B) the anterior cardiac border is formed by the right ventricle and is in close proximity to the sternum. Posteriorly, the cardiac border is formed by the left ventricle inferiorly and by the left atrium in its upper portion. The cardiac valves cannot be seen on the plain chest film unless calcified or prosthetic, but their positions are indicated. The aortic valve is located quite centrally in the heart, with the mitral valve leftward and somewhat inferior to the aortic valve. The pulmonic valve is superior and leftward to the aortic valve. The tricuspid valve is the most inferiorly located and in the PA projection overlies the spine. Figure 3 illustrates the location of the cardiac valves in a patient with three prostheses. Figure 4 emphasizes that in the frontal projection only the right atrium and left ventricle are cardiac border forming. The right ventricle is anterior and the left atrium is posterior and somewhat superior.

Cardiac Chamber Enlargement

Several means of measuring cardiac size and volume on the PA chest film have been devised. The most commonly used method is illustrated in Figure 5. This relates the transverse cardiac

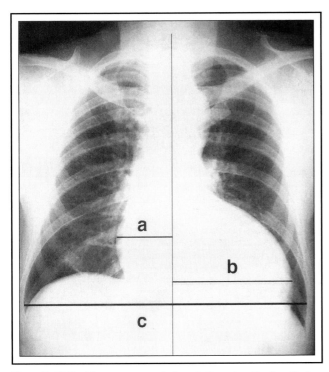

Figure 5. Method for measurement of cardiothoracic ratio. A vertical line at the center of the spine serves as a reference. The greatest distances of the right (a) and the left (b) cardiac borders from the reference line are measured. The transverse thoracic size is measured at its greatest dimension (c). The cardiothoracic ratio is (a + b) ÷ c (see text). Clinically this measurement is aided by drawing a vertical line on the X-ray view box with a wax pencil.

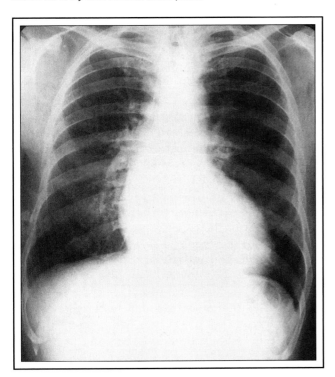

Figure 7. Moderately severe cardiomegaly in a 58-year-old man with rheumatic heart disease and predominant aortic regurgitation. Left ventricle is dilated as evidenced by elongation and leftward displacement of left ventricular segment. The right atrium is also enlarged.

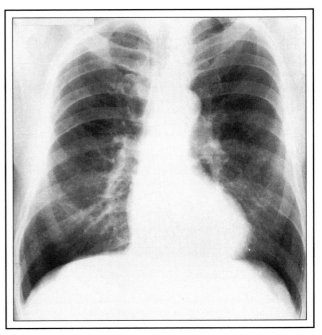

Figure 6. Concentric left ventricular hypertrophy in a 64-year-old male with severe calcific aortic stenosis (same patient as Figure 35). The left ventricular segment is rounded but the cardiothoracic ratio is not increased.

dimension to the transthoracic dimension and is termed the cardiothoracic ratio. Normally this value is less than or equal to 0.50. Usually, approximately one-third of the cardiac shadow is to the right of the midline, and two-thirds to the left. The cardiac apex generally remains medial to the mid-clavicular line.

The cardiac chamber most commonly showing enlargement is the left ventricle. Concentric hypertrophy without dilatation may produce little change in the cardiac silhouette in the frontal projection or may result in a more rounded and elongated left ventricular segment (Figure 6). Dilatation of the left ventricle (which generally implies hypertrophy) results in progressive leftward and sometimes caudad displacement of the left cardiac border (Figures 7 and 8). Overall cardiac size (cardiothoracic ratio) increases. The presence of a left ventricular aneurysm may distort the normally smooth left ventricular contour with a readily apparent bulge (Figure 9). The lateral projection also allows assessment of left ventricular size. From the point at which the inferior vena cava crosses the infero-posterior cardiac border, a 2 cm perpendicular line is drawn. The horizontal distance from the top of this line posteriorly to the cardiac border is normally <1.8 cm. A larger value indicates left ventricular enlargement (see Figure 2B).

There are several radiographic signs of left atrial enlargement. As the left atrial appendage enlarges,

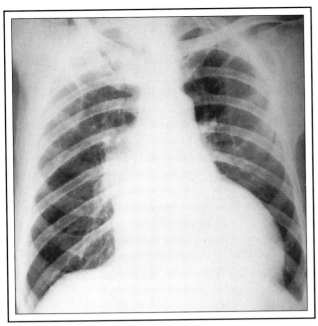

Figure 8. Cardiomegaly with left ventricular enlargement more marked than in Figure 7, also in a patient with predominant aortic regurgitation.

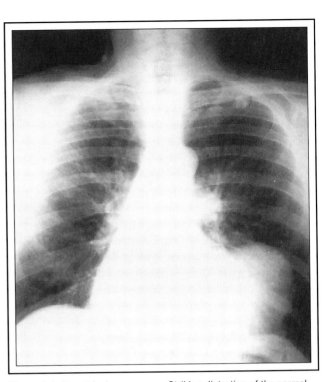

Figure 9. Left ventricular aneurysm. Striking distortion of the normal left ventricular silhouette is readily apparent.

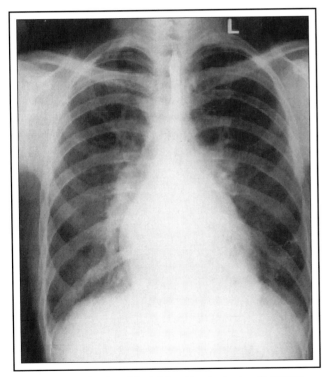

Figure 10. Straightening of the left heart border due to enlargement of the left atrial appendage in a patient with mitral stenosis and regurgitation.

it first fills in the indentation between the pulmonary artery segment and the left ventricle resulting in straightening of the left heart border (Figure 10). With progressive enlargement a frank bulge between the pulmonary artery segment and

left ventricular contour may occur, making four convexities apparent along the left cardiovascular border (aorta, pulmonary artery, left atrial appendage, and left ventricle; compare Figures 11 and 12 to Figure 2A). Another sign of left atrial enlargement is a double density, especially evident along the inferior portion of the right atrial silhouette (Figures 3 and 11). In some cases, the entire circumference of the left atrium may be identified. The carinal angle may become widened and the left mainstem bronchus elevated. With severe enlargement, the left atrium may extend to the right of the right atrial border. An extreme example is shown in Figure 13. In the lateral projection and with the esophagus filled with barium, left atrial enlargement results in a characteristic rounded posterior displacement of the esophagus (Figures 14, 15, and 16B). Echocardiography has largely replaced this formerly common means of assessing left atrial size. Right ventricular enlargement is difficult to identify on the PA chest film. It can result in rounding and elevation of the apex above the diaphragm. With marked right ventricular enlargement the left ventricle may be rotated leftward and posteriorly and the right ventricle may form a part of the left cardiac border. Right ventricular enlargement is better appreciated on the lateral projection, in which the right ventricle is border forming. Normally the right ventricle is in contact with the

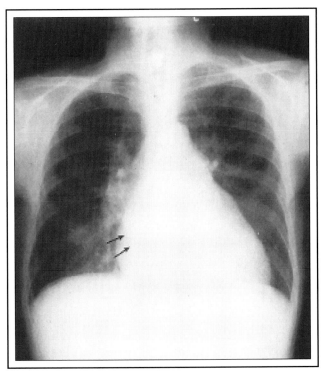

Figure 11. Left atrial enlargement evident as a fourth bulge along the left cardiac silhouette (left atrial appendage) and a double density in the right atrial shadow (arrows); double density of left atrial enlargement is more evident in Figure 3.

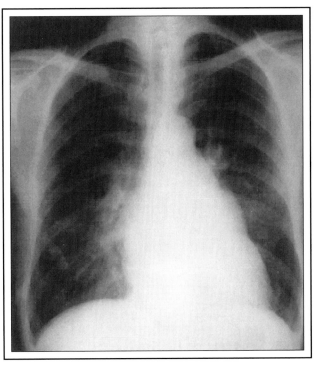

Figure 12. Prominent pulmonary artery and left atrial segments resulting in four convexities along the left heart border in a 48-year-old man with mitral stenosis and regurgitation. Enlargement of the left atrial appendage is more marked than in Figure 11.

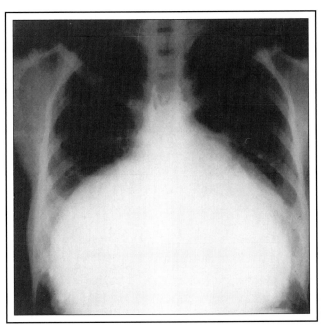

Figure 13. Giant left atrium in a young woman with rheumatic heart disease with predominant mitral regurgitation.

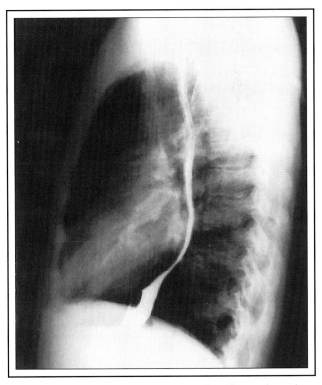

Figure 14. Lateral projection with barium swallow. The esophagus is posteriorly displaced by moderate left atrial enlargement.

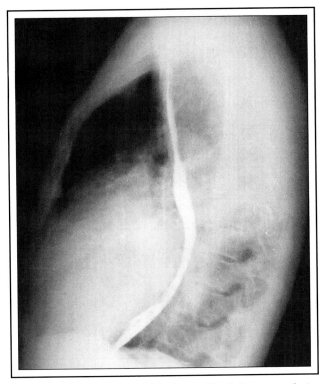

Figure 15. Lateral projection with barium swallow in the same patient as Figure 12. The esophagus is displaced posteriorly over a large portion of its length, indicating marked left atrial enlargement.

sternum only in its lower third. When the right ventricular silhouette is in contact with the sternum for more than one-half of its length, right ventricular enlargement is present (Figure 16B).

Right atrial enlargement is evidenced in the frontal projection by a rightward displacement of the right heart border (exceeding 3 cm from the spine) and an increase in its radius of curvature ("the right atrial sweep") (Figure 7). Elevation of right atrial pressure may also result in dilatation of the superior vena cava. Since the right atrial appendage curves anteriorly over the right ventricle and since right atrium and ventricle frequently enlarge together, a distended right atrial appendage may contribute to the retrosternal fullness of right ventricular enlargement on the lateral projection described before.

The Aorta

In the frontal projection, the ascending aorta is usually superimposed over the superior vena cava, which forms the upper right aspect of the cardiovascular silhouette, but may be border forming immediately superior to the right atrium. The transverse aortic arch displaces the trachea slightly to the right. The aortic portion of the silhouette

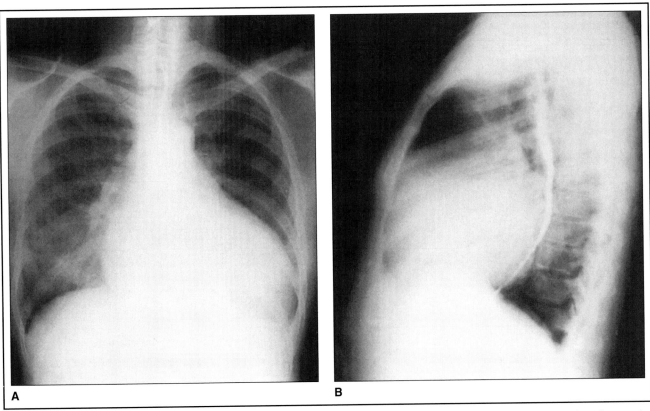

A

B

Figure 16. A: Marked cardiomegaly with left heart border almost reaching the thoracic wall. Right atrial enlargement and left ventricular enlargement are evident in the PA projection. **B:** Lateral view in the same patient shows posterior displacement of the barium-filled esophagus (left atrial enlargement) and right ventricular enlargement. The right ventricle is in contact with the sternum for more than one-half its length.

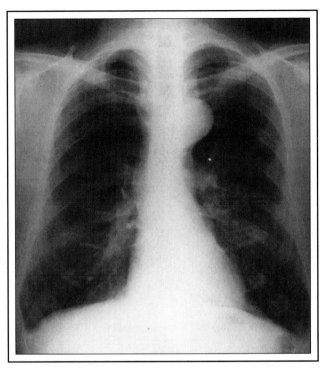

Figure 17. Fifty-one-year-old male with an elongated and tortuous ascending and transverse thoracic aorta. The ascending aorta is displaced to the right; aortic knob is very prominent.

(Figure 2A) is comprised of the posterior portion of the transverse aortic arch and is termed the "aortic knob". The descending aorta normally parallels the thoracic spine on its left.

A wide range of disease processes including hypertension, atherosclerosis, aortic stenosis and regurgitation, aneurysm formation, dissection, Marfan's syndrome, and syphilis result in dilatation of various segments of the aorta. Dilatation of the ascending aorta results in a convex deformity of the upper right cardiovascular silhouette (Figure 17). Enlargement of the aortic arch is evidenced by increasing prominence of the aortic knob, which may come to be the most striking feature of the cardiac silhouette (Figure 17). Rightward displacement of the trachea becomes more pronounced. Likewise, the normally inconspicuous descending aorta may become striking. The lateral or left anterior oblique projections allow the best assessment of the extent and distribution of aortic dilatation. The radiographic appearance of thoracic aortic aneurysms is varied, depending on location and degree of dilatation but is usually readily identified (Figures 18 and 19). The presence of aortic dissection is suggested by widening of the aortic shadow; diagnosis is made by computed tomography, magnetic resonance imaging, angiography, or trans-esophagaeal echocardiography.

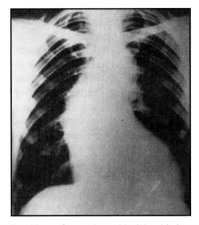

Fig A: X-Ray View - One patient with right-sided aortic diastolic murmurs. Note dilatation and rightward displacement of the aortic root.

CARDIAC PEARL

The great majority of murmurs of aortic regurgitation are heard louder at the left sternal border compared with the counterpart on the right. However, some aortic diastolic murmurs are best heard along the right sternal border rather than the left.

This "right-sided aortic diastolic murmur" is usually associated with dilatation and rightward displacement of the aortic root (Figure A).

W. Proctor Harvey, M.D.

The Pulmonary Vasculature

Careful analysis of the pulmonary vasculature provides important physiologic information in the cardiac patient. Increased pulmonary blood flow, pulmonary hypertension and elevation of the pulmonary venous pressure can each be inferred with reasonable certainty. Occasionally a paucity of pulmonary blood flow, either unilateral or bilateral, is evident.

The pulmonary hilar shadows are comprised primarily of the pulmonary arteries and veins, and to a lesser degree, bronchi and normal lymph nodes. The left hilum is usually slightly more cephalad than the right. The right hilum and right lower lobe vessels are better visualized than those on the left, which are partially obscured by the cardiac shadow. Normally, in the right hilum, the superior pulmonary vein and the inferior pulmonary artery form a sharply defined obtuse angle. When the film is taken with the patient upright, the peripheral lower lobe vessels are more prominent than upper lobe vessels due to hydrostatic forces. When the patient is supine, vascularity is more uniform. Vascular

249

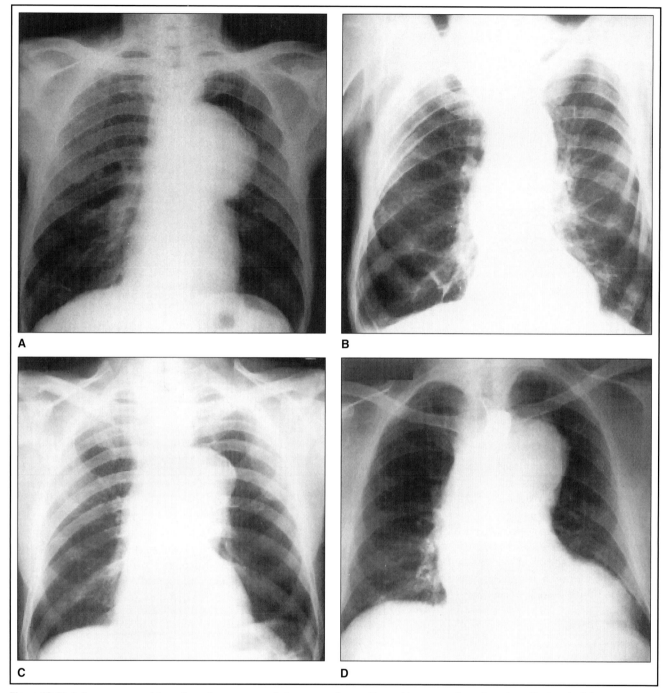

Figure 18. Varied appearances of thoracic aortic aneurysms. **A:** Aneurysm of ascending and transverse thoracic aorta; patient expired due to a rupture into the pericardium. **B:** Aneurysmal dilatation of ascending and transverse thoracic aorta, with prominent rightward displacement of ascending aorta. **C:** Thoracic aortic aneurysm. Note calcification in the markedly enlarged aortic knob. **D:** Aneurysm of thoracic aorta. Left ventricular enlargement is also present.

markings are normally quite inapparent in the lateral thirds of the lung fields. It is usually difficult to distinguish pulmonary arteries from pulmonary veins. However, in the lower lobes, the arteries follow a more vertical course, originating from the more cephalad pulmonary arteries, and the veins are oriented more horizontally as they course to the more caudad left atrium. In the upper lobes, veins are positioned lateral to the arteries and are more prominent than the arteries. Normally, pulmonary arteries and their accompanying veins and bronchi are of approximately the same size.

250

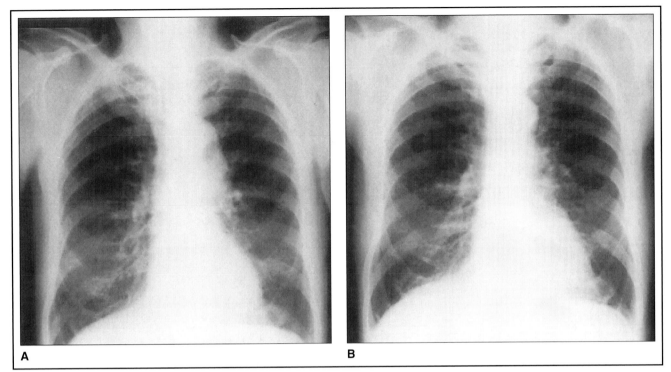

Figure 19. Ruptured descending thoracic aortic aneurysm, suggested by widening of the descending aortic shadow **(A)**, especially in comparison to a film taken several years before **(B)**.

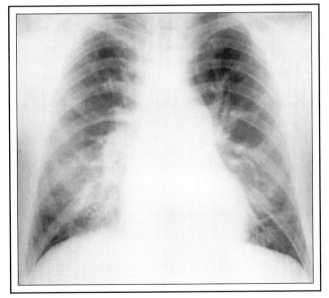

Figure 20. Increased pulmonary blood flow due to an atrial septal defect. Enlargement of pulmonary arteries and pulmonary vascular marking in the outer thirds of the lung fields are present.

Increased Pulmonary Blood Flow

Pulmonary arterial blood flow may be increased as much as five-fold to eight-fold when left-to-right shunting occurs, as with atrial and ventricular septal defects and patent ductus arteriosus. To accommodate this flow, pulmonary arteries become larger anatomically and radiographically, both centrally and peripherally (Figure 20). They become readily visible in the outer thirds of the lung fields. When a bronchus and accompanying pulmonary artery can be identified in transverse section, the pulmonary artery will be larger. Pulmonary venous blood flow must also increase in this setting, and will be reflected in the chest film, but changes in the pulmonary arterial size and distribution are more evident. These findings are also termed "shunt vascularity" and "pulmonary plethora".

Pulmonary Hypertension

In pulmonary hypertension (Figure 21), the central arteries become dilated (and occasionally calcified) but in contrast to the radiographic appearance with increased pulmonary blood flow, the peripheral vessels are quite inapparent and the outer thirds of the lung fields are lucent; medium-sized arteries may become tortuous. The disparity in size between the central and peripheral arteries has been compared to sharply trimmed tree branches and has been termed "pruning". Idiopathic dilatation of the pulmonary artery and pulmonary artery aneurysm can also result in prominence of the pulmonary artery segment (Figure 22).

Pulmonary Venous Hypertension

Pulmonary venous hypertension is the most commonly encountered abnormality of the pulmonary

251

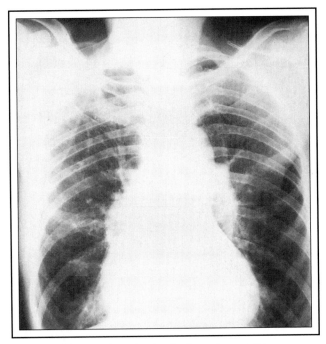

Figure 21. Pulmonary hypertension due to emphysema (cor pulmonale). Note prominent left pulmonary artery; enlarged right pulmonary artery is partially obscured by right atrial enlargement. Peripheral vascular markings are relatively well-preserved.

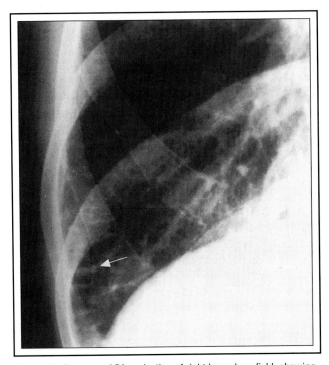

Figure 23. Close-up of PA projection of right lower lung field, showing Kerley B lines (one indicated by arrow). These linear densities, perpendicular to the pleural surface, are due to edema of interlobar septa and are evidence of elevated pulmonary venous pressure.

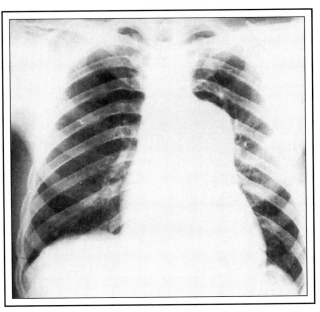

Figure 22. Prominent pulmonary artery segment due to pulmonary artery aneurysm.

vasculature, and its radiographic recognition is important in the care of many patients. Probably the earliest sign of chronic elevation of the pulmonary venous pressure (15 mmHg-18 mmHg) is an increase in the prominence of pulmonary veins in the upper lung fields, where they may be followed almost to the pleural surface. There is a concomitant decrease in the size of vessels to the lower lung fields, perhaps due to reflex of constriction of the pulmonary arteries and therefore reduced flow to the lower lobes in response to elevated hydrostatic pressure and to perivascular edema of the dependent arterioles and capillaries. This inversion of the normal vascularity has been termed "pulmonary vascular redistribution" or "cephalization of pulmonary blood flow" (Figure 39). When the upper lobe vessels are very prominent and those in the lower lobes very inconspicuous, the term "staghorn" has been applied. As pulmonary venous pressure rises further (20 mmHg to 25 mmHg) edema of the pulmonary interstitium and the walls of the arteries, veins and bronchi occurs. The medium sized arteries and veins appear wider when viewed either end-on or longitudinally, and their outer margins become indistinct. In the transverse view, this has been termed "perivascular cuffing". Likewise, the walls of medium sized bronchi become thicker when viewed in cross-section and their outline also loses sharp definition. This finding is termed "peribronchial cuffing". Interstitial edema is also evident in three patterns described by Kerley. The most commonly seen are Kerley B lines, which are 1 cm to 3 cm sharp linear densities perpendicular

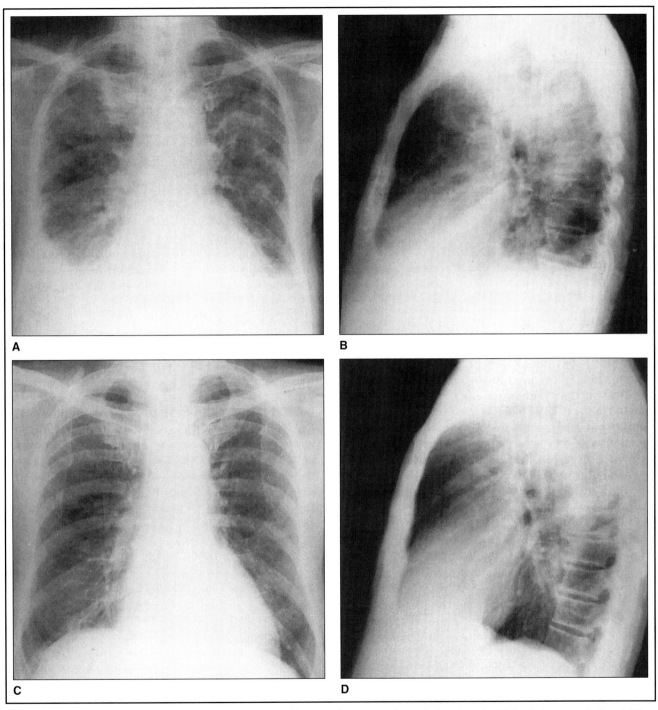

Figure 24. Moderate bilateral pleural effusion. **A:** Curvilinear densities extending up from the costophrenic angles bilaterally (more marked on right) identify pleural effusions. Pulmonary edema is also present. **B:** Pleural effusion causing blunting of posterior costophrenic sulcus (same patient as Panel A). **C** and **D:** Pleural effusions have cleared almost completely after diuresis.

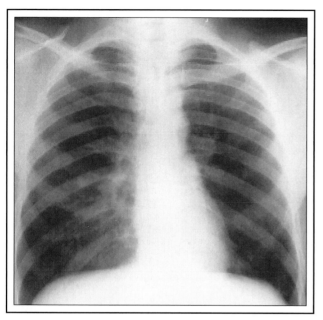

Figure 25. Hypoplastic left pulmonary artery; note absence of normal left pulmonary artery convexity and diminished left-sided pulmonary vascular markings (compare to Figure 1A).

to and abutting the pleural surface, usually appearing first in the right lower lung field (Figure 23) due to edema of interlobar septa. Kerley A lines are similar but longer, radiate from the hila, and may be slightly curved. They are often best seen in the lateral projection and represent edema in the perivascular connective tissue planes. Kerley C lines are a fine network of interlacing or reticular lines most commonly in the lung bases and possibly representing superimposed edematous interlobar septa. Subpleural thickening and perihilar and peripheral haze have also been described. Distention of the right superior pulmonary vein and perivascular edema in the right hilum can result in loss of the normally sharply defined hilar angle. With an increase in the pulmonary venous pressure to 28 mmHg to 30 mmHg pulmonary alveolar edema ensues (Figure 24). When of cardiac origin, the edema is most prominent in the inner two-thirds of the lung fields, giving rise to the so-called "butterfly" or "batwing" pattern. When alveolar edema is prominent peripherally, non-cardiac causes should be suspected.

Decreased Pulmonary Blood Flow

Decreased pulmonary blood flow results in increased radiolucency of the lung fields. In an adult population it is most commonly due to acquired lung disease and may be localized, as with emphysematous bullae or pulmonary embolic disease, or unilateral, as with pulmonary resection or pneumothorax. When decreased pulmonary blood

flow is of cardiac etiology it is usually congenital, as with pulmonary atresia, tricuspid atresia and Tetralogy of Fallot. These abnormalities result in a symmetrical decrease of blood flow to both lungs. Severity of the lesion can be judged from the reduction in size of the central pulmonary vessels. The peripheral vascular markings, of course, will also be diminished. Pulmonary blood flow may also be asymmetrical as with unilateral pulmonary atresia (Figure 25), pulmonary branch stenosis, or following a shunting procedure.

When pulmonary atresia is present, the lung parenchyma is supplied by collaterals from the bronchial circulation. These vessels do not radiate from the hilum (which is small), do not taper or branch, and appear tortuous and disordered, but may give the impression of normal or increased vascularity; careful inspection is therefore required.

Pleural Effusion

Fluid in the pleural space is visualized on the PA chest film first as a blunting of the normally sharp costophrenic angle. As the amount of fluid increases, a concave curvilinear density ascends progressively up the lateral thoracic wall (Figures 24 and 26). Small effusions may be inapparent in the frontal view, but readily seen in the lateral projection, as the lowest portion of the costophrenic sulcus is located posteriorly. The presence of small or moderate effusions can be confirmed by the appropriate lateral decubitus film, on which the fluid can be seen to layer against the dependent thoracic cage, with a nearly straight horizontal margin. Pleural fluid may accumulate in the diaphragm and the lung, following a "subpulmonic" pleural effusion (Figure 27), and in this location does not cause blunting of the costophrenic angle in the frontal projection, but gives the appearance of an elevated diaphragm. However, blunting of the posterior sulcus may be visible in the lateral view. Unless loculated, which is not usually the case, a subpulmonic effusion layers out on a lateral decubitus film. Pleural fluid may also accumulate in the minor fissure, forming an ovoid density simulating a tumor; fluid in this location is termed "pseudotumor" (Figure 28). When caused by congestive heart failure, it disappears with effective diuresis.

Pleural effusions are caused by a wide variety of diseases including pulmonary infarction, primary and metastatic tumors, hypoproteinemia, lupus erythematosus, tuberculosis, viral and bacterial infections, ascites, pancreatitis, and trauma. However, the most common cause of pleural effusion is congestive heart failure, in which the effusion may be bilateral or unilateral. A unilateral

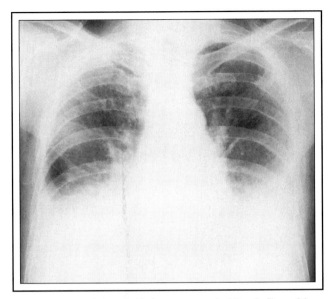

Figure 26. Bilateral pleural effusions more marked than in Figure 24.

effusion due to heart failure is almost always right-sided, the reason for which is unknown. Since the pleural veins drain into both systemic and pulmonary venous systems, pleural effusion due to heart failure usually implies the presence of both right and left heart failure, although occasionally marked elevation of the pressure in either venous system can result in pleural effusion.

Pericardial Effusion

Pericardial effusion causes an enlargement of the cardiac silhouette which may be subtle or massive (Figures 29 and 30). Although a triangular

flask-like or "water bottle" configuration is often described as classic, the enlargement may be quite globular and difficult to distinguish from cardiomegaly due to cardiomyopathy. Since the pericardial reflection extends to the bifurcation of the pulmonary artery, pericardial distention can obscure the hilar structures in the frontal projection, whereas cardiomegaly does not. The lateral projection is useful in diagnosing pericardial effusion in some patients. Normally, the epicardial fat pad and pericardium are in close apposition to the sternum. When an anterior pericardial effusion is present, the epicardial fat pad may appear as a radiolucent vertical stripe displaced posteriorly from the sternum by 1 cm to 2 cm. When pericardial effusion is suspected, an echocardiogram provides definitive information regarding its presence, size, distribution and suitability for percutaneous drainage, and replaces older, less accurate, and cumbersome diagnostic techniques.

Other Abnormalities of the Cardiac Silhouette

A variety of terms have been used to characterize abnormalities of the cardiac silhouette, especially those due to congenital heart disease. In Tetralogy of Fallot, the heart is frequently described as "boot shaped" because of right ventricular hypertrophy and a diminished pulmonary artery segment. In Ebstein's anomaly, the heart may be "box shaped" due to increased angulation at the junction of the superior vena cava and right atrium due to right atrial enlargement (Figure 31). In other instances

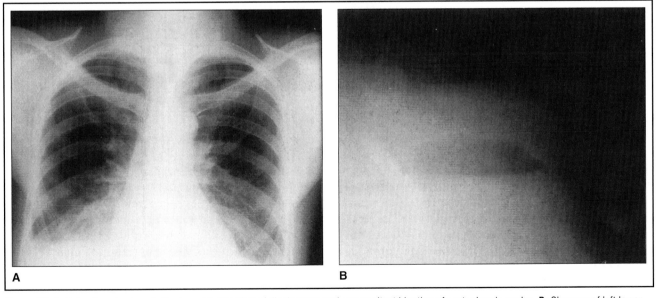

A

B

Figure 27. A: Subpulmonic pleural effusion with elevation of diaphragms and concomitant blunting of costophrenic angles. **B:** Close-up of left lower lung field and the left upper quadrant of abdomen with gas in stomach. Increased separation of stomach bubble from inferior margin of lung indicates presence of subpulmonic effusion.

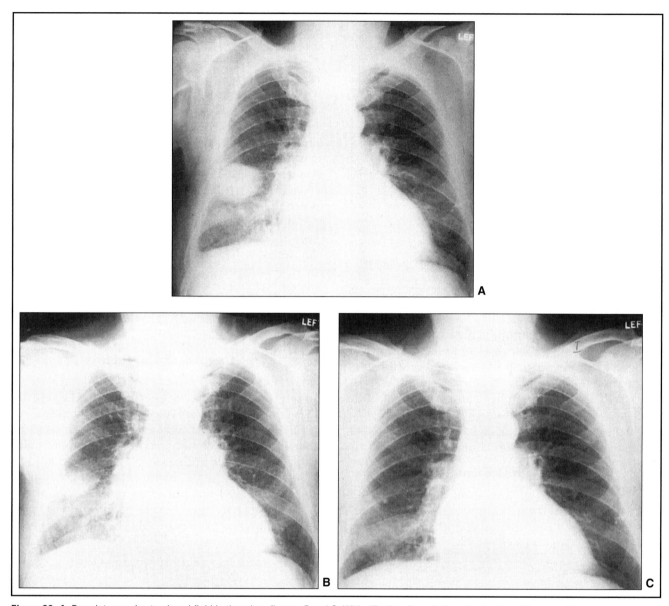

Figure 28. A: Pseudotumor due to pleural fluid in the minor fissure. **B** and **C:** With effective diuresis there is clearing of the pseudotumor over several days.

of Ebstein's anomaly, the heart may appear rounded or triangular (due to small pulmonary arteries). In coarctation of the aorta, a figure "3" pattern has been described in the region of the aortic knob, with the upper portion of the 3 due to dilatation of the aortic arch proximal to the coarctation, and the lower portion of the 3 due to post-stenotic dilatation of the aorta distal to the coarctation. Occasionally, the aortic arch develops on the right side and is seen to the right of the spine on the PA chest film (Figure 32).

Congenital complete and partial absence of the pericardium results in changes in the cardiac silhouette. "Complete" absence is actually unilateral and usually left-sided, and results in leftward dis-

placement of the heart, which may be striking. Partial absence of the pericardium involves the upper portion of either the right or left side of the pericardium and may result in herniation of the respective atrium through the defect, resulting in a bulge in the cephalad portion of the cardiac silhouette. Computed tomography can identify the defect.

Pericardial cysts usually occur as convexities along the middle or lower right heart border (Figure 33) but can occur on the left side as well. MRI or CT are useful in establishing the diagnosis.

Cardiovascular Calcification

The chest x-ray can show calcification of a number of intrathoracic structures including the pleura,

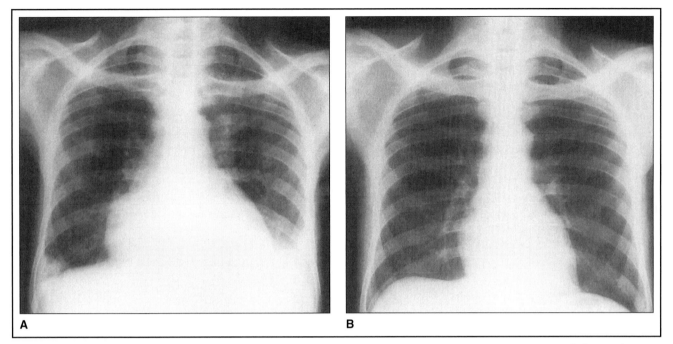

Figure 29. A: Pericardial effusion with a triangular configuration of cardiac silhouette. Bilateral pleural effusions are also present. **B:** Same patient following treatment for tuberculous pericarditis.

lymph nodes, and granulomata, as well as cardiovascular components. These include the pericardium, the aorta, the pulmonary arteries, the coronary arteries, the cardiac valve leaflets and annuli, the myocardium, and cardiac tumors. Image intensification fluoroscopy is many times more sensitive than the chest x-ray in detecting most cardiovascular calcification, in large part because characteristic patterns of motion aid identification but also because contrast and magnification can be adjusted and the field can be limited to an area of interest.

Valvular Calcification

Calcification of the cardiac valves always indicates a pathologic process but does not always indicate a functional abnormality. Mitral annular calcification occurs as a consequence of aging in some individuals and has a characteristic C, J, or flattened O-shaped appearance on chest x-ray (Figure 34). It is frequently associated with no abnormality of mitral valve function, but when marked can cause mitral regurgitation.

CARDIAC PEARL

Calcification of the mitral valve annulus, as noted on chest x-ray and fluoroscopy, was first described by the late Merrill Sosman of Boston, a master radiologist; he described the finding on fluoroscopy of the heart of a calcification resembling a letter "C" or "J". This cal-

cified annulus can occur in some patients with mitral valve prolapse and may be related to some of the auscultatory findings of prolapse, including a systolic murmur. In other patients having the calcification no murmur is present.

Calcification of the mitral annulus is associated with a spectrum of varied findings. Some patients are without symptoms entirely and may have no systolic murmur. Others may have a murmur in late systole that is typical of

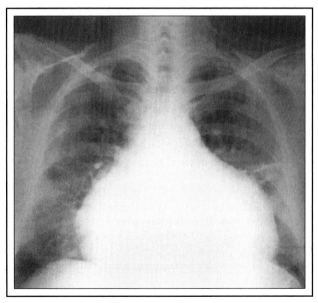

Figure 30. Large pericardial effusion. The heart shape is globular and the hilar structures are obscured (see text).

257

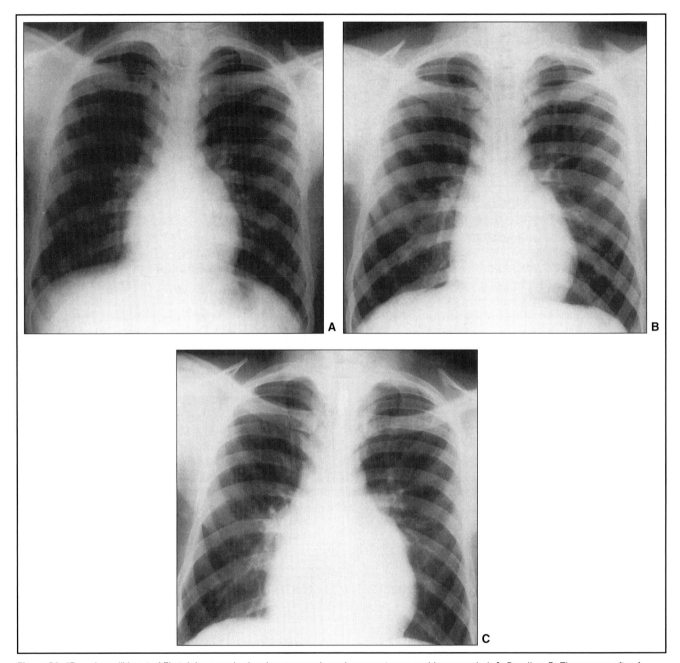

Figure 31. "Box-shaped" heart of Ebstein's anomaly showing progressive enlargement over an 11-year period. **A:** Baseline. **B:** Three years after A. **C:** Eight years after B.

mitral valve prolapse. Some patients may have mitral regurgitation in varying degrees, including very severe. This finding of "mitral stenosis" secondary to both "massive" mitral annulus calcific deposits and small hypertrophic left ventricles has been described. Therefore, it is apparent that the findings associated with mitral annular calcification are quite varied.

Uncommonly, the mitral valve annular calcification may form a complete circle like the letter "O".

A patient with calcification of the mitral valve annulus is more likely to have atrial fibrillation than a patient without calcification. This also applies to patients with mitral valve prolapse- those with calcification of the mitral annulus are more prone to have atrial fibrillation.

Therefore, as might logically be expected, emboli are more likely. Anticoagulant therapy as prophylaxis should be considered in this group.

W. Proctor Harvey, M.D.

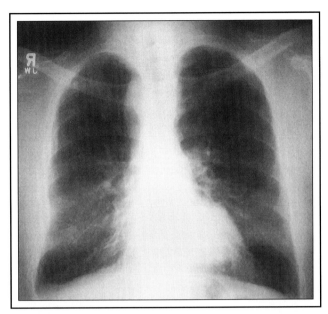

Figure 32. Right aortic arch. The ascending aorta and arch are seen to the right of the spine.

Calcification of the mitral valve leaflets almost always indicates presence of rheumatic heart disease and mitral stenosis or mixed mitral stenosis and regurgitation, although occasionally regurgitation may predominate.

Calcification of the aortic valvular apparatus usually begins in the valve leaflets and extends into the annulus and interventricular septum as the disease process becomes more severe. Calcification in the aortic valve leaflets usually indicates presence of aortic stenosis and the extent of calcification generally correlates with severity of obstruction. Mild calcification (1+) may be associated with trivial aortic stenosis ("aortic sclerosis") but heavy calcification (4+) almost always indicates severe stenosis (Figure 35), although severe aortic stenosis occasionally occurs with only minimal fluoroscopically visualized calcification. When calcification of the aortic valve is due to rheumatic heart disease, mitral valvular calcification is usually also present. Isolated aortic valvular calcification in an individual under 50 years of age generally implies aortic stenosis on a unicuspid or bicuspid valve. Isolated calcific aortic stenosis in a patient over 65 is usually due to a degenerative process on a previously normal tricuspid aortic valve.

Calcification of the pulmonary valve is rare but can occur with severe pulmonic stenosis. Tricuspid valvular and annular calcification also occurs rarely, is usually due to rheumatic heart disease, and when present is usually associated with marked hemodynamic abnormalities, especially right ventricular hypertension.

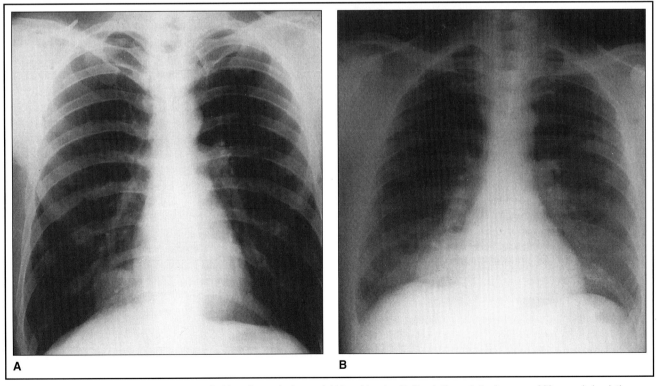

Figure 33. A: Pericardial cyst occurring in a typical location at the lower right heart border. **B:** Hernia through the foramen of Morgagni simulating a pericardial cyst.

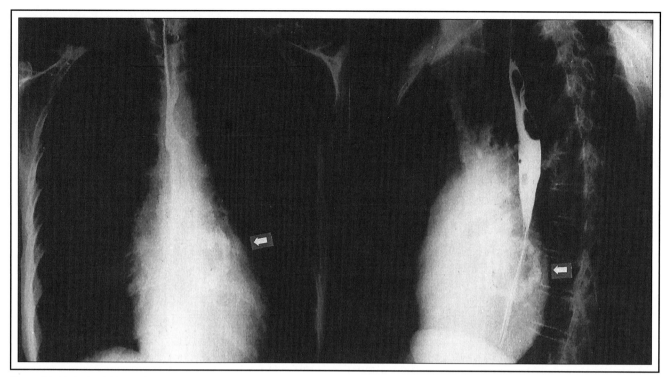

Figure 34. Marked calcification of annulus forming a complete "O". *(From Georgetown University Medical Center; permission Dr. W. Proctor Harvey.)*

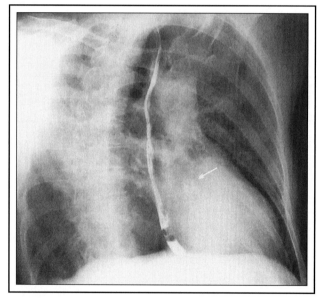

Figure 35. Right anterior oblique projection showing marked calcification of aortic valve (indicated by arrows) in a 64-year-old male with severe aortic stenosis. (PA projection appears as Figure 6).

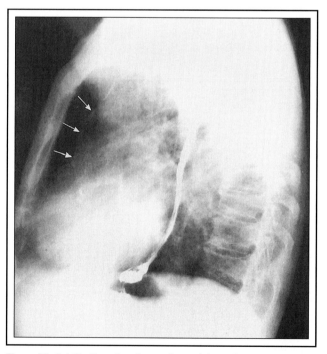

Figure 36. Calcification of aortic annulus and the entire ascending aorta (arrows). Serology was positive for syphilis.

Calcification of the Great Vessels

Thin linear calcification of the lateral aspect of the aortic knob best seen in the PA projection is the most commonly observed cardiovascular calcification on the chest x-ray and indicates the presence of atherosclerotic disease. Occasionally, this calcification can be extensive, and involve essentially the entire thoracic aorta, where it may be seen best in the lateral or LAO projections (Figure 36). Calcification in the anterior wall of the ascending aorta, best seen in the lateral projection, is classically observed in luetic aortitis and is frequently

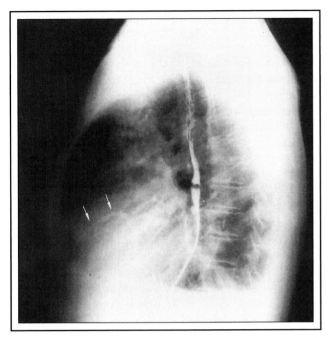

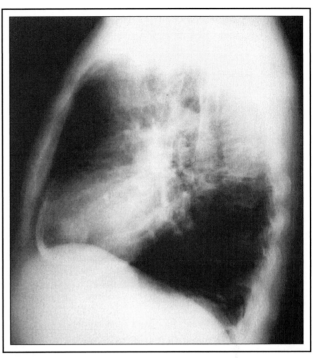

Figure 37. Calcification of left anterior descending coronary artery and diagonal branch (arrows).

Figure 38. Calcification of apical portion of pericardium.

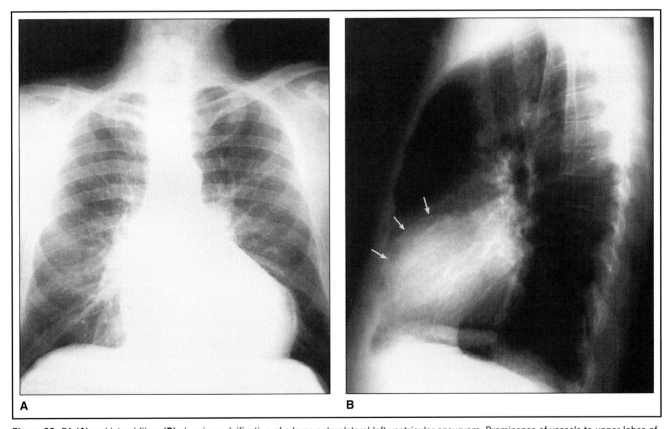

A

B

Figure 39. PA **(A)** and lateral films **(B)** showing calcification of a large anterolateral left ventricular aneurysm. Prominence of vessels to upper lobes of lungs indicates elevation of pulmonary venous pressure.

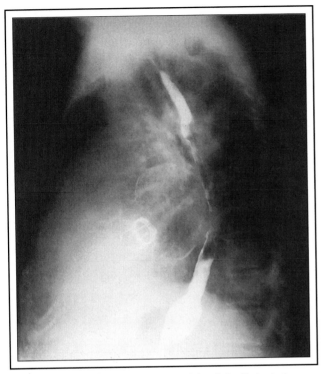

Figure 40. Eggshell calcification of left atrial wall. A mitral valvular prosthesis is present. *(From Vanden Belt RJ, Ronan JA: Cardiology: A Clinical Approach. 2nd edition. Chicago: Yearbook Medical Publishers Inc, 1987: used with permission of Mosby-Yearbook Inc.).*

associated with aortic regurgitation. Aortic calcification can also be seen in chronic dissection, sinus of Valsalva aneurysms, and Takayasu's arteritis. Inward displacement of the calcification from the radiographic aortic border may be a sign of aortic dissection.

Calcification of the pulmonary artery occurs in long-standing severe pulmonary hypertension and sometimes following surgery for correction of congenital abnormalities, such as Tetralogy of Fallot.

Coronary Artery Calcification

Coronary artery calcification is occasionally apparent on a plain chest film, especially the lateral projection, and when present is almost invariably associated with severe obstructive disease (Figure 37). Fluoroscopy is much more sensitive than radiography in detecting coronary arterial calcification and there is a close correlation between its presence and obstructive coronary disease, although its absence does not exclude significant disease. Ultrafast computed tomography is more sensitive than fluoroscopy in identifying coronary calcification *(vide infra).*

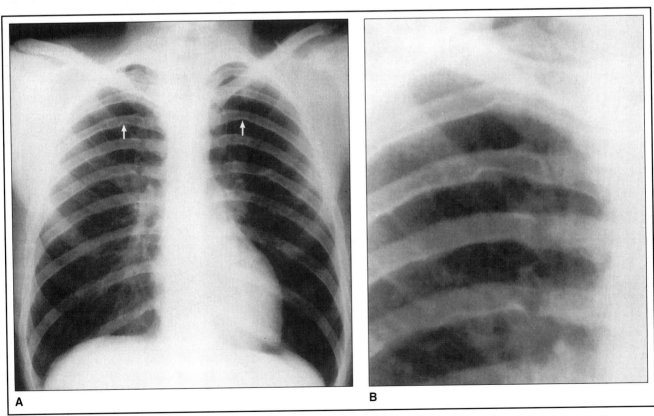

Figure 41. A: Notching of inferior margins of ribs due to coarction of aorta; (two areas are indicated by arrows; other ribs are also notched).
B: Close-up of upper right chest with rib notching evident.

262

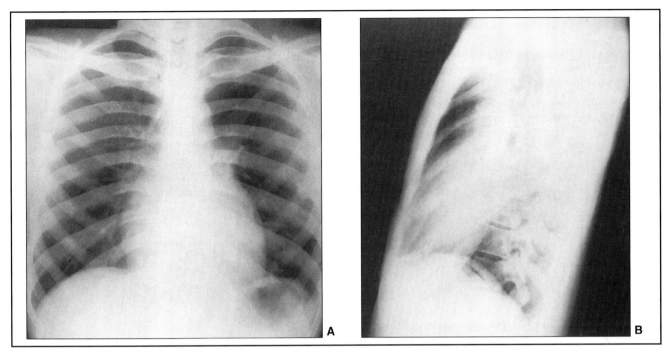

Figure 42. Apparent cardiac enlargement due to straight back syndrome; anteroposterior dimension on the lateral film **(B)** is less than one-third the transthoracic diameter on the PA projection **(A)**. No cardiac disease was identified.

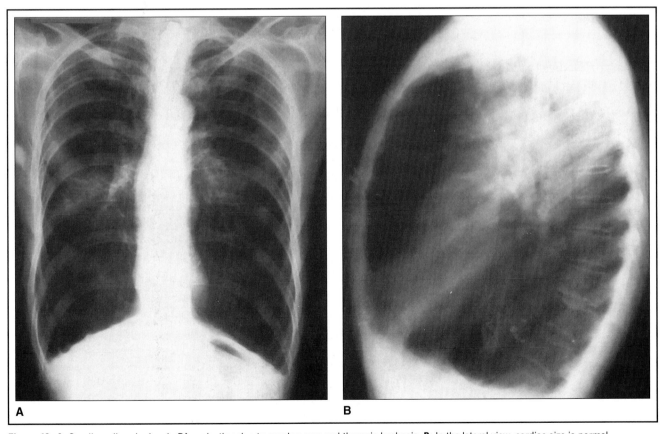

Figure 43. A: Small cardiac shadow in PA projection due to emphysema and thoracic kyphosis. **B:** In the lateral view, cardiac size is normal.

Pericardial Calcification

Pericardial calcification may follow any inflammatory process of the pericardium, including viral or tuberculous pericarditis, hemopericardium from trauma or rarely post-pericardiotomy syndrome or autoimmune disease. Pericardial calcification may appear radiographically first in the region of the right atrial and right ventricular borders and in the atrioventricular groove, but may be extensive, involving essentially the entire pericardium. Mild calcification may be most apparent in either frontal or lateral projections, so both should be inspected (Figure 38). Pericardial calcification is present in many patients with constrictive pericarditis, but is also frequently present without evidence of hemodynamic compromise.

Other Cardiac Calcification

Left ventricular aneurysms may become calcified and be visible as a thin curved rim outlining the aneurysm, most commonly involving the anterior or lateral walls or the apex (Figure 39). In rheumatic heart disease the left atrial wall may likewise acquire "eggshell" calcification, either due to rheumatic myocarditis or to calcification of thrombus along the left atrial endocardial surface (Figure 40). Finally, calcification may occur in cardiac tumors, most commonly atrial myxomas, but also fibromas, rhabdomyosarcomas, angiosarcomas and osteosarcomas. The pattern of calcification is variable and it is rarely detected first on the chest x-ray, but is more frequently found on fluoroscopy, CT or by echocardiography.

Pulmonary Parenchyma

The radiologic appearance of the pulmonary parenchyma may give important diagnostic information relating to the heart. Pulmonary embolism may present as chest pain or dyspnea and findings on the chest film may be subtle. Recurrent pulmonary embolism may be a cause of chronic right heart failure and may respond to anticoagulant therapy. Septic pulmonary emboli may be the first identified sign of tricuspid endocarditis. Findings of emphysema or pulmonary fibrosis may provide the explanation for chronic right heart failure (cor pulmonale).

Thoracic Cage

As indicated above, inspection of the chest x-ray for abnormalities of the thoracic cage can yield important diagnostic information. Coarctation of the aorta results in the development of collateral circulation to the lower portion of the body through intercostal and internal mammary arteries. As the intercostal arteries enlarge, they become tortuous and erode the inferior margins of the posterior aspect of the third to eighth ribs producing a characteristic scalloped or notched pattern (Figure 41). A similar pattern may be seen on the posterior surface of the sternum on the lateral film from dilated internal mammary arteries. Two abnormalities of the thoracic cage can result in a narrow anteroposterior dimension and possible abnormalities on the PA chest film which may be clarified by inspection of the lateral film. Pectus excavatum (funnel chest) can displace the heart leftward resulting in a prominence of the left heart border and pulmonary artery segment. When symptoms and equivocal physical findings are present, additional examinations, especially echocardiography, may be needed to rule out cardiac pathology. Marked pectus excavatum can occasionally produce impaired cardiac function. Straight back syndrome results from lack of the normal thoracic kyphosis with a resultant narrowing of the AP diameter. The criterion for this diagnosis is that the AP dimension (measured horizontally from the posterior surface of the sternum to the anterior aspect of the eighth thoracic vertebral body) is less than one-third of the transverse thoracic dimension at the superior aspect of the diaphragmatic domes. This condition may also result in a leftward shift of the heart with prominence of the pulmonary artery segment and apparent cardiac enlargement (Figure 42). It may be associated with mitral valve prolapse and/or a bicuspid aortic valve, but frequently no cardiac disease is present.

Pectus carinatum (pigeon chest), emphysema or an exaggerated thoracic kyphosis may result in a smaller than normal cardiac shadow in the frontal projection (Figure 43). Marked kyphoscoliosis can result in restrictive lung disease with cor pulmonale, and resultant radiographic changes. Ankylosing spondylitis is sometimes associated with aortic regurgitation, which can be marked.

CARDIAC PEARL

When we find on examination of our patients that there is a chest anomaly such as straight back, pectus excavatum, pectus coronatum, or chest asymmetry, we have a clue that mitral valve prolapse might be present. Perhaps 50% of patients with such anomalies may have mitral valve prolapse.

Pectus excavatum was described by Dr. William Evans of London as saucer, cup or funnel types.

A patient having the cup or funnel pectus can have the heart in the PA view displaced to

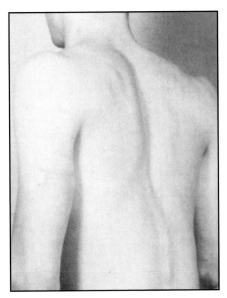
Fig A: Straight back.

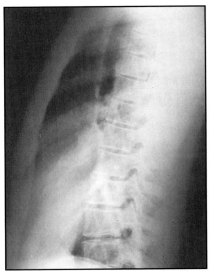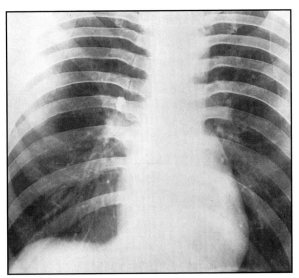

Fig B: Straight Back - Left: note "straight back" spine. In fact, it curves anteriorly rather than the usual normal posteriorly. The PA chest film (right) may show a "pancake" shape due to some compression of the heart between the spine and anterior chest wall.

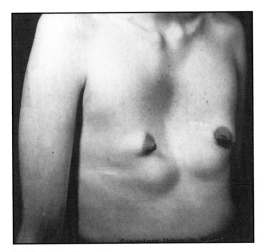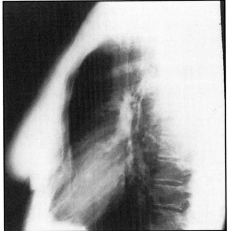

Fig C: Pectus Excavatum.

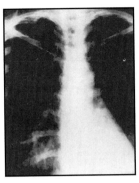

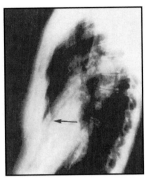

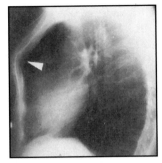

Fig D: Suspect Pectus excavatum when PA view shows little or no cardiac silhouette to right of spine as heart is displaced to the left.

Fig E: Lateral view shows pectus excavatum.

Fig F: Pectus Coronatum - The patient is a 30-year-old man with a congenital heart disease - pectus coronatum (arrow). He also has a mid-systolic click of mitral valve prolapse.

the left, showing little or no cardiac shadow on the right of the spine and a cardiac silhouette that can be misinterpreted as being enlarged. When one sees only this PA chest film, one can suspect pectus even before examining the patient.

These chest anomalies that cause compression on the heart cause no symptoms. Occasionally surgery for pectus is performed purely for cosmetic reasons (Figures A to F).

W. Proctor Harvey, M.D.

Prosthetic Devices

The chest x-ray can be used to identify various prosthetic devices which may have been implanted. Prosthetic valves from different manufacturers and different models from a single manufacturer often have a characteristic radiologic appearance. Porcine valves can be readily distinguished from mechanical valves. Charts available from manufacturers or in journal articles can be used for specific identification. Cardiac pacemakers and defibrillators can usually be identified by manufacturer and sometimes by model. Again, charts or other information from the manufacturer may be necessary for complete identification. Gross pacemaker lead displacement can be recognized easily and lead fracture (especially with unipolar leads) can sometimes be identified. The aortic anastomoses of saphenous vein-coronary artery bypass grafts are sometimes marked by surgeons with radio-opaque clips or loops, while certain coronary arterial stents are visible fluoroscopically.

Computed Tomography (CT) and Magnetic Resonance Imaging (MRI)

CT and MRI imaging provide clear tomographic images of the heart and great vessels. CT, which is

the older of the two techniques is more widely available and less expensive than MRI. However, the image quality and availability of multiple imaging planes with MRI lead many experts to prefer this technique.

Computed Tomography

CT imaging, although noninvasive, does expose the patient to ionizing radiation and frequently requires the use of contrast medium. It can provide clear images of the heart, great vessels and pericardium and is highly effective for the detection of cardiovascular calcification. A distinction must be made between conventional CT scanning and two more advanced techniques, ECG-gated CT and ultrafast CT scanning (which does not require ECG gating). Newer conventional CT scanners are useful in clinical evaluation of aortic dissection, pericardial disease, intracardiac tumors and thrombosis, and assessment of the patency of coronary arterial bypass grafts. Conventional CT is a rapid and quite accurate (±90%) method for diagnosis of aortic dissection, usually manifest as a lucent line (intimal flap) in the lumen of the aorta.

The pericardium can be seen on CT in most individuals as a thin stripe. Pericardial thickening, present in constrictive pericarditis, is readily detected by CT. Presence or absence of this finding can be very helpful in the often difficult differential diagnosis of constrictive pericarditis vs. restrictive cardiomyopathy. CT is also useful for evaluating pericardial cysts and neoplasms and clearly demonstrates pericardial effusions. Although echocardiography is the primary modality used for assessing pericardial disease, CT is sometimes useful when satisfactory echo images cannot be obtained. CT imaging is also fairly reliable for detecting patency of saphenous vein bypass grafts (left anterior descending grafts are seen better than right or circumflex grafts) but does not show distal graft stenosis or the runoff bed. Ultrafast CT scanners are not widely available, but have many potential applications. They have been used for evaluation of regional wall motion and thickening, left and right ventricular myocardial mass, determination of ventricular volumes, stroke volume, regurgitant fraction, and evaluation of complex congenital cardiac malformations. Ultrafast CT provides improved assessment of coronary artery bypass patency in comparison to conventional CT, and allows visualization of grafts to the right and circumflex coronary arteries. Ultrafast CT is much more sensitive in detecting coronary arterial calcification than fluoroscopy and there is ongoing research to evaluate the potential value of ultrafast CT as a screening tool for CHD.

Magnetic Resonance Imaging

MRI has the advantage of being completely non-invasive and does not require ionizing radiation. Because MRI inherently provides sharp delineation between cardiovascular structures and the blood pool, the use of contrast medium is not required. The availability of multiple imaging planes allows for 3-D visualization of cardiovascular structures. However, some patients are too claustrophobic to tolerate being surrounded by the large magnet, cardiac arrhythmias interfere with the necessary ECG gating and patients with pacemakers or certain other metallic implants cannot be placed in the magnet. Because of the duration of the procedure and the isolation of the patient in the magnet, MRI is less useful in the critically ill or unstable patient. Like CT, MRI produces excellent images of the heart and great vessels; however, MRI does not detect calcium well. MRI is highly accurate for the detection and delineation of aortic dissection. Nienaber and colleagues indicate their preference for MRI over CT for the reliable diagnosis of dissection. MRI is useful for the detection of coarctation of aorta and the follow-up of its surgical correction.

MRI effectively demonstrates the pericardium and has a utility similar to CT. It is especially useful for delineation of masses or neoplasms in and around the heart, pericardium, and great vessels. Congenital cardiac diseases, especially complex cyanotic malformations and those with great vessel abnormalities, are ideally imaged with this modality. Determination of pulmonary artery size in the presence of pulmonary atresia and assessment of the condition of surgically created shunts is well suited to imaging with MRI. MRI has been shown to be highly accurate for determination of left ventricular size, mass and function, including presence of myocardial infarction, and distribution of left ventricular hypertrophy. The patency of saphenous vein grafts and valvular function can also be assessed with MRI, but it is not widely used for these purposes.

Selected Reading

1. Beiser GD, Epstein SE, Stampfer M et al: Impairment of cardiac function in patients with pectus excavatum, with improvement after operative correction. *NEJM* 287 :267-272, 1972.
2. Carsky EW, Mauceri RA, Azimi F: The epicardial fat pad sign. Radiology 137:303-308, 1980.
3. Chait A: Interstitial pulmonary edema. *Circ* 45:1323-1330, 1972.
4. Daffner RH: *Clinical Radiology: The Essentials*. Baltimore, MD: Williams and Wilkins, 1993.
5. deLeon AC Jr, Perloff JK, Twigg H et al: The straight back syndrome. Clinical cardiovascular manifestations. *Circ* 32:193-203, 1965.
6. Dinsmore RE, Miller SW: The plain chest roentgenogram. In: Eagle KA, Haber E, DeSanctis RW, Austen WG, eds. *The Practice of Cardiology*. 2nd edition. Boston, MA: Little, Brown and Company, 1989: 1445-1464.
7. Felgin DS, Fenoglio JJ, McAllister HA et al: Pericardial cysts. A radiologic-pathologic correlation and review. *Radiology* 125:15-20, 1942.
8. Fleischner FG: The butterfly pattern of acute pulmonary edema. *AJC* 20:39-46, 1967.
9. Fulkerson PK, Beaver BM, Auseon JC et al: Calcification of the mitral annulus. Etiology, clinical associations, complications, and therapy. *AJM* 66:967-977, 1979.
10. Guthaner DF, Breen JF: Clinical aspects of chest roentgenology. In: Marcus ML, Skorton DJ, Schelbert HR, Wolf GL, eds. *Cardiac Imaging: A Companion to Braunwald's Heart Disease*. Philadelphia, PA: W. B. Saunders Co, 1991: 93-108.
11. Higgins CB: Newer cardiac imaging techniques (CT, MRI). In: Braunwald E, ed. *Heart Disease,* 4th edition. Philadelphia, PA: W. B. Saunders Co, 1992: 312-341.
12. Kerley PJ: Radiology in heart disease. *BMJ* 2:594, 1933.
13. Margolis JR, Chen JTT, Kong Y et al: The diagnostic and prognostic significance of coronary artery calcification. A report of 800 cases. *Radiology* 137:609-616, 1980.
14. Matsuyama S, Watabe T, Kuribayashi S et al: Plain radiographic diagnosis of thrombosis of left atrial appendage in mitral valve disease. *Radiology* 146:15-20,1983.
15. McHugh TJ, Forrester JS, Adler L, et al: Pulmonary vascular congestion in acute myocardial infarction: Hemodynamic and radiologic correlations. *Ann Int Med* 76:29-33, 1972.
16. Miller WT: *Introduction to Clinical Radiology*. New York, NY: Macmillan Publishing Co, Inc: 1982.
17. Nienaber CA, von Kodolitseh Y, Nicolas V et al: The diagnosis of thoracic aortic dissection by noninvasive imaging procedures. *NEJM* 328:1-9, 1993.
18. Perloff JK: *Clinical Recognition of Congenital Heart Disease.* 2nd edition. Philadelphia, PA: W. B. Saunders Co, 1978.
19. Rehr RB: Cardiovascular nuclear magnetic resonance imaging and spectroscopy. *Current Problems in Cardiology,* Mosby/Year Book 16:131-215, 1991.
20. Roberts WC: Structure of the aortic valve in clinically isolated aortic stenosis. An autopsy study of 162 patients over 15 years of age. *Circ* 42:91-97, 1970.

21. Roberts WC, Perloff JK, Costantino T: Severe valvular aortic stenosis in patients over 65 years of age. A clinicopathologic study. *AJC* 27:497-506, 1971.

22. Roberts WC, Waller BF: Mitral valve "anular" calcium forming a complete circle or "O" configuration: clinical and necropsy observations. *AHJ* 101: 619, 1981.

23. Squire LF, Novelline RA: *Fundamentals of Radiology*. 4th edition. Cambridge, MA: Harvard University Press, 1988.

24. Steiner RM, Levin DC: Radiology of the Heart. In: Braunwald E, ed. *Heart Disease: A Textbook of Cardiovascular Medicine*. 4th edition. Philadelphia, PA: W. B. Saunders Co, 1992:204-234.

25. Uretsky BF, Rifkin RD, Sharma SC et al: Value of fluoroscopy in the detection of coronary stenosis: Influence of age, sex, and number of vessels calcified on diagnostic efficacy. *AHJ* 115:323-333, 1988.

CHAPTER 13

The Role of Echocardiography in Clinical Practice

Julius M. Gardin, M.D.

With the increased emphasis on cost-containment in medicine, it is essential for any procedure to demonstrate medical validity, cost-effectiveness, and effect on outcome. *Medical validity* might be defined as accurately predicting the absence or presence of a disease state. *Cost-effectiveness* implies that the cost of detecting the desired finding is reasonable—e.g., not requiring the performance of 1,000 tests to detect one true positive result. These first two standards have generally been applied over the years by prudent clinicians to management of their patients. A third important requirement, perhaps less strictly adhered to in the past, is the need to demonstrate that tests and procedures will *affect medical decision-making* so as to promote a positive (or avoid a negative) *outcome.*

It is within this context that a responsible clinician today must reaffirm his or her commitment to the "five-finger approach" emphasized by Dr. W. Proctor Harvey throughout his teaching career. Specifically, it is important to demonstrate for echocardiography, as for other procedures, that it appropriately represents the "fifth finger" for each clinical situation in which it is applied.

CARDIAC PEARL

Without question, echocardiography is rightly "here with us" and "to stay". It is a great technique which provides valuable information in the diagnosis and treatment of our patients- and it is without risk or discomfort. Several decades ago, it became evident that echocardiography should be mastered and applied. I'm not inferring that one needs an echocardiogram with every cardiovascular evaluation, but knowledge of its usefulness and limitations does provide an extra dimension in diagnosis.

W. Proctor Harvey, M.D.

The formal science of outcomes research is still in its early-stages with regard to its application to the evaluation of medical procedures, including echocardiography. However, I would like in this chapter to adopt the approach of outlining how echocardiography may be useful in various clinical syndromes. A complete discussion of the various echocardiographic methods and their application in clinical practice is the subject of textbooks and beyond the scope of this chapter. Nonetheless, it is my goal to provide brief guidelines and selected examples of how echocardiography may be appropriately used in clinical practice. In 1990, a Joint Task Force of the American College of Cardiology and the American Heart Association published an important overview and "Guidelines" for the clinical application of echocardiography. This chapter follows the format of these guidelines and attempts to provide additional perspectives and illustrative clinical examples.

Echocardiography, as applied clinically, refers to the use of reflected ultrasound for the diagnostic evaluation of patients with known or suspected cardiovascular disease. Echocardiography comprises various modalities, including M-mode and 2-D echocardiography, as well as pulsed wave, continuous wave, and color flow Doppler. These ultrasound modalities may be applied from transthoracic, transesophageal, intravascular, or intracardiac approaches.

This chapter will focus on the use of *transthoracic* echocardiographic imaging and Doppler flow

TABLE 1

Causes of Dyspnea in Which Echocardiography May Be Useful for Evaluation

I. **Coronary artery disease**
   A. Myocardial infarction
   B. Left ventricular aneurysm
   C. Ventricular septal defect
   D. Papillary muscle dysfunction
   E. Ruptured chordae tendineae

II. **Myocardial disease**
   A. Dilated cardiomyopathy
   B. Concentric left ventricular hypertrophy
     1. Hypertensive heart disease
     2. Infiltrative cardiomyopathy
   C. Hypertrophic cardiomyopathy

III. **Pericardial disease**
   A. Restrictive pericarditis
   B. Cardiac tamponade

IV. **Valvular heart disease**
   A. Aortic or mitral stenosis
   B. Valvular regurgitation

V. **Congenital heart disease**

VI. **Left ventricular diastolic dysfunction**

recording as applied to common clinical conditions—i.e., symptoms, findings, or syndromes. In this application, echocardiography has the advantage over various other imaging techniques in being non-invasive—i.e., not requiring catheter insertion or, generally, injections; non-dependent on ionizing radiation; portable, and capable of providing information regarding both cardiovascular structure and function.

Shortness of Breath

Shortness of breath, manifested as dyspnea at rest or on exertion, orthopnea, or paroxysmal nocturnal dyspnea, may be related to cardiac or pulmonary disease and, in some cases, to renal or hematologic disorders, etc. In patients in whom there is a strong suspicion of a possible cardiac cause, echocardiography can provide invaluable information regarding etiology, anatomy, and function. Table 1 provides a summary of some conditions associated with dyspnea in which echocardiography may be useful. As a general rule, echocardiography can be helpful in differentiating regional or global left ventricular (LV) systolic dysfunction (Figure 1) from predominant LV diastolic dysfunction (Figure 2). LV diastolic dysfunction is

generally secondary to etiologies listed in Table 1, such as coronary artery or myocardial disease. Diagnosis of LV diastolic dysfunction is often difficult to make because Doppler transmitral filling patterns which suggest diastolic dysfunction are dependent on age, preload, afterload, heart rate, P-R interval, blood pressure, gender, etc. Nonetheless, LV diastolic dysfunction is an important cause of congestive heart failure, reportedly present in one-third to one-half of patients presenting with dyspnea and other symptoms of heart failure.

Myocardial Disease

Primary cardiomyopathies are diseases of the heart muscle of which the etiology is unknown. Three general categories have been defined: dilated (or congestive), hypertrophic (including concentric and asymmetric), and infiltrative (or restrictive).

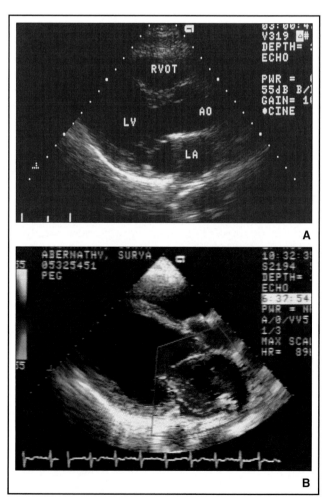

Figure 1. A: Parasternal long-axis view demonstrating normal left ventricle (LV), left atrium (LA), aorta (AO), and right ventricular outflow tract (RVOT) dimensions in a normal subject. **B:** Parasternal long-axis view demonstrating dilated left ventricle and left atrium with posteriorly directed mitral regurgitation jet (blue mosaic pattern) in a patient with dilated (congestive) cardiomyopathy.

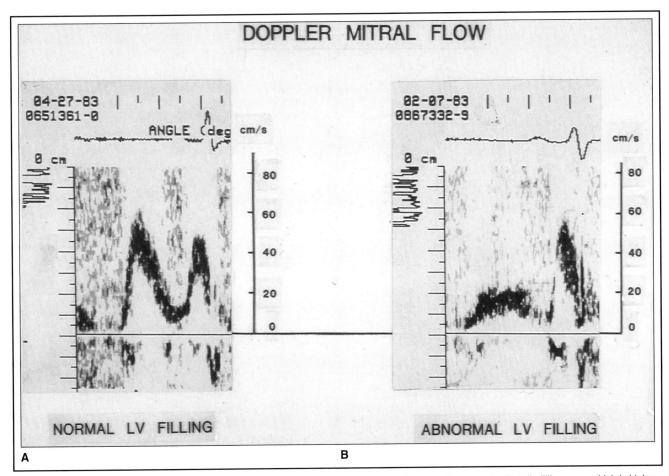

Figure 2. A: Pulsed Doppler mitral flow velocity recording in a younger normal individual demonstrating an early diastolic filling wave which is higher in velocity than is the late diastolic filling wave. **B:** Doppler mitral flow velocity recording demonstrating abnormally diminished early diastolic filling, peak filling velocity and deceleration, with an increased late diastolic peak filling velocity.

Echocardiography can define not only the cardiac anatomy, but also cardiac function and hemodynamics, in these disease states.

In dilated cardiomyopathies, echocardiographic imaging generally demonstrates ventricular dilation, reduced LV systolic function, and normal ventricular septal and LV posterior wall thickness. Figure 1B demonstrates typical findings of a dilated cardiomyopathy in a 45-year-old man with a history of alcohol abuse, hypertension, and a questionable history of a myocardial infarction. Occasionally, intraventricular or intra-atrial thrombi are detected. Doppler flow recording has been used to document mitral (and tricuspid) regurgitation, estimate systolic, diastolic or mean pulmonary artery pressure, and define patterns of left ventricular diastolic dysfunction. In addition, echocardiography can detect changes that occur after pharmacologic intervention—e.g., decreases in atrial or ventricular chamber dimensions, and changes in Doppler flow patterns.

Echocardiography is frequently used to differentiate *concentric* and *asymmetric* left ventricular hypertrophy. The causes for concentric hypertrophy include conditions such as hypertensive heart disease, infiltrative heart disease (see below), and aortic stenosis (see Figure 3). Primary *hypertrophic cardiomyopathy* is often characterized by asymmetric septal or LV free wall hypertrophy. The obstructive form can be detected by Doppler measurement of a gradient in the left ventricular outflow tract. Mitral regurgitation may also be detected by Doppler echocardiography. Figure 4 demonstrates typical echo-Doppler findings of hypertrophic cardiomyopathy and mild left ventricular outflow tract obstruction in a 28-year-old-man with a history of syncope and palpitations, a grade 3/6 systolic ejection murmur and a pseudo-infarction pattern on his electrocardiogram (Q waves in leads I, AVL and V_2 through V_6).

Restrictive cardiomyopathy may be produced by infiltrative diseases such as amyloidosis and hemachromatosis. Figure 3B demonstrates marked concentric left ventricular hypertrophy in a 52-year-old Vietnamese man with congestive heart failure and advanced amyloidosis. This condition is suggested

271

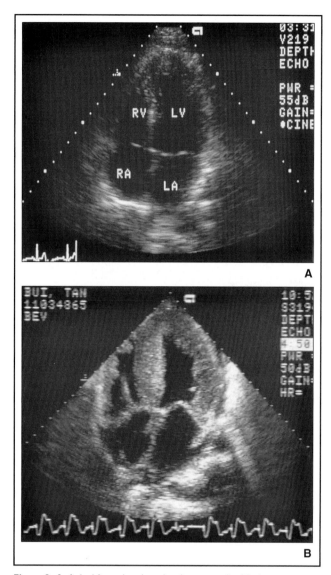

Figure 3. A: Apical four-chamber view in a normal subject demonstrating normal dimensions of the right and left atria and ventricles. **B:** Apical four-chamber view demonstrating marked concentric left ventricular hypertrophy in a patient with amyloidosis. Abbreviations as in Figure 1A.

by echocardiographically normal ventricular chamber dimensions, with normal-to-increased LV wall thickness. LV systolic function may be normal or abnormal. Doppler transmitral flow velocity recordings may show the characteristic restrictive pattern of *increased* peak early diastolic flow velocity, and reduced early diastolic deceleration time (in contrast to the *abnormal relaxation* pattern shown in Figure 2B). Echo-Doppler recordings can often help to differentiate this condition from constrictive pericarditis.

Pericardial Disease

Pericardial disease is usually characterized by *pericardial effusion,* pericardial thickening and/or

effusion, fibrous strands, etc., with or without tamponade or constriction. Pericardial effusions as small as 15cc in volume can be detected, and their size and location estimated (Figure 5). Whereas echocardiography is excellent at detecting even small effusions, it is not sufficiently specific in detecting increased pericardial thickness.

Echocardiography may help clarify a clinical suspicion of *cardiac tamponade.* Increased intrapericardial pressure occurring in this condition results in an increase in the distending force required for ventricular filling. Echocardiographic signs suggestive of tamponade include right atrial collapse at end-diastole—a sensitive but not specific sign; right ventricular compression in early diastole, a somewhat more specific sign; distention of the inferior vena cava not diminishing on deep inspiration. These findings can be augmented by pulsed Doppler flow recordings revealing marked inspiratory decreases in aortic and in transmitral peak early diastolic flow velocity, concomitant inspiratory increases in pulmonic and in transtricuspid early diastolic flow velocity; and a decrease in, or loss of expiratory diastolic transhepatic vein forward flow (Figure 6).

In *constrictive pericarditis,* echo and Doppler findings are often helpful in the diagnosis. Confirmatory, but nonspecific, findings include normal LV dimensions with abnormalities in ventricular septal and LV posterior wall motion in diastole, as well as mild atrial enlargement and premature opening of the pulmonic valve. Increased pericardial thickness is more specifically demonstrated by magnetic resonance imaging or ultrafast computed tomography than by echocardiography. Pulsed Doppler studies may reveal marked respiratory changes in the mitral and tricuspid velocity patterns, as well as increased peak transmitral early diastolic flow velocity with shortened deceleration time and often, decreased atrial filling velocity. These findings are helpful in establishing the pathophysiology of this disorder.

Native Valvular Heart Disease

Symptoms of valvular heart disease may include dyspnea, chest pain, murmur, syncope, etc.—in fact the whole clinical spectrum of cardiac symptoms. Echocardiography is useful in defining the etiology of the valvular lesion—e.g., rheumatic, degenerative, endocarditic, traumatic, etc.

Evaluation of valvular heart disease by echocardiography and Doppler techniques involves not only providing information about the intrinsic function of the valve, but also information about the anatomy of the atria, ventricles, and great vessels,

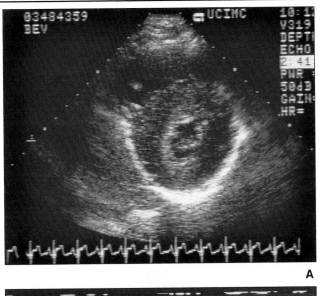

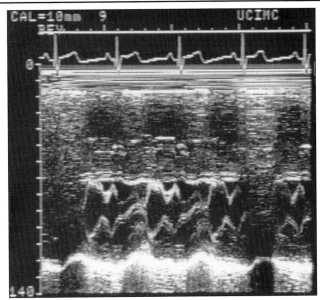

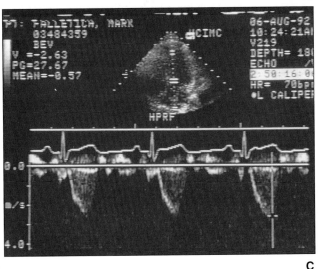

Figure 4. A: Parasternal short-axis view demonstrating diffuse increased thickness of the left ventricle, somewhat greater in the anteroseptal region, in a patient with hypertrophic cardiomyopathy. **B:** M-mode echocardiogram from the same patient revealing asymmetric septal hypertrophy and systolic anterior motion of the mitral valve. **C:** Pulsed Doppler recording in the left ventricular outflow tract in the same patient demonstrating a peak velocity of approximately 2.6 meters per second, corresponding to a subaortic gradient of approximately 28 mmHg. The late systolic peak of the flow velocity tracing is characteristic of the dynamic left ventricular outflow obstruction seen in hypertrophic cardiomyopathy.

as well as about possible concomitant findings such as thrombus, vegetation or effusion. With the addition of spectral and color Doppler techniques, very good estimates of valve gradients, areas, and degree of regurgitation are available from cardiac ultrasound.

In fact, in children or in adults in whom information regarding coronary artery anatomy is not necessary, Doppler echocardiographic data can often provide definitive information obviating the need for cardiac catheterization prior to cardiac surgery. Evaluation of *valvular stenosis* includes determining the degree of valve leaflet thickening, calcification, mobility, and subvalvular disease, as well as the valve area and gradient. This type of characterization may be extremely helpful, for example, in determining whether balloon catheter valvuloplasty is feasible in a patient with mitral stenosis. Specifically, increasing calcification and decreasing

leaflet mobility, as well as moderate or severe degrees of mitral regurgitation (determined by Doppler echocardiography), tend to make balloon valvuloplasty less feasible.

CARDIAC PEARL

Much information may be obtained from the echocardiogram concerning aortic valvular stenosis. The echocardiogram can frequently identify it as a bicuspid valve or an eccentric valve; this information is useful, of course, in establishing a congenital etiology rather than a rheumatic one. We have learned that a patient in the age group 50-55 years, particularly a man, with aortic stenosis (unassociated with a mitral valve lesion) has a high probability of having a congenital bicuspid valve. It was not too many years ago that many cases were erroneously diagnosed as

273

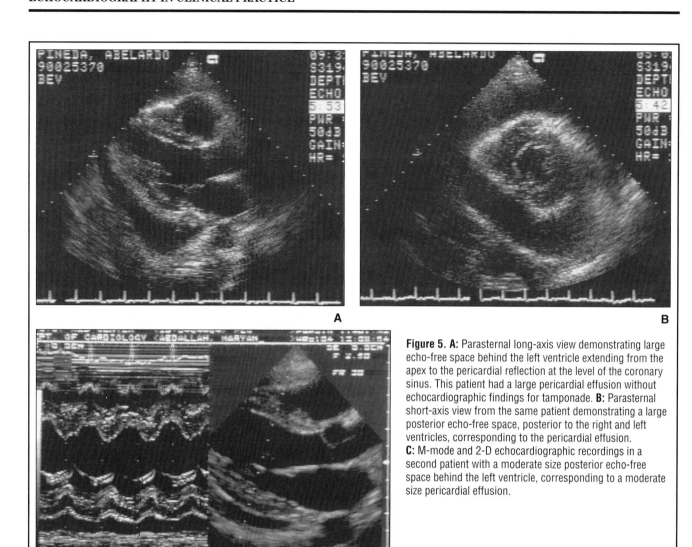

Figure 5. A: Parasternal long-axis view demonstrating large echo-free space behind the left ventricle extending from the apex to the pericardial reflection at the level of the coronary sinus. This patient had a large pericardial effusion without echocardiographic findings for tamponade. **B:** Parasternal short-axis view from the same patient demonstrating a large posterior echo-free space, posterior to the right and left ventricles, corresponding to the pericardial effusion. **C:** M-mode and 2-D echocardiographic recordings in a second patient with a moderate size posterior echo-free space behind the left ventricle, corresponding to a moderate size pericardial effusion.

rheumatic in etiology. Also, in this same age group, the possibility of calcification being present is quite high.

W. Proctor Harvey, M.D.

In *mitral stenosis,* the two most commonly employed ultrasound methods for quantitating valve area are direct planimetry from the parasternal short-axis view and the Doppler pressure half-time method (Figure 7). The latter method is based on the observation that the time required for the peak pressure gradient across the mitral valve to drop to one-half its peak value is the same time required for this peak Doppler velocity to fall to a velocity equal to this peak divided by the square root of two (based on the Bernoulli equation). Empirically, Holen and Hatle have found that the pressure half-time is 220 milliseconds for a mitral valve area of one square centimeter. Consequently, mitral valve area can be calculated as 220 millisec-

onds divided by the pressure half-time. Peak pressure gradients across native and prosthetic valves can be estimated using the Bernoulli equation, which in its simplified form states that:

$$\Delta P = 4V^2$$

where ΔP = transvalvular pressure gradient,
and V = peak velocity in the stenotic jet.

CARDIAC PEARL

Over the past several years, the unquestioned usefulness of the echocardiogram in diagnosis has become increasingly evident. This procedure is now firmly established as an extremely important diagnostic tool. I believe that all of us should become familiar with the technic of echocardiography and the tracings that result. Our diagnostic ability will improve without resorting to more sophisticated, often costly, laboratory proce-

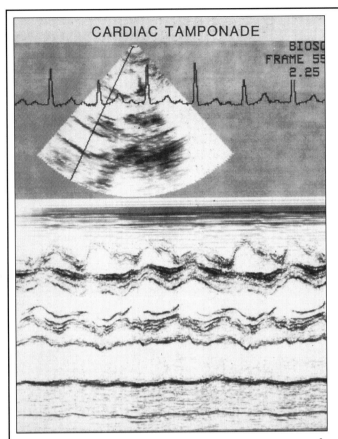

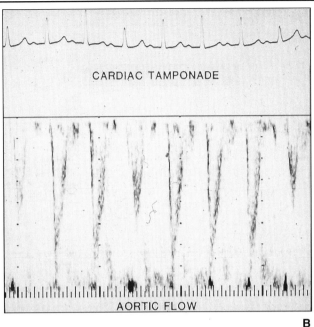

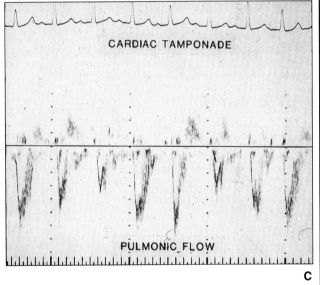

Figure 6. A: 2-D and M-mode echocardiographic images in a patient demonstrating: (1) large anterior and posterior echo-free spaces consistent with a large pericardial effusion, and (2) right ventricular compression (collapse) in early diastole. These findings are consistent with a diagnosis of cardiac tamponade. B: Markedly abnormal respiratory variation in pulsed Doppler aortic flow velocity (which is abnormally decreased during inspiration) in the same patient, characteristic of cardiac tamponade. C: Markedly abnormal respiratory variation in pulsed Doppler pulmonary artery flow velocity in the same patient.

dures that sometimes carry morbidity as well as mortality. This has certainly been true of echocardiography. In the past patients have been observed who had some features of a "tight" mitral stenosis. However, symptoms of dyspnea on effort suggested that these patients were still able to carry on fairly normal physical activities without significant complaint. Cardiac catheterization had been scheduled in both, but was cancelled when the echocardiogram revealed moderate degrees of mitral stenosis rather than the more advanced stenosis.

W. Proctor Harvey, M.D.

Figures 7A and 7B demonstrate echo-Doppler findings in a 40-year-old Hispanic male with mild rheumatic mitral stenosis and regurgitation who also demonstrated mild aortic stenosis and regurgitation. He presented with chest pain, dyspnea, and a systolic murmur. In *aortic stenosis,* although the Bernoulli equation can be applied to the estimation of peak and mean valvular gradients, the *continuity equation,* derived from Newton's principle of conservation of mass, is generally used to estimate aortic valve area. This equation is based on calculating the volumetric flow in the left ventricular outflow tract (by multiplying the mean or peak velocity times the outflow tract area) and dividing this

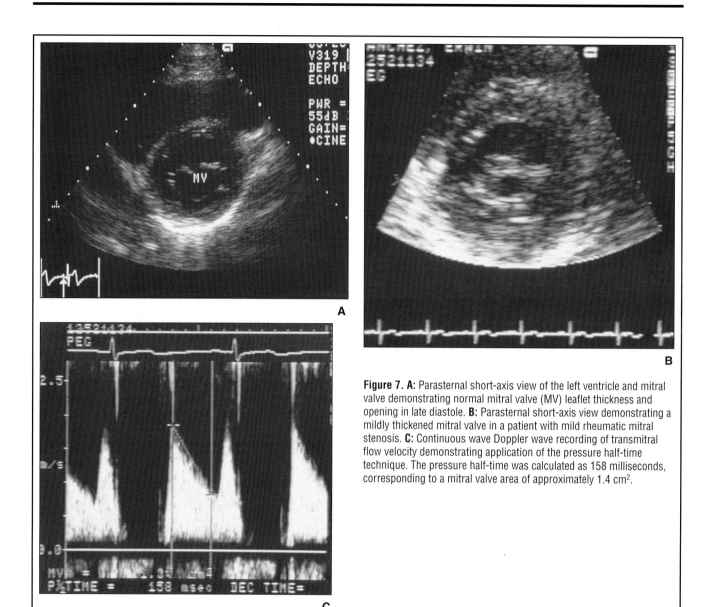

Figure 7. A: Parasternal short-axis view of the left ventricle and mitral valve demonstrating normal mitral valve (MV) leaflet thickness and opening in late diastole. **B:** Parasternal short-axis view demonstrating a mildly thickened mitral valve in a patient with mild rheumatic mitral stenosis. **C:** Continuous wave Doppler wave recording of transmitral flow velocity demonstrating application of the pressure half-time technique. The pressure half-time was calculated as 158 milliseconds, corresponding to a mitral valve area of approximately 1.4 cm².

quantity by the peak (or mean) velocity in the aortic stenotic jet. In general, these Doppler echocardiographic methods are quite accurate for estimating valve gradients and areas. Figure 8 presents two-dimensional echocardiographic findings in a 55-year-old Hispanic male with severe calcific bicuspid aortic valvular stenosis and concentric left ventricular hypertrophy.

The severity of *valvular regurgitation* can be estimated using spectral and color Doppler techniques. Such approaches as measuring the diameter or area of the color Doppler regurgitant flow jet—that is, the diameter of the aortic regurgitant jet at the aortic orifice, or the area of the mitral and tricuspid jets in the atrium—have been generally accurate in providing a semiquantitative estimate of regurgitation severity.

Other spectral Doppler techniques have also been useful in the quantitative or semiquantitative estimation of valvular regurgitation. These techniques include time velocity integral method, which estimates and compares volume flow calculated at different valves, comparison of areas under the reversed versus forward flow Doppler curves at the affected valve, and inspection of flows in the pulmonary veins for mitral regurgitation, and in the hepatic veins for tricuspid regurgitation. Figures 9A and 9B illustrate Doppler findings of moderate mitral regurgitation (posteriorly-directed jet) and severe aortic regurgitation in a 54-year-old man with a history of intravenous drug abuse and congestive heart failure who developed infective endocarditis on his aortic valve prosthesis. Figure 9C demonstrates two color Doppler aortic regurgita-

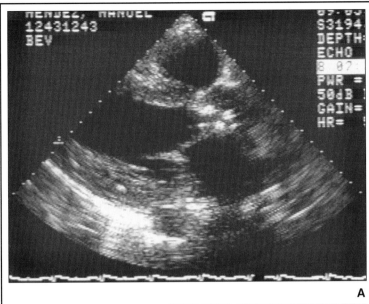

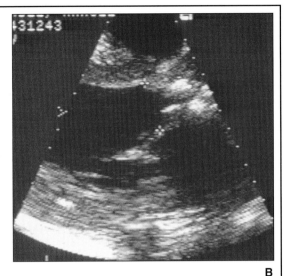

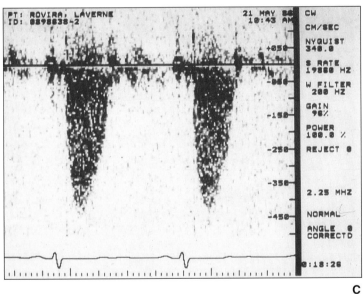

Figure 8. A: Parasternal long-axis view demonstrating calcified bicuspid aortic valve and concentric left ventricular hypertrophy in a patient with severe aortic stenosis. **B:** Method of measurement of diameter of left ventricular outflow tract at the level of the aortic anulus. This measurement is used in estimating the area of the left ventricular outflow tract in the calculation of aortic valve area using the continuity equation. **C:** Continuous wave Doppler recording in another patient revealing a peak flow velocity of 4.5 meters/sec, corresponding to a peak gradient of approximately 81 mmHg.

tion jets in a 61-year-old Vietnamese woman with calcific aortic stenosis and regurgitation, and concentric left ventricular hypertrophy, who presented in congestive heart failure.

Prosthetic Valve Dysfunction

Echocardiographic imaging can sometimes identify abnormalities of prosthetic valve function—e.g., reduced or erratic motion of a mechanical ball, disc, or bioprosthetic leaflet, or a vegetation or thrombus on the prosthetic valve or supporting structures. Echocardiographic imaging may also be useful in detecting the complications of native and prosthetic valve endocarditis, such as abscesses, fistulae, or ruptured chordae tendineae.

Figure 10 (Panels B, C, and D) presents an

example of a thickened and flail anterior porcine mitral valve leaflet, associated with severe mitral regurgitation. The patient is a 40-year-old Caucasian man with a past medical history of intravenous drug abuse and infective endocarditis. He presented most recently with a complaint of dyspnea and findings of congestive heart failure, and underwent a second mitral valve replacement after this endocardiographic study.

As is the case with native cardiac valves, spectral and color Doppler can be extremely helpful in identifying dysfunctional prosthetic valves. For example, gradients and effective orifice areas can be calculated using continuous wave (and sometimes pulsed) Doppler, applying the same equations as used for native valves—that is, the continuity

277

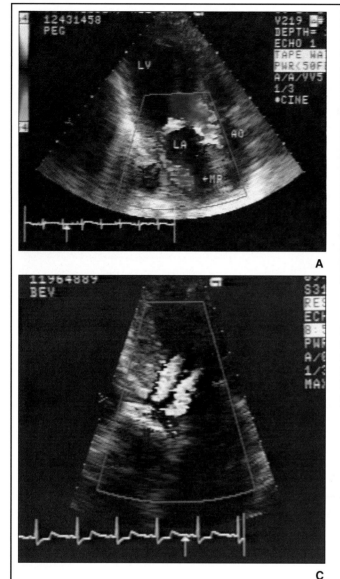

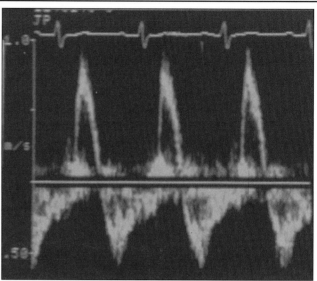

Figure 9. A: Apical long-axis view demonstrating a posteriorly directed color-Doppler mitral regurgitation jet in a patient with moderate mitral regurgitation. **B:** Pulsed Doppler abdominal aortic recording in the same patient as A, demonstrating holodiastolic flow reversal characteristic of moderate or severe aortic regurgitation. **C:** Color-Doppler recording in a different patient demonstrating two discrete aortic regurgitant jets. This patient also had severe calcific aortic stenosis.

equation for orifice areas in general, the pressure half-time method for mitral orifice area, and the velocity in the stenotic flow jet to estimate peak and mean transvalvular gradients. However, especially in the case of mechanical valves, vegetations, thrombi, or regurgitation may not be detected due to echocardiographic shadowing or reverberations which obscure structures behind the valve. In these cases, especially involving the mitral valve, transesophageal echocardiography may be helpful in imaging obstructive or regurgitant lesions.

It is important for the echocardiographer to become familiar with the different flow characteristics present for each class of mechanical and bioprosthetic valve. Specifically, "normal" transvalvular pressure gradients and effective orifice areas, as well as regurgitant characteristics, will vary among different valve types and sizes.

For example, it is not unusual for normally-functioning prosthetic tissue valves to exhibit mild central regurgitation. In contrast, detection of *bona fide* paravalvular regurgitation by color Doppler echocardiography suggests valvular dysfunction. Color Doppler jet areas may, for technical reasons, appear slightly larger when imaged from the transesophageal versus the transthoracic approach. In addition, recording of pulmonary venous flow, much more reliably performed from the transesophageal approach, may help in estimating the severity of mitral regurgitation.

Congenital Heart Disease

Echocardiography can provide essential information for the diagnosis and management of children

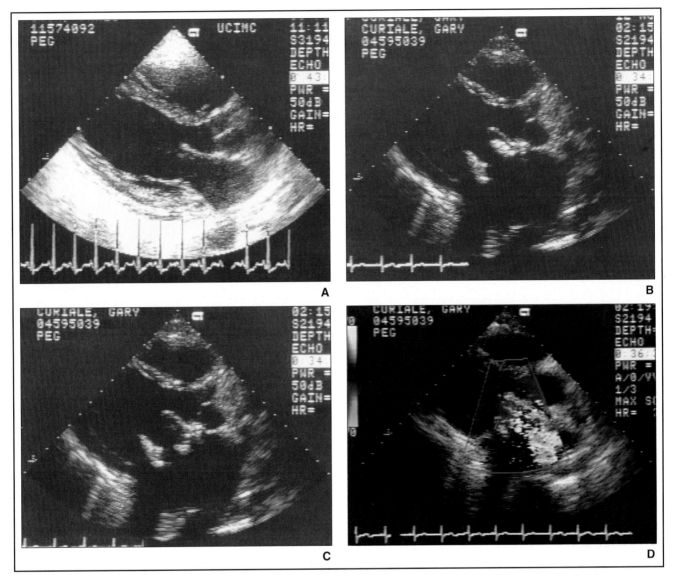

Figure 10. A: Parasternal long-axis view in a normal subject demonstrating normal opening of both native mitral valve leaflets in diastole.
B: Parasternal long-axis view demonstrating a prosthetic porcine mitral valve during diastole. Note the normal-appearing stents and the thickened tissue of the anterior leaflet. **C:** Parasternal long-axis view in systole from the same patient as in Panel B showing abnormal position of thickened, flail anterior porcine mitral leaflet. **D:** Color Doppler recording in parasternal long-axis view revealing color mosaic pattern occupying a large portion of the left atrium, probably reflecting severe regurgitation.

and adults with known or suspected congenital heart disease. In fact, some of the best-documented cost-effective indications for echocardiography occur in the context of congenital heart disease. This is true because echocardiography can often obviate the need for cardiac catheterization, as well as provide important serial information during the transition from fetus-to-newborn-to-infancy, or before, during, and after surgery, etc.

Although a detailed discussion of the uses of echocardiography in congenital heart disease is beyond the scope of this chapter, Figures 11, 12, and 13 demonstrate examples of three congenital conditions not uncommonly detected by echocardio-

graphy in the adult—namely, bicuspid aortic valve, subaortic membrane and patent ductus arteriosus. Figure 11, panels B and C, demonstrates a bicuspid aortic valve in a 34-year-old Caucasian male who also had moderate aortic regurgitation and mitral valve prolapse. Figure 12 displays echo-Doppler images from a man with a subaortic membrane and a peak subaortic gradient of nearly 90 mmHg. In Figure 13, spectral and color Doppler findings are illustrated in a baby girl with a patent ductus arteriosus. Table 2 lists generally agreed upon indications for echocardiography in the context of congenital heart disease, as cited by the American College of Cardiology/American Heart Association Task

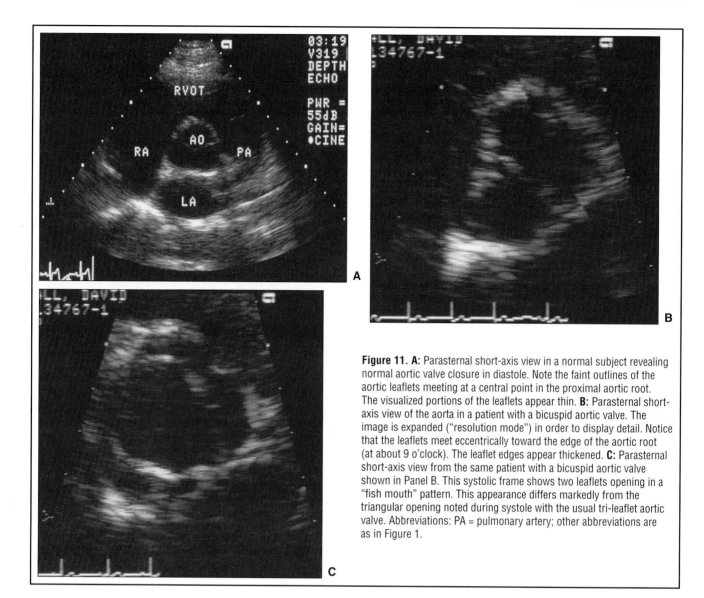

Figure 11. A: Parasternal short-axis view in a normal subject revealing normal aortic valve closure in diastole. Note the faint outlines of the aortic leaflets meeting at a central point in the proximal aortic root. The visualized portions of the leaflets appear thin. **B:** Parasternal short-axis view of the aorta in a patient with a bicuspid aortic valve. The image is expanded ("resolution mode") in order to display detail. Notice that the leaflets meet eccentrically toward the edge of the aortic root (at about 9 o'clock). The leaflet edges appear thickened. **C:** Parasternal short-axis view from the same patient with a bicuspid aortic valve shown in Panel B. This systolic frame shows two leaflets opening in a "fish mouth" pattern. This appearance differs markedly from the triangular opening noted during systole with the usual tri-leaflet aortic valve. Abbreviations: PA = pulmonary artery; other abbreviations are as in Figure 1.

Force on "Guidelines for the Clinical Application of Echocardiography."

Murmurs

In the evaluation of a cardiac murmur, the importance of a careful history and physical examination cannot be overemphasized. Information from these two of the "five fingers" can often establish whether a murmur is "innocent" (or functional) or has an organic basis. The electrocardiogram and chest x-ray, the third and fourth fingers, often add clarifying data. Echocardiography (a component of the large "fifth finger"!) may yield definitive diagnostic information, or important confirmatory information, regarding severity of disease, presence of concomitant disease, chamber sizes, ventricular function, etc. The echocardiogram often comprehensively delineates the pathoanatomy and severity of valvular stenosis and regurgitation, and shunt

---

TABLE 2
Indications for Echocardiography in Congenital Heart Disease

1. Cyanosis, respiratory distress, abnormal arterial pulses, or cardiac murmur in a neonate.
2. Loud or abnormal murmur or other abnormal cardiac finding in an infant or older child.
3. Failure to thrive in the presence of an abnormal or unusual cardiac finding.
4. Presence of a syndrome associated with cardiovascular disease and dominant inheritance or multiple affected family members.
5. Presence of a syndrome associated with heart disease, with or without abnormal cardiac findings, for which an urgent management decision is needed.
6. Cardiomegaly on chest radiograph.
7. Dextrocardia, abnormal pulmonary, or visceral situs.
8. Most ECG abnormalities.
9. Post-operative congenital or acquired heart disease.
10. Post-cardiac or cardiopulmonary transplant.

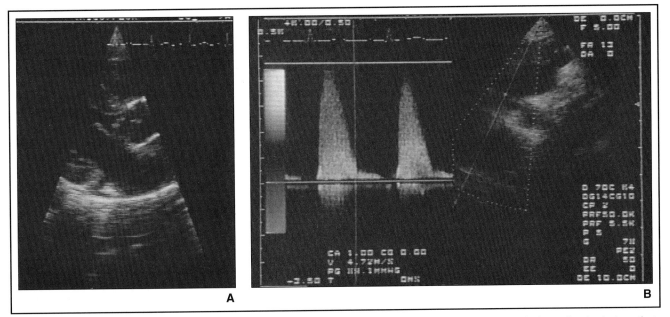

A

B

Figure 12. A: Parasternal long-axis view revealing a structure, corresponding to a subaortic membrane, in the left ventricular outflow tract of a patient with subaortic stenosis. **B:** Continuous wave Doppler recording of aortic flow in the same patient as in A. Peak velocity of 4.7 meters/sec corresponds to a peak subaortic gradient of approximately 89 mmHg.

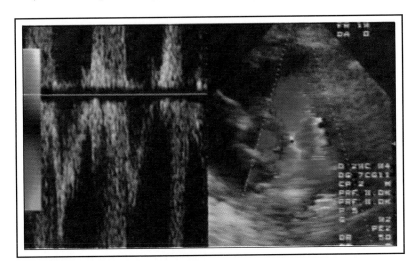

Figure 13. Right: Parasternal short-axis view demonstrating color Doppler flow in the main pulmonary artery in a patient with patent ductus arteriosus. The red region corresponds to shunt flow from the descending aorta into the main pulmonary artery. **Left:** Disturbed diastolic flow (increased spectral dispersion) in the main pulmonary artery, corresponding to the left-to-right shunt across the patent ductus arteriosus.

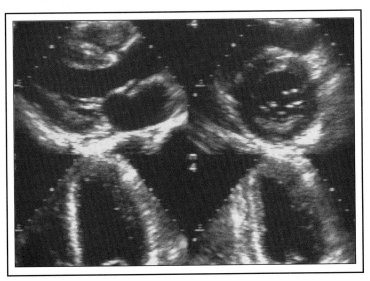

Figure 14. Quadrant screen display format in a subject at rest without ischemic heart disease. Left upper panel demonstrates the parasternal long-axis view, right upper panel depicts the parasternal short-axis view, left lower panel displays an apical four-chamber view, and right lower panel corresponds to an apical two-chamber view.

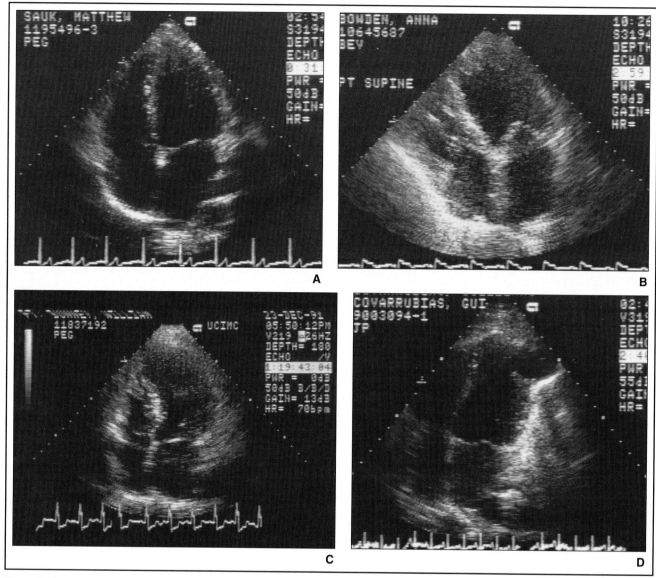

Figure 15. A: Apical four-chamber view from a normal subject recorded in systole and demonstrating normal chamber dimensions. **B:** Apical four-chamber view demonstrating an irregular thrombus at the apex of the left ventricle. **C:** Apical four-chamber view demonstrating apical dyskinesis consistent with a left ventricular apical aneurysm. **D:** Apical four-chamber view recorded in systole in a patient with a pseudoaneurysm of the left ventricular apex. Note the abrupt angulation of the out-pouching of the LV apex (at about 2 o'clock) compared with the smooth transition from normal LV to a true apical aneurysm in C. Not all layers of the ventricular wall are present in the pseudoaneurysm.

lesions, thus obviating the need for further invasive investigation.

Chest Pain

Echocardiography can be extremely helpful in diagnosis and management of patients with chest pain syndrome. Conditions in which echocardiography can provide suggestive or diagnostic findings include myocardial ischemia, aortic valvular or sub-valvular stenosis (including hypertrophic cardiomyopathy), mitral valve prolapse, pericarditis (pericardial effusion), aortic dissection, and acute pulmonary embolus.

In the case of myocardial ischemia, echocardiography has been used occasionally to image the coronary arteries—e.g., in Kawasaki's disease, or in atherosclerotic disease as a research tool from both transthoracic and transesophageal approaches. However, more commonly, echocardiography is used to image the *sequelae* of significant coronary arterial narrowing, either at rest or during exercise or pharmacologic stress imaging.

The typical myocardial ischemic sequelae detected by echocardiography include segmental left (and right) ventricular wall motion abnormalities, and absence of normal systolic thickening of

TABLE 3

Echocardiographically-Detectable Complications of Acute Myocardial Infarction

1. Pericardial effusion (pericarditis)
2. Intracardiac thrombus
3. Ventricular dilatation and remodeling, including infarct expansion or extension
4. Acute mitral regurgitation due to papillary muscle dysfunction or rupture, or rupture of chordae tendineae
5. Ventricular septal or left ventricular free wall rupture
6. Ventricular aneurysm or pseudoaneurysm

the affected myocardial regions. Various contrast agents are undergoing experimental animal and clinical trials and show promise for adding echocardiography to the array of techniques used to evaluate myocardial ischemia, perfusion, and viability.

Stress Echocardiography

Stress echocardiography is more sensitive than resting echocardiography in detecting myocardial ischemia. This is analogous to the situation in which exercise electrocardiography is more sensitive in detecting ischemic changes than is resting electrocardiography. Various modalities have been used to produce stress, including treadmill and (supine and upright) bicycle exercise, intracardiac pacing, and pharmacologic induction with dobutamine, dipyridamole, adenosine and other agents. The addition of digital recording and display of selected beats from multiple imaging views has greatly improved the diagnostic accuracy of all forms of stress echocardiography. Typically, images of the left ventricle obtained from the same view are displayed serially [e.g., at rest, during mild and peak stress, and post-stress in a four-image (quadrant) display mode]. Although judging subtle changes in segmental wall motion and wall thickening (e.g., worsening from hypokinesis to akinesis) is one of the most difficult distinctions made by the echocardiographer, viewing the images side-by-side at various stages of stress improves the ease and accuracy of diagnosis of ischemia.

Echocardiographic imaging adds to the cost of a stress electrocardiogram—although to a lesser extent than does radionuclide imaging. Therefore, it is important for there to be the *a priori* expectation that the addition of echocardiography to stress testing will provide accurate, cost-effective information which is useful in patient management. Clinical situations fulfilling these criteria include those in which the resting electrocardiogram is

abnormal and likely to obscure the diagnosis of exercise-induced ischemia—such as left bundle branch block or left ventricular hypertrophy with prominent ST-T wave changes. Figure 14 shows an example of a quadrant screen format display in a subject without ischemic heart disease.

Acute Myocardial Infarction

The ACC/AHA Task Force has summarized the potential indications for echocardiography in patients with acute myocardial infarction as follows: To assist in rapid diagnosis; to stratify patients into high- or low-risk categories; to monitor serial changes; to look for associated injury such as mitral regurgitation; and to diagnose complications of infarction. Figure 15 shows examples of patients with an LV apical aneurysm, an LV apical thrombus, and an apical pseudoaneurysm. Figure 15B, from a 69-year-old Caucasian woman who is status-post successful resuscitation from a cardiopulmonary arrest, demonstrates an LV apical thrombus in the presence of severe LV wall motion abnormalities. Figure 15C demonstrates an example of an LV apical aneurysm without a thrombus. Figure 15D depicts an LV pseudoaneurysm in a 29-year-old Hispanic man who had sustained multiple stab wounds and a ventricular laceration. Echocardiographic findings in acute myocardial infarction may include left or right ventricular segmental wall motion abnormalities, including diminished (hypokinesis), absent (akinesis), or paradoxical (dyskinesis) wall motion and/or decreased thickening, as well as decreased global LV function (ejection fraction). Other echocardiographically detectable complications of acute myocardial infarction are listed in Tables 1 and 3.

It should be noted that ventricular segmental wall motion abnormalities, and other findings detectable by echocardiography in acute myocardial infarction may be absent in patients with small infarcts. Furthermore, presence of these wall motion abnormalities may occur in the presence of acute or chronic ischemia (including myocardial *stunning or hibernation,* or scarring) and therefore are not diagnostic for infarction. Because segments adjacent to true myocardial infarction may be ischemic, stunned, hibernating, or tethered by the abnormally moving infarcted (scarred) myocardium, the *functional* infarct identified by echocardiography may overestimate the size of the true *anatomic* infarct in some patients. However, infarct size as measured by echocardiography has been shown to correlate with pathologic findings, thallium perfusion defects, contrast ventriculography and coronary angiography, peak creatinine kinase levels,

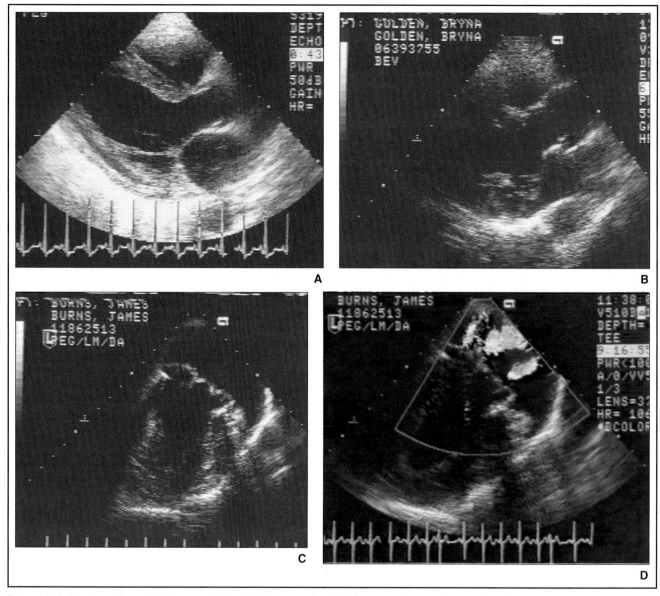

Figure 16. A: Parasternal long-axis view recorded in systole in a normal subject demonstrating normal coaptation of anterior and posterior mitral leaflets within the left ventricle. **B:** Parasternal long-axis view in a patient with mitral valve prolapse demonstrating coaptation of anterior and posterior leaflets within the left atrium, i.e., cephalad to an imaginary mitral annular line. **C:** Transesophageal echocardiogram recorded in a second patient from the longitudinal view and demonstrating definite prolapse of both anterior and posterior mitral leaflets behind an imaginary annular line. **D:** Color Doppler transesophageal recording in the same longitudinal plane from the same patient as in C demonstrating three distinct mitral regurgitation jets associated with mitral valve prolapse.

early and late complications, and mortality.

Serial echocardiography may be helpful in detecting changes occurring post-acute infarction, including infarct extension and expansion—both of which are associated with a worse prognosis. In addition, imaging of myocardial segments remote from those acutely infarcted can provide information regarding possible multivessel disease. Specifically, the absence of the expected compensatory hyperkinesis in apparently uninvolved remote segments suggests additional coronary artery involvement and is associated with an increased risk of post-infarction angina, progression in Killip classification, etc.

Mitral Valve Prolapse

Echocardiographic criteria for *mitral valve prolapse* have undergone extensive debate and evolution over the years. Most clinicians use a combination of either echocardiographic findings and/or the auscultatory presence of a mid-to-late systolic click (with or without a mid-to-late systolic murmur) as

T A B L E   4
Suspected Cardiac Sources of Embolism Detected by Echocardiography

1. Left ventricular thrombus
2. Left atrial (body or appendage) thrombus
3. Left atrial spontaneous contrast echos
4. Tumor (such as left atrial myxoma)
5. Valvular vegetation
6. Atrial septal aneurysm
7. Patent foramen ovale
8. Mitral valve prolapse
9. Calcific aortic stenosis
10. Protruding thoracic aortic (atherosclerotic) debris

evidence for the mitral valve prolapse syndrome. The most commonly accepted criteria for the diagnosis of mitral valve prolapse include the presence in the parasternal or apical long-axis views of *systolic superior displacement*—i.e, displacement into the left atrium of one or both mitral leaflets ≥3 mm above an imaginary annular line. In addition, some workers accept an additional M-mode echocardiographic criterion for prolapse, namely, the presence of late systolic displacement of one or both mitral leaflets ≥3 mm behind the C-D line. Previously used criteria, e.g., the displacement of one or more leaflets ≥3 mm into the left atrium in the apical four-chamber view, have been abandoned since it has been well-shown that the annulus is "saddle-shaped" and is actually non-planar in the apical four-chamber view. Workers have also shown by both M-mode and two-dimensional echocardiography that increased thickness of the body of the anterior or posterior mitral leaflet is associated with a higher incidence of complications, including death.

CARDIAC PEARL

Overdiagnosis and Underdiagnosis by Echocardiography- Some patients are diagnosed as having mitral valve prolapse because of misinterpretation of the echocardiogram.

We have seen a fair number of such patients. If a careful search for auscultatory findings of mitral valve prolapse fails to find any, repeat echocardiograms may also fail to show mitral valve prolapse.

A recent example was a 16-year-old high school football player who was evaluated because of a question as to whether he should play. History revealed that the echocardiogram taken by his physician was quoted as showing mitral valve prolapse. On physical examination, the patient was entirely asymptomatic and all findings were normal. When listening for auscultatory findings consistent with mitral valve prolapse, none were found. The echocardiogram was repeated at our institution with instructions to take extra time to search for any possibility of prolapse; the echocardiogram was completely normal. This made the decision about playing football quite easy.

The echocardiogram has been very useful in detecting mitral valve prolapse, but even in the best of hands, the echocardiogram may miss (or as pointed out previously, overdiagnose) mitral valve prolapse. When we were both participating in a medical symposium, I asked one of the country's experts in echocardiography how often echocardiography might miss the detection of mitral valve prolapse. He answered, "In about ten percent." I have seen many patients with mitral valve prolapse detected by the stethoscope, in whom the echocardiogram was interpreted as being normal. I have also seen a number of patients whose echocardiogram had initially been reported as negative, but the clinical auscultatory findings were diagnostic of prolapse, and on repeat echocardiogram positive findings of this condition were found.

W. Proctor Harvey, M.D.

Figure 16 displays images recorded in two patients with echocardiographic mitral valve prolapse. Figure 16B demonstrates mitral valve prolapse in a young (30-year-old) woman with a history of sleep apnea and arrhythmias. In contrast, Figures 16C and 16D depict definite mitral valve prolapse and mitral regurgitation in an older (78-year-old) Caucasian male with a history of a cerebrovascular accident.

Aortic Dissection

Transesophageal echocardiography has proven to be an extremely useful technique in the diagnosis of *acute aortic dissection.* In patients with this condition, time is of the essence in making a diagnosis and instituting (generally surgical) therapy.

In cooperative European trials, the sensitivity and predictive accuracy of transesophageal echocardiography for the diagnosis of aortic dissection were 98% and 99%, respectively. In addition to identifying the intimal flap, transesophageal echocardiography has been used to detect associated complications, e.g., pericardial effusion and aortic regurgitation, and to evaluate left ventricular size and function. Biplane and multiplane echocardiog-

285

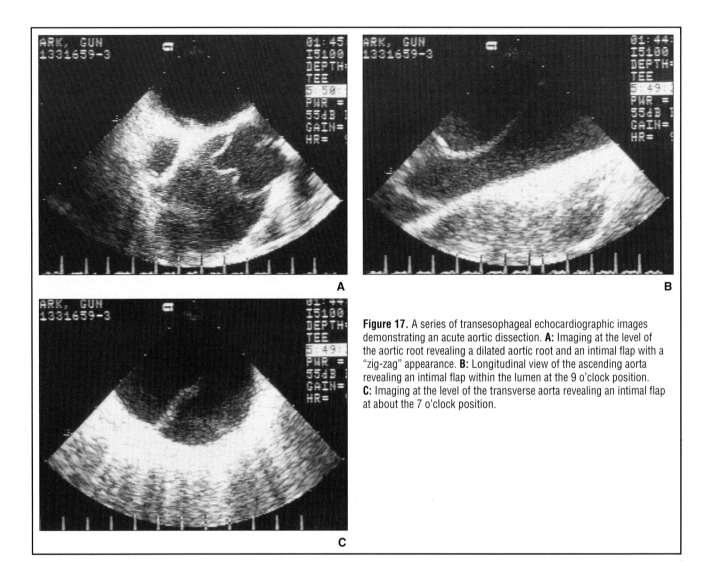

Figure 17. A series of transesophageal echocardiographic images demonstrating an acute aortic dissection. **A:** Imaging at the level of the aortic root revealing a dilated aortic root and an intimal flap with a "zig-zag" appearance. **B:** Longitudinal view of the ascending aorta revealing an intimal flap within the lumen at the 9 o'clock position. **C:** Imaging at the level of the transverse aorta revealing an intimal flap at about the 7 o'clock position.

raphy have offered an improvement over the single-plane technique, especially in delineating the proximal ascending aorta, which has proved, not uncommonly, to be a "blind spot" using the single-plane transducer.

Figure 17 shows transesophageal echocardiographic images in a 52-year-old Korean woman with an aortic dissection who presents with chest pain radiating toward her back, unrelieved by nitroglycerin, and absent pulses in her feet.

Stroke and Transient Ischemic Attack

It is estimated that cerebral embolism of cardiac origin is responsible for approximately 15% of ischemic strokes. Conditions which have been associated with a cardiac source for embolism, and which can be detected by echocardiography, include those outlined in Table 4.

Transthoracic 2-D echocardiography has a sensitivity of 75% to 95%, and a specificity of approximately 85%, for detecting *left ventricular* thrombi that are >4 mm in diameter. Although transthoracic echocardiography has a sensitivity and specificity of approximately 70% to 90% for identifying thrombi in the *body* of the left atrium, the sensitivity for thrombi in the left atrial *appendage* is <15 percent. On the other hand, transesophageal echocardiography has been reported to have a sensitivity for diagnosing *left atrial* and *atrial appendage thrombi* in the range of 95%. Figure 18 demonstrates a large left atrium with a large thrombus in a patient with mitral stenosis. In patients under 45 years of age, patent foramen ovale, atrial septal defect, and mitral valve prolapse may be important etiologies for cardiac embolic stroke or transient ischemic attack.

Spontaneous contrast echoes in the left or right atrium have been reported to be a pre-thrombus condition. Left-sided spontaneous contrast echoes are frequently seen in patients with mitral stenosis or prosthetic mitral valves. Figure 19A demonstrates spontaneous contrast echoes in the left

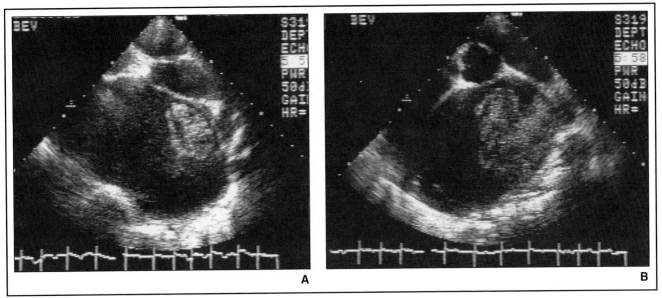

Figure 18. A: Parasternal long-axis view in a patient with mitral stenosis and a large left atrium which contains a large left atrial thrombus. **B:** Parasternal short-axis view in the same patient with mitral stenosis revealing the large thrombus in the large left atrium.

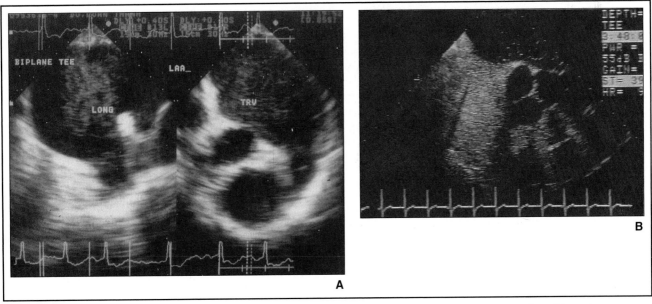

Figure 19. A: Biplane transesophageal echocardiographic images (longitudinal and transverse views) reveal a large left atrium with spontaneous contrast echoes in a patient with mitral stenosis. **B:** Transesophageal echocardiographic image in the transverse view reveals dense echo contrast in the right atrium (lower left) from a peripheral venous agitated saline injection. A few contrast "microbubbles" are seen to have crossed the atrial septum and to be present in the left atrium (center of image, just above the circular aorta).

atrium of a patient with mitral stenosis.

Preliminary data from Kichura and colleagues suggests a high incidence of recurrent cardiogenic embolic events (13%) during a 17+ month follow-up period in patients with patent foramen ovale. However, a recent study by Louie has shown that a patent foramen ovale can be detected by transesophageal echocardiography in 22% of patients *without* a prior stroke. Therefore, the prognostic importance of patent foramen ovale and the role of

treatment to prevent neurologic events remains to be further evaluated. Figure 19B demonstrates a right-to-left shunt of contrast microbubbles across a *patent foramen ovale* in a patient in whom a peripheral venous saline injection was performed in conjunction with a transesophageal echocardiogram.

Patients in whom an *atrial septal aneurysm* had been detected in association with a previous TIA or stroke reportedly had a 23% incidence of recurrent embolism over a 20-month period. Because of the

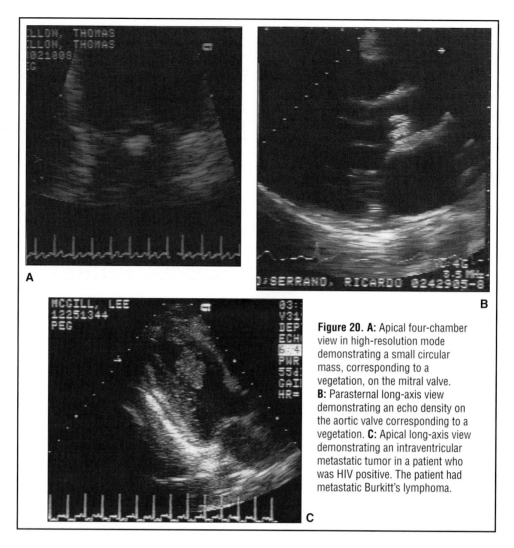

Figure 20. A: Apical four-chamber view in high-resolution mode demonstrating a small circular mass, corresponding to a vegetation, on the mitral valve. **B:** Parasternal long-axis view demonstrating an echo density on the aortic valve corresponding to a vegetation. **C:** Apical long-axis view demonstrating an intraventricular metastatic tumor in a patient who was HIV positive. The patient had metastatic Burkitt's lymphoma.

association of *protruding atherosclerotic debris* in the thoracic aorta with postoperative stroke, some surgeons are performing pre- or intraoperative transesophageal or epicardial echocardiography to identify these potential cardiac sources of embolus.

Syncope

It is often difficult to differentiate primary neurogenic (or other) causes of syncope from syncope of cardiac origin. Syncope of cardiac origin is most commonly the result of vasodepressor reflexes, or of cardiac tachyarrhythmias or bradyarrhythmias. Echocardiography is generally helpful in only relatively uncommon causes of cardiac syncope, all of which should be suggested by a murmur or other cardiac findings on the physical examination. The causes of cardiac syncope in which echocardiography may be helpful include severe aortic stenosis and hypertrophic obstructive cardiomyopathy, and masses such as atrial myxoma or vegetations. Figure 20A demonstrates a mitral valve vegetation in a 50-year-old Caucasian male with a history of

alcohol abuse, while Figure 20B demonstrates an aortic valve vegetation in another patient. A large (mobile) left ventricular mass, which was attached to the ventricular septum, is shown in Figure 20C. The patient was a 26-year-old Caucasian male with a history of HIV-positivity and Stage 4B Burkitt's lymphoma with widespread metastases (including to the heart).

In general, echocardiography may not be cost-effective if performed as an initial test in patients with syncope unless the physical examination suggests significant heart disease. In patients with unexplained syncope, after ruling out non-cardiac causes and after evaluating possible cardiac arrhythmias, the decision about performing echocardiography should be made on an individual basis since the yield is generally low.

Peripheral Emboli

The yield of echocardiography in patients with peripheral emboli is generally higher than it is in evaluation of patients with syncope, because the heart is the likely source for these relatively large arterial emboli. Both transesophageal and transthoracic echocardiography may have a role in the evaluation. Transesophageal echocardiography is especially helpful if the expected source of the embolus is a left atrial appendage thrombus, or there is suspicion of a paradoxical embolus passing through the right heart and across a patent foramen ovale (Figure 19B). Other causes for peripheral emboli in which echocardiography may be helpful include vegetative endocarditis, protruding ascending aortic atheroma, and aortic aneurysm or dissection

(Figures 17, 20, and 21). Figure 21 demonstrates two examples of thoracic aortic atheromata.

Edema

As is true for syncope, peripheral edema can also be caused by many cardiac and non-cardiac conditions. According to the ACC/AHA Task Force, echocardiography can be recommended in any patient who has evidence for an elevated central venous pressure, significant valvular or coronary artery disease, cor pulmonale, or pulsus paradoxus. In contrast, echocardiography "cannot routinely be recommended in patients with mild peripheral edema who have no evidence for an increase in central venous pressure, or clinical findings of heart disease, because the diagnostic yield in such patients is expected to be low." Uncommon cardiac disorders which may cause peripheral edema and can be detected by echocardiography in patients with abnormal physical findings include amyloid heart disease, restrictive cardiomyopathy, and constrictive pericarditis.

Arrhythmias

Echocardiography can define ventricular and atrial anatomy in patients with documented cardiac arrhythmias, information that may be useful in the management of these patients. For example, in a patient with atrial fibrillation, it is useful to know the left atrial size to help determine the likelihood that attempted cardioversion will be successful, as well as the likelihood for thrombus formation. Similarly, echocardiography helps to define left ventricular anatomy (such as presence or absence of left ventricular hypertrophy) and global and regional systolic function. This information can assist in selecting antiarrhythmic agents, deciding whether or not to perform invasive electrophysiologic studies, etc. Further, increasing degrees of ventricular dysfunction may be associated with a greater need to treat specific arrhythmias. A corollary of this observation is that minor arrhythmias, such as isolated premature ventricular beats, often occur without any structural heart disease and do not require any further evaluation. In such instances, the diagnostic yield of an echocardiogram may be low, except perhaps in revealing mitral valve prolapse, and unlikely to change management of the patient. Obviously, as in other cases, good clinical judgement is necessary to avoid unnecessary testing.

Conclusion

Echocardiography has proven to be an extremely useful noninvasive method for evaluating patients

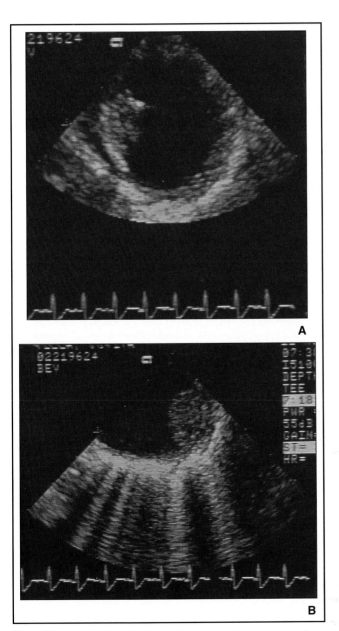

Figure 21. Transesophageal echocardiogram revealing examples of thoracic aortic debris in two patients. **A:** Protruding atherosclerotic debris can be seen at the 9 o'clock position. **B:** A protruding mass, most likely a thrombus, can be seen at the 3 o'clock position.

with known or suspected cardiac abnormalities. In its various applications, which include resting and stress echocardiography, and Doppler, transesophageal, epicardial, intracardiac and intravascular, echocardiography can provide accurate, and often unique information about cardiac structure and function. It is the challenge of the clinician to order echocardiographic studies in a cost-effective manner, while providing the best care for his or her patients.

Selected Reading

1. Adhar GC, Nanda NC: Doppler echocardiography: Part II: Adult valvular heart disease. *Echocardiography* 1:219-241, 1984.

2. Appleton CP, Hatle LK, Popp RL: Demonstration of restrictive ventricular physiology by Doppler echocardiography. *JACC* 11:757-768, 1988.

3. Benjamin EG, Levy SMD, Anderson KM, et al: Determination of Doppler indexes of left ventricular diastolic function in normal subjects (The Framingham Heart Study). *AJC* 70:508-515, 1992.

4. Brandenberg RO, Chazov E, Cherian G, et al: Report of the WHO/ISFC task force on definition and classification of cardiomyopathies. *Circ* 64:437A-438A, 1981.

5. Burstow DJ, Oh JK, Bailey KR, Seward JB, Tajik J: Cardiac tamponade: Characteristic Doppler observations. *Mayo Clin Proc* 64:312-324, 1989.

6. Cardiogenic brain embolism. Cerebral Embolism Task Force. *Arch Neurol* 43:71-84, 1986.

7. Castello R, Pearson AC, Lenzen P, Labovitz A: Effect of mitral regurgitation on pulmonary venous velocities derived from transesophageal echocardiography color graded pulsed Doppler imaging. *JACC* 17: 1499-1506, 1991.

8. Diebold B, Peronneau P, Blanchard D, et al:: Noninvasive quantification of aortic regurgitation by Doppler echocardiography. *BHJ* 49: 167-173, 1983.

9. Dressler FA, Sharma AK, et al: Short-term follow-up of patients with atrial septal aneurysm: incidence of cerebrovascular events. *Circ* 84:II-452, 1991.

10. Dougherty AH, et al: Congestive heart failure with normal systolic function. *AJC* 54:778-782, 1984.

11. Erbel R, Daniel W, Visser C, et al: Echocardiography in diagnosis of aortic dissection. *Lancet* 1:457-461, 1989.

12. Ewy GA, Appleton CP, DeMaria AN, et al: ACC/AHA Guidelines for the clinical application of echocardiography: A report of the American College of Cardiology/American Heart Association Task Force on Assessment of Diagnostic and Therapeutic Cardiovascular Procedures (Subcommittee to Develop Guidelines for the Clinical Application of Echocardiography). *JACC* 76:1505-1528, 1990. *Circ* 82:2323-2345, 1990.

13. Feigenbaum H: *Echocardiography* (Fifth Edition). Philadelphia: Lea & Febiger, 1994.

14. Feigenbaum H: Echocardio diagnosis of pericardial effusion. *AJC* 26:475-479, 1970.

15. Gibson RS, Bishop HL, Stamm RB, et al: Value of early 2-D echocardiography in patients with acute myocardial infarction. *AJC* 49:1110-1119, 1982.

16. Ginzton LE, Conant R, Brizendine M, Lee F, Mena I, Laks MM: Exercise subcostal two-dimensional echocardiography: A new method of segmental wall motion analysis. *AJC* 53:805-811, 1984.

17. Harvey JR, Teague SM, Anderson JL, et al: Clinically silent atrial septal defects with evidence for cerebral embolization. *Ann Intern Med* 105:695-697, 1986.

18. Hatle L, Angelsen B: *Doppler Ultrasound in Cardiology: Physical Principles and Clinical Applications* (Second Edition). Philadelphia: Lea & Febiger, 1985.

19. Hatle L, Angelsen B, Tromsdal A: Noninvasive assessment of atrioventricular pressure half-time by Doppler ultrasound. *Circ* 60:1096-1104, 1979.

20. Hatle LK, Appleton CP, Popp RL: Differentiation of constrictive pericarditis and restrictive cardiomyopathy by Doppler echocardiography. *Circ* 79:357-370, 1989.

21. Helmcke F, Nanda NC, Hsiung MC, et al. Color Doppler assessment of mitral regurgitation with orthogonal planes. *Circ* 75:175-83, 1987.

22. Holen J, Simonsen S: Determination of pressure gradient in mitral stenosis with Doppler echocardiography. *BHJ* 41: 529-535, 1979.

23. Kapoor WN, Karpf M, Weiand S, Peterson JR, Levey GS: A prospective evaluation and follow-up of patients with syncope. *NEJM* 309:197-204, 1983.

24. Klein AL, Oh JK, Miller FA, et al: Two-dimensional and Doppler echocardiographic assessment of infiltrative cardiomyopathy. *J Am Soc Echo* 1:48-59, 1988.

25. Kichura G, Camp A, Ofili EO, Castello R, Ploesser M, Labovita AJ: High incidence of cardiogenic embolic events during follow-up in patients with patent foramen ovale identified by transesophageal echocardiography. *Circ* 84 (4):II-451, 1991.

26. Klein AL, Hatle LK, Burstow DJ, et al: Doppler characterization of left ventricular diastolic function in cardiac amyloidosis. *JACC* 13:1017-1026, 1989.

27. Krivokapich J, Child JS, Dadourian BJ, Perloff JK: Reassessment of echocardiographic criteria for diagnosis of mitral valve prolapse. *AJC* 61:131-135, 1988.

28. Levine RA, Stathogiannis E, Newell JB, Harrigan P, Weyman AE: Reconsideration of echocardiographic standards for mitral valve prolapse: Lack of association between leaflet displacement isolated to the apical four-chamber view and independent echocardiographic evidence of abnormality. *JACC* 11:1010-1119, 1988.

29. Louie EK, Konstadt SN, Rao TLK, Scanlon PJ. Transesophageal echocardiographic diagnosis of patent foramen ovale in adults without prior stroke. *Circ* 84 (4):II-451, 1991.

30. Marks AR: Identification of high-risk and low-risk subgroups of patients with mitral valve prolapse. *NEJM* 320:1031-1036, 1989.

31. Matsamura M, Shah P, Kyo S, Omoto R: Advantages of transesophageal echo for correct diagnosis on small left atrial thrombi in mitral stenosis. *Circ* 80 (suppl II):II-678, 1989.

32. Meltzer RS, Visser CA, Fuster V: Intracardiac thrombi and systemic embolization. *Ann Intern Med* 104:689-698, 1986.

33. Mohr-Kahaly S, Erbel R, Rennollet H, et al: Ambulatory follow-up of aortic dissection by transesophageal two-dimensional and color-coded Doppler echocardiography. *Circ* 80:24-33, 1989.

34. Musewe NN, Smallhorn JF, Benson LN, Burrows PE, Freedom RM: Validation of Doppler-derived pulmonary arterial pressure with ductus arteriosus under different hemodynamic states. *Circ* 76:1081-1091, 1987.

35. Nixon JV, Narahara KA, Smitherman TC: Estimation of myocardial involvement in patients with acute myocardial infarction by two-dimensional echocardiography. *Circ* 62:1248-1255, 1980.

36. Otto CM, Pearlman AS: Doppler echocardiography in adults

with symptomatic aortic stenosis: Diagnostic utility and cost effectiveness *Arch Int Med* 148:2553-2560, 1988.

37. Peller OG, Wallerson DC, Devereux RB: Role of Doppler and imaging echocardiography in selection of patients for cardiac valvular surgery. *AHJ* 114:1445-1461, 1987.

38. Perry GJ, Helmcke F, Nanda NC, Byard C, Soto B: Evaluation of aortic insufficiency by Doppler color flow mapping. *JACC* 9:952-9, 1987.

39. Picano E, Lattanzi F, Masini M, et al: Usefulness of the dipyridamole-exercise echocardiography test for diagnosis of coronary artery disease. *AJC* 62:67-70, 1988.

40. Presti CF, Armstrong WF, Feigenbaum H: Comparison of echocardiography at peak exercise and after bicycle exercise in evaluation of patients with known or suspected coronary artery disease. *J Am Soc Echo* 1:119-126, 1988.

41. Rakowski H, Sasson Z, Wigle ED: Echocardiographic and Doppler assessment of hypertrophic cardiomyopathy. *J Am Soc Echo* 1:31-47, 1988.

42. Reid CL, Chandraratna AN, Kawanishi DT, Kotlewski A, Rahimtoola SH: Influence of mitral valve morphology on double-balloon catheter balloon valvuloplasty in patients with mitral stenosis: Analysis of factors predicting immediate and 3-month results. *Circ* 80 (3):515-524, 1989.

43. Reisner SA, Meltzer RS: Normal values of prosthetic valve Doppler echocardiographic parameters: A review. *J Am Soc Echo* 1:201-210, 1988.

44. Rokey R, Sterling LL, Zoghbi WA, et al: Determination of regurgitant fraction in isolated mitral or aortic regurgitation by pulsed Doppler two-dimensional echocardiography: *JACC* 7: 1273-1278, 1986.

45. Ryan T, Armstrong WF, O'Donnell JA, Feigenbaum H: Risk stratification after acute myocardial infarction by means of exercise two-dimensional echocardiography. *AHJ* 114: 1305-1316, 1987.

46. Ryan T, Vasey CG, Presti CF, O'Donnell JA, Feigenbaum H, Armstrong WF: Exercise echocardiography: Detection of coronary artery disease in patients with normal left ventricular wall motion at rest. *JACC* 11:993-999, 1988.

47. Schnittger I, Bowden RE, Abrams J, Popp RL: Echocardiography: Pericardial thickening and constrictive pericarditis. *AJC* 42:388-395, 1978.

48. Shah PM: Echocardiography in congestive or dilated cardiomyopathy. *J Am Soc Echo* 1:20-30, 1988.

49. Shen WK, Khandheria BK, Oh JK, et al: Quantitative correlation between echocardiographic wall-motion abnormalities and left ventricular infarct size determined by pathology. *Circ* 74(suppl II):II-479, 1986.

50. Shibata J, Takahashi H, Itaya M, et al: Cross-sectional echocardiographic visualization of the infarcted site in myocardial infarction: Correlation with electrocardiographic and coronary angiographic findings. *J Card* 12:885-894, 1982.

51. Soufer R, Wohlgelernter D, Vita NA, et al: Intact systolic left ventricular function in clinical congestive heart failure. *AJC* 55:1032-1036, 1985.

52. Talano JV, Gardin JM: *Two Dimensional Echocardiography.* New York, Grune and Stratton, 1983.

53. Tunick PA, Kronzon I. Protruding atherosclerotic plaque in the aortic arch of patients with systemic embolization: A new finding seen by transesophageal echocardiography. *AHJ* 120:658-660, 1990.

54. Wayne HH: Syncope: Physiologic considerations and an analysis of the clinical characteristics in 510 patients. *Am J Med* 31:418-438, 1961.

55. Weiss JL, Buckley BH, Hutchins GM, Mason SJ: Two-dimensional echocardiographic recognition of myocardial injury in man: Comparison with post-mortem studies. *Circ* 63: 401-408, 1981.

56. Weyman AE: *Echocardiography* (Second Edition). Philadelphia, Lea and Febiger, 1994.

291

Doppler Echocardiography: Appropriate Use in the Evaluation of the Patient with a Heart Murmur

Paul T. Cochran, M.D.

Since 1955, when Edler first reported the use of ultrasound in the diagnosis of heart disease, technologic advances have given us Doppler echocardiography which now is the most commonly used cardiac diagnostic imaging test. Initially, these studies were used only by cardiologists and were interpreted in the context of the "five-finger approach" made famous by Dr. W. Proctor Harvey to evaluating the patient. Today, widespread dissemination of the tools allowing high-resolution studies and the training of skilled ultrasonographers have resulted in many, if not most, tests ordered by primary care physicians and other specialists who are not cardiologists. The cardiologist's role thus may become that of a detached (from the patient) reporter of diagnostic impressions derived from looking at the imaging study in the abstract.

Considerable mischief can result whenever Doppler echocardiographic studies are either ordered or interpreted without the physician integrating the information derived into a "five finger approach" to the evaluation of the individual patient. By recognizing the strengths and limits of the Doppler echo assessment, the physician who has carefully reviewed the patient's history, performed a careful physical examination, and assimilated the electrocardiographic and radiographic findings is strongly prepared to derive a diagnosis and plan of management.

CARDIAC PEARL

Echocardiography is one of the great advances in the diagnosis of cardiovascular disease. However, there is also misuse-Echocardiography is often unnecessary or used for the wrong purpose.

Personally observed have been requests for a color Doppler echocardiogram and on the request sheet under "Reason for Request" was written "Question murmur". I have been told of similar situations in other echocardiographic laboratories. Sad, but true.

One's stethoscope is the obvious and accurate answer to determining the presence and cause of most murmurs. The aforementioned "Reason for Request" emphasizes the great need in medicine today to emphasize the basics of cardiovascular evaluation, the "five finger" approach, which includes a careful detailed history and physical examination, electrocardiogram, X-ray and simple laboratory tests that can be done in the physician's office or at the bedside. We need to bring the patient from the "back burner" up to the front.

W. Proctor Harvey, M.D.

Doppler Echocardiography

Strengths

1) The presence, severity, and etiology of valvular lesions can be defined.

2) Intracardiac shunts are evident and can be sized.

3) Size of cardiac chambers and thickness/ function of ventricles can be determined.

4) Complications of valvular lesions (left atrial thrombus, endocarditis) can be imaged.

5) Information about intracardiac hemodynamics can be inferred.

Potential Pitfalls

1) Good studies demand good tools and good ultrasonographers.

2) Some patients cannot be optimally studied due to body habitus.

3) Valvular regurgitation is evident by Doppler in many "normals."

4) Regurgitant lesion quantitation is difficult; doesn't correlate well with hemodynamic severity.

With these caveats in mind, this chapter will address the proper role of Doppler echocardiography in the examination of the patient with a heart murmur.

Systolic Murmurs

Systolic murmurs are the most commonly recognized in clinical practice; the physician hearing a systolic murmur must first decide if the murmur represents pathology or not with attention directed to defining precisely the characteristics of the murmur. Where is it best heard? Where does it radiate? Is it early, mid, late, or holosystolic? How does it respond to posture, Valsalva, respiration, or isometric tension? Are there "pearls" in the history, arterial or venous pulses, chest x-ray, or ECG that compel the examiner to reassess the auscultatory findings? Going back to the patient to listen again, the good clinician finds, is often more appropriate than ordering expensive diagnostic tests.

Mid-Systolic Murmurs

Innocent Systolic Murmur

The physiologic (innocent, functional) murmur and its characteristics have been detailed in earlier chapters. Doppler echocardiography is normal in these patients. It should be emphasized that when history, physical, ECG, and chest x-ray findings lead to the diagnosis of a physiologic murmur, it is not necessary to proceed to Doppler echocardiography to "prove" the clinician correct. Doppler echocardiography is indicated, however, in situations where careful examination leaves one with the sometimes difficult differential diagnostic possibilities of physiologic murmur versus mild obstructions to the right or left ventricular outflow tracts. Here, the Doppler echocardiogram may be critical in identifying mild valvular aortic or pulmonic stenosis and the need for endocarditis prophylaxis.

CARDIAC PEARL

The following features are characteristic of innocent murmurs. The murmur is short, occurring in the early to mid portions of systole or in midsystole. They may have a musical, vibratory "buzzing", "twanging" quality (Still's murmur). The innocent murmur is best heard over the pulmonic area or left sternal border, particularly the third left sternal border, but may also, in the same patient, be heard along the lower left sternal border, apex and aortic area. It is found very frequently in children and generally disappears in adulthood. However, an innocent murmur may be present in adults, including the elderly.

Uncommonly, an innocent murmur occurs in diastole related to low-frequency vibrations coincident with and following a physiological third heart sound. Also, filling sounds and atrial (S_4) and ventricular S_3 gallops in close proximity may produce a diastolic rumble that infrequently has been confused with mitral stenosis.

An innocent murmur may be continuous, as evidenced by the venous hum that is a common finding in children, pregnancy, anemia, thyrotoxicosis, etc. A continuous murmur (mammary hum) may also be heard over engorged breasts with pregnancy, particularly in the nursing breast. A continuous murmur (uterine souffle) is heard normally over the abdomen of the pregnant mother in the latter part of pregnancy. An innocent murmur may be heard with the cardiorespiratory murmur.

An innocent murmur may be heard as a normal finding over arteries (subclavian and/or carotid) in the neck, particularly when there is active blood flow that might occur with exercise in the hearts of children, pregnancy, thyrotoxicosis, etc. On the other hand, the murmur becoming more prolonged or continuous may be the first indication as to the presence of arterial occlusive disease. In instances in which there still is doubt as to whether the murmur is innocent or significant, the passage of time may aid in making the diagnosis. The otherwise asymptomatic patient, therefore, should be followed at intervals over the years; then time itself generally will aid in making the differentiation accurate. If the patient has an ejection sound in systole, this is an immediate clue that one is dealing with a murmur of significant pathology. The presence of abnormal splitting of the second heart sound (as with atrial septal defect) or the increase in intensity of the second heart sound indicating the presence of pulmonary hypertension may be another clue to underlying heart disease. Also, the presence of atrial and ventricular diastolic gallops may aid in affording additional clues as to the presence of associated heart disease. In brief, the careful total cardiovascular evaluation will afford evidence if the murmur is not innocent.

Too often, patients with innocent murmurs have been classified as having significant heart disease. One can cite numerous examples, particularly in past years, in which patients' lives have been severely altered and psychologically damaged because an innocent systolic murmur was thought to be significant heart disease. Because of the finding of this murmur, some patients have been restricted in physical activity, with the result that they have become "cardiac cripples." Remembered is a priest who, on the basis of a systolic murmur detected in his early teen age was diagnosed as having heart disease; he was also told that he probably would not live beyond the age of 25. With the passage of years, he had no cardiac symptoms and, until several years before the age of 25, apparently had been well adjusted. Then, he had numerous nonspecific cardiac complaints; subsequently, he was admitted to the hospital for evaluation, and it was at this time that an innocent systolic murmur was diagnosed. He had believed that at age 25 he would die, and this had become fixed in his mind. When told that he had no heart disease, he had very mixed emotions- one of great relief and, at the same time, one of great anger and resentment toward the physician who had made the diagnosis and prognosis. Another example was that of a young girl who was seen for evaluation of a systolic murmur. She now was in her late teens and had many nonspecific complaints. When asked to walk upstairs (I was accompanying her), she stated that she was not allowed to walk up stairs because of her heart. Despite this, we walked up the stairs without difficulty. Her evaluation revealed an innocent murmur; however, by this time, she had so much iatrogenic disease that, despite the reassurance, it was going to take considerable time to convince her that she had a completely normal heart and, therefore, could lead a normal life.

It is wise to tell the parents of a child, as well as the child, that a murmur is present, that it may well be detected on other examinations and that this murmur is innocent, of no significance.

It is evident and of great importance that the total cardiovascular picture must be evaluated carefully in diagnosing an innocent murmur. This entails a very careful detailed history and physical examination, electrocardiogram, x-ray and laboratory tests, often including echocardiogram. As a rule, most of this can be done by the physician in his office, and cardiac catheterization usually is not necessary to arrive at this diagnosis.

W. Proctor Harvey, M.D.

Left Ventricular Outflow Tract

The murmur of *left ventricular outflow tract obstruction* may be generated by valvular, subvalvular discrete, subvalvular dynamic, or supravalvular mechanisms. As discussed in earlier chapters, it is possible to distinguish valvular from subvalvular dynamic obstruction (hypertrophic obstructive cardiomyopathy) on the basis of the physical findings. Doppler echocardiography is essential in these conditions to define precisely the level of obstruction and provide excellent quantitation of the severity of obstruction.

• Valvular Aortic Stenosis

Doppler echocardiography is helpful in determining etiology: M-mode and 2-D imaging provide distinguishing features of degenerative, congenital, and rheumatic valvular deformity (Figure 1). The severity of obstruction can be reliably estimated: the aortic valve area (AVA) is the most important measure in the severity of aortic stenosis. In normal adults, AVA is 2.0-3.0 sq cm; in mild aortic stenosis, it measures greater than 1.0 sq cm, in moderate aortic stenosis it is 0.75-1.0 sq cm, and is less than 0.75 sq cm in severe aortic stenosis. The combination of 2-D echocardiography and continuous wave Doppler can be utilized to calculate the AVA in the great majority of patients with aortic stenosis (Figure 2 and Figure 3). The complications of valvular aortic stenosis, left ventricular hypertrophy, and dilatation as well as systolic and diastolic function can be measured, and presence or absence of pulmonary hypertension can be assessed.

CARDIAC PEARL

The use of Doppler echocardiography is rapidly increasing, as is the practical usefulness of this procedure. People are living longer today, and we are seeing more and more elderly patients with aortic stenosis whose degree of obstruction can be determined without performing cardiac catheterization.

W. Proctor Harvey, M.D.

In addition, coexisting lesions can be identified; unsuspected mitral valve disease, hypertrophic cardiomyopathy, or endocarditis can be recognized by

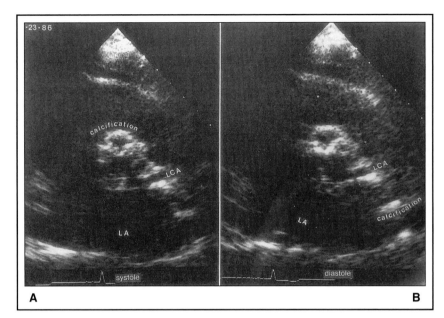

Figure 1-A. Degenerative valvular aortic stenosis: (A) The short axis echoes of the Ao show a calcified valve, and severely limited opening and closing. **(B)** There is a strong echo at the inlet of the left main coronary artery (LCA) which may also indicate calcification. *(From Wada)*

careful 2-D, colorflow, and Doppler evaluation (Figure 4).

There are several caveats to remember, however, in the Doppler echocardiographic study of valvular aortic stenosis. Inattention to careful technique allows the AVA to be overestimated (usually by failure to record the maximal velocity through the stenotic jet) or underestimated (by errors in measuring the left ventricular outflow tract). In certain patients, it may be very difficult to get diagnostic information due to body habitus — simply put, one should never attempt to make crucial measures of poorly visible data.

• **Hypertrophic Obstructive Cardiomyopathy (HOCM)**

Doppler echocardiography establishes the diagnosis of HOCM by defining the eccentric distribution of left ventricular hypertrophy, systolic anterior motion of the mitral valve, and localizing the intraventricular gradient in the left ventricular outflow tract (Figure 5). Continuous wave Doppler allows quantitation of the dynamic gradient across the outflow tract and the response of the gradient to provocative maneuvers as well as therapeutic efforts, with the need for cardiac catheterization to establish a diagnosis obviated. It has been shown that mitral regurgitation coexists in many patients with HOCM, occuring during mid-to-late systole and rarely is of independent hemodynamic significance. Pulsed Doppler confirms the reduced compliance of the left ventricle that effects symptoms of dyspnea in HOCM patients.

Pitfalls of Doppler echocardiography may be experienced if spurious measure is taken of the interventricular septum (by taking a tangential echocardiographic "cut" through the interventricular septum) and thus, may give an inappropriate diagnosis of asymmetric septal hypertrophy. "Pseudo"-systolic anterior motion of the interventricular septum may be seen in hyperdynamically contracting left ventricles and may be mistaken for the systolic apposition of the anterior mitral leaflet and the interventricular septum of HOCM. Also, the diagnosis may be missed unless the ultrasonographer is alerted to the possibility of the diagnosis

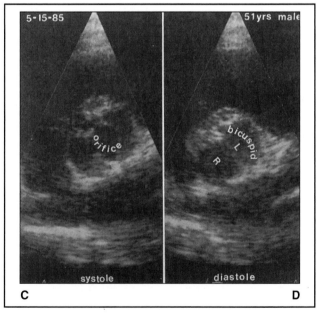

Figure 1-B. Bicuspid Aortic Stenosis: Short-axis 2D-Echos of the Ao show a vertical-type bicuspid valve and absence of the noncoronary cusp. **(C)** During systole the aortic orifice is vaguely seen. **(D)** In diastole, closure of the bicuspid valve is observed. *(From Wada)*

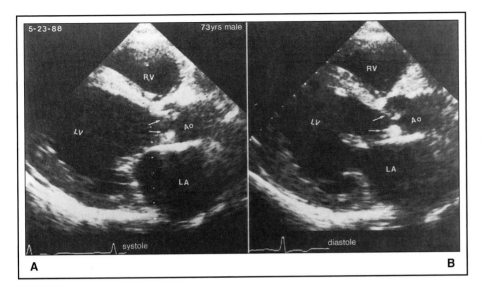

Figure 1-C. Rheumatic valvular aortic stenosis: Long-axis echoes from a 73-year-old man with rheumatic valvular heart disease. **(A)** During systole, limited opening of the aortic valve with heavy calcification can be seen. **(B)** During diastole, the aortic valve remains open (white arrows) suggesting the presence of aortic regurgitation. *(From Wada)*

and fails to perform a meticulous examination that may require provocative maneuvers like the Valsalva maneuver.

• Discrete Subaortic Stenosis

This uncommon congenital anomaly may be suspected on clinical grounds when a young patient with the signs of severe obstruction to left ventricular ejection has no response of the mid-systolic murmur to physical maneuvers. Also, there is almost always the coexistent murmur of aortic regurgitation that results from distortion of the aortic annulus by the thin membrane or subvalvular ridge that exists in the subaortic region. Doppler echocardiography is diagnostic in this situation by demonstrating, in the apical and parasternal long-axis views, the obstructing muscular ridge or thin membrane characteristic of this entity (Figure 6).

• Other Levels of Obstruction to Left Ventricular Ejection

Doppler echocardiography is the diagnostic test of choice in recognizing and defining other levels of obstruction, be they supravalvular or due to hypoplasia of the ascending aorta or coarctation. By careful study, this technique is definitive in most of the infants and children in whom this differential is most critical. Examination from the suprasternal, high parasternal, and subcostal areas is essential.

Right Ventricular Outflow Tract

• Valvular Pulmonic Stenosis

Congenital deformity of the pulmonary valve is responsible for an estimated 80% of the cases of obstruction to right ventricular ejection. The diagnosis is usually easily made based upon the physi-

cal findings, chest x-ray, and ECG. Doppler echocardiography is superb in definition and quantitation of the severity of the lesion as well as the differentiation of valvular from subvalvular or supravalvular sites of the obstruction.

• Atrial Septal Defect (ASD)

The pulmonic ejection murmur that is the result of increased pulmonary blood flow of an ASD often escapes detection in infancy and adulthood. If the examiner hasn't listened carefully to the second heart sound, or if the characteristic wide "fixed" splitting of the second heart sound has been muted by coexistent lung disease or obesity, this systolic murmur is often mistaken for that of a physiologic murmur. Doppler echocardiography becomes a major benefit in resolving this diagnostic question. In both pediatric and adult patients, the sensitivity and specificity of this technique are excellent. The location of the shunt is ostium secundum in the majority of adult patients and is generally easily identified by color flow Doppler (Figure 7). Associated right ventricular volume overload and abnormal interventricular septal motion are hallmarks of ASD, and transesophageal echocardiography with color flow imaging and contrast agents may be necessary to localize sinus venous defects, patent foramen ovale, and partial anomalous pulmonary venous connection.

Size of the defect imaged by subcostal views generally correlates closely with that measured at surgery; when correlated with the remainder of the "five fingers," most patients can be referred for surgery without the need for cardiac catheterization unless it is needed for evaluation of coexistent cardiac abnormalities.

The pitfall of diagnosing ASD by Doppler echo-

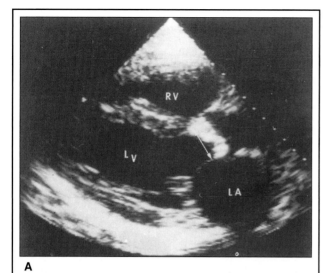

A

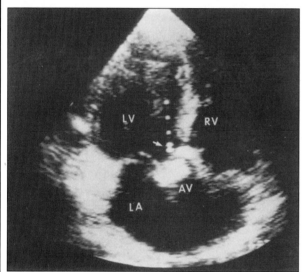

B

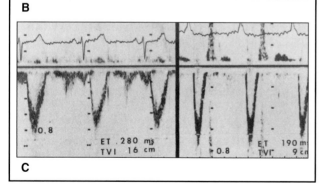

C

Figure 2. Stroke volume across the aortic valve needs to be calculated to determine aortic valve area. This is done by measuring the left ventricular outflow tract (LVOT) diameter and flow velocity. **A.** Measurement of LVOT diameter: from the systolic freeze-frame of the parasternal long-axis view, the distance from where the anterior aortic cusp meets the ventricular septum to the point where the posterior cusp meets the anterior mitral leaflet. The line between the two cusps is almost perpendicular to the anterior wall of the aortic root. **B.** Measurement of LVOT velocity from the apical long-axis view; the pulsed-wave sample volume *(arrow)* is located 3 to 5 mm proximal to the aortic valve (AV). If it is too close to the aortic valve, prestenotic acceleration jet velocity may be recorded. **C.** Determination of LVOT true velocity integral (TVI). Two examples of LVOT velocity spectra are shown. TVI is determined by tracing the velocity envelope, and is equal to the sum of individual velocities of the Doppler spectrum. Although both spectra show a similar peak velocity (0.8 m/sec), the TVI is markedly different due to the difference in ejection time (ET). Once the LVOT diameter (D) and TVI are determined, flow across the LVOT is calculated as follows:

$$LVOT = LVOT\ area \times LVOT\ TVI$$
$$= (D/2)^2 \times \pi \times LVOT\ TVI$$
$$= D^2 \times 0.785 \times LVOT\ TVI$$

The following table shows LVOT areas calculated from various LVOT diameters.

LVOT diameter (D) (cm)	Area ($D^2 \times 0.785$) (cm^2)
1.5	1.77
1.6	2.01
1.7	2.27
1.8	2.54
1.9	2.84
2.0	3.14
2.1	3.46
2.2	3.80
2.3	4.15
2.4	4.52
2.5	4.90

(From Seward JB, and Tajik AJ. The Echo Manual, Little Brown and Company. Boston, 1993.)

cardiography when no ASD exists has become unlikely with the advent of color flow imaging. Formerly, in imaging systems without color flow capability, it was possible to misinterpret the dropout of echoes in the thin atrial septum for a defect. Likewise, it is important to remember that the right ventricular volume overload pattern seen in ASD is also manifested by other causes such as pulmonic or tricuspid regurgitation. The greatest

potential source of misinformation from the Doppler echocardiographic evaluation comes from attempts to quantify the ratio of pulmonary to systemic blood flow (Qp/Qs). This derives from difficulties in the measurement of the diameter of the pulmonary artery. Any error in the measurement of the diameter of the pulmonary artery is squared in the final result; thus, Qp/Qs estimates are poor, at best, in many such reports.

Holosystolic (Pansystolic) Murmurs

Prototypes are those of mitral and tricuspid regurgitation and ventricular septal defect.

Mitral Regurgitation

• Strengths of Doppler Echocardiography

In those patients in whom careful history, physical exam, review of ECG, and chest x-ray have led to diagnosis of mitral regurgitation (MR), Doppler echocardiography is a powerful tool in:

1. Defining etiology: The echocardiographic characteristics distinguish congenital (cleft mitral leaflet), myxomatous degeneration, rheumatic, infectious, ischemic, cardiomyopathic, and traumatic (chordal rupture) causes of MR.

2. Documenting left ventricular size and func-

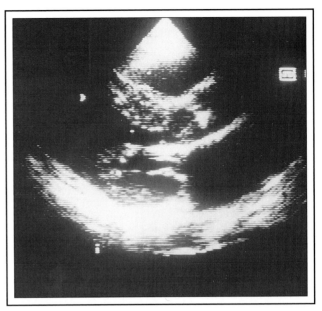

Figure 4. Still frames of 2-D echo from a parasternal long-axis view in a patient with clinical findings of hypertrophic obstructive cardiomyopathy. The echo shows asymmetric septal hypertrophy but also thickened and calcified aortic valve leaflets and marked thickening of the anterior leaflet of the mitral valve.

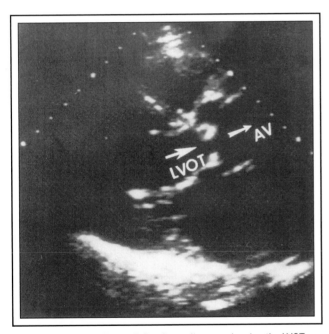

Figure 3. Still-frame from a 2-D echocardiogram showing the LVOT and the stenotic aortic valve (AV). The continuity equation states that the flow across the LVOT is the same as the flow across the aortic valve ("what goes in must come out"). Therefore,

LVOT flow = AV flow

LVOT D^2 x 0.785 x LVOT TVI = AVA x AV TVI

$$AVA = LVOT\ D^2\ x\ 0.785\ x\ \frac{LVOT\ TVI}{AV\ TI}$$

where D = diameter, and AVA = aortic valve area.

Since flow duration across the LVOT and the aortic valve is the same, the TVI ratio is similar to their peak velocity (V) ratio. Therefore, the continuity equation can be simplified to

$$AVA = LVOT\ D^2\ x\ 0.785\ x\ \frac{LVOT\ V}{AV\ V}$$

(From Oh JK, Seward JB, and Tajik AJ. The Echo Manual, Little Brown and Company. Boston, 1993.)

tion: This is especially true for clinical decision-making regarding the timing of surgery in a patient with few or no symptoms. As chronic MR causes progressive enlargement of the left ventricle, serial echocardiographic studies may document deteriorating left ventricular contractility (increasing left ventricular end systolic and end diastolic volumes and declining ejection fraction) portending a greater perioperative mortality and a poorer postoperative left ventricular function and survival.

3. Assessing severity of MR: Quantitation of the regurgitant volume and the regurgitant fraction can be obtained by technically demanding quantitative Doppler techniques (Figure 8). In routine clinical practice, semi-quantitative assessment is most common using the Doppler color flow jet area or the regurgitant jet area to left atrial area ratio. The clinician must recognize, however, that these semi-quantitative measures are variable depending on systolic arterial pressure, left atrial size, and left ventricular systolic function. Doppler color flow imaging is helpful in quantitating MR due to ischemic or functional causes where the regurgitant jet is central, but should not be used to quantitate MR in those patients where the regurgitant jet is eccentric.

4. Identifying complications of MR: Quantitation of left atrial enlargement and presence of atrial thrombus; availability of transesophageal echocardiography is of particular benefit in defining presence of vegetations on an already deformed mitral

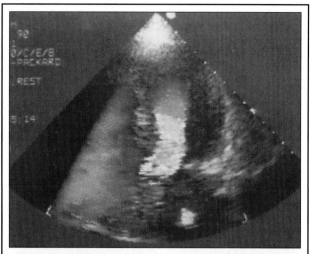

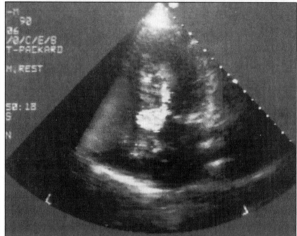

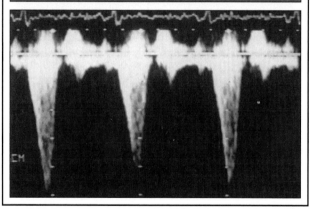

Figure 5. Demonstration of the dynamic character of an outflow tract obstruction by color-coded and continuous wave Doppler echocardiography. Narrowing of the jet during ejection from early systole (top) to late systole (middle) is shown. The site of end-systolic obstruction is characterized by the zone of flow acceleration (recognized by increasing brightness of blues that alias to red) just proximal to this zone and the turbulent jet (displayed as a mosaic of colors with admixtures of green) just distal to it. Note the angular deviation of the outflow tract and the gradual increase in jet diameter with increasing distance from the maximal septal thickening, which, in this case, is the site of mitral-septal contact (middle). Continuous wave Doppler recordings (bottom) show a gradual increase of velocity with a midsystolic acceleration and a sharp peak in late systole. Note the substantial beat to beat variability with maximal velocities between 4.0 and 4.9 m/s, corresponding to a variation of the pressure gradient between 64 and 96 mm Hg. *(From Schwammenthal, et al. Predication of the site and severity of hypertrophic cardiomyopathy. JACC 20;966, 1989.)*

valve. Findings of pulmonary hypertension, as estimated from the peak velocity of tricuspid regurgitation, is a helpful clue to severe MR.

5. Defining coexisting lesions: Particularly in patients with congenital mitral insufficiency, Doppler echocardiography may detect unsuspected coexistent intracardiac shunts or valvular abnormalities marked by the predominant lesion of MR. Careful attention to segmental wall motion may also provide clues to coexisting coronary disease that has damaged the left ventricle.

• Pitfalls of Doppler Echocardiography

1. Over-diagnosis of mitral regurgitation: Two factors contribute to an excessive reporting of "mitral regurgitation." First is the over-utilization of the technique of Doppler echocardiography in the assessment of patients with physiologic murmurs. Many studies are done "to rule out pathology." They are ordered by specialists other than cardiologists and, unfortunately, replace the careful cardiovascular physical examination that should be a rate-limiting step in the decision process preceding the deci-

sion to obtain a Doppler echocardiographic study. The second contributing factor to over-diagnosis is the exquisite sensitivity of Doppler ultrasound in detecting mitral regurgitation that is clinically silent through valves that appear echocardiographically normal. The term "physiological mitral regurgitation" conveys the concept that such a finding is present in the majority of healthy subjects. Unfortunately, the differentiation between physiological and mild pathological mitral regurgitation will not always be clear. Careful reporting of the Doppler echocardiography study and its integration into the individual patient's treatment plan are essential.

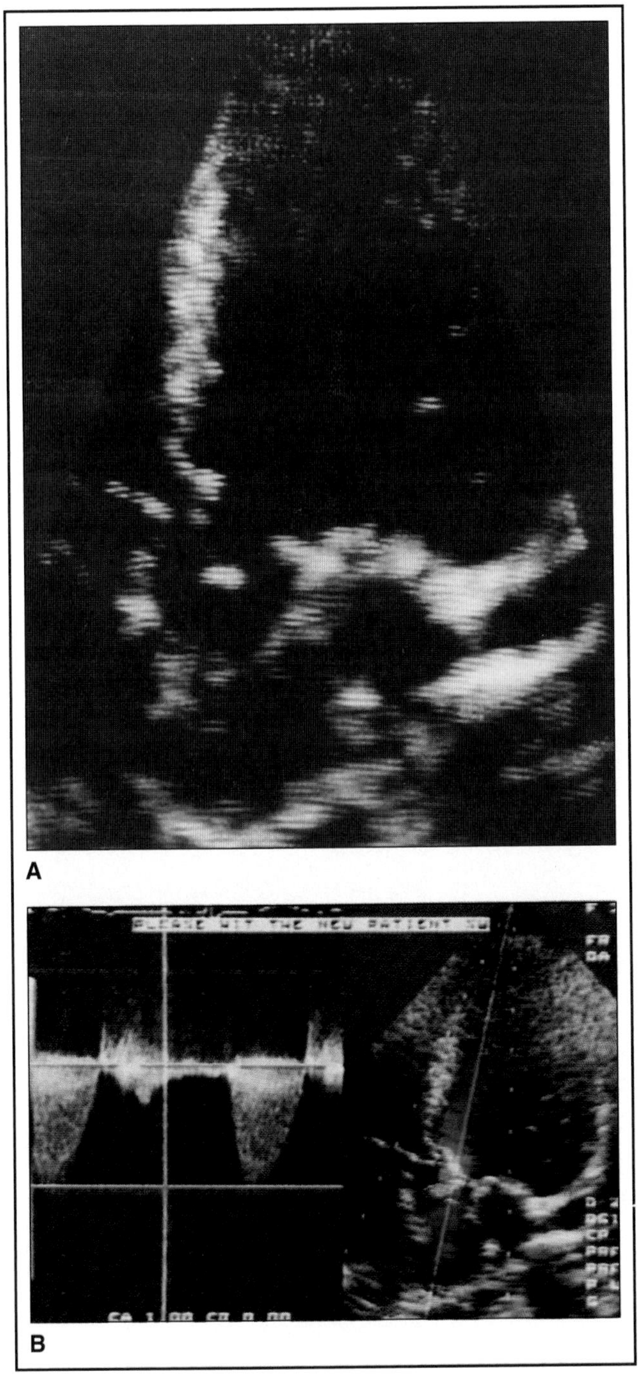

At times, too much can be read into an echocardiogram, which can be confusing to the physician. For example, the color Doppler echocardiograph may report the presence of tricuspid regurgitation and/or pulmonary regurgitation when there is no clinical evidence of this, and it does not represent any significance whatsoever as determined from a careful total cardiovascular examination. It should be stated in the report that these findings are frequently present and may be of no

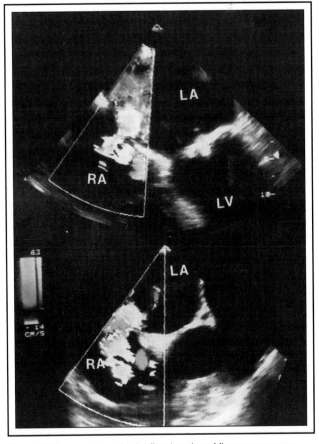

Figure 7. Transesophageal color flow imaging of flow convergence regions (FCRs) in two orthogonal planes - transverse (top) and longitudinal (bottom). FCR can be seen to be semicircular in both planes, justifying the hemispherical model used in the calculation of flow rate. LA, left atrium; RA, right atrium; LV, left ventricle. *(From Rittoo, et al. Flow convergence proximal to atrial septal defects. Circ 1993;87:1593.)*

Figure 6. (A) Apical 5-chamber view demonstrating horizontal membrane beneath the level of the aortic valve leaflets (courtesy of Dr. Julius M. Gardin). **(B)** Color Doppler and continuous wave Doppler demonstration of a gradient at the level of the subaortic membrane in the same apical 5-chamber view *(courtesy of Dr. Julius M. Gardin).*

importance if the clinical evaluation of the patient reveals no evidence of these conditions.

Too often the report of the presence of these conditions in the absence of any clinical evidence leads the physician who is not familiar with echocardiography to think that there is significant pathology in the values; unnecessary anxiety is thereby created for the patient and physician, leading to additional unnecessary and expensive tests.

The same was true of electrocardiography in its earlier days. The late Frank Wilson of the University of Michigan, along with his colleague Franklin Johnson, were instrumental in teaching electrocardiography directly or indirectly to hundreds of thousands of physicians over several decades. Physicians went to the "Mecca" in Ann Arbor, Michigan, to learn electrocardiography from these masters. I was one of them. I heard Dr. Wilson speak on several occasions, and he cautioned us physicians to be careful not to overinterpret the electrocardiogram, since he was aware of the problems that resulted when this was done. He stressed that the electrocardiogram should be part of the total clinical evaluation of a patient. The same problems exist today with the overinterpretation of the echocardiogram.

W. Proctor Harvey, M.D.

2. Overestimation of the severity of MR: There exist unresolved problems of quantitating regurgitant fractions and regurgitant volumes in clinical Doppler echocardiography laboratories. Compounding this is the lack of an acceptable "gold standard" for quantitation. The result is that many studies are being read as "severe" MR because the reader makes the error of viewing the study like an "ultrasonic angiogram." All too often, the clinician is confronted by a Doppler echocardiographic interpretation of severe MR, but normal dimensions of both left atrium and left ventricle in an asymptomatic patient who has a Grade 2/6 apical holosystolic murmur. It should not be surprising that regurgitant volume may not correlate with the measurements or visual estimates made from the color flow Doppler jet. Regurgitant volume is but one determinant; others include the differential in pressure between left atrium and left ventricle, the size of the regurgitant orifice, and the size and compliance of the left atrium. Perhaps of equal or greater importance are the many technical factors that may influence regurgitant jet size: Gain settings, attenuation of ultrasound energy, the angle of incidence, and limitations of instrumentation in recording varying flow velocities. Much needed research in quantitation of the severity of MR is under way. In the interval, the clinician must be especially wary

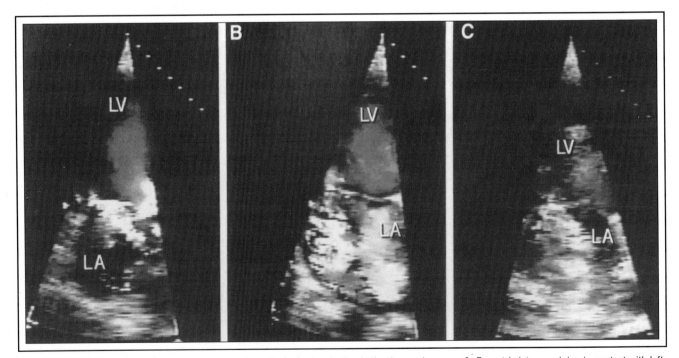

Figure 8. Examples of color flow Doppler imaging of jets of mitral regurgitation in the three subgroups. **A.** Eccentric jets remaining in contact with left atrial wall all along its border and occupying only a small portion of the left atrium (LA). LV = left ventricle. **B.** Central and organic mitral regurgitation. The jet is initially directed into the left atrial cavity but its main direction is toward the orifice of the left pulmonary veins, and it occupies only the external part of the left atrium. **C.** Central ischemic and functional mitral regurgitation. Jet is fully centrally directed into the left atrial cavity and occupies a large portion of the left atrium. *(From Enriquez-Sarano, et al. Severity of mitral regurgitation by Doppler study. JACC 1993;21:1218.)*

of accepting the Doppler echocardiographic report unless challenged by the "five-finger approach."

The typical holosystolic murmur of mitral regurgitation fills all of systole, starting with the first heart sound and continuing to the second sound. Sometimes, with more advanced regurgitation, it extends beyond the aortic valve closure (S_2), as some regurgitation continues across the incompetent mitral valve into the left atrium.

It is sometimes said that the systolic murmur of mitral regurgitation "obscures" or "masks" the first heart sound. This is not so because the first sound can be detected if the examiner carefully searches for it. The murmur begins with that first sound. A third heart sound (S_3) is an expected finding in the more advanced, more severe leaks of the mitral valve. A short diastolic rumble may also be heard in such patients. These auscultatory findings are caused by the large volume of blood in the enlarged left atrium filling the ventricle and producing the third sound plus low-frequency vibrations in the rapid filling phase. This rumble is usually not the result of stenosis of the mitral valve.

A giant left atrium, large enough to hold a grapefruit or small bowling bowl, can be identified on x-ray examination of the heart. Even if a diastolic rumble murmur is present in addition to the typical murmur of mitral regurgitation, no significant stenosis of the mitral valve exists. Cardiac pearl: giant left atrium + holosystolic murmur + diastolic rumble = no significant mitral stenosis.

Mitral regurgitation is also a cause of wide

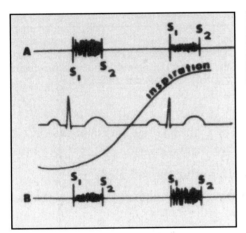

Fig A: The murmurs of mitral regurgitation and tricuspid regurgitation are holosystolic. The mitral murmur decreases in intensity with inspiration (A), whereas the tricuspid murmur increases with inspiration (B).

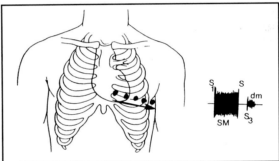

Fig B: Note bandlike radiation of holosystolic murmur (SM) of mitral regurgitation from the lower left sternal border to apex, axillary lines, and posterior lung base. Also, the murmur begins with the first sound (S_1), but does not mask it. A third heart sound (S_3) is present associated with short, low-frequency vibration of rumble quality (DM). No mitral stenosis is present.

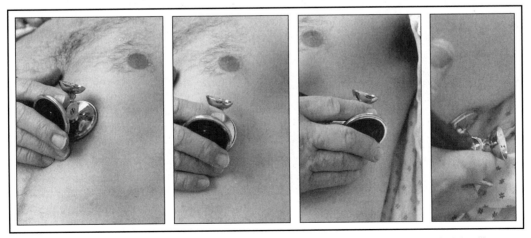

Fig C: "Band-like" radiation of a holosystolic murmur (SM) from the lower left sternal area (left) to the left axillary areas (right) and posterior lung base is characteristic of mitral regurgitation.

splitting of the second sound. With systole, blood is ejected through the usual aortic outflow track and simultaneously through the incompetent mitral valve into the left atrium. The left ventricular contents thereby empty earlier than usual, and the aortic valve closure (A_2) is earlier, which results in a wider split in both expiration and inspiration (Figs. A, B, and C).

W. Proctor Harvey, M.D.

Tricuspid Regurgitation

The bedside diagnosis of tricuspid regurgitation is often overlooked. The classic murmur is holosystolic, best heard at the lower left sternal border, and augments on inspiration. When this murmur occurs and one appreciates the associated findings of V waves in the jugular venous pulse and systolic pulsation of the liver, tricuspid regurgitation can be diagnosed with confidence. The Doppler echocardiogram then becomes most helpful in clarifying the etiology of the lesion. In the majority of adults, tricuspid regurgitation is secondary to pulmonary hypertension and/or right ventricular dilatation. Continuous-wave Doppler gives a good estimate of the pulmonary artery and the right ventricular systolic pressure (Figure 9). The echocardiogram may be definitive in defining tricuspid valve prolapse, rheumatic deformity (uncommon), Ebstein's anomaly, infective endocarditis, carcinoid (Figure 10), or connective tissue disorder as the causative agent. The greatest pitfall of the Doppler echocardiogram is over-diagnosis because of the great sensitivity of color flow in detecting tricuspid regurgitation. Because all three Doppler modes have been shown to detect tricuspid regurgitation in up to 100% of

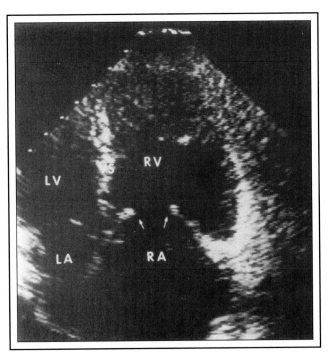

Figure 10. Right ventricular inflow view showing a systolic frame of the tricuspid valve *(arrows)*. It is held open due to carcinoid involvement of the valve. *(From Oh JK, Seward JB, Tajik AJ. The Echo Manual, Little Brown and Company. Boston, 1993.)*

normal healthy volunteers, it does not allow one to distinguish between physiologic and pathologic tricuspid regurgitation.

Ventricular Septal Defect

Ventricular septal defect (VSD) is among the most prevalent of congenital cardiac anomalies; the holosystolic murmur is the hallmark of VSD and is generally easily differentiated from that of mitral or tricuspid regurgitation or left ventricular outflow tract obstruction. Bedside clinical examination has proven remarkably accurate in identifying VSD; since clinical manifestations are determined by the size of the defect and pulmonary vascular resistance, Doppler echocardiography has become helpful in providing visualization of the size and location of the defect and in estimating the pulmonary artery pressures and size of the shunt. VSDs may be peri-membranous, muscular, subpulmonary, or of the atrioventricular canal type or the malalignment type, and the atrioventricular canal and malalignment types are usually large and easily identified. The apical four-chamber view is best for viewing the atrioventricular canal type, while parasternal and subcostal long-axis views best outline the peri-membranous and malalignment types. Color flow has been particularly helpful in finding small muscular and subpulmonary defects and in estimating the size of the defect by measuring the

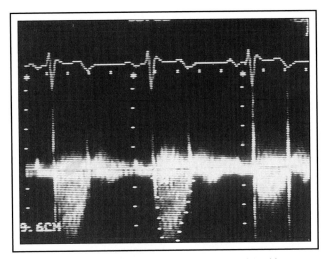

Figure 9. Continuous-wave Doppler recording of the tricuspid regurgitant jet in a 60-year-old man with cor pulmonale. The estimated pulmonary artery systolic pressure is 64 mm Hg plus the estimated right atrial mean pressure. (Also see Table 1.)

diameter of the color flow map (Figure 11). Natural history studies have shown the predictive value of Doppler echocardiography in infants and children with VSD. Two-dimensional echocardiography is essential in the assessment of chamber size and function in the patient with a VSD.

There are several potential pitfalls of Doppler echocardiography that the clinician who has made the diagnosis of VSD at bedside must recognize. The size of the defect on color flow mapping may be affected by many technical features, including gain, transmission, carrier frequency, pulse repetition frequency, wall filter display mode, and packet size. Unless the technician has been very careful to see that these factors are standardized, serial studies, in particular, may be prone to error. In the noninvasive quantitation of pulmonary artery pressures, the most commonly used indices are those of the peak systolic velocity of tricuspid regurgitation and the pulmonary regurgitation end diastolic velocity. Yet, both of these measures were detected in only a minority of patients studied at high volume centers. These technical/technician problems can be expected to be particularly serious when lower volume laboratories, imaging few patients with congenital defects of the heart, are asked to do the Doppler echocardiographic study. Caution also is appropriate in the interpretation of reports of the quantitation of the magnitude of the shunt as estimated by Doppler echocardiography. Although many investigators have reported the use of volumetric flow calculations using the area of the orifice on the two-dimensional echocardiogram and the time-velocity inte-

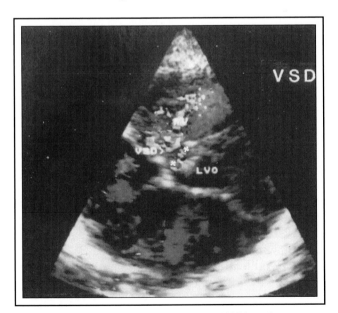

Figure 11. *(From Hornberger LK, Sahn DJ, Krabill KA, et al. Elucidation of the natural history of ventricular septal defects by serial Doppler color flow mapping studies. JACC 1989;13:1112.)*

gral, it is clear that there are many limitations to this technique. For clinical practice, estimates of pulmonary to systemic blood flow ratios by the present techniques are not helpful in the overall assessment of the patient with VSD.

Late-Systolic Murmurs

Late-systolic murmurs should focus the attention of the clinician on the possibilities of mitral valve prolapse, papillary muscle dysfunction, and, rarely, rheumatic valvular involvement. Usually, the bedside examination provides adequate clues to differentiate among these alternatives (presence or absence of a systolic click, history of angina or infarction, signs of coincident involvement of other valves, or history consistent with antecedent rheumatic fever). Doppler echocardiography has an important role in providing documentation of leaflet thickness, prolapse or lack thereof, as well as the size and function of the left atrium and left ventricle.

Mitral Valve Prolapse

Mitral valve prolapse has, as its hallmarks, the auscultatory findings of a mid-systolic click or clicks and a late-systolic murmur. Occasionally, these findings are present in papillary muscle dysfunction as well as rheumatic mitral regurgitation. Doppler echocardiographic demonstration of the mitral leaflet displacement from its normal position during systole has become the primary confirming study in the diagnosis of mitral valve prolapse. Careful research using rigid Doppler echocardiographic criteria for diagnosis indicates that mitral valve prolapse is present in 3%-5% of adults and has autosomal inheritance. Two-dimensional echocardiography is superb in imaging the plane of the mitral annulus and the point of coaptation of the mitral leaflets. It also allows a measure of the thickness of the mitral leaflets which is prognostically important, indicating perhaps as much as a tenfold increase in the risk of infective endocarditis, cerebral embolic events, and sudden cardiac death in those with thickened leaflets (Figure 12).

The mitral annulus is abnormally dilated in some patients with mitral valve prolapse; and in those with chronic severe mitral regurgitation, the systolic reduction in mitral annular area is less than normal. Complications such as chordal rupture or vegetations from associated endocarditis are often dramatically demonstrated (Figure 13). Color flow Doppler is useful in demonstrating the jet of mitral regurgitation which is seen in the majority of patients with mitral valve prolapse, but is hemodynamically significant in perhaps only 10% of patients studied.

The predominant pitfall of Doppler echocardiography in mitral valve prolapse is that of over-diagnosis; this has become less prevalent with the advent of two-dimensional echocardiography, but false positive (and occasionally false negative) studies remain a problem. Differentiation of functional from pathologic mitral prolapse continues to be difficult in many patients and has led to attempts to identify "rigid" (though still arbitrary) criteria for diagnosis. A reasonable set of guidelines has been proposed.

Definite mitral valve prolapse associated with clinically significant pathology and consequences requires that two or more of the following echocardiographic features be present:

1) Leaflet prolapse into the left atrium.
2) Thickened redundant valve leaflets.
3) Dilated mitral annulus.

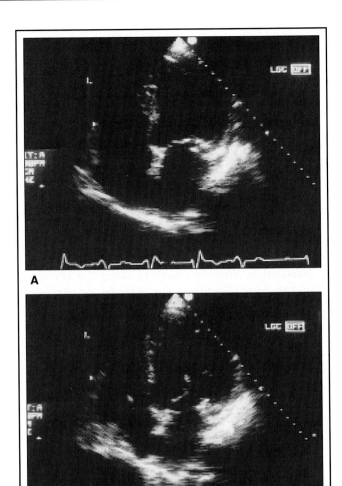

A

B

Figure 13. Still frames from systole **(A)** and diastole **(B)** of apical 4-chamber 2-D echocardiography in a patient with torn chordae tendineae with a flail tip of the anterior mitral leaflet.

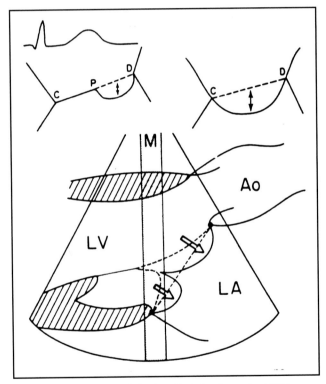

Figure 12. Currently accepted echo criteria for diagnosis of MVP. *Top,* two-dimensionally targeted M mode recordings of continuous mitral leaflet interfaces show *(top left)* late-systolic prolapse, with prolapse beginning in midsystole (P) and characterized by at least a 2-mm posterior displacement of leaflets behind the valve's C-D line; holosystolic prolapse *(top right)* is characterized by a 3-mm displacement of leaflets behind the C-D line and requires confirmation by demonstration of leaflet billowing in the two-dimensional, parasternal long-axis view. *Bottom,* two-dimensional parasternal long-axis view showing systolic billowing of mitral leaflets *(arrows)* into left atrium (LA), a motion the posterior component of which may be detected by the vertically oriented M mode beam (M, *central vertical bar). Dotted lines,* normal position of mitral leaflets and annulus: Ao = aorta; LV = left ventricle. *(From Devereux and colleagues; reproduced with permission of Annals of Internal Medicine 1989;111:305-317.)*

4) Associated tricuspid valve prolapse with dilatation of the tricuspid annulus; or

5) Associated aortic valve prolapse.

These patients usually have typical auscultatory features of systolic click and late systolic murmur.

Probable mitral valve prolapse is defined by two-dimensional echocardiographic evidence of leaflet prolapse plus the auscultatory signs but no other structural abnormalities on the Doppler echocardiographic study.

Possible mitral valve prolapse is diagnosed by the following features:

1) Trivial leaflet prolapse on Doppler echocardiography without auscultatory findings or leaflet thickening; or

2) Clicks, asthenic body habitus, and palpitations, but no echocardiographic abnormalities.

Because of the frequency of trivial mitral valve

prolapse, it is incumbent upon clinicians to carefully explain the implications of the diagnosis in terms of follow-up, endocarditis prophylaxis, long-term prognosis, and its differentiation from pathological mitral valve prolapse.

Diastolic Murmurs

The clinical recognition of a diastolic murmur equates to the recognition of pathology. When that pathology involves the semilunar valves, the characteristic murmurs of aortic or pulmonic regurgitation result. Because aortic regurgitation is the much more common culprit in adults, the physician must always be careful in assuring that the bedside features of pulmonary hypertension have not been ignored and pulmonary regurgitation is the source of the murmur. When pathology restricts the inflow

to the right or left ventricle, the diastolic rumbles of tricuspid or mitral stenosis ensue. Mitral stenosis is far more common, with tricuspid stenosis being a rare lesion today. Doppler echocardiography is a powerful tool in the assessment of patients presenting with these lesions.

Mitral Stenosis

Mitral stenosis should be apparent from the bedside examination in most patients with clinically significant disease. It is uncommonly truly "silent," presenting as a surprise to the ultrasonographer. Doppler echocardiography allows definition of leaflet anatomy, size of the left atrium and left ventricle, good quantitation of the effective mitral orifice, information about subvalvular disease, pulmonary artery pressures, as well as left ventricular

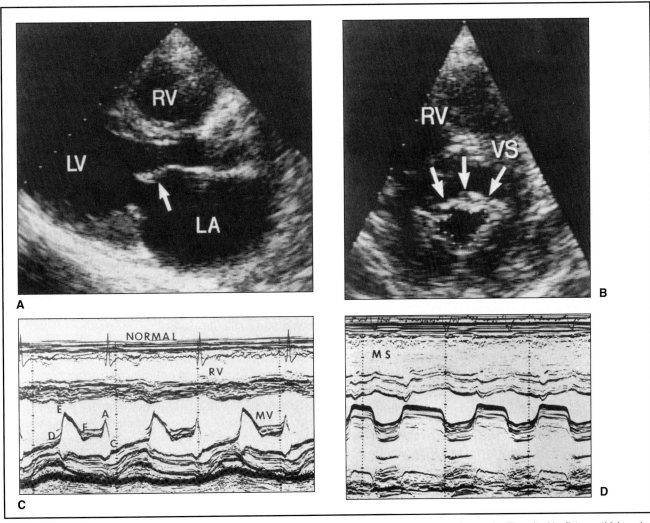

Figure 14. (A) 2D echocardiogram of the parasternal long-axis view during diastole in a patient with mitral stenosis. The mitral leaflets are thickened with the typical "hockey stick" appearance *(arrow)*. The left atrium (LA) is enlarged. **(B)** 2D echocardiogram of the parasternal short-axis view showing the "fish mouth" orifice *(arrows)* of the stenotic mitral valve. The orifice area is measured by manual tracing. **(C)** M-mode echocardiogram of a normal mitral valve. **(D)** M-mode echocardiogram of typical mitral stenosis. The mitral leaflet is thickened and the E-F slope is decreased. *(From Oh JK, Seward JB, Tajik AJ. The Echo Manual, Little Brown and Company. Boston, 1993.)*

307

function, and the degree of coincident mitral regurgitation and other valvular involvement (Figure 14). It provides essential information, beyond that of the clinical assessment alone, in the evaluation of patients for surgery.

Transesophageal studies are especially useful in determination of a patient's candidacy for percutaneous transvenous mitral commissurotomy. If there is no identifiable thrombus in the left atrium and the two-dimensional echocardiographic features of the valve (thickness, pliability, calcification, and subvalvular involvement) are appropriate, many patients with mitral stenosis can be treated by pervenous "balloon" technique. When combined with the remaining features of the clinical assessment of the patient, Doppler echocardiography obviates the need for cardiac catheterization in the majority of patients with mitral stenosis other than for the determination of coronary anatomy. Nonetheless, there are pitfalls of which one must be aware. It must be recognized that pressure gradient measurements, while helpful, are dependent on diastolic flow across the mitral valve and, when viewed alone, may not reflect the significance of the lesion. The more critical measure is that of the mitral valve area which can be determined either by planimetry of the orifice as outlined by two-dimensional echocardiography, or by the Doppler pressure half time, or continuity equation (Table 1).

Each requires meticulous attention to detail and, in the hands of experienced researchers, has been shown to correlate closely to invasive measurement (Figure 15). The performance of the measures by the community of ultrasonographers may be quite different. This demands that responsible physicians assure the reliability of their particular laboratory in the quantitation of mitral valve areas (as in all aspects of Doppler echocardiography).

Tricuspid Stenosis

Tricuspid stenosis is increasingly uncommon but should be thought of and carefully investigated in the patient who is recognized as having mitral stenosis. Doppler echocardiography is excellent in imaging the tricuspid valve thickness and mobility, and a lesion should be suspected when there is disproportionate enlargement of the right atrium noted on two-dimensional echocardiography. Transtricuspid valve gradients are often low and may not be evident without induced tachycardia or volume challenge. These gradients are amenable to Doppler measures and should be sought.

Aortic Regurgitation

In the patient who has a diastolic murmur or

T A B L E   1

Calculation of the Mitral Valve Area (MVA)

- **By pressure half time (PHT) method.**

  $$MVA = 220/PHT$$

- **By the continuity equation**

  $$MVA = LVOT\ D^2 \times 0.785 \times LVOT\ TVI/MV\ TVI$$

  Where LVOT D^2 = left ventricular outflow tract diameter squared

  LVOT TVI = left ventricular outflow tract true velocity integral

  MV TVI = mitral valve true velocity integral

---

aortic insufficiency, Doppler echocardiography should be ordered. Color flow Doppler is highly sensitive and specific for detecting aortic regurgitation and for judging severity in a semiquantitative way. Severity can also be estimated by the rate of deceleration of regurgitant blood flow velocity by continuous wave Doppler or maps of the regurgitant jet using pulsed wave or color flow Doppler (Figure 16). Two-dimensional echocardiography allows measurement of the dimensions of the left ventricle and permits serial studies in patients who remain asymptomatic but have evidence of substantial aortic regurgitation. Presently, the finding of a progressive increase in left ventricular end-systolic volume remains the best predictor (though imperfect) of the clinical course and is an indicator of the need for surgery, even in the asymptomatic patient. The technique is also helpful in determining the etiology of aortic regurgitation when characteristic features of bicuspid valve, annulo-aortic ectasia, endocarditis, dissection, or ruptured sinus of Valsalva may be evident. Recent advances hold promise that quantitative Doppler can be performed, allowing measures of regurgitant fraction and regurgitant volume. This may provide better answers to the problem of quantifying valvular regurgitation.

Pitfalls confronting the physician interpreting Doppler echocardiographic data on the patient with aortic insufficiency are commonly twofold. One is the problem of interpreting aortic insufficiency, seen by color flow Doppler, in a heart that is otherwise normal and in a patient with no audible murmur. Color flow is an exquisitely sensitive tool that in certain individuals may detect functional leakage of the aortic valve. Presently, there are no rigid criteria for differentiating physiologic from pathologic aortic regurgitation, nor are there likely to be. Careful integration of the Doppler echocardiographic information into the rest of the clinical

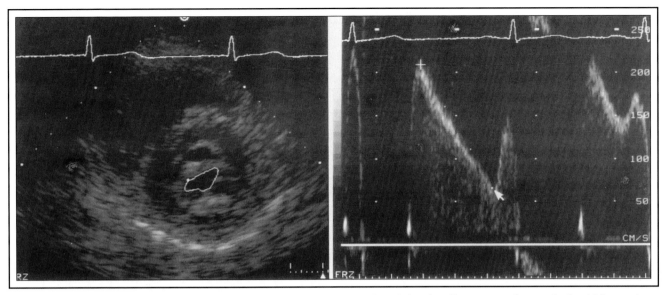

Figure 15. Echocardiographic data from a 73-year-old woman with New York Heart Association class III symptoms of congestive heart failure and clinical evidence of mitral stenosis. Left panel: Short-axis diastolic stop-frame image at level of mitral leaflet tips. Diastolic mitral orifice area has been traced and measures 0.95 cm². Right panel: Transmitral flow velocity recorded from cardiac apex by pulsed-wave Doppler sampling at mitral leaflet tips. Diastolic velocity decay is prolonged; half-time measures 209 msec, indicating that mitral orifice area is 1.05 cm². These concordant data confirm significant mitral stenosis. *(From Pearlman. Echocardiography in mitral and tricuspid stenosis. Circ 1991;84(Suppl):I-195.)*

examination will be essential in making specific recommendations to any particular patient. The second potential problem is that of over-estimation of the degree of aortic regurgitation by Doppler echocardiography; the difficulty in quantifying the severity of a regurgitant lesion by any of the current methods widely used in clinical cardiology is substantial. Unfortunately, many laboratories report studies as "severe aortic insufficiency" that may not have been done with the careful attention to the technical detail that is essential and they do not convey the caveat that quantitation is semi-quantitative, at best. The clinician is well advised to pay attention to the left ventricular size and systolic function as the more reliable parameters of the clinical significance of chronic aortic regurgitation. In the setting of acute aortic insufficiency, the clinical examination usually provides clues that are dramatic and the Doppler echocardiogram confirms the substantial regurgitant jet into a normal-sized left ventricle with early diastolic closure of the mitral valve.

Pulmonary Regurgitation Secondary to Pulmonary Hypertension

With severe pulmonary hypertension, the high-frequency diastolic murmur of pulmonary valve regurgitation characterized by Graham Steell is identical to that of mild aortic insufficiency; bedside clinical examination usually provides ample evidence of pulmonary hypertension. Color flow

Doppler is quite sensitive in detecting pulmonic valve insufficiency. Doppler echocardiography is helpful in determining the source of pulmonary hypertension by providing critical morphological information, especially in complex congenital heart disease. Color flow Doppler is especially useful in the detection of intracardiac shunts that, with progressive elevation of pulmonary artery pressures, have become bidirectional and no longer have the typical auscultatory features that allow bedside differentiation. Doppler echocardiography allows semi-quantitative measurement of the pulmonary artery pressure by several clinical techniques that are presently available (Table 2).

Of these techniques, the most widely used in clinical practice is that of the velocity measurement of the tricuspid regurgitant jet. Caution in integration of the Doppler echocardiographic data into the clinical management of the patient with pulmonary hypertensive pulmonary regurgitation is focused on the precision with which pulmonary pressures can be estimated. Though a precise number can be calculated, each of the previously mentioned techniques has its own problems. Since the presence of an audible murmur of pulmonary hypertension indicates moderate to severe pulmonary hypertension, it may be best to estimate the pulmonary pressures in those same terms, moderate or severe, from the Doppler echocardiogram.

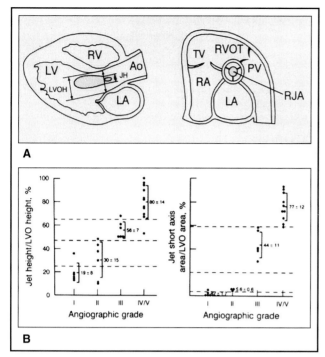

Figure 16-A. **(A)** Schematics of color-flow imaging to estimate the severity of AR, from the parasternal long- (left) and short- (right) axis views. LV outflow height (LVOH) and jet height (JH) are determined from the parasternal long-axis view. Regurgitant jet area (RJA) is measured from the parasternal short-axis view at the aortic valve level. **(B)** Jet height/LVO height ratio (left) and RJA/VLO area ratio (right) are plotted against angiographic grade of AR. When the ratios are greater than 60 to 65%, the AR is severe; when less than 30%, it is mild. *(A, B: From GJ Perry et al. Evaluation of aortic insufficiency by Doppler color flow mapping. JACC 1987;9:952-959.)*

Continuous Murmurs

Continuous murmurs always reflect a pathological communication between vessels or chambers of the heart that have pressure differences that persist throughout the cardiac cycle. *Patent ductus arteriosus* is the prototype. Rarely, coronary arteriovenous malformations or coronary to pulmonary artery malformations may be present with continuous murmurs. Doppler echocardiography has allowed for definitive imaging of patent ductus in childhood and for the identification of coexisting lesions. Cardiac catheterization may be unnecessary in many such patients prior to correction. Unless the examining ultrasonographer is inexperienced in the performance of studies in patients with congenital defects, there should be few false positive or false negative studies when the question of patent ductus arteriosus is raised (Figure 17).

Conclusion

Murmurs are one of the primary signs that lead to concern about or recognition of cardiac pathology. W. Proctor Harvey has devoted his professional

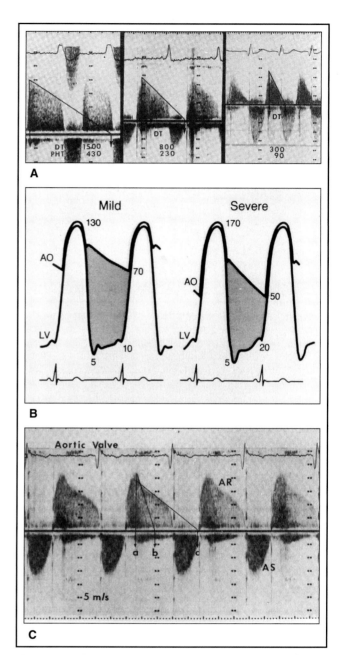

Figure 16-B. **(A)** Continuous-wave Doppler spectra of AR from three patients are shown to illustrate the decreased PHT with more severe AR. The left panel indicates mild AR with a PHT of 430 msec; the right panel indicates severe AR with a PHT of 90 msec, and the middle one indicates moderately severe AR. **(B)** The reason for shorter DT (or PHT) with severe AR is shown in the schematic of LV and aortic (AO) pressure curves. With more significant AR, the aortic pressure drop is more rapid as is the LV diastolic pressure rise with more regurgitant volume back into the LV. **(C)** Continuous-wave spectrum of the aortic valve demonstrating two separate slopes of the AR velocity curve. DT should not be measured from the initial steeper slope. Therefore, DT is the interval from a to c, not a to b. *(From Oh JK, Seward JB, Tajik AJ. The Echo Manual, Little Brown and Company. Boston, 1993.)*

career to teaching the skills and benefits of meticulous attention to the bedside examination and reinforcing that examination by appropriately used

TABLE 2

Doppler Measurements of Pulmonary Artery Systolic Pressure (PASP), Mean Pulmonary Artery Pressure (MPAP), and Pulmonary Artery Diastolic Pressure (PADP)

PASP = $4V^2 + 14$, where V is the peak systolic velocity of the tricuspid regurgitant jet obtained from continuous-wave Doppler

MPAP = $79 - 0.45 \times ACT$, where ACT is the pulmonary artery acceleration time measured by pulsed-wave Doppler.

PADP = $10 + 4V^2$, where V is the end diastolic velocity of the pulmonary artery regurgitation signal by continuous-wave Doppler.

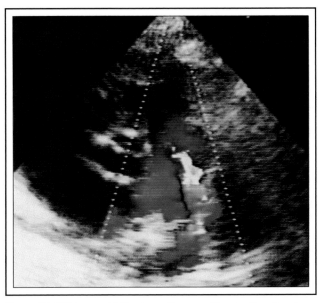

Figure 17. Still frame of 2-D echocardiogram with color flow Doppler defining patent ductus arteriosus in a neonate.

diagnostic tests. Of those tests, none has become more widespread in its availability to clinicians, nor provided more helpful information, than the Doppler echocardiographic study. Its realized potential to non-invasively provide measures of cardiac chambers, assess function, define anatomic relationships, detect shunts, estimate severity of lesions, and provide reference for serial follow-up of patients is phenomenal. Clinicians must be aware, however, of the real and potential shortcomings of the technique; not the least of these is the easy access of the patient to many laboratories and many ultrasonographers in a time of great expansion in medical technology. Great attention to technical detail, an awareness of what is being sought, and careful quality control should be demonstrated by the facility used for the test before information

from the study is accepted. A good study is just as essential as is appropriate integration of the Doppler echocardiographic information into the complete assessment of the patient and problem, and the development of a management plan. Only then will patients be maximally benefitted.

CARDIAC PEARL

The detection of a heart murmur is still one of the major causes for referral of a patient for evaluation of the possibility of heart disease. Regardless of what discipline of medicine the physician is engaged in, the evaluation of a murmur becomes of utmost importance. Is the murmur innocent or is it a murmur of significance indicating the presence of underlying heart disease? Unfortunately, today it still is often poorly understood as to how to differentiate between an innocent and a significant murmur. Certainly innocent murmurs are frequent findings in children, although they may be present in all age groups from infancy to old age. I am convinced that the physician can accurately make the diagnosis of an innocent murmur in the great majority of patients when he sees them in his office. This is accomplished by use of the "five-finger approach" in the diagnosis of cardiovascular disease, which includes a careful detailed history and physical examination, x-ray, electrocardiogram and laboratory findings. Included as a "non-invasive" laboratory technique might be an echocardiogram, which often can aid in differentiation between the innocent and the significant murmur. However, cardiac catheterization and angiography seldom are necessary.

Fortunately, there are fundamental characteristics of the innocent murmur concerning its intensity, quality and timing in systole, which are not difficult to master. Generally, taking the murmur out of the "ball park" of innocence are: the presence of extra sounds such as the ejection sound or systolic click, a very accentuated second heart sound (also palpable and accompanied by a right ventricular precordial impulse), abnormal splitting of the second heart sound, such as "fixed splitting".

W. Proctor Harvey, M.D.

Selected Reading

1. Barlow JB, Pocock WA, Marchand P et al: The significance of late systolic murmurs. *AHJ* 1963;66:443-452.
2. Bolger AF, Eigler NL, Maurer G: Quantifying valvular regurgitation: Limitations and inherent assumptions of Doppler techniques. *Circ* 1988;78:1316-1318.

3. Chandrarata PAN, Shah PM: Role of echocardiography and Doppler ultrasound in diagnosing mitral valve prolapse. In Boudoulas H., Wooley, C.F.: *Mitral valve prolapse and the mitral valve prolapse syndrome.* Futura Publishing Co., Inc. Mount Kisco, New York, 1988.

4. Cheitlin MD: Valvular heart disease management and intervention. *Circ* 1991;84 (Suppl I):I-259-I-264.

5. Devereux RVB: Mitral valve prolapse: Syndrome or valvular disease? *Card Rev* 1993;1:50-58.

6. Edler I: The diagnostic use of ultrasound in heart disease. *Acta Med Scand* 1955;308:32.

7. Enriquez-Sarano M et al: Quantitative Doppler assessment of valvular regurgitation. *Circ* 1993;87:841-848.

8. Hatle L, Angelsen B: *Doppler ultrasound in cardiology. Physical principles and clinical application.* Philadelphia: Lea and Febiger, 1982:161-2.

9. Hornberger LK, Sahn DJ, Krabil, KA et al: Elucidation of the natural history of ventricular septal defects by serial Doppler color flow mapping studies. *JACC* 1989; 13:1111-1118.

10. Houston AB: Doppler ultrasound and the apparently normal heart. *BHJ;* 1993;69:99-100.

11. Jaffe WM, Roche AHG, Coverdale HA et al: Clinical evaluation versus Doppler echocardiography in the quantitative assessment of valvular heart disease. *Circ* 1988;78:267-275.

12. Kidd L, Driscol, DJ, Gersony WM et al: Second natural history study of congenital heart defects. Results of treatment of patients with ventricular septal defects. *Circ* 1993; 87 (suppl):I-38-I-51.

13. Krozon I et al: Transesophageal echocardiography to detect atrial clots in candidates for transseptal mitral balloon valvuloplasty. *JACC* 1990;16:1320-1322.

14. Kurokawa S, Takahash M, Katoh Y, et al: Noninvasive evaluation of the ratio of pulmonary to systemic flow in ventricular septal defect by means of Doppler two-dimensional echocardiography. *AHJ* 1988.7;116:1033-1044.

15. Nishimura RA, McGoon MD, Shub C et al: Echocardiographically documented mitral valve prolapse. Long term follow-up of 237 patients. *NEJM* 1985;313:1305.

16. Ormiston JA, Shah PM, Tei C, Wong M: Size and motion of the mitral valve annulus in man. II: Abnormalities in mitral valve prolapse. *Circ* 1982;65:713.

17. Panidis IO, MacAllister M, Ross J, Mintz GS: Prevalence and severity of mitral regurgitation in the mitral valve prolapse syndrome. *JACC* 1986;7:975.

18. Pieroni DR, Nishimura RA, Bierman FZ et al: Second natural history study of congenital heart defects and ventricular septal defect: Echocardiography. *Circ* 1993;87 (Suppl I): I-80-I-88.

19. Yannick J, Slama M, Tribuoilloy C et al: Doppler echocardiographic evaluation of valve regurgitation in healthy volunteers. *BHJ* 1992;69:109-113.

CHAPTER 15

Cardiac Sound and Ultrasound: Echocardiographic and Auscultatory Correlations

James A. Ronan, Jr., M.D.

Cardiac auscultation has been a traditional method of evaluating the heart for the past two centuries, based on the principle that the mechanical activity of the heart and the blood flowing through it generate energy in the sound spectrum which can be detected and used to evaluate cardiac functions. Certain specific heart sounds and/or murmurs indicate valvular abnormalities, pericardial disease, congenital cardiac disease, and abnormalities of ventricular function. During the past 25 years echocardiography, both two dimensional and Doppler, has emerged as a major method of cardiac diagnosis and it is used to answer some of the same questions as auscultation. Furthermore, it is often used to interpret the findings of cardiac auscultation. Since both techniques, auscultation and echocardiography, are used to answer similar questions it is valuable to understand how each method reflects certain disease states, to know the strengths and limitations of each technique in the diagnosis of any disease state and to evaluate how the information obtained from auscultation relates to the information obtained from echocardiography.

Both methods have certain limitations in their diagnostic accuracy. These limitations are related to how well the disease expresses itself by sound or ultrasound, to what extent extrinsic factors interfere with the performance of the test (obesity, acutely ill patient, noisy surroundings, etc), and the skill and experience of the person performing and interpreting the test. The performance of auscultation or echocardiography is a skill and like any other skill, such as playing a sport or musical instrument, there is a great variability in the per-

formance levels of the users, determined to a large extent by training, practice, motivation, and organization. Auscultation is usually performed by a physician as a basic part of the physical examination but the method and extent of the examination is largely a matter of personal style. It is mainly for that reason that there is such variability between examiners in their reports of physical findings. There are no standards required to guarantee the quality of cardiac auscultation, and the examiner usually spends only a few minutes performing the examination. On the other hand, there is more consistency in the echocardiographic examination because it is usually performed by a specially trained sonographer who follows a standard protocol, collects data in a prescribed fashion over a period of 15 to 30 minutes, and is required to meet a certain performance standard. Furthermore, there is the distinct advantage that a second person, usually a cardiologist, reviews, critiques, and interprets the echocardiogram.

Since both techniques are directed at solving many of the same problems, it is helpful to see how each method reflects certain disease states. They each see things from different viewpoints. For example, in mitral stenosis the diagnosis can be made by auscultation, by 2-D echocardiography, or by Doppler echocardiography, but each of these methods detects the mitral stenosis in a different way using sets of diagnostic criteria specific for that method. Auscultation uses the opening snap and the diastolic rumbling murmur, the 2-D echocardiogram uses the doming of the anterior leaflet and the reduced mitral orifice size, while Doppler echocardiography uses the increased and prolonged mitral inflow velocity. However, in a given case all may not be equally helpful. It is not uncommon for auscultation to demonstrate an abnormality while echocardiography may be normal, or vice versa.

For example, cardiac auscultation may detect mild degrees of mitral regurgitation, the ejection sound of a bicuspid aortic valve, or a systolic click of mitral valve prolapse in patients in whom the echocardiogram does not display the abnormality. On the other hand, mild degrees of valvular regurgitation are frequently detected by echocardiography but are inaudible to even the most careful cardiac auscultation.

Heart Sounds

Echocardiographic Clarification of the Origin of Heart Sounds

It is important to verify the link between heart sounds and the cardiac events which produce them in order to appreciate the significance of those sounds. Echocardiography has contributed much to the knowledge of the meaning of those heart sounds. In order to have confidence that the findings on cardiac auscultation are valid and valuable the examiner must be confident that they accurately reflect important events within the heart and that modifications of those findings occur for definite reasons, most of which are related to cardiac function. The following shows some of the ways echocardiography has furthered our understanding of heart sounds.

• **First Heart Sound:** The first heart sound (S_1) has two components which occur simultaneously with closure of the mitral and tricuspid valves. This has been demonstrated by simultaneous echocardiography and phonocardiography (Figures 1 and 2). The normal first heart sound has a separation between mitral and tricuspid components of about 0.03 seconds.

The intensity of S_1 is related to ventricular contractility, particularly of the left ventricle. The peak rate of rise (dPdT) of left ventricular pressure at the instant of mitral valve closure is directly related to the amplitude of S_1. Factors which increase or decrease the rate of rise will correspondingly increase or decrease the intensity of the first heart sound. The first heart sound is loud in patients with a short PR interval, in those with mitral stenosis, and in those receiving sympathetic nervous system stimulation or taking catecholamine drugs. In these situations the mitral valve closes on the steep upslope of the left ventricular pressure curve so that the closing force of left ventricular contraction is increased. In mitral stenosis, the interval between ventricular contraction and mitral valve closure is prolonged because the valve can close only when left ventricular pressure is high enough to overcome the elevated left atrial pressure. The simultaneous echocardiogram and phonocardiogram clearly demonstrate the delay in mitral valve closure and the loud first heart sound. (Figure 3).

When rate of development of left ventricular pressure is slow at the instant of mitral valve clo-

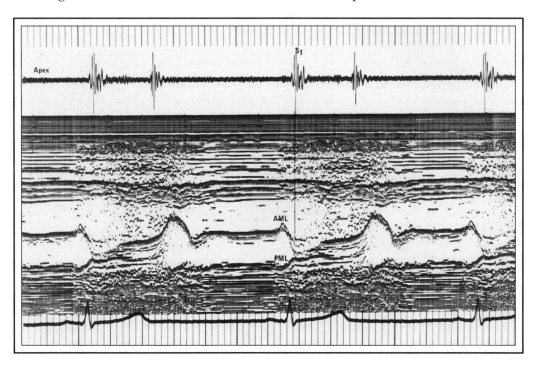

Figure 1. Simultaneous echocardiogram and phonocardiogram to compare timing of mitral valve closure with components of the first heart sound. Mitral valve closure is synchronous with first high frequency component of the first heart sound (S_1). AML = Anterior Mitral Leaflet. PML = Posterior Mitral Leaflet. *(Reproduced with permission. Ronan JA Jr. Cardiac sound and ultrasound. Current Problems in Cardiology 6:14; 1981.)*

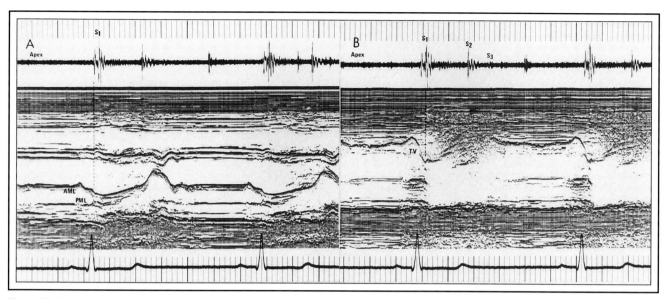

Figure 2A. A simultaneous phonocardiogram and echocardiogram of mitral valve. Mitral valve closure is synchronous with first high frequency component of first heart sound (S₁). QM1 interval is 0.06 seconds.

Figure 2B. Simultaneous phonocardiogram and echocardiogram of tricuspid valve in the same patient taken within one minute of recording A. Tricuspid valve closure is synchronous with second high frequency component of first heart sound. Q T1 interval is 0.09 seconds.

(Reproduced with permission. Ronan JA Jr. Cardiac sound and ultrasound. Current Problems in Cardiology 6:14; 1981.)

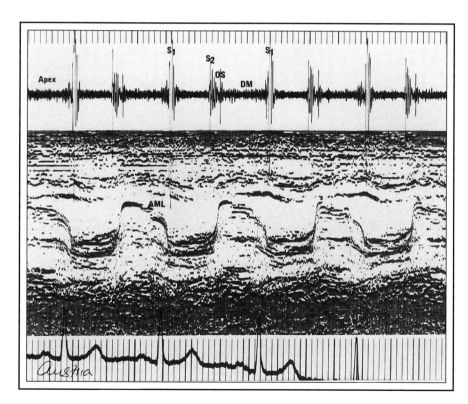

Figure 3. Timing of mitral valve closure in mitral stenosis. Mitral valve closure occurs 0.09 seconds after onset of Q wave. Opening snap (OS) and diastolic murmur (DM) of mitral stenosis are apparent.
(Reproduced with permission. Ronan JA Jr. Cardiac sound and ultrasound. Current Problems in Cardiology 6:15; 1981.)

sure the first heart sound is faint. Patients with a long PR interval have diastolic closure or semi-closure of the valve prior to ventricular contraction so that the interval between onset of left ventricular contraction and complete closure is brief and the closure occurs early on the left ventricular pressure curve at a time when the rate of rise (dPdT) is slow.

Those with depressed left ventricular function due either to disease or to agents such as beta-adrenergic blocking drugs also have a faint first heart sound because the rate of pressure development is reduced. In patients with severe mitral regurgitation, the rate of left ventricular pressure development may be reduced because of run-off into the

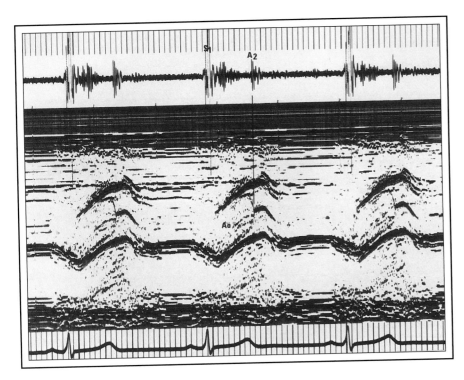

Figure 4. Timing of aortic valve closure in relation to second heart sound. Aortic valve closure is synchronous with first component of second heart sound (A_2). Valve closure can be clearly identified.
(Reproduced with permission. Ronan JA Jr. Cardiac sound and ultrasound. Current Problems in Cardiology 6:21; 1981.)

left atrium or because of reduced left ventricular contractility so the first heart sound may be faint.

In considering all of the causes of variation in the intensity of S_1, the most commonly encountered ones are related to variations in the interval between atrial and ventricular contractions, and these are reflected in variations of the PR interval on the electrocardiogram. This is most dramatically exhibited when there is dissociation between the atrial and ventricular rhythms. In any of the many forms of AV dissociation (complete heart block, ventricular tachycardia, AV junctional tachycardia with AV dissociation, etc), the intensity of S_1 fluctuates according to that interval between atrial and ventricular contractions.

• **Second Heart Sound:** Closure of the aortic and pulmonic valves produces the two components (A_2 and P_2) of the second heart sound (S_2) (Figure 4). The aortic and pulmonic valve closure sounds may be faint in valvular aortic stenosis or pulmonic stenosis. A loud P_2 is heard in pulmonary hypertension and wide fixed splitting of the second heart sound can be heard in atrial septal defect. When these auscultatory clues are detected, the echocardiogram can confirm the diagnosis.

• **Third Heart Sound:** The third heart sound is due to ventricular wall vibrations caused by the sudden completion of ventricular distention at the end of the rapid filling phase of early diastole. The sound is generated within the ventricle by the abrupt change in wall motion. Although there has been speculation that the sound might be related to

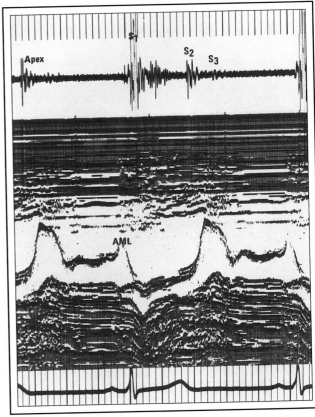

Figure 5. A physiologic third heart sound (S_3) occurs after maximum opening of mitral valve leaflet but is not related to any particular movement of the valve.
(Reproduced with permission. Ronan JA Jr. Cardiac sound and ultrasound. Current Problems in Cardiology 6:25; 1981.)

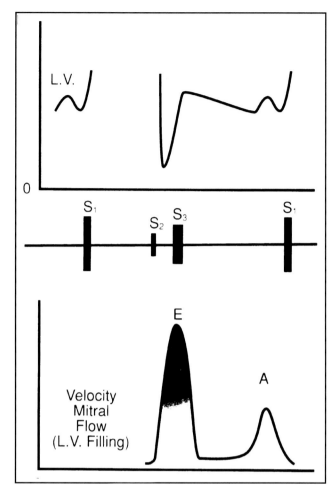

Figure 6. The third heart sound occurs immediately after the peak velocity of left ventricular filling and during the left ventricular rapid filling wave. Deceleration of left ventricular filling is just beginning when S_3 occurs. The upslope and downslope of the early filling wave (E) are rapid and the peak velocity is higher than the peak velocity of the late filling wave (A). LV, left ventricle; S_1, first heart sound; S_2, second heart sound; S_3, third heart sound. *(Reproduced with permission. Ronan JA Jr. Cardiac auscultation: the third and fourth heart sounds. Heart Disease and Stroke 1:268; 1992. Copyright 1992 American Heart Association.)*

mitral valve movement, echocardiography has proven that to be incorrect (Figure 5) and Doppler flow analysis of mitral inflow shows that S_3 occurs within 5 msec of the peak velocity of inflow (Figure 6). Patients with left ventricular systolic dysfunction and patients with mitral regurgitation frequently have high left ventricular inflow velocity due to elevated left atrial pressure and they usually have third heart sounds.

• **Fourth Heart Sound:** The fourth heart sound is a low-frequency sound in late diastole which is generated in the ventricle but is due to the atrium contracting and discharging blood into a ventricle which has reduced compliance. The poor compliance is usually due to factors such as ventricular

hypertrophy, scar or ischemia but may occur to a mild degree as a part of the natural aging process. Ventricular hypertrophy and/or scarring can easily be demonstrated on 2-D echocardiography and in such cases the mitral inflow Doppler studies usually show a high-velocity A wave after atrial contraction. In those individuals with ventricular hypertrophy and delayed early diastolic filling (diastolic dysfunction) the mitral Doppler flow pattern shows a low or normal peak rate of early diastolic filling (E wave), a slow deceleration time of the E wave and a high peak rate of late diastolic filling (A wave) (Figure 7).

• **Opening Snap:** The opening snap is a sharp sound in early diastole in patients with mitral stenosis and two dimensional echocardiography shows that it is due to the anterior mitral leaflet doming forward at the time the mitral valve opens (Figure 8). M-mode echocardiography shows the precise timing of this event (Figure 9).

• **Ejection Sounds:** Ejection sounds are distinct sounds produced at the onset of ejection from either the left or right side of the heart. They are usually due to a bicuspid aortic valve, or to mild aortic valve or pulmonic valve stenosis. In congenital valvular aortic stenosis, the ejection sound occurs

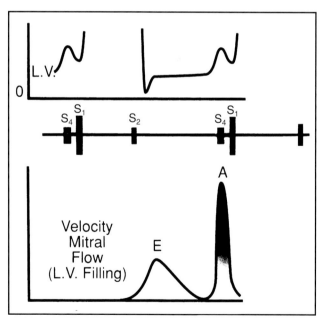

Figure 7. The fourth heart sound occurs at the time of high inflow velocity (A) after atrial contraction. The early diastolic filling wave (E) has low velocity and a slow downslope (prolonged deceleration time). The sharp increase in late diastolic filling velocity coincides with the abrupt rise in left ventricular diastolic pressure. A, late diastolic filling velocity; E, early diastolic filling velocity; LV, left ventricle; S_1, first heart sound; S_2, second heart sound; S_4, fourth heart sound.
(Reproduced with permission. Ronan JA Jr. Cardiac auscultation: the third and fourth heart sounds. Heart Disease and Stroke 1:269; 1992. Copyright 1992 American Heart Association.)

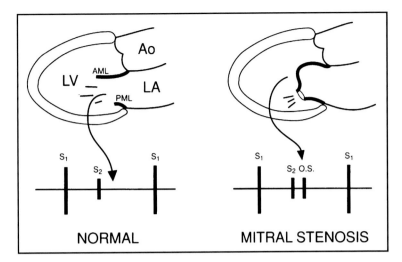

NORMAL   MITRAL STENOSIS

Figure 8. Diagram of the mitral valve at the onset of left ventricular (LV) filling. In the normal mitral valve, the anterior mitral leaflet (AML) and posterior mitral leaflets (PML) open widely and no sound is produced. In mitral stenosis the free edges of the leaflets are bound together but the belly domes forward. When it reaches its limit, the opening snap (O.S.) occurs. Ao, aorta; LA, left atrium; S_1, first heart sound; S_2 second heart sound.
(Reproduced with permission. Ronan JA Jr. Cardiac auscultation: opening snaps, systolic clicks, and ejection sounds. Heart Disease and Stroke 2:189; 1993. Copyright 1993 American Heart Association.)

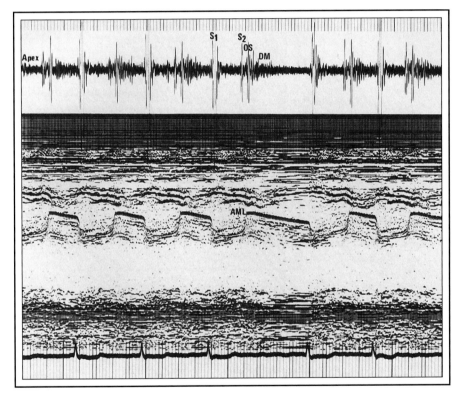

Figure 9. M-mode echocardiogram and phonocardiogram in mitral stenosis. The opening snap (OS) occurs synchronously with the rapid upstroke of the anterior mitral leaflet (AML) as it domes forward. Diastolic murmur (DM) follows.
(Reproduced with permission. Ronan JA Jr. Cardiac sound and ultrasound. Current Problems in Cardiology 6:33; 1981.)

when the dome-shaped aortic valve is abruptly checked in its upward movement at the onset of ejection (Figure 10). The fact that the sound and the valve movement occur simultaneously has been demonstrated by simultaneous M-mode echocardiography and phonocardiography (Figure 11). Two dimensional echocardiography can usually demonstrate the anatomy of the aortic valve and Doppler echocardiography can assess the severity of the stenosis or regurgitation. Occasionally an aortic ejection sound is caused by a dilated aortic root such as in Marfan's syndrome, luetic aortitis, or severe hypertension and that aortic root dilatation can be demonstrated by two dimensional echocardiography.

• **Systolic Clicks:** A systolic click is the hallmark of mitral valve prolapse (Figure 12). A click occurs when a segment or a scallop of a leaflet abruptly prolapses toward the left atrium (Figure 13).

Heart Murmurs

Individual valvular abnormalities produce specific heart murmurs, either systolic or diastolic. In each type of valvular heart disease, the murmur has characteristic features and there may be other auscultatory features such as an ejection sound, a systolic click, an opening snap, etc. Murmurs are created by turbulence of blood flow due to accelerated flow or regurgitant flow. The 2-D echocardio-

318

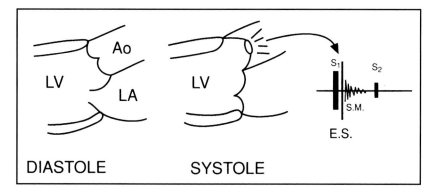

Figure 10. Diagram of the mechanism of the aortic valvular ejection sound (E.S.) in congenital valvular aortic stenosis. When the valve moves from its closed position in diastole to its open position in systole, a doming effect occurs because of restriction to complete opening. The E.S. occurs when the valve is checked at its maximally distended position. Ao, aorta; LA, left atrium; LV, left ventricle; SM, systolic murmur; S_1, first heart sound; S_2, second heart sound. *(Reproduced with permission. Ronan JA Jr. Cardiac auscultation: opening snaps, systolic clicks, and ejection sounds. Heart Disease and Stroke 2:190; 1993. Copyright 1993 American Heart Association.)*

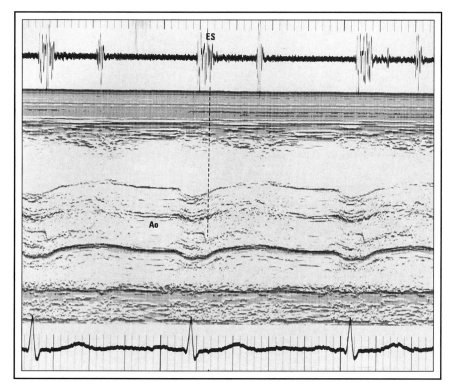

Figure 11. Echophonocardiogram in a patient with a bicuspid aortic valve (Ao). Posterior leaflet reaches its furthest extent at precise time of aortic ejection sound (ES). Aortic valve orifice size is reduced. Phonocardiogram shows ES in addition to the two components of the first heart sound. *(Reproduced with permission. Ronan JA Jr. Cardiac sound and ultrasound. Current Problems in Cardiology 6:29; 1981.)*

gram shows the structure of the heart and demonstrates many valvular abnormalities but it does not show the abnormalities of flow which generate the murmur. It is Doppler echocardiography which demonstrates the turbulent flow and provides the explanation for the murmurs. Abnormalities of high-velocity flow such as are seen in aortic stenosis can be demonstrated and quantitated by the spectral display of continuous wave Doppler, and abnormal flow patterns of lower velocity may be seen easily by pulsed wave Doppler either in spectral display or on color-flow Doppler patterns superimposed on the two dimensional image.

General Impressions Concerning Relationship of Heart Murmurs and Echocardiography

There may not be a precise correlation between auscultatory and echocardiographic findings because many factors may modify the findings of one method more than the other. Nevertheless, both methods provide useful information so we should compare and weigh the evidence found on auscultation with that found on echocardiography to obtain a more complete and accurate assessment of the patient. The following are general impressions gained from comparing both techniques:

1. Silent aortic and mitral regurgitation (Doppler study shows regurgitation but no murmur can be heard) usually is of no hemodynamic significance; regurgitation is usually so mild that no treatment is required.

2. When a heart murmur due to valvular regurgitation is faint (grades 1-2/6) *and is the only clinical evidence of regurgitation,* the regurgitation is usually mild. However, when there is other evidence of abnormality such as atrial or ventricular dilatation, heart failure, atrial fibrillation, etc. the

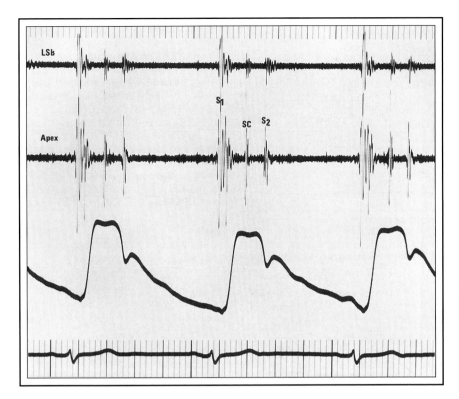

Figure 12. Phonocardiogram in mitral valve prolapse. There is a very loud mid systolic click and a prominently split first heart sound. *(Reproduced with permission. Ronan JA Jr. Cardiac sound and ultrasound. Current Problems in Cardiology 6:34; 1981.)*

regurgitation is at least of moderate degree. The assessment of the *severity* of the lesion usually can be made more accurately by echocardiography than by auscultation.

3. The murmur of aortic stenosis can be detected easily by auscultation so the diagnosis of aortic stenosis can be excluded if no murmur is present. However, the severity of the stenosis may be difficult to determine by auscultation alone and it is quantitated better by Doppler echocardiography, particularly in older persons.

4. Innocent pulmonic ejection flow murmurs usually can be clearly identified by cardiac auscultation because of their characteristic findings (Figure 14). These murmurs do not need echocardiographic confirmation as long as the examiner performs careful auscultation and has the experience necessary to distinguish an innocent murmur from a murmur due to a cardiac abnormality.

5. Routine diagnostic screening for valvular heart disease should be done by cardiac auscultation not by echocardiography. Auscultation is adequate for detecting significant valvular lesions so those individuals without auscultatory abnormalities can avoid the expense of echocardiography. The echocardiogram should not be used to "rule out a heart murmur" but if a murmur due to organic heart disease is detected, an echocardiogram may be helpful if there is doubt about the origin of the murmur or severity of the valvular lesion.

6. Tricuspid regurgitation and pulmonic regurgi-

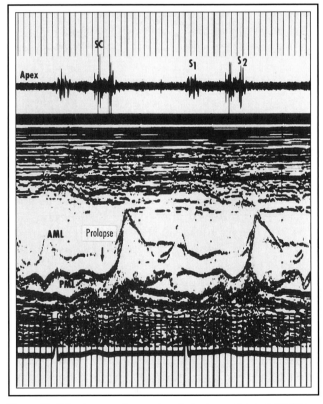

Figure 13. Echophonocardiogram in mitral valve prolapse. Posterior mitral leaflet moves posteriorly in late systole. Systolic click (SC) occurs at time of posterior movement of mitral valve. *(Reproduced with permission. Ronan JA Jr. Cardiac sound and ultrasound. Current Problems in Cardiology 6:35; 1981.)*

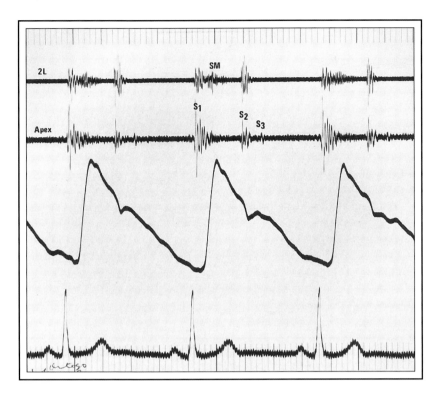

Figure 14. Phonocardiogram of innocent murmur in a 14-year-old boy. There is an early and midsystolic crescendo/decrescendo murmur (SM) which peaks in early systole. *(Reproduced with permission. Ronan JA Jr. Cardiac sound and ultrasound. Current Problems in Cardiology 6:48; 1981.)*

tation are detected by color flow Doppler in most normal patients, but the extent of regurgitation is mild. In almost all of those patients there is no murmur, i.e., silent regurgitation, and the echocardiographic regurgitation is considered of no significance. Occasionally moderate degrees of tricuspid regurgitation can be seen on echocardiography without producing a heart murmur. As a rule if those patients do not have pulmonary hypertension, right atrial or ventricular enlargement, or vena caval dilatation the regurgitation is not serious and does not require further evaluation.

Specific Disease States: Correlation Between Auscultation and Echocardiographic Findings

Aortic Stenosis

Aortic stenosis is a common form of valvular heart disease usually due to a degenerative process similar to atherosclerosis that slowly develops in a previously normal valve, usually in patients more than 60 years of age. On the other hand, patients with a congenital bicuspid valve, although they may have had no stenosis during their childhood years, eventually develop cusp thickening and calcification which becomes stenotic earlier than the degenerative form, commonly when the subjects are in their 40s.

• **Auscultatory Findings:** In aortic stenosis the main findings are a mid-systolic murmur at the base, a delayed or diminished aortic valve closure sound, a fourth heart sound, and occasionally an aortic ejection sound, particularly in those due to a bicuspid valve. The murmur is usually a diamond-shaped crescendo/decrescendo murmur (Figure 15). The more severe the stenosis the longer the murmur and the later it peaks in systole. The aortic ejection sound is due to the abrupt checking of the aortic valve when it domes upward and reaches the furthest extent of its opening. It identifies the aortic valve as the source of the ejection sound and murmur and it usually indicates that the valve is still movable and is not a rigid immobile calcified valve. A fourth heart sound is an indirect marker of the severity of aortic stenosis. It indicates reduced left ventricular compliance due to the left ventricular hypertrophy which has resulted from aortic valve obstruction. If left ventricular systolic dysfunction occurs and the left ventricle dilates, a third heart sound may be heard.

• **Echocardiographic Findings:** Two dimensional echocardiography shows thickening and decreased mobility of the individual valve leaflets and a reduced orifice size (Figure 16). Calcification usually is present. The severity of stenosis is reflected by the pressure gradient across the valve and the gradient can be estimated by determining the velocity of flow through the obstructed valve (Figure 17). According to the Bernoulli principle, the pressure gradient across an obstructed valve is related to the velocity of flow through the valve.

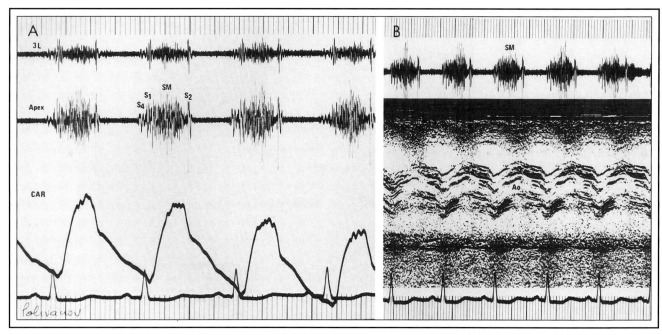

Figure 15A. Phonocardiogram in severe aortic stenosis. There is a very long systolic murmur (SM), which extends almost to second heart sound (S₂) and peaks late in systole. Fourth heart sound (S₄) is present. Carotid pulse tracing (CAR) shows a delayed peak and slow rate of rise.

Figure 15B. Echophonocardiogram in aortic stenosis. There is heavy calcification in aortic valve (Ao). SM, systolic murmur.

(Reproduced with permission. Ronan JA Jr. Cardiac sound and ultrasound. Current Problems in Cardiology 6:27; 1981.)

The simplified Bernoulli formula (Pressure Gradient = $4V^2$) means that in aortic stenosis the gradient across the valve may be calculated by squaring the aortic flow velocity, as measured in meters per second by continuous wave Doppler, and multiplying by 4. There has been a good correlation between gradients measured in this manner compared to those measured at cardiac catheterization.

The valve area itself can be calculated by the continuity equation. The continuity equation states that the volume of blood flowing through different areas of a continuously intact vascular system must be equal in all areas. Therefore, the blood flow proximal to a stenotic area ($V_1 \times A_1$) should equal the blood flow at the area of stenosis ($V_2 \times A_2$) (V = velocity, A = area). When this principle is applied to aortic stenosis the product of the area and flow velocity in the left ventricular outflow tract equals the product of the area and flow velocity through the aortic valve.

$$\text{AREA A.V.} = \frac{\text{AREA L.V.O. x VELOCITY L.V.O.}}{\text{VELOCITY A.V.}}$$

• Comparison of Methods

Auscultation: *Strengths:* Excellent for screening and diagnosing aortic stenosis. *Limitations:* May be difficult to estimate severity of the stenosis.

Echocardiography: *Strengths:* Excellent for

defining anatomy and establishing severity so that cardiac catheterization is not needed to judge severity. Ventricular function can be evaluated at the same time. *Limitations:* Cost.

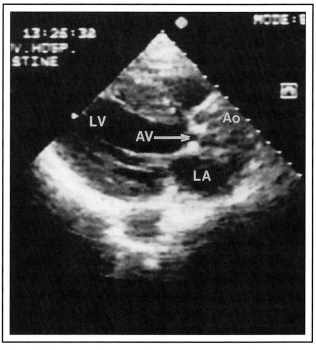

Figure 16. Parasternal long axis view of aortic stenosis. The aortic valve is calcified and has a narrow orifice (Arrow). AV = aortic valve; Ao = aorta; LV = left ventricle; LA = left atrium.

This is an excellent example of useful correlation of the echocardiogram with the clinical features, which may establish the diagnosis. It is now becoming well appreciated that congenital aortic stenosis is much more common than previously realized. We are indebted for this knowledge to physicians such as Jesse Edwards and William Roberts, who have correlated the pathology with clinical findings. As a matter of interest, the patient with the single valve lesion of aortic stenosis in the age group 40-50 years runs about an 80-90% chance of this being a bicuspid congenital valve. Also, we now know that the natural history of a patient with a bicuspid valve may, in some, be manifest in youth by only an aortic ejection sound. This may or may not be associated with a short midsystolic murmur. The ejection sound frequently is overlooked and the systolic murmur often is called innocent; however, the presence of an ejection sound almost always takes this out of the "ball park" of being innocent, despite the fact that the murmur itself is short and otherwise may sound like a typical innocent murmur. In addition, sometimes a faint aortic diastolic murmur may also be heard at an early age and no systolic murmur be present. Subsequently, in some there is progression over the years to the classic aortic stenosis (with or without aortic insufficiency). The valve may become calcific, and not uncommonly the diagnosis is made for the first time at the age of 50 or 60.

W. Proctor Harvey, M.D.

Bicuspid Aortic Valve

• **Auscultatory Findings:** An aortic ejection sound may be the earliest evidence of a bicuspid aortic valve (Figure 11) due to the sudden checking of the valve as it domes upward. A mild degree of aortic regurgitation is sometimes present but the murmur of regurgitation is usually very faint. Aortic stenosis due to a bicuspid aortic valve is usually not severe in younger individuals but may increase with age. The murmur tends to become louder, longer, and later peaking as the extent of aortic stenosis increases.

The natural history of a bicuspid aortic valve does not, of course, necessarily mean that every patient will have significant stenosis of that valve as years go by. It is well known that a bicuspid aortic valve without any degree of stenosis may be a surprise finding at autopsy. Often poorly appreciated is the fact that one of the early signs of bicuspid aortic valve is an ejection sound well heard at the apex and also at the base of the heart. This ejection sound is unaffected by respiration and may be confused with a split first heart sound. It can occur with or without a faint systolic murmur and may therefore be overlooked. Later, the same patient being followed may have a systolic murmur, which can progressively increase in intensity until the diagnosis of aortic stenosis is made. Also, the murmur of the bicuspid aortic valve stenosis has often been confused with that of an innocent murmur because it is a short murmur in early to midsystole or midsystole. One important clue often overlooked is the ejection sound, which immediately takes the systolic murmur out of the ball park of "innocence." Of course, the presence of a faint aortic diastolic blow in association with these auscultatory findings just described would be an immediate additional clue pinpointing the aortic valve pathology.

W. Proctor Harvey, M.D.

• **Echocardiographic Findings:** The two dimensional image on the parasternal short axis view shows two rather than three cusps (Figure 18). One cusp is usually larger than the other. Doppler study shows varying degrees of stenosis and usually mild aortic regurgitation.

• **Comparison of Methods**

Auscultatory Findings: *Strengths:* Ejection sound is the clue to diagnosis. Auscultation is a very adequate method to screen for significant obstruction or regurgitation. *Limitations:* Aortic ejection sound might be misinterpreted as the second part of a split first sound.

Echocardiographic Findings: *Strengths:* When the two-dimensional image of the bicuspid valve is clear it provides indisputable evidence that it is bicuspid. *Limitations:* Image of the individual cusps is often unclear enough to determine there are only two cusps. There may be a raphe in the larger cusp creating the false impression that there are three cusps.

The ejection sound is a hallmark of a congenital bicuspid aortic valve and occurs with "doming" of the valve in early systole. It, too, as with the systolic murmur, is generally well

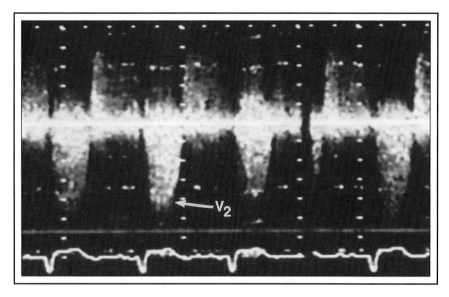

Figure 17. Spectral continuous wave Doppler recording of aortic flow velocity (V₂) in aortic stenosis. Peak flow velocity is 4.7 meters per second indicating severe aortic stenosis.

heard from the apex to the aortic area. It does not diminish in intensity with inspiration (as can occur with the ejection sound of congenital pulmonic stenosis).

If severe aortic stenosis is present, one readily hears a loud (grade 4 to 6) precordial murmur. However, aortic stenosis of a mild to moderate degree can easily be overlooked on a cursory physical examination, especially if the examining physician is not listening specifically for the tell-tale findings of an ejection sound and a systolic murmur. It is also worthwhile to remember that body build

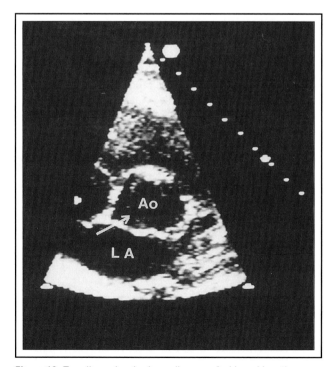

Figure 18. Two dimensional echocardiogram of a bicuspid aortic valve in the short axis view. Arrow points to one cusp. Ao = aortic valve; LA = left atrium.

(large frame, heavy weight, and highly developed chest musculature) can diminish the intensity of sounds and murmurs heard with the stethoscope. In contrast, murmurs in children and young people with thin chests will be more readily detected.

With increasing severity of stenosis due to a congenital bicuspid aortic valve, the systolic murmur usually becomes louder, harsher, and longer in duration. It may be well heard in the neck, supraclavicular area, and over the carotids. An aortic diastolic murmur is not an unexpected finding.

It is of great importance to differentiate the murmur of congenital aortic stenosis from an innocent systolic murmur. Early diagnosis can be readily accomplished in the physician's office.

The auscultatory findings in a patient with a congenital bicuspid aortic valve represent a spectrum. Most commonly, an early to mid-systolic murmur of grade 1 to 3 intensity is present. Frequently it has a harsh quality similar to the sound of clearing one's throat. In some, an early blowing, high frequency aortic diastolic murmur of grade 1 to 3 is heard. Firm pressure on the stethoscope's flat diaphragm chest piece should always be used to best detect this diastolic murmur, listening along the left sternal border, with the patient sitting upright, leaning forward, and breath held in deep expiration.

Since aortic events are usually well heard at the apex, the systolic murmur of aortic stenosis may be detected from the aortic area to the apex. This is also true of the aortic ejection sound that is another key to this condition.

W. Proctor Harvey, M.D.

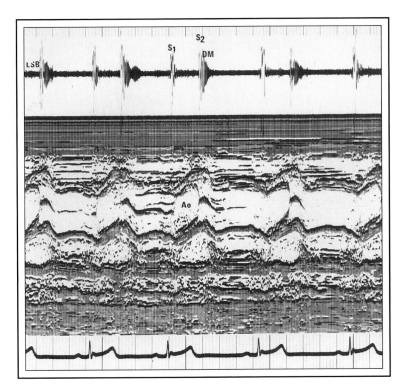

Figure 19. Echophonocardiogram in aortic regurgitation. Phonocardiogram showing the diastolic decrescendo murmur (DM) of aortic regurgitation. The aortic valve (Ao) opens normally. *(Reproduced with permission. Ronan JA Jr. Cardiac sound and ultrasound. Current Problems in Cardiology 6:34; 1981.)*

Aortic Regurgitation

Pure aortic regurgitation may be due to primary valvular disease (rheumatic, bicuspid valve, endocarditis, aortic valve prolapse) or due to diseases of the aorta itself (ascending aortic aneurysm, cystic medial necrosis of the aorta, hypertension, lues, dissection of the aorta). It may also occur in combination with aortic stenosis but in those cases the aortic stenosis is usually the dominant lesion.

• **Auscultatory Findings:** A diastolic decrescendo soft blowing murmur at the left sternal border is the classic murmur of aortic regurgitation (Figure 19). In some cases the aortic closure sound (A$_2$) may be diminished or indistinguishable from the beginning of the murmur. In severe aortic regurgitation there may be premature closure of the mitral valve leaflets due to the large volume of regurgitant flow which fills the left ventricle and moves the mitral leaflets to a closed or semi-closed position in late diastole even without ventricular contraction. In these cases the first heart sound is faint. A systolic ejection flow murmur is present when the regurgitation is of a moderate or severe degree. This does not imply that aortic stenosis is present, merely that there is a large and rapid flow because the regurgitation has produced a large blood volume in the left ventricle. The location of the diastolic murmur louder at the right sternal border than at the left border is a clue that the murmur may be due to aortic root disease, such as dissection of the aorta or ascending aortic aneurysm.

Generally, the best position to bring out the high-frequency diastolic blowing murmur of aortic regurgitation is with the patient sitting upright and leaning forward, with the breath held in deep expiration (Fig. A). The flat diaphragm of the stethoscope should be pressed firmly against the chest wall, which usually leaves a brief imprint of the chest piece. It is wise to tell the patient that firm pressure of the stethoscope will be used, and usually no discomfort is experienced, although the pressure will obviously be felt. Unless this position as just described plus the very firm pressure is used, the faintest aortic diastolic murmur may be overlooked. It should be carefully searched for in every patient.

Another valuable position to "bring out" a faint aortic diastolic murmur is by propping the patient on the elbows while he or she is lying on the stomach (Fig. B). Listen as just described. Most examiners are unaware of this maneuver, and it is seldom used. An initial clue might come from a slight "quick rise" or "flip" on palpation of the arteries, but this situation is not likely with the mildest degrees of aortic regurgitation.

W. Proctor Harvey, M.D.

An Austin-Flint murmur may be present in severe cases. It is a low frequency apical diastolic murmur which usually has both mid-diastolic and pre-systolic components and is indicative of aortic regurgitation of at least moderate degree. It is due to inflow across the mitral valve, which has been partially closed because of the aortic diastolic regurgitant jet. In very severe aortic regurgitation the Austin Flint murmur may be limited to mid-diastole because of premature closure of the mitral valve leaflets at end diastole.

• **Echocardiographic Findings:** 2-D echocardiography alone is not an accurate method of detecting aortic regurgitation. The image may give the false impression of separation of the leaflets even though the valve may be perfectly competent while, on the other hand, the leaflets may appear to close correctly but still be incompetent.

The most sensitive method for diagnosing aortic regurgitation is by Doppler echocardiography, including color-flow and pulsed-wave/continuous wave studies. There is no infallible way of measuring the extent of aortic regurgitation but it is probably best estimated by comparing the width of the regurgitant jet at the orifice of the valve to the width of the left ventricular outflow tract. If the ratio of the jet width to the left ventricular outflow diameter is less than 25%, the regurgitation is mild, if 25%-50% it is moderate, and if greater than 50% it is severe. This approach is only a guide to judging severity and there are many exceptions. In the past the most frequently used method had been to compare the area of the regurgitant jet to the area of the left ventricular cavity. However, that method has definite limitations because the size of the jet is easily altered if it impinges on the septum or mitral valve or if it mixes with mitral inflow. The direction of the jet corresponds to the radiation of the murmur. In most cases, the jet is directed near the interventricular septum into the body of the left ventricle and the murmur is heard along the left sternal border. In some cases the jet is directed more laterally and the murmur is heard better at the cardiac apex.

Continuous-wave Doppler analysis of the jet of aortic regurgitation demonstrates the velocity of the regurgitant jet and the duration that it persists in diastole (Figure 20). The velocity of the jet is a reflection of the pressure gradient between the aorta and left ventricle in diastole (Bernoulli principle). In mild aortic regurgitation, the aortic diastolic pressure is only minimally diminished so there is a large diastolic gradient between the aorta and left ventricle and it falls slowly; correspondingly, velocity of the regurgitant jet also diminishes slowly throughout diastole. The rate at which that flow velocity of the jet diminishes through diastole is related to the rate at which the diastolic gradient diminishes and to the severity of regurgitation. In mild aortic regurgitation the flow velocity diminishes at a slow rate (Figure 20A) whereas in severe aortic regurgitation it diminishes rapidly (Figure 20B). The pressure half time is an index of this function and it measures the time required for the pressure gradient to fall to half of its initial value. When this principle is converted from pressure gra-

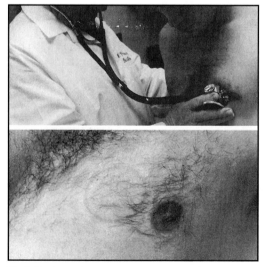

Fig A: To detect the murmur of aortic regurgitation, the physician has the patient sit upright, leaning forward, breath held in deep expiration. Listen along the left sternal border (top panel). Use firm pressure on the diaphragm of the stethoscope. If a brief imprint is not left on the skin, a faint aortic diastolic murmur can be missed (bottom panel).

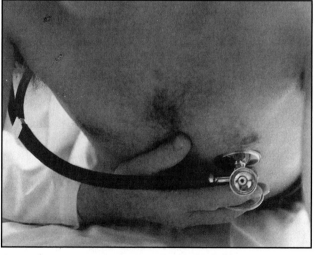

Fig B: Patient is propped up on the elbows. The diaphragm of the stethoscope is pressed firmly along the left sternal border. This seldom-used maneuver may be used to detect a faint aortic diastolic murmur or a pericardial friction rub.

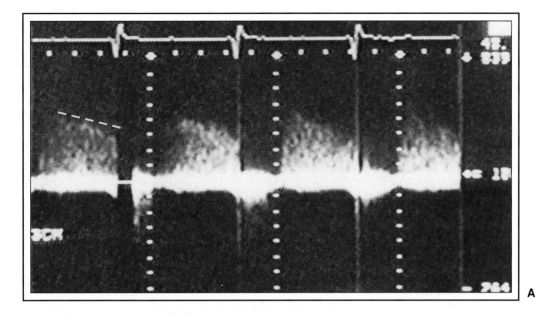

A

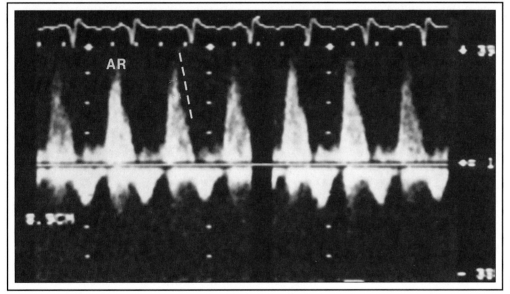

B

Figure 20. (A) Spectral continuous wave Doppler recording of aortic regurgitation. Dotted line shows a gradual decrease in flow velocity consistent with mild aortic regurgitation. (B) Continuous wave Doppler recording of severe aortic regurgitation. Dotted line shows rapid decrease in flow velocity of aortic regurgitation, consistent with severe aortic regurgitation.

dients to flow velocity the time required to fall to half the peak pressure gradient is the same as the time required to fall to 0.7 peak velocity of regurgitant flow. Therefore in aortic regurgitation the pressure half-time is the time required to reach 0.7 peak velocity of regurgitant flow. Values for mild degrees of aortic regurgitation generally are greater than 500 msec and for severe aortic regurgitation are less than 200 msec.

• Comparison of Methods

Auscultation: *Strengths:* The murmur of significant aortic regurgitation can usually be detected by auscultation and considered with the other clinical findings (arterial pulse pressure, heart size on chest x-ray, symptoms, etc.) allows a good estimation of lesion severity. Very mild degrees of aortic regurgitation frequently have a very faint murmur, or no murmur, but these lesions are usually of no hemodynamic significance, and the patient is not disadvantaged if it remains undetected. *Limitations:* Decisions about selecting the time for aortic valve surgery in patients with severe aortic regurgitation depend on serial evaluations of left ventricular function. If the left ventricle begins to fail, the valve should be replaced before failure is severe and irreversible. Auscultation alone is not a reliable method for measuring progressive myocardial deterioration, but it usually is consistent with the other evidence when all factors are considered.

Echocardiography: *Strengths:* Echocardiography is an excellent method to determine etiology of aortic regurgitation and is reasonably good for evaluating lesion severity. Left ventricular function can be measured well, a crucial factor for deciding the time for aortic valve surgery. *Limitations:* The Doppler method is so sensitive that it detects very minimal amounts of unimportant regurgitation. There is a risk of overestimating the importance of these small leaks.

CARDIAC PEARL

The echocardiogram is also useful in aiding evaluation of patients suspected of having severe aortic regurgitation, such as premature closure of the mitral valve. It is well appreciated today that in these acute cases one should move rapidly for aortic valve replacement.

W. Proctor Harvey, M.D.

Mitral Regurgitation

The mitral valve apparatus has five major components, each of which is important to proper functioning of the mitral valve. These include the anterior and posterior mitral leaflets, the chordae tendineae, the papillary muscles, the left ventricular myocardium, and the mitral annulus. Mitral regurgitation may be produced by abnormalities of any one or more of those components.

Acute rheumatic fever causes mitral valvulitis and regurgitation which sometimes persists and becomes chronic mitral regurgitation. Idiopathic degeneration of the mitral valve leaflets and/or elongation of the chordae tendineae leads to mitral valve prolapse and in the more severe cases, mitral regurgitation. Chordal rupture may occur spontaneously, particularly in patients with mitral valve prolapse, or from endocarditis. Papillary muscle dysfunction is due to ischemic heart disease, usually myocardial infarction, and is very common; papillary muscle rupture secondary to myocardial infarction is extremely rare. Left ventricular dilatation of any cause may produce mitral regurgitation if the mitral annulus dilates and if the papillary muscles become malaligned and prevent proper valve closure. Any disease which causes left ventricular dilatation such as the cardiomyopathies, extensive myocardial infarction, or aortic regurgitation can cause mitral regurgitation. Calcification of the mitral annulus commonly occurs in the elderly and in patients with hypertension, but it usually leads to only mild mitral regurgitation.

• **Auscultatory Findings:** A holosystolic apical murmur is the classic murmur of mitral regurgitation. The configuration of the murmur may vary (crescendo, decrescendo, crescendo-decrescendo, plateau-shaped, etc). In severe mitral regurgitation, a third heart sound usually occurs and in a few very severe cases there may be a short diastolic flow rumble after the third heart sound. In many patients with mitral valve prolapse the murmur does not begin until mid or late systole because the valve is competent in early systole and does not leak until the ventricle reaches a smaller critical size in mid or late systole to allow the prolapse to occur.

• **Echocardiographic Findings:** Doppler echocardiography illustrates mitral regurgitation both on color-flow Doppler and on spectral continuous-wave or pulsed-wave Doppler. The severity of mitral regurgitation is usually judged on color flow Doppler by comparing the area of the maximum regurgitant jet to the area of the left atrium. When the ratio of the jet area to the left atrial area is less than 20%, the regurgitation is mild. When it is 20%-40% it is moderate and if it is greater than 40% it is severe. Although this is the most widely-used method of quantifying mitral regurgitation there are some pitfalls inherent in that approach. If the jet is directed centrally into the left atrium the method is usually reliable but if the jet impinges on the atrial wall the flow velocity and direction will change and the area of the jet will appear falsely small. Variations in left ventricular loading conditions (pressure and volume) definitely influence the extent of regurgitation and the size of the jet area so that the significance of a certain amount of regurgitation is quite different if a patient is hypertensive or hypotensive, volume overloaded or hypovolemic. These factors must be considered when evaluating the importance of any mitral regurgitation. Technical factors such as the gain settings, the angle of the echo beam, and the carrier frequency of the ultrasound all may affect the jet size. Furthermore, in some patients it is difficult to evaluate the size of the area of the atrium so that the ratio of the area of the jet to the area of the atrium cannot be obtained.

Another method of estimating the severity of regurgitation is simply to measure the absolute size of the maximal jet area, disregarding the size of the atrium. Although there are certain limitations with the approach, particularly because it is sometimes difficult to determine the jet's borders, a reasonable clinical estimate of severity often can be made. If the jet is central in position with an area of <4 cm^2, the regurgitation is mild, if 4-8 cm^2 it is moderate, and if >8 cm^2 it is severe.

Specific Forms of Mitral Regurgitation

Rheumatic Heart Disease

The hallmark of rheumatic heart disease is mitral stenosis; in the patient with rheumatic

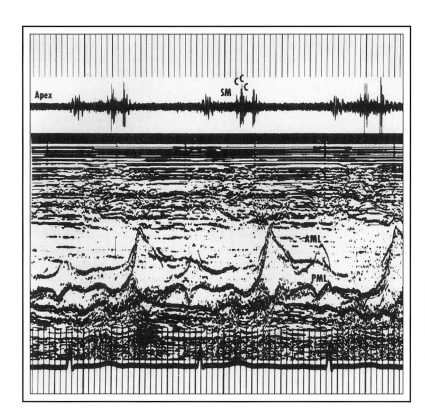

Figure 21. Echophonocardiogram in mitral valve prolapse. Prolapse begins in early systole but is accentuated in late systole. There are at least three systolic clicks (C) and a mid-late systolic murmur (SM). *(Reproduced with permission. Ronan JA, Jr. Cardiac sound and ultrasound. Current Problems in Cardiology 6:21; 1981.)*

mitral regurgitation the clue of the rheumatic etiology is the evidence of mitral stenosis.

• **Auscultatory Findings:** There is a typical apical holosystolic murmur and if the mitral regurgitation is severe there may be a third heart sound. However, if mitral stenosis is also present there is usually a loud first heart sound, an opening snap, and an apical diastolic low frequency murmur. Only in rare cases is there both a third heart sound and opening snap present because the third sound is due to rapid filling of the ventricle and that is usually prevented in mitral stenosis because of the obstruction to inflow.

• **Echocardiographic Findings:** On 2-D echocardiography, the mitral valve is thickened, has reduced mobility and usually has commissural fusion. The anterior leaflet domes forward in diastole with the classic "hockey stick" appearance. The left atrium is dilated. The left ventricular cavity size depends on whether the mitral regurgitation or mitral stenosis is the dominant lesion. When regurgitation is dominant the ventricle becomes dilated and when mitral stenosis is dominant, the ventricle remains small. The mitral regurgitation is evident on the Doppler study.

Mitral Valve Prolapse

The most common mitral valve abnormality is mitral valve prolapse. It occurs in up to 6% of the population and although the prolapsed valve may produce regurgitation, in most cases the prolapse occurs with little or no regurgitation.

• **Auscultatory Findings:** A systolic click is diagnostic of mitral valve prolapse and is due to the sudden checking of the valve when it reaches the limit of its distensibility as it prolapses into the left atrium in systole (Figure 21). Frequently, the systolic click is the only auscultatory evidence of mitral valve prolapse but in many cases there is also a systolic murmur due to mitral regurgitation. The classic murmur begins in mid or late systole because the prolapse itself does not occur until then. In the more severe cases, the prolapse begins at the beginning of systole and leads to a holosystolic murmur. The acoustic character of the classic click is often fine, sharp, and superficial, hence the name "click". However, in many cases the click has a medium frequency tone or may even be a faint low frequency sound. Most systolic clicks occur in mid or late systole and are not to be confused with an ejection sound which occurs in early systole at the onset of ejection. The vasoactive maneuvers can help differentiate between a click and an ejection sound. Any of the maneuvers that decrease ventricular size (sitting, standing, or the Valsalva maneuver), make the click appear earlier in systole whereas the maneuvers that tend to increase ventricular size (squatting, the supine position, or vasopressors) make the click appear later in systole. These maneuvers do not affect the timing of the ejection sound. Patients with mitral valve prolapse are frequently slender individuals who may have an innocent pulmonic ejection flow murmur. It is important to recognize the pulmonic ejection flow murmur and to distinguish it from the murmur of mitral regurgitation in mitral valve prolapse. The pulmonic ejection murmur is merely an innocent heart murmur and is unrelated to the mitral valve.

CARDIAC PEARL

Differentiating mitral valve prolapse from innocent systolic murmur generally is not difficult. The typical murmur of mitral valve prolapse is in mid to late systole, whereas the innocent murmur is in the early to mid portions of systole. A click (or clicks) frequently accompanies the murmur of mitral valve prolapse but is absent with an innocent murmur.

There are exceptions, of course. Occasionally, murmurs of mitral valve prolapse are heard in early or mid-systole with or without an associated click or clicks. The squatting maneuver is valuable in bringing out these systolic clicks and murmurs (generally late apical), because they can be altered on squatting.

At times, the squatting maneuver can also cause movement of clicks and/or murmurs in systole as a result of this change in position. A maneuver that increases volume to the left side of the heart, such as squatting, may delay these auscultatory findings, and therefore the click or murmur may move closer to the second heart sound (Figure A). On prompt standing and with a decrease in volume they may move in the opposite direction in systole-closer to the first heart sound. Also contributing is the bending of the knees and hips, which can increase peripheral arterial systolic pressure, and cause movement closer to the second sound, and closer to the first sound on standing.

The fact that there is a change in these auscultatory findings serves as additional evi-

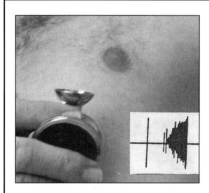

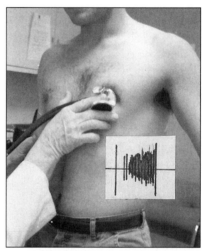

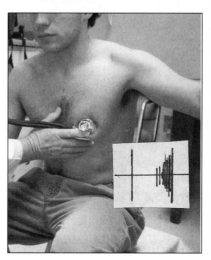

Fig A: Mitral Valve Prolapse - Movement of clicks and murmurs with change of position. Left: Patient lying on back. Note two systolic clicks in mid systole followed by late apical systolic murmur (SM). On standing (top right), the clicks move toward the first sound (S_1) as does the murmur, which becomes longer and often louder. On squatting (bottom right) the clicks and murmur move toward the second sound.

dence of the diagnosis of mitral valve prolapse. In some patients the clicks and/or murmurs might not be heard in either the standing or squatting positions.

W. Proctor Harvey, M.D.

• **Echocardiographic Findings:** On 2-D echocardiography the major criterion for the diagnosis of mitral valve prolapse is the displacement of one or both of the valvular leaflets to the atrial side of the atrioventricular plane (Figure 22). It is frequently difficult to make that judgment because the valve and the heart are both moving and the valve plane is only an imaginary line connecting the bases of the anterior and posterior mitral valve leaflets. Furthermore, on the apical four-chamber view, the plane of the mitral valve is in more of a saddle shape than that of a flat plane so that it is difficult to know the precise location of the valve plane. Other features sometimes seen in mitral valve prolapse are thickened, voluminous leaflets, enlargement of the annulus, and in some older individuals there may be thin linear calcification of a leaflet, sometimes fixing the leaflet in a cupped configuration. When mitral regurgitation is present, it usually is mild but in a very small minority of the cases there may be moderate or even severe mitral regurgitation. In very rare cases chordal rupture may result leading to a flail mitral leaflet which can be detected on 2-D images.

Papillary Muscle Dysfunction

• **Auscultatory Findings:** The murmur is usually a soft apical holosystolic murmur of grade 1 or 2 intensity, but in severe mitral regurgitation it may be louder. Since myocardial infarction usually is the cause of this mitral regurgitation there may be other evidences of systolic and/or diastolic left ventricular dysfunction such as third and/or fourth heart sounds.

• **Echocardiographic Findings:** In addition to the Doppler evidence of mitral regurgitation the 2-D images show a left ventricular wall motion abnormality of that segment involving the papillary muscle, most often the inferior wall at the base of the posteromedial papillary muscle. The wall motion abnormality includes a decrease in systolic thickening as well as a decrease in wall motion ranging from hypokinesis to dyskinesis. In chronic cases, scarring may result in a decrease in the mass of the papillary muscle. The mitral valve leaflets themselves are normal and have normal motion.

Mitral Annular Calcification

Mitral annular calcification is common in the elderly, particularly those with hypertension. Most

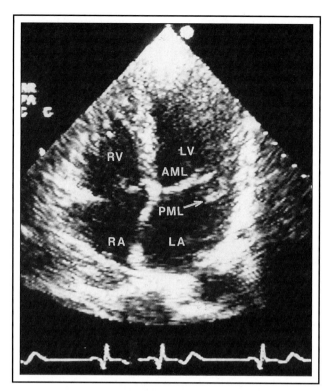

Figure 22. 2-D echocardiogram of mitral valve prolapse of the posterior mitral leaflet (PML). Arrow points to posterior mitral leaflet which has prolapsed posterior to the AV valve plane. AML, anterior mitral leaflet; LV, left ventricle; LA, left atrium; RV, right ventricle; RA, right atrium.

individuals over 80 years of age have significant annular calcification. The calcification probably interferes with the sphincter-like movement of the annulus during systole, but there also may be an extension of the calcification into the posterior mitral leaflet, which is directly adjacent to the annulus. The leaflet then becomes thickened and has decreased mobility; extent of mitral regurgitation is usually minimal.

In unusual cases, the annular calcification can become very heavy so that it may extend the length of the annulus and even protrude into the mitral orifice. In those rare cases when the anterior mitral leaflet also becomes thickened the net effect may be valvular obstruction, but invariably it is mild. It should be distinguished from rheumatic mitral stenosis because the pathology, the echocardiographic and auscultatory findings, and in some cases the treatment are different from the rheumatic form.

• **Auscultatory Findings:** The murmur of mitral regurgitation is usually holosystolic and of grade 1 or 2 intensity. The extent of mitral regurgitation is mild, and in some instances the murmur may only be mid and/or late systolic. Since aortic valve sclerosis or stenosis frequently accompanies mitral annular calcification there may be a separate systolic ejection murmur which must be identified in order to avoid confusion.

• **Echocardiographic Findings:** The 2-D echocardiogram shows the calcification of the annulus in all views but it is most easily identified in the parasternal long-axis view at the base of the posterior mitral leaflet. The parasternal short-axis view and the apical four chamber view display the entire length of the annulus and in those views the extent of involvement can be appreciated. Doppler study shows the mitral regurgitation. In those rare cases when mounds of calcification extend into the posterior leaflet and cause valve narrowing the Doppler study of mitral inflow can determine the extent of obstruction by the pressure half-time measurement. When aortic sclerosis, aortic stenosis, and/or left ventricular hypertrophy are present in the same patient with mitral annular calcification those abnormalities are easily detectable on 2-D echocardiography.

CARDIAC PEARL

It appears that the echocardiogram is an excellent means of diagnosing calcified mitral anulus. Radiographically this can be identified as a linear calcification assuming a C or J shape in the region of the mitral valve. This configuration is longer and is different from that of mitral valve calcification, which is more likely to be concentrated in a more circular or rosette formation. A mitral valve anulus may be present with or without a systolic murmur. At times it is present in patients with Marfan's syndrome and may be seen in some combination with prolapse of the mitral valve leaflet. It is good to know that the echocardiogram can identify the presence of mitral valve anulus calcification in a high percentage of cases.

W. Proctor Harvey, M.D.

• **Comparison of Methods**

Auscultation: *Strengths:* Auscultation is a practical and economical way to detect mitral regurgitation, and it is a simple method for detecting systolic clicks, an indicator of mitral valve prolapse. *Limitations:* Mild degrees of mitral regurgitation may be silent and when hypotension and/or congestive heart failure are present, even moderate degrees of regurgitation may be silent or difficult to hear. Occasionally the murmur can be confused with aortic stenosis, particularly if it radiates toward the base.

Echocardiography: *Strengths:* Excellent for detecting moderate and severe degrees of regurgitation. Mild mitral regurgitation is usually accurately detected. The mechanism of the regurgitation is usually apparent from the 2-D study. *Limitations:* There are occasional errors of both over-diagnosing and under-diagnosing minor degrees of regurgitation. Mild regurgitation can be missed if the scan-

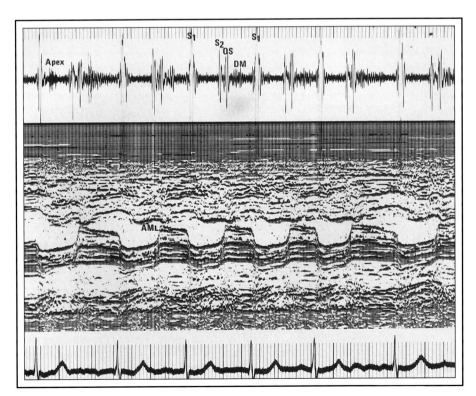

Figure 23. Echophonocardiogram in mitral stenosis showing marked decrease in early diastolic closing velocity, E-F slope and parallel movement of the anterior (AML) and posterior mitral leaflets. Phonocardiogram shows a loud opening snap (OS) simultaneous with doming of the anterior mitral leaflet. DM, diastolic murmur. *(Reproduced with permission. Ronan JA Jr: Cardiac sound and ultrasound. Current Problems in Cardiology 6:10; 1981.)*

ning does not cover the entire valve or because of technical considerations such as Doppler angle, system gain, frame rate, and pulse repetition frequency. The size of the jet area is also dependent on left ventricular pressure, valve orifice size, and jet geometry. Jets which impinge on the left atrial wall lose momentum and become smaller than if the jet had remained in the center of the atrium.

Mitral Stenosis

Mitral stenosis is due to rheumatic heart disease. It is the single valvular lesion that is diagnostic of rheumatic heart disease; all of the other valvular lesions that can be seen in rheumatic heart disease can also be attributed to other causes.

• **Auscultatory Findings:** A loud first heart sound, an opening snap, and a low frequency apical diastolic murmur are the classic findings of mitral stenosis (Figure 23). The first heart sound is loud because the mitral valve closure is delayed and occurs at a slightly higher point on the left ventricular pressure curve resulting in more forceful valve closure. The opening snap occurs when the anterior mitral leaflet domes forward and is abruptly checked in its anterior movement. The timing of the opening snap is related to the height of left atrial pressure; the higher the left atrial pressure the earlier the opening snap. The low-frequency diastolic

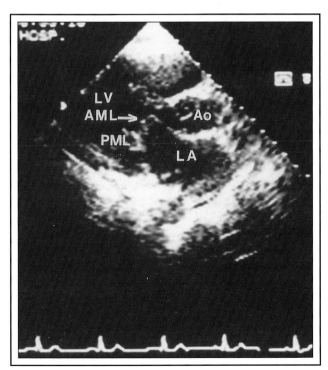

Figure 24. 2-D echocardiogram in mitral stenosis. Parasternal long axis view. Anterior mitral leaflet (AML) domes forward into the left ventricle in diastole. It is bound to the posterior mitral leaflet (PML) and cannot open freely. LV = left ventricle; LA = left atrium; Ao = aorta.

murmur is loudest at two separate times in the cardiac cycle corresponding to the times when the rate of ventricular filling is rapid. The first time occurs in early diastole immediately after the opening snap and the second time is in late diastole after atrial contraction and it produces a presystolic murmur immediately prior to the loud first heart sound.

• **Echocardiographic Findings:** The 2-D echocardiogram shows thickening of the mitral valve leaflets and anterior doming of the anterior mitral leaflet in early diastole (Figure 24). Leaflets also may have calcification and commissural fusion, and the chordae tendineae may become thickened and fuse together. The left atrium is dilated and the left ventricle is small (Figure 25). Mitral regurgitation frequently accompanies mitral stenosis and in those cases the left ventricle is usually larger than in pure mitral stenosis and the regurgitant jet is easily seen on color-flow Doppler. The valve area can be measured directly by planimetry or by the pressure half-time method which measures the time required for the mitral gradient to fall to half of its initial peak value. The smaller the valve area, the longer it takes the gradient to diminish.

• **Comparison of Methods**

Auscultation: *Strengths:* The classic findings are distinctive and make the diagnosis certain. *Limitations:* Sometimes findings can only be detected over a very small area at the cardiac apex so it requires careful evaluation.

CARDIAC PEARL

To "bring out" the diastolic rumble of mitral stenosis, as a rule, one does not have to try specific maneuvers such as having the patient exercise moderately by doing sit-ups in bed and listening afterwards. This can be done, if necessary, but generally all that is required is to find the localized spot, over the point of maximum impulse of the left ventricle. Also very helpful when the patient is in the left lateral position is to listen while he/she takes four or five deep breaths in rapid succession, or coughs several times. Immediately after either of these maneuvers it will be noted that the rumble may double or triple in intensity.

Indeed, the very act of turning can accentuate the rumble of mitral stenosis. I recall an illuminating personal experience that I had when I was a medical intern and was a member of a group on teaching rounds with a **Visiting Physician.** Our instructor listened to the patient just after turning him to the left

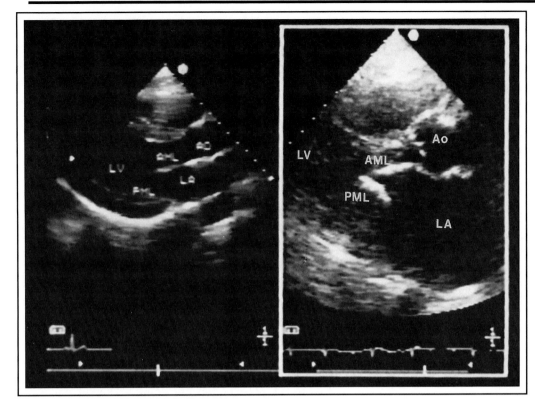

Figure 25. Parasternal long axis view of mitral valve in diastole. (Left panel, normal mitral valve. Right panel, mitral stenosis). The anterior mitral leaflet (AML) and the posterior mitral leaflet (PML) are thickened in mitral stenosis and the opening between the two leaflets is reduced. The left atrium (LA) is dilated.

lateral position and described the typical rumbling murmur of mitral stenosis. Several other physicians listened in succession, nodding their heads in agreement as to the presence of this typical murmur. I recall being about the fifth physician, but I could not hear what they had described. I did not hear the typical rumble even though I was apparently listening over the same area. This made some wonder if I was able to detect such a murmur; on the other hand, I also wondered if the others actually did hear it. Subsequent to this disappointment I had continuous recorded phonocardiograms made in other patients which showed how the murmur of mitral stenosis may change with the act of turning. The typical diastolic rumble with presystolic accentuation may appear or may be greatly accentuated coincident with turning and immediately afterwards, but then may wane in intensity after a few beats. By the time the fourth or fifth physician comes up to listen the murmur may not be audible although it was initially. It is of interest that one can turn the patient from the flat position to the right lateral position, and then back to flat and bring out this presystolic accentuation which seems to be initiated by the act of turning. It is important, therefore, to listen both during the act of turning, and, more importantly, to listen over the point of maximum impulse of the left ventricle after the patient has turned to the left lateral position.

W. Proctor Harvey, M.D.

Echocardiography: *Strengths:* Diagnosis can be made with absolute certainty on 2-D echocardiography and the severity of the lesion can be quantitated either by 2-D echocardiography or Doppler. Complicating factors such as mitral regurgitation, aortic valve disease, pulmonary hypertension, etc can also be detected so that the complete evaluation of mitral stenosis can be accomplished by echocardiography. *Limitations:* Cost.

Tricuspid Regurgitation

True organic tricuspid regurgitation may be due to rheumatic heart disease, endocarditis, carcinoid syndrome, or Ebstein's anomaly of the tricuspid valve, but these conditions are very uncommon. On the other hand, echocardiography has shown that tricuspid regurgitation is extremely common, usually of a mild to moderate degree, and in most cases is not clinically important. Significant tricuspid regurgitation may result from pulmonary hypertension of any cause (left ventricular heart failure, mitral valve disease, etc), and from right ventricular dilatation due to right ventricular failure or atrial septal defect. Right ventricular pacemaker leads usually cause a mild degree of tricuspid regurgitation. However, we now know that most normal individuals have very mild tricuspid regurgitation, which is not significant and without echocardiography would have been unrecognized.

• **Auscultatory Findings:** In moderate and severe tricuspid regurgitation, there is a long sys-

334

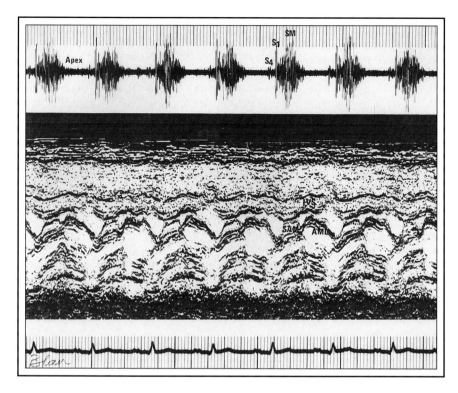

Figure 26. Systolic anterior motion (SAM) of anterior mitral leaflet (AML) producing left ventricular outflow tract obstruction. IVS, intraventricular septum. *(Reproduced with permission. Ronan JA, Jr. Cardiac sound and ultrasound. Current Problems in Cardiology 6:32; 1981.)*

tolic murmur, usually best heard at the lower left sternal border and it is louder on inspiration than on expiration. The murmur is sometimes not holosystolic, particularly if it is faint, but when it is loud it is almost always holosystolic. A third heart sound may be present and can be identified as originating in the right ventricle if it is louder on inspiration. The venous pulse contour in the neck has prominent V waves in severe cases, but in mild tricuspid regurgitation the peak V wave is of low amplitude and is usually unrecognized.

• **Echocardiographic Findings:** The jet of tricuspid regurgitation is easily seen on color flow Doppler; severity of regurgitation is estimated by comparing the area of the regurgitant jet with the area of the right atrium. The larger the jet area, the greater the degree of regurgitation. Estimation of the systolic pulmonary artery pressure can be made by measuring the velocity of the jet of tricuspid regurgitation and applying the Bernoulli principle. The gradient across the tricuspid valve is related to the velocity of tricuspid regurgitation (gradient = 4 x the velocity^2). The right atrial pressure is added to the gradient to calculate the right ventricular systolic pressure. Since the systolic right ventricular pressure and the systolic pulmonary artery pressure are identical, this technique is used to calculate systolic pulmonary artery pressure. It is a simple and effective method to measure pulmonary artery pressure.

• **Comparison of Methods**

Auscultation: *Strengths:* In moderate and severe tricuspid regurgitation there is usually a murmur, a parasternal right ventricular pulsation, and venous pulsations in the jugular venous pulse and/or liver. In such cases, diagnosis can be made at the bedside without requiring an extensive cardiac evaluation. Minimal and unimportant regurgitation usually is undetectable by auscultation, thus avoiding unnecessary concern. *Limitations:* Most cases of mild regurgitation and even many cases of moderate regurgitation do not have the "classic" holosystolic murmur which is louder on inspiration so it can either be unrecognized or misinterpreted as an ejection murmur.

Echocardiography: *Strengths:* Analysis of regurgitation by 2-D and Doppler echocardiography is usually technically easy and provides an accurate estimate of right ventricular function and severity of tricuspid regurgitation. Further, it usually identifies the cause of the problem (mitral valve disease, left ventricular heart failure, etc). Doppler analysis of hepatic venous flow is useful because in severe cases the regurgitant jet can be detected in the liver. The ability to estimate the pulmonary artery pressure by noninvasive means is extremely valuable for the complete cardiac evaluation. *Limitations:* It may be technically difficult to obtain clear images of the tricuspid valve in some individuals, particularly those with chronic lung disease.

Hypertrophic Cardiomyopathy

Hypertrophic cardiomyopathy is due to left ventricular hypertrophy (either concentric or localized), which can lead to left ventricular outflow tract obstruction, systolic anterior motion of the mitral valve, left ventricular diastolic dysfunction, and/or mitral regurgitation.

• **Auscultatory Findings:** There is usually a grade 2 or 3 ejection murmur along the left sternal border at the third left interspace due to rapid flow through a narrowed left ventricular outflow tract. It is loudest at a point lower than where valvular aortic stenosis is heard best and radiates both toward the aortic area and the cardiac apex. A fourth heart sound is usually present; a third sound is rare. An apical murmur of mitral regurgitation is present in many patients (Figure 26). There is no aortic ejection sound and no diastolic murmur of aortic regurgitation because the aortic valve is normal.

The left ventricular outflow tract murmur of hypertrophic cardiomyopathy can be identified by its characteristic response to vasoactive maneuvers at the bedside. Factors that decrease ventricular volume (sitting or standing or during the straining

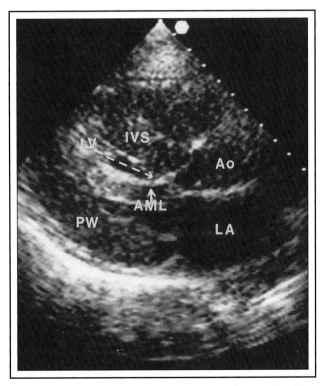

Figure 27. 2-D echocardiogram of hypertrophic cardiomyopathy with obstruction (parasternal long axis view). The anterior mitral leaflet (AML) has moved anteriorly and touches the interventricular septum (IVS). The left ventricular outflow tract (LV) is narrowed and the arrow points in the direction of outflow to the aorta (Ao). PW = posterior wall; LA = left atrium.

phase of the Valsalva maneuver) narrow the left ventricular outflow tract and intensify the murmur whereas maneuvers that increase ventricular volume (squatting, lying supine, hand grip, or during the release phase of the Valsalva maneuver) expand the left ventricular outflow tract and reduce the murmur intensity.

Components of the physical examination other than auscultatory findings may also be helpful. The carotid pulse is bifid, and is characterized by a brisk initial upstroke and a second slower peak (a "spike-dome" pattern) and apical impulse may have both a presystolic and late systolic pulsation.

• **Echocardiographic Findings:** Left ventricle is hypertrophied, either due to concentric hypertrophy or asymmetric septal hypertrophy. The left ventricular outflow tract is usually narrowed by the septum protruding into it even in those cases due to concentric, not asymmetric, hypertrophy. The left ventricular cavity size is normal or small, contractility is vigorous, and in many cases left ventricular end-systolic size is so small that the cavity is virtually obliterated. The anterior mitral leaflet may be displaced anteriorly into the outflow tract of the left ventricle during systole creating a partial obstruction (Figure 27). The extent of obstruction is related to the left ventricular cavity size so there is a dynamic progression of obstruction as cavity size diminishes during left ventricular contraction and the maximum obstruction occurs at end-systole. This can be shown by the Doppler study of flow through the left ventricular outflow tract, which shows a flow velocity pattern with a peak velocity near end-systole. Due to slow diastolic relaxation of the hypertrophied myocardium left ventricular diastolic dysfunction is commonly present. There is reversal of the E:A ratio and slow early diastolic filling as demonstrated by an E-wave deceleration time greater than 240 msec from peak of the E-wave to the baseline (Figure 28). Mitral regurgitation of a moderate degree is present in most cases, particularly those with systolic anterior motion of the anterior mitral leaflet.

• **Comparison of Methods**

Auscultation: *Strengths:* An ejection murmur is present whenever there is accelerated flow in the outflow tract, so if no murmur is heard, the diagnosis can be excluded. When outflow tract obstruction is present the murmur responds to the vasoactive maneuvers in a predictable way, confirming diagnosis. *Limitations:* Since the main murmur is an outflow tract murmur it is easily confused with valvular aortic stenosis. Furthermore mitral regurgitation frequently is present and because the out-

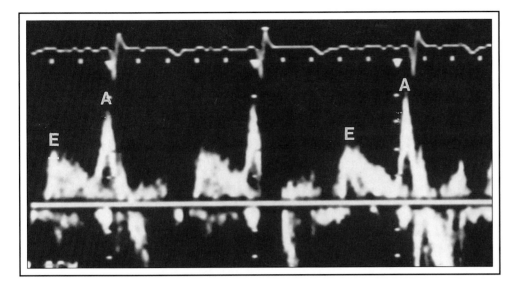

Figure 28. Pulse-wave Doppler of mitral inflow velocity in hypertrophic cardiomyopathy. The early diastolic wave (E) is of low amplitude and there is reversal of the E:A ratio. The downslope of the E wave is slow due to delayed ventricular filling.

flow tract murmur is not typical of valvular aortic stenosis, it is possible to attribute the entire clinical presentation to mitral regurgitation.

Echocardiography: *Strengths:* Echocardiography is the optimal way to establish the diagnosis because all the key elements can be demonstrated (ventricular hypertrophy, outflow tract obstruction, mitral valve abnormality, and diastolic dysfunction). *Limitations:* Patients with hypertrophic cardiomyopathy may not have all the classic features of the disease. When only a few of the abnormal findings are present it may be difficult to distinguish between marked left ventricular hypertrophy and hypertrophic cardiomyopathy. Ultimately, diagnosis depends on the preponderance of evidence, particularly whether there is outflow tract obstruction or systolic anterior motion of the mitral valve.

Heart Failure

Congestive heart failure is a common complication of many types of heart disease and is the most frequently used cardiovascular hospital discharge diagnosis (DRG) in the United States. In the past, physicians have relied heavily on auscultation (including pulmonary rales) to establish the diagnosis of heart failure but more recently echocardiography has played a major role. Now we recognize that there are two different types of heart failure, classified as either systolic or diastolic left ventricular dysfunction. In most patients with heart failure systolic dysfunction predominates. It is characterized by left ventricular dilatation, reduced contractility (either generalized or localized depending on the etiology), and by a reduced ejection fraction. On the other hand, in diastolic dysfunction, the ventricle is usually hypertrophied and the left ventricular cav-

ity size is normal or small (Figure 29). Contractility is normal or hyperdynamic but there is slow ventricular filling in early diastole during the period of passive filling. When there is a normal sinus rhythm there is rapid filling in late diastole after atrial contraction. Despite the dissimilarity of the mechanisms of these two types of heart failure, both can lead to identical degrees of elevation of mean left atrial pressure, severe pulmonary congestion, and even pulmonary edema. In some patients, there may be a combination of both systolic and diastolic dysfunction, particularly in ischemic heart disease, hypertensive heart disease, and aortic valve disease.

Left Ventricular Systolic Dysfunction

Many different types of heart disease, particularly coronary artery disease, myocardial disease, and valvular heart disease, damage or weaken the myocardium and eventually result in the clinical syndrome of heart failure produced by a dilated poorly contracting left ventricle whose pumping capacity is inadequate to meet the metabolic needs of the body, i.e., systolic dysfunction.

• **Auscultatory Findings:** The third heart sound is the major finding of systolic dysfunction. Because mean left atrial filling pressure is elevated, there is rapid left ventricular filling at a high velocity when the mitral valve opens in early diastole and the impact of that rapid filling creates the third heart sound.

Proper auscultatory technique is very important to detect the third heart sound. It is heard best with the bell of the stethoscope in a localized area at the point of maximal impulse of the cardiac apex. Ideally, the patient should be examined in a quiet room in a slight left decubitus position. However, in acutely ill patients the examining conditions may

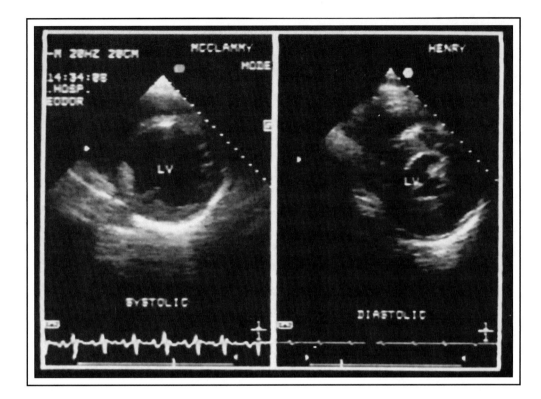

Figure 29. Left ventricular dysfunction, of the systolic and diastolic types. Two dimensional echocardiogram (short-axis view). LV, left ventricle with systolic dysfunction (left panel) and diastolic dysfunction (right panel). In systolic dysfunction, the left ventricle is dilated and the cavity:wall ratio is increased. In diastolic dysfunction, the left ventricular cavity is small and the left ventricle is hypertrophied.

be far from optimal, particularly if the patient is unable to lie comfortably, or if there are distracting background noises such as pulmonary rales, loud rapid breath sounds, or loud extraneous sounds from the area surrounding the patient.

In sinus tachycardia the third sound may be very loud because diastole is shortened and the ventricular filling due to atrial contraction (usually in late diastole) is superimposed on early diastolic filling to create a louder sound, the "summation gallop". When arrhythmias are present (premature atrial or ventricular beats, or rapid atrial fibrillation) it may be difficult to time the sound in early diastole and identify it as a third heart sound. In many cases there is a murmur of mitral regurgitation, but it is usually faint and of grade 1 or 2 intensity. The first heart sound may be faint.

• **Echocardiographic Findings:** 2-D echocardiogram shows reduced left ventricular contractility with a reduced ejection fraction. The left ventricle and atrium are usually dilated. Doppler study of mitral inflow velocity shows an early filling wave (E-wave) with an increased peak flow velocity, usually greater than 1 meter per second, and a rapid acceleration and deceleration. Mitral regurgitation frequently accompanies left ventricular systolic dysfunction because ventricular dilatation causes malalignment of the papillary muscles and mitral annular dilatation.

• **Comparison of Methods**

Auscultation: *Strengths:* The third heart sound is a reliable indicator of systolic dysfunction in most patients. The examination can be repeated frequently at low cost. *Limitations:* There are occasional false positives and false negatives. Infrequently, a third heart sound can be heard in healthy young adults, particularly slender individuals, so its presence is not absolutely diagnostic of systolic dysfunction. Further, in some patients with heart failure there are times when it may be impossible to hear the third sound, for a variety of reasons.

Echocardiography: *Strengths:* 2-D echocardiogram can show the cause of the heart failure, can indicate which ventricular segments are involved, and allows some quantitation of heart failure by calculation of an ejection fraction. Because of its simplicity and diagnostic accuracy, echocardiography is becoming the preferred method of diagnosing heart failure. *Limitations:* When the left ventricular endocardium cannot be seen clearly it is difficult to accurately measure ejection fraction. Because of the relatively high cost of echocardiography, frequent serial observations are usually not made.

Left Ventricular Diastolic Dysfunction

Left ventricular diastolic dysfunction is usually associated with left ventricular hypertrophy due to hypertension, but is also a major component in the clinical picture of hypertrophic cardiomyopathy and aortic stenosis. Coronary artery disease may cause myocardial ischemia, which interferes with myocardial relaxation and produces diastolic dysfunction and occasionally older persons may develop mild degrees of diastolic dysfunction even without left ventricular hypertrophy. Although left ventricular contractility is normal there is impaired filling of the left ventricle to such an extent that pulmonary congestion and even pulmonary edema may result. It is estimated that about one-third of patients over sixty-five years of age who have congestive heart failure have diastolic dysfunction as the basis of that heart failure.

• **Auscultatory Findings:** A fourth heart sound is the major finding and it is significant that the third heart sound is usually absent because early diastolic filling is slow. Older persons with hypertension, the major group with diastolic dysfunction, frequently have mitral annular calcification which produces a murmur of mild mitral regurgitation. In patients with hypertrophic cardiomyopathy, mitral regurgitation might be due to abnormal motion of the mitral valve.

• **Echocardiographic Findings:** 2-D echocardiography shows left ventricular hypertrophy without ventricular dilatation, but the left atrium is usually slightly dilated. Doppler study of mitral inflow velocity shows slow and prolonged early diastolic filling characterized by a low velocity E-wave with a slow downslope (prolonged deceleration). In many cases with this slow early filling there is compensatory rapid filling after atrial contraction, creating a tall A wave.

• **Comparison of Methods**

Auscultation: *Strengths:* A fourth heart sound is usually present and a good indicator of elevation of end-diastolic left ventricular pressure. Further, when considering other possible causes of heart failure, auscultation can help evaluate many other problems, such as valvular heart disease and systolic dysfunction. *Limitations:* In some cases, it may be very difficult to detect the fourth heart sound for a variety of reasons.

Echocardiography: *Strengths:* This is the most efficient and accurate way to make the diagnosis, using both 2-D and Doppler methods. *Limitations:* Cost.

Innocent Heart Murmur

An innocent heart murmur is one not due to any pathologic cause. Innocent murmurs are systolic and the most common types are the physiologic "pulmonic ejection murmur" and the vibratory, or Still's, murmur. They usually are present in childhood or young adulthood. Most children under 12 years old have had an innocent murmur. A type in older patients, generally in those more than 70 years of age, is an aortic ejection murmur due to sclerosis or thickening of the aortic valve, but without true stenosis, and it has been called "the innocent murmur of the elderly".

• **Auscultatory Findings:** The pulmonic ejection murmur is a mid-systolic, early peaking murmur usually heard best at the second and third left intercostal space and due to rapid flow of blood as it is being ejected through the right ventricular outflow tract into the pulmonary trunk. It is commonly found in children and adolescents and occasionally in young adults. It is usually soft and blowing in tone, although occasionally scratchy, and is of a grade 1 or 2 intensity. A physiologic third heart sound commonly accompanies it, and in some patients there may be a soft fourth heart sound. An ejection sound is not present because there is no abnormality of the aortic or pulmonic valve and no dilatation of the aorta or pulmonary artery. The pattern of second heart sound splitting is that of the normal physiologic response to respiration, wider on inspiration, narrower on expiration. The murmur decreases in intensity when the subject stands upright because of the decrease in venous return and ventricular filling.

Still's murmur, named after Dr. George Frederic Still, is an innocent murmur in children which usually has a vibratory tone, is heard best between the left sternal border and the cardiac apex, and occurs in early and mid systole. Dr. Still described it as "a twanging sound very like that made by twanging a piece of string". Still's murmur can vary markedly in intensity from day to day and even from beat to beat. In many patients it is difficult to distinguish between the pulmonic ejection murmur and Still's murmur because there may be features of each murmur heard in the same individual. A physiologic third heart sound is present in almost all children with the vibratory murmur.

• **Echocardiographic Findings:** The echocardiogram in children and young adults with an innocent murmur is entirely normal. Lesions which must be excluded in the differential diagnosis of this murmur are mild valvular pulmonic stenosis and atrial septal defect. The echocardiogram demonstrates that the features of those abnormalities are absent.

CARDIAC PEARL

The innocent systolic murmur is very common. It is a frequent finding in children and

339

teenagers and less likely in young adults. On one occasion, I had the opportunity to search carefully for the presence of a murmur in approximately 100 school children, average age 11 or 12. I found that approximately 60% of the students had an innocent systolic murmur. It is also of interest that in this particular group I found that 100% had a normal physiologic venous hum, which was detected listening over the right supraclavicular fossa, with the head turned "on a stretch" to the opposite direction. Short systolic murmurs (bruits) were noted in both the right and left supraclavicular fossae in about 25% to 30% of the students.

A venous hum generally is detected easily in children. As a rule, one needs to have the patient sitting upright, head turned to the opposite direction, placing the neck on a stretch. The bell of the stethoscope then is placed over the supraclavicular fossa. A specific position of the neck usually is necessary to obtain the optimal "stretch" before the venous hum is detected. As a rule, it is best heard over the right supraclavicular fossa rather than its counterpart on the left, presumably owing to the more direct flow from the jugular vein on the right to the superior vena cava. Occasionally, in some children a loud venous hum is present and may be heard over the base of the heart and be erroneously diagnosed as patent ductus arteriosus (when the venous hum is not listened for). Simple pressure over the jugular veins may result in the disappearance of the venous hum, thereby enabling medical correction of the "patent ductus arteriosus".

W. Proctor Harvey, M.D.

Innocent Murmur of the Elderly

The "innocent murmur of the elderly" is a grade 1 to 2/6 ejection murmur arising in the left ventricular outflow tract or the aortic valve. It is a very common finding and is due to sclerosis in and around aortic valve cusps, which does not cause true aortic valve obstruction, but does create some mild turbulent flow. It may also be due to septal hypertrophy or angulation of the septum (the "sigmoid system") which produces slight acceleration of flow and turbulence in the outflow tract.

• **Auscultatory Findings:** Auscultatory features are an early or mid-systolic murmur at the left sternal border radiating towards the second right interspace. There is no aortic ejection sound and no diastolic murmur. It may be difficult to distinguish this murmur from the murmur of mild aortic stenosis.

• **Echocardiographic Findings:** 2-D echocardiogram frequently shows thickening and sclerosis of the aortic valve often with decreased excursion of the cusps but still with an adequate opening and normal aortic flow velocity on Doppler study. The aortic flow velocity does not usually exceed 1.5 meters per second and the left ventricular outflow tract velocity is normal. In these patients with aortic sclerosis it is not uncommon for there to be a trivial amount of aortic regurgitation on Doppler study that cannot be heard on auscultation.

CARDIAC PEARL

Systolic murmurs in the elderly population are an expected and usually innocent finding.

The "innocent murmur of the elderly" has been a term used to describe a systolic murmur frequently heard in elderly patients in the age group of 60 and above. It has been termed innocent because it may represent an incidental finding in a number of asymptomatic patients. It generally is best heard over the aortic area, is of short duration and occurs around midsystole. No significant pathology may be noted at post mortem examination. It very likely is due to some sclerotic changes occurring in the aortic valve structure and/or the adjacent aorta. However, probably more frequently than realized, this may represent a mild or moderate stenosis of the aortic valve. Sometimes significant stenosis of the aortic valve may be present, and the systolic murmur may be musical, of a very high frequency, but on the faint side- grade 2 or grade 3. This is more likely heard in elderly patients with an increase in anteroposterior diameter of the chest, as with emphysema. Often it is well heard at the apex also. When one hears this peculiar type of high-frequency musical murmur, one always should think of aortic stenosis. It does not indicate the degree of stenosis. It is also apparent that some of these "innocent systolic murmurs" of the elderly are related to definite pathology of the aortic valve. It probably is true that auscultation often is not carried out as carefully in the elderly as in the younger age groups (or as carefully as one would like to see). For this reason, the murmur might be overlooked or, if heard, might be called "innocent," particularly when the other components of the total cardiac evaluation (the five fingers) are not put together.

Since people are living longer today, this murmur will be detected even more often if it is searched for. It is usually grade 1 to 3 in intensity and best heard over the aortic area or left sternal border, it may also be heard over the clavicles (bone transmission), in the suprasternal notch, supraclavicular areas of the neck, including over the carotid arteries.

The murmur frequently has a somewhat musical quality and can be transmitted down to the apex. Sometimes it can even be better heard at the apex. Occasionally a faint aortic diastolic murmur (grade 1 or 2) is heard in addition to the systolic murmur. If the patient is asymptomatic and the electrocardiogram and chest x-ray reveal no significant findings related to aortic valve disease, then no further diagnostic studies are needed at that time.

An aortic ejection sound is not a feature of aortic stenosis of the elderly as it is with the congenital bicuspid aortic valve. The murmur has been described as the "innocent murmur of the elderly" and is related to some minimal sclerosis or other alteration of the aortic valve; some of these patients have varying amounts of calcium in the valve leaflets, but the commissures are not fibrosed and fused, and the valve functions well. While many such patients remain stable for a number of years, others progress to more extensive fibrosis, calcium deposits, and stenosis of the valve leaflets, thereby resulting in significant signs and symptoms necessitating valve replacement.

W. Proctor Harvey, M.D.

Prosthetic Heart Valves

After an artificial heart valve has been placed it is important to make serial observations of that valve in order to detect complications. Major potential complications are valvular regurgitation, valvular obstruction due to thrombus or tissue ingrowth, and infection. Each of the individual types of prosthetic valve has unique properties depending on its size and construction and these properties must be considered when evaluating the valve. Therefore, it is important to establish a baseline auscultatory and echocardiographic evaluation of the valve shortly after surgery and then compare subsequent serial observations to that baseline observation. The major types of mechanical valves to be considered are the bi-leaflet valve (St. Jude Medical), the tilting disc valves (Medtronic-Hall and Bjork-Shiley), and the ball-cage valve (Starr-Edwards). The tissue valves are the porcine heterograft (Carpentier-Edwards and Hancock), the pericardial bioprosthesis (Carpentier-Edwards), and the human homograft valves.

• Normal Auscultatory Findings

Mechanical valves differ from tissue valves because a mechanical valve has a movable poppet or leaflets which create a distinct sound when the valve closes and often creates another sound when it opens. Each type of mechanical valve has different sound characteristics, some noisier than others, and the timing of the sounds is related to the valve location (aortic, mitral, or tricuspid). Character or pitch of the sound depends on the characteristics of the components of the valve (metal, plastic, cloth) and its design. The mechanical poppet valve in the aortic position opens at the onset of ejection and the poppet strikes the cage or strut producing a sound which has the timing of an aortic ejection sound, about 0.06 seconds after the first heart sound. When ejection has been completed it closes and produces the aortic component of the second heart sound when the poppet strikes the valve ring. In the mitral and tricuspid position, the mechanical poppet valve produces a sound when it opens in early diastole about 0.08 seconds after the second heart sound to allow ventricular filling. It closes at the time of ventricular contraction and creates the mitral or tricuspid part of the first heart sound.

The mechanical valves all produce fairly loud and metallic sharp sounds when they close (the poppet or the leaflet strikes the valve ring) but the opening sound is much more variable, sometimes faint. The ball-cage valve (Starr-Edwards) is a very noisy valve when the ball strikes the metal cage and there are even slight after-vibrations as the ball oscillates within the cage. The tilting disc valves (Medtronic-Hall and Bjork-Shiley) frequently have much fainter opening sounds, particularly in the mitral position when the flow rate through the open valve is slower than the flow rate in the aortic position. The bileaflet valve usually has a very faint, almost imperceptible, opening sound. Because of these individual variations in the sounds, it is important to make baseline observations of the intensity of these sounds soon after surgery so that there will be a reference point for later observations.

All prosthetic heart valves have effective valve areas smaller than normal native valves and all have small gradients across the valves. Since the transvalvular gradient is related to the flow rate across the valve, the faster the flow rate, the greater the gradient. Aortic valve prostheses have rapid flow rates and they have systolic gradients usually ranging from 6mmHg-20mmHg mean gradient or 15mmHg-40mmHg peak gradient. At surgery the size of the valve prostheses is selected to match the size of the native valve annulus and the prostheses range in size from 19mm-31mm in diameter. The smaller valves are inherently more stenotic than the larger valves. Because of these obstructions the prosthetic valves in the aortic position all are expected to have a systolic ejection murmur. In the mitral position, gradients are smaller, 2mmHg-8mmHg mean diastolic gradient and 5mmHg-18mmHg peak diastolic gradient. Mitral prostheses usually do not have a diastolic murmur, but occasionally a murmur is present. The timing of the opening sound of the mitral valve is influenced by the height of left atrial pressure and the diastolic gradient in early diastole. When left atrial pressure is high, the interval from aortic valve closure to the opening sound of the prosthesis is short. The normal range is from 0.06 to 0.12 seconds. This timing of the opening of the mitral valve prosthesis is comparable to the timing of the opening snap of mitral stenosis, occurring earlier in patients with more severe stenosis and elevated left atrial pressure.

Heart sounds of tissue valves are similar to native heart valves. They do not have extra or exaggerated sounds. Although these valves do not have any mechanical parts obstructing the orifice of the valve, they still have partial obstruction mainly because the valve rings are bulky and create some narrowing. The tissue valves in the aortic portion have ejection murmurs and in the mitral position there is usually no murmur, although occasionally there may be a faint diastolic apical murmur.

• Abnormal Auscultatory Findings

Regurgitation: Regurgitation may be due to thrombus or tissue ingrowth, which prevents the valve from closing, a defect in the closing mechanism of the valve, a ring abscess, or degeneration or infection of a leaflet of a tissue valve. In these cases there is usually a loud murmur of regurgitation. However, it should be recognized that many normally functioning valves may have a mild paravalvular leak and a faint regurgitant murmur.

Stenosis: Stenosis may be due to thrombus or tissue ingrowth into the valve or to a valve malfunction. The opening sound of the valve may be diminished if there is thrombus between the poppet and the cage or struts. In aortic obstruction the baseline murmur may become louder and in mitral obstruction a new diastolic murmur similar to mitral stenosis may appear, but it is usually faint.

• Echocardiographic Findings:
2-D echocardiographic evaluation of prosthetic valves is hampered by excessive reverberations from the metal and plastic components of the valve so that it is difficult to obtain a clear image. The extent of poppet or leaflet excursion cannot be clearly measured and it is difficult to distinguish vegetations, thrombus, or tissue ingrowth from the reverberation artifacts. Further, the highly echo-reflective metallic parts of

the valve produce shadowing behind those parts so that major parts of the heart may be in "blind spots" and cannot be seen. Transesophageal echocardiography has improved our ability to see these valves because the esophagus is much closer to the valves and shadowing is minimized. Higher frequency transducers are used so that image definition is much improved and vegetations, thrombi, abscesses, and torn cusps can be seen.

Doppler echocardiography has become the major method of evaluating valvular obstruction or regurgitation. Obstructions in prosthetic aortic and mitral valves are easily identified by transthoracic Doppler study, and obstruction is measured just like an obstruction in a native valve, i.e., use the modified Bernoulli equation for an estimate of aortic valve pressure gradient and use the pressure half-time method for estimation of mitral valve orifice size. There has been an excellent correlation between aortic valve gradients obtained by Doppler and by catheter measurement. The peak Doppler gradient may overestimate the degree of aortic stenosis, particularly in the bileaflet valve (St. Jude Medical) and in the Starr-Edwards ball-in-a-cage valve. In those valves there are localized high velocity jets which are not representative of the entire jet flow. In the bileaflet valve there is a small central orifice and two larger side orifices. The velocity through the smaller central orifice is faster than the average flow velocity for the entire valve so it is recommended that the mean gradient be used for clinical decisions.

Valvular regurgitation of a very mild degree can be a normal finding on color flow Doppler. There is a very small amount of physiologic regurgitation or backflow which occurs before the poppet or leaflets close the valve and some valves have a tiny built-in leak after the valve closes, particularly the St. Jude Medical valve. There are even tiny needle hole jets of regurgitation at the points where the sutures pass through the ring. None of these are significant.

Severity of aortic regurgitation can usually be evaluated by transthoracic Doppler study from the apical view. The pressure half-time method of analyzing the regurgitant jet and the color-flow Doppler analysis of the jet usually provide enough information so that transesophageal echocardiography is not needed.

Mitral regurgitation is usually difficult to evaluate by the transthoracic method, particularly from the apical views because the hardware masks the regurgitant jet behind the valve. The parasternal view creates less of a masking problem, but it may underestimate extent of regurgitation. Transesophageal echocardiogram provides the best evaluation of the mitral valve prothesis. A thrombus within the valve can often be identified indirectly by the decreased excursion of the poppet or leaflet opening. Vegetations, abscesses, and the location of the origin of regurgitant jets can be directly identified.

Conclusion

The cardiac sounds detected from the heart on auscultation and the ultrasound reflected from the heart on echocardiography provide valuable evidence about cardiac structure and function. Each method sees the cardiac events from its own perspective. Each has its own limitations, but both are based on reliable physical and physiologic principles. When cardiac auscultation or echocardiography are done carefully they usually lead to accurate conclusions.

Selected Reading

1. Barrington WW, Boudoulas H, Bashore T, Olson S, Wooley CF: Mitral stenosis: Mitral dome excursion at M1 and mitral opening snap - the concept of reciprocal heart sounds. *AHJ* 1988; 115:1280-1290.
2. Baumgartner H, Khan S, DeRobertis M, Czer L, Maurer G: Effect of prosthetic aortic valve design on the Doppler-catheter gradient correlation: An in vitro study of normal St. Jude, Medtronic-Hall, Starr-Edwards and Hancock valves. *JACC* 1992; 19:324.
3. Bouchard A, Yock P, Schiller NB, Blumlein S, Botvinick EH, Greenburg B, Cheitlin M, Massie BM: Value of color Doppler estimation of regurgitant volume in patients with chronic aortic insufficiency. *AHJ* 1989; 117:1099.
4. Burwash IG, Blackmore GL, Koilpillai CJ: Usefulness of left atrial and left ventricular chamber sizes as predictors of the severity of mitral regurgitation. *AJC* 1992; 70:774.
5. Chen C, Thomas JD, Anconina J, Harrigan P, Mueller L, Picard MH, Levine RA, Weyman AE: Impact of impinging wall jet on color Doppler quantification of mitral regurgitation. *Circ* 1991; 84:712.
6. Come PC, Riley MF, Carl LV, Nakao S: Pulsed Doppler echocardiographic evaluation of valvular regurgitation in patients with mitral valve prolapse: Comparison with normal subjects. *JACC* 1986; 8:1355.
7. Craige E: On the genesis of heart sounds: Contributions made by echocardiographic studies. *Circ* 1976; 53:207-209.
8. Craige E: The fourth heart sound. Physiologic Principles of Heart Sounds and Murmurs. Dallas, Texas, American Heart Association, Monograph No. 46, 1975, 74-78.
9. Curtiss EI, Matthews RG, Shaver JA: Mechanism of normal splitting of the second heart sound. *Circ* 1975; 51:157-164.
10. Devereaux RB, Kramer-Fox R, Kligfield P: Mitral valve prolapse: Causes, clinical manifestations, and management. *Ann Intern Med* 1989; 111:305.
11. Fortuin NJ, Craige E: Echocardiographic studies of genesis of mitral diastolic murmurs. *BHJ* 1973; 35:75.
12. Fortuin NJ, Craige E: On the mechanism of the Austin Flint murmur. *Circ* 1972; 45:558.
13. Geibel A, Gornandt L, Kasper W, Bubenheimer P: Reproducibility of Doppler echocardiographic quantification of aortic and mitral valve stenosis: Comparison between two echocardiography centers. *AJC* 1991; 67:1013.
14. Grayburn PA, Pryor SL, Levine BD, Klein MN, Taylor AL, Peters A: Day to day variability of Doppler color flow jets in mitral regurgitation. *JACC* 1989; 14:936.
15. Grayburn PA, Smith MD, Harrison MR, Gurley JR, DeMaria AN: Pivotal role of aortic valve area calculation by the continuity equation for Doppler assessment of aortic stenosis in patients with combined aortic stenosis and regurgitation. *AJC* 1988; 61:376.
16. Griffin BP, Flachskampf FA, Siu S, Weyman AE, Thomas JD: The effects of regurgitant orifice size, chamber compliance, and systemic vascular resistance on aortic regurgitant velocity slope and pressure half-time. *AHJ* 1991; 122:1049.
17. Hatle L, Angelsen B: *Doppler ultrasound in cardiology: Physical principles and clinical applications.* 2nd edition Philadelphia, Lea & Febiger, 1985.
18. Hatle L, Angelsen BA, Tromsdal A: Noninvasive assessment of aortic stenosis by Doppler ultrasound. *BHJ* 1980; 43:284.
19. Helmcke F, Nanda NC, Hsiung MC, Soto B, Adey CK, Goyal RG, Gatewood RP: Color Doppler assessment of mitral regurgitation with orthogonal planes. *Circ* 1987; 75:175.
20. Karp K, Teien D, Bjerle P, Eriksson P: Reassessment of valve area determinations in mitral stenosis by the pressure half-time method: Impact of left ventricular stiffness and peak diastolic pressure difference. *JACC* 1989; 13:594.
21. Labovitz AJ, Ferrara RP, Kern MJ, Bryg RJ, Mrosek DG, Williams GA: Quantitative evaluation of aortic insufficiency by continuous wave Doppler echocardiography. *J Am Coll Cardiol* 1986; 8:1341.
22. Labovitz AJ, Pearson AC, McCluskey MT, Williams GA: Clinical significance of the echocardiographic degree of mitral valve prolapse. *AHJ* 1988; 115:842.
23. Laniado S, Yellin EL, Miller H, Frater RWM: Temporal relation of the first heart sound to closure of the mitral valve. *Circ* 1973; 47:1006-1014.
24. Leon DF, Shaver JA: Physiologic principles of heart sounds and murmurs. New York, American Heart Association, 1975.
25. Levine RA, Stathogiannis E, Newell JB, Harrigan P, Weyman AE: Reconsideration of echocardiographic standards for mitral valve prolapse: Lack of association between leaflet displacement isolated to the apical four-chamber view and independent echocardiographic evidence of abnormality. *JACC* 1988; 11:1010.
26. Martin CE, Shaver JA, O'Toole JD, Leon DF, Reddy PS: Ejection sounds of right-sided origin: Physiological principles of heart sounds and murmurs. New York, American Heart Association, 1975, 35-44, AHA Monograph No. 46.
27. Oh JK, Taliercio CP, Holmes Jr DR, Reeder GS, Biley KR, Seward JB, Tajik AJ: Prediction of the severity of aortic stenosis by Doppler aortic valve area determination: Prospective Doppler-catheterization correlation in 100 patients. *JACC* 1988; 11:1227.
28. Otto CM, Nishimura RA, Davis KB, Kisslo KB, Bashore TM: Doppler echocardiographic findings in adults with severe symptomatic valvular aortic stenosis. *AJC* 1991; 68:1477.
29. Ozawa Y, Smith D, Craige E: Origin of the third heart sound: II. Studies in human subjects. *Circ* 1983; 67:399-404.
30. Panidis IP, Ross J, Mintz GS: Normal and abnormal prosthetic valve function as assessed by Doppler echocardiography. *JACC* 1986; 8:317.
31. Patel AK, Rowe GG, Thomsen JH, Dhanani SP, Kosolcharoen P, Lyle LEW: Detection and estimation of rheumatic mitral regurgitation in the presence of mitral stenosis by pulsed Doppler echocardiography. *AJC* 1983; 51:986.
32. Ronan JA, Perloff JK, Harvey WP: Systolic clicks and the late systolic murmur: Intracardiac phonocardiographic evidence of their mitral valve origin. *AHJ* 1966; 70:319-325.

33. Salerni R, Reddy PS, Sherman ME, O'Toole JD, Leon DF, Shaver JA: Pressure and sound correlates of the mitral valve echocardiogram in mitral stenosis. *Circ* 1978; 58:119-125.

34. Shah PM, Yu PN: Gallop rhythm: Hemodynamic and clinical correlation. *AHJ* 1969; 78: 823-828.

35. Shaver JA, Griff FL, Leonard JJ: Ejection sounds of left-sided origin: Physiological principles of heart sounds and murmurs. New York, American Heart Association, 1975, 27-34, AHA Monograph No. 46.

36. Smith MD, Grayburn PA, Spain MG, DeMaria AN, Kwan OL, Moffett CB: Observer variability in the quantification of Doppler color flow jet areas for mitral and aortic regurgitation. *JACC* 1988; 11:579.

37. Spain MG, Smith MD, Grayburn PA, Harlamert EA, DeMaria AN, O'Brien M, Kwan OL: Quantitative assessment of mitral regurgitation by Doppler color flow imaging: Angiographic and hemodynamic correlations. *JACC* 1989; 13:585.

38. Stevenson JG: Two-dimensional color Doppler estimation of the severity of atrioventricular valve regurgitation: Important effects of instrument gain setting, pulse repetition frequency, and carrier frequency. *JASE* 1989; 2:1.

39. Taylor R: Evolution of the continuity equation in the Doppler echocardiographic assessment of the severity of valvular aortic stenosis. *JASE* 1990; 3:326.

40. Thomas JD, Weyman AE: Doppler mitral pressure half-time: A clinical tool in search of theoretical justification. *JACC* 1987; 10:923.

41. Vancheri F, Gibson D: Relation of third and fourth heart sounds to blood velocity during left ventricular filling. *BHJ* 1989; 61:144-148.

42. Wranne B, Ask P, Lloyd D: Analysis of different methods of assessing the stenotic mitral valve area with emphasis on the pressure gradient half-time concept. *AJC* 1990; 66:614.

CHAPTER 16

Transesophageal Echocardiography: Clinical Applications

Steven A. Goldstein, M.D. and Louis Larca, M.D.

Remarkable advances have occurred in cardiovascular ultrasound over the past two decades. There has been a rapid evolution from M-mode echo (early 70s) to 2D-echo (late 70s) to conventional Doppler (early 80s) to color Doppler (mid 80s) and finally to transesophageal echo (late 80s). The last few years have seen the maturation of transesophageal echocardiography (TEE). With TEE, high resolution images can be obtained because of the proximity of the esophagus to the heart and because high frequency (5 MHz to 7.5 MHz) transducers can be used. Many of the limitations of precordial echocardiography are thereby overcome. Improvements in instrument design, including biplane and multiplane probes, and a growing recognition of the clinical applications have led to widespread use of this technique as a complement to transthoracic echocardiography (TTE). This chapter will focus on the clinical applications of this new and rapidly expanding technique.

CARDIAC PEARL

Over the past several years, the unquestioned usefulness of the transesophageal echocardiogram in diagnosis has become increasingly evident. This procedure is now firmly established as an extremely important diagnostic tool. I believe that all of us should become familiar with the technic of transesophageal echocardiography and the tracings that result.

W. Proctor Harvey, M.D.

Background

TEE was introduced in 1976, by Frazin and colleagues. They used a single crystal M-mode transducer for patients with poor precordial images. Although the thin coaxial cable of this M-mode transducer limited its steerability and views, this system represented a landmark in diagnostic ultrasound. Transesophageal 2-dimensional echocardiography was introduced one year later by Hisanaga. His mechanical sector scanner was limited by cumbersome probes and a limited field of view. Smaller transducers and electronic phased array technology from Germany led to the increased interest in TEE in the early 1980s.

TEE was initially used in the United States for intraoperative monitoring of regional myocardial function in high risk surgical patients and the recognition of intracardiac air during neurosurgical procedures. In Europe, however, investigators pioneered the use of TEE for diagnosis of cardiac disease in outpatients. Further improvements in transducer technology and the recognition of broader clinical applications by investigators in Europe and Japan led to a renewed interest in TEE in the United States in the mid 1980s. The addition to TEE of color flow and continuous wave Doppler and the development of biplane, multiplane, and pediatric transducers have led to widespread worldwide use of this technique.

Procedure

The transesophageal echocardiographic probe consists of a modified flexible endoscope containing a miniature mechanical or phased array ultrasound transducer (Figure 1) interfaced to a standard

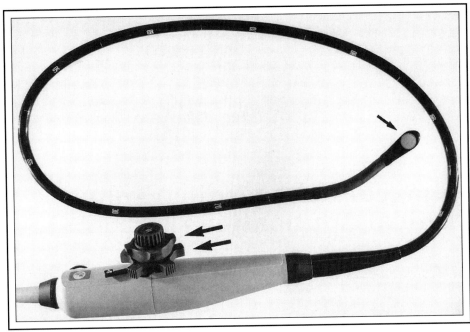

Figure 1. A commercially available multiplane transesophageal echocardiographic probe; two rotary knobs (large arrows) located on the handle permit the operator to control the mobility of the distal tip of the probe (small arrow) in the esophagus. The distal tip of the probe incorporates the transducer which transmits and receives the ultrasound beam, which can be electronically steered through an arc of 180°.

echocardiographic machine. Current transesophageal transducers are capable of M-mode and 2-dimensional imaging and pulse, continuous wave, and color flow Doppler. Controls at the proximal end of the scope allow anteroposterior and lateral flexion of the transducer at the distal end to optimize image quality and orientation. Biplane probes have 2 perpendicular scanning planes, transverse (horizontal) and longitudinal (vertical), to permit imaging of two separate cross-sections of the heart, although not simultaneously. Multiplane probes consist of a single imaging sector that can be rotated around the long axis of the ultrasound beam, typically in a 180° arc, producing a continuum of tomographic images. The commercially available TEE probes have a smooth, rounded distal end to minimize blunt trauma, as well as a variety of safety mechanisms to avoid overheating the surface of the transducer.

The procedure may be performed on fully conscious patients, but is most often performed using sedation with intravenous agents such as meperidine (Demerol), diazepam (Valium), midazolam (Versed), or fentanyl (Sublimaze). Patients should fast for a minimum of 4 to 6 hours to minimize risk of vomiting and aspiration. The procedure is described in detail to the patient and informed consent obtained. A brief medical history should be obtained to exclude contraindications to esophageal intubation, such as a history of esophageal disease, mediastinal radiation, recent gastrointestinal surgery, or active upper GI bleeding (Table 1). A drug and allergy history should also be obtained.

Dentures and oral prostheses are removed prior

to the examination. Blood pressure, heart rate, and respirations are routinely monitored; pulse oximetry is optional, but is recommended for patients receiving intravenous sedation. Topical oropharyngeal anesthesia is achieved using either aerosol sprays or liquid gargles. There are no established recommendations for infective endocarditis prophylaxis with antibiotics. With the patient in the left lateral decubitus position, the lubricated transesophageal transducer is introduced through the mouth and into the esophagus using standard techniques of probe insertion. The neck should be slightly flexed to facilitate entrance into the esophagus rather than the trachea. A bite guard avoids accidental biting and damage to the echo scope.

A comprehensive study usually requires 10 to 30 minutes. During the study, oral secretions are removed by suctioning, as needed. After the proce-

---

T A B L E 1
TEE: Relative Contraindications

1. Pre-existing esophageal pathology
   - Obstruction (cancer, stricture)
   - Esophageal diverticulum
   - Esophageal varices
   - Recent esophageal surgery
2. Active UGI bleeding
3. Perforated viscus (known or suspected)
4. Severe cervical arthritis
5. Profound oropharyngeal distortion
6. Unwilling or uncooperative patient

TABLE 2
Complications of TEE

1. Arrhythmia (V-tach; SVT; AV block)
2. Respiratory distress, hypoxia
3. Transient hypo-or hypertension
4. Aspiration
5. Laryngospasm, bronchospasm
6. Perforation of hypopharynx, esophagus
7. Laryngeal nerve damage

dure the patient should be observed until fully awake and should take nothing by mouth until the topical pharyngeal anesthetic has worn off (usually 30 to 60 minutes after the procedure). If sedatives are used, patients should be cautioned not to drive an automobile or to operate machinery for 12 to 24 hours. TEE can also be performed on anesthetized or unconscious patients in the operating room or in an intensive care unit. A respirator is not an obstacle. Such patients often must remain in the supine position. The left lateral position is not required. Temporary removal of naso-gastric or feeding tubes which may "crowd" the pharynx is sometimes required. In very agitated patients, paralytic agents such as Vecuronium (Norcuron) can be used. Cardiologists should have a low threshold for obtaining the assistance of intensivists, anesthesiologists, and anesthetists to assist with the introduction of the transducer in select patients.

In experienced hands, high quality images can be safely obtained in the outpatient, intensive care, and intraoperative settings. Despite its semi-invasive nature, TEE has an excellent safety record. Potential complications are listed in Table 2. Major complications (such as perforation of the hypopharynx or esophagus and bleeding) are exceedingly rare. Its safety has been documented in more than ten thousand patients in a cooperative study involving 15 European centers, and in several studies in the United States. In order to assure patient safety and maximum image quality, TEE should be performed only by specially trained physicians. The American Society of Echocardiography (ASE) Committee for Physician Training and Education has published a document that recommends guidelines for training to perform and interpret TEE. In general, physicians should have substantial experience with general precordial echocardiography, including M-mode, 2-D, spectral Doppler, color Doppler, and contrast echocardiography. Training in the TEE examination should include practical experience in four areas: introduction of the probe, manipulation of the transducer, optimization of the instrument controls, and interpretation of findings.

TEE should only be performed by physicians competent in upper GI endoscopy. The trainee should become familiar with the anatomy of the oropharynx and esophagus. Skillful introduction of the probe is best learned from a trained GI endoscopist or a cardiologist fully trained in the TEE procedure. To achieve competence, the average trainee should perform a minimum of 25 supervised esophageal intubations.

Once esophageal intubation is mastered, the trainee should understand the unique tomographic cardiovascular planes and learn the transducer manipulations necessary to obtain them. Physicians performing TEE must learn to recognize normal cardiac structures and blood flow patterns and distinguish them from pathologic structures and flow dynamics. In addition, the trainee should be familiar with the instrument knobs and controls in order to optimize the quality of the recorded data. The number of supervised TEE studies required to accomplish these goals will vary. The ASE has recommended that the trainee perform approximately 50 TEE examinations under the direct supervision of an echocardiographer who is expert in TEE procedures.

Experience with probe passage, TEE examination technique, and interpretation of study findings should be accomplished in outpatient, critical care, and cardiac surgical settings. Training should include information on the proper cleaning of the instrument following each use to avoid transmission of infection. In order to maintain competency,

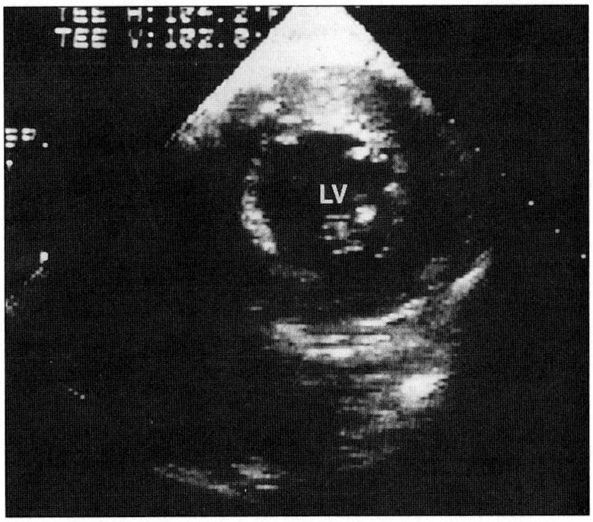

Figure 2. A transgastric view of the left ventricular cavity (LV) in the transverse plane. This short axis view is also used to monitor left ventricular function during non-cardiac surgery.

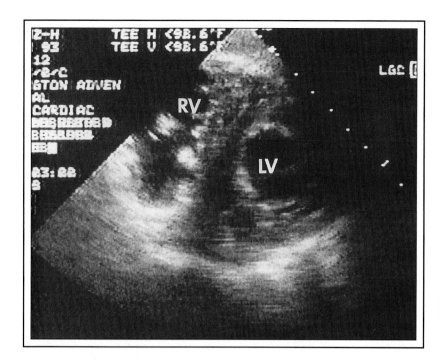

Figure 3. A transgastric view of the left ventricular (LV) and right ventricular cavity (RV).

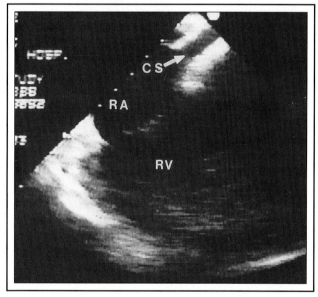

Figure 4. Transesophageal echocardiogram illustrating a systolic frame of the right ventricle (RV) and the right atrium (RA). The tricuspid valve is seen as a thin linear band separating the chambers. The coronary sinus (CS, arrow) opens into the right atrium.

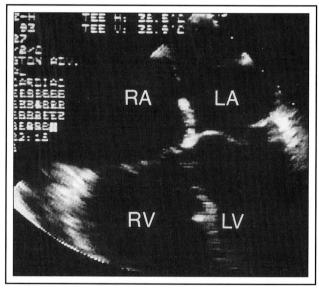

Figure 5. Transesophageal echocardiogram (transverse plane) illustrating 4-chamber view. The right atrium (RA) and ventricle (RV) are divided by a normal tricuspid valve. The left atrium (LA) and ventricle (LV) are divided by a normal mitral valve.

physicians who perform and interpret TEE studies should continue to perform a reasonable number of cases. The ASE recommends a minimum of 50 studies per year. In addition, ongoing education should be maintained by attending postgraduate courses and workshops, by reviewing pertinent textbooks, journals, and videotapes, and by reviewing random TEE studies with recognized experts. Granting of TEE privileges remains the purview of each individual hospital.

Anatomy

Performance of transesophageal echocardiography involves a thorough understanding of cardiac anatomy. The esophagus lies midline in the body posterior to the left atrium and anterior to the descending aorta; this location permits excellent imaging of the walls and chambers of the heart, the inferior and superior vena cavae, and the proximal segment of the aorta and pulmonary arteries. Because the heart is not a symmetrical structure,

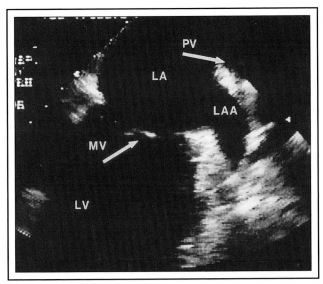

Figure 6. Transesophageal echocardiogram (longitudinal plane) of left ventricle (LV), mitral valve (MV, arrow), left atrium (LA) and appendage (LAA). The left upper pulmonary vein (PV - arrow) is visualized.

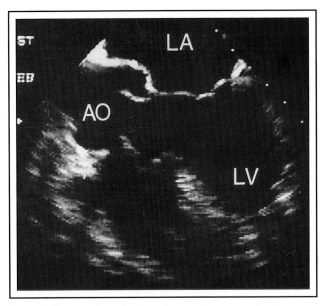

Figure 7. Transesophageal echocardiogram (transverse plane) illustrating a systolic frame of the left ventricle (LV), aortic valve (AO), and left atrium (LA).

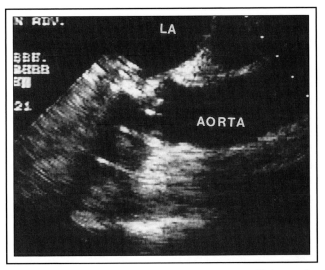

Figure 8. Transesophageal echocardiogram utilizing a multiplane probe demonstrates the capability of evaluating a significant portion of the ascending aorta (AORTA). The left atrium (LA) is visualized at the top of the screen.

and because the vertical and horizontal planes of the heart are neither parallel nor perpendicular to the esophagus, it is necessary to perform several maneuvers with the TEE probe. These include advancement and withdrawal of the scope in the esophagus, rotation of the shaft clockwise and counterclockwise, medial and lateral flexion of the tip, and anteflexion and retroflexion of the tip. At each position in the esophagus images are obtained in the horizontal or vertical transducer (biplane device) or by rotating the transducer through 0° to 180° for certain images (multiplane device). The

TEE probe has markers spaced 1 cm apart to determine the distance of the tip from the incisors. Images of the heart and great vessels are usually obtained when the probe is approximately 25 cm to 40 cm.

Performance of a complete transesophageal study requires the constant manipulation of the endoscope and controls. The following will serve as a guide to the standard views and the appearance of cardiac structures and chambers when imaged from the esophageal window. Images obtained with the biplane device in the horizontal plane generally correspond to 0° and the multiplane scope and vertical views correspond to 90°. Significant variability occurs. The scope is inserted into the esophagus as previously described and advanced to approximately 40 cm. An arbitrary preference is to begin imaging with a transgastric view in the horizontal plane. At this level the tip of the scope is usually in the stomach and retroflexion of the tip produces a transgastric short axis view of the left ventricle (Figure 2). With slight rotation of the scope portions of the right ventricle are seen (Figure 3). In the vertical plane a two chamber view is obtained. The apex can usually be imaged with this view. The mitral apparatus including papillary muscles, chordae and leaflets can be assessed. Left ventricular outflow tract, aortic valve and a portion of the proximal ascending aorta are sometimes visualized here. Withdrawal of the endoscope into the lower esophagus permits imaging of the right ventricle, tricuspid valve, right atrium, and coronary sinus in the horizontal plane (Figure 4). Use of the vertical

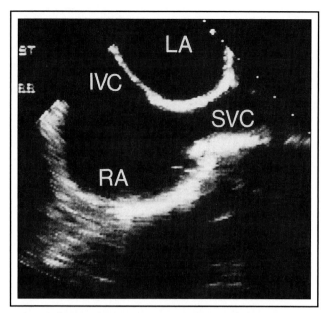

Figure 9. Transesophageal echocardiogram (longitudinal plane) of the right (RA) and left (LA) atria divided by the atrial septum. The superior vena cava (SVC) and the inlet of the inferior vena cava (IVC) are visualized.

lent view of the posterior leaflet of the mitral valve; the left atrium and its appendage are clearly imaged at this level (Figure 6). In the horizontal plane the aortic outflow can be visualized with slight rotation of the scope (Figure 7). In the longitudinal plane, the outflow tract, the aortic root and the ascending aorta are well imaged (Figure 8). Remaining in the vertical plane, clockwise rotation of the probe toward the right yields a view of the right atrium, superior vena cava, inferior vena cava and interatrial septum (Figure 9) and is suitable for detecting atrial shunts with intravenous contrast.

Additional withdrawal of the endoscope yields multiple images of the base of the heart. With minor manipulations of the probe (rotation, ante- and retroflexion, and the use of both horizontal and vertical planes) views of the left atrium, right atrium, aortic valve, atrial septum and appendage can be obtained. The left coronary artery can be easily visualized in almost all patients (Figure 10), but the right coronary artery is harder to view. Important views of the left atrial appendage are obtained.

An attempt should be made to identify all four pulmonary veins: the left upper pulmonary vein is usually easily identified in the horizontal plane; the left lower pulmonary vein is found by advancing the probe slightly. In the horizontal plane the right upper pulmonary vein is usually seen immediately posterior to the superior vena cava with the opening of the right lower pulmonary vein sometimes seen just above; the right upper pulmonary vein can also be imaged in the vertical plane (Figure 11). With slight withdrawal of the probe, additional

plane permits imaging of the tricuspid valve from a different viewing angle. This can provide an almost parallel alignment of a Doppler beam in order to measure the peak velocity of a tricuspid regurgitant jet. Further withdrawal of the probe to the mid-esophagus provides a four chamber view in the horizontal plane (Figure 5). With slight rotation, images of the mitral valve, ventricular septum, body of the left ventricle and papillary muscles are possible. Changing to the vertical plane provides the equivalent of a two chamber view and an excel-

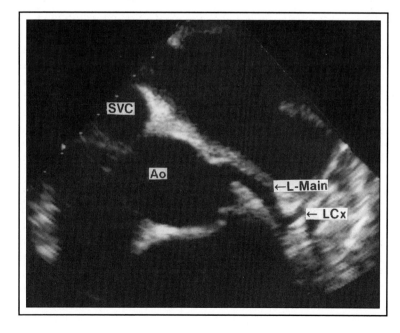

Figure 10. Transverse plane TEE view of left coronary artery illustrating its near parallel orientation to ultrasound beam. SVC = superior vena cava; Ao = aortic root; L-main = left main coronary artery; LCX = left circumflex artery.

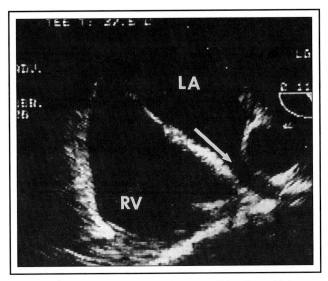

Figure 11. Transesophageal echocardiogram utilizing the multiplane probe demonstrates the opening of the right upper pulmonary vein (arrow). The atrial septum divides the left (LA) and right atrium (RA).

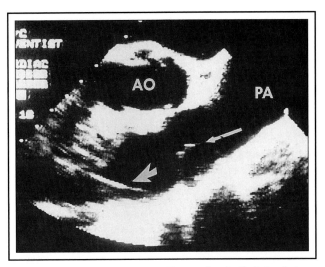

Figure 12. Transesophageal echocardiogram (longitudinal plane) at the base of the heart demonstrates the right ventricular outflow tract, pulmonic valve (thin arrow) and the main pulmonary artery (PA). The broad arrow is pointing to a Swan Ganz catheter. The aortic root (AO) appears distorted since the beam is not parallel or perpendicular at this level.

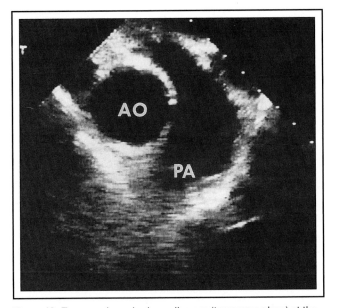

Figure 13. Transesophageal echocardiogram (transverse plane) at the base of the heart demonstrating the pulmonary artery (PA) and the aorta (AO). The superior vena cava is seen as a small circular structure at the upper left of the screen.

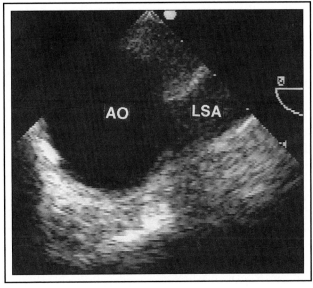

Figure 14. Cross-section view of the aortic arch (AO) illustrating the origin and proximal portion of the left subclavian artery (LSA).

images of the proximal portions of the great vessels are obtained (Figures 12 and 13).

A complete study also includes images of the thoracic aorta. The scope is advanced to the stomach and a transgastric view is obtained. The scope is then rotated counterclockwise until the aorta is visualized in cross-section. The depth of field can be adjusted at this point to provide a larger image. The scope is pulled back slowly with slight rotation to keep the aortic image centered. The intimal surface and lumen are observed for irregularities.

Horizontal imaging is adequate, but longitudinal views can provide better spatial orientation. In the region of the aortic arch, biplane and multiplane imaging often permit full examination of the arch as well as identification of the left subclavian (Figure 14) and carotid arteries. Imaging at this level is sometimes difficult because of discomfort to the patient. In addition, interposition of the trachea may prevent clear imaging of the distal ascending aorta and proximal aortic arch. Depending on the orientation of the heart in the chest, all of the stan-

TABLE 3
Major Clinical Applications for TEE

1. Infective endocarditis
2. Cardiac source of embolus
3. Native valve disease
4. Prosthetic valve disease
5. Thoracic aortic pathology
6. Intracardiac masses
7. Adult congenital heart disease
8. Coronary arteries
9. Critically ill patients
10. Intraoperative use
11. Guidance of interventional procedures

TABLE 4
Infective Endocarditis: Role of Echocardiography

1. Confirm diagnosis
2. Detect destructive consequences
3. Determine hemodynamic sequelae
4. Determine prognosis
5. Determine need for surgery and direct surgical approach

TABLE 5
Diagnosis of Infective Endocarditis: TTE and TEE

AUTHOR	YEAR	n	SENSITIVITY TTE (%)	SENSITIVITY TEE (%)
Erbel	1988	96	44	82
Daniel	1988	76	60	94
Chan	1989	29	55	90
Mugge	1989	80	58	90
Taams	1990	33	33	100
Shively	1991	62	44	94
Pederson	1991	24	50	100
Birmingham	1992	29	34	93

n = number of patients

dard views may not be obtainable and there will be considerable variability in the location and imaging plane best suited for a particular structure. With experience, a complete study can be performed very rapidly and additional time can be spent focusing on the specific clinical problem.

Clinical Applications

Development of transesophageal echocardiography has allowed major advances in diagnosis and evaluation of a large number of cardiovascular conditions. Although most cardiac abnormalities can be reliably evaluated with transthoracic echocardiography, TEE is being used with increasing frequency because of its unique advantages over standard TTE. TEE may be required in up to 10% of cases to enhance the limited diagnostic capability of transthoracic studies. The clinical applications for TEE are numerous and still expanding. TEE has already become the definitive noninvasive imaging modality for a broad range of cardiovascular disorders, including infective endocarditis and its complications, thromboembolism of cardiac and aortic origin, prosthetic mitral valve dysfunction, certain disorders of the aorta (such as aortic dissection and atherosclerosis), intra-atrial pathology, intracardiac masses, and certain congenital abnormalities. TEE is particularly useful for assessing the suitability for and the adequacy of certain surgical procedures, such as mitral valve repair. It has also proved useful as a means of intraoperative monitoring. It is being used increasingly in the ICU to evaluate patients who are being mechanically ventilated or who are otherwise difficult to image with TTE, and in the catheterization laboratory to assist a variety of procedures (such as transseptal puncture, balloon valvuloplasty, and catheter-ablation). This section contains a discussion of some of the commonly accepted clinical applications of TEE (Table 3).

Infective Endocarditis

Echocardiography has made a tremendous impact on both the diagnosis and management of infective endocarditis. Several important aspects of the role of echocardigraphy in evaluating infective endocarditis are listed in Table 4. Although physicians continue to rely on clinical features and characteristic bacteriologic findings for the diagnosis of infective endocarditis, the echocardiographic demonstration of vegetations is assuming increasing importance. Investigators from Duke University have recently proposed new criteria for the diagnosis of infective endocarditis that incorporate echocardiographic findings. In fact, the diagnosis of endocarditis may be based solely on echocardiographic findings when blood cultures are negative.

Transthoracic echocardiography has proven to be useful for the diagnosis of infective endocarditis, but suboptimal images in up to 20% to 30% of patients, limited image resolution, and limited accuracy in detecting abscesses and prosthetic valve endocarditis have been major obstacles. TEE, on the other hand, consistently yields high-quality images and has superior resolution which permits the detection of even small vegetations. A number

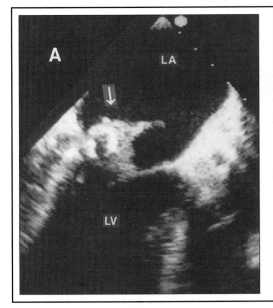

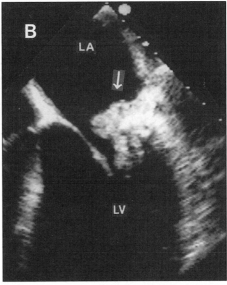

Figure 15. Very large, irregular vegetation on the posterior mitral leaflet (arrows) shown in both longitudinal plane (A) and horizontal plane (B). LA = left atrium; LV = left ventricle.

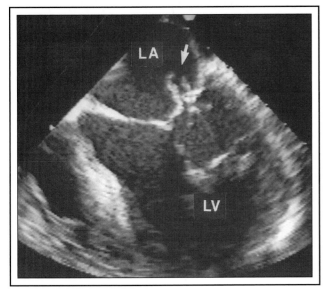

Figure 16. Several "stringlike" or filamentous vegetations (arrows) on both anterior and posterior mitral leaflets. LA = left atrium; LV = left ventricle.

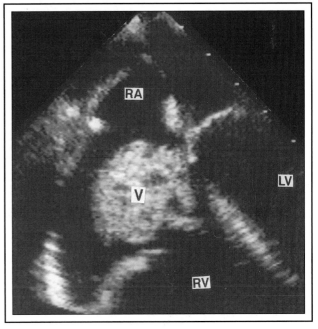

Figure 17. Very large vegetation (V) on the tricuspid valve. RA = right atrium; LV = left ventricle; RV = right ventricle.

of investigators have demonstrated improved diagnostic accuracy of TEE compared to TTE (Table 5). Figures 15 to 17 illustrate vegetations detected by transesophageal echo in three patients.

TEE has also proven to be superior to TTE in evaluating patients with suspected prosthetic valve endocarditis. In patients with prosthetic valves, especially mitral (Figure 18), TEE offers improved resolution and avoids shadowing and masking that obscure the atrial surface of the valve using TTE. Complications of infective endocarditis such as aortic and mitral valve ring abscesses are better detected by TEE (Figures 19 and 20). TEE is also

superior for the detection and characterization of other rare complications of endocarditis including sinus of Valsalva aneurysm, aneurysms of valve leaflets, aneurysm arising from the mitral-aortic intervalvular fibrosa (Figure 21) and aortic mycotic aneurysms (Figure 22).

Indications for TEE in patients with known or suspected endocarditis are currently controversial. Some echocardiographic experts have recommended TEE for all such patients. Others, partly influenced by a desire to contain medical costs, advocate TEE for select patients. Reasonable indi-

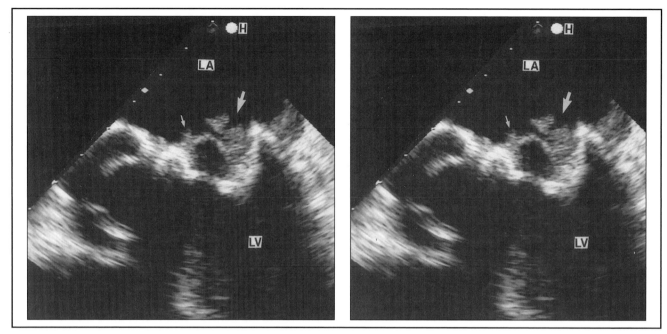

Figure 18. TEE illustrates multiple vegetations (arrows) on a porcine mitral prosthesis which could not be detected by transthoracic echo. Left panel is horizontal plane (H). Right panel is vertical plane (V). LA = left atrium; LV = left ventricle.

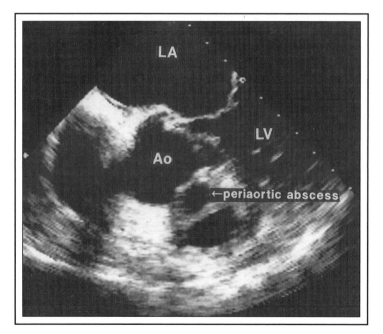

Figure 19. Transverse plane TEE illustrating a 1 cm anteriorly located periaortic abscess. LA = left atrium; LV = left ventricle; Ao = aortic root.

cations for TEE are listed in Table 6. TEE is probably not required when the clinical picture is clear, TTE reveals a small focal vegetation, and the patient is responding to treatment appropriately; and when there is a low index of suspicion for endocarditis (such as "fever workup" in the absence of a new regurgitant murmur, predisposing cardiac abnormalities, or clinical features of endocarditis); and certainly not for all patients with bacteremia.

Even with the high-resolution images provided by TEE, the definite diagnosis of a vegetation is not always possible. There are situations in which the echocardiographic findings can be particularly confusing or even misleading. Some of these situations include: differentiating vegetations from myxomatous thickening of mitral valves; ruptured chordae tendineae; focal, nonspecific thickening or calcium deposits; retained mitral leaflets and chordae with mitral valve replacement; Lambl's excrescences; sutures and other prosthetic materials for pros-

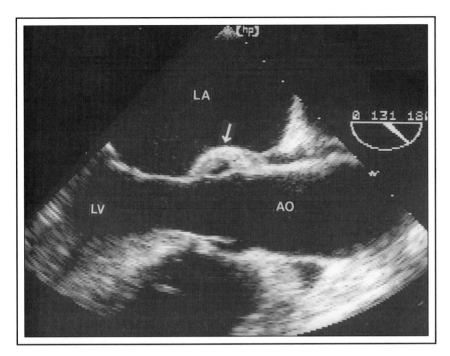

Figure 20. Multiplane TEE view (131°) of aortic root and ascending aorta (AO) which illustrates a posterior aortic root abscess (arrow) confirmed at surgery. LA = left atrium; LV = left ventricle.

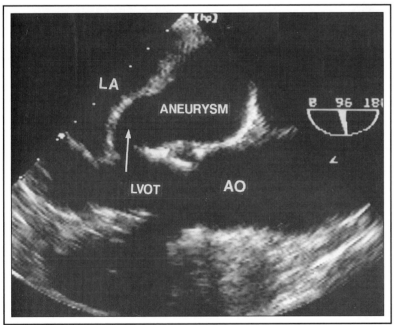

Figure 21. Longitudinal TEE view (96°) which illustrates a large aneurysm of the mitral-aortic intervalvular fibrosa region. Arrow is through the orifice connecting the left ventricular outflow tract (LVOT) with the aneurysm. AO = aortic root; LA = left atrium.

thetic valves; and small tumors. In these situations echocardiographic findings need to be carefully correlated and integrated with other clinical features.

In spite of these limitations, TEE is playing an expanding role in the evaluation of patients with infective endocarditis. Further use of TEE in this condition should provide greater insight into the natural history of endocarditis and the effects of antibiotic therapy on vegetation size. The effect of improved and earlier detection of vegetations by TEE on morbidity and mortality remains to be determined.

TABLE 6

Infective Endocarditis:
Indications for TEE

1. Strong suspicion for endocarditis and negative/nondiagnostic TTE
2. Persistent bacteremia (abscess suspected)
3. Suspected prosthetic valve endocarditis
4. Hemodynamic instability
5. Clinical embolic event
6. Immediately prior to surgery for IE
7. Staph aortic valve endocarditis
8. TTE reveals vegetation, but size, mobility, extent unclear

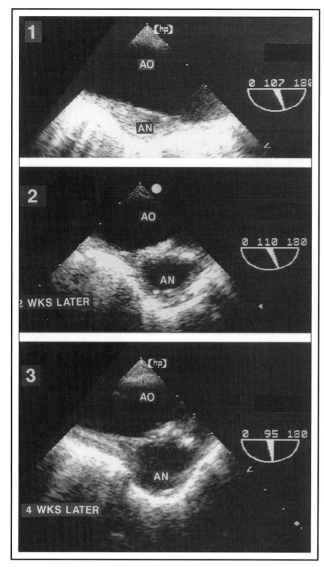

Figure 22. TEE views of the proximal descending thoracic aorta (Ao) in a 32 year-old dialysis patient with Staph Aureus aortic valve endocarditis. Top panel (1) shows a "mycotic" aneurysm (AN) detected by the first TEE at the time of initial diagnosis. Middle panel (2) shows enlargement of the aneurysm (AN) 2 weeks later noted at the time of aortic valve replacement. Bottom panel (3) shows further enlargement of the aneurysm (AN) 4 weeks later at the time of surgical resection.

Cardiac Source of Embolus and Intracardiac Masses

Evaluation of patients with unexplained arterial embolism is a challenging problem. In some patients, a cardiac source is suggested by clinical features such as those listed in Table 7. However, these features have not proved consistently to be reliable indicators of embolism from the heart. In other patients a cardiac source is suspected after exclusion of other causes for stroke following a thorough neurologic workup, including negative cerebral arteriography. TEE has proven to be useful for detecting cardiac sources of emboli in such

TABLE 7
Signs of Cerebral Embolus
1. Lack of prodromal symptoms
2. Abrupt onset of maximal deficit
3. Middle cerebral artery distribution
4. Multifocal signs
5. CT scan: Multiple defects
6. Angiography = No atherosclerosis

TABLE 8
Sources of Systemic Embolism Detectable by TEE
HIGH ASSOCIATED RISK
1. Left atrial/left atrial appendage thrombus
2. Left ventricular apical thrombus
3. Prosthetic valve thrombus
4. Intracardiac tumors
5. Protruding and/or mobile aortic atherosclerotic "debris"
UNCERTAIN RISK OF ASSOCIATION
1. Patent foramen ovale
2. Atrial septal aneurysm
3. Spontaneous echo contrast
LOW RISK OF ASSOCIATION
1. Mitral valve prolapse
2. Mitral annulus calcification

patients. As a result, an increasing number of patients are being referred for this indication. In fact, evaluation for "cardiac source of embolus" is the most common reason for referral for TEE in most laboratories.

Both transthoracic and transesophageal echo play an important role in evaluation of these patients. In most instances, transthoracic echocardiography is superior to TEE for detecting left ventricular mural thrombi, but there is general agreement that TEE is superior to TTE for detecting most other potential sources of unexplained systemic emboli. The major sources of emboli that can be accurately detected with TEE are listed in Table 8.

TEE is clearly superior to TTE for detecting thrombi in the left atrium since the majority are limited to the left atrial appendage, an area that is difficult to image by TTE. TEE, by providing excellent visualization of the left atrial appendage, is therefore the procedure of choice for the diagnosis of left atrial thrombi (Figure 23). Atrial thrombi are

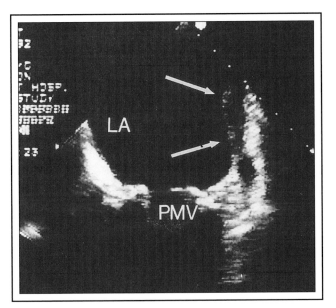

Figure 23. Transesophageal echocardiogram (transverse plane) demonstrates a thrombus (arrows) along the left atrial wall. The left atrium (LA) is enlarged. A prosthetic porcine mitral valve is present (PMV).

almost always associated with predisposing conditions such as mitral stenosis, prosthetic mitral valves, atrial fibrillation, and severe left ventricular dysfunction. While it is true that anticoagulation is recommended in these situations whether or not TEE detects atrial thrombi, their identification is particularly important when mitral balloon valvuloplasty is being considered. The presence of a clot in the body of the left atrium or near the "mouth" of the left atrial appendage is a contraindication to this procedure in this context. The significance of small, nonmobile thrombi near the apex of

the left atrial appendage is not clear at this time. The role of TEE for excluding atrial thrombi prior to cardioversion is under current investigation.

TEE is the most accurate method for detecting atrial septal aneurysms, another condition known to be associated with embolic events. An atrial septal aneurysm is a redundant atrial septum, usually located in the fossa ovalis region, which bulges 1.5 cm or more beyond the atrial septum at some point during the cardiac cycle (Figure 24). Atrial septal aneurysms may involve only the fossa ovalis region, or the entire atrial septum. Atrial septal aneurysms are identified in approximately 1% of all TTEs and up to 3% of all TEEs. The prevalence of this lesion is higher in patients with unexplained cerebral ischemia, suggesting an association, the mechanism of which is unclear. Two potential mechanisms have been postulated. One may be paradoxical embolization (Figure 25) through an accompanying patent foramen ovale, present in up to 75% of atrial septal aneurysms. Second, the atrial septal aneurysm may provide a nidus for thrombus formation, either within the aneurysm itself, or as tiny fibrin-thrombus tags attached to its roughened or wrinkled surface. Some authors have suggested that patients with atrial septal aneurysm and unexplained embolic disease should be anticoagulated, but such management issues will require further study.

A patent foramen ovale (PFO) is detected in up to 30% of patients at necropsy. Similarly, investigators from Mayo Clinic have identified PFO in 28% of 606 patients undergoing TEE. The extent to which paradoxical embolization by way of a PFO contributes to the incidence of embolic disease

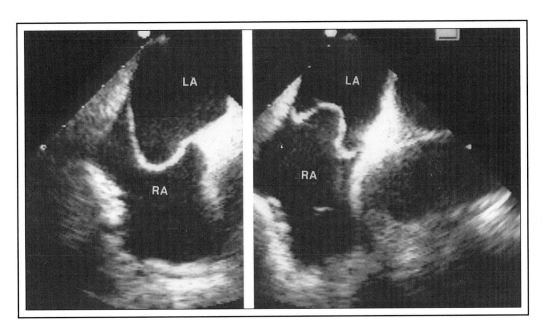

Figure 24. Transesophageal echo (transverse plane) illustrating an atrial septal aneurysm which oscillates back-and-forth between the right atrium (RA) as shown in the left panel and the left atrium (LA) as shown in the right panel.

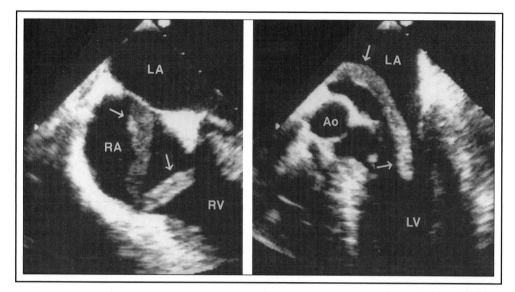

Figure 25. Transesophageal echocardiogram (transverse plane) illustrating a 21 cm long thrombus (arrows) that extended from the right atrium (RA) and right ventricle (RV) as shown in the left panel, through the atrial septum into the left atrium (LA) and left ventricle (LV). The thrombus was removed surgically and the patent foramen ovale was closed in this patient who had sustained both pulmonary and systemic emboli.

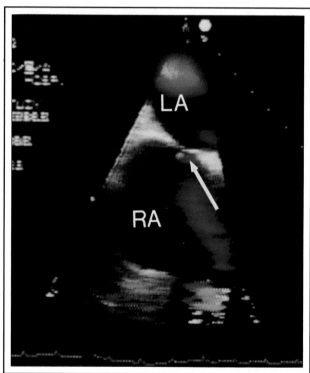

Figure 26. Transesophageal echocardiogram (transverse plane) of the atrial septum demonstrates a small color jet (arrow) suggesting a small shunt from the left (LA) to the right atrium (RA) through a patent foramen ovale.

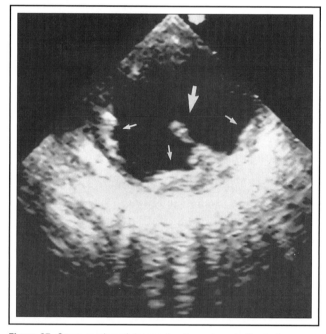

Figure 27. Cross-section of descending thoracic aorta illustrating a mobile thrombus (large arrow) overlying atherosclerotic plaque (small arrows).

remains speculative. Nevertheless, studies have suggested a higher prevalence of PFO detected by TEE in patients with cerebro-vascular events compared to populations with no evidence of such events. Several studies have documented that TEE is superior to TTE for detecting patent foramen ovale. If a PFO is the only abnormality detected by TEE, further workup, including a search for lower extremity venous thrombosis or pulmonary embolism, appears indicated to establish the likelihood of paradoxical embolism.

A PFO is often detected by color flow imaging of the atrial septum (Figure 26). However, contrast echocardiography has been shown to be more sensitive and should be routinely performed. Maneuvers that increase right atrial pressure such as cough or Valsalva maneuver enhance the detection of right to left shunting via a patent foramen ovale. The potential for paradoxical embolism also exists in patients with atrial septal defect (ASD). TEE is the procedure of choice for detection of ASD when this abnormality is suspected clinically but is not confirmed by conventional TTE. Spontaneous echo contrast ("smoke") can be detected by TEE in patients with mitral stenosis, prosthetic valves, atrial fibrillation, or low cardiac output. Because of the higher resolution of TEE as compared to TTE, this phenomenon is much more often recognized with TEE. This phenomenon is felt to be associated with an increased risk of thromboembolism since a greater prevalence has been demonstrated in patients with unexplained cerebral ischemia than in an unselected population.

TEE has provided a major advance in the evaluation of atherosclerotic lesions within the thoracic aorta. Several studies have reported an increased frequency of embolic events in patients with such plaques detected by TEE. This is particularly true with "complex" plaques as illustrated in Figure 27 ($\geq$ 5mm thickness and containing protruding and mobile components). Occasionally thin, filamentous, mobile projections from atherosclerotic plaques move freely within the bloodstream. TEE is the only imaging technique capable of imaging these small projections. The management of patients with embolic events and protruding atheromas is uncertain. Anticoagulation with coumadin, antiplatelet agents, and even surgical debridement in very select patients have all been considered.

TEE is uniquely helpful for detecting clots and vegetations associated with prosthetic valves. These may be responsible for systemic embolization. TEE is also superior to TTE for the detection of vegetations on native valves. There is data to suggest that the size of a vegetation, as determined by TEE, is directly related to its potential for embolization. Mitral valve prolapse (MVP), found in approximately 1% to 5% of the general population, may usually be detected by TTE, but can also be detected using TEE. To date, diagnostic criteria for MVP by TEE remain to be determined. Some patients with mitral valve prolapse have severe myxomatous degeneration and "redundant" or thickened leaflets. Although this subgroup more often has endocarditis, progressive mitral regurgitation, and ruptured chordae tendineae, an increased risk for stroke in this group has not been established.

Intracardiac tumors, although rare, do have the potential for systemic embolization. Atrial myxomas, the most common primary cardiac tumors, characteristically develop in the left atrium attached to the atrial septum (Fig 28). Myxomas occur with decreasing frequency in the right atrium, ventricles, multiple intracardiac sites, or as an isolated tumor on the mitral valve. While TTE and TEE have a similar ability to detect myxomas,

TEE provides useful additional information in the majority of instances because most tumors are located posteriorly where TEE image quality is clearly superior to TTE. TEE provides valuable information concerning the exact size, site of attachment, morphology, mobility, and acoustic characteristics. Other less common tumors such as sarcomas and fibromas can also be accurately evaluated by TEE.

CARDIAC PEARL

Myxomas are the most common of the intracavitary tumors, with the left atrial myxoma occurring more commonly than the right. Rarely, myxomas are bilateral. They also may occur in either ventricle, although much less commonly than in the atria. The myxomas represent a key group of tumors for which surgical removal is possible and often life-saving.

Depending on its size, a myxoma may present with various features. Some myxomas are small and, therefore, cause no obstructive symptoms. At times they are an incidental finding at autopsy, having produced no symptom in life. However, even though the myxoma is not large enough to cause obstruction, the danger that it will produce emboli is real. Systemic emboli represent a distinct hazard, at times involving even the coronary arteries and producing coronary pain and acute myocardial infarction. Evidence of peripheral emboli of unexplained origin may well be one of the first clues to alert the clinician to the possibility of an intracavity tumor. At other times hemiplegia or other cerebral vascular episode may be the first manifestation, or, in some patients, a larger embolus at the bifurcation of the aorta. Embolectomy in such cases has enabled the diagnosis by showing myxomatous thrombi on microscopic examination. Some emboli may go to other branches of the arterial system, including the mesenteric, splenic and renal arteries.

Peripheral emboli in association with fever and elevation of sedimentation rate in a patient with a variable heart murmur simulate endocarditis. Treatment with antibiotics in those patients whose condition is misdiagnosed as bacterial endocarditis is unsuccessful, and this negative result can alert the clinician to look for a different diagnosis.

W. Proctor Harvey, M.D.

In summary, the role of TEE for evaluating patients with suspected cardiac source of embolus is evolving. Although the superiority of TEE over TTE in detecting potential cardiac sources of

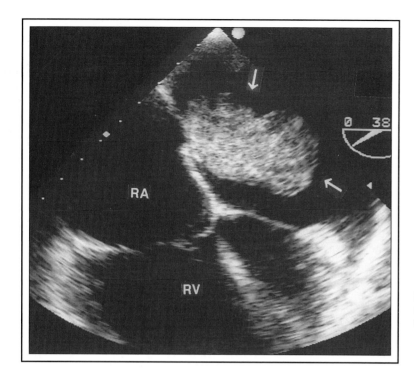

Figure 28. Multiplane TEE view (38°) illustrates a large (5 X 3 cm) left atrial myxoma (arrows) attached to the atrial septum. RA = right atrium; RV = right ventricle.

embolism is undisputed, assigning a cause and effect relationship is often difficult, if not impossible, in individual patients. Therefore, the role and cost-effectiveness of TEE for this purpose remains to be determined.

Native Valve Disease

Although the superior image quality of TEE provides a more detailed assessment of valve anatomy, most valvular abnormalities can be reliably diagnosed by TTE. In approximately 10% of cases, how-

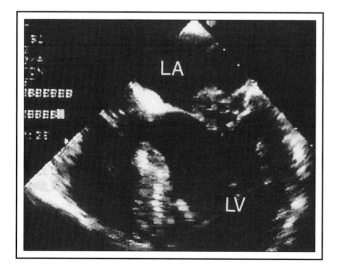

Figure 29. Transesophageal echocardiogram (transverse plane) 4-chamber view. The appearance of a mass on the mitral valve is caused by redundant myxomatous leaflets. At the time of surgical repair chordal structures were found to be intact. Evidence of endocarditis was not found. LA = left atrium; LV = left ventricle.

ever, TEE may be necessary because of suboptimal imaging by transthoracic studies because more detailed anatomic information is required for decision-making. This is more often true for mitral valve pathology than for aortic valve disease.

Due to the proximity of the esophagus to the mitral valve, and the higher frequency of the transducer, TEE provides more precise and detailed assessment of the mitral valve apparatus than TTE. For example, TEE is extremely helpful in determining the underlying mechanism of mitral regurgitation, including endocarditis, myxomatous degeneration (Figure 29), perforation (Figure 30), mitral valve aneurysm, ruptured chordae (Figure 31), and papillary muscle rupture (Figure 32). With the growing enthusiasm for operative repair of the mitral valve, TEE has provided an important tool for the preoperative assessment of the suitability of the valve as well as the immediate postoperative assessment of the repair.

CARDIAC PEARL

If moderate to severe mitral regurgitation as a single valvular lesion is present, the most common cause is mitral valve prolapse with rupture of a chorda tendineae or floppy valve. It is not rheumatic as was formerly thought.

Rupture of chordae tendineae is the most frequent serious complication of mitral valve prolapse. The clinical features of chordal rupture with mitral valve prolapse vary, usually relating to the size, number, or both. Chordal

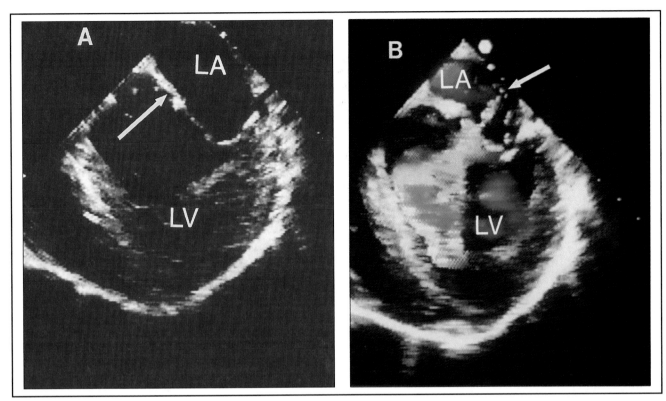

Figure 30. A: Intraoperative transesophageal echocardiogram in a patient with documented aortic valve endocarditis. The anterior leaflet of the mitral valve (arrow) appears thickened in comparison to the posterior leaflet. B: Color flow demonstrates a small high velocity jet through the anterior leaflet (arrow). A perforation of the leaflet was confirmed at surgery.

rupture can occur spontaneously or as a result of infective endocarditis. Many auscultatory variants of mitral valve prolapse exist. Any of these, including a single systolic click, can with chordal rupture become a holosystolic murmur of mitral regurgitation. It typically peaks in mid systole and decreases in the latter part of systole. This configuration of the murmur is due to a significant regurgitant leak of the mitral valve into a normal-sized left atrium, which occurs with chordal rupture. As pressure in the atrium builds up, it reaches a peak in mid systole because the atrium cannot continue to accommodate the large leak, and then the pressure decreases, as does the volume of blood in the last part of systole. The systolic murmur reflects this pressure change and gives the configuration as shown. On the other hand, with chronic significant mitral regurgitation an enlarged left atrium exists that can continue to accommodate the large volume of blood regurgitating into it.

W. Proctor Harvey, M.D.

Echocardiographic estimation of the severity of mitral valve regurgitation is difficult by any approach, including TEE, and remains semiquantitative. The area of the regurgitant jet displayed by both TTE and TEE is affected by the same factors, including heart rate, systemic blood pressure, preload, afterload, left atrial pressure and compliance, and jet location (i.e. central vs "wall-hugging"). Therefore, as with TTE, the quantitation of mitral regurgitation by TEE requires the integration of multiple factors (Table 9), such as maximal regurgitant color flow jet area in multiple planes, area of flow acceleration within the left ventricle, mitral inflow velocity profile, and pulmonary venous flow pattern (Figures 33 and 34) (Schiller has described twenty four signs of severe mitral regurgitation). TEE does offer some advantages over TTE for detecting mitral regurgitant jets in the left atrium. The precordial approach is sometimes limited because the left atrium is in the "far-field" resulting in diminished amplitude of Doppler signals over distance. "Flow-masking" of the left atrium from precordial apical imaging can occur due to a fibrotic or calcified mitral valve or annulus. TEE circumvents these problems as the transducer is positioned immediately behind the left atrium.

In general, severity of a stenotic lesion may be adequately assessed from the transthoracic approach. Nevertheless, estimation of the severity of mitral stenosis obtained by TEE correlates closely with results obtained from both TTE and

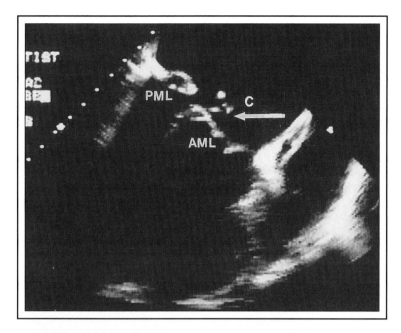

Figure 31. Transesophageal echocardiogram (longitudinal plane) demonstrates a systolic frame of a "floppy" myxomatous anterior (AML) and posterior (PML) mitral leaflet. Ruptured chordae tendinae (arrow) are seen above the valve plane in the left atrium.

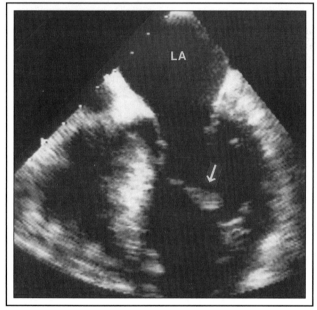

Figure 32. Transesophageal echo (transverse plane) illustrating a ruptured papillary muscle (arrow). LA = left atrium.

TABLE 9

Signs of Severe Mitral Regurgitation

1. Large mitral regurgitant jet area
2. Wall hugging jet
3. Jet circles the left atrium
4. Systolic reflux into pulmonary vein(s)
5. Wide jet at regurgitant orifice
6. Prominent flow acceleration on left ventricular side of mitral valve
7. High mitral inflow velocity

cardiac catheterization. On the other hand, TEE is far superior to TTE for detecting thrombi in the left atrium and left atrial appendage and for detecting spontaneous echo contrast ("smoke") in the left atrial cavity. TEE also provides better information regarding leaflet mobility and thickness. Such information is especially useful in selecting patients for balloon-catheter mitral valvuloplasty or open surgical commissurotomy. TEE has also been demonstrated to be helpful in guiding transseptal puncture, in assessing the extent of post-dilatation mitral regurgitation, in detecting procedure-related complications, and in detecting the presence of interatrial shunting as a result of transseptal puncture. Comprehensive TTE, including precordial, suprasternal, and abdominal windows is generally adequate for the semiquantitation of aortic regurgitation. TEE usually adds little except when TTE images are suboptimal. TEE is, however, superior for imaging the aortic valve leaflets and aortic root. Therefore, the mechanism of aortic regurgitation (such as dilated aortic root, aortic valve endocarditis, and proximal aortic dissection) is more accurately assessed with TEE than with TTE. Accurate Doppler evaluation of valvular aortic stenosis by TEE is often difficult to obtain because of difficulty in aligning the echo-beam parallel to the stenotic aortic jet. Similarly, continuous wave Doppler interrogation of tricuspid regurgitant jets is sometimes difficult using TEE. Moreover, tricuspid regurgitant jets are sometimes contaminated by flow from coexistent mitral regurgitation. However, details of tricuspid leaflet anatomy and right atrial structure are better depicted using

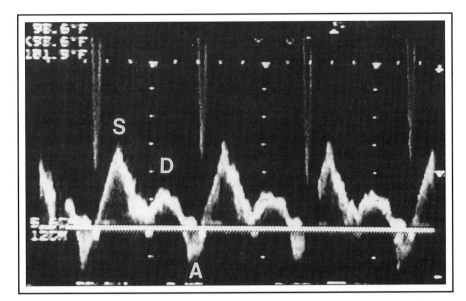

Figure 33. Pulse Doppler recording of flow in a pulmonary vein. A normal flow pattern into the left atrium consists of a large forward systolic flow(s) and a smaller forward flow in diastole (D). A normal presystolic reversal of flow is demonstrated (A).

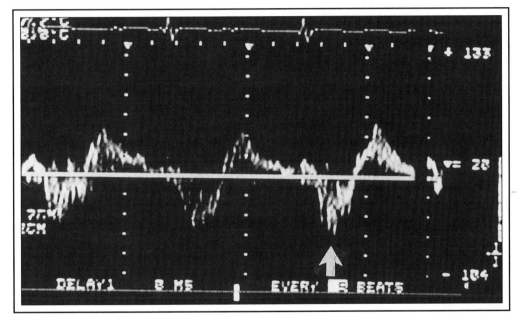

Figure 34. Pulse Doppler recording of flow in a pulmonary vein in a patient with severe mitral regurgitation. Reversal of flow in systole is demonstrated (arrow).

TEE. The right ventricular outflow tract, the pulmonic valve, and the pulmonary artery are better imaged with TEE than with TTE (Figure 12).

Prosthetic Valves

Although prosthetic valves have greatly improved prognosis and quality of life of many patients, all are imperfect and patients with them should not be considered free from heart disease. Echocardiography has played a major role in the evaluation of prosthetic valves. Confirmation of normal prosthetic function is important, but detection of complications and abnormal prosthetic function is critical. Listed in Table 10 are complications of prosthetic valves; such structural complications can lead to either prosthetic valve obstruction or regurgitation.

CARDIAC PEARL

Worthy of emphasis is that the prosthetic valve replacement procedure is a palliative one. Too many patients are under the erroneous impression that valve replacement will result in giving a person a new heart rather than repairing a damaged one.

W. Proctor Harvey, M.D.

Prosthetic valve obstruction is usually easily documented with a comprehensive standard transthoracic Doppler echogram. However, TTE has significant limitations in evaluating structural deterioration and prosthetic valve regurgitation, especially with mitral prostheses. In both paraster-

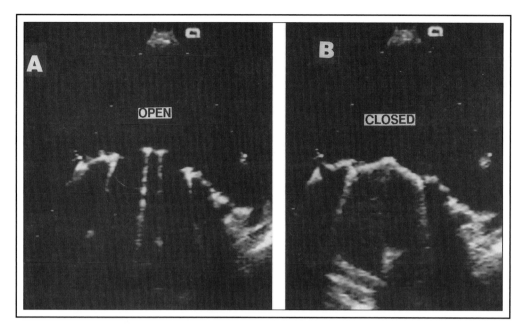

Figure 35. Illustrates the high-quality images obtained by TEE of a St. Jude mitral prosthesis. In the left panel (A) the two leaflets are aligned nearly parallel in open position. In the right panel (B) the two leaflets form an obtuse angle in the closed position.

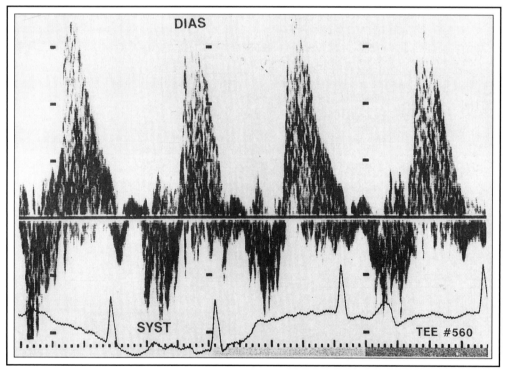

Figure 36. Pulsed wave Doppler of pulmonary venous flow illustrates systolic flow reversal (SYST) indicating severe mitral regurgitation. DIAS = diastole.

nal and apical TTE windows, the metallic sewing ring, stents, and poppets of prosthetic valves markedly attenuate ultrasound penetration beyond the prosthesis. This phenomenon of "flow-making" plus strong reverberations limit the assessment of flow in the left atrium, masking a central or paravalvular leak, or leading to underestimation of the degree of mitral regurgitation. This major limitation of TTE is circumvented by TEE, because the transducer lies immediately behind the left atrium, and therefore, provides a clear view of that cham-

ber without interference from the prosthesis itself (Figure 35). Several studies have documented the superiority of TEE over TTE for detecting and quantitating prosthetic mitral valve regurgitation. In fact, the assessment of a mitral prosthesis and the quantitation of mitral regurgitation are among the most frequent indications of TEE. Pulmonary venous flow pattern, detectable by TEE in almost all patients, provides supplemental information for quantitating mitral regurgitation. Reduction of forward systolic flow and systolic flow reversal (Figure

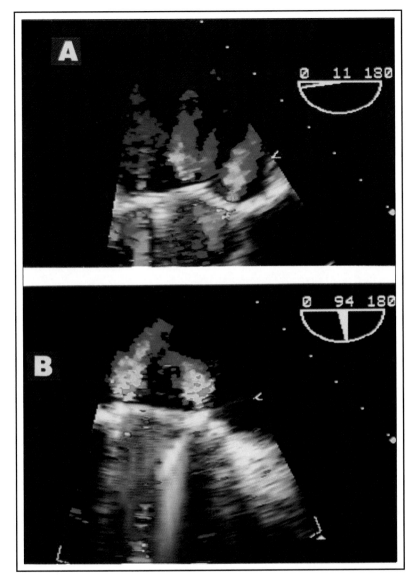

Figure 37. Close-up view of a St. Jude mitral prosthesis illustrating physiologic trivial mitral regurgitation. Top panel (A) illustrates diverging jets in the transverse plane. Bottom panel (B) illustrates two converging jets.

36) are indications of the presence of severe mitral regurgitation.

All types of normally functioning mitral prosthetic valves have been shown by TEE with color Doppler to produce systolic regurgitant jets into the left atrium. Each prosthetic type generates its own specific pattern of "physiologic leak" (Figure 37). TEE is superior to TTE in differentiating these "physiologic" leaks from pathologic regurgitation. TEE is useful not only for detecting and quantitating prosthetic mitral regurgitation and helping to differentiate "physiologic" from pathologic regurgitation, but also for detecting vegetations (Figure 18), thrombi in the left atrium and left atrial appendage, and spontaneous echo contrast or "smoke." A mild degree of "smoke" or "swirling" is detectable in the left atrium in more than half the patients with mitral prostheses, especially in those with an enlarged left atrium and atrial fibrillation.

However, marked "smoke" may indicate an increased potential for thromboembolism.

TEE is less accurate for evaluating prosthetic aortic regurgitation than for mitral prosthetic regurgitation. Attenuation of the ultrasound beam as it traverses the aortic prosthesis results in "flow-masking" of the left ventricular outflow tract and incomplete visualization of bioprosthetic leaflets and mechanical disks. Nevertheless, TEE is of diagnostic value in the majority of patients. Moreover, TEE is superior to TTE for detecting vegetations, periprosthetic abscesses, aneurysms, sewing ring dehiscence and fistulas, especially when posterior or in the mitral-aortic intervalvular fibrosa.

Although seldom necessary, evaluation of obstruction of mitral prostheses is also possible with TEE using continuous wave Doppler. Elevated mean diastolic gradient, increased antegrade flow velocity, prolonged pressure halftime and decreased

```
T A B L E   1 0
```
Complications of Prosthetic Valves

1. Thrombosis
2. Thromboembolism
3. Fibrous tissue ingrowth
4. Infection
5. Dehiscence
6. Degeneration (Bioprostheses)
7. Structural deterioration (Mechanical prostheses)
8. Prosthetic and periprosthetic regurgitation
9. Obstruction

```
T A B L E   1 1
```
Indications for TEE Evaluation of Prosthetic Valves

1. Suspected embolic event
2. Suspected endocarditis
3. Discordance between clinical and TTE findings
4. Inadequate imaging using TTE

effective orifice area suggest obstruction. In addition, restriction of leaflet or poppet motion is usually better demonstrated by TEE than by TTE. On the other hand, the Doppler hemodynamic evaluation of aortic prostheses by TEE is limited because of difficulty in aligning the continuous wave Doppler beam parallel to flow through aortic prostheses. Multiplane probes and the use of the deep transgastric transducer position sometimes help to overcome this problem.

In summary, TEE provides more detailed structural information than TTE. TEE is usually superior to TTE for detecting and quantitating mitral prosthetic regurgitation and marginally superior to evaluating aortic prosthetic regurgitation. In addition, TEE is superior to TTE for detecting masses such as thrombi and vegetations, periprosthetic abscesses, and sewing ring dehiscence. Nevertheless, abnormal gradients across prosthetic valves are adequately estimated by TTE and therefore TEE should always be used in conjunction with standard TTE when evaluating prosthetic valves. Indications for TEE evaluation of prosthetic valves are listed in Table 11.

Thoracic Aortic Pathology

Examination of the thoracic aorta is one of the most important applications of TEE. TEE is ideally suited for imaging the thoracic aorta because of the proximity of the esophagus to the aorta and the high resolution of TEE transducers. The transesophageal window avoids many of the limitations of precordial echocardiography and provides images that are superior to those obtained by TTE. The entire thoracic aorta, except for the distal portion of the ascending aorta where the trachea and left-mainstem bronchus intervene, can be clearly imaged in almost all patients. TEE, therefore, is playing an increasingly important role in the evaluation of aortic diseases, including aortic dissection, aortic aneurysm, and aortic atherosclerosis. Rapid and accurate diagnosis of aortic dissection is critical to effective patient management. Four important diagnostic methods are available, including aortography, computed-tomography (CT), magnetic resonance imaging and transesophageal echocardiography. Numerous publications have touted the merits of each of these. In truth, each diagnostic test has strengths and weaknesses (Table 12). The evaluation of patients with suspected aortic dissection requires the acquisition of certain information (Table 13). TEE routinely provides almost all of the necessary clinical information about aortic dissection. It is most important to establish the diagnosis with a high level of sensitivity and specificity. In recent publications, TEE has been demonstrated to be highly accurate. Erbel and colleagues, from the European Cooperative Study Group, published the results of a multicenter study of 164 patients with suspected dissection. Eighty two patients had an independently proven diagnosis by necropsy, surgery, angiography, and/or CT-scan. Sensitivity and specificity of uniplane TEE were 99% and 98% respectively, and a positive predictive value of 98%.

```
T A B L E   1 2
```
Disadvantages of TEE (Including TEE for Aortic Dissection)

DISADVANTAGES

1. Can miss dissection of upper ascending aorta (especially with uniplane probe)
2. May not define branch vessel involvement
3. Semi-invasive, with a small potential for morbidity

ADVANTAGES

1. Very prompt diagnosis, even at bedside
2. Easily performed on critically ill patients, even those on ventilators
3. Can usually define intimal flaps, entry, and reentry sites
4. Can detect and quantitate aortic regurgitation
5. Can detect involvement of coronary orifices
6. Can detect pericardial effusion
7. Can assess left ventricular function

T A B L E   1 3
Aortic Dissection: Useful Information

1. Confirmation of the diagnosis
2. Type of dissection (location)
3. Location of primary or entry site
4. Location of secondary or reentrant site(s)
5. Involvement of major branch vessels
6. Presence, severity, and cause of aortic insufficiency
7. Blood flow dynamics within true and false lumens
8. Involvement of coronary arteries
9. Left ventricular function

T A B L E   1 4
Goals of Imaging Thoracic Aortic Aneurysms

1. Confirm diagnosis
2. Measure maximal diameter of the aneurysm
3. Define longitudinal extent of the aneurysm
4. Determine involvement of the aortic valve
5. Determine involvement of arch vessels(s)
6. Detect periaortic hematoma or other sign of leakage
7. Differentiate from aortic dissection
8. Detect mural thrombus

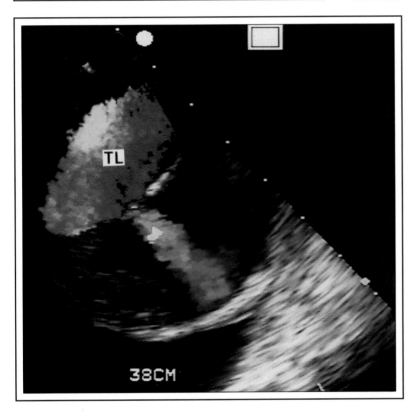

Figure 38. Cross-section view of the descending thoracic aorta 38cm from incisors. Orange color represents flow in true lumen (TL). A re-entry site is detected by the blue jet from the true lumen to the false lumen.

This large study leaves little doubt about the accuracy of TEE in the diagnosis of acute dissection. Seventeen patients in that study underwent operation without any other investigative procedure. The diagnosis of dissection was confirmed in all 17. Subsequent studies have confirmed the accuracy of TEE. However, there have been a few reports of failure to recognize type II dissection, presumably due to the limited imaging of the distal ascending aorta by TEE.

Use of color flow Doppler with TEE helps to identify entry and reentry sites (Figure 38). True and false lumens can almost always be distinguished (Figure 39). TEE is not only useful for detecting and quantitating aortic insufficiency, but also can assist the preoperative planning of the surgical procedure by determining the mechanism of aortic insufficiency. In addition, echocardiography is the choice for detection of pericardial effusion. Left ventricular function and other significant valvular disease can also be readily assessed.

CARDIAC PEARL

Right-Sided Murmurs of Aortic Regurgitation: Most murmurs of aortic regurgitation are heard louder on the left sternal border as compared with the counterpart on the right. However, some aortic diastolic murmurs are best heard along the right sternal border as

compared with the left. Cardiac pearl: this "right-sided aortic diastolic murmur" is usually associated with dilation and rightward displacement of the aortic root. This murmur has been associated with aortic aneurysm, aortic dissection, hypertension, arteriosclerosis, rheumatoid spondylitis, Marfan's syndrome, a variant of Marfan's syndrome, osteogenesis imperfecta, and ventricular septal defect with aortic regurgitation. The key interspaces are the third and fourth right as compared with their counterparts, the third and fourth left interspaces. The third interspaces are most likely to show the more definitive difference. The detection of the aortic diastolic murmur louder at the right sternal border as compared with the left immediately suggests the diagnosis of the abnormality just described. This valuable "cardiac pearl" has stood the test of time but is frequently overlooked because we have not trained ourselves to listen to every patient along the right sternal border as well as the left. Many of the conditions that are listed as causing a "right-sided murmur" can also have the murmur louder on the left side as compared with the right.

When the "right-sided aortic diastolic murmur" is present, it represents an immediate clue about one of these conditions. When the murmur is of equal intensity on both the left and right sides, the physician can still suspect the diagnoses as listed.

Another "cardiac pearl" concerning right-sided aortic diastolic murmurs is what we term a "formula": diastolic hypertension plus aortic regurgitation plus a right-sided aortic diastolic murmur equals aneurysm and/or dissection of the first portion of the ascending aorta. Even when an aortic diastolic murmur develops in a patient with hypertension, the possibility of aneurysm, dissection, or both should be considered.

W. Proctor Harvey, M.D.

TEE has become the diagnostic method of choice for evaluating aortic dissection in many centers worldwide. It is favored since it can be performed rapidly (within 10 minutes), and on critically ill patients in the intensive care unit, the emergency room, and the operating room. Aortography may be required in instances when the diagnosis is still unclear after TEE and in situations in which there is a need to delineate blood supply to vital organs or the coronary arteries.

TEE is also an excellent technique for the serial follow-up of patients with aortic dissection. It is well-tolerated and can be performed on an outpatient basis without exposing patients to radiation or contrast agents. Follow-up by TEE can document healing and stability, and can detect changes, progression, and complications. Items to be evaluated include: diameter of the aorta at various levels (with careful attention to progressive dilatation); aneurysm or pseudoaneurysm formation; competence of aortic valve after surgical reconstruction; prosthetic aortic valve function; and development of aneurysm or aneurysms of the sinuses of Valsalva, especially in patients with Marfan's syndrome.

The role of TEE for detecting and evaluating thoracic aortic aneurysms is currently evolving. The major goals of imaging thoracic aortic aneurysms are listed in Table 14. Both CT-scan and angiography, the most firmly established methods for evaluating thoracic aortic aneurysms, have limitations. TEE promises to overcome some of these limitations and appears to be at least as accurate in identifying the size and location of aneurysms (Figure 40). Although several case studies have been reported, there has been only one "large" study using TEE to evaluate thoracic aortic aneurysms. In this study by Taams and colleagues, 15 patients with thoracic aortic aneurysms were diagnosed by TEE, whereas three of these were missed by CT scan. TEE provides detailed information of intraluminal structures such as thrombus and atherosclerotic plaques (Figures 41 and 42). TEE can detect compression of adjacent structures such as the pulmonary artery and the left atrium. Moreover, color Doppler may be used to detect complications of aneurysms such as fistulae.

Before TEE, there was no reliable technique for detecting thoracic aortic atherosclerosis. Recently, several authors reported the effectiveness of TEE for the detection, characterization, and embolic potential of atherosclerotic plaques in the thoracic aorta (Figure 27). Karalis and colleagues identified aortic atheromas in 36 (6%) of 556 patients undergoing TEE. Eleven (31%) of those 36 patients had embolic events. They concluded that atheromatous embolization from the thoracic aorta may be a more common occurence than is generally recognized. However, their data do not reflect the incidence of atheromas in the general population because of referral bias. Moreover, the significance of their presence as a predictor of future events has not been determined. Nevertheless, important therapeutic issues have been raised. What is the optimal management of either asymptomatic or symptomatic patients in whom intra-aortic atherosclerosis (especially protruding and maybe a protruding and mobile atheroma) has been detected? Should cardiac catheterization be avoided? Is there a role for

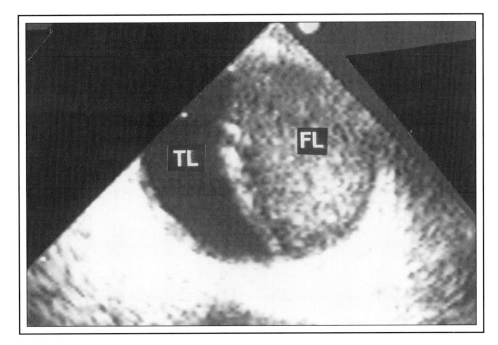

Figure 39. Cross-section of the descending thoracic aorta in a patient with aortic dissection. The false lumen (FL) contains thrombus which helps distinguish it from the true lumen (TL).

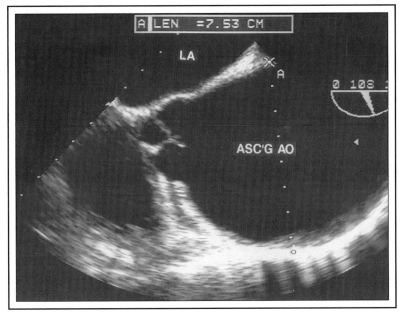

Figure 40. Longitudinal TEE view (108°) of the aortic root and proximal ascending aorta illustrates a large (7.5 cm) aneurysm of the proximal ascending aorta. LA = left atrium.

surgical removal of a protruding atheroma associated with multiple embolic events? The ability of TEE to detect and characterize atherosclerosis may provide a better understanding of this disease via prospective clinical trials that will address these important issues.

Congenital Heart Disease

Transthoracic echocardiography with Doppler has become an indispensable tool for the evaluation of congenital heart disease and has reduced the need for cardiac catheterization in most pediatric centers. Infants and children with un-operated congenital heart disease usually have excellent images with precordial transducers. However, post-operative patients and adults with congenital heart disease may have suboptimal images. Moreover, congenital heart disease may be associated with malpositioning of the heart and skeletal abnormalities which can compromise transthoracic imaging. Transesophageal echo now plays a significant role in the evaluation of these patients. In addition, TEE provides superior imaging of posterior structures such as the atrial septum, pulmonary veins, main and branch pulmonary arteries, and the atrial appendages. TEE also has improved the ability to detect small lesions which require greater resolution.

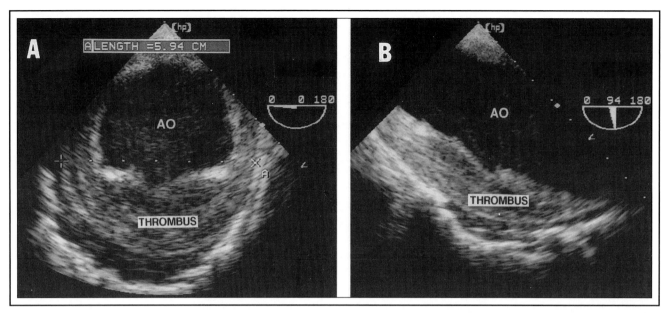

Figure 41. Transverse (A) and longitudinal (B) views of a 6 cm. fusiform aneurysm of the descending thoracic aorta (AO) which is lined with thrombus.

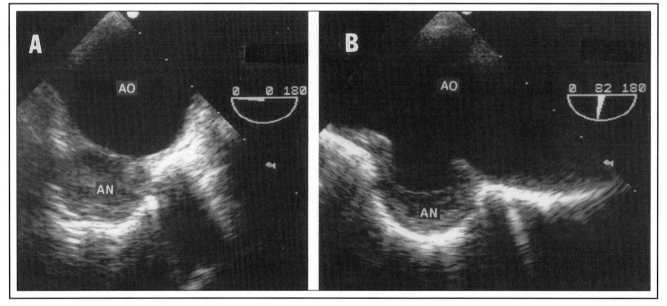

Figure 42. Transverse (A) and longitudinal (B) views of a small saccular aneurysm (AN) of the descending thoracic aorta (AO) which is lined with thrombus.

The proximity and orientation of the TEE probe to the atrial septum makes TEE a reliable technique for the detection of atrial septal defects (ASDs) and the differentiation of secundum, primum, and the more difficult sinus venosus defects. Transthoracic echo can detect approximately 90% of ostium secundum, nearly 100% of ostium primum and up to 75% of sinus venosus ASDs. Therefore, TEE may not be necessary when the diagnosis is clearly established by TTE. However, the superb imaging of the atrial septum by TEE permits the diagnosis of all 3 types in almost 100% of patients. Moreover, the size of the atrial septal defect measured by TEE correlates well with surgical measurements. TEE is particularly useful for detecting sinus venosus ASDs (Figure 43), which are notoriously difficult to detect with TTE. Figure 44 shows an example of a secundum ASD in a patient in whom the precordial echo was suboptimal. Figure 45 illustrates an example of a septum primum atrial septal defect. Other congenital heart diseases in which TEE has an important role include

Ebstein's anomaly, bicuspid aortic valve (Figure 46), discrete subaortic stenosis, cortriatriatum (Figure 47), supramitral valve ring, left superior vena cava, coarctation of the aorta, and coronary anomalies and fistulas. TEE also has an important role in the operating room to assist the determination of adequacy of surgical repair procedures. TEE combined with color Doppler and contrast is used to detect residual shunting after repair of atrial or ventricular defects and valve competence. Further details and discussion of less common entities are available in more specialized textbooks and journals dealing specifically with congenital heart disease.

Coronary Arteries

Visualization of the coronary arteries by conventional transthoracic echocardiography (TTE) has been well-documented, but the image quality is generally inadequate to consistently permit reliable anatomic details in adult patients. Moreover, TTE-imaging of the coronary arteries is time consuming because the arteries are small and rapidly move in and out of the image plane. The superior imaging ability of TEE permits higher resolution and imaging of longer lengths of the coronary arteries than by TTE.

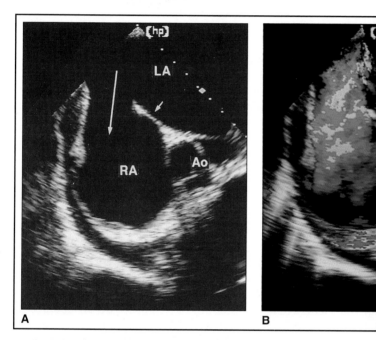

Figure 43. Transesophageal echocardiogram (transverse plane) illustrates a sinus venous atrial septal defect (ASD). Left panel (A): Large defect (long arrow) in the postero-superior portion of the atrial septum near the entrance of the superior vena cava into the right atrium (RA). Small arrow indicates the fossa ovalis region of the atrial septum, the site of the more common septum secundum ASD. Right panel (B): Color Doppler shows the left-to-right shunt across the ASD. LA = left atrium; Ao = aortic valve.

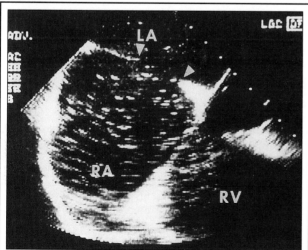

Figure 44. Transverse plane transesophageal echocardiogram at the level of the right atrium (RA) and left atrium (LA). A 1.5 cm defect in the atrial septum is imaged (arrows). Contrast study reveals "bubbles" passing from the RA into the LA via the secundum atrial septal defect. RV = right ventricle.

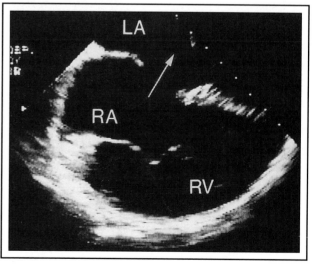

Figure 45. Transverse plane TEE at the level of atrial septum, right atrium (RA), and left atrium (LA) reveals a septum primum atrial septal defect (arrow).

371

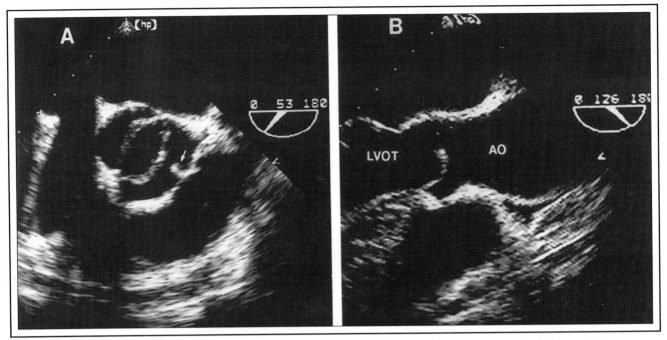

Figure 46. Left panel (A): Cross-section multiplane view (53°) shows a bicuspid aortic valve. Small arrow points to raphe. Right panel (B): Longitudinal view (126°) of the ascending aorta illustrates doming of the bicuspid aortic valve in systole. Ao = aortic root; LVOT = left ventricular outflow tract.

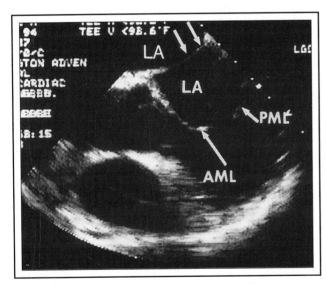

Figure 47. Transverse plane transesophageal echocardiogram illustrates a thin membrane (2 parallel arrows at top of image) which divides the left atrium into 2 portions. The upper portion (thin LA) receives the pulmonary veins (not shown). The lower portion (thick LA) is immediately above the mitral valve. AML = anterior mitral leaflet; PML = posterior mitral leaflet.

The coronary arteries are imaged just above the level of the aortic valve. The left-main and left circumflex coronary arteries are nearly perpendicular to the echo beam and are easily imaged in most patients. The left main coronary artery may be followed to the bifurcation in almost all patients. The left circumflex coronary artery can sometimes be visualized over a distance of 3 cm to 4 cm. The left anterior descending (LAD) and right coronary (RCA) arteries are nearly parallel to the echo beam. The proximal LAD is usually well seen. The proximal RCA, further from the TEE echo beam, is more difficult to image, but is often visible for about 3 cm. Variable success rates for visualizing the different coronary arteries have been reported: the left main coronary artery is visualized in 54% to 100%; and the RCA in 7% to 100%.

The proximal LAD coronary artery lies almost parallel to the interrogating Doppler beam (Figure 10). This favorable orientation permits adequate pulsed wave Doppler recordings of coronary blood flow velocity (CBFV) in up to 75% of patients. The normal velocity flow profile is biphasic with a larger diastolic component and a smaller systolic component (Figure 48). Although evaluation of CBFV by TEE is feasible, its clinical value remains to be determined. Certain limitations must be recognized: velocity and not flow is measured (the latter requires accurate measurement of the vessel diameter); the angle between the Doppler beam and the coronary artery may not be 0° resulting in underestimation of the true velocity; this method is limited to assessing flow in the LAD artery; a clear flow-velocity signal during systole is often not suitable for analysis because cardiac motion prevents a stable position of the sample volume within the

| T A B L E 15 ||||
| **Safety of TEE in the Critically Ill** ||||
AUTHOR	NUMBER	MEAN AGE (YEARS)	COMPLICATIONS
Oh	51	63	2
Font	112	59	0
Pearson	61	58	0
Foster	83	57	0

| T A B L E 16 |
| **Indications for TEE in Critically Ill Patients** |

1. Unexplained hypotension
2. Low output state
3. Acute pulmonary edema
4. Left and right ventricular function
5. Source of cerebral and peripheral emboli
6. Unexplained sepsis, suspected endocarditis
7. Suspected prosthetic valve dysfunction
8. Mechanical complications post-myocardial infarction
9. Suspicion of pericardial tamponade or mediastinal bleeding
10. Suspected aortic dissection
11. Cardiovascular trauma
12. Superior vena caval obstruction

| T A B L E 17 |
| **Intraoperative TEE: Major Indications** |

1. Monitoring of the non-cardiac surgical patient
2. Pre-and post-operative assessment of mitral valve repair
3. Pre-and post-operative assessment of aortic and tricuspid valve repair, hypertrophic cardiomyopathy, congenital defects
4. Assessment of difficulty weaning from cardiopulmonary bypass
5. Detection of retained intracardiac air

coronary vessel. Nevertheless, TEE has the advantage of being less invasive and associated with fewer complications than cardiac catheterization and has proven useful to estimate coronary flow reserve and changes in coronary flow with various drugs. TEE is also useful in evaluation of coronary artery aneurysms, coronary saphenous vein bypass graft aneurysms, coronary arteriovenous fistulae, and abnormal origin of the coronary arteries.

Critically Ill Patients

Use of TEE now extends to assessment of critically ill patients. Studies have documented the utility and safety of performing TEE in critical care settings (Table 15). A major advantage of TEE compared to other imaging techniques (CT-scan, magnetic resonance imaging, cardiac catheterization) is the ability to rapidly evaluate patients at the bedside with portable equipment obviating the need to transport the patient from the critical care setting. A transthoracic study should be quickly attempted first, and if the clinical question is satisfactorily answered, then TEE is not necessary. However, TTE has been disappointing and limited in the critical care setting, especially in intubated patients.

Common indications for TEE in critically ill patients are listed in Table 16. Imaging obtained from a TEE performed on a young patient on a ventilator for pulmonary edema is shown in Figure 49. TEE documented the etiology to be acute, severe

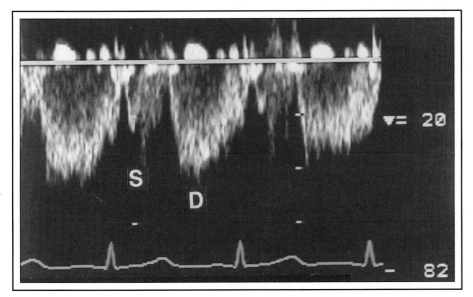

Figure 48. Normal pulsed wave Doppler profile of flow in the proximal left anterior descending coronary artery illustrating a large diastolic component (D) and a smaller systolic component (S).

373

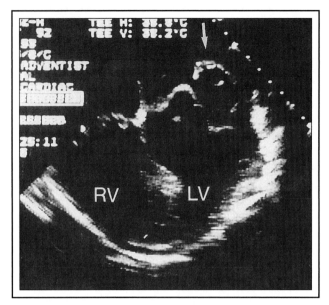

Figure 49. Transverse plane TEE illustrates a partially flail posterior mitral leaflet (arrow) due to a ruptured chordae tendinae in this patient with acute pulmonary edema. RV = right ventricle; LV = left ventricle.

mitral regurgitation. Figure 50 is an illustration from a patient evaluated for severe hypotension after coronary artery bypass surgery.

Intraoperative Applications

TEE has become a valuable tool in the operating room for patients undergoing either cardiac or non-cardiac surgery. Some of the major applications of intraoperative TEE are listed in Table 17. TEE is being used in some hospitals to supplement traditional monitoring (ECG, arterial and pulmonary capillary wedge pressures) of potentially "high-risk" patients with known or suspected cardiac disease

undergoing cardiac or noncardiac surgery. The transgastric short-axis view provides an excellent view for directly monitoring left ventricular function (Figure 2). Additional views obtained with biplane and multiplane probes should provide additional detail regarding left ventricular size and function. Continuous TEE-monitoring may allow detection of abnormalities of global or regional left ventricular dysfunction and myocardial ischemia earlier than traditional monitoring. This is true since regional wall motion abnormalities appear to be more sensitive markers for myocardial ischemia than ECG or hemodynamic data. In addition, there is evidence to suggest that monitoring changes in left ventricular and left atrial dimensions and pulmonary venous and mitral flow patterns provide more reliable information than pulmonary capillary wedge pressure for assessing left ventricular pressure during general anesthesia.

An important role of TEE in the operating room is the pre-operative assessment of mitral valve anatomy, feasibility of repair, and the post-operative assessment of the adequacy of such repairs. TEE is superior to the conventional surgical methods of assessing residual mitral regurgitation, including fluid filling of the arrested left ventricle, measurement of the left atrial V-wave, and digital palpation of the mitral regurgitant jet. There has been growing interest in mitral valve repair (Figure 51) because it results in lower operative mortality and greater preservation of left ventricular function. Moreover, it avoids use of prosthetic valves with their inherent risk of thromboembolism, and greater risk of endocarditis. Intraoperative echocardiography has played a significant role in the rapid

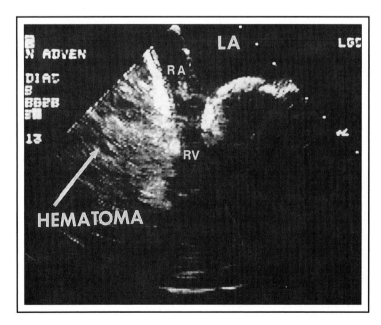

Figure 50. Transesophageal echo (transverse plane) illustrates a large intrapericardial hematoma (arrow - HEMATOMA) which compresses the right atrium (RA) and right ventricle (RV). LA = left atrium.

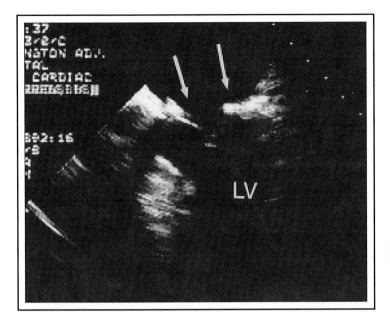

Figure 51. Intraoperative transesophageal echocardiogram of a patient who has undergone mitral valve repair. A Carpentier ring is in place (arrows). The native valve leaflets and the mitral apparatus are preserved.

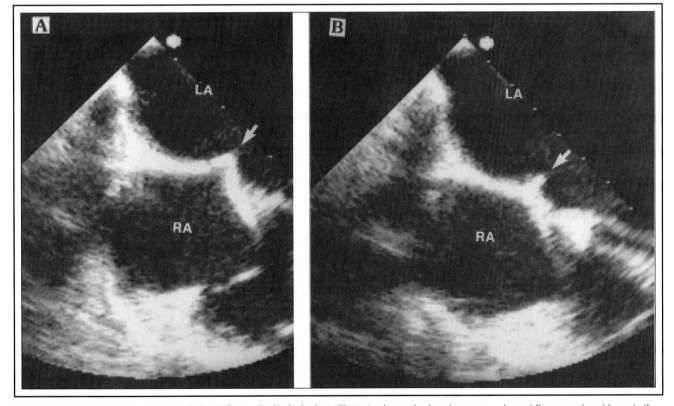

Figure 52. Transesophageal echo done during balloon mitral valvuloplasty illustrates how echo-imaging can supplement fluoroscopic guidance in the cardiac catheterization laboratory. Left panel (A) illustrates "tenting" or bowing of the atrial septum toward the left atrium (LA) due to contact with the advancing transseptal needle. Right panel (B) illustrates the tip of the transseptal needle (arrow) in the left atrium. RA = right atrium.

advances in surgical repair of the mitral valve. Epicardial imaging, which was used prior to TEE, has several important drawbacks, including invasion of the sterile surgical field and delay of the operation. TEE, by avoiding these problems, has become the procedure of choice in most centers. TEE

is also useful for determining the adequacy of a variety of other surgical procedures such as tricuspid annuloplasty, myotomy-myectomy for hypertrophic cardiomyopathy, congenital defects, aortic valve repair or resuspension following aortic root surgery.

TEE, with its high-frequency transducers is

┌───┐
│ **T A B L E   1 8**   │
│ **Interventional Echocardiography**   │
│   │
│ **1.** Intraoperative echocardiography   │
│ **2.** Intravascular ultrasound   │
│ **3.** Echo-guided pericardiocentesis   │
│ **4.** Guide endomyocardial biopsy   │
│ **5.** Guide balloon and blade atrial septostomy │
│ **6.** Guide catheter-based closure of ASD and VSD │
│ **7.** Transvenous "rescue" of intracardiac foreign bodies │
│ **8.** Monitor high-risk or complex coronary interventions in the │
│   cardiac cath lab   │
│ **9.** Guide catheter ablation of cardiac arrhythmias │
│ **10.** Guide percutaneous balloon valvuloplasty │
└───┘

extremely sensitive for detecting intracardiac air. Microbubbles as small as 10 µm may be visualized. TEE has been used to detect intracardiac air during neurosurgical procedures, in which paradoxical venous air embolism has been observed in patients in an upright position. During cardiac surgery, intracardiac air bubbles may be observed in 40% to 80% of cases. The clinical significance of this high incidence of intracardiac microbubbles is not yet clear. It is uncertain whether TEE can differentiate these microbubbles from larger and potentially more dangerous air emboli.

Guidance of Interventional Procedures

Although the primary purpose of cardiac ultrasound remains diagnostic, the evolution in technology has permitted the expansion of cardiac ultrasound into what has been termed *interventional echocardiography*. Examples of interventional echocardiography, that is, the use of echocardiography to guide invasive techniques are listed in Table 18.

TEE can provide superb imaging quality continuously during positioning of catheters and other devices, delineating their relationship to intracardiac structures without interrupting or interfering with catheter manipulation or fluoroscopy. Thus, it is a useful technique during a variety of invasive procedures. For example, during balloon mitral valvuloplasty, TEE may guide transseptal puncture (Figure 52) and balloon positioning, may immediately assess results, and may detect or prevent complications. Application of on-line TEE guidance to facilitate the success and safety of a number of interventional procedures is expected to increase.

Selected Reading

General

1. Daniel WG, Erbel R, Kasper W, et al: Safety of transesophageal echocardiography. A multicenter survey of 10,419 examinations. *Circ* 83:817-821,1991.
2. Daniel WG, Mugge A: Medical Progress. Transesophageal Echocardiography. *NEJM* 332:1268-1279, 1995.
3. Pandian NG, Hsu TL, Schwartz SL, et al: Multiplane transesophageal echocardiography: imaging planes, echocardiographic anatomy, and clinical experience with a prototypic phased array omniplane probe. *Echocardiography* 9:649-666, 1992.
4. Pearlman AS, Gardin JM, Martin RP, et al: Guidelines for physician training in transesophageal echocardiography: Recommendations of the American Society of Echocardiography Committee for Physicians Training in Echocardiography. *JASE* 5:187-194,1992.
5. Seward JB, Khandheria BK, Edwards WD, et al: Biplanar transesophageal echocardiography: anatomic correlations, image orientation, and clinical applications. *Mayo Clin Proc* 65:1193-1231,1990.
6. Seward JB, Khandheria BK, Freeman WK, et al: Multiplane transesophageal echocardiography: Image orientation, examination technique, anatomic correlations, and clinical applications. *Mayo Clin Proc* 68:523-551,1993.
7. Seward JB, Khandheria BK, Oh JK, et al: Critical appraisal of transesophageal echocardiography: limitations, pitfalls, and complications. *JASE* 5:288-305,1992.
8. Seward JB, Khandheria BK, Oh JK, et al: Transesophageal echocardiography: technique, anatomic correlations, implementation, and clinical applications. *Mayo Clin Proc* 63:649-680,1988.

Infective Endocarditis

1. Daniel WG, Mugge A, Martin RP, et al: Improvement in the diagnosis of abscess associated with endocarditis by transesophageal echocardiography. *NEJM* 324:795-800,1991.
2. Durack DT, Lukes AS, Bright DK: New criteria for diagnosis of infective endocarditis: utilization of specific echocardiographic findings. *AJM* 96:200-210,1994.
3. Karalis DG, Bansal RC, Hauck AJ, et al: Transesophageal echocardiographic recognition of subaortic complications in aortic valve endocarditis: Clinical and surgical implications. *Circ* 86:353-362,1992.
4. Mugge A, Daniel WG, Frank G, et al: Echocardigraphy in infective endocarditis: reassessment of prognostic implications of vegetation size determined by the transthoracic and the transesophageal approach. *JACC* 14:631-638,1989.
5. Shively BK, Gurule FT, Roldan CA, et al: Diagnostic value of transesophageal compared with transthoracic echocardiography in infective endocarditis. *JACC* 18:391-397,1991.
6. Sochowski RA, Chan KL: Implications of negative results on a monoplane transesophageal echocardiographic study in patients with suspected infective endocarditis. *JACC* 21:216-221,1993.

Cardiac Source of Embolus and Intracardiac Masses

1. Castello R, Pearson AC, Labovitz AJ: Prevalence and clinical implications of atrial spontaneous contrast in patients undergoing transesophageal echocardiography. *AJC* 65:1149-1153,1990.
2. DeRook FA, Comess KA, Albers GW, et al: Transesophageal echocardiography in the evaluation of stroke. *Ann Intern Med* 117:922-932,1992.
3. Hausmann D, Mugge A, Becht I, et al: Diagnosis of patent foramen ovale by transesophageal echocardiography and

association with cerebral and peripheral embolic events. *AJC* 70:668-672,1992.

4. Pearson AC, Labovitz AJ, Tatineni S, et al: Superiority of transesophageal echocardigraphy in detecting cardiac source of embolism in patients with cerebral emboli of uncertain etiology. *JACC* 17:66-72,1991.

5. Pop G, Sutherland GR, Koudstaal PJ, et al: Transesophageal echocardiography in the detection of intracardiac embolic sources in patients with transient ischemic attacks. *Stroke* 21:560-565,1990.

6. Schneider B, Hanrath P, Vogel P, et al: Improved morphologic characterization of atrial septal aneurysm by transesophageal echocardiography: Relation to cerebro-vascular events. *JACC* 16:1000-1009,1990.

7. Strom JA: Myxoma of the mitral valve detected by transesophageal echocardiography. *AHJ* 125:1449-1451,1993.

Native Valve Disease

1. Devereux RB, Kramer FR, Kligfield P: Mitral valve prolapse: causes, clinical manifestations, and management. *Ann Intern Med* 111:305-317;1989.

2. Hoffmann R, Flackskampf FA, Hanrath P: Planimetry of orifice area in aortic stenosis using multiplane transesophageal echocardiography. *JACC* 22:529-534,1993.

3. Marks AR, Choong CY, Sanfilippo AJ et al: Identification of high risk and low-risk subgroups of patients with mitral valve prolapse. *NEJM* 320:1031-1036;1989.

4. Nishimura RA, Tajik AJ: Follow-up observations in patients with mitral valve prolapse. *Herz* 13:326-334;1988.

5. Schiller NB, Foster E, Redberg RF: Transesophageal echocardiography in the evaluation of mitral regurgitation. *Card Clinics* 11:399-408,1993.

Prosthetic Valve Disease

1. Daniel LB, Grigg LE, Weisel RD, et al: Comparison of transthoracic and transesophageal assessment of prosthetic valve dysfunction. *Echocard* 9:83-95,1990.

2. Khandheria BK, Seward JB, Oh JK, et al: Value and limitations of transesophageal echocardiography in assessment of mitral valve prostheses. *Circ* 83:1956-1968, 1991.

3. Khandheria BK: Transesophageal echocardiography in the evaluation of prosthetic valves. *Card Clinics* ll:427-443,1993.

4. Nellesen U, Schnittger I, Appleton CP, et al: Transesophageal two-dimensional echocardiography and color Doppler flow velocity mapping in the evaluation of cardiac valve prostheses. *Circ* 78:848-855,1988.

Thoracic Aortic Pathology

1. Ballal RS, Nanda NC, Gatewood R, et al: Usefulness of transesophageal echocardiography in assessment of aortic dissection. *Circ* 84:1903-1914,1991.

2. Erbel R, Engberding R, Daniel W, et al: The European Cooperative Study Group for Echocardiography in the diagnosis of aortic dissection. *Lancet* i:457-460,1989.

3. Goldstein SA, Mintz GS, Lindsay JL: Aorta: comprehensive evaluation by echocardiography and transesophageal echocardiography. *JASE* 6:634-659, 1993.

4. Karalis DG, Chandrasekaran K, Victor MF, et al: Recognition of embolic potential of intraaortic atherosclerotic debris. *JACC* 17:73-78,1991.

5. Mohr-Kahaly S, Erbel R, Rennollet H, et al: Ambulatory follow-up of aortic dissection by transesophageal two-dimensional and color flow Doppler echocardiography. *Circ* 80:24-33,1989.

6. Taams MA, Gussenhoven WJ, Schippers LA, et al: The value of transesophageal echocardiography for diagnosis of thoracic aortic pathology. *EHJ* 9:1308-1316,1988.

7. Tunick PA, Perez JL, Kronzon I: Protruding atheromas in the thoracic aorta and systemic embolization. *Ann Intern Med* 115:423-427,1991.

Congenital Heart Disease

1. Essop MR, Skudicky D, Sareli P, et al: Diagnostic value of transesophageal versus transthoracic echocardiography in discrete subaortic stenosis. *AJC* 70:962-963,1992.

2. Kronzon I, Tunick PA, Freedberg RS, et al: Transesophageal echocardiography is superior to transthoracic echocardiography in the diagnosis of sinus venous atrial septal defect. *JACC* 17:537-542,1991.

3. Marelli AJ, Child J, Perloff JK, et al: Transesophageal echocardiography in congenital heart disease in the adult. *Card Clinics* 11:505-520,1993.

4. Morimoto K, Matsuzake M, Tohma Y, et al: Diagnosis and quantitative evaluation of secundum type atrial septal defect by transesophageal Doppler echocardiography. *AJC* 66:85-91,1990.

5. Weintraub R, Shiota T, Elkadi T, et al: Transesophageal echocardiography in infants and children with congenital heart disease. *Circ* 86:711-722,1992.

Coronary Arteries

1. Samdarshi TE, Nanda NC, Gatewood RP, et al: Usefulness and limitations of transesophageal echocardiography in the assessment of proximal coronary artery stenosis. *JACC* 19:572-580,1992.

2. Yamagishi M, Miyatake K, Beppu S, et al: Assessment of coronary blood flow by transesophageal two-dimensional pulsed Doppler echocardiography. *AJC* 62:641-644,1988

Critically Ill Patients

1. Font VE, Obarski TP, Klein AL, et al: Transesophageal echocardiography in the critical care unit. *Cleve Clin J Med* 58:315-322,1991.

2. Foster E, Schiller NB: Transesophageal echocardiography in the critical care patient. *Cardiology Clinics* 11:489-503,1993.

3. Khoury AF, Afridi I, Quinones MA, et al: Transesophageal echocardiography in critically ill patients: Feasibility, safety, and impact on management. *AHJ* 127:1363-1371,1994.

4. Oh JK, Seward JB, Khandheria BK, et al: Transesophageal echocardiography in critically ill patients. *AJC* 66:492-1495,1990.

5. Pearson AC, Castello R, Labovitz AJ: Safety and utility of transesophageal echocardiography in the critically ill patient. *AHJ* 119:1083-1089,1990.

Intraoperative Use

1. Maurer G, Siegel RJ, Czer LS: The use of color flow mapping for intraoperative assessment of valve repair. *Circ* 84 (Suppl I):250-258,1991.

2. Sheikh K, Bengtson J, Rankin J, et al: Intraoperative transesophageal Doppler color flow imaging used to guide patient selection and operative treatment of ischemic mitral regurgitation. *Circ* 84:594-604,1991.

3. Stewart WJ, Currie PJ, Salcedo E, et al: Intraoperative Doppler color flow mapping for decision-making in valve repair for mitral regurgitation: Technique and results in 100 patients. *Circ* 81:556-566,1990.

Guidance of Interventional Procedures

1. Goldstein SA, Campbell AN: Mitral stenosis: Evaluation and guidance of valvuloplasty by TEE. *Card Clinics* 11:409-324,1993.

CHAPTER 17

Clinical Exercise Testing

Guillermo B. Cintron, M.D.

Exercise testing is an extension of the initial patient evaluation by the "five finger" approach. As discussed in previous chapters, the purpose of the physician-patient encounter is to establish or exclude the presence of disease and evaluate its severity and prognosis; management plans and therapeutic interventions would then follow in logical sequence. Frequently, the initial and subsequent patient visits may leave some unresolved questions even after a thorough use of the history, physical examination, and routine resting electrocardiogram (ECG). An exercise test may then be a diagnostic option worth exploring. By subjecting selected patients to progressive levels of physical exertion the clinician can use the same basic tools, symptoms (history), physical examination, ECG, ultrasound, or radionuclide scanning to detect abnormalities in cardiovascular function which were not apparent in the resting state. In patients with known cardiovascular disease, the exercise test may help the clinician establish a cause and effect relationship between symptoms and the disease process, and may help evaluate the impact of the disease upon cardiac reserve.

When a clinician is considering a diagnostic test several questions should be posed:

1. Do the benefits justify the risk and cost?

2. Will the results provide information that will influence medical management?

3. Are there other tests that will provide a better risk/benefit or cost/benefit ratio?

A clinical example illustrating this last principle is the 55-year-old male smoker with a family history of premature coronary disease admitted to the hospital for evaluation of recent onset progressive episodes of chest discomfort. In such a setting, the physical examination and resting ECG may be normal and the diagnosis unclear. An ECG performed while the patient is experiencing spontaneous chest discomfort or an exercise stress test may yield the required information (ST segment depressions indicative of myocardial ischemia) thus obviating the need for further diagnostic tests and allowing the clinician to initiate therapy without delay.

In choosing a diagnostic test it is important to keep in mind several principles. After the initial history and physical examination the skillful and experienced clinician usually narrows the diagnostic possibilities to a carefully selected few. The diagnostic laboratory tests are then used first to confirm the most likely diagnosis rather than to exclude all the other numerous less likely diagnoses. It is easier, quicker, and more cost effective to prove what a patient has than to exclude or "rule out" the almost limitless possibilities of what he/she does not have. In addition, based on the bedside evaluation, the clinician should have a clear idea of what the diagnostic test is likely to show so as to better hone his skills. Whenever possible, the primary clinician should perform the test or review the test with the person who performed it so as to provide clinical insight and discuss the diagnostic and therapeutic possibilities. The test results will rarely surprise the experienced clinician since he/she will already have a clear idea of the possible results and to proceed thereafter.

The Exercise Test

The purpose of an exercise test is to attain a level of physical exertion high enough to impose upon the heart and circulatory system a physiologic load that will challenge cardiac reserve. Certain definitions adopted by investigators in the field of exercise testing should be reviewed.

Predicted Maximal Heart Rate (MHR)

Heart rate is one of the determinants of myocardial oxygen consumption and thus peak attained heart rate is used as an indirect index of the work load imposed upon the heart during exercise. Tables and formulas are available which provide the expected peak heart rate that should be attained during an exercise test carried out to a maximal effort. These tables have been derived from progressive maximal exercise tests performed in healthy individuals, are adjusted for age and may vary among different investigators. The maximal achieved heart rate is usually expressed as percentage of maximal predicted heart rate. A test which is limited by non-cardiac factors (i.e. gait difficulty or orthopedic problems) at an attained heart rate less than 85% of MHR may not have challenged the circulatory cardiac reserve enough to attain predictive validity. The percent of MHR at which symptoms or electrocardiographic evidence of myocardial ischemia occurs is an indicator of severity of the cardiac impairment, the individual's disability, and a rough index of prognosis.

Total Exercise Time

Since the majority of exercise test protocols impose a progressive physical load, total exercise time is an index of the intensity of physical and cardiac work attained. When exercise tests are performed by standardized protocols, total exercise time is a rough index of functional capacity. The observed total exercise time is determined by the specific exercise protocol used, familiarity with the exercise equipment, cardiac status, and physical conditioning. During serial, frequent exercise testing, an increase in total exercise time is frequently noted. This increase in exercise time is not necessarily due to an improvement in cardiac status or medications but to the effect of progressive physical conditioning ("training effect").

Metabolic Equivalent (METS)

The definition of a unit of metabolic equivalent (1 MET) is the total O_2 consumption measured in ml O_2/kg body weight/minute for an adult individual sitting quietly at rest and has been measured at approximately 3.5 ml/kg/min. METs can be measured by sophisticated expired gas analyzers or from published tables (Figure 1). METS can be used as work equivalent when comparing the level of physical work attained during different activities or different exercise protocols (Table 1).

VO₂ Max and Anaerobic Threshold

Maximal O_2 consumption (VO_2 max) is the highest level of O_2 consumption a subject can achieve during maximal exercise. During exercise, a physically fit subject will progressively increase his O_2 consumption, cardiac output, and pulmonary venti-

Figure 1. The oxygen cost per stage of some commonly used protocols. Total exercise time is not as important a value as is the estimated oxygen consumption value of the protocol stage or workload reached. MPH = miles per hour; %GR = percent grade; KPDS = kiloponds. *(From Cardiology Clinics, May 1993, WB Saunders.)*

TABLE 1

Energy Cost (METS) of Various Activities for Convalescent Cardiac Patients*

SELF-CARE ACTIVITIES

1.2	Sitting quietly
1.1–1.5	Standing quietly
1.5–2.0	Eating, conversation
1.5–2.0	Washing hands and face, brushing teeth
1.6–3.4	Washing and dressing, moving about (women)
2.6–4.3	Washing and dressing, moving about (men)
3.7–4.4	Showering

DIVERSIONAL ACTIVITIES

1.5–2.0	Knitting, sewing, listening to radio
1.5–2.0	Playing cards, watching TV
1.8–2.8	Playing a musical instrument – piano, strings
2.8–4.0	Playing organ or drums
2.0–3.0	Light woodworking

LIGHT WORK AT HOME

1.5–1.9	Office work at a desk, standing, moving about
1.5–2.0	Typing and using office business machines
1.2–3.6	Driving (depends on traffic)
3.1–4.2	Gardening – weeding, using trowel, edging borders, raking
5.3–5.7	Cutting hedges, mowing lawn

HOUSEWORK

1.6–2.0	Sweeping floors, preparing vegetables
2.1–3.0	Preparing and serving a meal, washing dishes
2.1–3.0	Dusting, polishing, ironing
3.1–4.1	Bedmaking, vacuuming, shopping (light load)
4.2–5.3	Scrubbing floors, shopping (heavy load)

PHYSICAL EXERCISE

2.6–2.7	Walking 2.0 mph
3.1–3.2	Walking 2.5 mph
3.6–3.8	Walking 3.0 mph
4.1–4.4	Walking 3.5 mph
2.0–3.4	Light calisthenics (trunk bends, knee raises, arm circles)
2.3–4.4	Bowling
2.0–3.0	Golf with power cart
4.0–7.0	Golf pulling cart
2.5–5.0	Volleyball
4.0–5.0	Table tennis
4.0–5.0	Climbing down stairs
6.0–8.0	Climbing up stairs
4.0–6.0	Sexual activity with familiar partner

* Rest, supine but not basal equals 1.0 MET (metabolic unit). These values are based on average weights of 55 kg (female) and 65 kg (male). All values are approximate since speed of performing activity, proficiency, climatic conditions, and emotional pressure can induce significant variation. *(From the American Journal of Cardiology, April 1983, Vol. 51.)*

bic metabolism, lactic acid production, and metabolic acidosis. The anaerobic threshold is characterized by a flattening of the O_2 consumption and a rise in CO_2 production measured in expired air, and usually occurs at 40% to 60% of VO_2 max. There are several methods for measuring anaerobic threshold, all of them subject to several sources of error.

Functional Aerobic Impairment (FAI)

The difference between predicted VO_2 max (from tables for healthy individuals according to age and gender) and the attained VO_2 max as measured or calculated from tables is a measurement of the inability of any given individual to attain his predicted workload. This deficit of work capacity or FAI is usually expressed as a percent of predicted VO_2 max by the formula:

$$\frac{\text{Predicted VO max} - \text{attained VO}_2 \text{ max x } 100}{\text{Predicted VO}_2 \text{ max}}$$

Maximal Double Product

During progressive exercise performed by normal subjects, heart rate and systolic blood pressure progressively increase. The product of the maximal achieved heart rate and blood pressure is called "double product" and serves as an index of the myocardial O_2 consumption. At rest, a normal subject may have a heart rate of 70 beats/minute and a systolic blood pressure of 120mmHg; thus his double product is 8,400; however during exercise, the double product may exceed 30,000. When a subject cannot achieve a double product of 18,000 without signs or symptoms of cardiac disease, his cardiac reserve is markedly impaired usually indicating a poor prognosis.

A normal or negative test is one where the endpoints are achieved without the appearance of symptoms, signs, ECG or cardiac imaging findings that suggest or confirm the presence of cardiac disease. A negative test usually indicates a low statistical probability for the presence of clinically important cardiac disease and/or adverse events.

Probability Analysis

An abnormal or positive test is one where symptoms, signs, ECG or imaging findings appear that suggest or confirm the presence of heart disease with or without attainment of clinical endpoints. This indicates an increased statistical probability for the presence of cardiac disease and adverse clinical events. The severity of the abnormalities and the hemodynamic workload attained are rough indications of severity of disease.

A nondiagnostic or inadequate test is one where

lation as the circulatory system provides blood and O_2 to the exercising tissues. When the physical effort exceeds the circulatory capacity to provide O_2 to the working musculature (anaerobic threshold), a metabolic deficit ensues with subsequent anaero-

the preset endpoints were not achieved, and there were no symptoms, signs, or ECG or imaging findings suggestive or confirming the presence of heart disease. A statement regarding probability of disease cannot be made with such a test.

Sensitivity of a test is the percentage of subjects with disease who have an abnormal test (TP/TP+FN) and specificity is the percentage of subjects without disease who have a normal test (TN/TN+FP).

• *TP true positive* = abnormal test in a subject with disease.
• *FN false negative* = normal test in a subject with disease.
• *TN true negative* = normal test in a subject without disease.
• *FP false positive* = abnormal test in a subject without disease.

The diagnostic accuracy of a test is an expression of both sensitivity and specificity. Positive predictive accuracy expresses the probability of disease in a subject with an abnormal test, and negative predictive accuracy is a statement of the probability that a subject with a negative test has no disease.

Pre-test probability is the likelihood for presence of disease prior to the diagnostic test. This is determined by disease prevalence in specific population groups and presence or absence of predisposing risk factors. Post-test probability is the likelihood for the presence of disease after the diagnostic test is performed. A clinically useful test will prove major likelihood for the presence of disease. This predictive impact is maximal in patients with intermediate pre-test probability (i.e. 50%) where the post-test probability for the presence/absence of disease will be converted to 80% or better.

The Bayesian concept of probability is named after Thomas Bayes (1702-1761), who tried to predict the presence of a condition between two degrees of probability. Bayesian analysis uses the pre-test probability, sensitivity, and specificity of a given test to calculate the post-test probability. The use of Bayes' theorem in making predictive statements is illustrated in Figure 2. From the graph in this figure it is apparent that the clinical usefulness of a given test is greatly influenced by the pre-test probability. In individual cases where the clinical situation indicates a very high or very low probability for the presence of disease the likelihood that the specific diagnostic test will change the clinical management is low. In such cases, when the presence of disease is highly probable, the clinician may opt to proceed with direct therapeutic interventions. On the other hand, the clinician may choose to omit or postpone a diagnostic test or

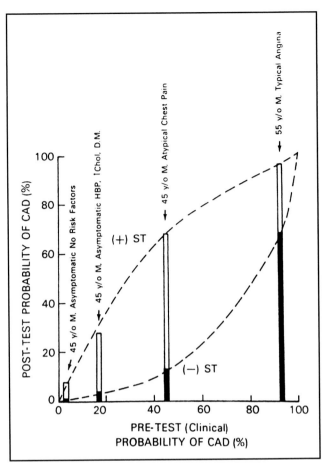

Figure 2. Use of Bayes' theorem to calculate the probability of coronary artery disease (CAD). Clinical data (pretest probability, increasing from left to right) are combined with results of exercise electrocardiography (positive [+] or negative [–] ST segment response) to yield final posttest probability (increasing along the vertical axis). Four specific patient examples are shown by vertical bars, where the height of the solid dark bar shows the results for a negative exercise electrocardiogram (ECG) (–) ST, and the clear bar shows the results for a positive exercise ECG (+) ST. *(From Patterson et al, JACC 1989 V13 P1653-65.)*

intended therapy and clinically observe the patient when the probability for the presence of disease is very low.

Physiology of Exercise

The maximal amount of physical exercise any given subject can attain is determined by the efficiency of the circulatory and oxygen transport systems, his musculo-skeletal architecture and level of physical training. During progressive exercise the function of the circulatory system is to keep up with the incremental metabolic demands imposed by the working tissues. Prior to the actual start of physical activity there is an anticipatory phase characterized by a heightened adrenergic output. This can become clinically manifest by a slight increase in heart rate which may occur during the preparation for the exercise session, when the exercise treadmill machine is activated or upon the arrival of the physician. I have had the infrequent patient whose coronary status is so precarious, that this mild anticipatory adrenergic stimulus is enough to provoke an anginal episode. Obviously such patients should not be exercised, and the antianginal management should be aggressively optimized.

Once the actual physical exercise begins, a series of integrated changes in cardiac and circulatory function ensue. At low to moderate levels of exercise, there is a withdrawal in vagal tone and an increase in adrenergic drive. This is mediated both by increased sympathetic tone and neuro-hormonal activation, with increases in circulating levels of norepinephrine, aldosterone, argininine, vasopressin, renin and angiotensin. The end result is an increase in heart rate, myocardial contractility, cardiac output and systolic blood pressure. In addition, the increase in sympathetic tone and circulating cathecholamines produce a moderate diffuse vasoconstriction which is counterbalanced by potent local vasodilatory responses in the working skeletal musculature and coronary circulation. Local metabolic, mechanical, and circulatory stimuli combine to augment the local production of vasodilatory substances such as adenosine and endothelial derived relaxing factor (EDRF), resulting in a decrease in total systemic and pulmonary vascular resistance. As the intensity of exercise increases, this vasodilatory effect serves to direct a large amount of blood flow to the working musculature. Peripheral circulatory and mechanical factors also help to optimize the mechanical efficiency of the heart during intense exercise. Contracting limb and abdominal muscles increase venous return to the heart, thus increasing cardiac preload. Venous return is further augmented by the increase in negative thoracic pressure generated by the increased excursion of the respiratory muscles and the vasoconstrictor influence of cathecholamines upon the systemic venous capacitance vessels. Thus, during heavy exercise, cardiac function is enhanced by the Frank-Starling mechanism with an increase in end diastolic volume. End systolic volume is reduced by the combined effects of cathecholamines and tachycardia both of which increase myocardial contractility. The decrease in total systemic peripheral resistance produced by exercise induced vasodilation also facilitates systolic emptying. Maximal cardiac output is therefore achieved by both an increase in heart rate and stroke volume, and can attain levels four-to-six times higher than the resting cardiac output. At peak physical effort, heart rate usually reaches the MHR and systolic blood pressure is usually around 200mmHg, while diastolic pressure increases only minimally. Pulmonary artery pressures increase only mildly, indicating a decrease in pulmonary resistance. During maximal exercise, arterial-venous oxygen difference is increased as a result of enhanced O_2 extraction by the working musculature.

The normal subject who attains his maximal level of exercise on a motorized treadmill is usually walking briskly, jogging or running with a flushed appearance, skin glistening with perspiration (first apparent by palpation over the lower back, forehead or forearms), flaring nostrils, and vigorous respiratory movements. At palpation, the skin is moist and warm, the pulse rapid but full. At this exertion level, it is my practice to tell the subject that all the information needed has been obtained and there is no need to continue. We then start a gradual decrease in treadmill velocity and elevation and proceed with the cooling-off period.

If the subject exercises beyond his physiologic limit the physical effort will exceed anaerobic threshold and the capacity of the circulatory system to provide oxygen to the working tissues. The subject who has exceeded his circulatory reserve may appear anxious, a pale color may replace the facial rubor seen at peak tolerable exercise, the gait may become unsteady and the hands will blanch as the subject tightly clenches the support bars in a futile effort to keep up the pace. The heart rate may exceed the MHR, the pulse may become thready and the systolic blood pressure may actually fall. The prudent clinician will avoid "pushing" subjects to this level of effort.

Exercise in Cardiac Disease

Coronary Disease

The normal physiologic response to exercise may be altered by a number of cardiac diseases, the most common of which is coronary atherosclerosis. Coronary atherosclerosis limits the dilatory capacity of the coronary arteries and thus restricts the amount of blood available to the myocardial muscle. In addition to the mechanical obstruction produced by the atheroma, the atherosclerotic process produces endothelial vascular dysfunction which limits or abolishes the local vasodilatory effects of exercise and thus restricts the amount of blood available to the myocardium. Heart rate, blood pressure, myocardial contractility, left ventricular chamber diameter and wall thickness all determine myocardial oxygen demand. The increase in heart rate, systolic blood pressure and myocardial contractility induced by exercise is balanced by an increase in myocardial blood flow. Since myocardial oxygen extraction is almost maximal, even at rest, an imbalance between O_2 demand and blood supply quickly leads to myocardial ischemia and its clinical counterparts, angina, electrocardiographic changes, transient myocardial mechanical dysfunction and occasionally cardiac rhythm disorders.

The most common objective finding in patients with physiologically limiting coronary atherosclerosis subjected to exercise testing is electrocardiographic ST segment depression with or without anginal symptoms. As part of the subjective response to myocardial ischemia the patient may develop what I call "the angina look" so well depicted by Dr. F. Netter in his classic illustration of a middle aged heavy-set man, clutching his chest in a snow covered sidewalk stairwell. The patient who experiences angina during an exercise test may show a facial expression of anguish, his color may turn pale and he may describe a feeling of discomfort in the chest, shoulder, arms or neck. Occasionally the patient will develop auscultatory signs of myocardial dysfunction such as the appearance of new S_4 gallop rhythm, a new mitral insufficiency murmur, an S_3 gallop or new pulmonary rales. Precordial palpation may likewise show an abnormal apex beat with a palpable presystolic distention (S_4 equivalent) or rarely an early diastolic impulse (S_3 equivalent). This transient, exercise induced myocardial dysfunction has been demonstrated by radionuclide techniques with left ventricular cavity dilatation and increased pulmonary uptake of the radioisotope due to pulmonary congestion. During the episode of myocardial ischemia the heart rate and blood pressure may remain unchanged, may increase due to the additional angina-induced catecholamine surge or may ominously decrease as a sign of ischemic chronotropic incompetence and systolic myocardial dysfunction. Exercise induced bradycardia and hypotension due to severe myocardial ischemia are signs of impending circulatory collapse and the exercise session should be stopped immediately. When this happens the patient should be taken off the treadmill and moved to the adjacent examining table or recliner, nitroglycerine and nasal O_2 should be administered and vital signs must be closely monitored. In our institution, such a response is an indication for hospitalization and subsequent cardiac catheterization.

Heart Failure

In patients with chronic heart failure, exercise testing is used to objectively document exercise intolerance and to obtain prognostic information. Patients with chronic heart failure develop abnor-malities in cardiac function, peripheral circulation and skeletal muscle function, which may severely limit exercise capacity. This exercise limitation has proven to be an independent predictor of survival in these patients. The patient with severe myocardial systolic dysfunction and chronic heart failure may be able to increase his heart rate as a response to exercise. These patients, however, usually lack the myocardial reserve needed to increase the stroke volume and cardiac output is thus dependent mainly on heart rate response, which may already be impaired due to the chronic neurohormonal activation characteristic of patients with heart failure. This same neurohormonal activation accounts for the chronic vasoconstriction and the blunted vasodilatory response to exercise which further impairs both cardiac performance and blood flow to the working skeletal muscles of patients with heart failure. The skeletal muscles in patients with chronic heart failure have intrinsic metabolic and structural abnormalities which, when combined with physical deconditioning and limited blood flow, place a further limit on physical work.

The patient with severe chronic heart failure characteristically exhibits a blunted or flat blood pressure response during exercise. Heart rate response may be normal or blunted, and the exercise induced increase in heart rate and cardiac output is obtained at the expense of high ventricular filling pressures. Although, traditionally, heart failure has been a contraindication for exercise testing, these patients, when adequately screened and clinically stable, tolerate submaximal and symptom limited exercise testing well. Exercise may accentuate the palpatory and auscultatory evidence of systolic dysfunction (palpable and audible S_3) but rarely do patients develop new pulmonary rales. Complex ventricular arrhythmias are present in approximately 30% of patients with moderate to severe chronic congestive heart failure and yet, if carefully selected it is rare for these patients to develop lethal ventricular arrhythmias during exercise testing.

Valvular Disease

Exercise testing is occasionally used to evaluate functional capacity in patients with valvular heart disease. Patients with chronic valvular heart disease may slowly and subtly modify their lifestyle in an effort to adapt to the symptomatic limits imposed by the disease. In such patients, the history may not accurately reflect the true physiologic limitations and exercise testing is an objective method to evaluate the work capacity. Patients with severe, symptomatic obstructive valvular heart disease traditionally have poor exercise tolerance and exercise testing is best avoided in such patients. The exercise induced increase in heart rate and cardiac contractility will produce large increases in the cardiac pressures proximal to the valvular obstruction, even in patients with mild-to-moderate valvular stenosis. The exercise-induced vasodilatation, together with the limit imposed on stroke volume by the valvular obstruction, may induce peripheral hypotension in these patients.

Patients with chronic valvular regurgitant lesions have better exercise tolerance than patients with obstructive lesions; those with chronic moderate or severe aortic insufficiency may have unimpaired exercise tolerance until late in the disease. The peripheral vasodilatation and shortening of diastolic time associated with exercise have a favorable effect on the hemodynamic load imposed by the aortic regurgitant lesion. The diminution in diastolic time decreases the time available for the aortic leak into the left ventricular cavity and the exercise-induced peripheral vasodilatation facilitates forward flow.

On the contrary, patients with chronic, moderate or severe mitral regurgitation, minimal symptoms, and normal resting pulmonary pressures frequently develop severe pulmonary hypertension during exercise. These findings support the clinical observation that chronic aortic insufficiency is well-tolerated for years, and that stenotic lesions produce symptoms earlier in the course of the disease.

Patients with hypertension will demonstrate accelerated and exaggerated blood pressure response to exercise, even when baseline resting blood pressures are in the normal range. Exercise testing can be used to monitor the effect of therapy in hypertensive patients who frequently engage in moderate to severe physical exertion.

Indications and Contraindications for Exercise Testing

As a clinician-scientist, the practicing cardiologist should have a clear hypothesis to be tested. The main purpose of a diagnostic test is to establish a statistical probability as to the validity of the hypothesis. In addition, the clinician should be aware of the risks, cost, and possible pitfalls of the diagnostic test upon which he and his patient are about to embark.

The indications for exercise testing have been tabulated by the ACC/AHA task force into the now classic 3 groups: class I is patients with a clear indication; class II is patients with a probable indication (Table 2) and class III is patients in whom the indications, if any, are questionable (Table 3). Class I

TABLE 2
Indications for Exercise Testing
CLASS I (clearly indicated)
• To assist in diagnosis of coronary disease (CAD).
• To assess functional capacity and prognosis of those with known CAD.
• To evaluate patients with symptoms of exercise-induced arrhythmias.
• To evaluate functional capacity of selected patients with congenital, valvular or hypertensive heart disease or chronic heart failure.
• To evaluate possible heart transplant candidates.
CLASS II (possibly indicated)
• To evaluate asymptomatic middle aged subjects with some risk factors for CAD.
• To evaluate females with atypical chest pains and risk factors for CAD.
• To assist in the diagnosis of CAD in subjects taking digitalis or with ECG abnormalities which would hinder interpretation.*
• To evaluate response to drug therapy.
• To evaluate serially (1-2 yr interval) those with known CAD.
* Stress testing with nuclear or ultrasound imaging is a reasonable option in these patients.

indications include those patients in whom the clinical picture suggests the presence of coronary disease, but no objective evidence documents its presence. In such patients, the purpose of the test is to establish a diagnosis; thus, they should be encouraged to exercise to a point where the test attains statistical predictive validity (85-90% of MHR). Also included as a class I indication are patients with known, documented coronary disease in whom the test is being performed to establish their functional capacity and thus to obtain a prognostic indicator. Included in this group are patients with recent uncomplicated myocardial infarction, patients with chronic stable angina who present to a physician for the first time, and patients who have undergone revascularization procedures when it is important to establish the effect of such therapy.

Patients with class II indications encompass a group of subjects with or without known coronary disease in whom, for one reason or another, the electrocardiographic response may be equivocal, or patients in whom the result of the test is unlikely to change medical management. Patients with class III indications are those in whom it has been demonstrated that this test is of no diagnostic or prognostic value. In patients who fall in group II and III due to an abnormal resting ECG or with conditions or medications which may alter the ST segment response to exercise, the use of an imaging modality such as ultrasound or perfusion imaging with radionuclides will greatly enhance the diagnostic accuracy of this test. Additional groups of subjects in whom exercise testing has clinical utility include patients being considered for heart transplantation and selected patients with congenital heart disease, valvular heart disease or hypertension.

The number and types of contraindications to exercise testing have changed since its inception. It was not that long ago when a recent myocardial infarction (<3 wks) was listed as a contraindication to exercise testing. The principle behind the list of conditions that are possible contraindications to exercise testing is based on risk/benefit ratio. Any condition, cardiac or otherwise, which would place the patient at risk, especially if the possible benefit of the test is limited, should be considered a contraindication. Several absolute contraindications remain, the most important of which is operator/equipment dependent. In patients with cardiovascular disease, exercise testing should always be performed by experienced, adequately trained personnel, with adequate monitoring equipment and cardiopulmonary resuscitation equipment available in the exercise room. This clinician has found that in addition to blood pressure and electrocardiographic monitoring equipment, pulse oximetry for continuous analysis of tissue oxygenation ($\%O_2$ saturation) offers additional valuable information. Table 3 lists some of the conditions which are thought to be contraindications to exercise testing.

The listed contraindications are a general guide, subject to change according to clinical setting and individual laboratory. In a suburban or rural office distant from a major medical facility, the list of contraindications would be more extensive than in an exercise laboratory within a major referral hospital located adjacent to a critical care unit. The complications that may arise from exercise testing include cardiac arrest, pulmonary edema, myocardial infarction or severe prolonged myocardial ischemia, CNS events such as strokes or transient neurologic deficits, symptomatic hypotension, falls, trauma, and death.

In our laboratory, complications have arisen in patients with recent "uncomplicated" myocardial infarction who have denied recurrent myocardial ischemic symptoms during the pre-exercise screening, and in patients with severe congestive heart failure and previous cardiac rhythm disturbances.

Methods

In the United States, the preferred method for exercise testing is the motor-driven treadmill. The disadvantage of this system is that patients with musculo-skeletal conditions affecting the weight-bearing limbs are unable to tolerate the test. Arm ergometry with a variable resistance apparatus which the patient rotates with both arms have been used with variable results. Bicycle exercise testing, widely used in Europe, has also been well standardized and allows some patients with musculoskeletal diseases to perform an adequate amount of exercise. Bicycle tests, however, have failed to gain popularity in the United States except in some research laboratories. Standard pre-test instructions include use of comfortable attire and shoes, abstention from heavy exercise, smoking, or large meals for at least 3 hours prior to the exercise session, and continuation of the usual medications. When patients undergo diagnostic exercise tests to confirm or exclude presence of myocardial ischemia, the clinician may opt to wean those medications which blunt the heart rate response in order to attain the appropriate target heart rate. In addition, patients who are taking digitalis should be screened and, if appropriate, digitalis preparation should be stopped at least four days prior to testing. Decisions to wean or stop such medications as noted above should be performed by or in consultation with the referring physician.

In order to minimize risks, it is of utmost importance for the individual performing and supervising the test to obtain a brief past and recent cardiovascular history and to perform a screening cardiac exam. In addition, if available, the medical record should be reviewed. The technical aspects of lead selection, preparation and placement have been described in numerous publications. Prior to the

---

T A B L E   3

Conditions Generally Thought to be Contraindications for Exercise Testing

- Signs/symptoms of uncontrolled myocardial ischemia such as resting angina with ECG changes.
- Hemodynamically unstable patients.
- Decompensated heart failure (Class IV).
- Severe aortic stenosis/mitral stenosis.
- Uncontrolled, potentially lethal cardiac arrhythmias.
- Acute myocarditis/pericarditis.
- Deep venous thrombosis or acute thrombophlebitis.
- Neuromuscular/musculoskeletal conditions that preclude exercise or produce dangerous gait instability.
- Uncontrolled arterial hypertension diastolic >110, systolic >180.
- Lack of desire or patient consent.

exercise session a 12 lead resting ECG should be performed in the supine and erect position, to assess the baseline ECG and ST segment stability. Vital signs should be obtained and recorded in both positions, and the patient should be instructed in use of the treadmill. If necessary, a brief trial may be performed prior to the exercise session where the patient is allowed to walk on the treadmill at a low speed in order to mitigate his fears. During testing, the ECG is continuously monitored in a multi-lead format, and blood pressure is obtained and recorded at least at the end of every stage, and more often if clinically indicated.

This clinician prefers manual blood pressures with a mercury manometer because it provides closer contact with the patient for manually identifying brachial pulse. It is important that whoever is not obtaining the blood pressure maintains a close observation of the patient and the ECG.

Endpoints

Endpoints to exercise testing can be clearly defined such as heart rate or onset of angina with ischemic ST segment changes, but may also be subjective and require clinical judgement. It is just as important to know when to stop the exercise test to prevent an unfavorable outcome as to know when to encourage a patient to continue in order to obtain a valid test.

When the test is performed to document the presence of myocardial ischemia, the usual endpoint are the onset of angina with ST segment depression, the attainment of target heart rate, or a near-maximal perception of exertion by the subject. Target heart rate in diagnostic submaximal stress testing is 85%-90% of MHR or MHR ± 5% during a maximal effort test. Patients with known coronary disease who have experienced a recent uncomplicated major ischemic event such as myocardial infarction or unstable angina, may be candidates for limited exercise testing. The goal of such an exercise test is not diagnostic, but rather to identify high risk patients for further diagnostic or therapeutic interventions. Target heart rate in such cases is 70% to 80% of MHR. In subjects where the purpose of the test is to evaluate the physical restraints imposed by cardiac disease, symptom or effort-limited endpoints would be the goal. During the exercise test, the appearance of abnormalities noted in Table 4 may of themselves be an indication to stop the test.

If the test is terminated due to the occurrence of an untoward event the subject should be expeditiously assisted off the treadmill or exercise equipment into a recliner or examining table and the appropriate measures should be instituted. When

---

T A B L E   4

Reasons to Terminate an Exercise Test Prior to Target Heart Rate or Workload

- Unexpected ventricular tachycardia.
- Progressive decrease in systolic blood pressure.
- Ataxia.
- Mental confusion or any neurologic change.
- Progressive ischemic ST elevation in non-infarct lead exceeding 1.5mm.
- Severe fatigue, dyspnea or chest discomfort.
- Ischemic ST segment depression >3mm.
- Sustained supraventricular tachycardia.
- Abnormal elevation of blood pressure.
- Inability to monitor ECG or blood pressure.
- Patient wishes to stop.
- Appearance of any sign or symptom which in the clinicians judgement places the patient at risk.

---

the test is terminated due to the attainment of a pre-established endpoint the velocity and incline of the treadmill should be progressively reduced until a 0% incline and a 1.0 to 1.5 MPH velocity is attained. At this level, a 1 to 2 minute "cool down" period is continued and the patient is moved to the observation chair or table.

Sudden cessation of intense maximal exercise with the patient in the supine position should be avoided since it may lead to symptomatic hypotension. The usual subject should have the ECG and vital signs monitored for a minimum of 6-10 minutes after the exercise is stopped, or until all signs or symptoms of myocardial ischemia have resolved.

The Abnormal Exercise Test

Abnormal Duration

The functional aerobic impairment (FAI) is a rough estimate of the exercise limitation. This limitation may be imposed by non-cardiac factors such as musculo-skeletal problems, cardiac factors such as myocardial ischemia, or a combination of both. In subjects with heart disease, exercise limitation is frequently related to the severity of heart disease. In patients with ischemic heart disease, exercise duration is thus a predictor of future coronary events, and in patients with heart failure the maximal attained VO_2 and the simple 6 minute walk test have been shown to be independent predictors of mortality. In general, patients who are able to complete the equivalent of a standard Bruce 3 stage have a low probability for developing major adverse cardiovascular events as compared to patients who are unable to complete stage 2. Serial changes in total exercise duration have been used as indices of drug efficacy in patients with ischemic heart disease or chronic heart failure. Small changes in exercise duration, however, are difficult to interpret since variables such as time of day, motivation and training effect may also influence exercise duration.

Abnormal Symptoms & Physical Signs

When an exercise test is being performed to establish the diagnosis of myocardial ischemia in a subject with a high pre-test probability for the presence of coronary disease the reproduction of angina offers strong confirmatory evidence even in the absence of electrocardiographic signs of ischemia. A more difficult situation exists in the subject who has an intermediate probability for the presence of coronary disease and whose exercise test may reproduce some chest discomfort, but the ECG fails to show evidence of myocardial ischemia. In such patients, physical assessment can occasionally uncover signs of myocardial ischemia such as the appearance of an S_4 or S_3 gallop or the transient mitral regurgitant murmur of ischemic papillary muscle dysfunction. When such findings are not present other imaging modalities may demonstrate either exercise induced myocardial contraction abnormalities (echocardiography or radionuclide ventriculography), perfusion abnormalities (radionuclide perfusion imaging) or metabolic abnormalities (positron emission tomography). The clinician, however, has to put into balance the cost and may opt to go directly to coronary arteriography which may be a more cost effective strategy. The clinician and the patient must realize, however, that coronary arteriography may by itself modify the perception of the disease to the extent that revascularization techniques may be considered as a very seductive alternative even when scientific proof is lacking that such techniques offer a clinical advantage when compared to medical therapy.

In patients with either valvular heart disease or heart failure the expected limiting symptoms are either fatigue, dyspnea or leg discomfort. Such symptoms usually appear without any noticeable changes in the ECG. In the patient being evaluated for recurrent, symptomatic exercise induced arrhythmias, the appearance of symptoms in the absence of demonstrable arrhythmias will also help the clinician in deciding if antiarrhythmic therapy is justified.

Abnormal Heart Rate Response

Subjects undergoing exercise test may develop an accelerated heart rate response, a blunted heart rate response (chronotropic incompetence) or a decrease in heart rate. An accelerated heart rate response is a sign of excessive sympathetic activation due to anxiety, physical deconditioning, hypoxia, anemia, heart failure, thyrotoxicosis or adrenoreceptor sensitization secondary to recent beta blockade withdrawal. Partial or complete chronotropic incompetence can be due to cardiac sympathetic denervation as seen in heart transplant recipients' drugs such as beta blockers and calcium channel inhibitors, advanced age, intrinsic SA node disease, or may be an indicator of myocardial ischemia.

Abnormal Blood Pressure

The usual exercise induced elevation of blood pressure may be accelerated, exceeded, or blunted by pharmacologic interventions or by pathologic changes. An accelerated or excessive hypertensive response can be observed in hypertension, anxiety, and high catecholamine states such as pheochromocytoma and recent beta blockade withdrawal.

A blunted blood pressure response may be the result of sympathetic denervation (diabetic autonomic neuropathy) adrenoreceptor blockade (beta blockade) inadequate cardiac output (heart failure) or excessive vasodilatation. In the absence of these, the appearance of a hypotensive response associated with signs of myocardial ischemia speaks for an extensive severe coronary disease.

ECG

For over 50 years, ECG analysis during stress testing has remained as the most reproducible objective sign in the evaluation of the patient with possible ischemic heart disease. In normal subjects, the measured ECG intervals shorten progressively during exercise and the J point is displaced downward with a gradual upsloping deviation of the ST segment. The usual electrocardiographic sign of ischemia consists of horizontal or downsloping ≥1mm ST segment depression lasting at least .08 seconds after the J point. These changes may occur during the exercise portion or during the recovery phase of the exercise test. ST segment depression may precede, occur concurrently, or occur after the onset of angina or may appear and resolve in the absence of angina. The 1mm horizontal depression criteria has been arbitrarily chosen as a compromise between marked (2mm) ST segment depression which is highly specific but yields a poor sensitivity (rarely false positive, frequently false negative) and mild (0.5-0.75mm) ST segment depression which is very sensitive but yields a low specificity (rarely false negative, frequently false positive). ST segment changes are not an all or none, positive or negative issue and should be considered a continuum from the normal response to the grossly abnormal (Figure 3). The intensity of the ST segment abnormality has been used as a marker for functionally severe disease. The early appearance of ischemic ST changes (heart rate >120; double product >18,000), the number of leads demonstrating the ECG abnormality, the severity of the ST segment depression (≥2mm), and the persistence of ischemic ST segment changes into the recovery phase have all been associated with the extent and severity of the coronary disease. Occasionally, a subject may demonstrate electrocardiographic ST segment elevation rather than depression. The majority of instances where this occurs the leads demonstrating the ST segment elevation are leads also demonstrating evidence of prior Q wave myocardial infarction. Angiographic studies performed in patients with exercise induced ST segment elevation have demonstrated abnormal myocardial systolic contraction in the segments that correspond to the ECG leads where the ST segment elevation is noted. Such patients also have more ventricular dysfunction than patients without ST segment elevation during exercise. The electrocardiographic explanation for the abnormal exercise induced ST segment elevation in patients with prior Q wave infarction is unclear and is possibly related to abnormal systolic contraction, scar tissue formation and changes in depolarization sequence. Patients may develop exercise induced ST segment elevation in the absence of Q waves when the prior infarcts have lost the electrocardiographic Q waves with time. This is more likely to occur in patients with inferior as compared to anterior wall myocardial infarction.

ST segment elevation during exercise in the absence of prior infarction usually indicates severe, transmural myocardial ischemia and may be a manifestation of the same phenomenon which is responsible for the ECG changes observed in Prinzmetal's variant angina. This uncommon finding is a marker for either severe obstructive coronary disease or less frequently for exercise induced vasospasm in a patient with normal coronary arteries.

Other electrocardiographic signs of ischemia including changes in R wave amplitude, normalization of resting ST or T wave abnormalities, isolated T wave changes, new premature ventricular beats or precordial U wave inversion have been associated with the presence of coronary disease. Such changes, however, lack adequate specificity or sensitivity and have not withstood the test of time. The appearance of major cardiac arrhythmias such as atrial flutter, atrial fibrillation, coupled multiformed premature ventricular beats or nonsustained ventricular tachycardia are a cause of concern and are more likely to occur in patients with heart disease. The appearance of complex ventricular arrhythmias during exercise testing has a negative impact on prognosis and usually indicates cardiac abnormalities such as ventricular dysfunction or prior myocardial infarction. Such arrhythmias, however, are not specific for the presence of coronary disease and also occur in subjects with hypertensive, valvular or primary cardiomyopathic disease. Frequently isolated PVC's are suppressed by the tachycardic response to exercise. This "overdrive suppression" has been thought to be a sign of benign PVC's but this phenonenom has been observed both in normal subjects and in patients with coronary disease. The presence of rate-related bundle branch block or AV conduction abnormalities although not normal, lack specificity for the presence of coronary atherosclerosis.

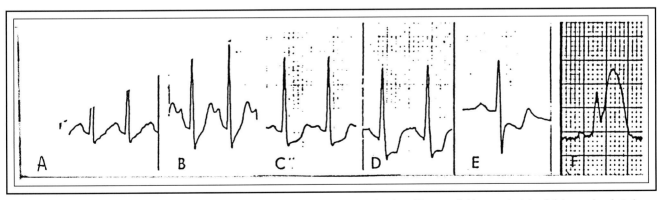

Figure 3. The S-T segment response to exercise. *A,* Minimal J point depression, isoelectric at 80 msec. *B,* More marked J point depression, but also isoelectric at 80 msec. *C* = Slowly upsloping S-T segment depression, remaining depressed more than 1 mm at 80 msec. *D* = Horizontal S-T segment depression. *E* = Downsloping S-T segment depression. *F* = S-T segment elevation. *(From Glasser, 8.)*

Modifiers of ST Segment Depression

Exercise-induced ST segment depression must be interpreted within the clinical context where it occurs. Table 5 outlines a number of factors that may alter the ST segment response to exercise.

Any condition where ST segment depression exists prior to exercise will facilitate or magnify the appearance of further ST segment shifts and thus decrease the diagnostic accuracy of this electrocardiographic sign. It has been recommended that in patients with underlying "primary" ST segment abnormalities an additional 1.5mm horizontal or downsloping segment depression beyond the baseline tracing be used as a criterion for the presence of exercise induced myocardial ischemia. Abnormal left ventricular depolarization sequence such as seen in left bundle branch block, right ventricular pacemakers or accessory pathways will also produce diffuse ST segment abnormalities which may temporarily persist even after the conduction abnormality has disappeared. In subjects with such conditions it is best not to use exercise induced ST segment changes as an index of myocardial ischemia but rather to use other noninvasive imaging techniques or to go directly to invasive diagnostic testing. Left ventricular pressure overload, and less commonly volume overload, may also induce ST segment abnormalities in the absence of obstructive coronary disease. These abnormalities in repolarization are possibly related to abnormalities in subendocardial perfusion. Thus, in addition to the increased risk associated with exercise testing in patients with uncorrected systemic hypertension or severe aortic stenosis the information obtained from such may not help the clinician confirm or exclude the presence of obstructive coronary disease.

Presence of left ventricular hypertrophy, whether identified by electrocardiographic or echocardiographic methods, will also increase the prevalence of false positive tests. The exact mechanism of this is unclear but does not appear to be related to the presence of electrocardiographic signs of left ventricular hypertrophy.

Cardioactive and neuroactive drugs may alter the myocardial cellular ion concentrations or cellular membrane depolarization and thus may also affect the ECG response to exercise. Digitalis drugs have been shown to facilitate exercise induced ST segment depression even in the absence of ST segment abnormalities in the resting ECG.

Diuretics have also been associated with false positive exercise test. The use of diuretics, however, when not associated with hypokalemia does not appear to alter the ST segment response to exercise

---

T A B L E   5

Conditions Producing Abnormal ST Segment Changes in the Absence of Obstructive Coronary Disease

- Preexisting ST segment abnormalities
- Pressure overload
- Electrolyte imbalance
- Drugs
- Mitral valve prolapse
- Left ventricular hypertrophy
- Sudden intense exercise
- Abnormal ventricular depolarization sequence
- Hyperventilation

---

in normal subjects. Psychotropic drugs such as tricyclic antidepressants and lithium have been reported to produce electrocardiographic changes. It seems prudent to discuss the discontinuation of such medications with a psychiatric consultant prior to a diagnostic stress test. Electrolytic or metabolic imbalances may also alter resting and exercise ST segment. Severe hypokalemia with extracellular concentrations of potassium below 3.0 mEq/liter will produce electrocardiographic changes with prominent U waves, flattened T waves, prominent P waves and ST segment depression. When serum potassium is between 3 and 4mEq/liter the resting ECG changes may not be apparent but the clinician should be very cautious in interpreting exercise induced ST segment changes in such patients. Large glucose loads, severe alkalosis and hyperventilation have also been mentioned as possible causes of false positive exercise test.

Gender is a strong modifier of the interpretation of the ST segment response to exercise. Since the prevalence of coronary atherosclerosis is lower in ovulating females the prevalence of false positive tests is higher (Baye's Theorem).

CARDIAC PEARL

Exercise testing: Certainly exercise testing is with us and is "here to stay."

It is good to know the "false negative" as well as the "false positive" possibilities of the treadmill exercise test. A "false positive" test may occur in patients, particularly in women who have prolapse of the mitral valve. I have seen, as a result of serendipity, of a woman with chest discomfort who had an exercise treadmill test that was interpreted as positive for ischemic heart disease. Because of this,

390

the patient was admitted to our hospital for coronary arteriograms, which were negative. The important clue in this middle-aged woman was the presence of several midsystolic clicks, indicating the syndrome of prolapse of the mitral valve.

W. Proctor Harvey, M.D.

Prognostic Implications of Exercise Testing

Although exercise testing was initially used as a diagnostic tool, it soon became obvious that exercise testing was also a powerful predictor of subsequent cardiac events and survival. In coronary artery disease, the two most important predictors of morbidity and mortality are the number and severity of the vessels involved and left ventricular systolic function. Exercise testing reflects the impact of the disease process upon the functional capacity of the heart and thus provides additional prognostic information.

In asymptomatic middle aged males with elevated serum cholesterol, a strongly positive exercise test ($\geq$2mm ST depression) predicts a five fold increase (5% vs <1% at 3 years) for the development of a coronary event; however, the low overall event rate demonstrates that in asymptomatic populations, the prognostic value of exercise testing depends on the prevalence of the disease in the group being tested. Thus, an abnormal exercise test in an asymptomatic subject may not necessarily have a major impact on survival. In contrast, patients with known coronary disease who on exercise testing develop severe ischemia or ischemia at a low work load have a higher mortality than similar patients with minimal or no ischemia on exercise testing. Of the patients with known stable coronary disease who can undergo exercise testing, those who are able to complete a stage 3 Bruce protocol without evidence of ischemia have a good prognosis with yearly mortality $\leq$2%. Patients with known stable coronary disease and evidence of ischemia prior to completing stage 1 of the Bruce protocol, have a yearly mortality $\geq$5%.

Patients with recent myocardial infarction or unstable angina are at high risk of subsequent ischemic events. Once stabilized and medically treated such patients may also be risk stratified by exercise testing. Patients with recent uncomplicated MI and a negative pre-discharge exercise test have a good 1-2 year prognosis with a $\leq$2% mortal-

ity while similar patients with an ischemic response during pre-discharge exercise testing have a 1-2 year mortality between 5 to 15%.

Exercise duration has been used in patients with heart failure as an index of drug efficacy. As the experience with exercise testing in patients with heart failure increased it became apparent that exercise performance could not be reliably predicted by measurements of ventricular function. Several large multicenter studies have demonstrated that exercise tolerance as measured by VO_2 max or by a six minute walking test is a powerful independent predictor of mortality in patients with heart failure. Patients with moderate to severe heart failure who cannot exceed a VO_2 max of 10 mLO_2/kg/min have a yearly mortality of 20% while similar patients who exceed a VO_2 max of 18 have a yearly mortality $\leq$10% Likewise patients with moderate heart failure who are unable to walk a distance <300 meters within six minutes have an eight month mortality of 10% as compared to 3% in similar patients who are able to walk >450 meters within six minutes.

Selected Reading

1. AHA Medical Scientific Statement. Special Report. Guidelines for Clinical Exercise testing laboratories. *Circ* 1995; 91:912-921.
2. Bittner V, Weiner DH, Yusuf S, et al: Prediction of Mortality and Morbidity with a 6-Minute Walk Test in Patients with Left Ventricular Dysfunction. *JAMA* 1993; 270:1702-7.
3. Chaitman BR: *Exercise Testing in Heart Disease.* Braunwald, E. ed., pg 161-79, 4th ed. W.B. Saunders, 1992.
4. Clinical Competence in Exercise Testing. A statement for physicians from the ACP/ACC/AHA task force on clinical privileges in cardiology. *Circ* 1990; 82:1884-8.
5. Cohn JN, Johnson GR, Shabetai R, et al: Ejection Fraction, Peak Oxygen Consumption, Cardiothoracic Ratio, Ventricular Arrhythmias and Plasma Norepinephrine as Determinants of Prognosis in Heart Failure. *Circ* 1993:87 (Suppl VI):V5-16.
6. Fletcher GF: Exercise Testing and Rehabilitation. *Cardiology Clinics,* May 1993; WB Saunders.
7. Fletcher GF and Schlant RC: The Exercise Test. In: *Hurst's The Heart;* Shlant RC, Alexander RW, Pg 423-40, 8th ed. McGraw Hill, 1994.
8. Glasser SP, Clark PI: *The Clinical Approach to Exercise Testing;* Harper & Row, 1980.
9. Glasser SP: Clinical Exercise Testing. *Cardiology Clinics,* Aug 1984: WB Saunders.
10. Guidelines for Exercise Testing. A report of the ACC/AHA task force on assessment of cardiovascular procedures. *JACC,* 1986, 8:725-38.
11. L'Abbate A, Picano E: Stress Testing for the Diagnosis of Coronary Artery Disease. (Circulation Supplement), *Circ* 1991; 83 (Suppl III), 333.

Nuclear Cardiology: Clinical Applications

Michael R. Nagel, M.D.

The "five finger approach" of Dr. W. Proctor Harvey has all the necessary elements to guide us in establishing a diagnosis of cardiovascular disease and thus lead to a successful therapeutic triumph. While Dr. Harvey stresses the necessity of utilizing the history, physical examination, electrocardiogram, chest x-ray, and other ancillary laboratory testing in evaluating patients with cardiac problems, his real emphasis was on continuing education in order to keep up with new developments in the field of Cardiology.

The technological advances in nuclear cardiology over the past 25 years have had a significant impact on our clinical assessment of patients. Incorporation of these newer technologies into the "five finger approach" has helped us to be more accurate in our diagnostic and therapeutic interventions.

Initially, utility of radionuclides in cardiac diagnosis was limited to localization of areas of acute infarction, evaluation of valvular heart disease with regurgitant fractions, cardiac output, ejection fraction determinations, and detection of significant intracardiac shunts (greater than 1.3 to 1). Currently, however, the main application of nuclear cardiology is in the evaluation of patients with ischemic coronary artery disease, which continues to be the most prevalent cause of death in the United States.

This chapter will trace the historical landmarks in nuclear cardiology, including a discussion of the pharmacokinetics of newer radiopharmaceutical agents that have emerged, advances in computer technology, and new software programs that have made possible the introduction of first-pass nuclear radioangiography (FPNRA) and SPECT imaging.

These innovations have led to greater sensitivity and specificity in our ability to diagnose coronary artery disease. Recent studies support the role of cardiac nuclear scintigraphy in not only diagnosing the presence or absence of coronary ischemia vs. infarction, but also in the risk stratification of patients with established coronary artery disease.

CARDIAC PEARL

Most patients with ischemic heart disease can be diagnosed on the basis of a careful evaluation of the total clinical picture, including a complete history and physical examination, ECGs, X-ray studies, and less complicated, often routine, laboratory tests. The history in particular is often still the most important key in making the correct diagnosis. On the other hand, some patients obviously need more specialized tests, such as are outlined in this chapter. These newly developed noninvasive techniques have not only been ingenious and imaginative, but highly accurate.

W. Proctor Harvey, M.D.

In the final section of this chapter, a case presentation format will be used to illustrate the practical utility of nuclear cardiology in the daily management of clinical problems.

Nuclear Myocardial Scintigraphy (NMS)

The specific developments that truly stand out in nuclear cardiology include the introduction of radiopharmaceuticals, such as Thallium-201(^{201}Tl) and Technetium-99m Sestamibi(^{99m}Tc-Sestamibi) and the widespread utility of Single Photon Emission Tomography (SPECT). The advent of Single Photon Emission Tomography (SPECT) has enabled us to obtain three dimensional, triangulated, images of perfusion defects. Based on these technological advances, differentiation of atypical chest pain, especially when coupled with a "positive" treadmill stress test, has been much easier. It needs to be stressed that the perfusion abnormalities detected by nuclear myocardial scintigraphy result from a discrepancy in blood flow and develop sequentially before any EKG abnormalities, wall motion abnormalities, or symptoms of angina pectoris are noted (Table 1). The detection of the discrepancy in myocardial perfusion seen with nuclear scintigraphy will become apparent before any wall motion abnormalities appear on stress echocardiography. This makes nuclear myocardial scintigraphy a diagnostic tool with a very high sensitivity and specificity for the diagnosis of myocardial ischemic syndromes.

Clinical assessment of patients with chest pain can often be quite perplexing, even when we have electrocardiographic data to complement a careful history and physical examination. This is particularly true in patients whose electrocardiograms are abnormal at baseline as a result of drug therapy, e.g. digoxin, the presence of left bundle branch block, left ventricular hypertrophy, cardiomyopathy, or previous EKG evidence of infarction with persistent ST-T abnormalities. Treadmill stress testing is of little use in this population since the ST-T abnormalities often worsen with exercise or the repolarization abnormalities make it impossible to detect the presence of ischemia. The other dilemma is that 30% to 40% of the normal population, with normal resting EKGs, particularly women, may develop ST-segment abnormalities with exercise stress testing without having underlying coronary ischemia.

The need to verify the clinical impression of "atypical", non-ischemic, chest pain often results in a "positive" exercise stress test. Prior to the advances in nuclear myocardial scintigraphy, the clinician was faced with the quandary of exposing the patient to an "invasive" procedure, namely coronary angiography, to clarify the diagnosis.

Ellestad et al. have demonstrated that the predictive value of treadmill stress testing alone has a rather low sensitivity in detecting coronary artery disease in unselected patients, averaging only 64% (range=38%-80%). Average specificity of treadmill stress testing is 85% (range=50-97%), and the positive predictive value is 90% (range 72%-96%). The lower sensitivity and specificity was noted particularly in patients with single vessel coronary artery

---

T A B L E   1

Pathophysiology of Angina Pectoris

1. Discrepancy between coronary blood flow and myocardial oxygen demand
2. EKG abnormalities suggestive of ischemia
3. Wall motion abnormalities
4. Angina Pectoris

---

disease, especially if the circumflex coronary artery was involved. Sensitivity of treadmill stress testing is dependent on the patient's ability to exceed 85% of his/her age-predicted maximal heart rate. This correlates to the finding that the onset of anaerobic metabolism and lactate production begins when the heart rate exceeds 85% of the maximal predicted value. Both treadmill stress testing and nuclear myocardial scintigraphy are at their highest sensitivity and specificity when the stress test is symptom limited, and the heart rate achieved exceeds 85% of the maximum age-predicted heart rate for the patient. A rough estimate of the maximum age-predicted heart rate can be calculated quickly by subtracting the patients age from 220. Even in patients following acute myocardial infarction who undergo treadmill stress testing one week following their infarct, the yield of positive findings increases if symptom-limited exercise vs. submaximal exercise stress testing is carried out, e.g. chest pain in 20% vs 13%, ST-depression in 89% vs 56% and exercise time 9 vs 7 minutes. No increase in morbidity or mortality was seen in this subset of patients by carrying out a symptom limited stress test.

Benefits of NMS

It was, therefore, a significant advance in our armamentarium when a "noninvasive" procedure such as nuclear myocardial scintigraphy was introduced into clinical practice to augment the sensitivity, and thus the negative predictive value, of our diagnostic assessment of patients with suspected coronary artery disease. The additional potential to detect myocardial ischemia by use of pharmacologic stress with nuclear myocardial scintigraphy, in patients who are unable to exercise or to reach 85% of their maximum age-predicted heart rate, is a distinct advantage over treadmill stress testing alone. The "negative" treadmill stress EKG study, if confirmed by a normal myocardial perfusion study, carries a very favorable prognosis, with the annual cardiac event rate being less than 1%. This, however is

T A B L E   2

Candidates for Pharmacologic Stress NMS

1. **Patients unable to exercise**
    a) Orthopedic problems of the lower extremities
    b) Rheumatologic illnesses
    c) Neurologic illness
        (1) Paralysis secondary to cerebrovascular accidents
        (2) Severe neuritis involving the lower extremities
        (3) Primary skeletal muscle disorders
2. **Peripheral vascular disease**
    a) Claudication of the lower extremities
    b) Large abdominal aortic aneurysms
    c) Venous insufficiency with severe edema of the lower extremities
3. **Severe cardiovascular deconditioning**
4. **General debility**
5. **Drug therapy** with calcium channel blockers or beta blockers which may prevent heart rate increases above 85% of maximum predicted for age.

not true if the heart rate achieved during exercise is low (under 60% of maximum predicted heart rate). Likewise, a rapid heart due to "deconditioning", atrial fibrillation, emotional stress, or atrial pacing is not associated with a rise in blood pressure or cardiac work which would be comparable to the workload achieved with physical exercise. Under these circumstances, it would be desirable to carry out pharmacologic stress testing with myocardial perfusion scintigraphy (Table 2). Generally, patients who would routinely be candidates for pharmacologic stress testing associated with nuclear myocardial scintigraphy include patients with: 1) orthopedic problems of the lower extremities: 2) rheumatologic illness of lower extremities; 3) neurologic illness, including cerebrovascular accidents, neuritis, or primary skeletal muscle disorders; 4) peripheral vascular disease with claudication or aortic aneurysms; 5) severe deconditioning due to obesity or postoperative status or; 6) general debility due to acute non-cardiac illness or age. Recent surveys have found that pharmacologic stress testing is utilized in 30%-40% of all patients undergoing nuclear myocardial scintigraphy. Shaw and colleagues in 1992 described the utility of pharmacologic stress myocardial scintigraphy in stratifying risk of patients with coronary artery disease who need to undergo non-cardiac surgery. They found that the presence of combined fixed and partially reversible perfusion defects during adenosine pharmacologic stress and ^{201}Tl scintigraphy as being the most powerful predictor for subsequent cardiac events.

Developments in Nuclear Cardiology

Developments in the field of nuclear myocardial imaging have been explosive in the past 20 years. The first clinical application, however, dates back to 1927 when Blumgart and Weiss carried out an experiment to measure circulation time by injecting a salt of Radium into an arm vein and measuring the appearance of radioactivity in the opposite arm. Using this principle, subsequent investigations were carried out in the late 1940s to measure cardiac output. It was not until the development of rectilinear scanners, however, which produced a line by line static image, and then gamma cameras, that we began to have some greater promise from this new emerging technology. Recent advances in computer-software applications to the field of nuclear cardiology has, however, been making the greatest impact on the improved images and acquisition of functional data which makes this technology so valuable in the management of patients with ischemic heart disease.

Cameras

While there are some obvious differences in the final format which planar and SPECT imaging yields, the underlying principle is the same; namely, the ability to count radioactivity in a given organ and display it as an indicator of concentration or function of that organ. The radiation detection single crystal camera designed originally by H.O. Anger in 1956 has served as the basis for planar imaging and has changed very little since that time (Figure 1). By modifying the raw data obtained by

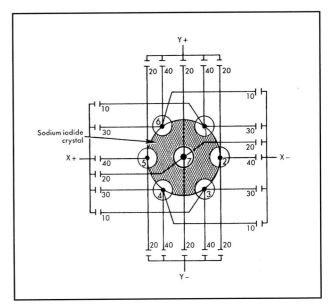

Figure 1. Anger Camera – H.O. Anger's original camera design using seven photomultiplier tubes. *(Courtesy of Paul Early: The Principles & Practice of Nuclear Medicine; The C.V. Mosby Company, 1985)*

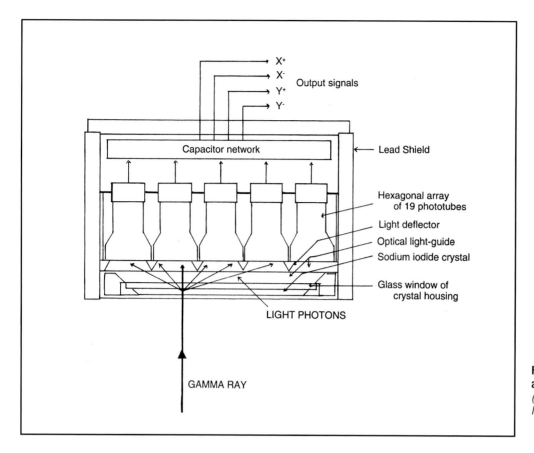

Figure 2. Scintillation Counter and Photomultiplier Tubes
(Courtesy of Paul Early, NMA Manual, 1993)

the scintillation camera, the information can be formatted either as planar or tomographic images. All the imaging systems employed in cardiac work utilize collimators in front of sodium iodide crystals for more accurate detection and localization of the gamma rays from the radioactive source (Figure 2). Transparent 'lightpipes' then carry the photon energy generated by interaction of the gamma rays and the sodium iodide crystal to an array of photomultiplier tubes. The amplified electrical pulses from the photomultiplier tubes then are sent to a complex capacitor network which converts the information into 'pulse-height' data, as well as four output signals needed for spatial localization of the original source of the gamma energy. The 'pulse-height' signal is the Z signal, whereas the spatial data from the four output signals is designated as the X^+, X^-, Y^+, Y^- signals. The Z signal is fed to a pulse-height analyzer which either accepts or rejects the signal, depending on the 'window' parameters set for the radionuclide being scanned.

Planar Imaging

As the name implies, all of the data collected from a radioactive source is displayed as if it were originating from a single plane (Figure 3); there is no tomographic display of the data. The original rec-

tilinear scanners, which required movement of the detector or the patient to allow the acquisition of counts from the target organ of interest, has no utility in cardiac work and has been replaced by the scintillation camera. This latter camera can be configured as a single crystal scintillation camera, or Anger camera, or a multicrystal camera, with the matrix of separate crystal separated from each other by lead septae. This separation of the crystal by the lead separators prevents crossover of gamma rays and photon rays from traveling to neighboring crystals. The presence of collimators arranged to correspond to each crystal further prevents 'cross talk' between the crystals. This further enhances the localization of the origin of gamma rays.

Single Photon Emission Tomography (SPECT)

Advances in computer technology and software products have allowed the emergence of SPECT myocardial scintigraphy to acquire, store and process the planar images (Figure 4). The camera detector utilized in cardiac work acquires the data transaxially, by rotating 180° to 360° around the patient's torso and acquiring data at 128, 64, or 32 equal angles around the circumference of the torso. Images are stored on a 64x64 matrix, with each image consisting of 125,000 counts. A desirable

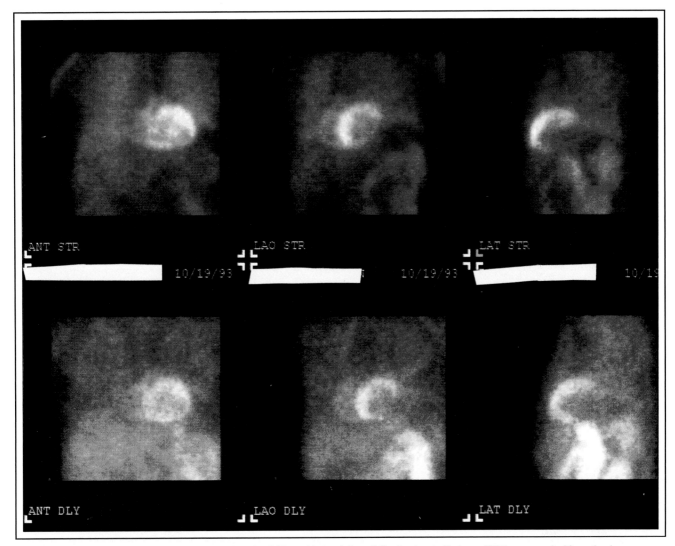

Figure 3. Planar Imaging – Planar images in the Anterior, LAO, and Lateral views following treadmill stress (STR) compared with resting images, showing a fixed infero-lateral perfusion defect diagnostic of infarction.

count per study is 8 million counts; this allows for the more accurate reconstruction of the heart images by the computer in a three-dimensional format. This type of presentation permits the triangulation of defects which improves the sensitivity and specificity of nuclear myocardial scintigraphy (Table 3 and Figure 5). The introduction of high resolution, multipinhole, collimators has also improved the acquisition of sharper planar images by removal of scatter radiation and allows processing of these images, with the assistance of computer software programs, to reconstruct tomographic slices of the heart.

Radiopharmaceuticals

Development of radiopharmaceuticals has allowed us to get clearer functional data pertaining to the myocardial blood flow, viability of the myocardium, and the contractile pattern of the myocardium. The two major radiopharmaceuticals currently used in Nuclear Cardiology are Technetium-99m (^{99m}Tc) and Thallium 201 (^{201}Tl).

Myocardial Infarction Localization

^{99m}Tc pyrophosphate was initially used to diagnose transmural myocardial infarction during the first 16 hours to 6 days of an acute infarct (Table 4). Its use was based on the incorporation of some of the phosphate molecules into the matrix of inorganic phosphate laid down along with amorphous calcium and crystalline hydroxyapatite into newly infarcted tissue. This "hot spot" imaging of infarcted tissue has its greatest application when the EKG and enzyme tests were ambiguous or conflicting. Other applications of this radionuclide included the diagnosis of myocardial infarction fol-

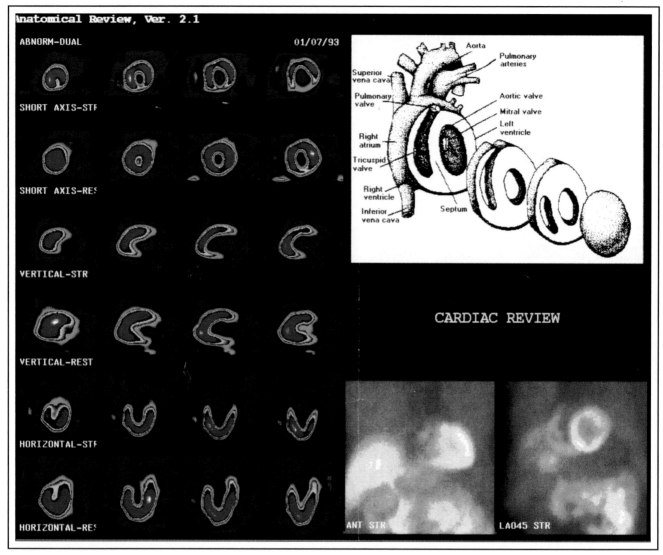

Figure 4. SPECT Imaging – (Courtesy of Adac, Inc.) – SPECT images in the Short Axis, Vertical Axis, and Horizontal Axis are displayed after processing the raw data acquired on planar imaging. The top images in each view are following exercise stress (STR) and are compared with the delayed rest (RST) images. A reversible inferior wall perfusion defect is noted, which is diagnostic of ischemia of the inferior wall.

lowing coronary revascularization surgery, the localization of infarcts in patients with bundle branch block patterns or who are electrically paced, and possibly in identifying right ventricular infarctions. While some images may be obtained as early as 10 to 12 hours following infarction, the greatest uptake of the radionuclide occurs during the first 40 to 72 hours. Since ^{99m}Tc pyrophosphate has such a high affinity for calcium, and 50% of the administered dose is taken up by bone, its first application was in bone scanning. This bone uptake has made the interpretation of ^{99m}Tc pyrophosphate scans more difficult due to the interference by rib uptake of the radionuclide. Furthermore, since the myocardial uptake of ^{99m}Tc pyrophosphate is dependent on both blood flow and tissue damage, large infarcts

may not show uptake in their centers, since perfusion of these areas is compromised. Abnormal ^{99m}Tc pyrophosphate scans can also be found in patients

---

T A B L E   4

Myocardial Infarct Localization with ^{99m}Tc Pyrophosphate

1. Nonspecific EKG and enzymes in patient with classical symptoms of infarction
2. Complete left bundle branch block is present
3. Patient has electrical paced rhythm
4. Immediately following coronary revascularization surgery
5. Patient with right ventricular infarction

TABLE 3

Sensitivity and Specificity of ^{99m}Tc Sestamibi vs TI-201 for Detection of CAD in Patients: SPECT

REFERENCE (n)	SENSITIVITY (%)		SPECIFICITY (%)		NORMALCY (%)	
	TI-201	Tc-99m SESTAMIBI	TI-201	Tc-99m SESTAMIBI	TI-201	Tc-99m SESTAMIBI
Kiat	80	93	75	75	77	100
Iskandrian	82	82	82	100	—	—
Kahn	84	95	—	—	—	—
Overall	83	90	80	93	77	100

Kiat et al. AHJ 1989;117:1.
Iskandrian et al. AJC 1989;64:270.
Kahn et al. Circ 1989;79:1282.

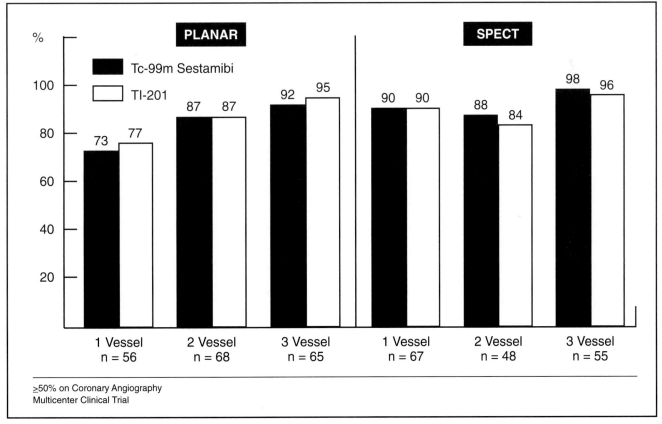

Figure 5. ^{99m}Tc Sestamibi vs TI-201: Sensitivity According to CAD Extent

with myocardial contusion, cardiomyopathy, ventricular aneurysm, valvular calcification, infective endocarditis, skin lesions, breast tumors, rib fractures, calcified costal cartridges, and following electrical cardioversion. While ^{99m}Tc may still have a role in confirming diagnosis of myocardial infarction, newer radiopharmaceuticals and advances in echocardiography have displaced the use of ^{99m}Tc pyrophosphate in clinical practice.

Ventricular Function Assessment

The ejection fraction (EF) is widely utilized as a measure of left ventricular function. The EF ratio represents the amount of blood ejected with each beat [EF=stroke volume (end-diastolic volume minus the end-systolic volume) divided by the end-diastolic volume](Figure 6). The EF may be used as a prognostic tool since mortality from coronary artery disease, cardiomyopathy, and valvular heart

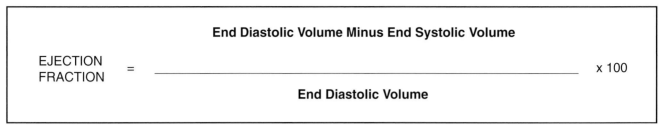

$$\text{EJECTION FRACTION} = \frac{\text{End Diastolic Volume Minus End Systolic Volume}}{\text{End Diastolic Volume}} \times 100$$

Figure 6. Ejection Fraction Formula.

disease is increased when the EF is reduced. Prognosis is poorer in patients with a depressed EF and an increased end-diastolic volume, as compared to patients with a depressed EF who have a normal end-diastolic volume. The EF may remain normal, for a time, in some patients with valvular regurgitant lesions, at the expense of a rise in the end-diastolic volume, since this is the basis for compensation of a failing heart by increase in the preload according to Starling's Law; this is usually associated with a concomitant increase in left ventricular hypertrophy. In patients with obstruction to left ventricular outflow, e.g., systemic hypertension or aortic stenosis, the ventricle also compensates to the increased peripheral resistance by concentric hypertrophy and shows signs of failure when increased end-diastolic volume becomes associated with a fall of EF. Use of the predictive value of the EF in patients with coronary artery disease is predicated on the normal response of the heart to exercise. Normal individuals who are exercising decrease their end-systolic volume while maintaining their end-diastolic volume, which results in an increase of the EF (Figure 7).

Patients with significant coronary artery disease, who become ischemic with exercise, drop their

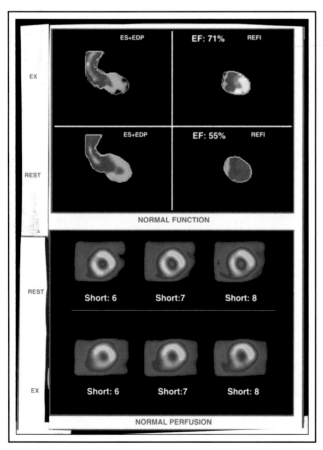

Figure 7. First Pass Radionuclide Angiography – Normal Response
(Courtesy of Scinticor Inc.) – The normal response to exercise is demonstrated with an increase in the ejection fraction (EF). Associated myocardial perfusion scan is normal.

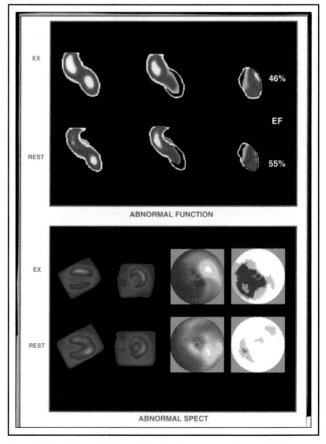

Figure 8. First Pass Radionuclide Angiography – Abnormal Response
(Courtesy of Scinticor Inc.) – Ejection fraction (EF) falls with exercise in this patient with evidence of ischemia of the inferoseptal and apical walls.

EF with exercise due to an increase in the end-diastolic volume as well as the end-systolic volume (Figure 8). They may be able to maintain their stroke volume at the expense of an increase in preload. Diagnosis of CAD can be made by use of exercise first pass radionuclide angiography to detect an increase in end-systolic volume and a failure to increase the EF by more than 5% during submaximal exercise. At the same time, patients with ischemic heart disease develop segmental wall abnormalities following exercise which can be detected with gated SPECT studies.

Multiple Gated Acquisition Studies (MUGA)

Multiple gated acquisition studies have been carried out for a number of years and labeled by various names, including gated cardiac blood pool studies, or gated equilibrium studies. They were initially carried out by use of labeled human serum albumin (HSA) and more recently by *in vivo or in vitro* labeling of red cells by ^{99m}Tc. Indication for the MUGA studies have been for 1) determination of the EF (LVEF or RVEF), 2) the demonstration of wall motion abnormalities, 3) assessment of cardiac output, 4) detection of ventricular aneurysm, 5) quantification of regurgitant fraction in aortic or mitral regurgitation, 6) followup of chemotherapy with Adriamycin for cardiotoxicity, 7) and evaluation of results of medical or surgical interventions on cardiac function.

First Pass Radionuclide Angiography (FPRNA)

^{99m}Tc has also been utilized to obtain real time wall motion and systolic function studies of the right and left ventricles, with quantitative ejection fractions at rest and with exercise. These studies can be carried out utilizing the first-pass technique, with images acquired during the first 25 to 60 seconds following an intravenous bolus of 10 to 30 mCi of ^{99m}Tc pertechnetate into the external jugular vein or the antecubital vein and followed immediately by an intravenous "flush" of 10 to 20 cc of normal saline. The scintigraphic images are recorded as the bolus travels through the cardiac chambers. This allows separate visualization of the right sided cardiac chambers, the lungs, and the left sided cardiac chambers. This technique lends itself to the use of short lived radionuclides and the acquisition of real-time peak exercise ejection fractions due to the rapid acquisition time.

In addition, determination of right ventricular function can add valuable information in patients with chronic obstructive pulmonary disease, congenital heart disease, pulmonary hypertension, and

coronary and valvular heart disease. Data derived regarding diastolic performance includes peak filling rate, time to peak filling rate, and the filling fraction can assist in the detection of patients with diastolic left ventricular dysfunction. Up to 30% of patients with congestive heart failure have diastolic dysfunction and can respond adversely if treated with inotropic or vasodilating drugs.

Recent developments in multicrystal camera technology allows the acquisition of high count rates, ranging between 450,000 counts per second to 1 million counts per second. The multicrystal arrays can be composed of between 290 to 400 individual sodium iodide crystals. Each of these is in turn connected to 35 to 115 photomultiplier tubes which allows rapid detection of photoelectric events and eliminates "dead" time in the acquisition of the data. Data is stored on a high speed magnetic disk at 20 to 25 frames per second. The frame rate is dependent on the heart rate in order to maintain good spatial resolution.

With exercise, the higher heart rates require a faster frame rate, as well as high-sensitivity collimators and adequate doses of the radiopharmaceutical. Lee and colleagues have reported the value of the exercise ejection fraction in prognosticating survival free of myocardial infarction over a 7-year period. Patients with a greater than 50% EF had an 80% survival rate at 7 years and a 75% chance of being free of an infarct during that 7 year period. This is in contrast with patients with a 30% EF who had a 55% survival and 50% infarct-free survival at 7 years (Fig 9). The exercise test can be carried out on either the bicycle or the treadmill, with an americium marker used on the chest wall to cor-

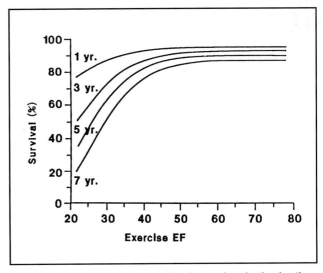

Figure 9. Survival curves as a function of exercise ejection fraction (EF). (Reprinted from Lee et al.[16] by permission of the American Heart Association, Inc.)

rect for chest wall motion artifact and to align the images properly. Use of ^{99m}Tc sestamibi as the radiopharmaceutical during FPRNA allows the acquisition of not only functional data from the first pass study but also affords the acquisition of flow data from the subsequent SPECT perfusion study.

Gated SPECT Studies

Another approach is to apply the gated-EKG technique following a submaximal stress study. The cardiac cycle (R-R interval) is divided into 64 frames and the computer stores the scintillation counts in each "frame". Software reconstruction allows these frames to be played back in a "video" format, as real time motion in systole and diastole, enabling us to analyze wall motion of both the right and left ventricles simultaneously. Additionally, the computer reconstructions yield three views of the cardiac chambers, including the left anterior oblique, the right anterior oblique, and the left lateral view, which facilitates better definition of the segmental wall motion abnormalities. This ability to view the motion of the myocardium in systole and diastole from different slices gives a higher sensitivity and specificity in the detection of segmental wall motion abnormalities. The acquisition of images displaying regional wall thickening with gated-SPECT appears to offer some additional data, which will allow for better discrimination between artifact, scar, and "hibernating" myocardium. The wall motion abnormalities can then be correlated with the standard perfusion SPECT images that would demonstrate either reversible or fixed defects, compatible with either ischemia or infarction. Additionally, a very valuable quantitative piece of data derived from gated-SPECT radionuclide angiography is the ejection fraction (EF). This technology is still relatively new, and additional experience will define its contribution to the management of patients with coronary artery disease.

Myocardial Perfusion With Thallium-201

In 1973 Lebowitz and colleagues were able to produce Thallium- 201 (^{201}Tl) by proton bombardment of naturally occurring targets, such as Thallium-203, in a cyclotron, resulting in the Thallium 203 (p,3n) Pb-201 reaction. The Pb-201 was separated from the target Thallium and decayed within a 9.4 hour half-life to its 'daughter' isotope Thallium-201. These investigators suggested the use of ^{201}Tl as a myocardial imaging agent since it had many advantages over potassium-43, cesium 129, or rubidium 81, which were in limited use for study of regional myocardial blood flow at that time.

^{201}Tl, a monovalent cation, is available in clinical practice as thallous chloride and has proven to be the principal radionuclide in the evaluation of patients with ischemic heart disease since the late 1970s (Maddhi). ^{201}Tl has a reasonable myocardial extraction ratio, a low photon energy that is acceptable for imaging with ordinary gamma cameras and collimators, a slower myocardial clearance than K-43 or RB-81, and a half-life of 73 hours, which allows for shipment over distances so that an adequate dose could be delivered without excessive exposure to radiation. ^{201}Tl decays by electron capture to Mercury (Hg)-201 and emits gamma rays of 135 kev (3% abundance) and 167 kev (10% abundance) and x-rays with a photon energy of 69-83 kev (with 95% abundance).

The renal medulla is the organ that receives the greatest radiation exposure, at 1170 mrad/mCi, following an intravenous injection of ^{201}Tl. The thyroid receives 1030 mrad/mCi, while the heart only receives 340 mrad/mCi. After an intravenous injection, Tl-201 is rapidly cleared from the circulation, with 90% of the injected dose being removed from the circulation within the first minute.

^{201}Tl is an element found in group IIIA of the periodic table and exhibits biologic properties similar to potassium. Similar to potassium's distribution in the body, the thallous ion has its greatest concentration intracellularly following an intravenous injection. A mechanism of active intracellular transport across the cell membrane, which is partly blocked by quabain, has been reported and is presumed to be the Na-K ATPase pump. As a result, Tl-201 concentrates rapidly in heart muscle following an intravenous bolus injection. Because the influx of ^{201}Tl is in large part mediated by metabolically generated ATP, the concentration of ^{201}Tl in myocardium can be used as a marker of tissue viability.

Studies have demonstrated that the regional myocardial uptake of ^{201}Tl correlates directly to the regional blood flow. Gould, in 1978, demonstrated that the coronary reserve, the ability to increase blood flow in response to an increase in metabolic demand, is decreased in arteries with occlusions greater than 50%. The myocardial uptake of ^{201}Tl also is dependent on the myocardium's ability to remove the tracer from the blood (the extraction fraction), which is reported to be 87%-95% at normal blood flow rates (Bellar). In animal studies, extraction fraction is higher relative to flow rates when blood flow rates decrease below 10% of normal, since the slower blood transit time allows for greater than normal extraction of the radionuclide by the myocardium (Nielsen). On the other hand, at flow rates that exceeded twice the control levels, such as induced by dipyridamole infusion, the extraction fraction may be decreased. If, however, the increased flow rate is a result of increased metabolic demand of the myocardium then the extraction fraction does not decrease, and the linear relationship between ^{201}Tl uptake and blood flow is maintained. Experimental studies, by Weich and colleagues and McCall and colleagues, have demonstrated a decreased myocardial extraction fraction of Tl-201 in the presence of hypoxia or inhibition of oxidative phosphorylation or glycolytic pathways. Drugs like diphenylhydantoin have been shown by Schachner and colleagues in experiments with rats to decrease myocardial ^{201}Tl uptake by decreasing the myocardial extraction fraction. In humans, the role of myocardial ischemia and drug effects appear to be a minor consideration in the initial scintigraphic defects seen with ^{201}Tl imaging.

It is, rather, the regional differences in myocardial blood flow distribution that account for the defects seen after injection of the ^{201}Tl dose intravenously, either at rest, at peak exercise, or following the use of coronary vasodilators such as adenosine or dipyridamole.

Pohost and colleagues, in 1977, demonstrated that following ^{201}Tl intravenous injection, the initial perfusion defects in patients with ischemia, but without infarction, would disappear on delayed imaging. Beller suggested that the distribution of ^{201}Tl was a dynamic process which changed with time, and led to the concept of redistribution of the radionuclide on the delayed images. This redistribution of ^{201}Tl results from the accumulation of the radionuclide in areas that were previously underperfused and also from the release of the radionuclide from the normal myocardium.

With exercise stress protocols injecting the ^{201}Tl at peak exercise enhances the demonstration of the discrepancy in blood flow between the normally perfused myocardium and the areas supplied by obstructed coronary arteries. The normally perfused area will show a higher uptake of radionuclide when compared with the ischemic zone, which will appear on film as having fewer "counts" and therefore look like a "cold spot".

Since ^{201}Tl will attempt to equilibrate with the blood pool with the passage of time, the ischemic zone will eventually take up sufficient ^{201}Tl to equal concentration in the normally perfused myocardium. Thus, the delayed, redistribution images will show a reversible perfusion defect, which will confirm and localize the region of ischemia. One can also make a judgement on SPECT images as to the amount of myocardium at risk; in order to

enhance the redistribution images, particularly in regions of "hibernating" myocardium, it is the standard of practice now to inject an additional 1 mCi of ^{201}Tl just before the acquisition of the delayed images. Patients with severe ischemia might also be brought back for delayed images at 24 hours to insure that viable myocardium is not misdiagnosed as infarct. Mahmarian and colleagues reported the sensitivity and specificity of ^{201}Tl myocardial imaging SPECT-scintigraphy to be 92% and 87%, respectively, in patients with multivessel coronary artery disease. The sensitivity of ^{201}Tl-SPECT in single vessel disease was lower and depended on the vessel involved, being highest, at 83%, for the right coronary artery, 80% for the left anterior descending coronary artery, and falling off to 72% for the circumflex coronary artery. Most studies support the finding that the sensitivity falls off in cases of single vessel coronary artery disease, small branch or distal artery stenosis, circumflex coronary artery stenosis, non-jeopardized well-collateralized arteries, in the presence of low work-loads and submaximal heart rates, and in the presence of certain drugs, e.g. beta blockers or calcium channel blockers, which blunt the heart rate response.

There is ample evidence to suggest an increased risk for development of future coronary events if there is evidence for 1) increased lung uptake; 2) reversible cavitary dilatation; 3) multivessel involvement; and 4) male gender.

It is noteworthy that in patients with multivessel disease we do not see global hypoperfusion with ^{201}Tl, since the degree of ischemia is not exactly identical throughout the perfused myocardium. It has also been demonstrated that in the presence of only 6% to 14% fibrosis of the myocardium, one may see hypokinesia, or even akinesia, of a ventricular segment. This finding on stress echocardiography might lead to the misdiagnosis of an infarct, whereas the ^{201}Tl perfusion scan would correctly identify these zones as having viable myocardium which would benefit from revascularization surgery.

Thallium's pharmacokinetics are unique and allow for the determination of functional data that is not readily available with Technetium-99 (^{99m}Tc) Sestamibi. The presence of increased lung uptake following stress testing has been shown to correspond to ventricular dysfunction associated with an increase in pulmonary capillary wedge pressure, which may be secondary to coronary ischemia, mitral valve regurgitation or stenosis, decreased left ventricular compliance associated with left ventricular hypertrophy, or from non-ischemic dilated cardiomyopathy (Boucher and colleagues, 1980). Caution must be utilized, therefore, in interpreting this finding as an indicator of significant coronary artery disease, unless other supporting evidence is present to suggest perfusion defects. If increased lung uptake is associated with the presence of reversible cavitary dilatation, which has been established as evidence of severe ischemia, diagnosis of significant multivessel coronary artery disease is more firmly established (Stolzenber 1980).

Technetium-99m Sestamibi

[99m]Tc-Sestamibi (Cardiolite) is an isonitrile compound (2-methoxy isobutyl isonitrile) which was released for commercial use as a myocardial imaging radiopharmaceutical in 1991. It has ideal physical properties for myocardial imaging, including a 140 Kev photopeak, and a relatively short half-life of 6 hours, allowing larger dose administration. The ability to elute the ^{99m}Tc from a molybdenum-technetium generator makes it a radiopharmaceutical that can be readily available, 24 hours a day. While it is an excellent marker of myocardial perfusion, being distributed in proportion to the regional blood flow, it is taken up by the myocardium by passive diffusion, unlike the active transport seen with [201]Tl. There is a 90% clearance of ^{99m}Tc-Sestamibi from the blood stream within four minutes following intravenous injection. More than 80% of the drug remains bound to the mitochondrial membrane in the myocyte. There is no significant myocardial redistribution, and the drug clears very slowly from the myocardium. Because of its short half-life and its rapid hepatobiliary clearance, ^{99m}Tc-Sestamibi can be injected at doses up to 30 mCi (1110 MBq)/70 Kg; this results in improved image resolution because of the high image count density. Sensitivity and specificity of ^{99m}Tc-Sestamibi

myocardial perfusion SPECT-imaging is 89% and 90%, respectively (Table 5). Because of its favorable dosimetry, ^{99m}Tc-Sestamibi can be used for ejection fraction measurements, utilizing first-pass radionuclide angiography (FPRNA), as well as for myocardial perfusion imaging in the same study, through SPECT-myocardial scintigraphy.

The ability to acquire regional wall motion information, ejection fractions, and ventricular volume data from ^{99m}Tc-Sestamibi first-pass radionuclide angiography, in addition to the perfusion data, improves the sensitivity and specificity of the diagnosis of single vessel coronary artery disease to 93%. It should be stressed that the ejection fraction acquired during peak exercise by the first-pass radionuclide angiography protocol has been found to yield 80% of the prognostic data obtained from this technique. Risk stratification can be carried out from this data, since patients with a peak-exercise FPRNA ejection fraction greater than 50% have less than a 1% annual mortality.

By gating the perfusion acquisition data, the regional wall thickening in systole and the relaxation phase in diastole can be displayed in a cineformat. Computer programs also allow the calculation of ejection fractions from this gated data. While this post-exercise gated-SPECT ejection fraction does not have the same prognostic significance as the exercise ejection fraction acquired by first-pass radionuclear angiography, it nevertheless adds important data for prognosticating future morbidity and mortality. Gated-SPECT will have wider appeal since first-pass radionuclear angiography (FPRNA) requires the use of specialized cameras that can record 150,000 counts/second in the designated photopeak window, using a collimator that gives optimum spatial resolution. Currently, this implies use of multi-crystal gamma cameras,

---

TABLE 5

Sensitivity and Specificity of [99m]Tc Sestamibi vs Tl-201 for Detection of CAD in Patients: Planar

| REFERENCE | SENSITIVITY (%) | | SPECIFICITY (%) | | NORMALCY (%) | |
	TI-201	Tc-99m SESTAMIBI	TI-201	Tc-99m SESTAMIBI	TI-201	Tc-99m SESTAMIBI
Wackers	97	89	100	100	—	—
Kiat	73	73	50	75	88	94
Najm	70	88	—	—	100	100
Overall	81	86	67	83	93	97

Wackers et al. J Nucl Med 1989;30:301.
Kiat et al. AHJ 1989;117:1.
Najm et al. Int J Cardiol 1990;26:93.

since only one or two of the available single-crystal cameras have the count rate capability and the required software needed to obtain diagnostic quality first-pass imaging.

A dual-isotope protocol has been proposed by Berman and colleagues, whereby a resting ^{201}Tl SPECT acquisition study begins 10 minutes after the radionuclide is administered. A treadmill stress test follows, as soon as the resting ^{201}Tl SPECT study is completed, and the ^{99m}Tc-Sestamibi SPECT study follows 15 minutes after the dose of ^{99m}Tc-Sestamibi is administered at peak exercise. A total dose of 3 mCi of ^{201}Tl, given as Thallous Chloride, and 25-30 mCi of ^{99m}Tc-Sestamibi is administered intravenously, giving a total radiation exposure to the patient of only 5 rads. By counting at the separate photopeak windows of the two isotopes and using high resolution collimators we can acquire excellent quality images with SPECT technology. This approach allows for faster through-put of patients, with the total study lasting 90 to 120 minutes. This is a definite advantage when compared with the 4.5 to 5 hours required to complete a rest/stress ^{201}Tl protocol.

An additional benefit is the ability to obtain delayed 24 hour images of the ^{201}Tl redistribution in patients suspected of having hibernating myocardium. A variant of this dual-isotope protocol is to inject the ^{201}Tl the evening before the resting imaging study is acquired to allow for adequate redistribution and unmask hibernating myocardium. The rationale for not acquiring data simultaneously from the separate photopeak windows of ^{99m}Tc and ^{201}Tl has been elegantly demonstrated by Kiat and colleagues with phantom studies demonstrating 'crosstalk' by the higher energies of ^{99m}Tc spilling over to the lower energy window of the ^{201}Tl and resulting in a decreased ability to discriminate the ^{201}Tl defect from the normally perfused region. There is, however, very little effect from the ^{201}Tl photon energies on the ^{99m}Tc window, which makes it possible to use the resting ^{201}Tl /stress ^{99m}Tc data acquisition protocol without concern of crosstalk between the two radionuclides. Berman pointed out, at the Society of Nuclear Medicine meeting in Toronto, Canada in 1993, that visual analysis allows excellent accuracy in the detection of coronary artery disease (CAD) by this protocol, with an overall sensitivity of 91% in the CAD population without a history of myocardial infarction. The specificity was 75% in patients with normal coronary angiograms while the normalcy rate was 95% in 107 patients with a low probability of having CAD. Furthermore, he cited a correlation of 97% with studies utilizing a rest/stress ^{99m}Tc-Sestamibi

protocol. With the use of pharmacologic stress, it is suggested that an hour interval be allowed following the injection of ^{99m}Tc-Sestamibi before beginning the stress SPECT acquisition study. This delay will compensate for the slower hepatobiliary clearance noted following pharmacologic stress.

There are, however, some pitfalls in the comparison of the images obtained with the dual isotope technique; namely, the apparent smaller cavity size of the left ventricle and the thicker myocardial walls which are seen normally with the resting ^{201}Tl SPECT images in comparison to normal, sharply defined myocardial walls seen on the ^{99m}Tc-Sestamibi SPECT images.

The disadvantage of using just ^{99m}Tc-Sestamibi, in patients with coronary artery disease, for both stress and delayed imaging is the need to utilize a 2-day protocol, since ^{99m}Tc-Sestamibi does not redistribute. This is quite inconvenient for most patients who have to give up two days in a row to complete the test. If the patient has a normal stress study, there is no need to return on the following day for a rest study.

Proponents of the dual-isotope protocol stress the ability to get "late" images at 12 or 24 hours to check for viable, "hibernating" myocardium, based on the known redistribution of ^{201}Tl. But some recent reports espouse the view that viability data can also be obtained from ^{99m}Tc-Sestamibi perfusion studies by a quantitative analysis of the ^{99m}Tc content within a defect, e.g. utilizing a cut point of 60% of peak radionuclide activity. The studies suggest resting ^{99m}Tc-Sestamibi, when viewed in this quantitative manner, yielded similar predictive results of viability as seen with ^{201}Tl. Correlation with PET evidence of viability has also been cited.

Experimental Radiopharmaceuticals

Several experimental radiopharmaceuticals are being investigated and hold promise for clinical release. The first is ^{99m}Tc-Tetrofosmin, which has a 0.87 correlation with blood flow and clears very rapidly from the blood stream. It has a favorable heart-to-liver ratio, making it useful for pharmacologic stress protocols. It has been compared to ^{201}Tl studies and has an 82-90% accuracy, being able to detect normally perfused myocardium with a 93% accuracy.

The second agent is ^{99m}Tc-Q-12; this agent has a good correlation with coronary blood flow but exhibits "roll-off" at higher flow rates. A related agent to ^{99m}Tc-Q-12 is ^{99m}Tc-Q-3, which exhibits an excellent correlation to blood flow, showing no "roll-off" at higher flow rates. It has a stable ischemic/non-ischemic ratio in the myocardium, with no significant washout for over 4 hours. It has more hepatic uptake than ^{201}Tl, which may lead to problems in interpretation of inferior wall and diaphragmatic perfusion abnormalities. The sensitivity of ^{99m}Tc-Q-3 is 84% when compared with 90-95% for ^{201}Tl perfusion studies. The total time for a rest-stress study with this radiopharmaceutical is 120 minutes, utilizing 7 mCi at rest and 23 mCi following stress, which would allow for a very rapid "through-put" of patients.

Exercise Stress Protocols

The most common protocols utilized with ^{201}Tl are standard treadmill or bicycle exercise protocols, with injection of 2 to 3 mCi of the ^{201}Tl radionuclide intravenously at peak exercise. The endpoint of exercise should be either exhaustion at a heart rate greater than 85% of maximum predicted for the patient's age, or signs or symptoms suggestive of myocardial ischemia. Planar and SPECT images are obtained immediately following exercise, and the patient returns in four hours for redistribution planar and SPECT imaging. As noted above, Berman and colleagues have demonstrated that IV reinjection with 1 mCi of ^{201}Tl on the resting SPECT study, four hours after the stress study, enhances the uptake of the radionuclide in regions of myocardium that are severely ischemic, and which might appear as fixed defects suggesting "scar" tissue on routine 4 hour redistribution study. In fact, 49% of the "irreversible" defects seen on routine 4-hour redistribution SPECT perfusion studies were shown to improve or normalize their uptake of radionuclide when reinjection of ^{201}Tl was utilized. Clinically, revascularization has shown that 50% of the "irreversible" regions on routine ^{201}Tl redistribution studies will improve function. The reinjection at 4 hours, therefore, enhances our ability to discriminate between viable and infarcted tissue. There is also a 3% increase in sensitivity for detecting viable myocardium when the delayed reperfusion images are acquired at 24 hours. The detection of viable myocardium by use of the reinjection technique at 4 hours following stress have been confirmed by FDG (fluorine-18, fluorodeoxyglucose) uptake studies on PET scans, which measures metabolic activity in myocardial tissue. This is based on the finding that myocardium that is ischemic or "hibernating" utilizes glucose as its metabolic substrate in preference to fatty acids or lactate. As a result of this reinjection ^{201}Tl protocol, there is a reported 87% concordance between FDG uptake PET scanning and ^{201}Tl scanning in the ability to identify infarcted tissue.

Without any question, PET scanning remains the more sensitive, though much more expensive and less accessible, method for detection of metabolically active, viable myocardium, with a positive predictive value of 78%-85% and a negative predictive value of 78%-92%.

Pharmacologic Stress Protocols

In those unable to exercise to a workload greater than 3 METS or achieve a maximum age-predicted heart rate greater than 85% because of vascular, neurologic, orthopedic, or arthritic problems, we now have pharmacologic stress protocols with dipyridamole (Persantine), adenosine (Adenocard), or dobutamine (Dobutrex). The dobutamine protocol seems particularly well-suited for individuals with histories of bronchial asthma or chronic obstructive lung disease with bronchospasm. However, the most commonly utilized pharmacologic stress protocol is with dipyridamole. Dipyridamole acts by blocking the receptor site where adenosine is metabolized, thus enhancing the vasodilatory effect of adenosine on the coronary arteries. Adenosine has also been utilized directly as the pharmacologic agent, and because of its potent direct vasodilatory effects has been reported to have a higher incidence of side effects. In one series, 79% of patients receiving adenosine infusion had side effects, particularly facial flushing (35%), chest pain (34%), headache (20%) and dyspnea (19%) (Abreu 1991). Because of the stimulation of the A1 receptors in the proximal parts of the AV node, atrio-ventricular block was noted in nearly 15% of patients, including 10% with first degree AV block, 4% with second degree AV block, and <1% with third degree AV block. The effects of adenosine are very fleeting and rarely require any specific therapy. On the other hand, dipyridamole has a more sustained effect on the adenosine receptor site, with a resulting blockade lasting from 10 to 30 minutes. Since the normal coronary arteries will respond by increasing their flow to a much greater degree than significantly obstructed vessels, the discrepancy in flow can precipitate angina or evidence of ischemia on the EKG tracing and on the nuclear myocardial scintigraphy scan.

With the patient's EKG monitored continuously, after acquiring a baseline 12 lead tracing, an intravenous infusion is started with 5% dextrose and water. A calculated dose of dipyridamole (Persantine), 0.142 mg/kg/min, is administrated intravenously over four minutes, with blood pressure determinations and 12 lead EKG recordings at each minute. [201]Tl or ^{99m}Tc-sestamibi is injected at the 6th minute of the test as a bolus. The patient is then observed with blood pressure checks and 12 leak EKGs every 2 minutes. At the 8th to 12th minute of

T A B L E   6

**Endpoints for
Dobutamine Infusion**

---

1. Angina Pectoris
2. Ischemic ST segments greater than 2 Mv below baseline
3. Achieving a heart rate exceeding 85% of maximum predicted for age
4. Nonsustained ventricular tachycardia
5. Hypotension

the test, aminophylline 50 mg may be given over 2 minutes intravenously to reverse the dipyridamole (Persantine) effect. If the patient has additional symptoms of flushing, nausea, headache or chest pain, additional aminophylline may be given slowly intravenously at a rate of 25 mg/min, the dose rarely needing to exceed 100 mg. We are utilizing submaximal exercise stress, e.g. lifting the legs or raising 2 pound weights with the arms, in addition to the pharmacologic stress, since a 30% increase in cardiac double product (heart rate x systolic blood pressure) further enhances the resultant ischemia and may reduce the noncardiac IV dipyridamole vasodilator side effects. In addition, the submaximal exercise decreases the blood flow to the splanchnic bed resulting in better visualization of the diaphragmatic wall of the left ventricle on the myocardial perfusion scan. The myocardial images may also be enhanced since more tracer is available in the myocardium since less blood flow is diverted to the splanchnic bed. A desired end-point from the dipyridamole infusion is an increase in the heart rate of at least 10% above baseline. Rarely one sees hypotension of greater than 20 mm Hg following dipyridamole infusion. It would be best to avoid physical exercise in this latter subset of patients.

The same dose calculations can be utilized with adenosine. Because of its rapid metabolism, with a half-life of only 10 to 15 seconds, there is no need to reverse its effect with aminophylline at the end of the test.

Dobutamine infusion may also be utilized for pharmacologic stress because of the induction of an increase in myocardial oxygen consumption by increasing contractility, blood pressure and the heart rate. Mason and colleagues, in 1984, first described the use of dobutamine infusion stress in combination with nuclear myocardial scintigraphy and reported a sensitivity of 94% and a specificity of 87% in detecting significant coronary artery disease. Pennel, in 1991, reported a 97% sensitivity and 80% specificity and Hays and colleagues in

1993 reported a 85% sensitivity and 90% specificity with the use of the dobutamine stress protocol.

The protocol involves starting the infusion at 5 to 10 micrograms/kg/min, with an increase in the infusion dosage by 5 micrograms/kg/min every 3 minutes. Blood pressure and 12 lead EKG recordings are obtained every 3 minutes. A maximum infusion dosage of up to 40 micrograms/kg/min has been reported (normal range 5 to 20 micrograms/kg/min) (Zanet). At the higher doses, Zanet reported a 78% incidence of side effects, including chest pain in 31%, palpitations in 29%, headache in 14%, flushing in 14%, and dyspnea in 14%. Dysrhythmias, including atrial fibrillation and nonsustained ventricular tachycardia, are also reported with the use of dobutamine. The radionuclide is injected when the end-point is reached. The end-points used are 1) angina pectoris 2) ischemic ST segment changes greater than 2 mV below baseline 3) greater than 85% of age-predicted heart rate 4) nonsustained ventricular tachycardia and 5) hypotension (Table 6). If the heart rate fails to rise adequately at dobutamine doses above 25 mcg/kg/min, the use of atropine sulfate at 0.5 to 1.0 mg intravenously has been helpful.

The effect of the dobutamine infusion will dissipate rapidly in 4 to 6 minutes, if side effects are noted. Volume repletion for hypotension and nitroglycerin for ongoing angina can be utilized. As noted above this protocol is suited for patients with asthma, bronchospasm, or allergy to Persantine.

Pitfalls in Interpreting NMS

The most common preventable potential error made in the interpretation of nuclear myocardial scans is to try to read a scan when the exercise level was insufficient to elicit an ischemic response (Table 7). As noted in the text of this paper, a minimum target level of 85% of the maximum predicted heart rate must be reached in order to allow the stress test to be considered adequate for interpretation. If a patient has no evidence of ischemia and is unable to exert to this level, it is far better to cancel the nuclear scan and reschedule the patient for pharmacologic stress testing either with dipyridamole/adenosine or with dobutamine.

On the other hand, if the amount of ischemia is so extensive as to be global, the uptake of radionuclide may appear homogenous due to software enhancement of the reduced counts throughout the myocardium. This phenomenon makes it difficult to identify the myocardium as being ischemic. In this setting, other clues need to be utilized, such as the presence of increased lung uptake and reversible

---

TABLE 7

Factors Adversely Affecting Sensitivity of Nuclear Perfusion Scans

1. **Single vessel coronary artery disease**
   a) Circumflex coronary artery branches or small distal obstructions
2. **Obstructed, but nonjeopardized, well-collateralized arteries**
3. **Low workloads on exercise**
4. **Heart rates less than 85% of maximum predicted for age with exercise**

---

cavitary dilatation on the planar scan, to make the correct interpretation. The same difficulty is encountered when anterior wall and inferior wall defects coexist on a short axis view, but are difficult to see on the vertical slices due to the computer software's enhancement of the two ischemic areas.

It has also been established that a zone of ischemia representing less than 5 grams of myocardium, approximately 1/20 the weight of the left ventricle, will not be detectable on a scintigram. This is particularly true in the evaluation of the left ventricular apex, which in some patients is only a few millimeters thick and results in an "apical slit" which is a normal finding and not representative of an ischemic zone.

Other reported causes for possible errors in interpretation have been in patients with complete left bundle branch block, where basal septal defects have been noted (Hirzel HO and colleagues, 1984).

Technical problems often arise that make the interpretation of scans more difficult (Botvinick and colleagues, 1980). The most common problems are due to soft tissue attenuation of the radionuclide counts by extracardiac structures such as breast tissue, liver, or diaphragm. Motion artifacts occurring during the acquisition of the raw data

can also give the appearance of perfusion defects. This stresses the importance of adequate supervision of the patient by the nuclear technologist during the data acquisition process. Improper processing of the raw data by the nuclear technologist can also lead to erroneous interpretation of a study, particularly if the slices are not accurately aligned to the ventricular cavity, as pointed out in a recent paper by Starksen and colleagues, where basal septal defects can be "created" by improper selection of the angle of the cuts (Figure 10).

It must again be stressed that incomplete redistribution at 4 hours may be interpreted as a fixed defect suggestive of an infarction, whereas additional acquisition of data at 24 hours may show a more complete redistribution of counts into a very ischemic zone of myocardium which is still viable. It is this attribute of ^{201}Tl to redistribute from non-ischemic to ischemic zones that makes it so useful.

Finally the presence of interobserver error has been found to be as high as 33% in the interpretation of equivocal studies, whereas there is only a 10%-15% interobserver variability in normal or clearly abnormal scan interpretations (Trobaugh and colleagues, 1978).

Positron Emission Tomography (PET)

Regional myocardial metabolic activity, as well as myocardial blood flow, can be best evaluated noninvasively through positron emission tomography (PET). The regional changes in the metabolism of various substrates as a result of ischemic injury can be accurately demonstrated by PET and allows the differentiation of viable vs. nonviable tissue. Metabolic studies with PET have been used as the "gold standard" for determination of myocardial viability. These metabolic abnormalities exist in stable and unstable coronary artery disease, in the early phases following an acute infarction, as well as following spontaneous or interventional revascu-

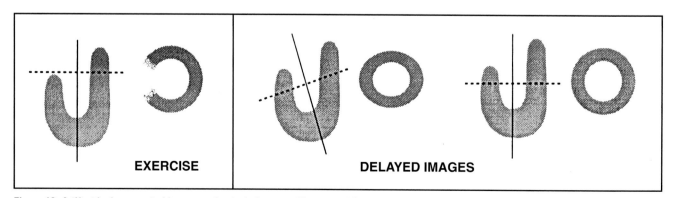

EXERCISE

DELAYED IMAGES

Figure 10. **Artifact lesions created by processing techniques.** – *(Courtesy of Starksen, et al)* – Image malalignment leading to inaccurate slice selection on the delayed images results in a false basal septal reversible defect. The drawing depicts the ventricle in long axis and short axis views, with the septum being on the left side of the images.

larization (Schelbert, 1989). The higher energy level (511Kev) of the photons counted with PET decreases the amount of soft tissue attenuation and allows better collimation which leads to better image resolution.

Distinct clinical patterns have emerged with the use of N-13 ammonia or rubidium-82 to determine regional blood flow and the use of F-18 2-deoxyglucose (FDG) for evaluation of glucose metabolism (Marshall and colleagues, 1983). Healthy myocardium takes up fatty acids as its main source of fuel, while ischemic myocardium uses glucose as its metabolic substrate. Studies have demonstrated that decreases in N-13 ammonia concentration can be associated with concomitant decreased, normal, or even increased FDG uptake. When this data is viewed from a functional perspective, the finding of decreased "blood-flow and glucose metabolism matches" corresponds to irreversibly injured (scarred) myocardium, and the presence of "blood-flow to glucose metabolism mismatches" corresponds to ischemic but viable myocardium. These studies have correlated the return of normal myocardial contractility following revascularization, in segments that were dyskinetic but "viable" by PET criteria preoperatively. PET has been shown to be more accurate than ^{201}Tl in predicting viability. Of partially reperfused defects by ^{201}Tl myocardial scintigraphy, 64% were shown to be normally viable by PET criteria, and 58% of fixed ^{201}Tl defects were found to be viable by PET criteria. Even modification of the ^{201}Tl myocardial scintigraphy protocol to assess late redistribution at 24 hours was less successful than PET in the identification of viable myocardium (Brunken and colleagues, 1988).

PET identified viability in 53% of "^{201}Tl fixed defects" at 24 hours and 61% viability if partial redistribution was noted at 24 hours by ^{201}Tl. It is readily apparent from these studies that PET would be extremely useful in determining the candidacy for revascularization procedures of patients with extensive previous ischemic injury. PET can also be utilized to differentiate between idiopathic congestive dilated cardiomyopathy and ischemic cardiomyopathy and may aid in selecting patients for revascularization procedures vs. cardiac transplantation. The myocardial blood flow and glucose metabolism has been shown to be normal in the patients with idiopathic congestive cardiomyopathy.

Schelbert and colleagues demonstrated in patients undergoing PTCA the rapid reversal of blood flow-metabolism mismatches following the intervention. On the other hand, improvement in segmental wall motion was delayed by 2 to 3 months, pointing out the danger of relying on the mobility of myocardial segments as an indication of viability shortly after revascularization procedures. It would appear that ^{201}Tl would be more predictive than echocardiography, although less sensitive than PET, in the identification of myocardial viability. PET's ability to assess myocardial viability accurately and noninvasively assures it an important role in the clinical decision making process for selection of patients for revascularization procedures, where this information cannot be ascertained by use of other diagnostic modalities. The expense of the PET equipment and a cyclotron to generate the positron emitting radionuclides, however, makes its widespread use impractical, particularly in today's cost-driven medical care environment.

To bring the above data into clinical focus, the following case histories will illustrate practical utility of nuclear cardiology in daily management of patients.

Case 1: Bundle Branch Block with Abnormal Treadmill

History

DB is a 76-year-old woman with a one year history of "spells" characterized by substernal pressure associated with shortness of breath and weakness; episodes are more related to emotional stress rather than physical exertion. The patient also notes feeling lightheaded with these episodes, but is not aware of any palpitations. She sleeps on 2 pillows and claims to walk 2 miles in divided walks each day.

Physical Exam

Examination reveals an elderly woman who is in no acute distress. Blood pressure was 132/90 mm Hg with a regular pulse of 66 beats per minute. Lungs are clear to percussion and auscultation; cardiac examination reveals no jugular venous distention and arterial upstroke is normal. No cardiomegaly is appreciated, and first and second heart sounds are normal. No S4 or S3 is heard. No ejection sound is present, and midsystolic murmur is noted at the left sternal border and base; no diastolic murmurs are heard.

EKG

EKG reveals a right bundle branch block pattern with secondary ST-T abnormalities. An initial treadmill stress test is carried out with the patient only completing 2.5 METs at a submaximal heart rate of only 64%. No chest pain or significant change in baseline ST-T abnormalities is precipitated by the treadmill stress test.

Echocardiogram

Normal left ventricular contractility pattern with slight left ventricular hypertrophy is noted on echo. Mild aortic valve sclerosis is noted, but no significant gradient is documented across the aortic valve by doppler study.

NMS

The patient was rescheduled for a pharmacologic stress test, because of her inability to reach 85% of her maximum predicted heart rate on treadmill stress testing, and myocardial imaging utilizing ^{201}Tl was carried out. A total dose of 35.1 mg of Persantine was infused intravenously over 4 minutes, followed by 3.0 mCi of ^{201}Tl. At the 8th minute of the test, aminophylline was given slowly intravenously at 25 mg/min for a two-minute interval to reverse the Persantine effect. The patient's heart rate rose from a baseline of 56 beats per minute to 84 beats per minute. Blood pressure at baseline was 120/80 and rose to 160/100 after the Persantine. Both the heart rate and blood pressure returned to baseline after the aminophylline infusion. The patient had no complaints of chest dis-

comfort or dyspnea during or following the test. No ST-T changes or dysrhythmias were noted; myocardial scintigraphy was then performed. The format for analysis consisted of planar images in the anterior and LAO views following stress and comparison views acquired at rest.

The planar images revealed normal lung uptake. No cavitary dilatation of left ventricle was noted. Symmetrical uptake of radionuclide was evident, with no perfusion defects identified.

SPECT images revealed uniform uptake of the radionuclide in the short axis, horizontal axis, and vertical axis. No perfusion defects were identified (Figure 11).

Clinical Outcome

The patient was taken off her nitroglycerin patches since no myocardial ischemia could be confirmed; she was maintained on her Cardene for hypertension control. This case illustrates the use of pharmacologic stress with myocardial scintigraphy to rule out significant coronary ischemia, in a patient with chest pains and resting ST-T abnormalities due to BBB who is unable to exercise to an adequate heart rate.

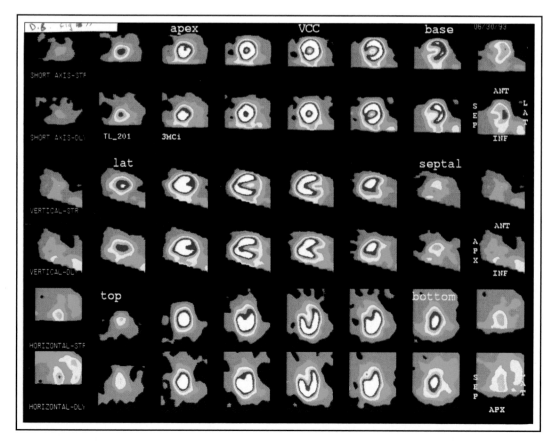

Figure 11. Patient DB: Normal perfusion myocardial scan in the face of RBBB and ST abnormalities.

Case 2: Resting ST-T Abnormalities on EKG and Family History of Coronary Heart Disease

History

SB is a 32-year-old woman with atypical chest pains that were non-exertional, but were of considerable concern to her because of a strong family history of coronary artery disease.

Physical Exam

BP 122/74 Pulse 68. Cardiopulmonary exam was within normal limits; no clicks, murmurs, rubs, or gallops were detected.

EKG

EKG revealed mild nonspecific ST-T abnormalities at rest which became more depressed (greater than 1 mV) on treadmill stress testing.

Echocardiography

Echocardiography demonstrated trivial mitral regurgitation which was not heard clinically. No myopathy was found on echocardiography to explain the ST-T abnormalities noted on the resting tracing.

Nuclear Myocardial Scintigraphy

Treadmill stress testing with ^{201}Tl myocardial scintigraphy was carried out. The patient's ST segments became depressed below the baseline level (> 1 mV), but she had no chest discomfort during or following exercise.

The nuclear myocardial scintigram revealed a small cardiac silhouette with exercise and no perfusion abnormalities were detected on either the planar or the SPECT scintigrams.

Clinical Outcome

The patient was reassured that her pains appeared to be non-cardiac and that no significant obstructive coronary disease was present.

Case 3: Effort Angina Pectoris with Normal Treadmill

History

WP is a 52-year-old single man with a 3-month history of exertional substernal chest pains associated with shortness of breath. He has never smoked, denies diabetes mellitus or hypertension, and claims a cholesterol check six months prior to his visit was OK. Medical history of his mother and father are not known.

Physical Exam

WP is a thin, well developed, white male in no acute distress. Blood pressure was 140/70; heart rate 72 per minute and regular, respirations 12 per minute. Jugular venous pressure was normal at 20 degrees elevation of the head of the bed, and carotids were 2+ and free of bruits. No thyromegaly was noted; lungs were clear to percussion and auscultation. Cardiac examination revealed no abnormal heaves and no cardiomegaly could be demonstrated. Heart tones were normal. No S4 or S3 was noted in the left lateral decubitus position, at the apex. Abdomen was free of tenderness or guarding. Extremities were free of edema and 2+ posterior tibialis pulsus were present bilaterally.

EKG

Resting electrocardiogram was normal. A treadmill stress test was carried out to a workload of 10 METS and a heart rate of 171 beats per minute, which represented greater than 100% of the maximum predicted heart rate for his age. The patient developed substernal chest pressure and dyspnea but no electrocardiographic (EKG) abnormalities (Figures 12, 13, 14).

NMS

Nuclear myocardial scintigraphy was then carried out with baseline resting planar and SPECT imaging after an injection of 3.0 mCi of ^{201}Tl, followed by pharmacologic stress with an intravenous Persantine infusion. Substernal chest pressure associated with nausea and vomiting was precipitated without any EKG evidence for ischemia at a peak heart rate of only 107 beats per minute (from a baseline heart rate of 80 beats per minute). The patient was given 30 mCi of ^{99m}Tc Sestamibi intravenously and repeat planar and SPECT imaging was carried out following the pharmacologic stress. Extensive reversible ischemia of the anteroseptal and apical segments of the left ventricle, extending to the inferior apical wall, was demonstrated (Figure 15).

Clinical Outcome

Subsequent coronary angiography revealed a critical 95% proximal left anterior descending coronary artery (LAD) obstruction, involving a moderate sized first diagonal branch. Apical segment of the LAD was receiving retrograde collateral filling from the dominant right coronary artery (RCA), which was free of any significant atherosclerosis.

Because the very proximal location of the LAD obstruction is associated with a 50% restenosis rate following percutaneous coronary angioplasty and

411

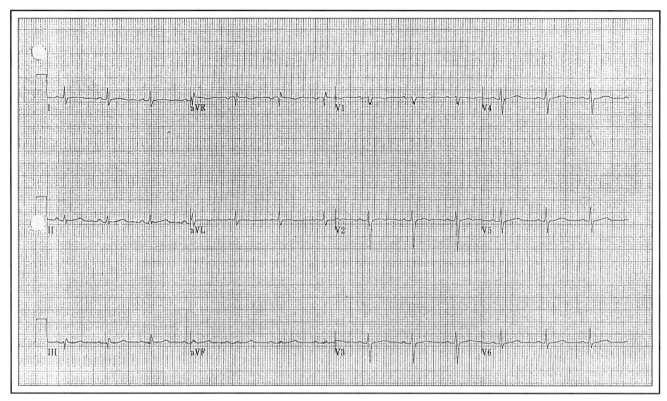

Figure 12

Figures 12, 13, 14 – WP: Baseline EKG, Peak Exercise EKG, and Post Exercise EKG are normal in the presence of angina pectoris.

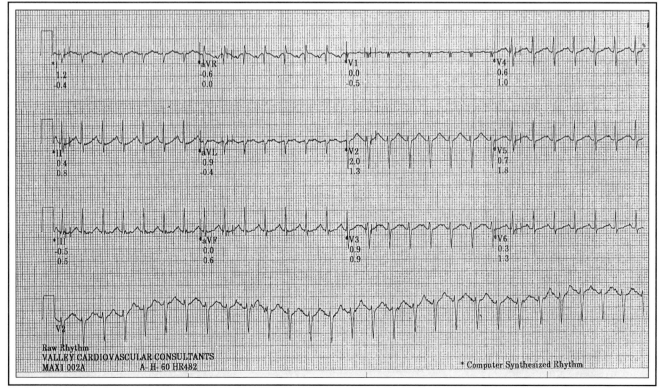

Figure 13

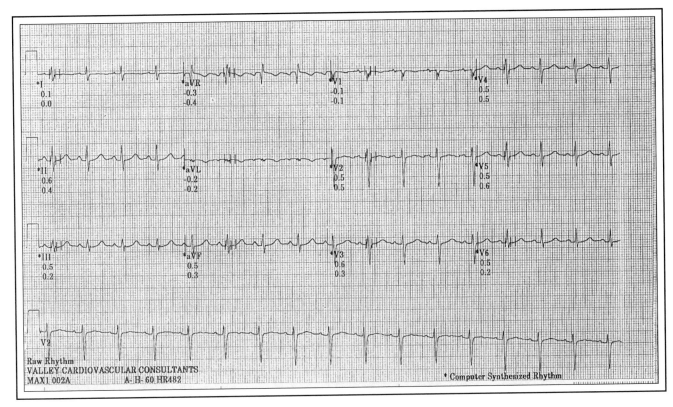

Figure 14

the risk of main left coronary artery occlusion and possible dissection during balloon inflation, the patient was referred for surgical revascularization with a left internal mammary graft to his LAD and a saphenous vein graft to his diagonal branch. Subsequent post-operative treadmill stress testing failed to precipitate any symptoms of chest discomfort or EKG evidence of ischemia.

This case clearly demonstrates the utility of nuclear myocardial scintigraphy in establishing the diagnosis of ischemia in patients with normal treadmill stress tests but with symptoms that are suggestive of effort angina.

Case 4: Absence of Angina with Abnormal Treadmill

History

JA is a 60-year-old man, with insulin dependent diabetes mellitus, who was referred by his internist for treadmill stress testing with a history of progressive fatigue on exertion. He denied any associated chest or arm discomfort, and had a history of hypertension and dyslipidemia. His total cholesterol was 208, triglycerides were 283, LDL was 121, and his HDL was low at 30 mg per deciliter. He smoked for 5 pack years, stopping at age 34. There was no family history of coronary artery disease.

Physical Exam

Exam revealed an overweight, alert, white male with a BP of 152/96 on the left arm and 150/98 on the right arm. Pulse was 75 and regular, lungs were clear, and cardiac exam revealed the left border of cardiac dullness to be 10 cm to the left of the mid-sternal line. Heart tones were normal and no S4 or S3 was noted. No murmurs were heard and abdomen was free of bruits. Peripheral pulses were symmetrical and 2-3+. No bruit was noted over the femoral arteries and no edema was present.

EKG

Resting electrocardiogram revealed only borderline T changes in AVL, but otherwise appeared normal. A symptom limited treadmill stress test was carried out, with the patient stopping due to fatigue at a workload of 7 METS and a heart rate of 137 beats per minute, representing 86% of his maximum predicted heart rate. Non-diagnostic upsloping ST segments were noted at peak exercise, with "evolutionary ST-T" abnormalities developing in the recovery phase, though these never exceeded 1 mV of ST depression. Blood pressure rose from 140/90 to 200/100.

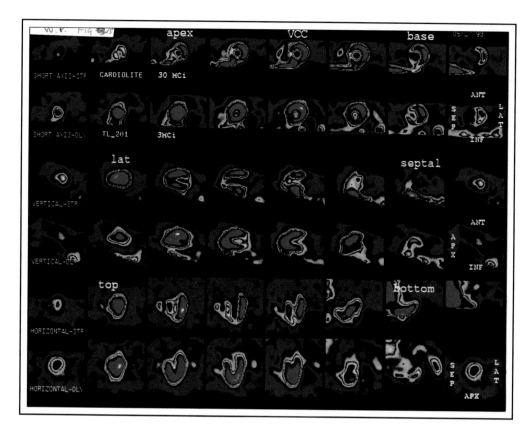

Figure 15. Patient WP: Abnormal myocardial perfusion SPECT scan, utilizing dual isotope technique, with normal EKG after persantine pharmacologic stress.

An anteroseptal perfusion defect involving the apex is seen following pharmacologic stress. Normal perfusion of the myocardium is noted on the rest study. This is diagnostic of reversible ischemia despite the normal EKG present during and following the pharmacologic stress with Persantine.

NMS

Because of his coronary risk factors and the suggestive treadmill result and symptoms, a repeat treadmill stress test with nuclear myocardial scintigraphy was carried out. ^{201}Tl was injected at peak exercise and planar and SPECT imaging was carried out. Four hours later, the patient returned for redistribution planar images and an additional 1 mCi of ^{201}Tl was administered prior to the acquisition of redistribution SPECT images. Planar stress images revealed normal lung uptake with left ventricular cavitary dilatation being apparent on both the LAO and anterior stress views. Reversible perfusion defects were present over the anteroseptal and inferior walls. SPECT images confirmed the anteroseptal and inferior wall perfusion defects which reversed on the redistribution images and suggested ischemia involving at least two vessels (Figure 16).

Coronary Angiography

The patient underwent cardiac catheterization and coronary angiography and was found to have left ventricular hypertrophy with a normal ejection fraction of 81%. The main left coronary artery had only mild irregularities, and left anterior descending (LAD) coronary artery gave off a moderate sized first diagonal branch, which had a 90% obstruction near its origin. A second diagonal branch of moderate size was given off and then the LAD became totally obstructed. Right to left collaterals were seen to fill the diffusely sclerotic LAD. The circumflex coronary artery had a large obtuse marginal branch which had a 50% to 60% obstruction, while the right coronary artery (RCA) had 60% to 70% obstructive lesions in its proximal third, and a 50-60% tubular narrowing before the distal bifurcation into the posterior descending branch and the distal inferolateral branch. The inferolateral branch had a 50% to 69% obstruction shortly after its origin.

Clinical Outcome

The patient was advised to undergo coronary revascularization surgery, but elected to try medical management. He was treated with vigorous dietary counseling, as well as placed on Mevacor. The Mevacor dose was gradually raised to 40 mg per day. He was also maintained on Cardizem CD 240 mg per day and ASA 80 mg per day, and did not tolerate topical nitrates, due to headaches. He continued to use Humulin Insulin for control of his diabetes mellitus. His lipid panel revealed a cholesterol of 161, triglycerides of 142, LDL of 97 and an HDL of 36; he did well clinically and had no angina while exercising on a treadmill.

414

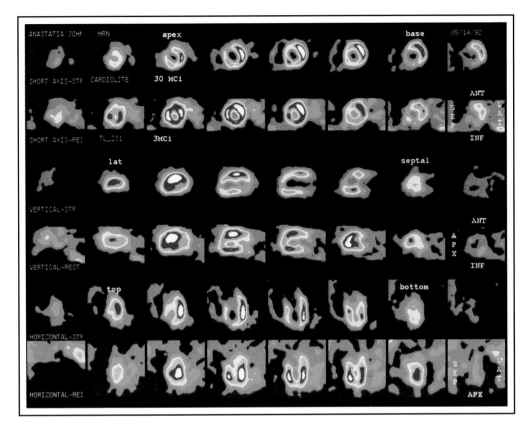

Figure 16. Patient JA: Extensive ischemia is documented involving the anteroseptal, apical, and invferior walls of the left ventricle, utilizing a dual-isotope technique, in the presence of ischemic ST changes on the EKG but in the absence of any complaints of angina.

Case 5: Chest Pain and Normal Treadmill Following PTCA

History

LS is a 50-year-old white woman who was referred for treadmill stress testing with a 3-month history of angina. Her treadmill stress test was negative for ischemia, but she developed classical symptoms of angina pectoris on exertion.

NMS

Thallium myocardial scintigraphy following stress was carried out and disclosed a large reversible perfusion defect over the anteroapical wall of the left ventricle, diagnostic of ischemia (Figure 17). Coronary risk factors included a family history of CAD and BP of 160/80. No other significant findings were present in the history or the physical examination; the patient did not smoke.

Coronary Angiography

Coronary angiography demonstrated a 90% obstruction of the left anterior descending coronary artery (LAD), proximal to the takeoff of the first diagonal branch. A successful PTCA of the lesion was carried out, with only a 20% residual obstruction noted at conclusion of the procedure.

Followup Myocardial Scintigraphy

The patient began to note recurrence of her symptoms of angina with exertion. A repeat Thallium myocardial perfusion scan following stress was carried out; again the patient developed angina with exertion but no EKG evidence of ischemia.

Her myocardial perfusion scintigram, however, showed unequivocal evidence of reversible ischemia of the anteroapical wall, suggesting restenosis at the PTCA site.

Clinical Outcome

Based on findings of demonstrable ischemia at the time of the initial and followup myocardial perfusion scans, the patient was advised to undergo cardiac catheterization leading to percutaneous coronary angioplasty on each occasion. The treadmill stress tests were not helpful by themselves in establishing the diagnosis.

Case 6: Idiopathic Cardiomyopathy with Reduced Ejection Fraction

History

MH is a 54-year-old woman presenting to her

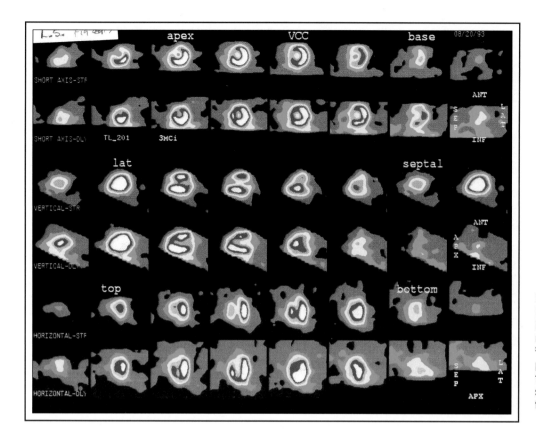

Figure 17. Patient LS: Reversible anteroseptal ischemia, involving the apex, noted on SPECT study with ^{201}Tl, in the presence of angina pectoris but no EKG evidence for ischemia. Patient subsequently had a PTCA of the proximal LAD.

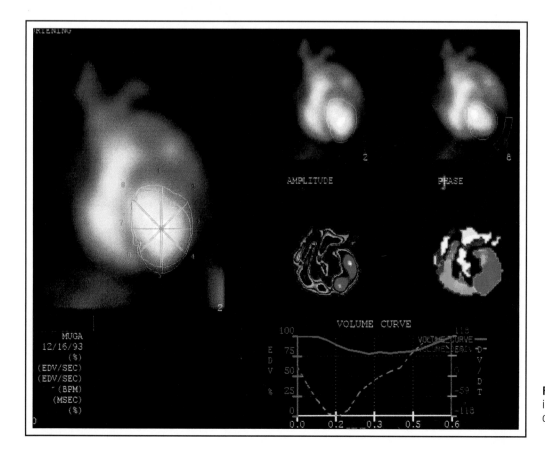

Figure 18. MUGA study in patient with idiopathic cardiomyopathy (E.F.=22%).

internist with a two-week history of fatigue, progressive dyspnea on exertion, development of paroxysms of nocturnal dyspnea and a 20-pound weight gain.

Physical Exam

Examination revealed a slightly overweight white woman with a resting pulse of 114, blood pressure of 124/70 bilaterally, and a respiratory rate of 32 per minute. Jugular venous distention was noted with an estimated elevation of the venous pressure to 14 cm above the right atrium; lungs were clear to percussion; auscultation and cardiac rhythm was regular. No heaves were noted. Left border of cardiac dullness was displaced 12 cm to the left of the midsternal line, and an S_4 and S_3 gallop were audible at apex. Faint holosystolic murmur was noted at apex.

Echocardiogram

Echocardiogram confirmed a severely dilated cardiomyopathy with a reduced ejection fraction of 17%. Moderately severe (3+) mitral regurgitation was seen on color flow doppler exam.

MUGA Study

Baseline MUGA ejection fraction study was carried out to enable subsequent documentation of clinical improvement following start of preload and afterload reduction therapy (Figure 18).

Clinical Outcome

The patient responded dramatically to diuretic and ace inhibitor therapy, with a 12-pound weight loss in the first 72 hours of hospitalization. Her venous pressure was normal, and only an S_4 gallop was audible at apex the day of discharge. A repeat MUGA ejection fraction will be carried out after three months of medical therapy.

Selected Reading

1. AHA/ACC Task Force Report. Guidelines for clinical use of cardiac radionuclide imaging. *Circ* 91:1278-1303, 1995.
2. Baily IK, Come PC, Kelly DT, et al.: Thallium-201 myocardial perfusion imaging in aortic valve stenosis. *Am J Cardiol* 40:889, 1977.
3. Beller GA, Prohost GM: Mechanism for Tl-201 redistribution after transient myocardial ischemia. *Circ* 56:141, 1977.
4. Beller GA, Watson DO, Pohost GM: Kinetics of thallium distribution and redistribution: Clinical applications in sequential myocardial imaging, in Straps H.W., Pint B. (ed.): Cardiovascular Nuclear Medicine. St Louis, *C.V. Mosby Co*, pp.243-252, 1979.
5. Blumgart HL, Weiss S.: Studies on the velocity of blood flow. II. The velocity of blood flow in normal resting individuals, and a critique of the method used. *J Clin Invest* 4:15-31, 1972.
6. Bonow RO, Berman DS, Gibbons RJ, et al: Cardiac positron emission tomography. A report for health professionals from the committee on advanced cardiac imaging and technology of the council on clinical cardiology, AHA. *Circ* 84(1):447, 1991.
7. Botvonick EH et al: A consideration of factors affecting the diagnostic accuracy of Thallium-201 myocardial perfusion scintigraphy in detecting coronary artery disease. *Semin Nucl Med* 10:247, 1980.
8. Botvinick EH, Dunn RF, Hattner RS, et al: A consideration of factor affecting the diagnostic accuracy of thallium-201 myocardial perfusion scintigraphy in detecting coronary artery disease. *Sem Nucl Med* 10:247-257, 1980.
9. Boucher CA et al: Increased lung uptake of Tl-201 during exercise myocardial imaging; Clinical hemodynamic and angiographic implications in patients with coronary artery disease. *AJC* 46:189, 1980.
10. Boucher CA, Brewster DC, Darling RC et al: Determination of cardiac risk by dipyridamole-thallium imaging before peripheral vascular surgery. *NEJM* 312:389, 1985.
11. Brunken RC et al: Positron Tomography detects glucose metabolism in segments with 24-hour tomographic Thallium defect (abstr). *Circ* 78: suppl II;91, 1988.
12. Diamond GA, Forrester JS: Analysis of probability as an aid in clinical diagnosis of coronary artery disease. *NEJM* 300:1350-1355, 1979.
13. Dilsizian V, Rocco TP, Freedman NMT, et al: Enhanced detection of ischemic but viable myocardium by reinjection of thallium after stress-redistribution imaging. *NEJM* 323:141-146, 1990.
14. Early PJ: Radiation detection. Principles and Practices of Nuclear Medicine. *CV Mosby Company*, pp 207-287, 1985.
15. Francisco DA, Collins SM, Go RT, et al: Tomographic Thallium-201 myocardial perfusion scintigram after maximal coronary artery vasodilation with intravenous dipyridamole. *Circ* 66:370-379, 1982.
16. Garcia E, Maddahi J, et al: Space/time quantitation of thallium-201 myocardial scintigraphy. *J N Med* 22: 309-317, 1981.
17. Gould KL: Noninvasive assessment of coronary stenoses by myocardial perfusion imaging during pharmacologic coronary vasodilatation: Physiologic basis and experimental validation. *Am J Card* 41:267, 1978.
18. Gresnahan JF, Bresnahan DR, et al: Measurement of myocardium at risk by technetium-99m sestamibi: correlation with coronary angiography. *JACC:* 19:67-73, 1992.
19. Hamilton GW, Narahara KA, Yee H: Myocardial imaging with thallium-201: Effect of cardiac drugs on myocardial images and absolute tissue distribution. *J N Med* 19:10-16, 1978.
20. Hirzel HO, Senn M. Nuesch K, et al: Anormal thallium-201 scintigram in left bundle branch block. *AJC* 53:764-769, 1984.
21. Ideker RE, Behar VS, Wagner GS et al: Evaluation of asynergy as indicator of myocardial fibrosis. *Circ* 57:715-725, 1978.
22. Kiat H, Berman DS, Maddahi J, et al: Late reversibility of tomographic myocardial thallium-201 defects: an accurate marker of myocardial viability. *JACC* 12:1456-1463, 1988.
23. Kiat H, Germano G, Van Train K, et al: Quantitative assessment of photon spillover in simultaneous rest ^{201}Tl /stress ^{99m}Tc sestamibi dual isotope myocardial perfusion SPECT. *J N Med* 33:854-855, 1992.
24. Kushner FG, Okada RD, Kirshenbaum HD et al: Lung thallium-201 uptake after stress testing in patients with coronary artery disease. *Circ* 63:341, 1981.

25. Lebowitz E, Green MW, et al: Thallium-201 for medical use. *I J Nuc Med.* 16:151, 1975.

26. Lee KL, Pryor DB, Pieper KS, et al: Prognostic value of radionuclide angiography in medically treated patients with coronary artery disease: A comparison with clinical and catheterization variables. *Circ* 82:1705, 1990.

27. Maddahi J, Garcia EV, Berman DS, et al: Improved noninvasive assessment of coronary artery disease by quantitative analysis of regional stress myocardial distribution and washout of thallium-201. *Circ* 64:924, 1981.

28. Maddahi J, Rodrigues E, Berman D: Assessment of myocardial perfusion by single photon agents. Chapter 7. The technology of cardiovascular imaging. pp245-285.

29. Mahmarian JJ, Boyce TM, Goldberg RK, et al: Quantitative exercise thallium-201 Single Photon Emission Computed Tomography for the enhanced diagnosis of ischemic heart disease. *JACC* 15:318-329, 1990.

30. Marshall RC, et al: Identification and differentiation of resting myocardial ischemia and infarction with positron computed tomography F-18 labeled fluorodeoxyglucose and N-13 ammonia. *Circ.* 67:766, 1983.

31. Mason JR, Palac RT, Freeman ML, et al: Thallium scintigraphy during dobutamine infusion: nonexercise-dependent screening test for coronary disease. *Am H J* 107:481,1984.

32. Massie BM, Botvonick EH, Brundage BH: Correlation of thallium-201 scintigrams with coronary anatomy: factors affecting region by region sensitivity. *Am J Card* 44:616, 1979.

33. Parker J.A., Treves S.: Radionuclide detection, localization and quantitation of intracardiac shunts and shunts between the great arteries. *Prog Card Dis* 10:121-150. 1977.

34. Pennell DJ, Underwood SR, Swanton RH, et al: Dobutamine thallium myocardial perfusion tomography. *JACC* 18:1471, 1991.

35. Pohost GM, Zir LM, Moore RH, et al: Differentiation of transiently ischemic from infarcted myocardium by serial imaging after a single dose of thallium-201. *Circulation* 55:294, 1977.

36. Rozanski A, Berman DS: Efficacy of cardiovascular medicine exercise studies. *Sem Nuc Med* 2:104-120, 1987.

37. Schachner ER et al: Effect of diphenhydantoin (Dilantin) on Tl 201 uptake. *J Nuc Med* 21;57, 1980.

38. Schelbert HR: Myocardial ischemia and clinical applications of positron emission tomography. *Am J C* 64:46, 1989.

39. Schelbert HR, Ingwall J, Sybers H, et al: Uptake of Tc-99m pyrophosphate and calcium in irreversibly damaged myocardium. *Cir Res* 39:860-868, 1976.

40. Sharpe DN, Botvonick EH, Shames DM, et al: Noninvasive diagnosis of right ventricular infarction. *Circ* 57:483-490, 1978.

41. Shaw L, Miller DD, Kong BA, et al: Determination of preoperative cardiac risk by adenosine thallium-201 myocardial imaging. *AHJ* 124:861, 1992.

42. Stalzberg, J: Dilatation of the left ventricular cavity on stress thallium scan as an indicator of ischemic disease. *Clin N Med* 5:289, 1980.

43. Starksen NF, O'Connel W, Dae MW, et al: Basal interventricular septal thallium-201 defects: real or artifact? *Clin N Med.* 18:291-297, 1992.

44. Trobaugh GB, Wackers FT et al: Thallium-201 myocardial imaging: An interinstitutional study of observer variability. *J Nuc M* 19:359, 1978.

45. Verani MS: Thallium-201 Myocardial Scintigraphy: An Overview. *Clin N Med* 8:276-287, 1983.

46. Verani MS, Mahmarian JJ, Hixon JB, et al: Diagnosis of coronary artery disease by controlled coronary vasodilation with adenosine and thallium-201 scintigraphy in patients unable to exercise. *Circ* 82:80-87, 1990.

47. Weich HF, Strauss HW, Pitt B: Extraction of Tl-201 by the myocardium. *Circ* 56:188, 1977.

48. Yang LD, Berman DS, Kiat H, et al: Frequency of late reversibility in SPECT thallium-201 stress-redistribution studies. *JACC* 15:334-340, 1990.

49. Zaret BL, Wackers FJT, Soufer R: Nuclear Cardiology. In:Braunwald E. (ed) *Heart Disease: a textbook in cardiovascular medicine. 4th ed Vol 1.* Philadelphia: *W.B. Saunders,* 276-311, 1992.

CHAPTER 19

Diagnostic and Therapeutic Cardiac Catheterization and Coronary Angiography

Bruce Genovese, M.D. and Richard A. Walsh, M.D.

In the mid-nineteenth century, Claude Bernard performed experiments which form the foundation of modern cardiac catheterization techniques; for example, he introduced probes into the canine heart through the jugular vein and the carotid artery. Soon after, Chauveau and Marey recorded intracavitary pressure tracings. The ensuing years saw other developments in hemodynamics and physiology, including the principle of cardiac output measurement by Fick.

However, it was not until the report in 1929 by Werner Otto Forssmann of self-catheterization of the right atrium that these experimental principles could be applied to people. Forssmann, in his training years, performed a venous cutdown on his left arm and advanced a catheter to the right atrium, documenting the procedure with an x-ray. Subsequent rapid progress in the technique of intravascular access and data recording was made by Dickinson Richards, Andre Cournand, Lewis Dexter, and others into the 1940s. Refinements of the technique occurred during the following two decades, but the major modern development resulting in the widespread use of catheterization was the technique of coronary angiography fortuitously developed by Sones and later by Judkins.

While development of catheterization techniques was initially stimulated by scientific inquisitiveness and subsequently by the desire for diagnostic insight, the popularization of the procedure resulted from the advent of therapeutic technique, which made possible use of data obtained for the benefit of the patient. This remains the guiding principle in use of cardiac catheterization - that the

technique be used not just for its diagnostic value, but to guide therapy.

CARDIAC PEARL

It is always interesting to use the "retrospectoscope" in the analysis of present day situations, procedures, and events. The development and clinical application of cardiac radiology has been exciting and remarkable. An important application is today's coronary bypass surgery. This is now recognized as one of the outstanding advances in the field of medicine that has evolved in the past several decades. Just think each day of the thousands of patients all over the world who are receiving benefits from this surgery. Skilled surgeons are able to perform this almost miraculous surgery with a mortality rate of approximately 1% to 2%. Certainly, coronary bypass surgery is "here to stay." Unquestionably, it has improved the quality of life in appropriately selected patients and, in addition, has increased longevity.

It is, of course, obvious that without coronary arteriography, and the specific and accurate techniques of identifying coronary lesions, coronary bypass surgery, as we know it today, would not have developed.

W. Proctor Harvey, M.D.

Indications for Cardiac Catheterization

Cardiac catheterization is a technique intended to confirm and refine a diagnosis previously made on clinical grounds and through use of noninvasive techniques. Risk of catheterization is relatively small, but a definite mortality and morbidity rate exists, and a certain degree of patient discomfort is involved in the procedure. Also, catheterization is a relatively costly procedure in comparison to other forms of diagnostic evaluation. As a result, catheterization should not be employed as a "screening" procedure in patients without suspected significant underlying heart disease.

Occasionally, a definite pre-catheterization diagnosis cannot be made, but at least a general notion of the type of information sought is necessary to adequately plan the procedure. Unsuspected associated findings may also be found during a procedure intended to confirm another diagnosis. The primary indication for the test remains confirmation of a suspected diagnosis and it should not be employed in the manner of a "fishing expedition."

An additional indication for the procedure is to quantify severity of disease. With availability of various noninvasive studies to confirm clinical diagnoses, this may be said to be the primary indication. This is true both from the hemodynamic and angiographic standpoints. As a result, catheterization should generally be reserved for those patients in whom a therapeutic as well as diagnostic decision needs to be made.

It is imperative that indications for any particular catheterization be understood prior to undertaking the procedure. This is important from the standpoint of weighing the risks vs. the potential benefits to the patient. It is also necessary in order to adequately plan the study, as cardiac catheterization is not a "generic" procedure; the technique is tailored to each particular case. Careful thought about and screening for possible associated abnormalities other than the primary diagnostic concern should be undertaken to be sure that all the appropriate data are collected at the time of the study. If a procedure is planned to evaluate the severity of coronary artery disease, for example, an adequate assessment of the severity of coexistent aortic valve disease may not be made if this abnormality is not suspected and planned for as part of the procedure. Cardiac catheterization is an extremely valuable tool in the diagnosis and evaluation of the severity of heart disease. It should be employed in a well-integrated plan in the management of a patient, with realization of its risks and limitations.

Technique of Cardiac Catheterization

Catheterization studies are carried out in specialized facilities, usually in a hospital. The generally accepted requirements for such facilities have been described by national bodies and include ade-quate hemodynamic and electrocardiographic monitoring, fluoroscopic and cineangiographic capability, and adequate safety and emergency treatment equipment. A specially trained staff, including technical, radiologic, and nursing personnel should be available. Adequate post-procedure care and monitoring must also be available as many of the complications which may occur develop in this period. While a significant proportion of procedures are performed on an outpatient basis, use of laboratories which are not physically associated with an inpatient facility remains controversial. Though uncommon, complications which require inpatient monitoring or operative intervention do occur and immediate access to the hospital setting (either through geographic proximity or reliable, monitored, rapid transport) is needed. Likewise, the role of mobile laboratories which visit institutions intermittently is unclear. It may not be possible to maintain adequate volume (see below) and experienced personnel in this setting to insure that safe and technically adequate studies can be performed.

In general, two types of data are accumulated during catheterization procedures, hemodynamic and angiographic. Hemodynamic data include measurement of pressure and cardiac output from which further calculations can be made. As a result, pressure gradients, valve areas, intracardiac shunt determinations, and other parameters can also be derived. Pressures are generally measured using fluid-filled catheters inserted into appropriate chambers and vessels and connected to a transducer. Using a Wheatstone bridge, variations in pressure transmitted to the transducer are converted into electrical potentials, which are then displayed by an appropriate amplifier. Intrinsic to this system is some element of error related to time lag of pressure transmission from the tip of the catheter back to the transducer, damping of the wave form, and catheter motion artifact. There is also a need for careful positioning of the transducer and "zeroing" of the baseline which, if not carefully performed, can lead to errors in measurement.

Some laboratories make use of manometer-tipped catheters to eliminate some of these sources of error and obtain more precise data. This technique presently is used primarily in the research setting. While use of the standard system is adequate in the clinical setting, careful attention to detail in its use is required in order to obtain accurate data.

Right Heart Catheterization

Catheterization of the right heart is accomplished through venous access from either a

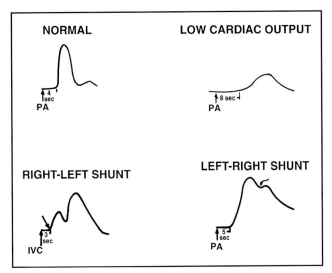

Figure 1. Green Dye Curves. Injection in the pulmonary artery or inferior vena cava (as noted) with peripheral arterial sampling. The appearance time is delayed in patients with low cardiac output. Early appearance is noted in right to left shunting when dye is injected proximal to the shunt. Early recirculation is noted with left to right shunting.

brachial, subclavian, or femoral vessel. While a cut-down and venotomy can be performed using the upper extremity, the most common approach is some modification of the Seldinger technique. In this method, the vessel is entered with a needle (after administration of appropriate anesthetic) of sufficient caliber to accept a guidewire of small caliber. The guidewire is inserted into the vessel when adequate entry has been insured (by the character of blood return) and advanced several centimeters. The needle is then removed and a small (2mm-3mm) incision in the skin is made (if not performed previously) at site of entry. Hemostasis is obtained with manual pressure throughout. A sheath (usually with a sideport to enable flushing) is then passed over the wire into the vein using a twisting motion and countertraction on the wire. The wire (and a dilator which is usually part of the sheath assembly) is then removed and the sheath flushed with heparinized saline.

With venous access established, an appropriate right heart catheter is then advanced under fluoroscopic visualization to the right atrium. A variety of catheters can be used, but the most common is the balloon-tipped variety *(Swan-Ganz)*. This catheter can be "floated" with the balloon inflated to the heart easily without the need for much manipulation. Usually, a multilumen model is used with the capability of being used for thermodilution cardiac output determinations.

The pressures in the right atrium, right ventricle, and pulmonary artery are measured and recorded. Blood samples for oxygen saturation can be obtained in each position with both fluoroscopic and hemodynamic confirmation of location. If an intracardiac shunt is suspected, an attempt to cross the anatomic defect should also be made. Once in the pulmonary artery, a measurement of pulmonary capillary wedge pressure is made either by advancing the catheter to the "wedge" position (thus occluding a smaller divisional vessel) or inflating the balloon and advancing the catheter to occlude a larger branch vessel ("pulmonary artery occluded pressure"). The pressure obtained in this position is the reflected pulmonary venous pressure which generally indicates the left atrial pressure.

In most laboratories, cardiac output determinations are made using the thermodilution principle in the right-sided circulation. Cold or room temperature indicator is injected into the right atrium through one lumen of the catheter and the temperature change is sensed by a thermocouple in the pulmonary artery. A specialized computer attached to the thermocouple calculates the cardiac output by sensing the time of the temperature change and constructs an output curve.

In addition, cardiac output determinations can also be made by the *Fick principle* (often considered the "gold standard"). Oxygen consumption is determined by determining the difference between the oxygen content of room air and that of expired air which is collected from the subject. Arteriovenous oxygen difference is calculated by subtracting the oxygen content of mixed venous blood (sampled in the pulmonary artery) from post-pulmonary capillary blood (sampled in the left ventricle or aorta). Then using the Fick equation:

$$\text{Cardiac Output} = \frac{\text{Oxygen Consumption}}{\text{arteriovenous oxygen difference}}$$

cardiac output is calculated. This can then be corrected for body surface area to determine the cardiac index.

Indocyanine green has been used as an indicator to calculate cardiac output (in a similar fashion to the thermodilution method). The dye is injected in the pulmonary artery and arterial blood is withdrawn through a densitometer to sense its appearance in the periphery. A cardiac output curve is thus inscribed and a numeric value can be calculated using a variant of the Fick principle. Early appearance of a recirculation "bump" on the curve is also helpful in determining the presence of intracardiac shunts (Figure 1).

Bedside catheterization of the right heart for the purpose of managing patients in a critical care unit can also be performed. Because of the need to maintain these catheters for several days, access is usually gained by introduction in the brachial, subclavian, or internal jugular vein. The femoral vein is avoided because of the possibility of triggering deep venous thrombosis. Balloon-tipped flotation catheters are used exclusively in this setting. Bedside monitoring of pressure, recording of wave forms, and determinations of cardiac outputs can be made on a serial basis in this way. The fidelity of the hemodynamic measurements is usually somewhat reduced, however, due to the nature of bedside amplification equipment.

Endomyocardial biopsy can be carried out through sheaths introduced into either the femoral or internal jugular vein. A small biopsy tome is introduced through a specialized sheath and guided to the right ventricle. Samples of small amounts of endocardium and myocardium are obtained in various positions, taking care to avoid the tricuspid apparatus.

Angiography of right-sided structures (with late demonstration of the left heart as well) can also be performed (see below). Demonstration of right-sided inflow, right atrium and ventricle, and pulmonary artery structure is thus possible.

Left Heart Catheterization

Generally, left heart catheterization is performed utilizing a femoral approach. This is true because of the ease of this method when compared with the brachial approach as well as the more ready performance of therapeutic maneuvers. The brachial approach is usually reserved for those patients with difficult femoral access (related to iliofemoral vascular disease, recent surgical intervention, massive obesity, or local cutaneous problems).

Access to the femoral artery is obtained by *Seldinger technique* (as described above). In most cases, a sheath is used and catheters are introduced through the sheath and passed up the iliac artery, the descending aorta, and around the aortic arch using a guidewire. Alternatively, the catheter can be introduced over the guidewire directly into the artery without use of a sheath. In either situation, a pigtail catheter is used for pressure measurement and angiography in the ascending aorta and left ventricle (although occasionally other catheters are used because of difficulty encountered crossing the aortic valve). The left ventricle is entered by passing the catheter (with or without the help of the guidewire) retrograde across the aortic valve. This is accomplished easily in most cases by causing the catheter to bend back on itself in the proximal aorta, advancing it at the level of the valve, and then withdrawing it. In patients

with dilated aortic roots or aortic stenosis, manipulation of the catheter with the guidewire protruding from the tip may be necessary to cross the valve.

Careful positioning of the catheter in the left ventricle is important to prevent ectopy and assure adequate angiographic technique. Pressures are recorded in the left ventricle prior to angiography in order to assure that no hemodynamic changes occur as a result of the injection of contrast material (which can have several effects: increasing intravascular volume, decreasing peripheral resistance, and diminishing left ventricular contractility). If mitral stenosis is suspected, simultaneous measurement of pulmonary capillary wedge pressure and left ventricular pressure is made. If aortic stenosis is suspected, then simultaneous measurement of left ventricular and aortic pressure (using two catheters, a double lumen pigtail catheter, or a peripheral arterial pressure line with appropriate correction for the increased pulse pressure in the smaller peripheral vessels compared to the central aorta) is made.

Two other methods of left heart catheterization are used less commonly. The brachial approach is employed frequently when access through the iliofemoral vessel is difficult (or sometimes as the operator's choice). Traditionally, the brachial artery is isolated by performing a cutdown just above the antecubital fossa. An anterior arteriotomy is performed and the appropriate catheter is passed to the level of the ascending aorta and left ventricle. A pigtail catheter can be used for the pressure measurements and angiography by employing a guidewire to straighten the tip, but "straight" catheters are also used. Following left heart catheterization and angiography the arteriotomy and then the antecubital cutdown are closed.

An alternative method is to obtain access to the brachial artery by use of a sheath in a similar fashion to the technique used for the femoral approach. This obviates the need for a cutdown and arteriotomy with the attendant risk of infection. Because there is less supporting connective tissue surrounding the brachial artery, obtaining adequate hemostasis with the percutaneous brachial approach is more difficult and requires extra attention.

Catheterization of the left heart using the *transseptal approach* is a third method. This approach is often used when there is a mechanical aortic valve prosthesis or as a part of balloon valvotomy for mitral stenosis. In this technique, the right femoral vein is entered by needle puncture percutaneously and a guidewire is advanced up the inferior vena cava to the right atrium and then the superior vena cava. A catheter or long sheath is then advanced over the wire and the wire is withdrawn. A long, specially constructed needle with a curved tip and an arrow at the proximal end indicating the direction of the needle tip is then advanced through the catheter or sheath (with the needle tip just inside). The entire assembly is then withdrawn into the right atrium (over the protrusion of the aorta) and can usually be seen to engage the foramen ovale (with the indicator arrow held at the "4 o'clock" position). With continuous pressure monitoring and under fluoroscopic control, the needle is then advanced until a left atrial wave form is noted. Sampling of blood for oxygen saturation is then carried out to confirm left atrial position.

The catheter, or sheath, and needle are then advanced together until they are positioned in the mid-atrium. The needle is then withdrawn and the catheter (or a catheter passed through the sheath) is then used for pressure measurements and oxygen saturation sampling in the left atrium. The catheter is then advanced across the mitral valve to the left ventricle where pressures are measured and angiography is performed. The apparatus is then withdrawn across the septum and removed from the femoral vein.

In addition to hemodynamic measurements, angiography is performed using catheters placed as described above. Cineangiography of the right atrium, right ventricle, and pulmonary artery are performed using catheters with multiple side holes and often with a balloon tip. The catheter is connected to an injector which can be set to deliver a specific amount of contrast material (usually in the range of 30cc-50cc) in a specified period of time (usually about 3 seconds). A record is made on videotape and usually on 35mm x-ray motion picture film at a speed of 60 frames per second. However, many laboratories now store images on high resolution videotape or optical discs instead of film. When injection of contrast material is made in the right heart, a levophase of contrast opacification can be recorded as the material transits through the pulmonary circulation and to the left heart structures.

Similarly, angiography of the left ventricle and aortic root can be carried out using a pigtail catheter (or, alternatively, a straight catheter with side holes such as a Sones catheter or multipurpose catheter). In either right or left-sided angiography, a variety of views are used to particularly image certain structures (Figure 2). These are obtained by changing the axis of the x-ray beam and sometimes using a system of dual beams (biplane imaging). A lateral projection best demonstrates the pulmonary outflow tract, left and right anterior oblique projec-

tions are used to demonstrate the left ventricular wall motion, and so forth. Analysis of regional and global wall motion can be made from these angiographic studies. Using traced outlines of the left ventricle in systole and diastole and by employing the equation for the volume of an ellipsoid, ventricular volume can be obtained and global ejection fraction can be calculated.

In addition, using these volumes multiplied by the heart rate, a calculation of left ventricular cardiac output can be made. By subtracting the systemic cardiac output (as noted above) from the angiographic cardiac output, an estimate of the

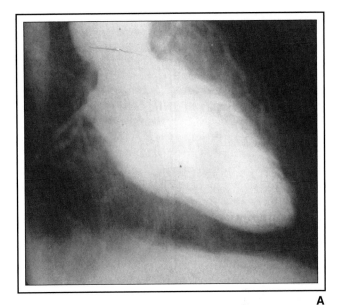

A

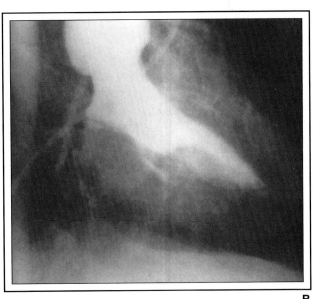

B

Figure 2. Normal left ventriculograms (RAO projection) in diastole and systole (A). Posterior papillary muscle shadow can be seen in the systolic frame (B).

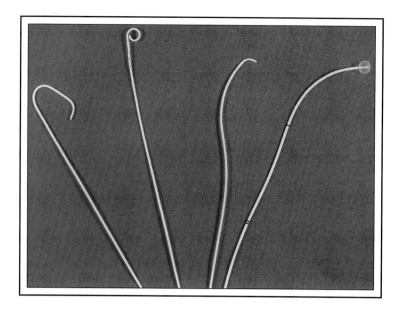

Figure 3 Catheters used for routine right and left heart catheterization. L to R: Left coronary catheter (Judkins), pigtail catheter, right coronary catheter (Judkins), Swan-Ganz multilumen catheter.

regurgitant volume and fraction in patients with aortic regurgitation can be made. Angiographic confirmation of intracardiac shunts can also be made by appropriate positioning of the catheters.

Coronary angiography is the most frequently performed catheterization technique. It is most commonly performed using the femoral approach and usually in combination with retrograde left heart catheterization and left ventriculography. Coronary angiograms are obtained for the definitive diagnosis of suspected coronary artery disease as well as to diagnose unsuspected coronary abnormalities in patients who may require cardiac surgery for other reasons.

Specially formed catheters are usually used to selectively catheterize the right and left coronary vessels (Figure 3). The tip of the catheter is manipulated into the ostium of the vessel and hand injections of contrast material are made. Visualization by fluoroscopy and cineangiographic recording of the coronary tree in various radiographic projections is thus possible. The degree of detail which can be obtained depends on the patient's size, adequacy of the equipment used, and the ability to effectively engage the coronary ostium. Obese patients, those with very ectatic aortic roots, and those with ostial coronary lesions (preventing safe catheter placement) present problems which may result in less than adequate visualization.

If the brachial approach is used for coronary angiography, preformed catheters can also be employed. However, straight catheters (Sones, multipurpose) are frequently employed. Some skill is required to appropriately form these catheters in the aortic root so they engage the coronary ostia. Use of the percutaneous approach from the right or left side has become more frequent, enabling operators without experience in the traditional brachial approach to successfully perform coronary angiography by this route.

Information regarding presence of obstructive lesions in the coronary tree and their severity and location is obtained through this method. Estimates of severity (expressed in terms of percentage of diameter obstruction) are made, although the use of electronic calipers, edge detection programs, and other computer-based techniques have made these estimates more precise in many laboratories.

Complications

As with any "invasive" procedure, cardiac catheterization carries with it a definite risk of morbidity and mortality (Table 1). In experienced laboratories, complication rate is less than 1% for serious events (excluding vasovagal episodes and local vascular problems). It is well accepted that higher complication rates occur in laboratories with low volumes of procedures and among operators with low case loads. The Intersociety Commission on Heart Disease Resources has recommended minimum volume standards for laboratories and physicians, which will be updated periodically. Presently it is recommended that adult catheterization laboratories perform at least 300 procedures and operators perform at least 75 procedures yearly.

Incidence of death related to cardiac catheterization is in the range of 0.1%-0.2%. The exception is in patients with documented left main coronary obstruction in whom risk has been reported to be as high as 5%, but is probably in the 1% range currently. Serious rhythm disturbances such as ventricular tachycardia and fibrillation occur infre-

TABLE 1
Major Complications of Cardiac Catheterization

Local vascular problems
- bleeding
- vascular occlusion or dissection

Major vessel problems
- dissection
- occlusion
- plaque dislodgement (cholesterol emboli)

Embolic complications
- cerebrovascular
- renal
- splanchnic
- peripheral

Left ventricular
- perforation
- ventricular arrhythmia

Coronary arteries
- dissection
- air or thromboembolism

Contrast
- allergic reaction
- anaphylaxis
- renal failure

quently and are usually readily treated. Development of transient bundle branch block or atrioventricular block has occurred. Of specific concern is the performance of right heart catheterization in the setting of left bundle branch block. A resulting right bundle conduction disturbance leading to complete heart block in this setting has occurred requiring emergency temporary pacing. Nonfatal myocardial infarction as a result of a diagnostic catheterization procedure is exceedingly rare. Transient neurologic events and strokes associated with the procedure occur in about 0.1% of cases. Cardiac perforation (usually associated with use of the guidewire in crossing the aortic valve) is rare.

It occurs more frequently, however, using the transeptal approach. Injection of air, either systemically or intracoronary, during angiography (or catheter flushing) can occur. Major complications may result, depending on the volume injected. Reactions to the contrast material used (containing iodine) are not uncommon. Hypersensitivity resulting in hives or very rarely anaphylaxis does occur. Occasionally a pyrogen reaction with resulting fever develops. Pulmonary edema related to hypertonicity of the contrast material and resultant intravascular volume increase can also occur. Rarely, staining of the myocardium occurs with extravasation of contrast into the pericardial space. Many of these contrast-related complications are

less common with use of nonionic contrast material, although it is used generally only in selected cases because of its expense (Figure 4).

A variety of vascular complications may occur; local thrombosis or dissection of a peripheral vessel at the site of catheter entry may occur. This is more common in the brachial approach. Distal vascular occlusion (particularly in the lower extremity) may occur as a result of thromboembolism from this site. Systemic heparinization is often used in an attempt to prevent thrombus formation (Figure 5). Dissection of the aorta or the promulgation of cholesterol emboli as a result of catheter passage may also occur. Dissection of a coronary artery during coronary angiography occurs rarely, but may be associated with myocardial infarction. Phlebitis (in the upper or lower extremity) rarely occurs following transvenous procedures if the catheter is not left in place subsequent to the procedure. Infection at the site of catheter entry is rare using the percutaneous route, but occasionally occurs if a brachial cutdown is performed which requires surgical closure.

Rupture of a pulmonary vessel as a result of inflation of the pulmonary artery catheter balloon is frequently fatal. Great care must be taken, particularly at the bedside when fluoroscopy is not available, to be sure that the catheter is in an appropriate position prior to inflating the balloon. Suspicion that the catheter is too distal in a pulmonary vessel by pressure tracing damping or fluoroscopy requires that the operator reposition the catheter prior to inflation.

Vagal reactions are not uncommon with catheterization. Adequate sedation beforehand helps to prevent many of these. In patients with severe aortic outflow tract obstruction or significant underlying conduction disturbances, associated hypotension and bradycardia may be life-threatening. Pretreatment with atropine may be indicated in such patients, and atropine usually is effective in treating those patients who experience profound vagal episodes.

A variety of methods have been employed with varying success to prevent some complications. Use of nonionic contrast agents was mentioned above. The role of systemic heparin is not universally accepted but has been employed in an attempt to prevent embolization which may result in peripheral, coronary, or central nervous system embolization and local thrombosis. Certainly, most agree that the duration of the procedure may be directly proportional to the incidence of some complications. Those patients considered to be at higher risk might benefit from having their procedures performed by more experienced operators.

Angiographic contrast material may cause pro-

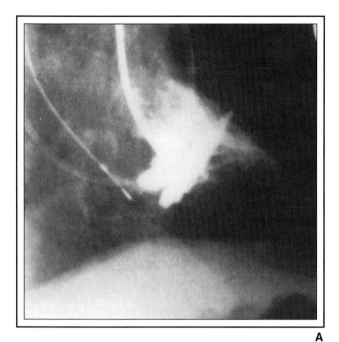

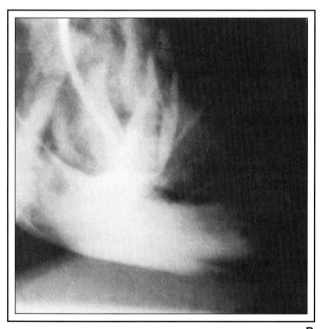

Figure 4. Frames of a left ventriculogram (RAO projection) documenting intramyocardial injection of contrast (myocardial staining) through an end hole catheter (A). Extravasation into the pericardium (with subsequent risk of tamponade due to the osmotic effect of the contrast) develops (B).

gression of renal failure, transiently or permanently, in patients with underlying renal dysfunction. The most accurate predictor of this occurrence is the severity of underlying renal dysfunction. Attempts to limit this risk by use of less contrast material, pre-catheterization hydration, use of osmotic diuretics, and use of nonionic contrast

material have been only marginally successful. Careful consideration must be given to the potential benefit of the information obtained using angiography in relation to this risk.

It is questionable whether truly informed consent can be obtained from most patients regarding any medical procedure. However, an attempt at educating the patient and family as to the potential risks and the risk/benefit ratio must be made regarding the catheterization procedure. Having the patient (or guardian) sign a legal consent form does not substitute for an honest discussion of the potential complications and the justification for taking the risk that those complications may occur. While catheterization has become almost "routine" in some clinical situations, it is vital that those involved recognize the potential hazards.

Pitfalls of Data Interpretation

Hemodynamic findings determined at catheterizations should be interpreted in light of the patient's state when compared with that under which their symptoms and other evaluation have occurred (Table 2). Therefore, if the patient is very anxious during the procedure, heart rate and left ventricular function may be altered by their hyperadrenergic state. Likewise, the onset of a new arrhythmia at the time the data are collected could result in misleading findings (such as changes in left ventricular filling pressure brought about by new onset of rapid atrial fibrillation, or the effect of atrial fibrillation on the accuracy of the gradients determined in valvular stenosis). On the other hand, the patient with mitral stenosis and symptoms of pulmonary congestion with exercise may not exhibit elevated pulmonary capillary wedge pressures in the sedated, resting state. Exercise during the procedure may be needed to mimic the clinical setting.

Interpretation of pressure data requires careful attention to variations related to respiratory variation. Particularly in the bedside use of right heart catheterization, these variations may result in misleading information used to make therapeutic decisions. Visually inspecting pressure curves and correcting for respiratory variation or recording pressures in mid-expiration is necessary. Left ventricular pressure obtained using a straight catheter are occasionally inaccurate due to catheter entrapment (the tip of the catheter abutting the ventricular wall causing an artifactual pressure reading). It is necessary to obtain simultaneous pressure readings in calculating valve gradients. Pressures obtained by pulling the catheter through the aortic valve from left ventricle to aorta do not always

426

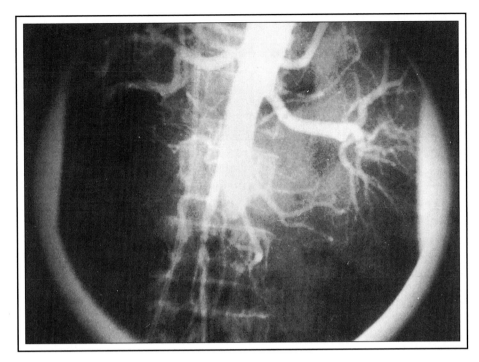

Figure 5. Complication of femoral artery catheterization. Occlusion of the abdominal aorta.

accurately reflect the true gradient, especially if there is any variation in heart rate. The end diastolic pressure measured after angiography does not reflect the baseline state and can be misleading. Other sources of error include "catheter whip" (changes in pressure related to catheter tip motion), use of a peripheral arterial pressure as a substitute for central aortic pressure, and problems with transducer calibration and leveling.

In those patients in whom cardiac output (and, therefore, aortic valve flow) is reduced due to left ventricular failure or hypovolemia, the aortic valve gradient will be reduced. Estimation of severity must be made on the basis of aortic valve area determination and not on the severity of the gradient, or a hemodynamic underestimation of severity may occur.

Several problems can occur in interpreting angiograms. Estimates of left ventricular function using the formula for an ellipsoid (as noted above) contain inherent inaccuracies. In large, more spherical, poorly functioning ventricles, the calculations tend to underestimate ejection fraction. In small, elongated, hypercontractile ventricles, the calculations overestimate level of left ventricular function. Left ventricular function by ejection fraction calculation in patients with significant mitral regurgitation may underestimate the level of left ventricular impairment because of the unloading effect of ejection into the low impedance left atrium. The presence of segmental wall motion abnormalities which alter ventricular morphology injects a source of error into both visual and calculated estimates of

left ventricular function. The validity of visual estimates of left ventricular function in comparison with calculated ejection fraction has been questioned.

The severity of aortic regurgitation as estimated by aortic root angiography is influenced by the peripheral vascular resistance at the time of the study. If vasodilation has occurred as a result of contrast use just before the angiogram, the degree of aortic regurgitation may be less than in the baseline state. A similar phenomenon may also occur in mitral regurgitation to a lesser extent.

Valvular Heart Disease

Aortic Stenosis

In the patient with history compatible with angina pectoris, congestive heart failure, or syncope/pre-syncope, careful evaluation for aortic stenosis should be undertaken. In most patients, a careful physical examination will reveal this diagnosis and permit an estimate of severity. Noninvasive studies, particularly echocardiography and cardiac Doppler, can be of significant help in establishing and quantifying diagnosis. However, in patients in whom an intervention such as valve replacement is contemplated, catheterization to confirm the severity of the lesion and to exclude other unsuspected abnormalities such as coronary artery disease should be undertaken (Table 3).

Several aspects of the physical examination may suggest severe aortic stenosis and, therefore, justify consideration of catheterization and corrective

427

TABLE 2

Factors Leading to Misinterpretation of Data

- Lack of "steady state" blood pressure and cardiac output
- Arrhythmia
- Volume alterations
- Inadequate attention to zeroing, leveling, and balancing transducers
- Artifact on pressure tracings

intervention. These include a markedly diminished carotid pulse (which may not be present in older patients with systolic hypertension), a prolonged, late peaking outflow murmur, and absence of the aortic component of the second heart sound. A narrow pulse pressure obtained by cuff may also be present. Some of these findings may not be as obvious in the patient with significant heart failure.

CARDIAC PEARL

A worthwhile reminder is that the typical findings of significant aortic stenosis may be masked. It is well to remember that a loud systolic murmur of aortic stenosis such as grade V intensity may become very insignificant when advanced cardiac decompensation is present and may become grade I or II. I have personally observed a patient with a classic grade V aortic systolic murmur with a palpable thrill who subsequently had advanced cardiac decompensation. No aortic systolic murmur was evident, causing physicians who saw the patient for the first time not to suspect the presence of aortic stenosis. In fact, I recall 1 patient who had no murmur, but had a severe "tight" aortic stenosis; he presented more as a case of right-sided heart failure, causing some observers to raise the possibility of constrictive pericarditis. However, the patient had a previously known grade 5 typical aortic stenosis murmur before the onset of failure.

W. Proctor Harvey, M.D.

Echocardiographic analysis of aortic valve structure and function can help confirm diagnosis. Doppler estimates of the gradient and valve area are usually accurate, although technical imaging problems sometimes inhibit both echo and Doppler accuracy. When the combination of symptoms, physical findings, and noninvasive evaluation suggest that severe aortic stenosis warranting intervention is present, then cardiac catheterization (with coronary angiography in most cases) is indicated.

When this diagnosis is considered, both right and left heart catheterization are needed to quantify severity of obstruction. Retrograde left heart catheterization is often difficult and occasionally impossible in aortic stenosis due to the valve narrowing and deformity. The transeptal approach may be used in this setting. Simultaneous central aortic and left ventricular systolic pressure measurements are required to quantify the gradient (Figure 6). Measurements of peak gradient and mean gradient are made (the latter by hand or, more commonly, computerized planimetry).

Using the Gorlin formula for valve orifice size,

$$\text{Aortic Valve Area} = \frac{\text{Aortic valve flow}}{44.3\sqrt{\text{aortic valve mean gradient}}}$$

the aortic valve flow is calculated using the cardiac output, systolic ejection period and heart rate *at the time of gradient determination*. The calculated valve area can be divided by the body surface area and expressed as the aortic valve area/meter^2, or aortic valve index, for comparison. In addition, determination of left ventricular end diastolic pressure, pulmonary capillary wedge pressure, and left ventricular ejection fraction help to assess left ventricular function and the risk of a surgical procedure. The catheterization may also reveal unsuspected coexistent mitral regurgitation and coronary artery disease.

At times, severity of the findings at cardiac catheterization may not correlate with the clinical setting. Areas of possible misinterpretation of the results of catheterization are several. The use of peak rather than mean aortic valve gradients in the Gorlin formula can lead to erroneous results. Using non-simultaneous aortic and left ventricular pressures, particularly in the setting of atrial fibrillation, can be misleading. Using cardiac output obtained at a time distant from gradient determination introduces a potentially significant source of error, and catheter tip damping or entrapment (if a straight catheter is used) may result in a false pres-

TABLE 3

Findings in Aortic Stenosis

- Diminished cardiac output
- Possibly elevated right heart pressures
- Aortic valve gradient and reduced area
- Elevated left ventricular diastolic pressure with prominent A-wave
- Fluoroscopic calcification of aortic valve
- Possibly associated aortic regurgitation
- Diminished left ventricular function

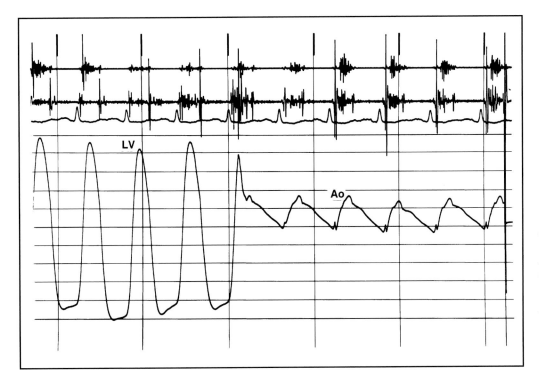

Figure 6. "Pullback" with continuous pressure recording in aortic stenosis. A 70mm gradient is noted. Simultaneous catheter tip phonocardiographic recording (lower phonocardiogram tracing) documents the site of murmur generation during pullthrough.

sure reading. Using an uncorrected peripheral arterial pressure rather than central aortic may falsely reduce the gradient, while presence of coexistent aortic regurgitation can influence hemodynamic findings (see below).

Calculated aortic valve areas of 0.7cm² or less are consistent with severe aortic stenosis and should correlate with other findings suggesting that level of severity. Areas in the range of 0.8cm to 1.2cm suggest moderate disease but should be used in conjunction with other clinical parameters.

Aortic Regurgitation

Appropriate timing of surgical intervention in patients with chronic aortic regurgitation is more difficult than in aortic stenosis. Patients may have physical findings and noninvasive studies consistent with severe regurgitation and marked cardiac enlargement without significant symptoms. Therefore, the role of catheterization is limited to those patients with symptoms of congestive heart failure and noninvasive parameters consistent with advanced disease. Echocardiographic criteria have been helpful in predicting which symptomatic patients may benefit from aortic valve replacement. Physical findings and historical data suggesting congestive heart failure in patients with aortic regurgitation suggest the need for operation. Presence of the associated wide pulse pressure, typical bounding bifid carotid pulse, and a long diastolic murmur help to confirm the etiology.

Catheterization in this setting can add to the

assessment of left ventricular function by determination of left ventricular filling pressure and by use of left ventricular angiography. Catheterization is probably most helpful in determining the presence of otherwise undetected coronary disease to help in planning a complete operation.

Right and left heart catheterization are carried out with determination of cardiac output, pulmonary capillary wedge pressure, and left-sided studies (Table 4). Occasionally, undiagnosed aortic stenosis may be noted during the study. An estimate of the severity of aortic regurgitation can be made by aortic root angiography. This quantification is quite subjective. 1+ severity connotes mild reflux of contrast into the left ventricle during diastole without residual opacification. 2+ and 3+ connote increased severity of regurgitant flow with increasing opacification of the ventricle. 4+ severity is associated with rapid reflux of contrast and opacification of the ventricle in the first diastole.

T A B L E 4	
Severe Aortic Regurgitation	
ACUTE	**CHRONIC**
"Normal" aortic pressure tracing	Wide aortic pulse pressure
Marked early elevation of LV diastolic pressure	Elevated end diastolic LV pressure
Angiographic aortic regurgitation diminished in late diastole	Pan-diastolic aortic regurgitation

429

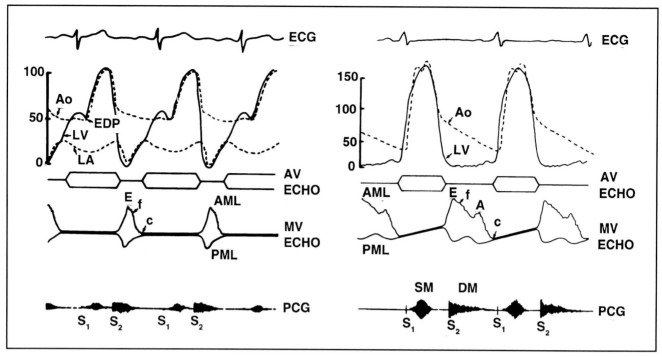

Figure 7. Left ventricular, aortic and left atrial pressure wave forms in acute (left) and chronic (right) aortic regurgitation (accompanied by echo and phonocardiogram tracings). In acute aortic regurgitation, left ventricular diastolic pressure rises abruptly to systemic aortic level. As a result, early mitral valve closure occurs (see echo tracing) as the left atrial and left ventricular diastolic pressures cross. In the right panel, the low aortic diastolic pressure of chronic aortic regurgitation is seen without the abrupt rise in left ventricular diastolic pressure. Early closure of the mitral valve does not occur.

In acute aortic regurgitation (e.g., aortic root disssection, native valve endocarditis), the left ventricle has not had time to dilate substantially. As a result, left ventricular diastolic pressure rises abruptly and to higher levels. The "reverse gradient" between aortic diastolic pressure and left ventricular diastolic pressure narrows quickly and the systemic diastolic pressure is "supported" by the left ventricular diastolic pressure at a higher level than would be ordinarily found in chronic aortic regurgitation of the same severity. This phenomenon may result in a diastolic blowing murmur of brief duration despite severe aortic regurgitation (Figure 7).

CARDIAC PEARL

During the past several months, we evaluated a patient in our hospital who had such a severe leak of his aortic valve that the left ventricular diastolic pressure quickly exceeded left arterial pressure, resulting, thereby, in a very early closure of the mitral valve in diastole. This produced a quite loud sound; in fact, it was louder than either the first or second heart sound. The echocardiogram easily identified this premature closure

of the mitral valve. The need for operation for aortic valve replacement was urgent and was performed successfully. As in many cases of severe, acute aortic insufficiency, the diastolic pressure was not low, as it generally is in the chronic cases of severe aortic insufficiency. Instead, it was normal. The physician, not recognizing that the diastolic pressure in some patients with acute severe aortic insufficiency may be normal, fell into a trap because of this. Operation, as in the patient just cited, should be performed promptly.

W. Proctor Harvey, M.D.

Angiographic severity of aortic regurgitation varies with the state of the peripheral vascular resistance and diastolic aortic pressure. Adequate time must be allowed for the patient to return to baseline state following maneuvers which might affect diastolic pressure (such as left ventricular angiography) prior to aortic root angiography. Careful positioning of the catheter just above the aortic valve is also important. Too low a position may result in increased regurgitant flow due to catheter interference with valve closure. Too high a position will result in apparently less severe regurgitation.

Aortic Stenosis and Regurgitation

Clinical assessment of mixed aortic valve disease may present some difficulty. If only mild stenosis or regurgitation is present when the alternate lesion is severe, the diagnosis may be straightforward. However, when both regurgitation and stenosis are moderately severe, gauging the severity of each lesion on clinical grounds may be misleading. Coexistent aortic regurgitation increases aortic valve systolic flow as the regurgitant volume and the forward cardiac output cross the aortic orifice during systole. This may lead to physical and Doppler findings consistent with artificially more severe obstruction. The pulse and blood pressure findings will likewise be altered from those usually present when the lesions are found in isolation.

Similarly, the catheterization findings can be altered. The aortic gradient obtained at catheterization is a reflection of the increased aortic valve flow due to the regurgitant fraction as well as severity of obstruction. Since the usual methods for determining cardiac output and those deriving aortic valve flow do not take into account the regurgitant fraction, the calculation of aortic valve area (see Gorlin formula above) will result in an underestimation of the orifice size. Using the true left ventricular output, as calculated by angiography, in the Gorlin formula will result in a more valid estimate of aortic valve area.

Mitral Stenosis

Patients with mitral stenosis are evaluated for intervention when symptoms become significant enough to limit activity, when uncontrollable systemic embolization occurs, or when signs of pulmonary hypertension and early right ventricular failure develop. Dyspnea and fatigue are the most common symptoms. A narrowing of the A_2-O.S. interval, a long diastolic rumble, and development of atrial fibrillation are associated with increased severity of mitral obstruction. The resulting increases in pulmonary and right ventricular pressures are manifested by an elevated jugular venous

pressure with large A-waves, a right ventricular lift, a loud pulmonic component of the second heart sound, right-sided filling sounds, and evidence of tricuspid regurgitation.

However, examination findings in the resting state may not account for exertional symptoms. Echocardiography and cardiac Doppler have aided significantly in the diagnosis and quantification of severity. This technique is generally performed at rest and, as in the case of the physical examination, may not correlate with activity-related symptoms.

In those patients in whom the clinical and noninvasive findings do not correlate with the symptom state, a preliminary right heart catheterization can be carried out. If a significantly elevated pulmonary capillary wedge pressure is not found, supine bicycle exercise or arm ergometry (or rapid pacing) can be performed with the catheter in place. This may demonstrate a significant rise in right-sided pressures, explaining exercise-related symptoms. As a preparation for surgery, right and left heart catheterization (sometimes employing the transeptal approach), with coronary angiography in appropriate patients, is performed (Table 5). Simultaneous measurement of left atrial pressure (as reflected in the pulmonary capillary wedge position or directly by transeptal technique) and left ventricular pressure is made. This can also be done with exercise as described above. Using the mitral constant in the Gorlin formula, the mitral valve area can be calculated:

$$MVA = \frac{\text{Mitral valve flow}}{37.7\sqrt{\text{mean mitral gradient}}}$$

The mean gradient is obtained by hand or computer planimetry of the diastolic gradient. The mitral valve flow is calculated by dividing cardiac output by the product of the heart rate and the diastolic filling period. The area can be standardized to an index by dividing by the body surface area (in meters). Many patients with severe mitral stenosis are in atrial fibrillation. In these patients, an average gradient over several cardiac cycles should be used as the gradient will vary significantly depending on the diastolic filling intervals (both of the cycle of interest and the preceding cycle) (Figure 8).

Determination of the degree of pulmonary hypertension is made by pressure measurements. In addition, analysis of the right atrial wave form may demonstrate large V-waves consistent with tricuspid regurgitation. As mitral stenosis is almost always due to rheumatic fever in adults, a thorough evaluation for associated other valvular disease should be made. This includes evaluation of the

431

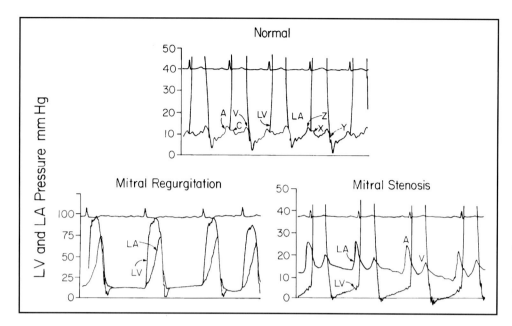

Figure 8. Simultaneous left atrial and left ventricular pressure tracings in the normal situation and in mitral valve disease. In mitral regurgitation, huge early V-waves are noted (which may not be apparent in the pulmonary capillary wedge tracing in chronic mitral regurgitation). In mitral stenosis, the diastolic gradient is noted. Large A-waves, associated with decreased right ventricular compliance, are seen.

right-sided pressure curves for tricuspid regurgitation, inspection of the left ventricular and aortic curves for aortic stenosis, and an aortic root angiogram for aortic regurgitation.

While the valve area calculation in mitral stenosis is a reliable indicator of severity of the obstruction, intervention (surgery or balloon valvuloplasty) may be based on other factors as well. A high pulmonary capillary wedge pressure, at rest or with exercise, consistent with symptoms may indicate the need for intervention in patients with less than critical stenosis (valve area greater than $1cm^2$). The presence of significant pulmonary hypertension, especially if it is disproportionate to the elevation of pulmonary capillary wedge pressure, is another indicator for intervention despite only a moderate degree of mitral obstruction.

There are potential pitfalls in analyzing data in mitral stenosis. Because the pressure levels recorded in the left ventricle, the left atrium, and pulmonary wedge position during diastole are low, errors in calibration and zeroing have a more significant effect in this setting than in the evaluation of aortic stenosis. When pulmonary capillary wedge pressure is used in the gradient determination, a temporal lag in pressure transmission is present and must be corrected; presence of atrial fibrillation makes accurate calculations more difficult, and presence of associated mitral regurgitation will cause an overestimation of severity, as in aortic valve disease. Right ventricular failure due to pulmonary hypertension may reduce preload sufficiently to lower pulmonary capillary wedge pressure, resulting in an underestimate of the severity of valvular obstruction. Likewise, previous treatment with diuretics may cause sufficient decrease in preload to alter pulmonary capillary wedge (or left atrial) pressure sufficiently to result in an underestimation of severity. When the hemodynamic findings do not correspond to the severity of symptoms in these settings, acute volume loading followed by repeat hemodynamic measurements is appropriate.

Mitral Regurgitation

Like aortic regurgitation, the timing of surgical intervention and, therefore, the need for diagnostic cardiac catheterization in chronic mitral regurgitation is a difficult judgement to make. Certainly, the patient who presents with significant symptoms of congestive heart failure should be considered for evaluation. However, the nature of chronic left ventricular volume overload lesions is such that intervention in the symptomatic patient may come too late to ensure improvement or even prevent progression of left ventricular failure. This is particularly true in mitral regurgitation because the mitral leak itself acts as an "afterload reducing" mechanism and correction may lead to worsening of left ventricular function. Patients with signs of significant mitral regurgitation characterized by evidence of left ventricular decompensation (loud third heart sound, cardiomegaly with a hyperdynamic apical impulse) or pulmonary hypertension (jugular venous pressure elevation with prominent A-waves, right ventricular lift, loud P_2, right-sided gallop, evidence of tricuspid regurgitation) should be evaluated for corrective intervention. Doppler echocardiography has been helpful, as in aortic regurgitation, in estimating the severity of mitral regurgitation and in the prediction of benefit from intervention.

432

TABLE 6	
Severe Mitral Regurgitation	
ACUTE	**CHRONIC**
Severe pulmonary hypertension	Pulmonary hypertension with right ventricular dysfunction and tricuspid regurgitation
Large V-waves in the PCWP tracing	Elevated mean PCWP
Hyperdynamic LV function	Diminished LV function

Cardiac catheterization has a role in confirming severity of mitral regurgitation both directly and by assessing right-sided hemodynamics. Additionally, further evaluation of left ventricular function can be carried out, which can be particularly important in patients in whom echocardiography and cardiac Doppler are technically difficult. Information regarding possible coexistent coronary artery disease (in preparation for surgical intervention) is also obtained.

Right and left heart catheterization are performed when surgical intervention is planned. Findings include elevated right heart pressures in passive or reactive pulmonary hypertension, as well as elevated pulmonary capillary wedge pressure or pulmonary artery occluded pressure. Evidence of tricuspid regurgitation may be present either due to intrinsic tricuspid valve disease or, more commonly, related to right ventricular failure. Large V-waves in the reflected left atrial pressure may be present (2-3 times mean pulmonary wedge pressure) (Figure 8). In chronic mitral regurgitation, the increase in left atrial size may act as a buffer to transmission of large V-waves and these are not commonly seen. Left heart catheterization will demonstrate elevated end diastolic pressure if left ventricular failure has developed. Left ventricular angiography demonstrates reflux of contrast from left ventricle to left atrium. Reflux of contrast into the pulmonary veins corresponds to severe (4+) mitral regurgitation. Filling of the left atrium in one systole is considered moderately severe (3+) regurgitation. 2+ mitral regurgitation is characterized by progressive atrial opacification. In mild (1+) regurgitation, contrast clears the left atrium during diastole. A regurgitant fraction can be calculated by subtracting the systemic cardiac output (determined by Fick, green dye, or thermodilution techniques) from the angiographically determined left ventricular output. A regurgitant fraction of 50% corresponds to severe mitral regurgitation.

Careful attention should be paid to the pressure curves to be sure that associated aortic stenosis is not overlooked. An aortic root angiogram should be performed to exclude aortic regurgitation (unless these conditions have *definitely* been excluded by echocardiographic and Doppler studies).

As mentioned above, the unloading effect of mitral regurgitation on the left ventricle can cause an underestimate of impairment of function of this chamber. Patients with apparently normal or even hypercontractile left ventricular function may actually have already suffered left ventricular impairment.

Evaluation of severity of regurgitation may be difficult in patients with arrhythmia, either baseline atrial fibrillation or catheter-induced ventricular arrhythmia. Peripheral vascular resistance can influence the degree of mitral regurgitation during catheterization (if vasodilation has occurred, regurgitant volume will be less and vice versa). As mentioned above, measurement of the V-wave height in chronic mitral regurgitation is frequently not helpful. Patients with acute, severe mitral regurgitation present with the abrupt onset of symptoms. Because of the sudden onset of the regurgitant leak, they generally do not have significant left atrial enlargement. As a result, the left atrial pressure rises abruptly during ventricular systole and regurgitant flow is diminished in late systole. The murmur generated tapers or ends in late systole rather than being the plateau-shaped, holosystolic murmur of chronic mitral regurgitation. Because of preserved left atrial size and contractility, a fourth heart sound is prominent, and a third heart sound is uncommon.

At catheterization, right heart pressures may be significantly increased. The pulmonary capillary wedge pressure is increased and large V-waves are seen associated with the abrupt rise in left atrial pressure. Left ventricular diastolic pressure may not be significantly elevated. Severe mitral regurgitation is seen on left ventriculography. Left ventricular volume is usually not significantly increased. Left ventricular contractility is vigorous (hypercontractile) and ejection fraction is elevated (Table 6). Patients with combined mitral stenosis and mitral regurgitation can present clinical difficulties in the estimation of severity of the lesions. Significant symptoms may develop even though the severity of each lesion is only moderate. Because of the increased diastolic mitral valve flow resulting from the systolic regurgitant fraction, the mitral rumble will be more prolonged and louder than would be expected from the degree of stenosis alone; increased elevation of left atrial pressure resulting from mitral regurgitation also narrows the A_2-OS interval further than would be expected.

At catheterization, the mitral valve gradient will be relatively increased because of the increased

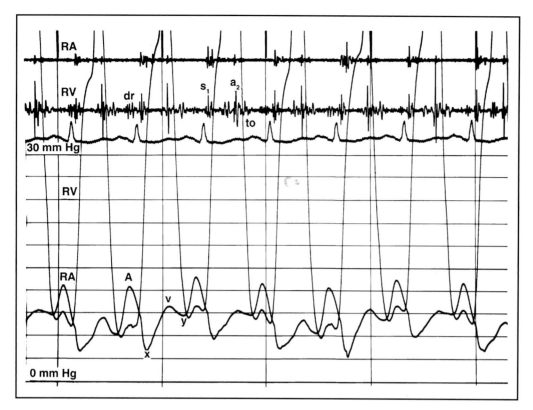

Figure 9. Simultaneous right atrial and right ventricular pressure tracings in tricuspid stenosis. Note the diastolic gradient. The simultaneous phonocardiogram documents the associated diastolic rumble.

diastolic mitral valve flow. If the systemic cardiac output is used in the mitral valve area calculation, severity of mitral obstruction will be overestimated. Using the cardiac output calculated from left ventriculography will result in a more reliable valve area estimation. A correlation between symptoms and level of pulmonary capillary wedge pressure (either at rest or with exercise) should be present. The severity of left ventricular dysfunction may be underestimated (both by left ventricular end diastolic pressure and by left ventricular angiography) because of diminished left ventricular filling due to the diminished mitral valve orifice.

Tricuspid Valve Disease

Primary tricuspid valve disease is uncommon, usually associated with rheumatic heart disease (although involvement with carcinoid syndrome, Ebstein's anomaly, and endocarditis occurs). Intervention is rarely undertaken primarily for correction of tricuspid abnormalities. Evidence of systemic venous hypertension is the clinical correlate of tricuspid valve disease along with diminished forward cardiac output secondary to decreased left ventricular filling. Fatigue rather than dyspnea predominates, and pleural effusions, elevated jugular venous pressure, edema, ascites, and hepatic failure are the major physical findings. Large jugular venous A-waves may be seen in tricuspid stenosis, and large V-waves are noted in tricuspid regurgitation.

Diagnosis of tricuspid stenosis by catheterization is difficult, as the gradient is generally small. Either two catheters, one in the right atrium and one in the right ventricle, or a double lumen catheter with an appropriately positioned proximal side hole, are required (Figure 9). A tricuspid gradient can thus be determined, and orifice calculations are not performed. A 5mm of mercury or greater tricuspid gradient is considered significant (requiring precise hemodynamic measurements). The diagnosis of tricuspid regurgitation can be confirmed by analysis of the right atrial pressure wave form for V-wave height (Figure 10). In addition, right ventricular angiography can be performed, although some degree of tricuspid regurgitation may be induced by catheter position across the tricuspid valve.

Secondary tricuspid valve regurgitation is more common and is usually the result of the right ventricular reaction to pulmonary hypertension. Findings consistent with tricuspid regurgitation as well as pulmonary hypertension are present. Pulmonary disease or significant left heart disease are usual etiologies. Catheterization demonstrates the findings of tricuspid regurgitation mentioned above. In addition, the etiology of the right ventricular dysfunction will be apparent from measurement of pulmonary artery pressure and analysis of left-sided hemodynamics.

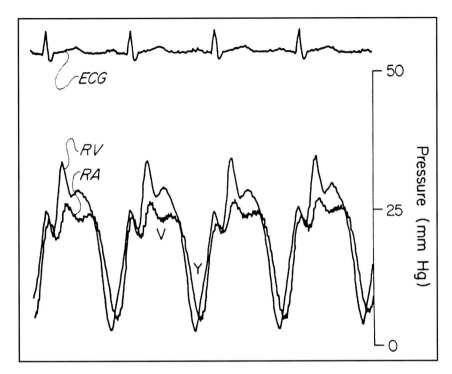

Figure 10. Simultaneous right atrial and right ventricular pressure tracings in severe tricuspid regurgitation.

Pulmonic Valve Disease

Pulmonic valve disease in adults is rarely a primary abnormality and almost never requires intervention. Pulmonic regurgitation occurs in the setting of pulmonary hypertension and occasionally due to endocarditis. It can be demonstrated by pulmonary angiography with the radiographic axis positioned in the lateral position. Since right heart catheters are passed antegrade, the degree of pulmonic regurgitation is enhanced by catheter position. In the rare instance that primary pulmonic regurgitation is clinically significant, evidence of its hemodynamic effect may be seen on parameters of right ventricular function (elevation of diastolic pressure, tricuspid regurgitation).

Coexisting Valve Disease

Coexisting mitral and aortic valve disease may present confusing clinical data in relation to severity. Preload reduction as a result of mitral stenosis may alter hemodynamics of aortic stenosis and the left ventricular volume overload of aortic regurgitation. Increased outflow resistance due to aortic stenosis may exaggerate the severity of mitral regurgitation. Similarly, allowance for these interactions needs to be made in interpreting the catheterization data. Severity level of left ventricular dysfunction in aortic stenosis may appear to be less than it actually is if there is coexistent mitral regurgitation. The degree of mitral regurgitation may appear more severe as a result of the aortic outflow obstruction. Left ventricular preload reduc-

tion due to mitral stenosis may make the aortic valve gradient appear less severe.

Catheterization in the setting of endocarditis presents special concern. The possibility of the catheter dislodging friable vegetations resulting in septic emboli must be considered. This is especially true in right-sided and aortic valve endocarditis. Because of the inability of noninvasive studies to pinpoint the presence and location of coexistent coronary artery disease, coronary angiography may have to be performed without complete invasive evaluation of the valvular lesion.

Congenital Heart Disease

Various forms of congenital heart disease may be found in adults. Aortic stenosis is frequently of congenital origin and has been described above. Other commonly encountered abnormalities include atrial septal defect, ventricular septal defect, and coarctation of the aorta.

Atrial Septal Defect

Atrial septal defect is a volume overload lesion of the right ventricle which also may be associated with pulmonary hypertension. The patient may ultimately develop symptoms and signs of right ventricular failure with systemic venous hypertension (manifested by edema, ascites, and hepatic failure) as well as low systemic output state due to diminished left ventricular filling. When severe reactive pulmonary hypertension develops (Eisenmenger's physiology), reverse shunting with

435

cyanosis may occur. Common physical findings are a persistent or fixed split second heart sound and pulmonary outflow tract murmur. Findings of pulmonary hypertension (loud P_2, right ventricular lift), as well as elevated jugular venous pressure, edema, ascites, and tricuspid regurgitation, may be present.

CARDIAC PEARL

Not uncommonly, atrial septal defect has been overlooked because close attention was not given to auscultation of the splitting of the second heart sound. A wide, so-called fixed splitting of the second sound provides an immediate clue, and atrial defect must be ruled out as one of the causes of a wider split of S_2. In the uncomplicated, usual type of atrial defect (ostium secundum type) the occurrence of a single second sound with expiration is rare, but it does occur. "Never say never" in medicine.

A systolic murmur heard over the pulmonic area and/or third left sternal border is almost always present and will be found if carefully sought. It is usually a grade 2 or 3, early to mid, or midsystolic murmur; however, it may be a grade 1 or, rarely, grade 4 (a palpable systolic thrill may be associated).

I recall seeing only one patient with proved atrial septal defect in whom I was unable to hear a systolic murmur- and this was shortly after cardiac catheterization; subsequently, I heard a systolic murmur in this patient. Again, "never say never."

W. Proctor Harvey, M.D.

Right and left heart catheterization (and coronary angiography when appropriate) are performed. Measurement of right-sided pressures may demonstrate elevated right atrial pressure (with prominent A- waves if right ventricular hypertrophy is present) and large V-waves, if tricuspid regurgitation has developed. Right ventricular diastolic pressure may be elevated and pulmonary artery pressure may also be high. Generally, left-sided pressures are normal in the absence of other cardiac disease. Attempts to cross the defect to the left atrium from the right are frequently successful with documentation by oxygen saturation and contrast injection. Oxygen saturation is measured on samples obtained from the inferior and superior venae cavae, the high, mid, and low right atrium, right ventricle, the pulmonary artery, and a systemic arterial site (usually the left ventricle, aorta, or left atrium). The mixed venous oxygen saturation is determined by adding three times the infe-

rior vena cava saturation to the superior vena cava saturation and dividing by four. An oxygen "step up" of 2 volumes % per chamber progressively from right atrium to pulmonary artery is indicative of left-to-right shunting. Shunting can also be demonstrated using the green dye cardiac output curve with the presence of an early recirculation phase and by the inhalation of H_2 with early appearance in the right atrium noted by using a platinum-tipped electrode. The levophase of pulmonary artery angiography can enable visualization of the shunt in most cases, aiding in determining the anatomic location.

Quantification of the shunt is made by determining the pulmonary flow (right-sided cardiac output) and systemic flow (left-sided cardiac output) as noted above. The two are then subtracted and net shunt flow is determined. A ratio of pulmonary to systemic flow (Q_p/Q_s) is also determined and this shunt ratio is used for therapeutic decisions. An abbreviated method for determining the ratio is:

$$\frac{Q_p}{Q_s} = \frac{\text{arterial saturation - mixed venous saturation}}{\text{pulmonary venous saturation - pulmonary arterial saturation}}$$

Saturation determinations should be made with the patient in a steady state, breathing room air. Samples must be drawn at the various sites in rapid succession to ensure validity. Small (probably hemodynamically insignificant) shunts may not be detected by all techniques; it's preferable that shunts be documented by at least two techniques.

Ventricular Septal Defect

Large congenital ventricular septal defects are generally discovered early in life. A VSD is primarily a volume overload lesion of the left ventricle as the majority of left to right shunting occurs during systole (the left ventricle essentially shunting blood through the right ventricle into the pulmonary artery). As a result, left ventricular failure results. Reactive pulmonary hypertension can develop which may become severe and fixed (Eisenmenger's physiology). Clinical findings include evidence of left ventricular dysfunction such as dyspnea, rales, S_3, left ventricular enlargement, and functional mitral regurgitation. A holosystolic murmur usually associated with a thrill is heard at the lower left sternal border with wide radiation; evidence of pulmonary hypertension may be present and cyanosis occurs in severe cases. Lack of second sound splitting may be noted.

Catheterization technique is similar to that for atrial septal defects. Pressure measurements may demonstrate elevated right-sided pressures if pul-

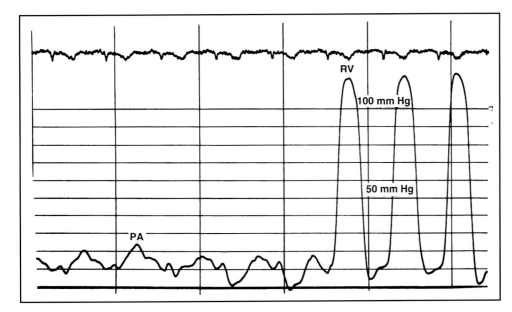

Figure 11. Pulmonic stenosis with a large pressure gradient noted on "pullback" from pulmonary artery to right ventricle. Note the massively elevated right ventricular systolic pressure and the damped appearing pulmonary artery pressure tracing.

monary hypertension has developed. Left ventricular end diastolic and pulmonary capillary wedge pressures will be elevated when left ventricular failure has developed. Oximetry will demonstrate a "step up" at right ventricular level. The defect may be crossed with the catheter, but because of the tendency for ventricular ectopy, persistent attempts are not made. Left ventricular angiography in the LAO projection will demonstrate contrast flow across the ventricular septum and into the pulmonary artery. Pulmonary and systemic blood flow calculations (as noted above) are made with calculation of shunt flow and shunt ratio (Q_p/Q_s).

Partial Anomalous Pulmonary Venous Return

Partial anomalous pulmonary venous return may occur in isolation or in combination with an atrial septal defect. Clinical findings are similar to those in an ASD, but the diagnosis may be suggested by findings on chest x-ray or echocardiography. Catheterization technique is similar to that employed for an atrial defect and careful measurement of oxygen saturation in various positions in the right atrium is of critical importance. The anomalous vein(s) may be entered directly with the catheter as documented fluoroscopically and by oximetry. The levophase of pulmonary arteriography may also be helpful in identifying this anomaly.

Pulmonic Valve Disease

Congenital pulmonic valve disease may be discovered in adulthood. Clinical findings of pulmonic stenosis include an outflow murmur and ejection sound (more apparent in expiration); chest x-ray film may demonstrate right ventricular enlargement and poststenotic pulmonary artery dilation,

and valvular pulmonic regurgitation (frequently a secondary abnormality due to previous surgery for pulmonic stenosis) is characterized by a middiastolic murmur of mid-frequency.

Catheterization entails pressure and cardiac output measurements on the right side, as well as a thorough search for other congenital abnormalities (particularly shunt lesions) (Figure 11). Right ventricular angiography in the lateral projection is helpful in demonstration of pulmonary outflow tract and pulmonic valve anatomy. Outflow tract hypertrophy may be seen (particularly in patients with forms of tetralogy of Fallot) and valvular "doming" is often noted. Pulmonary arteriography in the same projection is used to demonstrate pulmonic regurgitation (taking into account catheter interference with valve closure). Left heart catheterization and coronary angiography, in the appropriate setting when operative intervention is contemplated, are also performed.

Decisions regarding intervention in pulmonic valve disease rely primarily on the secondary effects of the lesions on right ventricular hemodynamics. In pulmonic stenosis, the level of right ventricular systolic pressure is a determining factor, rather than the pulmonic valve gradient. Balloon valvuloplasty frequently may be employed when intervention is required. Right ventricular dysfunction indicated by elevated right atrial pressure and right ventricular end diastolic pressure, along with evidence of tricuspid regurgitation, might indicate need for surgery in patients with pulmonic regurgitation.

Ebstein's Anomaly

Ebstein's anomaly of the tricuspid valve is associated with evidence of right ventricular dysfunction and significant arrhythmias. Jugular venous pulse evidence of tricuspid regurgitation is frequently lacking, while systemic venous pressure elevation may be present. Tricuspid regurgitation is noted on auscultation and characteristic electrocardiographic abnormalities may be present. Right heart catheterization demonstrates findings of tricuspid regurgitation and right ventricular dysfunction. Using an electrode tipped hemodynamic catheter, simultaneous recordings of right atrial pressure and a right ventricular electrogram at the same position document diagnosis. Right ventricular angiography is also helpful in demonstration of the anatomy.

Coarctation of the Aorta

Coarctation of the aorta is often found in conjunction with congenital aortic stenosis. Clinically, findings of unequal upper extremity blood pressure measurements, radial-femoral pulse lag, diminished lower extremity blood pressure, a posterior thoracic murmur, and abnormalities of the aortic shadow on chest film may be present. Pressure measurements documenting a gradient at the site of coarctation, along with aortic angiography (preferably with rapid sequence "cut film" recording) document the diagnosis. As an alternative to surgical correction, balloon dilation has been useful in some cases.

Other Syndromes

A variety of other congenital syndromes may rarely be found in adults and require detailed precatheterization diagnostic evaluation as well as careful, thorough planning of the catheterization protocol. The availability of balloon tipped catheters has made catheterization technically more feasible in many of these instances; availability of partially corrective surgical procedures in the pediatric age group has resulted in large numbers of adult patients with residual abnormalities who would not have previously survived. As a result, adult catheterization laboratories will be seeing more of these patients in the future. Very careful precatheterization assessment and thorough hemodynamic and angiographic evaluation are necessary in order to make appropriate therapeutic decisions.

Coronary Artery Disease

Suspected coronary artery disease is probably the most frequent indication for cardiac catheterization. Indications for this procedure have included symptoms suggestive of myocardial ischemia (classical angina pectoris, chest pain of uncertain etiology), the finding of an abnormal noninvasive indicator of ischemia with or without associated symptoms, and previously documented myocardial injury. Unlike other forms of heart disease, there are presently no universally accepted, highly accurate, noninvasive methods for determining the presence and severity of coronary artery stenosis. As a result, coronary angiography remains the "gold standard" for the diagnosis and risk profiling of coronary disease. Other techniques are available to gauge the functional consequences of ischemia. Echocardiography and cardiac Doppler are helpful in assessing ischemia-related left ventricular dysfunction and mitral regurgitation. Stress testing with or without concommitant myocardial perfusion imaging (exercise or pharmacologic) can help determine functional reserve. But only coronary arteriography can accurately determine the extent of coronary obstructions.

As in other disease states, catheterization in this setting should generally be reserved for those patients in whom an intervention is contemplated. Unlike the situation in valvular heart disease, gauging the timing of intervention is not always possible based on symptoms or noninvasive studies. As a result, many noninvasive studies may be performed in order to make a decision regarding need for intervention. A decision should be made prior to invasive study, however, that the patient is a candidate for either surgery or an intravascular procedure such as coronary angioplasty. Such a decision is based on a combination of factors, including the patient's overall medical condition, the estimate of the state of left ventricular function, and, importantly, the patient's own desires regarding intervention. These should be considered prior to undertaking an invasive diagnostic procedure.

Catheterization assessment of coronary disease includes left-sided hemodynamics, left ventriculography, and coronary arteriography. In addition, right heart catheterization is performed if severe left ventricular dysfunction or mitral regurgitation is suspected. Aortic root angiography may be performed if there is suspicion of aortic disease which would complicate coronary bypass surgery. Visualization of the internal mammary arteries by direct cannulation is sometimes performed to assure that they are of sufficient caliber to be used as conduits. If previous bypass surgery has been performed, visualization of the grafts by direct injection is also carried out. This may be difficult, particularly if radiopaque markers were not placed at the time of surgery or if the grafts are occluded proximally.

Left Ventriculography

Left heart catheterization is performed in a standard manner as noted above; left ventricular hemo-

TABLE 7

Coronary Artery Anomalies

Origin from the opposite aortic cusp

Origin from the pulmonary artery

Absent vessel

Arteriovenous malformation

dynamic recordings are made. Left ventriculography is performed, preferably in two planes (left and right anterior oblique projections), if there is evidence of segmental left ventricular dysfunction. Estimates of diminished ejection fraction are difficult because of the segmental nature of left ventricular dysfunction; use of the ventriculogram to calculate the ejection fraction using the formula for ellipsoid volumes is subject to error because of changes in ventricular shape.

Coronary Arteriography

Coronary arteriography is performed in the manner described above using either straight or, more commonly, preformed catheters. Multiple views of the right and left coronary arteries are recorded with "special" views to evaluate the left main coronary artery as well as the proximal left anterior descending and circumflex vessels.

- **Coronary Artery Anatomy:** The right coronary gives rise to the posterior descending vessel, the posterolateral vessel, and the vessel to the A-V node. Other right coronary vessels include the atrial branch and infundibular branches proximally, and the acute marginal branch supplying the right ventricle. The left coronary artery usually bifurcates into circumflex and left anterior descending branches but, not infrequently, an intermediate branch *(ramus intermedius)* is present and of variable size. The left anterior descending vessel characteristically is located in the interventricular groove anteriorly and reaches to or just beyond the cardiac apex, where it generally bifurcates into two small terminal branches. The vessel gives rise to several septal perforating branches, the first of which is larger than the rest and supplies the proximal portion of the distal conduction system as well. There are usually several diagonal branches which supply the anterior surface of the left ventricle. In some instances, the left anterior descending vessel terminates well proximal to the apex and its usual distal territory is supplied by the posterior descending coronary artery or the circumflex and intermediate branches. In some patients, the left anterior descending vessel reaches well beyond the

apex and supplies a significant portion of the inferior wall. The circumflex vessel runs in the A-V groove (easily identified by visualization of the coronary sinus) running posteriorly. It gives rise to one or more obtuse marginal branches which supply the lateral left ventricular wall. When a left dominant circulation is present, the circumflex vessel gives rise to the posterior descending coronary artery, a posterolateral branch, and the artery to the A-V node. When an intermediate vessel is present, it arises between the left anterior descending and circumflex vessels and supplies to a greater or lesser extent the left ventricular free wall between diagonal and obtuse marginal branches.

In the right dominant circulation, the right coronary artery is as described above. The posterior descending vessel supplies the inferior wall of the left ventricle and the posterolateral branch supplies that territory. In the left dominant circulation, the right coronary artery supplies its more proximal branches with supplying any significant portion of the left ventricle. However, a "balanced" or "codominant" situation exists in some patients in which portions of the posterior and inferior left ventricle are supplied by both the right and left circumflex coronary arteries.

- **Coronary Artery Anomalies:** Anomalies of the coronary circulation also occur in up to 2% of patients (Table 7). Separate origins of the proximal branches of the left coronary artery (circumflex and anterior descending) may be present. Unrecognized, this situation can lead to the erroneous interpretation that one of these vessels is occluded. The conus branch of the right coronary artery occasionally arises as a separate vessel in the right coronary cusp; direct injection of this branch with a large amount of contrast may result in ventricular fibrillation. Anomalous origin of the left coronary artery or a major branch from the right coronary vessel (or cusp) may occur. The vessel may then pass between the pulmonary artery and aorta as it runs a course toward the left ventricle. This may lead to compression of the left vessel when the great vessels stretch to accommodate higher cardiac output or pressure. A similar situation can occur with anomalous origin of the right coronary artery from the left. Rarely, a coronary artery may arise from the pulmonary artery. Usually, this results in myocardial infarction with left ventricular dysfunction or death in infancy or early childhood. Coronary artery arteriovenous fistulas may also be seen, but these usually involve small branch vessels and are clinically insignificant (although larger vessels may be involved in the acquired form secondary to trauma).

- **Coronary Artery Spasm:** In addition to clas-

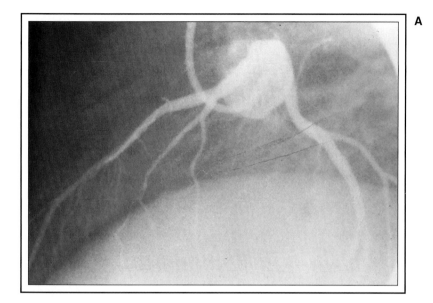

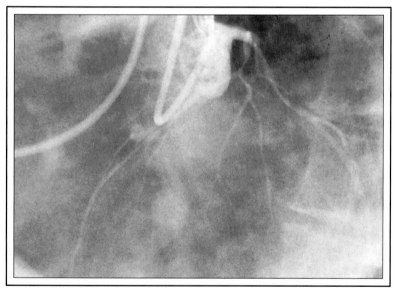

Figure 12. The left coronary artery (LAO projection) before (A) and after (B) administration of ergonovine. Note diffuse spasm.

sic coronary artery disease, occasionally diagnosis of coronary artery spasm is entertained, either in the appropriate clinical setting (variant or Prinzmetal angina) or in patients with no or trivial coronary disease on baseline angiography (Figures 12, 13). Techniques can be employed to stimulate spasm while monitoring symptoms, the ECG, and performing repeat coronary arteriography. Sometimes injection of contrast material may itself cause spasm. Immersion of a hand in cold water or the injection of an ergot alkaloid peripherally in incremental doses of 0.2mg to 0.6mg (after a small test dose) may cause discrete spasm. Parenteral nitroglycerin used intravenously or intracoronary must be available to reverse spasm if it occurs; diffuse narrowing of the coronary tree usually occurs, but an abnormal test is characterized by localized high grade spasm (along with symptoms of charac-

teristic chest discomfort and ECG changes).

• **Severity of Coronary Stenosis:** Abnormalities found during coronary arteriography range from minimal plaque formation, characterized by irregularities noted in the lumen, to complete obstruction of one or more major epicardial vessels. Localized stenosis of the coronary vessels is generally estimated as percentage of diameter narrowing by visual inspection of the segment on cineangiograms (or on tape or disc) in various projections. Use of manual calipers or computerized measurement can increase the precision of this estimate. Less than 50% diameter obstruction is not considered hemodynamically significant, while greater than 70% obstruction is felt to be critical, capable of causing ischemic syndromes. Also, 50%-70% obstruction is moderate and correlation with the clinical findings is necessary. Because lesions may

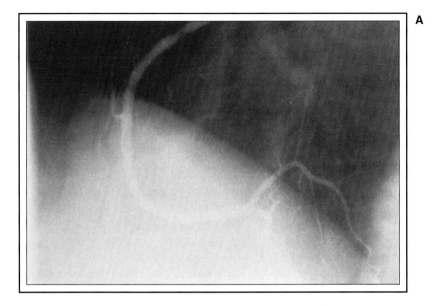

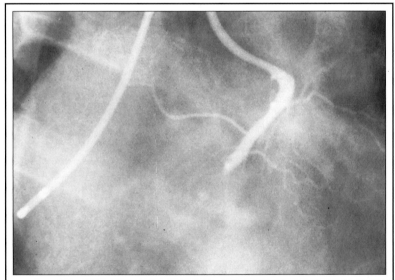

Figure 13. The right coronary artery (LAO projection) before (A) and after (B) ergonovine administration. Complete "obstruction" due to spasm has occurred in the mid portion, which is normal on baseline angiography.

be eccentric, multiple views are needed to be sure that the axis demonstrating the maximal degree of luminal obstruction is clear. Multiple views are also needed to eliminate overlap of vessels and to correct for radiographic shadowing due to tortuosity of vessels.

• **Coronary Lesion Morphology:** In addition to severity of coronary stenosis, the character of the coronary lesions should be observed. Ulcerated lesions may be more prone to thrombus formation, and they result in more acute coronary syndromes. The appearance of thrombus in a vessel is also of significant additional concern. This may be characterized by a hazy appearance to the lesion, the uptake of contrast by the lesion, or the presence of a mobile filling defect. Again, this finding is often associated with acute coronary syndromes. Other research level coronary diagnostic techniques are

currently under development. These include fiberoptic angioscopy, which permits direct visualization of coronary lesions and intracoronary ultrasound imaging. These techniques supply information regarding coronary lesions as well as their severity.

Complications of coronary disease, such as evidence of previous infarction characterized by areas of decreased wall motion (hypokinesis), lack of wall motion (akinesis), or paradoxical wall motion (dyskinesis) may be found on left ventriculography (Figure 14). Because wall motion abnormalities do not always indicate permanent myocardial damage, but sometimes result from chronic ischemia (hibernating myocardium), maneuvers may be performed to document functional reserve including analysis of wall motion during a systole following a premature beat (spon-

441

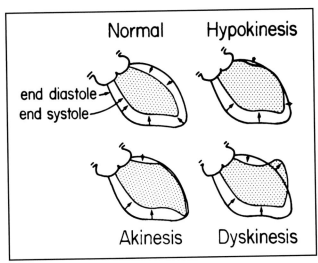

Figure 14. Diagramatic representation of the systolic and diastolic frames of the left ventriculogram depicting normal function and segmental wall motion abnormalities of varying degree.

taneous or stimulated) and response of the segment to nitroglycerin administration.

Acute Myocardial Infarction

In the setting of acute myocardial infarction, wall motion abnormalities in the zone of myocardium supplied by the infarct-related vessel may be related to myocardial "stunning" and are potentially reversible. Overall impairment of left ventricular function and ejection fraction decrease are analyzed as mentioned above. Other complications noted by ventriculography include associated mitral regurgitation (also associated with large V-

waves in the pulmonary artery occluded pressure tracing) and ventricular septal rupture (which may be confirmed by techniques mentioned above for the diagnosis of left to right shunts at the ventricular level) (Figures 15, 16, 17).

Right Heart Catheterization

Bedside right heart catheterization can be helpful in patients with complications related to coronary artery disease. In patients with severe left ventricular dysfunction, right heart hemodynamics, cardiac output determinations, and wedge pressure readings can guide therapeutic maneuvers such as intravenous inotropic support, afterload reduction, and intra-aortic balloon assist. Diagnosis of right ventricular infarction can also be made by right heart catheterization, which reveals elevated and equalized right-sided diastolic pressures, and appropriate therapy can be instituted. Acute mitral regurgitation, as characterized by large V-waves in the pulmonary artery occluded pressure tracing, may be noted. If ventricular septal rupture is suspected, analysis of O_2 saturations from the proximal and distal lumens of the catheter for a step-up in the pulmonary artery may confirm the diagnosis.

Pitfalls in Data Interpretation

Pitfalls in the interpretation of catheterization data in coronary artery disease exist. As mentioned above, ejection fraction calculation may be imprecise because of the regional nature of left ventricular dysfunction. Associated mitral regurgitation may result in an overestimate of left ventricular

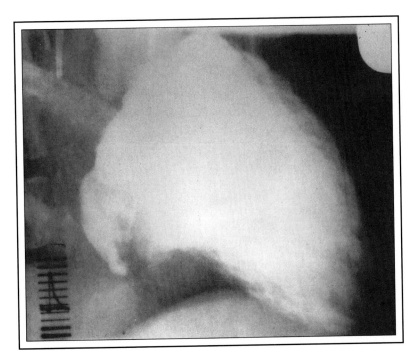

Figure 15. Left ventriculogram in the RAO projection demonstrating anteroapical aneurysm formation. Filling defects which may reflect thrombus formation are seen.

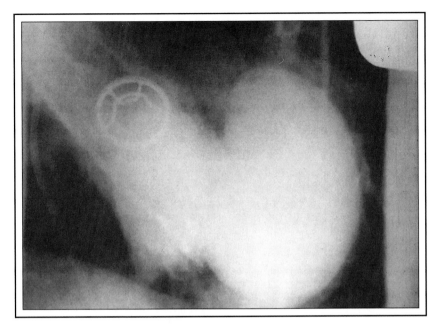

Figure 16. A pseudoaneurysm of the left ventricle following mitral valve replacement. Note the "neck" connecting the left ventricular chamber with the smoothly outlined aneurysmal "sac" comprised of pericardial tissue.

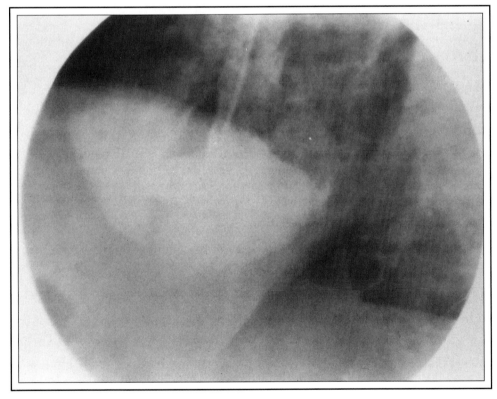

Figure 17. Ventricular septal defect (acquired). Left ventriculogram in the LAO projection demonstrating contrast shunting to the right ventricle through a well-outlined mid-septal defect.

function. Interpretive errors in coronary arteriography include masking of lesions due to an incomplete set of angled views, poorly seen lesions at the origin of the major coronary arteries, and overlapping of vessels. Overestimation of severity can result from shadowing due to overlap of vessels and using views where tortuosity creates the same effect (viewing the vessel *en face*). Lesions may be "created" by spasm at a site of contact with the tip of the catheter and by myocardial bridges (areas where

an epicardial coronary artery passes intramyocardial for a portion of its course) (Figure 18).

Interventional Catheterization Techniques

In addition to being a site for diagnostic procedures, the catheterization laboratory has increasingly become the arena for therapeutic maneuvers (Table 8). The development of a percutaneous method for insertion of the balloon and catheter

443

system used for intra-aortic balloon pump support has allowed initiation of that therapy in the catheterization laboratory. Pericardiocentesis under fluoroscopic and pressure guidance is likewise performed in the catheterization laboratory setting.

Transluminal Balloon Valvuloplasty

Transluminal balloon valvuloplasty is a recently developed therapeutic maneuver with application primarily in patients with aortic and mitral stenosis. In the case of aortic stenosis, the technique has shown limited usefulness because of the marginal improvement in hemodynamic state, and short duration of effect. Its role now is limited to patients who are critically ill as a "bridge" to prepare them for a surgical procedure.

The procedure can be performed using either the retrograde arterial approach or by use of the transseptal technique. A double-length wire is used to cross the aortic valve, using an additional loop in the ventricle in the retrograde technique or with the wire extending into the ascending and preferably descending aorta in the transseptal method. A catheter with a large caliber balloon (up to 20mm) is then advanced over the wire and across the valve. The balloon is inflated with diluted contrast one or more times, with an attempt to reduce or abolish the "waist" at the site of the stenotic aortic orifice. When successful, the procedure generally results in a gradient decrease of 50% and a two-fold increase in the valve area. However, this effect is usually lost in six months time. Complications of the procedure include local arterial problems related to the large gauge of the associated catheters and sheaths, disruption of the aortic annulus and aorta, and the other complications mentioned above in association with catheterization. In addition, development of or increase in severity of aortic regurgitation frequently occurs and the procedure must be limited to those patients with mild or no baseline aortic regurgitation.

Balloon valvuloplasty of the mitral valve has proven to be a more definitive procedure. In appropriate cases, the technique can produce excellent, long-lasting results. Patients with mitral stenosis who have mobile, minimally calcified valves and little or no mitral regurgitation are candidates. Using the transseptal approach, two double length wires are passed across the septum, through the stenotic valve orifice, and preferably through the left ventricle and into the aorta (although frequently passage across the aortic valve is not always possible and the wires are looped in the left ventricle). The atrial septum is dilated with a balloon catheter and two appropriately-sized large

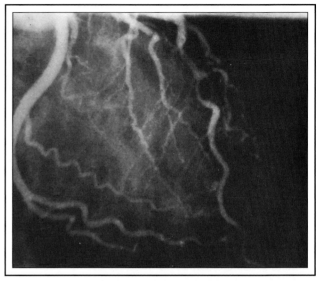

Figure 18. The left coronary artery (RAO projection) demonstrating an intramyocardial segment (myocardial bridge) simulating an intrinsic coronary lesion. Significant obstruction can be seen during systole.

caliber balloons are passed across the septum and positioned to straddle the mitral orifice. The balloons are simultaneously inflated with diluted contrast one or more times to diminish or eliminate the indentation caused by the stenotic orifice. Successful balloon dilation of the mitral valve can result in virtual elimination of the gradient with minimal enhancement of mitral regurgitation in appropriately selected patients. Complications, in addition to those for transseptal catheterization, include disruption of the mitral annulus due to inappropriate balloon sizing, increased severity of mitral regurgitation, and, rarely, left-to-right shunting through the enlarged atrial septal orifice (usually only in those with persistently elevated left atrial pressure due to significant residual mitral obstruction).

Percutaneous Transluminal Coronary Angioplasty

The greatest advances in interventional techniques in the catheterization laboratory have taken place in the field of coronary artery therapy. Initial efforts in this arena were limited to intracoronary drug infusions, such as thrombolytic agents and nitroglycerin. The popularization of balloon angioplasty by Grüntzig has led to the unprecedented development and application of transluminal coronary interventional techniques. Transluminal coronary angioplasty has found wide application in a variety of coronary syndromes.

Indications for angioplasty are not universally accepted; patients with intractable symptoms and

TABLE 8
Interventional Catheterization Techniques

Intra-aortic balloon assist

Coronary angioplasty

Coronary lesion ablation (atherectomy extraction, rotoblation, laser)

Coronary stenting

Transcatheter valvuloplasty

Shunt ablation devices

who would otherwise require bypass surgery are candidates; patients with multivessel disease who have accepted anatomic indications for intervention are also considered. A more controversial group of patients are those with coronary artery obstructions of critical severity (70% diameter obstruction or greater) who would not be considered surgical candidates based on severity or distribution of their obstructions. In patients with unstable coronary syndromes, angioplasty of the "culprit" vessel as an initial strategy has become widely accepted. In the setting of acute myocardial infarction, angioplasty is a well-accepted reperfusion strategy.

The technique of coronary angioplasty is similar to retrograde coronary arteriography. Guiding catheters, of similar design to coronary angiographic catheters but of larger bore, are advanced (by use of previously described techniques) to the appropriate coronary or bypass graft ostium. A fine wire is advanced across the lesion to be opened and an appropriately sized balloon catheter is advanced into the lesion; the balloon is then inflated with dilute contrast material under fluoroscopic control. Reduction or abolition of the "waist" demonstrates improvement in the severity of the lesion. Pre- and post-dilation angiography are performed to document initial findings and therapeutic result. Lesions of critical severity, including totally obstructed vessels, can be treated with a high degree of success (85% or greater) initially. Unfortunately, there is an approximately 30%-45% rate of restenosis or closure in the first six months after treatment. Repeat angioplasty has been effective in most of those patients and, therefore, the more complex and costly surgical approach avoided. In multiple vessel angioplasty, this reocclusion rate applies to each lesion dilated.

New Interventional Techniques and Devices

Alternative techniques to standard balloon angioplasty, e.g. atherectomy, rotary ablation or laser vaporization, have been developed but major improvements in the restenosis rate have not resulted. Directional atherectomy employs a circular rotating cutting device in a hollow cylinder which exposes the blade on one side. A balloon is also part of the device and is used for stabilization. The material carved out of the atheroma is packed into the cylinder and can then be extracted. This technique, like most of the alternative techniques, is limited in its applicability to proximal coronary lesions in areas of minimal tortuosity. The transluminal extraction catheter utilizes a rotating blade accompanied by a suction device which extracts the fragments of plaque. The Rotoblator employs a rotating burr which drills through the plaque material and produces minuscule particles which are carried downstream. Laser devices are also available. Laser energy is employed in some of these devices to heat either the tip of a catheter or an angioplasty balloon; other laser devices use light energy to ablate the plaque. All these alternative methods require traditional methods of guiding catheter use and crossing the obstruction with a wire. Intracoronary stents are thin metallic scaffolds that mechanically support the vessel wall. By virtue of size, stenting may help reduce restenosis in selected patients by creating a much larger lumen especially in native vessels greater than 3 mm in diameter with de novo lesions. Coronary stents may also play a beneficial role as a "bail-out device" in restoring or maintaining vessel patency in the setting of abrupt (or threatened) closure and acute dissection during failed interventional procedures.

Complications of interventional coronary procedures include those associated with standard coronary angiography. Spasm, dissection, and thrombus formation leading to occlusion, can occur at the site of angioplasty or other alternative interventions. These problems may develop during the course of the procedure or in the first several hours afterwards. Intravenous anticoagulation with heparin or a Hirudin analog is used to prevent thrombus formation. Complications are often amenable to correction by intravascular techniques such as repeat angioplasty. However, 1%-3% of patients require emergent coronary bypass surgery as a result of acute coronary obstruction. Possibility of late restenosis is discussed above.

Cardiomyopathies

Dilated Cardiomyopathy

Patients with dilated cardiomyopathy may undergo cardiac catheterization to evaluate the possibility of an underlying correctable cause. Occasionally these patients may have such processes as valvular heart disease or coronary artery disease with hibernating myocardium as the etiology of their ventricular dysfunction. Likewise, patients with infiltrative or inflammatory myopathy may be candidates for specific medical intervention and, therefore, ventricular biopsy may be indicated. In the majority of patients with classic idiopathic dilated cardiomyopathy, standard cardiac catheterization offers little benefit. Right heart catheterization for purposes of vasodilator or inotropic therapy has a role in many patients with advanced disease.

Findings at right and left heart catheterization usually include elevated right-sided pressures (due to either direct right ventricular involvement or secondary to passive pulmonary artery pressure elevation), tricuspid regurgitation, elevated pulmonary capillary wedge pressure, elevated left ventricular diastolic pressure, diminished cardiac output (in advanced stages), and diminished left ventricular function by angiography. Frequently, some degree of mitral regurgitation may be present. It may be difficult to judge whether the valvular dysfunction is caused by or results from the left ventricular abnormality. As noted above, significant degrees of mitral regurgitation may result in an underestimation of ventricular impairment. The left ventricular and aortic pressure tracings may exhibit an alternating level of systolic pressure in far advanced cases which corresponds to the clinical finding of *pulsus alternans.*

CARDIAC PEARL

Pulsus alternans can be one of the most subtle signs of heart failure, but we must look for it. We must then specifically search for the ventricular (S_3) gallop and alternation of the sounds and murmurs. A method personally used is as follows: place the stethoscope along the patient's lower left sternal border, thereby providing an overview; listen specifically to the first sound, then the second sound, and then systematically listen for sounds in systole, murmurs in systole, sounds in diastole, and murmurs in diastole. In this way we are dissecting, so to speak, the various heart sounds and murmurs of the heart cycle. We are not trying to listen to everything at once. it is analogous to listening to the music played by a symphony orchestra. The listener is able to pick out a particular instrument, such as a violin, horn, piano or kettle drum, by concentrating on it.

After detecting a pulsus alternans, focus on listening for a sound occurring in early to mid systole. A faint third heart sound is present, which has the timing of a ventricular (S_3) gallop. A simple but important cardiac pearl is to now turn the patient to the left lateral position and palpate with the index and middle fingers of the left hand to locate the point of maximum impulse of the left ventricle. Hold that spot with the fingers and place the bell of the stethoscope lightly over this localized area; the ventricular (S_3) gallop may now be louder and clearly heard. The gallop may also alternate in intensity with every other beat. Pressure on the stethoscope can eliminate this gallop. We now have noted in this patient pulsus alternans of the radial pulse observed when first greeting our patient, alternation of the second sound and systolic murmur, and a ventricular (S_3) gallop, also alternating in intensity. With these clinical cardiac pearls, we have definitely diagnosed cardiac decompensation. This diagnosis has been accomplished in the office or at the bedside, without having to use expensive procedures.

With advanced degrees of cardiac decompensation (the ejection fraction is low), these physical signs are more easily detected, as might be expected. They become more difficult to find as improvement takes place (the ejection fraction is higher). If they are no longer present, the decompensation has been eliminated (the ejection fraction is now likely in a normal range). The ejection fraction determined in the diagnostic laboratory is a way of determining the degree of cardiac decompensation. At times, it is a helpful test; however, it can be used too frequently, adds expense for the patient, and might be spared if the physician pays close attention to these clinical findings Figures A and B).

W. Proctor Harvey, M.D.

Right ventricular biopsy may be performed as above and a pulmonary artery balloon catheter may be left in place for manipulation of therapy (generally not from the femoral position). Coronary angiography is performed in appropriate settings.

Hypertrophic Cardiomyopathy

Catheterization in the setting of hypertrophic cardiomyopathy (an abnormality best evaluated by Doppler echocardiography) is performed in patients with symptoms of coexistent coronary artery disease, as well as in those in whom left ventricular outflow tract obstruction is suspected (and the possibility of a therapeutic intervention exists).

Right and left heart catheterization are carried out in the usual fashion and coronary angiography is performed if otherwise indicated. Right sided pressures may be elevated ("passively" if the pulmonary capillary wedge pressure is substantially

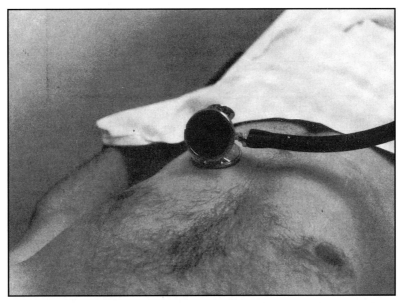

Fig A: The stethoscope is placed over the lower left sternal border, providing an overview.

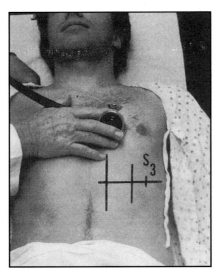 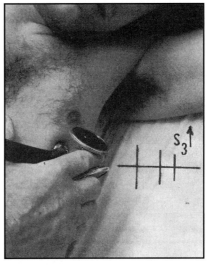

Fig B: A faint ventricular (S₃) diastolic gallop louder and clearer when the patient turns from the supine position (left panel) to the left lateral position (right panel), with the physician listening with the bell of the stethoscope held lightly over the point of maximal impulse of the left ventricle.

elevated) but are usually normal. Wedge pressure and left ventricular end diastolic pressure are frequently elevated reflecting reduced diastolic compliance. An intraventricular pressure gradient exists in those patients with left ventricular outflow obstruction. Careful positioning of the catheter will reveal a reduction in systolic pressure in the outflow tract in comparison to the body of the ventricle (lower systolic pressure being at the same level as a simultaneously-recorded aortic root pressure). This gradient may be enhanced or provoked by Valsalva maneuver, amyl nitrite, isoproterenol, exercise, and during the systole following a pause caused by a premature beat. The systolic pressure in the aorta may paradoxically fall during a post-extrasystolic cycle due to the enhanced obstruction (Brockenbrough effect) (Figures 19, 20). Because of the relatively small size of the ventricle in this condition, "catheter entrapment" (alluded to above), with resultant misinterpretation of the pressure curves in the left ventricle, must be carefully eliminated as the cause of a pressure gradient. Analysis of the left ventricular pressure curve in diastole may reveal a retarded drop in early diastolic pressure as well as a large A-wave consistent with impaired diastolic function. Left ventricular angiog-

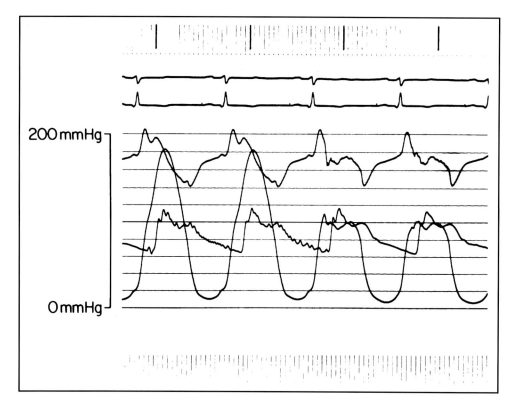

Figure 19. Hypertrophic obstructive cardiomyopathy. Continuous aortic pressure tracing with left ventricular pressure from the apex (first two cycles) and the area above the obstruction (second two cycles). Note the "spike and dome" configuration of the aortic pressure tracing. An apex cardiogram is also present.

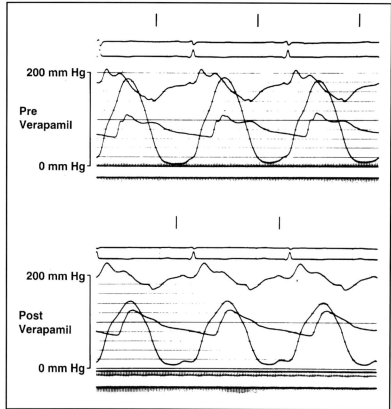

Figure 20. The gradient in hypertrophic obstructive cardiomyopathy before and after infusion of a calcium channel blocking agent. Virtual disappearance of the gradient occurs with normalization of the aortic pressure contour.

raphy usually demonstrates a small, hypercontractile ventricle (Figure 21). The lateral or left anterior oblique projection may demonstrate a "banana" shape with visualization of the hypertrophied portion of the proximal septum. Systolic anterior motion of the mitral valve leaflets and some degree of mitral regurgitation may be present in the obstructive variety.

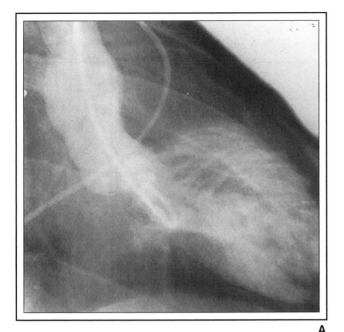

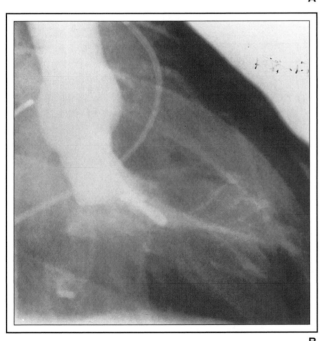

Figure 21. Left ventriculograms (RAO projection) in hypertrophic cardiomyopathy during diastole and systole. Note near cavity obliteration in the systolic frame.

Restrictive Cardiomyopathy

The differentiation between restrictive cardiomyopathy (an abnormality not correctable by surgical intervention) and constrictive pericarditis (abnormality potentially correctable by surgery) is not always certain on clinical and Doppler echocardiographic grounds. As the need for a major, invasive therapeutic decision may be present, cardiac catheterization with appropriate interventions is necessary. Restriction may result from infiltrative diseases such as amyloidosis or hemachromatosis, or may be idiopathic. The patient suffers from low forward cardiac output and elevated systemic venous pressure, both related to diminished filling.

Findings on right and left heart catheterization include elevated right atrial and right ventricular diastolic pressures. There is a rapid Y-descent noted on the right atrial pressure tracing and an early diastolic "dip" with abrupt rise and then plateau on the ventricular pressure wave form ("square root" sign). Right ventricular end diastolic and left ventricular end diastolic pressures are identical or nearly so. Left ventricular systolic function by angiography is usually normal.

To differentiate restrictive from constrictive disease, an attempt should be made to widen the difference between right and left ventricular end diastolic pressure (which will occur in restriction but not constriction). Maneuvers which may cause this differentiation include exercise and rapid volume loading. In constriction, the left ventricular end diastolic pressure will generally rise disproportionately higher than the right. In addition, right ventricular biopsy, by demonstrating an infiltrative process, may be helpful.

Pericardial Disease

Cardiac catheterization may be indicated in the setting of pericardial constriction and cardiac tamponade. In both of these instances, an appropriate therapeutic intervention (pericardiectomy or pericardial drainage) may result from the hemodynamic findings (Figure 22).

Constrictive Pericarditis

In patients with pericardial constriction, evidence of "low" output state along with systemic venous hypertension (unless the patient has undergone significant diuresis) is prevalent. Clinical findings include elevation of jugular venous pressure with Kussmaul's sign (inspiratory augmentation of the height of the venous pressure) and a rapid, prominent Y-descent of the jugular venous wave form. A pericardial knock may be present and edema, ascites, and hepatomegaly are frequently seen. The systematic blood pressure may be low with a narrow pulse pressure; infrequently *pulsus paradoxus* is present. Evidence of pericardial calcification may be seen on chest film and Doppler echocardiography demonstrates diastolic filling abnormalities.

Catheterization demonstrates elevation of right and left atrial pressures and ventricular end diastolic pressures with all filling pressures being

449

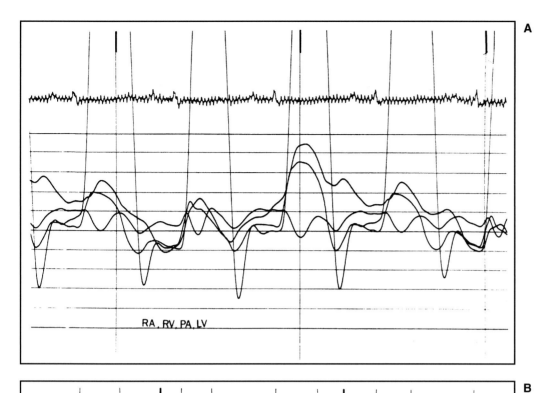

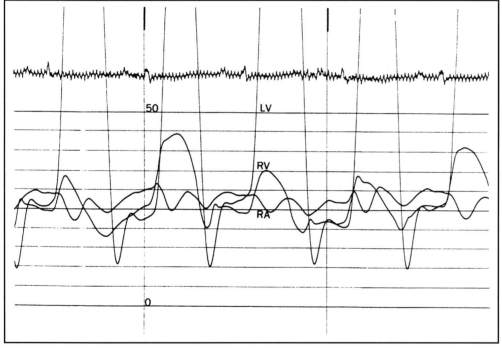

Figure 22. The "monotony" of end diastolic pressures in constrictive pericarditis. Note the dip and plateau ("square root sign") on the diastolic right and left ventricular pressure tracings.

equal. As venous return increases during inspiration, right atrial pressure rises because the constricting pericardium prevents distention of the atrial wall. Steep X and Y descents are noted as well. The early diastolic "dip" and then pressure plateau (also present in restriction) is seen in the ventricular pressure tracing. The cardiac output is diminished while left ventricular ejection fraction is increased as measured by angiography. Left ventricular volume is normal. Maneuvers to distinguish constriction from myocardial restriction are described above (Table 9).

Cardiac Tamponade

Cardiac tamponade can result from any cause of pericardial effusion. Common etiologies include malignancy, trauma, idiopathic (probably viral), infectious, and autoimmune disease. Depending on rapidity of development of the effusion, symptoms and hemodynamic findings may develop with modest

TABLE 9
Restriction to Ventricular Filling

RESTRICTIVE CARDIOMYOPATHY	PERICARDIAL CONSTRICTION	PERICARDIAL TAMPONADE
Atrial and ventricular diastolic pressures nearly equal	Equal ventricular and atrial diastolic pressure	Ventricular diastolic, atrial, and intrapericardial pressure equal
Volume infusion and exercise separate right and left-sided pressures	No separation with volume or exercise	
Kussmaul's phenomenon (right atrial pressure elevation with inspiration)	Kussmaul's phenomenon	Kussmaul's phenomenon uncommon
Paradoxic pulse uncommon	Paradoxic pulse uncommon	Paradoxic pulse apparent
Prominent X and Y descents on atrial wave form	Prominent X and Y descents on atrial wave form	Elevated atrial pressure
Ventricular diastolic dip and plateaus	Ventricular diastolic dip and plateau	Normal ventricular wave form

as well as larger effusions. Factors affecting pericardial distensibility will also alter the amount of effusion required to produce hemodynamic compromise (a relatively small amount, for instance, in seroconstrictive disease). Patients with tamponade exhibit symptoms of dyspnea and low output state (occasionally characterized by syncope). Clinically, with cardiac enlargement on chest x-ray and dyspnea, their syndrome may be mistaken for congestive heart failure. Physical findings include pulsus paradoxus of over 10mm of mercury and elevated venous pressure (occasionally with Kussmaul's sign). In patients with large effusions, the heart sounds are distant and the apical impulse quiet. Echocardiography and Doppler cardiography are extremely helpful in patients with suspected tamponade (except in patients in whom technical difficulties are present).

Intracardiac filling pressures are governed by the intrapericardial pressure in tamponade. As a result, filling of the ventricles and, therefore, cardiac output are diminished. Atrial pressures and ventricular filling pressures are the same when measured simultaneously, and are elevated in most cases; they are equal to the intrapericardial pressure (which may be determined directly by measurement through a catheter inserted in the pericardial space for pericardiocentesis). Rarely, patients who have been treated with diuretics or are volume-depleted for other reasons may have normal intracavitary pressures. If the patient under study for tamponade is a candidate for surgical pericardial removal, left ventriculography and coronary angiography should be performed after stabilization of the hemodynamics by pericardiocentesis.

Pericardiocentesis

Pericardiocentesis is frequently performed in the catheterization laboratory in conjunction with right heart catheterization when the diagnosis of tamponade has been confirmed. The lower chest and upper abdomen are prepped in the usual fashion for sterility. A pericardiocentesis needle (usually 6cm-10cm and 18 gauge) is connected to a three-way stopcock and syringe. Frequently, a unipolar electrogram is recorded from the needle using alligator clips to connect it to the ECG monitor to observe for current of injury if the myocardium is contacted. In many laboratories, this technique has been supplanted by echocardiographic guidance. With the patient in the semirecumbent (45°) position, the needle is inserted in the left xypho-costal angle and advance superiorly and slightly posteriorly with continuous aspiration. When the pericardium is entered, pressure measurements may be immediately made through the stopcock and then a guidewire is advanced into the pericardial space. A pigtail catheter is then inserted and allowed to drain actively by aspiration and then passively, observing the patient for ventricular ectopy. Care must be taken to observe fluoroscopically that the wire and catheter are not intracardiac. Recently, balloon pericardiotomy, similar to balloon valvuloplasty, has been described as another, longer-term drainage procedure.

Conclusion

Diagnosis and management of patients with known or suspected cardiac disease requires orderly accumulation of appropriate information. The history and physical examination set direction for the use of other diagnostic studies, and the ever-expanding armamentarium of noninvasive techniques has made definitive diagnosis in cardiac disease more readily available. However, catheterization remains the definitive diagnostic technique in patients requiring an interventional therapeutic maneuver.

Selected Reading

1. Alpert JS, Sloss LJ, Cohn, PF: The diagnostic accuracy of combined clinical and noninvasive cardiac evaluation: Comparison with findings at cardiac catheterization. *Catheterization and Cardiovascular Diagnosis* 6: 359-370, 1980.

2. Ambrose JA, Hjemdahl-Monsen CE: Arteriographic anatomy and mechanisms of myocardial ischemia in unstable angina. *JACC* 9(6): 1397-1402, 1987.

3. Antman EM, Marsh JD, Green LH, Grossman W: Blood oxygen measurements in the assessment of intracardiac left to right shunts: A critical appraisal of methodology. *AJC* 46: 265-271, 1980.

4. Baim DS: New technologies in interventional cardiology. *Cur Op Card* 8: 637-644, 1993.

5. Bernard Y, Etievent J, Mourand J: Long-term results of percutaneous aortic valvuloplasty compared with aortic valve replacement in patients more than 75 years old. *JACC* 20 (4): 796-801, 1992.

6. Boyd KD, Thomas SJ, Gold J: A prospective study of complications of pulmonary artery catheterizations in 500 consecutive patients. *Chest 84* (3):245-249, 1983.

7. Brockenbrough EC, Braunwald E: A new technic for left ventricular angiocardiography and transseptal left heart catheterization. *AJC* 6: 1062-1064, 1960.

8. Cannon RO, Bonow RO, Bacharach SL: Left ventricular dysfunction in patients with angina pectoris, normal epicardial coronary arteries, and abnormal vasodilator reserve. *Circ* 71 (2): 218-225, 1985.

9. Click RL, Holmes DR, Jr, Vlietstra RE: Participants of the Coronary Artery Surgery Study: Anomalous coronary arteries: Location, degree of atherosclerosis and effect on survival. *JACC* 13 (3): 531-537, 1989.

10. Cohen MV, Gorlin R: Modified orifice equation for the calculation of mitral valve area. *AHJ* 84 (6): 839-840, 1972.

11. Cournand A: Cardiac catheterization. Development of the technique, its contributions to experimental medicine, and its initial application in man. *Acta Med Scand Suppl* 579: 1-32, 1975.

12. Dyke SH, Cohn PF, Gorlin R, Sonnenblick EH: Detection of residual myocardial function in coronary artery disease using post-extra systolic potentiation. *Circ* 50: 694-699, 1974.

13. Freed MD, Miettinen OS, Nadas AS: Oximetric detection of intracardiac left-to-right shunts. *BHJ* 42: 690-694, 1979.

14. Fischman DL, Leon MB, Baim DS, et al: A randomized comparison of coronary stent placement and balloon angioplasty in the treatment of coronary artery disease. *NEJM* 331:496-501, 1994.

15. Gaines PA, Kennedy A, Moorhead P: Cholesterol embolisation: A lethal complication of vascular catheterisation. *Lancet* 1 (8578): 168-170, 1988.

16. Greene DG, Carlisle R, Grant C: Estimation of left ventricular volume by one-plane cineangiography. *Circ* 35: 61-69, 1967.

17. Grossman W, Baim DS: *Cardiac Catheterization, Angiography and Intervention.* 5th ed. Baltimore: Williams and Wilkins, 1995.

18. Helfant RH, Pine R, Meister SG: Nitroglycerin to unmask reversible asynergy. Correlation with post coronary bypass ventriculography. *Circ* 50: 108-113, 1974.

19. Heupler FA, Jr, Proudfit WL, Razavi M: Ergonovine maleate provocative test for coronary arterial spasm. *AJC* 41 (4): 631-640, 1978.

20. Hillis LD: Percutaneous left heart catheterization and coronary arteriography using a femoral artery sheath. *Cath Card Diag* 5: 393-399, 1979.

21. Johnson LW, Lozner EC, Johnson S et al: Registry Committee of the Society for Cardiac Angiography and Interventions: Coronary arteriography 1984-1987: A report of the registry of the society for cardiac angiography and interventions. I. Results and complications. *Cath Card Diag* 17:5-10, 1989.

22. Judkins MP: Selective coronary arteriography. Part I: A percutaneous transfemoral technic. *Rad* 89: 815-824, 1967.

23. Judkins MP, Kidd HJ, Prische LH, Dotter CT: Lumen-following safety J-guide for catheterization of tortuous vessels. *Rad* 88: 1127-1130, 1967.

24. Kern MJ: *The Cardiac Catheterization Handbook.* St. Louis: Mosby Year Book, Inc. 1991.

25. Kosmorsky G, Hanson MR, Tomsak RL: Neuro-ophthalmologic complications of cardiac catheterization. *Neurology* 38: 483-485, 1988.

26. Mason JW, O'Connell JB: Clinical merit of endomyocardial biopsy. *Circ* 79 (5): 971-979, 1989.

27. Mehan VK, Meier B: Conventional coronary angioplasty. *Cur Op Card* 8: 645-651, 1993.

28. Mosseri M, Yarom R et al: Histologic evidence for small-vessel coronary artery disease in patients with angina pectoris and patent large coronary arteries. *Circ* 74 (5): 964-972, 1986.

29. NHLBI balloon valvuloplasty registry participants: percutaneous balloon aortic valvuloplasty: acute and 30-day follow-up results in 674 patients from the NHLBI balloon valvuloplasty registry. *Circ* 84 (6): 2383-2397, 1991.

30. Oliva A, Scherokman B: Two cases of occipital infarction following cardiac catheterization. *Stroke* 19 (6): 773-775, 1988.

31. Parfrey PS et al: Contrast material-induced renal failure in patients with diabetes mellitus, renal insufficiency, or both. A prospective controlled study. *NEJM* 320 (3): 143-149, 1989.

32. Pepine CJ,, Hill JA, Lambert CR: *Diagnostic and Therapeutic Cardiac Catheterization.* 2nd ed. Baltimore: Williams & Wilkins 1994.

33. Rackley CE, Hood WP, J.: Quantitative angiographic evaluation and pathophysiologic mechanisms in valvular heart disease. *Prog Card Dis* 15 (5): 427-447, 1973.

34. Raizner AE, Chahine RA, Ishimori T et al: Provocation of coronary artery spasm by the cold pressor test. Hemodynamic, arteriographic and quantitative angiographic observations. *Circ* 62 (5): 925-932, 1980.

35. Roberts WC: No cardiac catheterization before cardiac valve replacement - a mistake. *AHJ* 103 (5): 930-933, 1982.

36. Ross J, Jr, Brandenburg RO et al: Coronary angiography: A report of the American College of Cardiology/American Heart Association task force on assessment of diagnostic and therapeutic cardiovascular procedures. *Circ* 76 (4): 963A-977A, 1987.

37. Roubin GS, Califf RM, O'Neill WW, et al (eds.): *Interventional Cardiovascular Medicine Principles and Practice.* Churchill Livingstone, New York 1994.

38. St. John Sutton MG et al: Valve replacement without preoperative cardiac catheterization. *NEJM* 305 (21): 1233-1238, 1981.

39. Schoonmaker FW, King SB: Coronary arteriography by the single catheter percutaneous femoral technique. *Circ* 50: 735-740, 1974.

40. Selzer A, Sudrann RB: Reliability of the determination of cardiac output in man by means of the Fick principle. *Circ Res* 6: 485-490, 1958.

41. Serruys PW, de Jaegere P, Kiemeneijf, et al: A comparison of balloon-expandable stent implantation with balloon angio-

plasty in patients with coronary artery disease. *NEJM* 331:489-495, 1994.

42. Sheehan FH, Mitten-Lewis S: Factors influencing accuracy in left ventricular volume determination. *AJC* 64: 661-664, 1989.

43. Spears JR, Sandor T et al: Computerized image analysis for quantitative measurement of vessel diameter from cineangio-grams. *Circ* 68 (2): 453-461, 1983.

44. Sprung CL, Elser B, Schein RMH et al: Risk of right bundle-branch block and complete heart block during pulmonary artery catheterization. *Critical Care Medicine* 17 (1): 1-3, 1989.

45. Topol EJ: New devices for coronary revascularization. *J Myocard Ischemia* 7:51-55, 1995.

46. Vignola PA et al: Guidelines for effective and safe percutaneous intraaortic balloon pump insertion and removal. *AJC* 48:660-664, 1981.

47. Weisel RD et al: Measurement of cardiac output by thermodilution. *NEJM* 292 (13): 682-684, 1975.

48. Wisneski JA, Gertz EW, Dahlgren M et al: Comparison of low osmolality ionic (ioxaglate) versus nonionic (iopamidol) contrast media in cardiac angiography. *AJC* 63: 489-495, 1989.

49. Wyman RM, Safian RD et al: Current complications of diagnostic and therapeutic cardiac catheterization. *JACC* 12(6):1400-1406, 1988.

CHAPTER 20

Coronary Angiography and Intravascular Ultrasonography: Anatomic and Physiologic Correlates

Jeffrey M. Isner, M.D.

The development of efficacious therapies such as bypass surgery and percutaneous revascularization have required critical appraisal of the accuracy of coronary angiography. Certain liabilities associated with this technique have been identified, studied, and in some cases solved. In patients with coronary heart disease studied at necropsy, for example, it was observed that the residual nonoccluded lumen was often eccentric in location and slit-like in shape; because such lumens may allow contrast opacification of most or all of the luminal diameter in a given plane, severity of luminal narrowing could be underestimated. Attempts to solve this issue led to the routine recording of multiple (including orthogonal) views.

It was subsequently recognized, however, that variations in coronary anatomy, body habitus, and lesion location often precluded accurate angiographic depiction of a putative lesion in its narrowest dimensions due to overlap with other vessels and foreshortening of the vessel of interest. This issue was answered in large measure by the development of more versatile angiographic gantries allowing a greater range of nonaxisymmetric views.

Even when a lesion could be successfully isolated and depicted in its most severely narrowed orientation, visual estimates of the resulting degree of luminal narrowing were shown to vary significantly among different observers, leading not only to occasional inaccuracies, but limited reproducibility as well. Quantitative coronary arteriography, proposed initially by Brown and colleagues, validated by Gould and colleagues, and subsequently modified to include computer-assisted automated edge-detection resulted in more objective angiographic analyses and thereby aided the deducibility of lesion assessment.

Necropsy examination initially constituted the most widely employed means by which to study the accuracy of coronary angiography. Subsequently, intraoperative physiologic assessment was used to evaluate the results of preoperative coronary angiography. More recently, the advent of intravascular ultrasound (IVUS) has provided an in vivo equivalent to the cross-sectional area analysis available previously only at necropsy examination; this consideration has proved to be particularly useful in the era of interventional cardiology for assessment of irregular lumen geometry. This chapter will attempt to outline the manner in which necropsy, physiologic, and IVUS examinations have clarified the utility and limitations of coronary angiography.

Necropsy Studies

Necropsy studies have varied in their assessment of the accuracy of coronary angiography, but all have indicated at least some degree of inaccuracy inherent in this technique. Kemp and associates compared angiographic and post-mortem findings in 131 major coronary arteries in 29 patients and concluded that although the degree of narrowing had been underestimated by angiography in 16 coronary arteries, the degree of underestimation was functionally significant in only three. Vlodaver and associates compared angiographic with necropsy narrowing in 134 coronary arterial segments and found that the degree of luminal narrowing had been significantly underestimated in 44 (33%) of the coronary segments. Grondin and associates compared the angiographic and necropsy findings in 23 patients who died after coronary bypass operations within 30 days of selective coronary cineangiography: in nine patients, coronary arterial narrowings had been significantly underestimated, and in four patients, this resulted in incomplete myocardial revascularization. Schwartz and associates compared angiographic with necropsy narrowing in 226 coronary segments and found that the degree of narrowing had been significantly underestimated in 34 (15%). Hutchins and associates compared the degree of luminal narrowing seen on selective cineangiograms with the degree observed on post-mortem angiograms in 28 patients who died after cardiac operations. By this method, they found that in 15 of the 315 coronary artery segments, the pre-mortem cineangiogram underestimated the degree of narrowing by more than 50%.

Arnett and associates attempted to improve upon the preceding necropsy investigations by altering both the manner in which the coronary angiograms were reviewed and the manner in which the coronary arteries were examined at necropsy. The coronary angiograms were independently assessed by three experienced angiographers in order to account for problems related to interobserver variability. Furthermore, serial (5-mm) histologic examination of the coronary arteries at necropsy was used in preference to either gross examination or post-mortem angiography employed by previous investigators. The percentage of cross-sectional area narrowing by atherosclerotic plaque was quantified by a videoplanimetry system interfaced with a light microscope; elastic tissue stains of the internal elastic membrane were used to demonstrate the native coronary arterial lumen. A total of 61 coronary arteries or their subdivisions in 10 patients were analyzed by the three angiographers, none of whom was aware of the results of necropsy examination. Because for any degree of diameter reduction (by angiography) there is a greater degree of cross-sectional area narrowing (by histologic examination), an *angiographic error* was defined as a difference of more than 25% between the degree of narrowing found by cineangiography during life and that found by histologic examination after death.

In all 10 patients, a significant narrowing in at least one extramural coronary artery was underestimated by at least one or more angiographers. Of eight arteries shown by histologic examination to be narrowed 51% to 75% in cross-sectional area, underestimation of the degree of luminal narrowing by one or more angiographers occurred in seven. Of 42 arteries narrowed 76% to 100% in cross-sectional area by histologic examination, underestimation of the degree of luminal narrowing by angiography occurred in 17. The coronary segments most frequently misinterpreted were the left main and proximal left circumflex coronary arteries. Of the 24 coronary arteries or their subdivisions in which the degree of narrowing was underestimated by angiography, two angiographers erred in nine, and all three angiographers erred in three.

Quantitative histologic examination of the coronary arteries performed at necropsy examination of these 10 patients disclosed two principal morphologic features that accounted for the tendency to underestimate degrees of coronary narrowing. First, the coronary atherosclerotic process is diffuse rather than focal, a fact that has been emphasized by Roberts and colleagues. Of the total 465 5-mm segments of coronary artery examined histologically in the 10 patients, 209 (45%) were narrowed 76% to 100% and 139 (29%) were narrowed 51% to 75%; remarkably, only 45 of the total 465 sections (<10%) were narrowed less than 26% in cross-sectional area by atherosclerotic plaque. Such diffuse narrowing forces the angiographer to compare sites of maximal narrowing with sites that may be less, but still severely narrowed rarely, then, does the angiographer have a truly normal uncompromised lumen on which to base estimates of percentage of luminal diameter reduction.

Second, the residual non-occluded lumen is usually eccentric in location and often slit-like in shape. Vlodaver and Edwards studied the shapes and positions of the residual lumens in 200 coronary arteries from patients with severe coronary atherosclerosis. In only 30% of the sections studied were the residual lumens central in location; in 69% the lumens were eccentric, and in 29% eccentric lumens were slit-like. In the 10 patients described earlier, eccentric lumens were found in 17 of the 24 coronary arterial segments in which there was a lack of correlation between the angiographic and histologic estimates of coronary narrowing.

One of the angiographic techniques now routine in an attempt to deal with the problem of slit-like lumens and luminal eccentricity is the recording of two orthogonal views of a lesion. Spears and coworkers have delineated mathematically the extent to which the maximum potential error in

456

area estimation increases rapidly as the angle between a given pair of orthogonal views decreases from 90 degrees. Furthermore, the maximum potential error in estimating luminal narrowing is proportional to the degree of ellipticity. For example, when ratio of major to minor axes of the stenotic lumen is 2, the calculated maximum error is 25%; when the ratio increases to 5, calculated error becomes 160%; as a result, Spears and associates have recommended that more than two views of a given lesion need to be obtained in cases in which the coronary arterial lumen is more than mildly elliptical. Parenthetically, it is worth noting that unless post-mortem angiography is performed in multiple obliquities relative to each major extramural vessel, it, like its pre-mortem counterpart is subject to misinterpretations related to diffuse narrowing and slit-like, eccentric lesions. In the case of the left main coronary artery (LMCA), the difficulties created by the diffuse nature of the atherosclerotic process and the presence of slit-like lumens are exacerbated by its short length and unpredictable course. The LMCA is the shortest of the four major epicardial coronary arteries. For atherosclerotic narrowing to involve the LMCA diffusely, it need only extend over a length of 3 mm to 12 mm; such narrowing would obliterate any portion of "normal" or relatively unobstructed lumen for comparison.

If the proximal left anterior descending and left circumflex coronary arteries are severely narrowed as well, the angiographer may be deprived of any reasonable standard for comparison. Furthermore, the LMCA is the only major epicardial coronary artery without a "fixed anchorage." The left anterior descending coronary artery, for example, generally follows the course of the ventricular septum, and the proximal left circumflex and right coronary arteries lie within the subepicardial adipose tissue of the atrioventricular grooves. Although the lengths of these arteries may be variable, their locations are relatively constant. In contrast, the LMCA may arise at an unpredictable angle from the aorta and may follow one of three axes in each of the horizontal and frontal planes before bifurcating into the left anterior descending and left circumflex branches. Previous studies have in fact noted that when the LMCA was unusually short, diffusely diseased, or obscured by overlapping vessels, significant interobserver disagreement resulted.

Because LMCA stenosis generally is considered to be an indication for coronary artery bypass surgery, regardless of the symptomatic status of the patient, accurate identification of LMCA narrowing is critically important. In an attempt to determine the extent to which the aforementioned anatomic considerations affected angiographic evaluation of the LMCA, coronary angiograms obtained shortly before death in 28 patients studied at necropsy were analyzed in a manner analogous to that employed by Arnett and associates.

The angiograms were evaluated independently by three experienced angiographers. In 20 of the 28 patients (71%), degree of LMCA narrowing was either underestimated (13 patients) or overestimated (10 patients) by two or three of the three angiographers; of 84 angiographic judgments made by the three angiographers in the 28 patients, 54 (64%) were underestimates (33 judgments [33%]) or overestimates (21 judgments [35%]) of LMCA narrowing. Of 12 LMCAs narrowed 51% to 75% in cross-sectional area at necropsy, all 12 were either underestimated or overestimated angiographically by two or three of the three angiographers; of four LMCAs narrowed 26% to 50% in cross-sectional area at necropsy, two were overestimated by two of three angiographers. Thus, angiographic determination of the degree of LMCA narrowing during life is subject to considerable error. Analysis of factors contributing to these documented misinterpretations indicated that failure to obtain an adequate number of projections was a common problem. Of the six patients in whom LMCA narrowing of >75% in cross-sectional area (at necropsy) was underestimated, none was viewed in the anteroposterior projection, and only three patients were examined in very shallow obliquities. Of the seven patients in whom the LMCA was narrowed 51% to 75% in cross-sectional area and was underestimated angiographically, only two were viewed in the anteroposterior projection, and only five patients were examined in a very shallow obliquity. None of the 13 patients in whom the LMCA was narrowed >50% in cross-sectional area were studied in all three projections (anteroposterior, very shallow right anterior oblique, and very shallow left anterior oblique).

Although recommendations have varied widely regarding the number of views necessary for satisfactory angiographic evaluation of the LMCA, more recent experience suggests that all three projections (one flat and two shallow oblique) are mandatory for complete examination of the LMCA. Lipton and coworkers found that when these three views were routinely used, the angiographic frequency of LMCA stenosis was considerably higher (74 of 500 cases [15%]) than that reported in most studies. Nath and associates performed 120 consecutive coronary angiograms of the LMCA in all three views and found eight patients with LMCA steno-

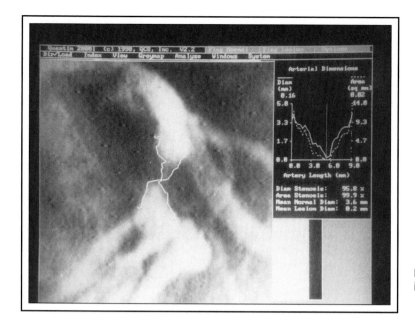

Figure 1. Patient 1. Quantitative analysis of focal stenosis in the proximal left anterior descending coronary artery.

sis, five of whom were recognized only in the anteroposterior projection. Because any one of the three views may result in angiographic foreshortening of the LMCA, depending on its course, it would seem prudent to accept the recommendation that all three views be used routinely for adequate angiographic analysis of the LMCA. Even with an adequate number of projections, technical problems may complicate assessment of ostial stenosis. Specifically, failure to perform non-selective cusp injections may obscure a critical stenosis. Angiographic overestimation of LMCA narrowing may occur owing to a variety of factors. Technical problems such as injecting contrast material too slowly or through a catheter with excessive length may inadequately opacify the LMCA. Even when these technical problems are avoided, the funnel-shaped origin of the LMCA occasionally compromises LMCA filling. Spasm of the LMCA has been well-documented and may on occasion contribute to angiographic overestimation.

It is fair to point out that all of the aforementioned angiographic-necropsy correlative investigations were performed prior to the widespread availability of x-ray tube-image intensifier configurations with triaxial motion capability. The advent of such systems has now made use of angulated views for coronary angiography routine and has permitted unequivocally improved definition of lesions that might otherwise constitute a potential source of diagnostic inaccuracy. On the one hand, this capability for angulated viewing would almost certainly improve the angiographic-morphologic correspondence in a subsequent angiographic-necropsy study. On the other hand, the very fact

that angulated views are now regarded as essential for defining degrees of luminal narrowing that appear equivocal in standard projections supports observations made in the angiographic-necropsy studies cited previously.

The angiographic and necropsy findings in the three patients whose angiograms and necropsy findings are illustrated in Figures 1 to 4 document that previous concerns regarding coronary narrowing which remains occult by virtue of diffuse distribution extend to the evaluation of patients being considered for coronary angioplasty. The angiographic finding of focal narrowing has long been regarded as the sine qua non for coronary angioplasty. Because of the limited number of patients studied at necropsy shortly following angioplasty, prevalence of diffuse disease masquerading as a nearly normal baseline remains undetermined. These cases, however, suggest that such anatomy may be more common than previously recognized. As the cases illustrate, unless the absolute luminal dimensions can be interpreted to distinguish non-obstructed, diminutive arteries from arteries diffusely and severely narrowed, extent of coronary disease in patients undergoing coronary angioplasty may nevertheless be underestimated. The extent to which diagnostic angiography failed to reflect severe, diffuse coronary artery disease may have contributed to the demise of these three patients. Not only was coronary narrowing more diffuse and more severe than anticipated in the artery selected for angioplasty, but so too were other extramural arteries similarly affected. As a result, the ischemic burden at time of balloon inflation was underestimated in these three patients.

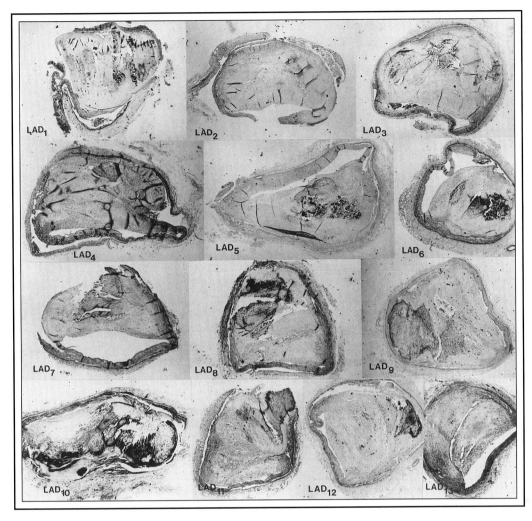

Figure 2. Patient 1. Serial 5-mm histologic sections of the left anterior descending (LAD) coronary artery. The sections are arranged in sequence from proximal (LAD$_1$) to distal (LAD$_{13}$).

Had each been recognized to have diffuse three-vessel coronary arterial narrowing, it is questionable whether angioplasty would have been recommended.

Physiologic Studies

Another independent source of inferential support for the findings derived from angiographic-necropsy investigations is composed of attempts to assess physiologic significance of angiographically-documented stenoses. Using a Doppler velocity flow probe applied to an epicardial coronary artery at the time of open-heart surgery, Marcus and coworkers have evaluated the coronary reactive hyperemic response to measure coronary vasodilator reserve. With the chest open, the Doppler probe is positioned on the artery of interest; blood flow is then measured at rest and following transient occlusion of the artery, produced with vascular forceps applied proximal to the probe (distal to the stenosis). As coronary narrowing becomes progressively more severe, the magnitude of hyperemia observed following release of the forceps diminishes. Using this technique, these investigators showed no sig-

nificant correlation between percentage of stenosis determined angiographically and magnitude of the peak/resting velocity ratio.

Further, for coronary stenoses causing <60% diameter narrowing, both overestimation and underestimation of lesion severity were observed. These results, like those of the angiographic-necropsy studies, raise serious questions regarding accuracy of coronary angiography in depicting the extent to which blood flow to the myocardium may be compromised.

Additional studies performed by the same group have demonstrated that the magnitude of the hyperemic response correlates better with measurements of minimal cross-sectional area than with the measurements of the percentage of stenosis. Such necessarily precise measurements of cross-sectional area have been performed using computerized quantitative coronary angiography, as originally described by Brown and colleagues. Although published necropsy validation of this approach has been limited to the study of 12 arteries in three post-mortem hearts, canine experiments have

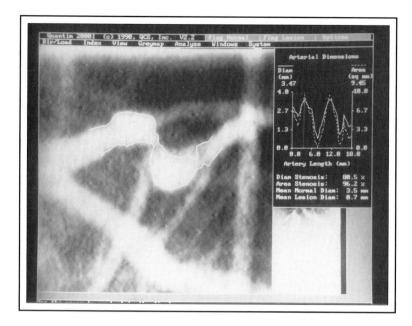

Figure 3. Patient 2. Quantitative analysis of the right coronary artery.

demonstrated that the approach of Brown and associates may be used to compute experimentally created stenosis resistance. A major virtue of the technique of Brown and coworkers is that it obviates the documented interobserver variation characteristic of non-quantitative coronary angiography, even though edge detection is manual.

Intravascular Ultrasound (IVUS)

Intravascular ultrasound (IVUS) imaging offers a potential solution to many of these limitations inherent in conventional contrast angiography. IVUS is unequivocally superior to contrast angiography in its ability to demonstrate detailed characteristics at the lumen/vessel wall interface, as well as to depict structures within the plaque and vessel wall. Several investigators have demonstrated that lVUS is exquisitely sensitive in detecting plaque and other details that are angiographically "silent". IVUS now provides the opportunity for the first time to accurately assess qualitative and quantitative effects of interventional therapy *in vivo*. As such, the mechanisms by which balloon angioplasty increases luminal patency, as well as the device-specific effects of directional and rotational atherectomy, laser angioplasty, and stent deployment, may be more clearly elucidated.

Utility of IVUS for Quantification of Vessel Dimensions

The most critical advantage of IVUS for clinical work derives from its unequivocally superior capability to define luminal dimensions, particularly cross-sectional area. Early *in vitro* studies by Nishimura and colleagues demonstrated the accu-

racy (correlation coefficient=.98) of IVUS lumen measurements compared to histology. Nissen and colleagues, using animals, found a correlation for diameter between quantitative angiography and IVUS of .98 for normal sites, and .89 for experimentally-induced concentric stenoses. Subsequent studies in humans found similarly close correlations (.80 to .95) between cross-sectional area in normal or near-normal vessels measured by IVUS versus quantitative angiography. Diseased, non-dilated vessels demonstrated a lesser, but still respectable correlation (r=.86). While these data demonstrate a good *correlation* between cross-sectional area measured by IVUS and those derived by quantitative angiographic algorithms, *absolute* values for area may differ substantially. Furthermore, since algorithms developed for quantitative angiography fail to address problems posed by diffusely diseased vessels, relative degree of compromise of a given site may be better determined by IVUS.

To the extent that IVUS may directly demonstrate luminal cross-sectional area in cases in which angiography is complicated by certain anatomical factors, IVUS may be useful as a diagnostic tool. Angiographic assessment of the left main coronary artery, for example, has been a well-documented source of angiographic ambiguity. IVUS imaging has been useful in such cases for elucidating extent of luminal compromise. IVUS may also resolve lesion severity in instances in which bends, vessel overlap, or branch points obscure the border of contrast during angiography. IVUS can also be particularly helpful in circumstances where it is necessary to define components of the arterial wall. While difficulty in assessing pathology is not uncommon in

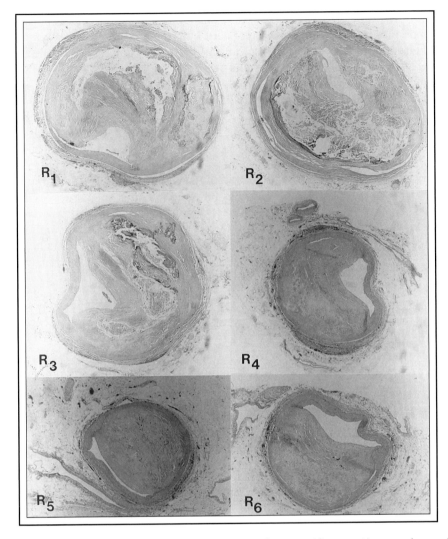

Figure 4. Patient 2. Serial 5mm histologic sections of the right coronary artery. The sections are arranged in sequence from proximal (R_1) to distal (R_6) orientation.

the tortuous coronary tree, IVUS may be specifically useful for defining severity of aorto-ostial lesions in renal and mesenteric vessels; stenoses at these sites are often difficult to visualize angiographically, due to their proximity to the aorta, brisk flow of contrast, and abundance of calcium.

Post-interventionally, there is significantly more discrepancy between vessel dimensions determined by IVUS and angiography. This was graphically demonstrated in the assessment of 13 consecutive patients in whom the results of balloon or laser angioplasty were quantified by both quantitative angiographic analysis and intravascular ultrasound. Minimal luminal diameter and cross-sectional area were calculated for interventional sites and nearby reference sites. Corresponding ultrasound frames from both interventional and reference sites were digitized and the minimal luminal diameter was measured directly; cross-sectional area was obtained by tracing the perimeter of the lumen. Luminal diameter for reference sites measured 3.9 mm by IVUS, versus 3.3 mm by quantitative angiography ($p < 0.05$). Regression analysis disclosed a correlation coefficient of 0.87. For cross-sectional area of reference sites, the absolute difference between ultrasound and angiography (12.6 vs 9.6 mm^2) was also statistically significant ($p < 0.05$). Regression analysis disclosed a correlation coefficient of .92, similar to that calculated for analysis of luminal diameter. Luminal diameter for *interventional sites* measured 2.8 mm by IVUS, vs 1.8 mm by angiography ($p < 0.01$). Regression analysis disclosed a poorer correlation, .62 than that calculated for reference sites. Similarly, for cross-sectional area of interventional sites, there was a statistically significant difference between absolute measurements made by ultrasound (6.9 mm) versus quantitative angiography (2.8 mm; $p < 0.01$).

There is reason to believe that cross-sectional area measurements are more accurate by IVUS than by quantitative angiography, especially post-interventionally. First, IVUS provides accurate delineation of luminal borders and obviates the need for multiple orthogonal angiographic views.

461

Secondly, IVUS provides the ability to directly plan the cross-sectional area, eliminating dependence on algorithms which derive area from diameter measurements and which make potentially incorrect assumptions about luminal geometry. Thirdly, in quantitative angiography, the catheter used for calibration may be located at a distance from the segment being measured; yet with IVUS, the calibration instrument is, by definition, within the plane of measurement. Fourth, with IVUS, the area being measured occupies nearly the entire field of view on the screen; in contrast, for angiographic analysis, the vascular region of interest involves only a small fraction of the cine frame from which it is measured.

Utility of IVUS to Define Mechanism of Balloon Angioplasty

The most extensive clinical experience with IVUS to date, and the application in which IVUS appears to offer the greatest practical clinical utility, has been in the assessment of intravascular effects of percutaneous therapy in coronary and peripheral vessels. Contrast angiography, while routinely performed pre- and post-instrumentationally, provides only a profile of luminal diameter, rather than depiction of cross-sectional area; this fact, along with other methodological limitations described previously, compromises its usefulness for study of angioplasty mechanisms. *In vitro* studies have demonstrated that IVUS consistently provides exquisite detail regarding morphologic alterations in the arterial wall and subjacent plaque resulting from the barotrauma of balloon inflation.

Experience with *in vivo* imaging post-dilation has confirmed *in vitro* data. In the few patients studied at necropsy post-PTA in whom IVUS had also been performed, IVUS images displayed identical morphologic abnormalities seen by light microscopy. The fact that IVUS routinely depicts tomographic full-thickness images of the arterial wall, allows one to gain *(in vivo)* a perspective similar to that achieved by histologic examination. Furthermore, the ability to perform serial examinations *in vivo* enables documentation about pathologic alterations attributable to specific instrumentation employed. These unique features of IVUS have been used to good advantage to study mechanisms by which balloon angioplasty improves luminal patency. Observations from IVUS at our own institution and others suggest that plaque fracture and/or dissection is associated with balloon dilation in the overwhelming majority of angiographically and hemodynamically successful procedures. Recent data suggest that at least some degree of

plaque fracture must be seen by IVUS in order to achieve a successful long-term result; vessels which display no tearing may be much more prone to recoil or restenosis.

The relative contribution of plaque fractures, as opposed to other factors, to the overall increase in luminal area seen following balloon angioplasty has been elucidated by IVUS. Tobis and colleagues demonstrated *in vitro* that diseased vessels subjected to balloon dilation tended to tear longitudinally at the thinnest region of the plaque; they suggested that these tears account for the enlargement of luminal cross-sectional area. Losordo and colleagues evaluated IVUS images obtained before and after PTA performed in 40 patients, and quantified the relative contributions of plaque fracture, plaque compression, and arterial stretch to the enhanced overall luminal area. Luminal cross-sectional area more than doubled, from 11.5 mm^2 pre-PTA to 25.4 mm^2 post-PTA. The neolumen created by plaque fractures accounted for the majority (72%) of total increase in luminal area. Compression of plaque was seen in all treated vessels and made an important but quantitatively less significant contribution to post-angioplasty increase in luminal area. Arterial stretching was demonstrated in only 25% of patients and, even in this group, its contribution to increased area was minimal. These data confirm previous observations suggesting that plaque fracture constitutes the principal mechanism reponsible for increased luminal patency after balloon angioplasty. These results consequently contradict conclusions based on prior in vitro studies and a smaller in vivo study which implicated stretching of the vessel wall as a major factor contributing to increased lumen size.

In an attempt to categorize degree of plaque fracture observed by IVUS following balloon angioplasty, Honye and colleagues have identified six characteristic morphologic patterns of vessel disruption. In their proposed scheme, patterns A through D represent increasing degrees of plaque tearing and separation from subjacent structures, while pattern E represents stretching without obvious tearing. Of 66 coronary lesions subjected to balloon dilation, Honye and colleagues observed fairly equal distribution of the different morphologic subtypes, with a slight predominance in types B, C, and especially E. Interestingly, in their preliminary analysis, Type E1 lesions displayed a greater tendency towards restenosis at 6-month follow-up.

Calcified plaque is detected by IVUS in most vessels undergoing angioplasty, a feature under-appreciated by angiography and which may be important in understanding mechanism of PTA. Honye and

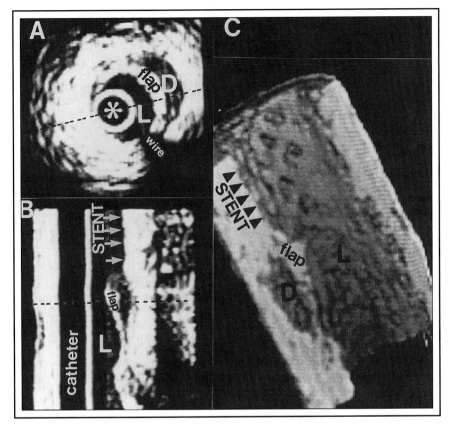

Figure 5. Three-dimensional reconstruction of endovascular stent. Panel A: representative two-dimensional intravascular ultrasound (IVUS) image obtained before percutaneous transluminal angioplasty from nonstented portion of iliac artery immediately distal to stent. IVUS catheter (asterisk) is within true lumen (L): as a result of balloon dilation, a large flap separates true lumen from dissection (D) tract in underlying vessel wall. Shadowing artifact is seen from wire. Dashed black line indicates plane of sagittal view in panel B, where sagittal reconstruction illustrates a smooth endoluminal border at site of stent deployment: distal to stent, however, flap and subintimal dissection are evident. Note increased luminal diameter in stented portion of vessel compared with nonstented segment. Dashed black line in panel B indicates level of two-dimensional image shown in panel A. Panel C: Cylindrical reconstruction with region of interest drawn to encompass at 180° hemisection of same segment of iliac artery shown in panels A and B; note cobblestoned appearance imparted by stent struts. Adjacent dissection and intimal flap are seen below. IVUS catheter has been eliminated from this image using mask function of the software.

colleagues, for example, identified calcific deposits in 14% vs 83% of patients studied by angiography and ultrasound, respectively. Our experience has been similar. Waller and colleagues have previously suggested that tears and fractures typically occur along the border between calcific plaque and softer tissue; assuming that is the case, the increased sensitivity of IVUS in detecting calcific deposits may be clinically relevant. Recent observations lend further support to the notion that presence of calcium may predict location and extent of plaque fracture. Fitzgerald and colleagues, for example, imaged 41 patients following angioplasty and found that in 87% of patients with focal deposits of calcium who also demonstrated dissections, fracture site was located adjacent to the calcified plaque. Furthermore, extent of dissection was greater in the patients with calcified than in those with non-calcified vessels.

To the extent that large dissections may portend a poor angioplasty outcome, including specifically a higher risk of abrupt closure, detection and localization of calcium may become an important, practical application of IVUS. Further studies are necessary, however, to discriminate characteristic features or patterns of calcific deposition that might be a harbinger of a poor PTCA result. Preliminary evidence from *in vivo* IVUS studies

has also provided insight regarding mechanisms by which directional atherectomy, stent deployment, and laser angioplasty enhance luminal area. In contrast to vessels undergoing balloon angioplasty, vessels in which directional atherectomy is performed demonstrate less prominent plaque-arterial wall disruption; instead, the perimeter of the neolumen is typically smooth and uninterrupted. In our initial series of patients, no plaque cracks were observed on post-atherectomy IVUS examination. Rather, discrete "bites" corresponding to individual passes of the cutting blade were often observed, consistent with tissue removal. Similar findings have been reported by Yock and colleagues, Smucker and colleagues, and Tenaglia and colleagues, all of whom reported a relatively low incidence of plaque fracture. Controversy persists regarding the extent to which inflation of eccentric balloon of the Simpson Atherocath contributes to increased luminal area; indeed, angiographic studies have suggested that the amount of tissue retrieved is not enough to account for the resultant increase in luminal diameter, and in certain cases the Dotter effect of the catheter and effects of balloon inflation have been documented to produce the majority of luminal patency. Signs of arterial wall trauma are most completely effaced on IVUS images recorded following delivery of an endovascu-

463

lar stent: the fact that extensive trauma is observed at these same sites post-balloon (pre-stent) suggests that stent implantation acutely ameliorates arterial wall pathology (Figure 5).

Selected Reading

1. Arnett EN, Isner JM, Redwood DR, et al: Coronary artery narrowing in coronary heart disease: Comparison of cineangiographic and necropsy findings. *Ann Intern Med* 1979; 91:350.

2. Baptista J, di Mario C, Escaned J, et al. Intracoronary two-dimensional ultrasound imaging in the assessment of plaque morphologic features and the planning of coronary interventions. *Am Heart J* 1995; 129:177-187.

3. Brown BG, Bolson E, Frinner M, et al: Quantitative coronary arteriography: estimation of dimensions, hemodynamic resistance, and atheroma mass of coronary artery lesions using arteriogram and digital computation. *Circ* 1977; 55:329.

4. Brown BG, Bolson E, Petersen, RB, et al: Mechanism of nitroglycerin action: Stenosis vasodilation as a major component of drug response. *Circ* 1981; 64:1089.

5. Cabin HS, Roberts WC: Comparison of amount and extent of coronary narrowing by atherosclerotic plaque and of myocardial scarring at necropsy in anterior and posterior healed transmural myocardial infarction. *Circ* 1982; 66:93.

6. DeRouen TA, Murray JA, Owen W: Variability in analysis of coronary arteriograms. *Circ* 1977; 55:324.

7. Detre KM, Wright E, Murphy ML, et al: Observer agreement in evaluating coronary angiograms. *Circ* 1975; 52:979.

8. Donaldson RF, Isner JM: Intercoronary continuity: An anatomic basis for bidirectional flow distinct from coronary collaterals. *AJC* 1984; 53:351.

9. Esente P, Gensini GG, Giambartolonei A, et al: Bidirectional blood flow in angiographically normal coronary arteries. *AJC* 1983; 51:1237.

10. Fitzgerald PJ, Ports TA, Yock PG. Contribution of localized calcium deposits to dissection after angioplasty: an observational study using intravascular ultrasound. *Circ* 1992; 86:64-70.

11. Grondin CM, Dydra I, Pasternac A, et al: Discrepancies between cineangiographic and postmortem findings in patients with coronary artery disease and recent myocardial revascularization. *Circ* 1974; 49:703.

12. The Guide Trial Investigators. Discrepancies between angiographic and intravascular ultrasound appearance of coronary lesions undergoing intervention: a report of Phase I of the GUIDE Trial. *JACC* (Abstract) 1993; 21:118 A.

13. Harrison DG, White CW, Hiratzka LF, et al: Can significance of coronary stenosis be predicted by quantitative coronary angiography? *Circ* 1981; 64:160.

14. Hausmann D, Erbel R, Alibelli-Chemarin MJ, et al: The safety of intracoronary ultrasound. A multicenter survey of 2207 examinations. *Circ* 1995; 91:623-629.

15. Honye J, Mahon DJ, Jain A, et al: Morphological effects of coronary balloon angioplasty in vivo assessed by intravascular ultrasound imaging. *Circ* 1992; 85:1012-1025.

16. Hutchins GM, Bulkey BH, Ridolfi RL, et al: Correlation of coronary arteriograms and left ventriculograms with post-mortem studies. *Circ* 1977; 56:32.

17. Isner JM, Lee SS: Clinicopathologic conference. *NEJM* 1983;309: 1233.

18. Isner JM, Kishel J, Kent KM: Accuracy of angiographic determination of left main coronary arterial narrowing. Angiographic-histologic correlative analysis in 28 patients. *Circ* 1981; 63:1056.

19. Isner JM, Rosenfield K, Losordo DW, et al: Combination balloon-ultrasound imaging catheter for percutaneous transluminal angioplasty: Validation of imaging, analysis of recoil, and identification of plaque fracture. *Circ* 1991; 84:739-754.

20. Isner JM, Virmani R, Jones AA, et al: Comparison of degrees of coronary arterial luminal narrowing determined by visual inspection of histologic sections under magnification among independent observers compared to that obtained by video planimetry: Analysis of 559 5mm segments of 61 coronary arteries. *Lab Invest* 1980;42:566.

21. Kelly K, Gould L: Validation of computerized quantitative coronary angiography. *Circ* 1981; 64:107.

22. Kemp HG, Evans H, Elliott WC, et al: Diagnostic accuracy of selective coronary cinearteriography. *Circ* 1967; 36:526.

23. Levin DC, and Fallon JT: Significance of angiographic morphology of localized coronary stenosis: histopathologic correlations. *Circ* 1982; 66:316

24. Lipton, MJ, Pfeifer JF, Murphy ML, et al: Dangers of left main coronary artery lesions: angiographic technique and evaluation. *Invest Radiol* 1977; 12:447.

25. Marcus ML, Doty DB, Hiratzka LF, et al: Decreased coronary reserve: a mechanism for angina pectoris in patients with aortic stenosis and normal coronary arteries. *NEJM* 1982; 307:1362.

26. Marcus ML, Wright C, Doty D, et al: Measurements of coronary velocity and reactive hyperemia in the coronary circulation of humans. *Circ Res* 1981; 49:877.

27. Nath, PH, Velasquez, G., Castaneda-Zuniga, WR, et al.: An essential view in coronary angiography. *Circ* 60:101, 1979.

28. Nissen SE, Gurley JC, Grines CL, et al: Intravascular ultrasound assessment of lumen size and wall morphology in normal subjects and patients with coronary artery disease. *Circ* 1991; 84:1087-1099.

29. Roberts WC: Coronary arteries in fatal AMI. *Circ* 1972; 45:215.

30. Roberts WC, Jones AA: Quantitation of coronary arterial narrowing at necropsy in sudden coronary death: analysis of 31 patients and comparison with 25 control subjects. *AJC* 1979; 44:39.

31. Roberts WC, Jones AA: Quantification of coronary arterial narrowing at necropsy in acute transmural myocardial infarction: analysis and comparison of findings in 27 patients and 22 controls. *Circ* 1980; 62:786.

32. Schwartz JN, Kong Y, Hackel DB: Comparison of angiographic and post-mortem findings in patients with coronary artery disease. *AJC* 1975; 36:174.

33. Spears JR, Sandor T, Baim DS, et al: Minimum error in estimating coronary luminal cross-sectional area from cineangiographic diameter measurements. *Cathet Cardiov Diag* 1983; 9:119.

34. Tenaglia AN, Buller CE, Kisslo KB, et al: Mechanisms of balloon angioplasty and directional coronary atherectomy as assessed by intracoronary ultrasound. *JACC* 1992; 20:685-691.

35. Tobis JM, Mallery J, Mahon D. Intravascular ultrasound imaging of human coronary arteries in vivo. *Circ* 1991; 83:913-926.

36. Vlodaver Z, Frech R, Van Tassel RA: Correlation of the antemortem coronary arteriogram and the post-mortem specimen. *Circ* 1973; 47:162.

37. White CW, Wright CB, Doty DB, et al: Does visual interpretation of the coronary arteriogram predict physiologic importance of coronary stenosis? *NEJM* 1984; 310:819.

CHAPTER 21

Clinical Electrophysiology: Techniques For Recording, Interpretation, and Ablation

Ross D. Fletcher, M.D., Cynthia M. Tracy, M.D. and
Albert A. Del Negro, M.D.

Clinical electrophysiology received a major impetus in 1969 when Scherlag and Damato reported a technique for recording electrical potentials from the bundle of His in man. Since then, a wide array of tests and approaches have been developed to help solve problems and expand our knowledge of clinical heart block, bradyarrhythmias and tachyarrhythmias.

This chapter will emphasize not only the technical aspects of obtaining electrophysiological information with intracavitary recording and pacing catheters, but also the interpretation of that information. The anatomy of the conduction system, the choice of catheters, recording principles, and validation techniques will be discussed. Pacing principles used to reveal conduction defects and to induce arrhythmias and assess the efficacy of acute and chronic pharmacological intervention will be reviewed. The progression from diagnostic techniques to therapeutic ablation techniques will be reviewed. Many clinical applications are obvious, but several remain controversial. The technical details are most important for the electrophysiologist, but awareness of these details also allows the practicing clinician to critically evaluate the complex reports and elaborate recordings now routinely available in the clinical record after electrophysiological studies. Studying clinical arrhythmias with the knowledge gained from intracavitary tracings improves the clinician's diagnostic accuracy and allows one to request invasive electrophysiology only when strongly indicated.

Anatomy

The sinus node, located adjacent to the superior vena cava, forms impulses that spread through specialized internodal tracts of the right atrium to the AV node (Figure 1). Simultaneously, the impulse propagates across Bachmann's bundle to the left atrium. Internodal tracts coalesce at the AV node where conduction is delayed until it emerges in the narrow bundle of His. This single tract to the ventricles is 15mm long and gives off the fibers forming the left bundle as it passes the insertion of the tricuspid valve. The last left bundle branch fibers are given off beyond the tricuspid valve insertion, after which remaining fibers continue as the right bundle branch. The right and the left bundle branch fascicles continue to the middle third of the ventricles where conducted impulses then spread through the muscle.

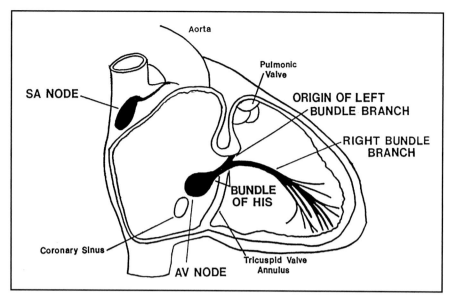

Figure 1. Electrophysiological anatomy of the right atrium and ventricle.

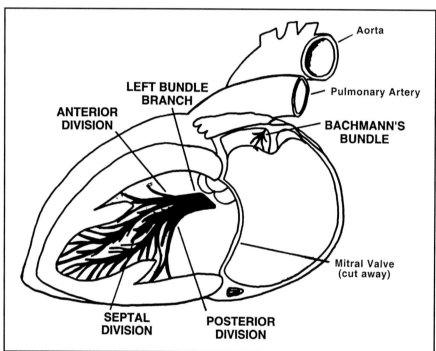

Figure 2. Electrophysiological anatomy of the left atrium and ventricle.

The main right bundle branch is longer (45mm) than the left (30mm). The left bundle passes as a sheet over the left ventricles with three areas of early activation representing anterior superior, posterior inferior, and septal fascicles (Figure 2). In abnormal states, accessory tracts can connect atrium and ventricle at virtually any site in the right or left atrio-ventricular sulcus (Figure 3). Branches can bypass the AV node to the His bundle (James fibers) or bypass the His Purkinje system through Mayhem fibers. Connections can also occur from the right lateral AV sulcus to the apical right bundle branch, and may contain nodal tissue.

Several anatomic sites are capable of automatic

impulse formation. The fastest automatic impulse starts the propagation wave which resets all slower automatic cells. The laddergram in Figure 4 represents normal propagation from the automatic SA node to the sinoatrial junction, the high right atrium, the internodal atrial tracts, the low right atrial septum AV node, the His bundle, and the specialized ventricular conduction system to the ventricle.

The external electrocardiogram (Figure 4, Panel B) measures onset of atrial activity, usually in the high right atrium, and onset of ventricular activity. Common intracavitary recording sites include electrodes in the high right atrium adjacent to the

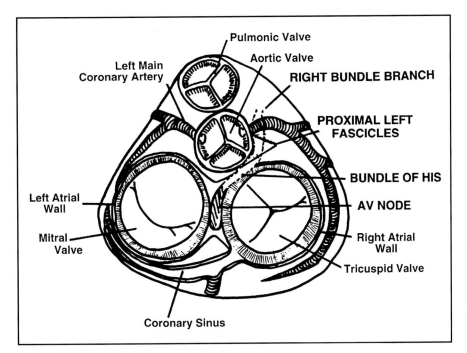

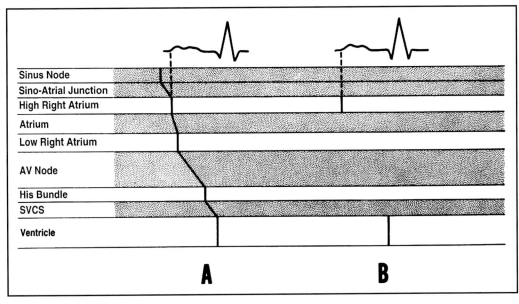

Figure 3. Transection at valve level showing relationship of the coronary sinus to the posterior AV groove and the relationship of the atrioventricular (AV) node and His bundle to the AV sulcus and the aortic valve.

Figure 4. The unshaded rungs of the intracavitary laddergram in A display the information obtained with standard intracavitary recording catheters from the high right atrium, low right atrium, His bundle and ventricle. By contrast, onset of P wave and ventricle from external ECG are in B.

sinoatrial node. The low septal right atrium adjacent to the AV node, the His bundle, and high right ventricle are sampled by a single catheter in the His bundle position.

The left atrium through the coronary sinus, other areas of right atrium, right ventricle and at times left ventricle are less commonly recorded. A typical recording format includes at least 6 external leads (I, II III V_1, V_3 and V_6,) and intracavitary leads such as the high right atrium, the His bundle, and the right ventricle. Time marking is at 10msec intervals (Figure 5A/B). Arrival times of these commonly recorded structures permit one to see the conduction system in the unshaded areas of the

laddergram (Panel A); the PR interval seen on the external trace can be divided into specific subintervals. Standard PR subintervals represent conduction times from onset of atrial activity to low right atrium (P-A), low right atrium through the AV node to the His bundle (A-H), and His bundle to ventricle (H-V).

Basic recordings of spontaneous electrophysiological events, accurate measurement of conduction times, and relationships of the His bundle deflection to ventricular and atrial activation are important for baseline analysis. Stimulation studies are essential for diagnosis and quantitation of electrophysiological deficiencies, but when they induce

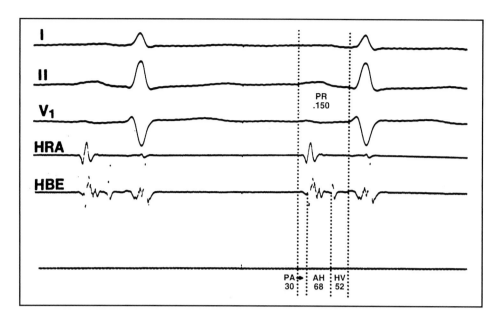

Figure 5A. The PR subintervals include: the P-A measured from onset of P wave to onset of sharp, low atrial deflections on the His bundle electrogram (HBE); the A-H measured from the low A to earliest His deflection; and the H-V, measured from earliest His to earliest ventricular depolarization in any external or internal lead.

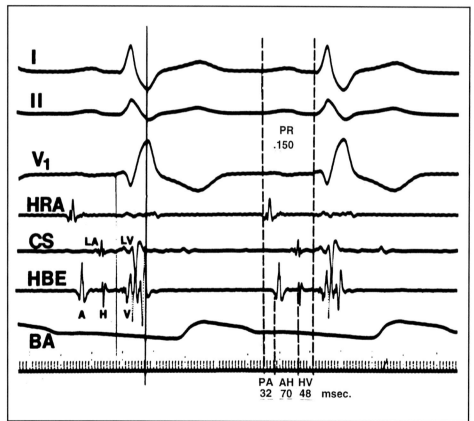

Figure 5B. The PR subinterval of 150msec in this patient with RBBB is composed of P-A 32, A-H 70 and H-V of 48msec, all within normal limits.

arrhythmias, they also provide a useful target for therapeutic interventions. Ability to suppress catheter-induced supraventricular and ventricular arrhythmias with pharmacological therapy in the acute study shows a strong correlation with clinical control over subsequent months. Further, accurate diagnosis of SVT, in particular, permits catheter ablation.

Components of the Electrophysiological Study

An effective study requires careful preparation of the patient, a proper selection of catheters, a versatile recording and playback system, and a stimulator for dynamic testing. Clinical indications and techniques for interpretation of the spontaneous records and stimulation studies will follow a

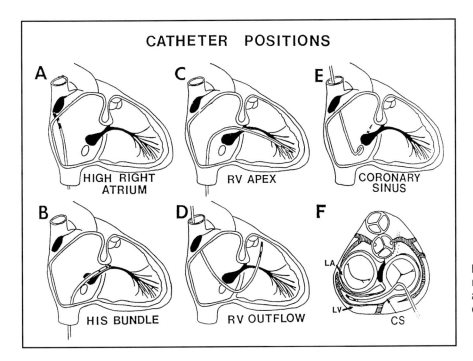

CATHETER POSITIONS

A HIGH RIGHT ATRIUM

B HIS BUNDLE

C RV APEX

D RV OUTFLOW

E CORONARY SINUS

F

Figure 6. Common catheter positions for recording electrical events in the high right atrium (A), His bundle (B), RV apex (C), RV outflow (D), and coronary sinus (E&F).

description of the components necessary to perform the basic study.

The Patient

Meaningful results require careful integration of the patient's history, physical examination, and ECGs, including new tracings, old tracings, and long rhythm strips. All noninvasive ECG studies such as exercise testing, Holter monitoring, and drug interventions should be available. The design of the electrophysiological study will carefully follow the clinical indications as in any heart catheterization study; several principles for preparing the patient and the recording area apply to all procedures. The patient must remain at a physiological baseline and therefore be comfortable and as relaxed as possible. Comfortable radiolucent mattresses and arm boards, and pleasant professional conversation are the best tranquilizers. Agents, such as morphine and meperidine, are avoided because of their cholinergic and anticholinergic action. Intravenous midazolam HCl should be used for anxiety or discomfort. Catheterization laboratory tables are traditionally used, but fluoroscopic beds will provide comfort for long procedures.

Patient safety mandates frequent monitoring of systemic pressure, with a brachial artery needle if necessary. An intravenous line is mandatory for pharmacological correction of arrhythmias or vagal reactions, and will also be used to correct induced arrhythmia. The table and equipment must be checked for a common ground and electrical safety, and a frequently tested synchronized defibrillator

must be available. The procedure should be well planned so that it will progress with speed so as to avoid patient fatigue and obtain information before physiological variables change.

Catheters

Catheters are selected according to the site of the conduction system to be recorded. Knowledge of catheter characteristics, as well as means of insertion into the vascular system, and accurate placement in the heart, are vital to all recording pacing studies. The design characteristics of the catheter including size, number of electrodes, inter-electrode distance, shape, and polarity will vary with the recording site and the clinical arrhythmia. Catheters are inserted percutaneously by modified Seldinger technique, passed transvenously to several important recording and pacing areas:

• **High Right Atrium:** The venous approach can be through the right arm or the femoral area to the junction of the superior vena cava and lateral high right atrial wall (Figure 6A). Use of four electrodes allow the distal two to be attached to the atrial pacemaker and the proximal two to be attached to the recording system.

• **His Bundle Area:** Difficulty may be encountered passing the catheter from the right atrium to the His region. Temporary shaping of a curve in the atrium aids passage there. Alternatively, a deflectable tip catheter can facilitate His recordings. Medial clockwise motion to a superior position, proximal to the tricuspid valve orifice, is the best position for the His bundle recording (Figure 6B).

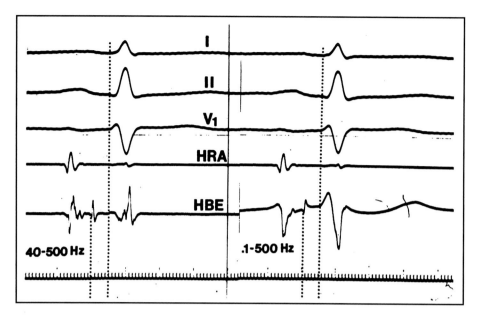

Figure 7. (Left:) His bundle electrogram recorded at the usual frequency (40Hz-500Hz) which filters low frequency ECG events such as the T wave, (Right:) unfiltered (1Hz-500Hz).

This positioning should be guided by the actual His recording. During a study, the His spike may diminish, but can be brought back with minor clockwise torque, withdrawal, or advancement.

• **Ventricle:** A ventricular recording and pacing catheter is required for studies assessing retrograde atrioventricular conduction and other ventricular stimulation studies from the RV apex (Figure 6C) or RV outflow tract (Figure 6D). Supraventricular tachycardia studies will require a catheter in the right ventricle. On occasion, a left ventricular catheter for mapping as well as for stimulation is used.

• **Coronary Sinus:** Catheter placement is easiest from the left subclavian vein. In addition to a 120° curve at 5cm, the catheter shape should include an upward bend in the last centimeter to facilitate passage upward in the main coronary sinus instead of the inferior cardiac vein (Figures 6E, 6F). The coronary sinus allows recording of the atrium and the basal left ventricle in the AV sulcus. While the ventricle can be paced in the distal coronary sinus, the left atrium is paced in the proximal coronary sinus. Use of an electrode catheter with lumen facilitates coronary sinus placement as both simultaneous pressures or use of contrast material help guide the catheter into the coronary sinus.

Recording Technique and Equipment

Recording systems should have a large selection of external and internal ECG amplifiers. At a minimum, three external ECGs such as leads I, II, and V1 are recorded. Six or twelve external leads are valuable and available in modern computer-based recorders. Three internal ECGs are a minimum and require high-gain amplifiers with input filters to record intracavitary signals such as high right atrium, His bundle, coronary sinus, and right ventricle. A low frequency filter at 40Hz and a high frequency filter at 500Hz are standard. Use of the low frequency filter differentiates the signal, making the high frequency local deflections obvious, eliminating the low frequency ST and T wave, remote QRS, and baseline changes (Figure 7). Most intracavitary signals (His bundle, high right atrium, coronary sinus and ventricle) are recorded at the 40Hz to 500Hz setting. Whenever an unusual signal appears on a filtered record, it is good practice to record this signal without filtering. Simultaneous recording of unipolar unfiltered tracings from the tip monitors ST elevation which denotes contact with the endocardium and reveals perforation if the ST elevation becomes depressed. In addition to ECG recordings, direct current inputs are necessary for catheters recording monophasic action potentials and for recording telemetry from pacemaker analyzers or defibrillation testing equipment. Time lines every msec are available in all modern systems. Two pressure amplifiers are used for simultaneous arterial and venous pressure monitoring, and the screen should display a minimum of eight channels. A triggered freeze capability allows assessment during a study but is not standard. A screen and recorder capable of speeds up to 200mm/sec should be available.

An analog tape recorder or online storage to optical disc allows playback or retrieval of events which are transient and not initially recorded on paper. This feature is particularly important when dealing with tachyarrhythmias. Accurate diagnosis often depends on capturing the onset and offset of spontaneous arrhythmias.

470

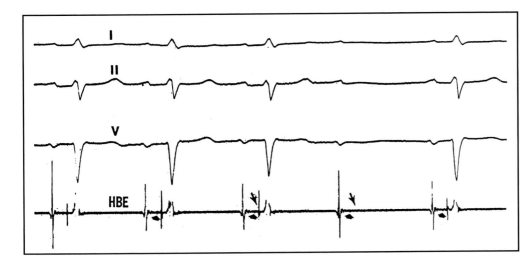

Figure 8A. Despite the Mobitz second degree heart block, the intracavitary tracing showed apparent absence of conduction to the His Bundle on the blocked beat (large arrows). Closer inspection revealed a consistent small deflection after all low atrial deflections implicating possible intra His block (small arrows).

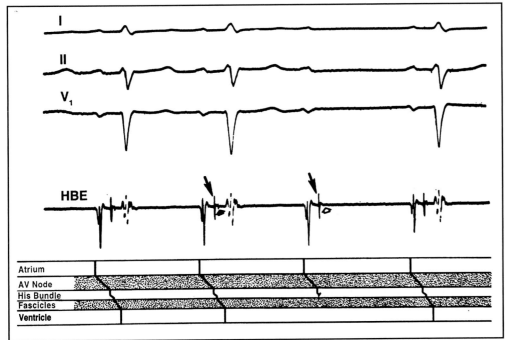

Figure 8B. Withdrawing the His bundle catheter revealed large proximal His deflections after each conducted and nonconducted P wave, with absence of distal His deflection after intra His block (open arrow).

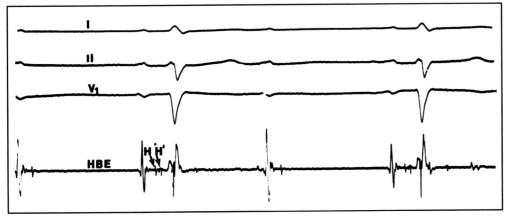

Figure 8C. Intra-His block with discrete His, His1 (H, H1) are seen at an intermediate catheter position.

A standard 12-lead ECG for immediate analysis of induced arrhythmias is useful and can be online in computer based EP systems. Sixty cycle interference in an electrophysiological laboratory can greatly prolong cases and distort interpretations and is reduced by the use of adequately shielded cables.

471

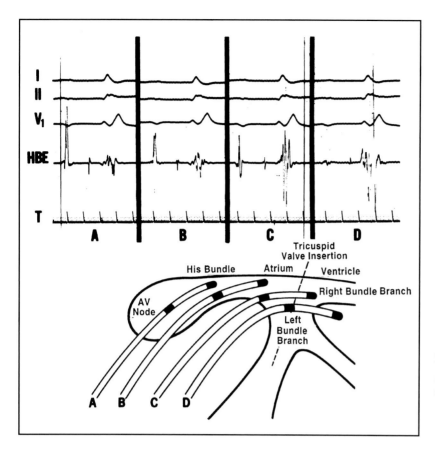

Figure 9. Panels A,B,C and D represent recordings at increasingly distal positions in the AV junction. The most proximal position with largest atrial deflection and smallest V is where the H-V interval should be measured.

Stimulators

While many tests required of an electrophysiological laboratory can be achieved with standard pacemakers, all laboratories have the capability of rapid stimulation to revert rhythms that would otherwise require external synchronized cardioversion. Programmed stimulators are valuable both for induction and rapid use of antitachycardia pacing. They all can pace at rapid rates (up to 400bpm) in both standard pacing and pacing using extrastimulus technique. They should have constant current pacing output to at least 20 mamp and at least 2msec pulse width.

Validation and Recording

Once catheters are placed in their approximate sites, they are connected to the recorder and programmed stimulator. Polarity should be consistent, but recording polarity may be the opposite of that used for pacing. The positive electrode should be distal in the conduction system for recording. Since cathodal (-) thresholds are lower, the negative pole for pacing should be closest to the surface being paced. Since this is often the distal electrode its polarity may be negative during pacing and positive during recording.

Validation that the recorded His deflection is the most proximal part of the His bundle potential eliminates errors in H-V times averaging 10-15msec. Errors as long as 20msec-30msec are possible if recordings are made when the His bundle catheter is in a distal position toward the right bundle branch. More importantly, a distal position may not show a His deflection after a non-conducted P-wave (Figure 8A), and be falsely interperted as proximal AV nodal block. With a more proximal position (Figure 8B/C), the His deflection is seen after the same blocked P-waves indicating serious distal intra-His block.

Our technique for validation is to seek the most proximal position, which records the His bundle (Figure 9). Once the most proximal His bundle is seen, an attempt to pace the His bundle is made. Since the effect of pacing from the proximal electrode is desired, pacing polarity is negative for the most proximal electrode and positive for the distal electrode. Pacing is performed close to threshold. At times, excellent His pacing is seen (Figure 10A), but low atrial pacing with good His potentials are accepted as indicating a proximal His bundle recording (Figure 10B). High right ventricular pacing revealed by a paced QRS with LBBB configuration, and an inferior frontal plane axis, indicates an unacceptable distal recording site (Figure 10C).

When it becomes necessary to separate the His deflection from atrial deflections, incremental atrial

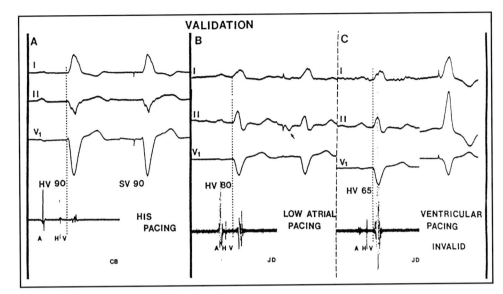

Figure 10. Validation of the abnormally long H-V interval (90msec) is achieved by pacing from the His bundle catheter, reproducing the conducted QRS morphology with a pacing spike to ventricle (SV) equal to the HV (90msec) as in panel A. When His bundle pacing cannot be achieved, pacing the atrium with a negative P in lead II indicates a very proximal position with an H-V interval of 80msec (panel B). When the ventricle is paced, in the same patient producing inferior axis with left bundle branch block morphology, the catheter is in an abnormally distal position. In that position, it will record an inaccurately short HV interval of 65 (panel C).

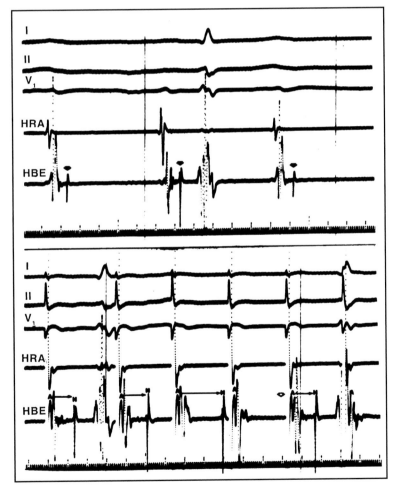

Figure 11. The His bundle deflections (dark arrows) in the upper panel are validated by atrial pacing, which routinely increases the AH nodal conduction time. In the lower panel the A-H interval progressively lengthens before it blocks (open arrow), then resumes conduction at a shorter pacing typical of Wenckebach periodicity.

pacing will increase A-H interval. Seeing the His deflection move away from the low atrial deflection identifies and confirms appropriate physiology of the intervening AV node (Figure 11). With WPW, the His may not be easily seen because the preexcited ventricle is superimposed on the His activity.

When the refractory period of the bypass is reached by incremental pacing or timed premature atrial beats, an uncluttered A-H is revealed (Figure 12). The His may be seen even with ventricular tachycardia during AV dissociation (Figure 13) and accurate identification of the His deflection is valuable

473

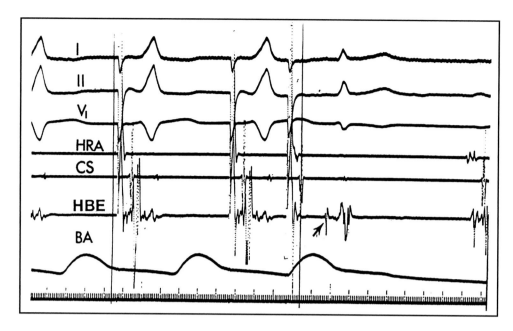

Figure 12. The patient has preexcitation on the first two atrial paced beats. The atrial premature extrastimulus finds the bypass refractory, thus revealing a clear His bundle deflection (arrow).

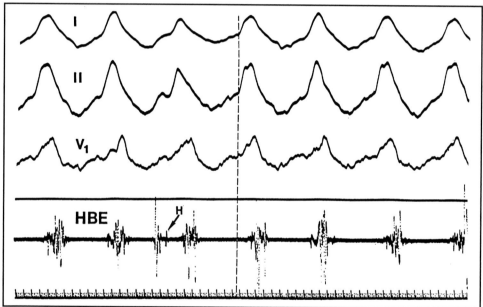

Figure 13. Ventricular tachycardia shows His recordings well within the onset of the QRS (dotted line) except when the disassociated atrium captures the His bundle (arrow).

during normal and abnormal rhythms. Absence of a His deflection even from beat to beat can be artifactual, but presence of a typical deflection in the proximal His position behaving physiologically allows accurate diagnoses.

After placement of the quadripolar high right atrial catheter, the two distal electrodes are connected to the stimulator, while the two proximal electrodes are attached to the filtered recorder. Appropriate recording occurs when the high atrial deflection from the high right atrial area appears earlier than the low atrial deflection in the His recording area. Pacing threshold should be assessed and the output of the stimulator set at double the threshold with a 2msec pulse duration. Thresholds can change with minor changes in catheter position and should be rechecked whenever the stimulation interval approaches refractory periods. Additional catheters for recording or pacing should be adjusted according to need.

Once catheters have been accurately positioned and validated, the patient's spontaneous rhythms should be recorded at rapid speeds (e.g., 100-150mm/sec. The standard conduction times (subintervals) are more accurate when measured from the fast recordings. His relationships to blocked P waves and anomalous beats can be satisfactorily seen at 100mm/sec and slower.

T A B L E   1

Diagnostic Pacing

STRAIGHT PACING TECHNIQUES

- Sinoatrial recovery times
- Incremental pacing
- Reversion of atrial and ventricular tachycardias

EXTRA STIMULUS TECHNIQUE

A. Paced Set-up Intervals

- Antegrade challenge – pace atrium
  Refractory periods, SVT induction, dual pathway detection
- Retrograde challenge – pace ventricle
  Refractory periods, detect concealed bypass tracts with unidirectional block
- 1, 2, and 3 extra stimuli
  Ventricular tachycardia induction
- Paired pacing – one paced set-up interval
  Reproduce aberrant conduction

B. Sensed Set-up Intervals

- Sinoatrial conduction times – sense and pace atrium
- Coupled pacing – one sensed set-up interval
  a. Maximum test of distal system
  b. Reproduce aberrant conduction

Pacing Technique

While spontaneous recordings of complex arrhythmias frequently provide the most valuable information, many times the disturbance in question subsides during the recording. A wide array of dynamic challenges with pacemakers and drugs have been developed to provide quantitative information at the time of the study. While the chamber being paced and the intervals differ, even the most sophisticated pacing challenge is a variation on one of two pacing sequences: straight pacing or the use of a test stimulus. The test stimulus is placed at decreasing intervals after a predetermined number of paced or sensed setup intervals. When the setup intervals are paced the term extra stimulus technique is used (Table 1).

Straight pacing is used in obtaining sinoatrial recovery times (SART). After straight pacing for one minute, the pacemaker is turned off. Rates are increased in steps of 10bpm from 90 to 150 in the ideal SART. At each level, the baseline interval, the pacing rate, and the recovery intervals are recorded. Straight pacing is also used in incremental pacing of the atrium. The pacing rate is decreased by 10msec and allowed to pace at least 10 consecutive beats before being further increased, until atrial ventricular block is observed. The rate at which Wenckebach occurs and the rate of 2:1 block are noted. In addition, aberrantly conducted beats and reentrant

supraventricular tachycardia can be produced by straight pacing, especially during the Wenckebach periods. Intermittent incremental pacing is used when a sustained fast rate cannot be tolerated by the patient. After ten paced beats, the pacer is turned off to return the patient to baseline before increasing the rate and restarting.

Straight pacing with sudden cessation is used for reversion of SVT, atrial flutter, and ventricular tachycardia. Pacing is begun at 10bpm-20bpm above the baseline arrhythmia. The period of pacing can be varied, from 3 beats to a minute, before sudden turn-off depending on the arrhythmia. The pacing interval is gradually shortened, and atrial flutter can be reverted 70% of the time to sinus rhythm with this technique. If care is taken not to exceed pacing above 375 beats/min, the patient does not revert to atrial fibrillation. Atrial fibrillation in this setting frequently reverts to normal sinus rhythm or back to flutter within the next 24 hours.

Use of a test stimulus after paced setup cycles, called the extra stimulus technique is the standard for measuring refractory periods. The paced area is driven at a constant rate for eight or ten beats (S_1's) followed by a test extra stimulus (S_2). Pacing is terminated after the test stimulus for several normally conducted beats and then resumed for another train of eight beats and an extra stimulus. The test stimulus should begin at an interval nearly equal to the driving rate and be decreased gradually by decrements of 10msec-20msec until refractoriness to pacing occurs. In the case of extra stimulus technique of the atrium, if atrial refractoriness occurs before AV block, the atrial catheter should be either repositioned or the stimulus increased in amplitude beyond its usual level of double the threshold. Caution should be taken, since the stimuli four- to ten-times the threshold are more likely to cause atrial fibrillation.

A second (S_3) and third (S_4) extra stimulus, may be programmed to follow the first. This technique has been useful in inducing ventricular tachycardia. Each stimulus is brought in to ventricular refractoriness. As stimulation protocols become more aggressive, they become less specific for induction of clinical tachycardias. Inductions in the ventricle are also attempted at more than one site, usually the RV apex and the RV outflow. Following these principles, investigators usually begin at the RV apex. A progressively shorter S_1-S_2 interval will be delivered after an S_1-S_1 drive of 600msec. The S_1-S_1 drive will be decreased to 500msec, then 400msec, with the S_2 extra stimulus decreased each time to refractoriness. The S_3 challenge will resume at the longer drive, 600msec with the S_1-S_2 interval

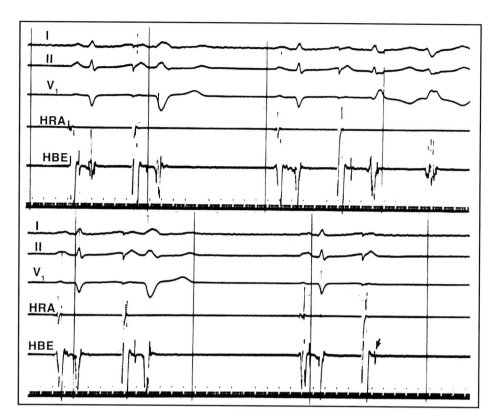

Figure 14. Atrial pacing coupled to each sensed sinus P wave produces the longest setup intervals and is therefore most likely to reproduce aberrant functional bundle block. In this instance, the block typically alternates between left bundle branch block and right bundle branch block. When both bundles block individually, as in this patient, it is not uncommon to see both bundles block simultaneously to produce distal infranodal second degree block (arrow).

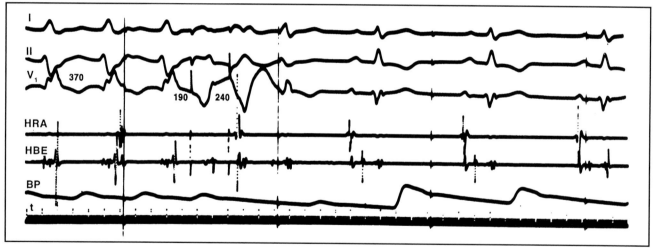

Figure 15. Two paced premature ventricular beats are coupled to sensed ventricular tachycardia, after which the rhythm reverts to normal.

10msec to 20msec above the refractory period. As before, the S_1-S_1 drive will be decreased from 600msec to 500msec, then to 400msec.

Several protocols exist for delivery of extra stimuli. Some protocols advise positioning the ventricular catheter at a second site and repeating the S_2 then S_3 challenge before adding an S_4. The challenge is complete when two sites have been stimulated with two to three S_1-S_1 drive intervals, with extra stimuli of one (S_2), two (S_2, S_3), and three (S_2, S_3, S_4) paced beats.

For atrial pacing, a variation on the extra stimu-

lus technique involves sensing a native depolarization and coupling a test stimulus to this. This allows the longest setup cycles before the premature stimulus to the atrium. Since refractory periods in the distal system are lengthened by long setup cycles, this technique is more likely than any other to produce aberration or distal block (Figure 14). Tachycardia can often be reverted this way, and may require several coupled beats in rapid succession (Figure 15).

When arrhythmias can be induced and reverted in the laboratory, a target is available for both acute

TABLE 2			
Physiologic Testing			
DRUG	ROUTE	DOSE	THERAPEUTIC LEVEL
Atropine	IV	0.5 - 2.0 mg	
Propanolol	IV	0.1 - 0.15 mg/kg Administer 1 mg IV Q2 min	50 - 100 mg/ml
Digoxin	IV	0.75 - 1.5 mg	0.5 - 2.0 mg/ml
Adenosine	IV	6 - 12 mg	—
Verapamil	IV	2 - 10 mg	—
Diltiazem	IV	10 - 20 mg	—
Lidocaine	IV	loading 2 - 3 mg/kg then 2 - 4 mg/min	2.5 mg/ml
Procainamide	IV	10 -12 mg/kg Administer 50 mg Q2 min	4 - 8 mg/ml
Quinidine	IV	600 - 800 mg	2.5 - 5.0 mg/ml

and chronic drug therapy. When drugs are used acutely, the time to test is governed by the pharmacokinetics, and should be confirmed by drawing a drug level whenever possible. Dosing and therapeutic levels are listed for many of the commonly used agents (Table 2), and effects on conduction times and refractory periods are noted (Table 3). While effects listed are correct for the majority of subjects, the individual patient may have an unpredictable and individual response.

Recording Measurements and Interpretations

Recording of spontaneous rhythms, especially during active arrhythmia, can provide the most valuable information in an intracavitary study. Measurements of PR subintervals reveal abnormal intracavitary conduction times, even when the external conduction times appear normal. Onset of atrial activity is the earliest P-wave in any of the three external leads. Onset of low atrial deflection in the AV nodal region is the beginning of rapid electrical activity at a position from which one can also record the proximal His potential. The His bundle activation time is measured from the onset of electrical activity in the His bundle, not from peak of the deflection. The initial ventricular activation time is measured from its earliest onset in any external lead.

Conduction Times

In normal conduction and pacing challenges, arrival of the depolarization wave immediately proximal to a structure (input) is compared with arrival of the depolarization wave distal to the structure (output). Conduction time is the time required for the propagated impulse to go from input to output (Table 4). Intra-atrial conduction time is measured from the onset of the P-wave to the low medial right atrial deflection (P-A) (Figures 5A/B). The AV node conduction time is measured from onset of rapid electrical activity in the low medial right atrium (A) to onset of the deflection in the His bundle (H) referred to as the A-H interval. Normal A-H intervals are .06 to .12. sec (or 60 to 120 msec). Measuring from the onset of depolarization in the proximal His bundle (H) to the first depolarization in the ventricle (V) defines the conduction time for the His bundle and the specialized ventricular conducting system, often referred to as the His Purkinje system. Normal values for the H-V interval average 35msec to 55msec (Table 5).

TABLE 3								
Effects of Pharmacologic Agents During Electrophysiologic Testing								
DRUG	RESTING INTERVALS			LENGTH OF ERP				
	Sinus Cycle	A H	HV	Atrium	AVN	HPS	Vent.	Accessory Pathway
Atropine	–	–	0	0/–	–	0	0	0
Digoxin	+/–	+	0	+/–	+	0	+/–	0/–
Lidocaine	0	0	0	+/–	0 / sl. –	0 / sl. –	+	+/0
Procainamide	sl. +/0	sl. +/–	+	+/0	+/–	+	+	+
Quinidine	sl. –/0	0	+	+/–	+/–	+	+	+
Propanolol	+	+	0	+/–	+	0	+/0	0
Diltiazem	+	+	0	0	+	0	0	0/–
Adenosine	+	+	0	–	+	0	0	0

– = decreased, + = increased, 0 = no change, sl = slightly

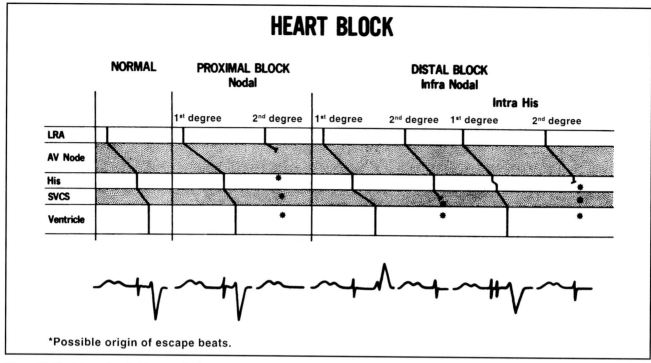

Figure 16. The intracavitary laddergram displays conduction times and area of block for proximal nodal, distal infranodal, 1st and 2nd degree block. Infranodal block includes intra-His block. The possible origin of escape beats is also denoted, as well as stylized external ECG with superimposed His bundle deflections.

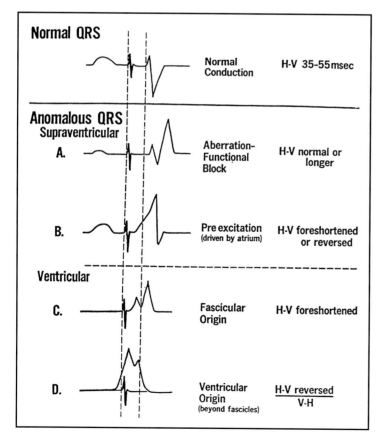

Figure 17. The H-V relationship and relationship of A to V in a normally conducted QRS is compared with supraventricular aberrant functional block (normal or long H-V), preexcitation (short H-V), ventricular fascicular beats (short H-V) or standard ventricular beats (H-V reversed).

478

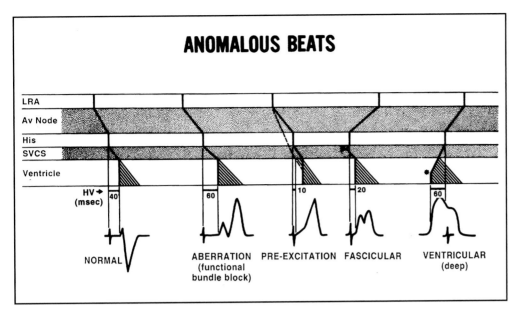

ANOMALOUS BEATS

LRA

Av Node

His

SVCS

Ventricle

HV→ (msec)   40   60   10   20   60

NORMAL   ABERRATION (functional bundle block)   PRE-EXCITATION   FASCICULAR   VENTRICULAR (deep)

Figure 18. The intracavitary laddergram depicts a comparison of normal conduction with four types of anomalous beats. Aberration of functional bundle branch block has normal or prolonged H-V intervals. Beats with foreshortened or reversed H-V but related to atrial rhythm are preexcited. Beats of fascicular origin arrive at the His after conduction has started toward the ventricle producing fore-shortened H-V intervals. The QRS can be relatively narrow, while standard wide ventricular beats have reversed H-V or a V-H. Stylized external tracings depict the relative position of the His bundle deflection to the QRS.

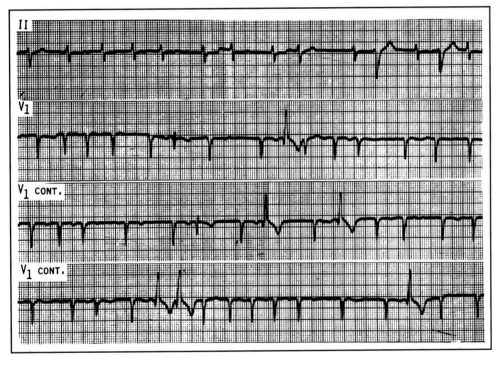

II

V₁

V₁ CONT.

V₁ CONT.

Figure 19A. The patient has atrial fibrillation with wide QRS beats individually and as couplets. The beats have left axis deviation and a RBBB morphology. While not triphasic, the initial vector in V1 or wide QRS is similar to narrow QRS. Intermediate less wide forms are also present. The ventricular rate is 125/min.

Relationship of His Bundle, Blocked P Waves, and Anomalous Beats

More meaningful than conduction time is the relationship of the His bundle to blocked P waves (2nd and 3rd degree block/Figure 16). First degree block denotes prolonged conduction times, where 2nd degree block results from an attempt to conduct during the effective refractory periods of the AV node, His bundle, or specialized ventricular conducting system. Proximal or nodal block records no His deflection as the wave front is extinguished within the AV node, and distal or infranodal block has conducted through the AV node to the initial His deflection. Distal block, except in the presence of a long, short cycle sequence, carries a bad prognosis because of lack of stable escape pacemakers beyond the block area.

Relation of His potentials to anomalous beats is also of value during spontaneous recordings. Figure 17 and the laddergram in Figure 18 demonstrate the distinction between aberrantly conducted supraventricular beats, preexcitation syndrome, fascicular, and deep ventricular premature beats. The aberrantly conducted beat has a normal or longer than normal H-V interval, caused by a functional delay of at least a portion of the distal system. The wide QRS beats in

479

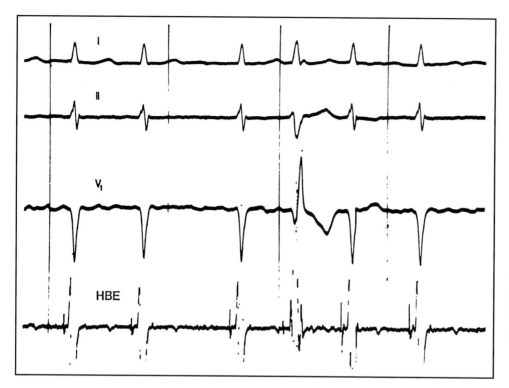

Figure 19B. Simultaneous external leads I, II and V1 as well as His bundle electrogram, show the right bundle branch block morphology beats to have left axis deviation and to have a longer than normal H-V interval, confirming functional bundle branch block. Intermediate forms are likely to be incomplete bundle branch block.

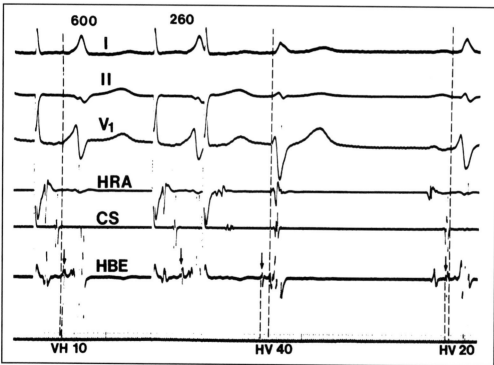

Figure 20. Atrial pacing produces QRS initially with a reversed H-V or V-H of 10msec at 600msec pacing interval. This indicates preexcitation through an accessory pathway. A premature extrastimulus at 260msec blocks the accessory pathway, conducts through the AV node and then through His Purkinje system, with a normal HV interval of 40 msec. The first sinus beat is less preexcited, with an HV interval foreshortened to 20msec.

Figure 19A are shown to have a longer-than-normal H-V in Figure 19B; bypass fibers in WPW allow excitation of the ventricle before conduction has proceeded through the His Purkinje system, thus shortening or reversing normal H-V time. In Figure 20, the H-V is 10msec when delta waves are present and becomes 40msec when a prematurely paced atrial beat finds the accessory pathway refractory.

The two types of ventricular beats differ from WPW in that there is no evidence for control by the atrium. The fascicular premature beat arises proximally enough in the specialized conducting system to conduct retrograde to the His bundle while conducting antegrade to the ventricle. The beats appearing like incomplete RBBB, in Figure 21A, are parasystolic with fusion on beat 1 and increased

TABLE 4

PROXIMAL INPUT		STRUCTURE	DISTAL OUTPUT	CONDUCTION TIME (input to output interval)
Conduction Times				
P-wave		Right atrium	Low right atrium (His area)	PA
P-wave		Left atrium	Low left atrium (Coronary Sinus)	P - LA
Low right atrium		AV node	His	AH
His		His and specialized ventricular conduction system	Ventricle	HV
Refractory Periods				
Effective Refractory Period: Input - Input Longest input interval which fails to conduct			Functional Refractory Period: Output - Output Shortest output interval which conducts	
Stimulator	$S_1 - S_2$	Atrium	High Right Atrium	$A_1 - A_2$
Low Right Atrium	$A_1 - A_2$	AV Node	His Bundle	$H_1 - H_2$
Initial His Bundle	$H_1 - H_2$	His Bundle and specialized ventricular conducting system (His Purkinje System)	Ventricle	$V_1 - V_2$
Local Atrium	$A_1 - A_2$	Bypass	Onset of Delta	$D_1 - D_2$

right bundle aberration on beat 4. While the His deflection in Figure 21B is in front of the V, the H-V interval (40msec) is foreshortened compared to the H-V of the normally conducted beats (60msec), indicating the origin of the beat to be in the proximal left bundle branch as shown in Figure 21C. The usual ectopic beat of ventricular origin has the retrograde His within or following the ventricular complex. On occasion the antegrade His follows dissociated P-waves during ventricular rhythm.

Response to Pacing Studies

After conduction times are measured and the His relationship to blocked P-waves and anomalous QRS is determined, response to pacing studies should be determined. The tests performed with straight pacing techniques are relatively simple to execute, measure and interpret. The laddergram in Figure 22 shows the pacing intervention and calculation for sinoatrial recovery times. The atrial pacer is turned on for one minute at a time at rates of 90, 100, 110, 120, 130 and 150 bpm respectively and abruptly shut off. The time from last paced A to first sinus A is the sinus node recovery time. This is corrected for underlying sinus rate by subtracting the baseline A_1-A_1 interval from the recovery time (A_2-A_3), then the longest recovery time is reported. Many labs shorten the procedure by pacing at slower rates, for example 130 or 120 bpm only.

These rates usually yield the longest recovery time.

Incremental pacing interpretation merely cites the rate at which Wenckebach of the AV node and 2:1 block are first seen. Wenckebach occurring at a rate of less than 130beats/min is abnormal. Block distal to the initial His deflection should be noted. Incremental pacing in Figure 23A, from 430msec to 410msec produced distal block, indicating need for permanent pacing. Distal block occurs after a pause produced by AV nodal block in Figure 23B. This does not have the same prognosis as distal block during ramp pacing in the absence of a long setup cycle (Figure 23A).

The extra stimulus technique controls refractory periods with constant setup cycles before the test stimuli; driving rate or setup cycle can be varied. Reproducible baseline refractory periods can be established and compared before and after drug intervention. Refractory periods can be estimated on spontaneous tracings any time failure to conduct occurs, but the extra stimulus technique allows the most reproducible measure of refractoriness.

Refractoriness is understandably confused with conduction times. Conduction times are a measure of the time from input to output of a given structure, while refractory periods are a measure of the interval between two successive inputs when conduction time is delayed (relative refractory period), or when conduction is blocked (absolute refractory

481

TABLE 5
Electrophysiologic Normal Values

(1) RESTING INTERVALS		
PA	**AH**	**HV**
18 - 36 msec. (Rosen)	73 - 111 msec. (Rosen)	37 - 49 msec. (Rosen)
24 - 45 msec. (Narula)	50 - 120 msec. (Narula)	35 - 45 msec. (Narula)
	60 - 140 msec. (Gallagher)	30 - 55 msec. (Gallagher)
		42 - 60 msec. (Damato)
Average: 20 - 40 msec	60 - 120 msec.	35 - 55 msec.

(2) INCREMENTAL PACING
AV Node Wenckebach
Onset: 130 / min (Narula)
Average onset: 133 / min (Damato)

(3) REFRACTORY PERIODS (ROSEN)

(CL 850 - 600, 70 - 100 bpm)

	Effective Refractory Period	Functional Refractory Period
Atrium	235 (150 - 360)	278 (190 - 390)
AV Node	303 (250 - 265)	421 (350 - 495)

(4) SINUS NODE RECOVERY TIME

Sinus Node Recovery Time	Corrected Sinus Node Recovery Time
1041 ± 56 msec. (Mandel)	110 - 525 msec. (Narula) mean 260 ± 95 msec.
1044 ± 216 msec. (Breithardt) 1029 ± 37 msec. (Rosen; Atropine)	66 - 508 msec. (Breithardt) mean 270 ± 112.5 msec.
Average: 1040 ± 75	265 ± 100

(5) SINO - ATRIAL CONDUCTION TIME

40 - 153 msec.	Mean 92 ± 60 msec. (Rosen)
39.5 - 97.5 msec.	Mean 70 ± 30 msec. (Mosini)
48 - 112 msec.	Mean 82 ± 19.2 msec. (Breithardt)
Average: 80 ± 40 msec.	

period). The longest input-to-input where propagation fails to occur is the effective refractory period (ERP). Any input interval shorter than the ERP meets refractory tissue and fails to conduct.

Refractory Periods

Relative refractoriness of a structure begins when impulse conduction is delayed. The effective refractory period defines the largest coupling interval at which tissue can receive impulses and fail to conduct. The functional refractory period is the shortest interval seen distal to the conducting structure. It is the shortest output-to-output. The common structures where both refractory periods and conduction times are calculated are the atrium,

the AV node, the His bundle, and specialized ventricular conducting system (Table 4).

A detailed analysis of the intracavitary tracings in Figure 24 A-D included measurement of all input intervals and output intervals (Table 6). In panel A, whose intervals are at the top of the table, the S_1-S_2, High A_1-A_2, Low A_1-A_2, H_1-H_2 and V_1-V_2 intervals were the same (500msec). Thus, no relative or absolute refractory periods were challenged. When the H_1-H_2 entered the His Purkinje system at an interval less than 400msec, no V_2 resulted indicating the ERP of the distal purkinje system. As the stimulus interval S_1-S_2 in the atrium was further reduced to 330msec, the A_1-A_2 lengthened to 335, indicating the relative refractory period in the

Set-up Cycle Length: 600/msec				TABLE 6				
S₁ S₂	ATRIUM	HIGH A₁ A₂	LOW A₁ A₂	AV NODE	H₁ H₂	HIS PURKINJE SYSTEM	V₁ V₂	
500		500	500		500		500	Panel A
480		480	480		480		480	
460		460	460		460		460	
440		440	440		440		440	
420		420	420		420	RRP	430	
400		400	400		400	↓	420	
390		390	390	RRP	400	ERP	—	
380		380	380		400		—	
370		370	370		395		—	
360		360	360		*380		—	
350		350	350		390		—	
340		340	340		395		—	
330	RRP	335	335		385		—	
320		330	330		400		—	
310		325	325		405	RRP	505	Panel B
300		320	320		400	ERP	—	Panel C
300		320	320		410	RRP	**415	
280		315	315		410	↓	420	
270		310	310	ERP	—		—	
260		310	310		—		—	Panel D
250	↓	310	310		—		—	
240	ERP	—	—		—		—	
230		—	—		—		—	
220		—	—		—		—	

* FRP AVN   ** FRP His Purkinje

RRP – Relative Refractory Period
ERP – Effective Refractory Period
FRP – Functional Refractory Period
S – Stimulus   A – Atrium
H – His   V – Ventricle

atrium. The relative refractory period in the AV node began at input intervals (Low A₁-A₂) less than 390msec. At 325msec in the low atrium, the H₁-H₂ was 400msec or less as in panel C. At an A₁-A₂ interval of 310msec, the AV node failed to conduct, as in panel D. The laddergram of a typical driving rate and four separate test stimuli are portrayed in Figure 25 A-D.

Input intervals are often graphed against output intervals; ERP and FRP are easily seen on such a graph (Figure 26/upper panel). The input interval plotted against conduction time helps reveal the relative refractory period and dual pathways (Figure 26 lower panel). Typical input vs. output intervals are plotted in Figure 27 as seen for normal, for AV node delay, for dual AV nodal pathways and for various physiological types of WPW.

Retrograde extrastimulus technique is performed in the same manner as antegrade studies except that the ventricle is paced rather than the atrium (Figure 29). Frequently the His bundle is obscured by the ventricular deflections, but V-A curves can be constructed in the same way as the antegrade A-V curves with the longest V₁-V₂ interval which fails to capture the ventricle representing the ventricular refractory period. Plotting V₁-V₂ against A₁-A₂ is valuable for revealing retrograde bypass tracts or dual retrograde pathways through the AV node. The bypass tract exhibits no relative refractory period before complete block, showing no increase in V-A conduction time.

Coupled pacing for sinoatrial conduction times (SACT) is a simple pacing technique which at times produces responses which are difficult to interpret. The technique is depicted as a laddergram in Figure 30, which shows the last of ten sensed atrial deflections followed by a test stimulus whose interval is gradually shortened until the atrial refractory period is reached. When the A₁-A₃ starts to shorten to less than twice the sinus cycle (A₁-A₁), the sinus node is being reset. The reset zone can be best determined by plotting test intervals corrected

483

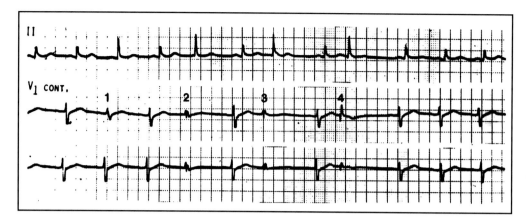

Figure 21A. The interectopic interval for beats 1, 2, 3 and 4 is the same, suggesting parasystole. The narrow RSR1 of beats 2 and 3 have a larger R1 when the beat has a close coupling interval as in beat 4, and fuses with the sinus beat in beat 1. Fusion supports ventricular origin despite the narrow QRS.

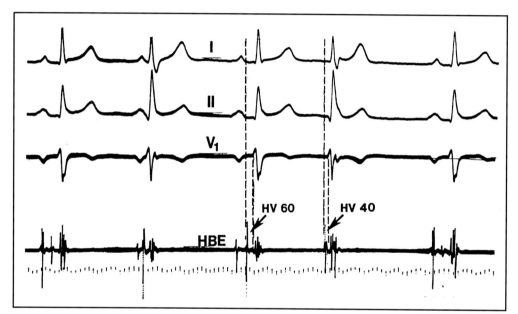

Figure 21B. The normal H-V interval of 60msec is foreshortened to 40msec for the narrow premature beats, indicating fascicular origin.

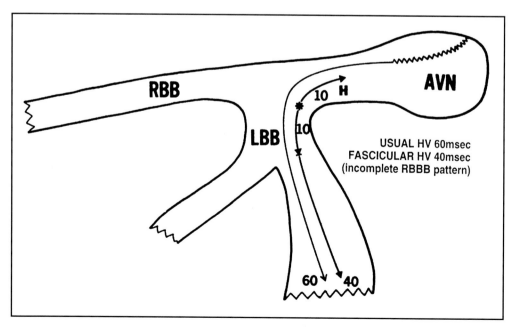

Figure 21C. The fascicular origin in the left bundle branch allows conduction further toward the ventricle before the His deflection. The remaining conduction time produces the foreshortened HV of 40msec for these fascicular beats.

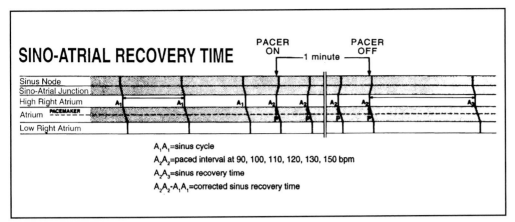

Figure 22. Sinoatrial recovery time as depicted by intracavitary laddergram shows an A 1- A1 sinus cycle before straight pacing A2 at predetermined intervals, usually to include 130 beats per minute. After 30 seconds or 1 minute, pacing is stopped and the interval to the first recovery atrial beat is measured as A2-A3. The A2-A3 is the sinoatrial recovery time (SART). The corrected SART is the A2-A3 minus the A1-A1 sinus interval.

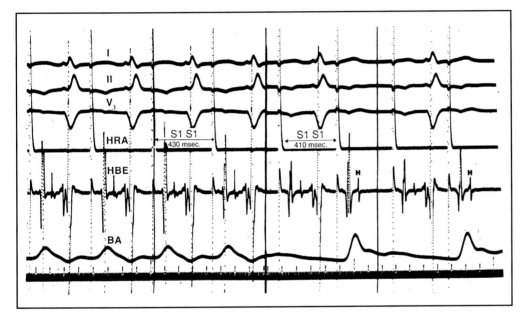

Figure 23A. Incremental ramp pacing shows distal infranodal block occuring after the atrial pacing interval was decreased from 430msec to 410msec.

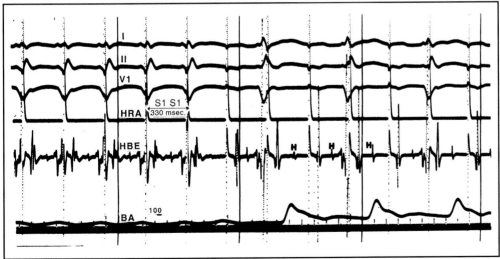

Figure 23B. Incremental ramp pacing shows proximal nodal block at 330msec. After the Wenckebach episode, the next atrial stimulus fails to conduct in the distal infranodal structures, which continues as 2:1 distal block. Distal block after a pause is interpreted as functional and of no prognostic importance. Distal block during ramp pacing which is not preceded by a pause denotes need for pacing as in 23A.

for sinus rate (A_1-A_2/A_1-A_1) against return cycles corrected for sinus rate (A_2-A_3/A_1-A_1).

When the A_2-A_3 plateaus, the sinus node is being reset and sinus conduction times can be measured (Figure 31). During the reset zone, the test stimulus in the sinus node region causes atrial depolarization which travels through the sinoatrial junction to the SA node. After a sinus cycle, a sinus impulse exits

485

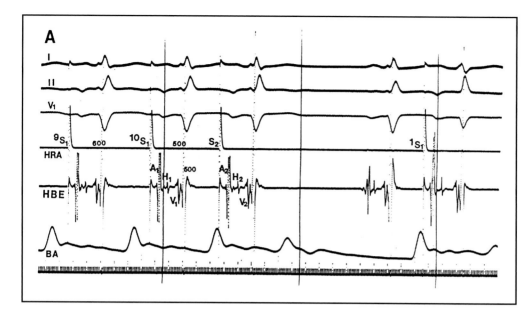

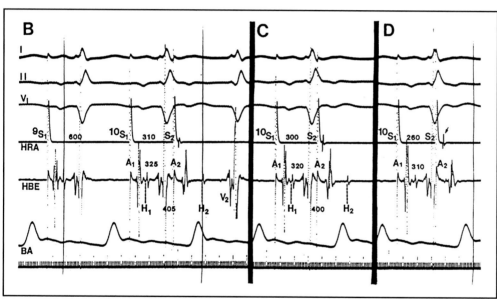

Figure 24. Panels from standard extrastimulus atrial pacing. The drive S1 or setup cycles were at 600msec. In each case they end with the 10th S1 , followed by a sequentially shorter S2 extrastimulus. Panel A displays an S2 of 500msec A1-A2 = H1-H2 = V1-V2. When the atrial S2 is decreased to 310msec in panel B, delay in conduction from stimulus to atrium produces an A1 -A2 of 325msec. Delay in AV nodal conduction produces a lengthened H1 -H2 of 405msec, which meets the relative refractory period of the distal system and which increases HV interval and the V1- V2. A further decrease in S1- S2 to 300 msec produces an A1 -A2 of 300msec. The shorter H1 - H2 finds the distal system refractory. When S1 -S2 is decreased in panel D to 260msec the stimulus to atrium time further lengthens (arrow). This results in minor decrease in A1 -A2 to 310msec, which finds the AV node refractory.

through the sinoatrial junction to the atrium to produce A_3. The test stimulus to return cycle $(A_2\text{-}A_3)$ thus represents one sinus cycle and two periods of travel through the sinoatrial junction. Two sinoatrial conduction times then are equal to $A_2\text{-}A_3$ minus $A_1\text{-}A_1$. Since the retrograde and antegrade conduction time may not be equal, the number is often reported as two sinoatrial conduction times, but by convention, half this interval represents one sinoatrial conduction time. Unfortunately, many patterns appear which do not follow simple expectations, some of which prevent accurate measure of SACT, such as complete block to the sinus node.

A summary of definitions for the tests described above is on Table 7. Normal values for the tests vary with the laboratory and patient population. A list of values for conduction times, sinus node func-

tion tests and refractory periods are present in Table 5. Patients with ERPs greater than 400msec are usually symptomatic.

Clinical Applications

Anatomy, catheter selection, recording and pacing technique, measurement and interpretation of data have been detailed. The techniques clearly document and distinguish rhythm disturbances and types of block clinically meaningful. Since intracavitary recordings are invasive, they are used only when the information cannot be obtained in any noninvasive way and further, when it is likely to alter prognosis or therapy. When pacing catheters are used therapeutically, diagnostic recordings can be easily obtained and will support, or occasionally negate, therapeutic decisions.

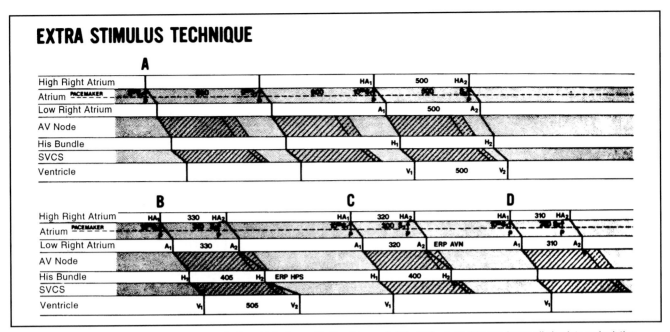

Figure 25. A laddergram arrow depicts panels A, B, C and D in figure 24. The drive cycle S1 of 8 beats to 10 beats keeps all absolute and relative refractory periods constant before the test stimulus S2. The subsequent panels depict enlargement of the distal relative refractory period (B), the distal effective refractory period (C), and proximal A-V nodal effective refractory period (D).

AV Conduction Delay

Clinical applications are listed in Table 8. In the area of AV conduction delays or block, to categorize second degree block as proximal (nodal) or distal (infranodal) is particularly useful when diagnosis is unclear from clinical tracings. Proximal AV nodal block can masquerade as distal block when the conducted beats have a bundle branch block and the PR interval is long (Figure 32A). In this patient, after second degree block, the escape beats are of the opposite bundle branch morphology (RBBB). The intracavitary tracing shows a long AH normal HV and second degree block in the AV node without conduction to the His bundle (Figure 32B).

Clinically the diagnosis of proximal rather than distal block was made using the bedside maneuver of gentle carotid massage.

Each time the carotid was massaged, the second degree block often followed by a ventricular escape was reproduced. A vagal source for the block was suspected in part because of pancreatitis causing nausea, but also because the second degree block was always associated with sinus slowing.

Another less common cause for apparent AV nodal block is concealed His bundle extrasystoles. The first portion of the ECG in Figure 33A shows a 4:3 AV block as classic Mobitz II. The fifth P-wave in lead II is unexpectedly inverted, indicating a possible His bundle extrasystole. This suspicion is further supported later in the tracing by premature His beats conducting to the ventricle. The intracav-

itary tracing in Figure 33B confirms a premature His extrasystole prior to the nonconducted antegrade P-wave followed by two His extrasystoles, one conducting retrograde to produce the inverted P-wave in lead II. His extrasystole conducts antegrade to produce the last QRS.

When distal infranodal block masquerades as proximal AV nodal block, intracavitary traces can clarify the diagnosis. The patient in Figure 34A begins with 2:1 AV block followed by periods of 3:2, 4:3, and 5:4 Wenckebach periods. The patient has RBBB with left-axis deviation on most conducted beats, but on the lowest tracing it changes from RBBB to LBBB before the second-degree block. Intracavitary tracings show a very narrow A-H with a long H-V interval (70msec) becoming longer (120msec) before complete distal infranodal block (Figure 34B). Pacing was indicated in this patient, who had marked calcification of the mitral annulus extending to the septum. Another case of distal Wenkebach is present in Figure 35. The increment in the second PR interval of 15msec is less than the increment for the final PR interval of 55msec. Classic Wenckebach of the AV has decrementing increments, while distal block may have increasing increments. Thirty-five percent of patients with Wenckebach and bundle branch block have block in the distal infranodal region.

Long pauses with atrial fibrillation are commonly due to AV nodal block. In the presence of bundle branch block, especially bifascicular block,

---

TABLE 7
Definitions of Measured Intervals

I. CONDUCTION TIMES

A. General time from input or output of a structure
B. Specific
   1. Right atrium – PA
     Input – onset of sinus P-wave (P)
     Output – Low right atrium (A)
   2. AV Node – AH
     Input – low right atrium (A)
     Output – His (H)
   3. His and Specialized Ventricular Conducting System – HV
     Input – His (H)
     Output – Ventricle (V)

II. REFRACTORY PERIODS

A. General
   1. Relative Refractory Period (RRP)
     The longest proximal input interval (1_1-1_2) that causes
     prolonged conduction (input or output 1_1-0_2)
   2. Effective Refractory Period (ERP)
     Longest input interval (1_1-0_2), which fails to produce an output
   3. Functional Refractory Period (FRP)
     Shortest output interval (0_1-0_2), fastest interval that can be
     seen distal to a structure
B. Specific
   1. Atrial Refractory Period
     Input – stimulus (S) double threshold
     Output – high right atrium (A)
     RRP – the longest $S_1$1-S_2 that causes prolongation of S_2-A_2
     ERP – longest A_1-S_2 that fails to produce an A_1-A_2
     FRP – shortest H_1-H_2
   2. AV Node Refractory Periods
     Input – low right atrium (A), output – His (H)
     RRP – the longest A_1-A_2 that causes prolongation of A_2-H_2
     ERP – longest A_1-A_2 that fails to produce an H_1-H_2
     FRP – shortest H_1-H_2
   3. His Purkinje System
     Input – His (H), output – ventricle
     RRP – the longest H_1-H_2 that causes prolongation of H_2-V_2
     or aberration
     ERP – longest H_1-H_2 that fails to produce a V_1-V_2
     FRP – shortest V_1-V_2
   4. Accessory Pathway
     Input – Atrium (A), Output – Onset of Delta in Ventricle (D)
     ERP – longest A_1-A_2 that fails to produce D_1-D_2 (RRP almost
     never occurs therefore FRP=ERP)
   5. Ventricle
     Input – Stimulus (S), Output – Ventricle (V)
     ERP – longest S_1-S_2 that fails to produce a V_1-V_2
     FRP – shortest V_1-V_2

---

minute (Figure 36B). Only 4 of the 11 beats conducting to the His bundle conducted to the ventricle. The other seven were blocked infranodally in the remaining anterior superior fascicle.

The patient in Figure 37A had a right-bundle branch block with left-axis deviation on most conducted beats. After pauses, the beats conducted with minor variation of the RR interval with left-bundle-block configuration. The shift from right to left bundle makes an infranodal block probable. The intracavitary tracing on Figure 37B shows an impulse at a coupling interval of 620msec failing to conduct to the ventricle, while coupling at 1240msec, 760msec, and 670msec successfully conducted to the ventricle with increasing H-V intervals of 55msec, 95msec, and 115msec. The shorter H-V after the longest coupling was associated with left bundle branch block while shorter coupling produced longer H-V and right bundle branch block.

The apparent contradiction of previously blocked bundles becoming able to conduct is explained by the diagram in Figure 37C. In the top panel, delay down the left bundle was equal to conduction down the right plus transseptal conduction time, and apparent left bundle branch block was seen. When the right bundle was blocked, the previously delayed left bundle branch conducted to the ventricle with its longer H-V interval. This patient with 2nd degree distal block requires pacing. Complete heart block is easier to analyze. Distal infranodal heart block confirmed by intracavitary tracings (Figure 38) was suspected from the wide QRS escape rhythms and absence of conducted beats. Intracavitary tracings showing a His bundle after each P wave (arrow) confirmed infranodal block and the need for pacing. Narrow conducted beats and narrow escape beats on the other hand do not confirm proximal block. This is particularly true for the patient in Figure 39A who presented with 2:1 block and a conducted QRS of .10 sec. The lower panel reveals narrower escape beats of .09 sec. The last QRS was captured by the atrium.

The shift in QRS configuration during escape suggests fascicular and therefore ventricular escape, and makes distal infranodal block a likely possibility. Intracavitary tracings in Figure 39B demonstrate a long H-V interval of 100msec on conducted beats, a short A-H indicating brisk conduction through the AV node and frequent second degree distal infranodal block. The narrow escape QRS with a shorter H-V of 40msec is originating from fascicles in the ventricle. This patient who complained of dizziness for 9 months was suspected to have digitalis intoxication. Distal block which could not be due to digitalis excess was documented and

infranodal block is the cause of the pause in 30% of cases. The conducted beats in Figure 36A display right bundle branch block and right axis deviation, suggesting posterior inferior hemiblock as well as right bundle branch block. Intracavitary recordings showed excellent conduction through the AV node to produce His bundle deflection at 150beats/

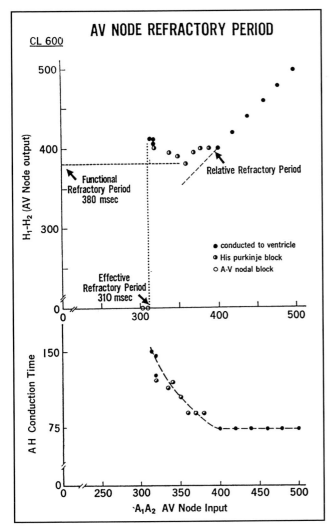

AV NODE REFRACTORY PERIOD

CL 600

- conducted to ventricle
- His purkinje block
- A-V nodal block

Figure 26. The intervals from Table 5 can be graphically presented. The input interval of a given structure such as the AV node can be plotted against the output interval (in the upper panel), or against the input to output conduction time (lower panel). Note that all H1 - H2 output intervals longer than 400msec conduct to the ventricle, while shorter intervals cause distal infranodal block (half shaded dots).

required permanent pacing. She has lived 20 additional years to the age of 96.

Distal infranodal heart block can occur suddenly without ventricular escape. One clue for predicting future distal block is the conduction time of the distal system, or H-V interval. Normal intervals are rarely seen with 2nd degree distal block (2.5%-5%). The patient with acute myocardial infarction and new right bundle branch block virtually never goes to complete heart block if the H-V interval is normal, but there is a high incidence of distal block when the H-V is long (Table 9). Note that the patients in Table 9 with long H-V and distal heart block all had PR intervals longer than .15. Thus, while a PR less than .20 does not exclude a long H-V, a PR of .15 or less makes it so unlikely in this

---

TABLE 8

Clinical Applications

I. AV Conduction
- Localize site of block and refractory periods
  Identify cases masquerading as distal infranodal block
    Bundle branch block with proximal AV nodal block and ventricular escape
    Concealed His bundle extrasystoles simulating Mobitz II
  Identify cases of distal block masquerading as AV nodal proximal block
    Wenckebach periods with bundle branch block – 35% are distal Wenckebach
    Atrial fibrillation with bundle branch block and pauses – 30% are due to distal block
    Intra His block with narrow conducted beats and fascicular escape beats
    Wide conducted beats with identical morphology for escape beats originating from the distal conduction system
- Localize and quantitate prolonged conduction times

II. Identify origin of anomalous beats (especially with atrial fibrillation or in sustained tachycardia)
- Supraventricular functional block – aberrancy
- Preexcitation
- Ventricular – fascicular origin
- Ventricular – deep

III. Preexcitation – WPW
- Precise diagnosis when:
  – simulating myocardial infarction
  – atypical – long PR, latent antegrade conduction
  – unidirectional block
- Mechanism for tachycardia and response to specific pharmacological agents
- Define shortest R - R with atrial fibrillation < 205 msec is associated with ventricular arrhythmias and sudden death
- Identify site of bypass for ablation therapy

IV. Integrity of A-V conduction prior to permanent atrial pacing

V. Test integrity of the sinus node

VI. Determine mechanism for supraventricular tachycardia and response to pharmacological intervention

VII. Induce ventricular tachycardia for mapping source and determine response to therapy

VIII. Reversion of reentrant PAT, atrial flutter, ventricular tachycardia – test for pacing solutions to intractable arrhythmias

IX. Ablation – AV node, accessory pathways, atrial tachycardia, atrial flutter, ventricular tachycardia

setting that His recording or pacing therapy is unnecessary.

In chronic symptomatic patients with suspected distal block because of bundle branch block, a normal H-V interval virtually excludes intermittent distal block and leads one away from pacing therapy. The symptomatic patient with long H-V has an

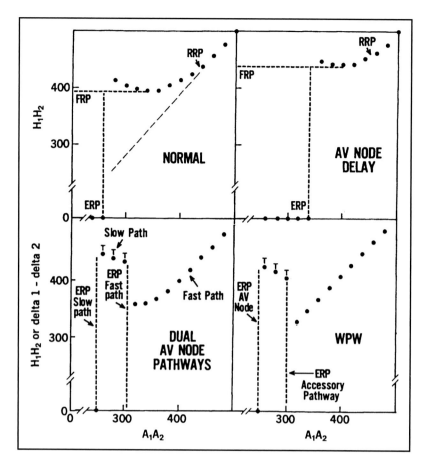

Figure 27. Typical input-interval to output-interval curves across the AV node for normal (A), AV node delay (B), dual pathways (C) and accessory pathways (WPW) (D). Tachycardia with either dual AV node or accessory pathways can begin with the effective refractory period of the faster pathway.

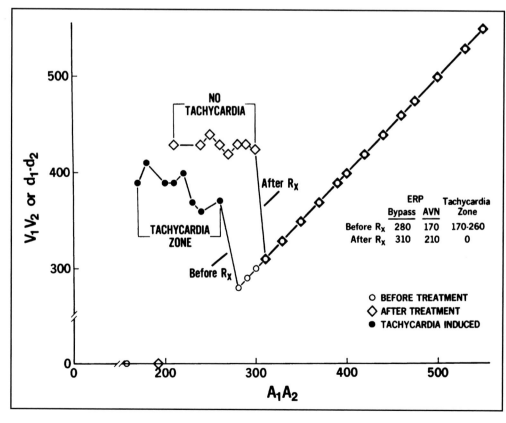

Figure 28. A typical input-interval (A1-A2) to output-interval (V1-V2) curve in WPW shows active tachycardia after the ERP of the accessory pathway. When the ERP is lengthened for both the accessory pathway and the AV node, the two pathways conduct anterogradely and tachycardia fails to occur, thus closing the tachycardia window, indicative of efficacious therapy.

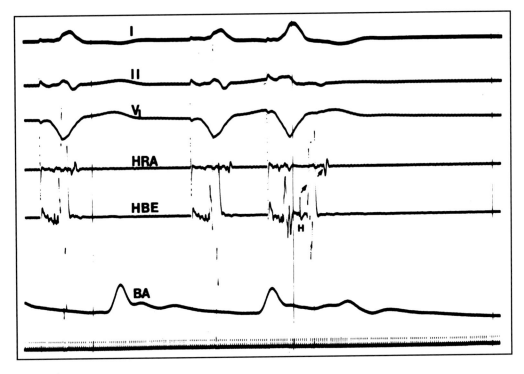

Figure 29. Retrograde extrastimulus technique shows the drive S_1-S_1 and S_2 pacing the ventricle and reveals a retrograde His bundle deflection followed by a low A then the high right atrial deflection (arrows).

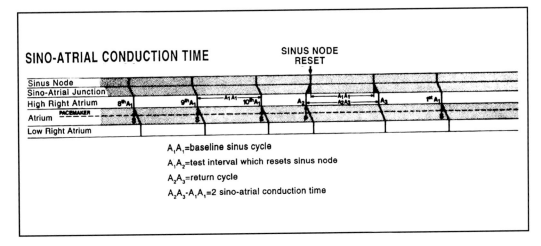

SINO-ATRIAL CONDUCTION TIME

SINUS NODE RESET

Sinus Node
Sino-Atrial Junction
High Right Atrium
Atrium
Low Right Atrium

A_1A_1=baseline sinus cycle

A_1A_2=test interval which resets sinus node

A_2A_3=return cycle

A_2A_3-A_1A_1=2 sino-atrial conduction time

Figure 30. Pacing coupled to the sensed atrium is used to determine the sinoatrial conduction time (SACT) when sinus node reset is present. The paced A_2 to sensed A_3 represents the combination of the A_1-A_1 sinus cycle and conduction into and out of the sinus node. Thus A_2-A_3 minus A_1-A_1 calculates the conduction time into and out of the sinus node, which is reported as 2 SACTs or when divided by 2 is one SACT.

TABLE 9

HV with Right Bundle Branch Block with Acute Myocardial Infarction

	JOSEPHSON (1993)	ARONSON (1973)	LIE *ET. AL.* (1974)	TOTAL
Number of patients	40	70	35	145
Normal HV	15	31	19	65
(Progressed to CHB)	2	0	1	3 (5%)
Prolonged HV	25 (HV > 55)	39 (HV > 55)	16 (HV > 60)	80
(Progressed to CHB)	16	27	11	54 (68%)
minimum PR		0.17 sec	0.16 sec	0.16 sec

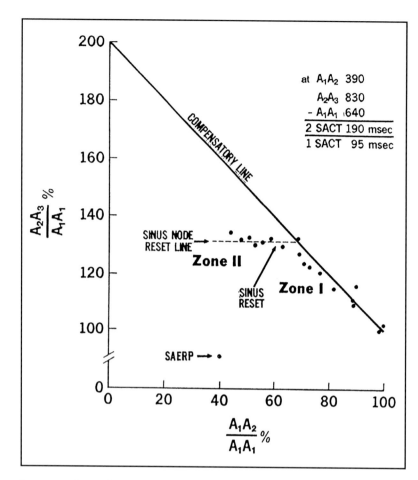

Figure 31. All responses to coupled atrial pacing can be graphed after intervals normalizing the input interval A_1-A_2 the output interval A_2-A_3 to the immediate sinus interval A_1-A_1. When compensatory intervals cease and a sinus node is reset, the A_1-A_1 minus the A_2-A_3 equals 2 SACTs, which can be divided by 2 for one SACT. Further decrease in A_1-A_2 might not penetrate the SA node, producing interpolated atrial beats, thus defining the sino-atrial effective refractory period.

increased incidence of distal heart block and sudden death, and may be helped by pacing therapy. The asymptomatic patient with bundle branch block and long H-V intervals has an increased mortality rate, which is not clearly due to heart block. Electrophysiological evaluation has also been useful in determining the integrity of the AV node in candidates for atrial pacing.

Identify Origin of Anomalous Beats

Identifying the origin of beats with anomalous QRS has been useful in specific patients, especially when antecedent atrial activity cannot be found. Previous cases presented in this text discuss the ability to distinguish between beats which are wide or different from normally conducted beats (Figure 17, 18). The H-V intervals for beats with functional bundle block or aberration are equal to or longer than the H-V of normally conducted beats. Fascicular beats can have a narrow QRS but have an H-V less than the normally conducted beat, while ventricular ectopy usually has a reversed H-V, or V-A. The run of wide QRS beats of a left bundle branch configuration in Figure 40A was difficult to diagnose.

The fact that the patient has atrial fibrillation and that the narrowly conducted beats are at the same rate as the wide anomalous beats suggests that these beats could be conducted with left bundle functional block. The cycle sequence for intervals 1 and 2 compared with 3 and 4 favored ventricular ectopy. The long, short cycle sequence (intervals 1 and 2) without bundle block after interval 2 was compared to the shorter setup interval in 3. The same or longer coupling in interval 4 was unlikely to produce functional block and therefore supported the wide QRS after interval 4 as due to ventricular ectopy. The intracavitary tracing shows His deflections in front of both narrow and wide QRS complexes in Figure 40B and also shows unexpected distal block. The distal block is seen better in Figure 40C for this patient. The longer H-V interval of the aberrantly conducted beat (80msec vs 50msec) explains why an externally measured R-R interval can appear longer than the H-H interval that engaged the His Purkinje system. Note in Figure 40D that an H_1-H_2 interval of 400msec will produce a V_1-V_2 of 400msec if no H-V lengthening occurs (lower panel).

When the shorter H_1-H_2 of 390msec caused left bundle branch block, the longer H-V of 80msec resulted in an externally measured R-R interval, of 420msec, 20msec longer than the previous normally

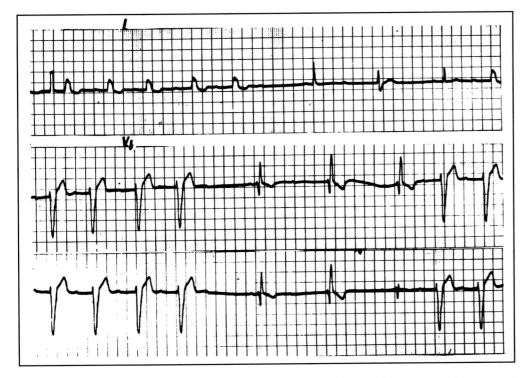

Figure 32A. Initial conduction with a long PR interval and left bundle branch block is followed by a non-conducted P wave and an escape beat which has a right bundle branch pattern. When a P wave is close to the escape, QRS narrows in various degrees of fusion, revealing a shorter PR interval during the return cycle characteristic of Wenckebach second degree block. This sequence was reproduced with carotid massage, making proximal nodal block most likely.

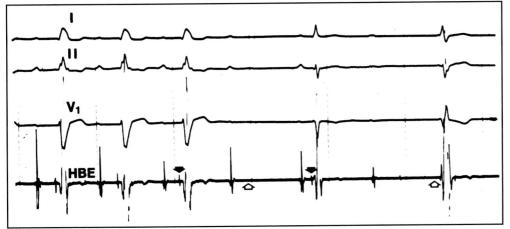

Figure 32B. The intracavitary His bundle electrogram reveals a long A-H and normal H-V with conducted beats and no His bundle deflection with non-conducted P waves (open arrow). Following the block, a short AH and fusion are seen. That last QRS has no His in front (second open arrow) and represents ventricular escape from the left bundle branch.

conducted R-R interval without LBBB. Thus the true short coupling interval at the proximal site of the blocked bundle branch will be concealed and be shorter than the external R-R to the same extent that the H-V prolongs in the unblocked but delayed bundles which conduct the abberrant beat. Prolonged H-V intervals can be seen in all forms of abberration but are routine in patients with left-bundle-branch block abberation.

The patient with wide QRS tachycardia in Figure 41A has a similar left bundle configuration. Intracavitary tracings for this patient show a more rapid dissociated atrial rhythm, with His bundle deflections associated retrogradely with each QRS (Figure 41B). The patient's atrial and ventricular tachycardias were due to digitalis intoxication.

Preexcitation – WPW Syndrome

In preexcitation (WPW syndrome), the diagnosis, mechanism of tachycardia, site of bypass, and maximum ventricular response to atrial fibrillation are valuable in prognosis and treatment. Figure 42A is from a patient with a history of rapid heart action during exercise and a short PR interval. Anomalous beats 1 and 2 were seen after the onset of atrial fibrillation on the treadmill. Intracavitary tracings revealed functional right bundle branch and left anterior fascicular block to be responsible for morphology 2 (Figure 42B). While atrial pacing continues to control the ventricle in Figure 42C, the His bundle is within the QRS and then absent, indicating pure preexcitation of the ventricle from an accessory pathway for beats of morphology in beat 1.

493

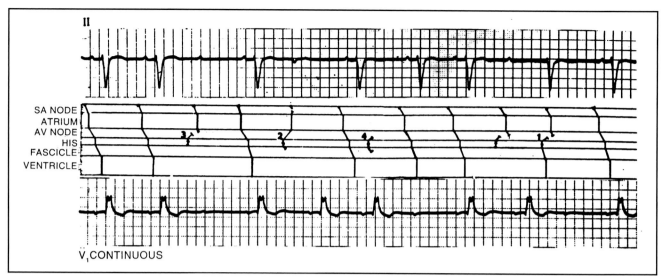

Figure 33A. The ventricular response to the first four P waves is a classic 3:2 Mobitz II pattern. The fifth P wave is unexpectedly inverted and the seventh QRS occurs after a blocked P wave but unexpectedly early for an escape QRS. A His extrasystole could be responsible, conducting retrogradely but not anterogradely in the first instance and conducting anterogradely in the second. The laddergram depicts these two extrasystoles (3,1) which suggest a concealed His extrasystole which neither conducts to the atrium or the ventricle but blocks anterograde conduction. The laddergram so depicts a completely concealed His extrasystole (4) which does not affect the tracing.

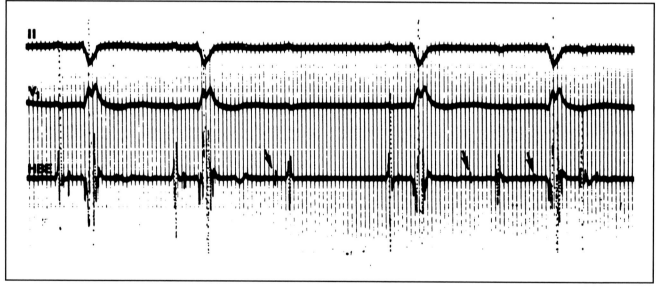

Figure 33B. The intracavitary tracing confirms the His extrasystole (1st arrow) and a more premature His extrasystole (2nd arrow), which conducts retrogradely to the atrium as denoted by the inverted P wave. The last QRS is probably caused by a third His extrasystole (3rd arrow).

Test Integrity of Sinus Node

Sinus node function tests are useful for confirmation of clinical suspicions but have not yet been used as absolute indicators of pacing therapy.

Determine Mechanism for SVT and VT

Patients with intractable SVT can receive distinct benefit from knowledge of the mechanism of the arrhythmia and its response to pharmacological agents or pacing. In most instances, the arrhythmia can be induced and subsequently reverted by pac-

ing catheters (Figure 43). The ability of pharmacological agents to suppress catheter-induced arrhythmias predicts successful long-term therapy. This technique is successful against chronic ventricular arrhythmias as well.

While these studies are usually performed using temporary electrode catheters, virtually the same data can be obtained using most standard implanted pacemakers and their electrodes, and by most modern pacing defibrillators. The pacemaker output should be 2 times, then 4 times diastolic threshold.

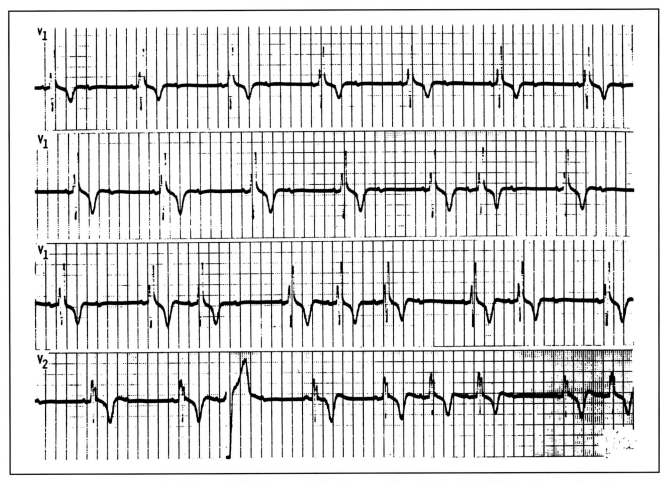

Figure 34A. An external V1 shows 2:1AV block with RBBB in conducted beats in association with 3:2 and 4:3 AV block . Later complexes show progressive increase in PR interval before the blocked beat of Wenckebach. The lower V_2 tracing suggests a change from right to left bundle branch block before the block.

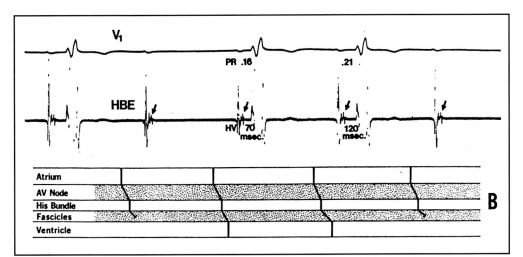

Figure 34B. The intracavitary tracing shows progressive lengthening of the H-V interval from 70msec to 120msec before AV block, typical for distal infranodal Wenckebach.

The full range of setup drive cycles (600-400 msec) and 3 premature beats minimizes false negatives because only one right ventricular position is used for testing. Reentrant supraventricular tachycardia, atrial flutter, and ventricular tachycardia can be successfully reverted by intracavitary pacing.

Intracavitary recording of electrical potentials has provided a large body of useful information on bradyarrhythmias, tachycardias, and pharmacological effects on the human heart. Much of the information was suspected by extension from animal data and elegant deductive reasoning by workers

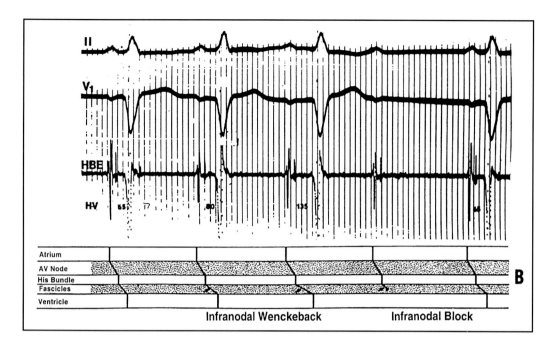

Figure 35. The 4:3 Wenckebach period in the presence of left bundle branch block is shown by intracavitary tracing to be due to progressive lengthening of the H-V interval from 65msec to 80msec, then 135msec. The last increment is frequently the largest in distal infranodal Wenckebach.

such as Wenckebach, Mobitz, Langendorf, and Pick. Deductive reasoning is still necessary to complete the links in between the shaded areas of the more detailed intracavitary laddergram. Seeing the additional rungs has not only helped patients under study, but has improved our interpretation and concepts of clinical arrhythmias. While the discipline of viewing the surface ECG in terms of what would be found with intracavitary recordings and electrophysiological testing has improved our interpretations, even the most alert clinician can be surprised by the actual recording in individual patients. On occasion, more specific therapy and avoidance of overzealous pharmacological and pacemaker therapy are the rewards of intracavitary recordings. Diagnostic electrophysiology has progressed to therapeutic electrophysiology with the widespread use of catheters for ablation. As the risk of antiarrhythmic pharmacological agents becomes increasingly clear, ablative therapy is used earlier in the course of a patient's arrhythmia history. This field remains dynamic, promising new insights and options.

Ablation in Treatment of Cardiac Arrhythmias

Historic Perspectives

The details of electrophysiologic testing outlined above have been refined to an extent which permits therapeutic intervention for cardiac arrhythmias. Initial definitive therapy for cardiac arrhythmias in the 1960s and 1970s was limited to the surgical interruption of anomalous pathways. The first reported successful division of an AV bypass tract by John Sealy in 1968 opened the door to these definitive interventions. Rapid expansion in the understanding of the pathophysiology of arrhythmias and improved tools for localization have resulted in the development of non-surgical methods of ablating myocardial tissue. Initially, DC ablation was performed using high energy (100 joules to 400 joules) and was used to ablate the AV node by Scheinman and Galagher. Scheinman later applied DC ablation to posterior septal accessory pathways.

Energy was delivered between an intracardiac cathode and an indifferent skin patch anode. A large vapor globe formed and resulted in electrolysis. This globe typically expanded and resulted in a small intracavitary explosion. The ablative effects of direct current energy were related to the high energy discharge and the resultant barotrauma. Direct current ablation gave rise to unpredictable lesion sizes. While success rates warranted its use over surgical thoracotomy the complication rate limited applicability. In 1987, Frank Marcus used radiofrequency current to ablate the AV node and Mark Borggrefe in 1989 first reported the results of radiofrequency ablation in Wolff-Parkinson-White syndrome. The early success rates were again marginal, but rapidly improved by techniques of catheter placement and enlarging the size of the catheter tip to over 4mm.

Biophysics of Radiofrequency Energy Lesion Formation

Radiofrequency ablation involves the delivery of a high frequency alternating current in the range of 300 to 1,000kHz. Current flows from the distal electrode to the low resistance tissue while ablative

496

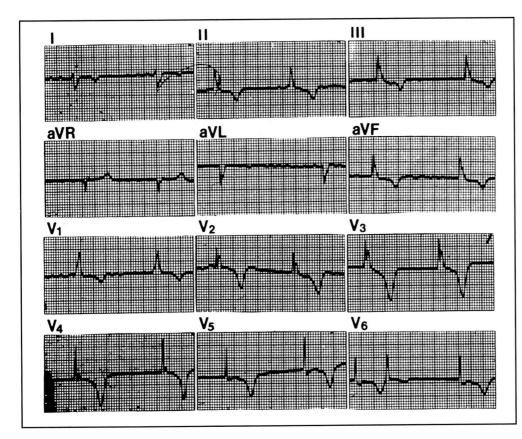

Figure 36A. The 12 lead ECG shows atrial fibrillation with variable RR intervals up to 1.6 seconds. The right bundle branch block is associated with marked right axis suggestive of posterior hemiblock. A premature QRS in V6 is suggestive of supranormal conduction. Distal infranodal H-V block is suggested as the cause of the patient's slow heart rate.

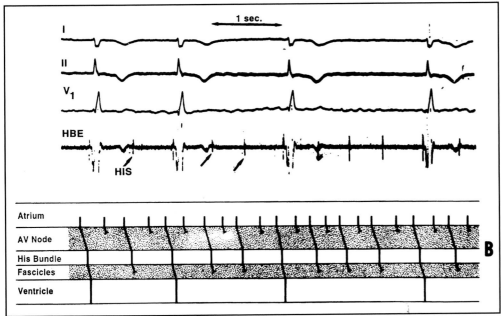

Figure 36B. The intracavitary tracing for the patient in 36A shows His bundle deflections at a relatively rapid rate. While AV nodal conduction to the His bundle occurred eleven times, conduction beyond the His bundle was successful only 4 times. This confirms serious 2nd degree distal infranodal block.

effects derive from tissue heating. Desiccation occurs as heat rises and water is driven out of the tissue. Lesion size and morphology is much more predictable with radiofrequency application than with direct current ablation. Lesion size and depth depend on several variables, including total energy delivered (a factor of the power and duration of energy application), tissue contact, electrode size, convective heat loss, and impedance of the patient-electrode system. Performance of successful radiofrequency ablation is critically dependent on accurate localization of and adequate contact with target tissues.

A variety of catheters have been developed for energy delivery to the myocardium. It is critical that the catheter be non-porous, to prevent coagu-

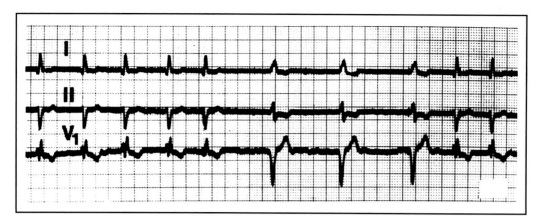

Figure 37A. The external ECG shows atrial fibrillation. The conducted beats are initially right bundle branch block with left axis deviation. After a one-second pause the QRS changed to left bundle branch block. Since the slower RR interval was variable, these beats with left bundle branch block probably were also conducted from the atrium.

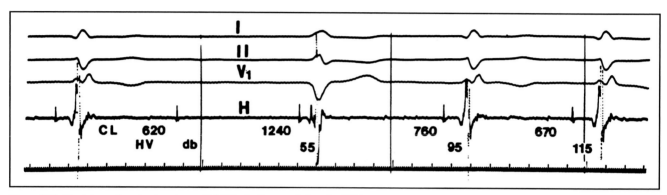

Figure 37B. The intracavitary tracing shows distal block after a cycle length of 620 msec, conduction with H-V interval of 55msec after a 1240 msec pause. After cycle length of 760msec, conduction with right bundle branch block occurred with an H-V of 95msec. The H-V interval is further lengthened to 165msec when the interval shortened to 670msec.

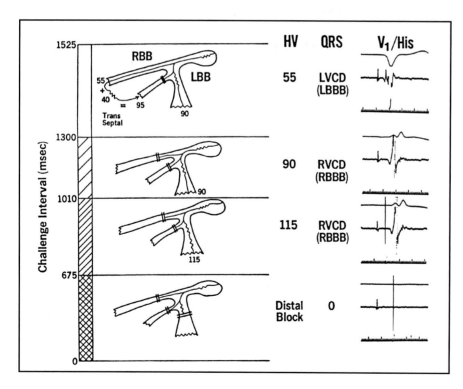

Figure 37C. The events on Figure 37B are summarized using the challenge interval, the HV, the recorded data, and a diagram of the areas in the conduction system of block and delay. Note that left bundle branch pattern after intervals greater than 1300msec may be because delay down the left bundle branch is slower than the time to conduct both down the right bundle branch and then transeptally to the left ventricle. The delayed left bundle branch becomes the only conducting bundle after the right bundle branch blocks at challenge interval less than 1010msec. At challenge intervals less than 675msec, the left bundle also blocks producing bilateral bundle branch block with no conduction to the ventricle.

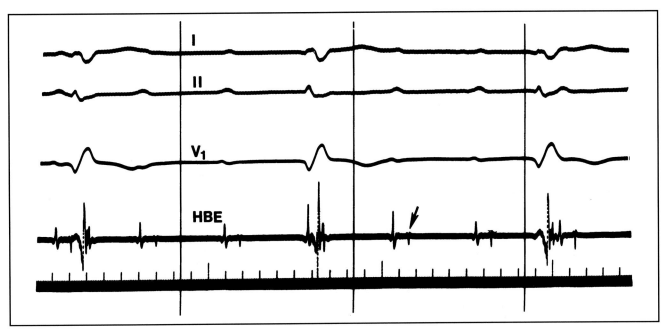

Figure 38A. The regular slow ventricular escape is dissociated from the atrium. The His bundle electrogram shows excellent conduction through the AV node to the His bundle but not beyond (arrow). The patient therefore has complete distal infranodal heart block.

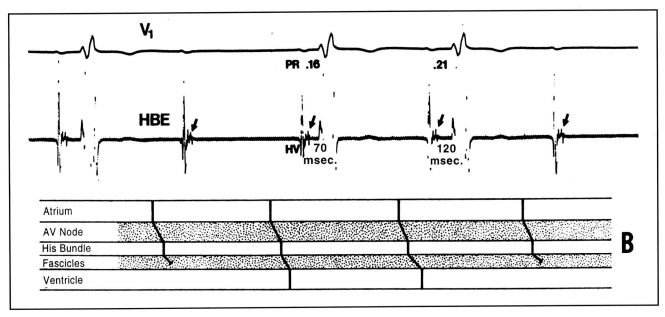

Figure 38B.

lum formation as heating occurs on the myocardial surface. Ideally, the catheter tip should be large enough to allow adequate tissue contact and the catheter shaft rigid enough to transmit torque. Bidirectional tip deflection or highly flexible unidirectional deflectability facilitate catheter manipulation. Clinically, the ability to measure the temperature reflected back to the catheter by use of an imbedded thermistor bead has proven useful in assuring adequate tissue contact.

Typically, during the performance of a catheter ablation in our laboratory, multiple parameters, including temperature and impedance, will be observed during each application of radiofrequency energy. Abrupt rises in temperature or impedance suggest coagulum formation. Observations of this sort result in the need to remove the catheter to ensure that no coagulum has formed at the tip. Currently available power sources permit adjustment of features such as power delivered (watts) and duration of energy application. Some include feedback mechanisms, which automatically cut off

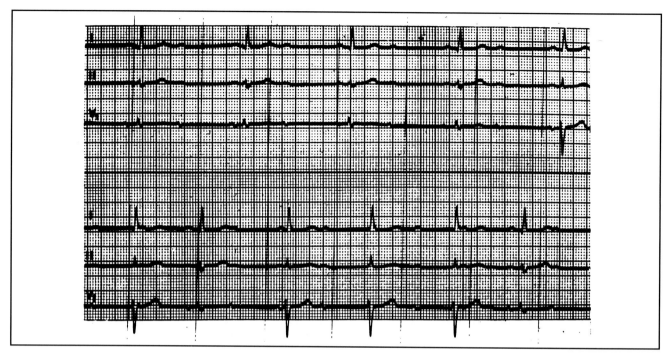

Figure 39A. The simultaneous rhythm of leads I,II and V1 show 2:1 block followed by an escape QRS on the lower tracing. The conducted QRS is .10sec while the escape QRS is .09msec. While all QRS durations are normal the marked difference in QRS morphology suggests distal infranodal block rather than proximal AV nodal block. The fixed duration for the PR, whether the R-P is long as in the upper tracing, or shorter as in the lower, suggests a Mobitz II equivalent.

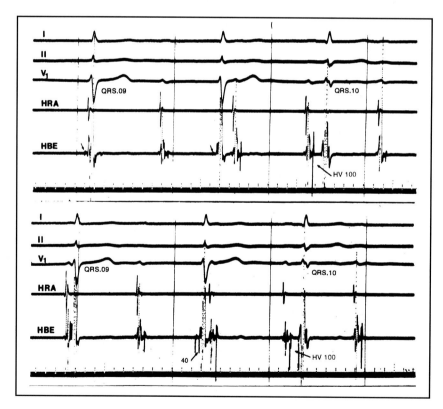

Figure 39B. The two intracavitary tracings show 2 narrow escapes followed by one conducted QRS. Conducted beats have a HV of 100msec while nonconducted P waves block after the His bundle deflection confirming distal infranodal block.

energy delivery if impedance rises occur. Future models of generators may include a similar temperature feedback.

Parameters utilized for therapeutic radiofrequency ablation typically include 3 to 5 energy deliveries at power settings between 25 watts and 35 watts; usual duration is between 30 seconds and 60 seconds. Depending on the target tissue, the temper-

TABLE 10

Evolving Indications for Radiofrequency Catheter Ablation of Supraventricular Arrhythmias

	ACCESSORY PATHWAY ABLATION	AV NODE MODIFICATION	AV NODE ABLATION
Drug refractory arrhythmia	25.3%	40.0%	69.6%
Arrhythmia had malignant potential	54.9%	39.2%	39.3%
Excessive surgical risk	35.9%	38.6%	26.8%
Patient drug intolerant	86.9%	85.0%	71.4%
Patient anticipated pregnancy	2.7%	5.5%	3.6%

EP Technologies, multicenter trial. Ages ranged from 7-89 years and arrhythmia substrates were accessory pathways (n = 288), AV node modifications (n = 129) and AV node ablation (n = 56).

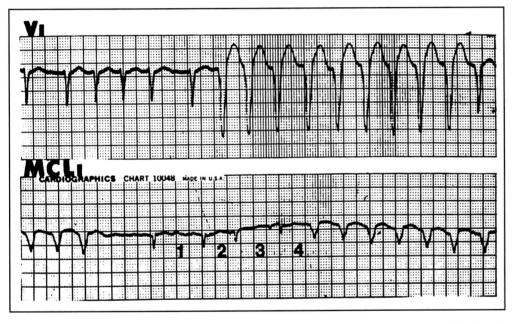

Figure 40A. Atrial fibrillation with a rapid ventricular response, with narrow QRS. An irregular wide rapid QRS follows, with a left bundle branch block morphology. The last QRS on the upper tracing is an intermediate form. Intervals 1, 2, 3 and 4 were measured carefully. The first setup interval (1) was challenged by short interval (2) with a narrow QRS. A larger setup interval 3 was challenged by an interval equal to interval 2 with a wide QRS. This suggested ventricular origin. However, the irregularly irregular response at a rate comparable to the narrow QRS suggest, left bundle branch aberration as the reason for the wide QRS beats.

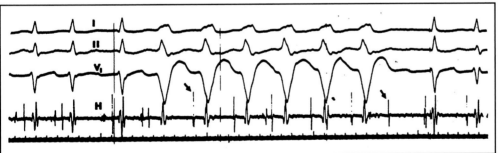

Figure 40B. The intracavitary tracing shows a His bundle deflection before all wide QRS beats, as well as nonconduction after the His deflection resulting in a brief pause.

ature as reflected back to the thermistor bead ranges between 50 degrees and 60 degrees C.

Clinical Indications for Radiofrequency Ablation

Since the advent of radiofrequency catheter ablation, indications continue to evolve. In one large multicenter trial, indications varied somewhat with target tissue, but included drug refractoriness, arrhythmias with malignant potential, unacceptable surgical risk, inability to take drugs, or a reluctance to take drugs in anticipation of pregnancy (Table 10). Prior to the advent of radiofrequency ablation, definitive therapy had been limited to patients with life-threatening arrhythmias. While fairly extensive follow-up is available in the surgical literature on patients who have undergone surgical ressection, followup is still limited in

501

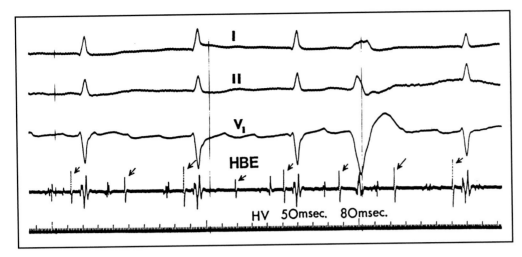

Figure 40C. Distal infranodal block is confirmed. The H-V interval of 50msec when the QRS is narrow increases to 80msec when QRS has a LBBB morphology.

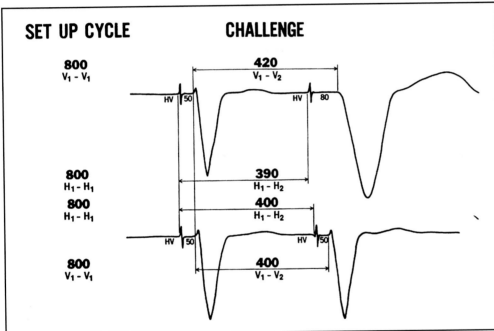

Figure 40D. This 30msec extension of the HV from 50msec to 80msec during bundle branch block explains why an external RR with left bundle branch block of 420msec would have a challenge A_1-A_2 interval of 390msec. A longer challenge H1-H2 of 400msec might produce normal conduction and a narrow QRS with the shorter RR of 400msec.

patients who have undergone radiofrequency catheter ablation.

Targets for Catheter Ablation

• **Atrioventricular Node Modifications:** The ability to direct radiofrequency energy selectively at a very small focal area, and the improved manipulability of catheters, has allowed us to expand not only the clinical indications for ablation, but also appropriate target sites for ablation. Atrioventricular nodal reentrant tachycardia is the most common paroxysmal supraventricular tachycardia; its physiology involves anatomically distinct pathways at the atrioventricular junction. Huang and others first demonstrated that the titratability of radiofrequency application could be used to create selective lesions at the AV junction and to create modification on AV node physiology, without causing interruption of anterograde conduction. Selective radiofrequency energy application permits performance of AV node modifications by specifically directing energy against either the slow pathway or fast pathway. Success rates for this procedure are on the order of 90%.

A good deal has been written regarding appropriate mapping techniques for performance of AV node modifications. Generally, one relies on an anterior superior location for a fast pathway modification, and a posterior inferior location for a slow one. Typically, for fast pathway ablations, mapping is performed both anterograde and retrograde, with retrograde mapping being utilized to define earliest retrograde atrial activation as the impulse travels up the fast pathway and exits into the atrium. However, energy is more prudently delivered during sinus rhythm, with observations made regard-

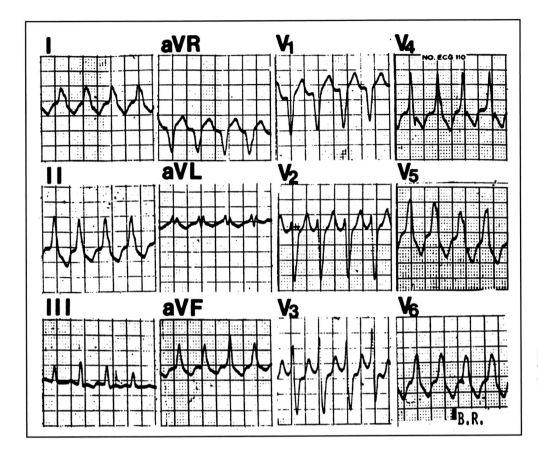

Figure 41A. Twelve lead ECG with a wide QRS tachycardia with LBBB morphology.

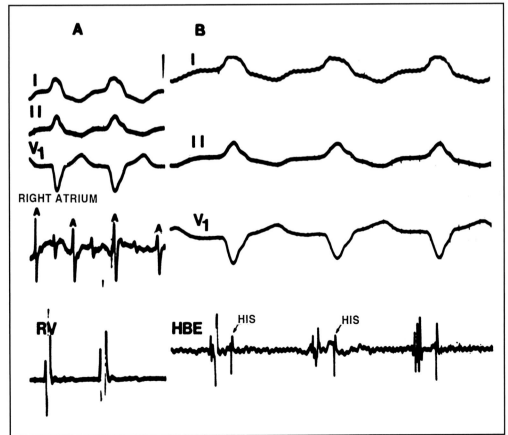

Figure 41B. Intracavitary tracing shows rapid atrial rhythm (A) dissociated from less rapid ventricular arrhythmia with retrograde His deflection (B). This double tachycardia resolved after digoxin was withdrawn.

503

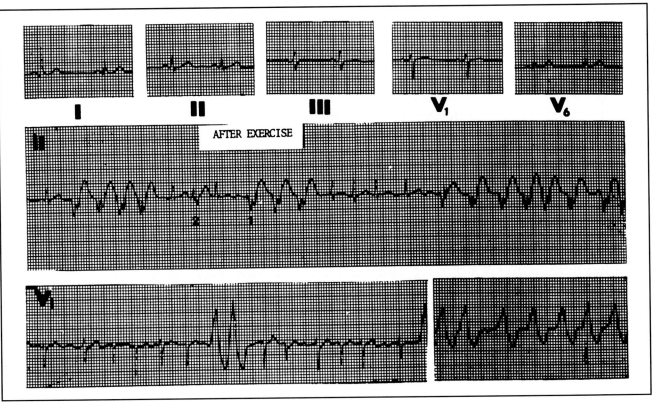

Figure 42A. The twelve lead ECG represented by I, II, III, V1 and V6 shows a short PR interval with a narrow QRS. After a treadmill test, leads II and V1 reveal atrial fibrillation with a narrow QRS ventricular response, as well as wide QRS beats with two morphologies in lead II, a "W" pattern (1) and an RS (2).

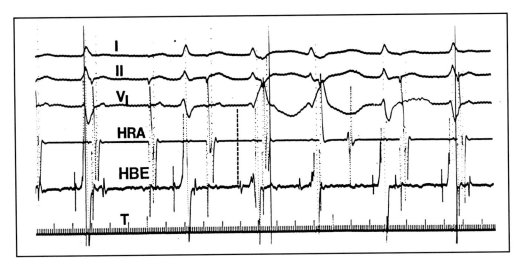

Figure 42B. Intracavitary tracings with atrial pacing show a pause due to AV nodal Wenckebach followed by a normal QRS, and then wide QRS which is triphasic RSR1 in V1 and which is preceded by His bundle deflection with an HV as long or longer than the normal QRS. These beats are like beat 2 and represent functional right bundle branch block with block of the left anterior superior fascicle.

ing the local amplitude of atrial, His, and ventricular deflections.

Energy delivery is typically made in sinus rhythm for either slow or fast pathway ablations to ensure that continued anterograde conduction is maintained. During fast pathway ablation, one anticipates approximately a 50% increase in the AH interval and loss of retrograde fast pathway conduction. For slow pathway modifications, slow pathway potentials are sought, but are not critical

to the performance of a successful ablation. If the patient has atypical AVNRT, observations of retrograde atrial activation during atypical AVNRT are invaluable in determining the atrial exit from the slow pathway.

Initially, incidence of complete heart block was reported to be between 2% and 8%. With further refinement of the procedure and a better understanding of appropriate endpoints to ablation, the incidence is now between 1% and 3%. With more

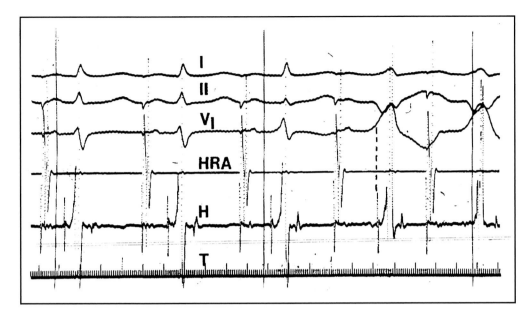

Figure 42C. Intracavitary tracings with atrial pacing. As the PR interval prolongs in Wenckebach of the AV node, HV interval becomes short, then reverses (dotted line), then fails to conduct to the His bundle. The last two beats are fully preexcited, however, with a morphology in lead II similar to beat 1 on the post exercise tracing. Thus, all wide beats on the exercise tracings were supraventricular, due either to preexcitation or functional bundle branch block (B).

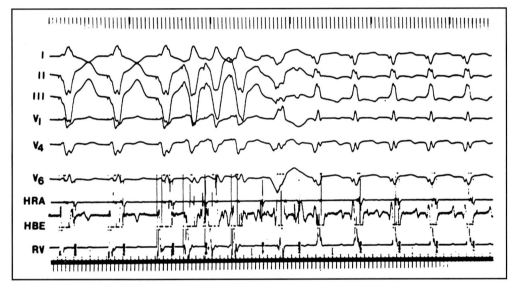

Figure 43. Typical S1-S1 drive, with S2,S3 and S4 prematurely paced beats, initiates a sustained monomorphic ventricular tachycardia. Drugs which prevent this tachycardia from being induced predict efficacy.

prudent energy deliveries, there does not appear to be a difference in the incidence of complete heart block for slow pathway versus fast pathway modification. However, there does remain the theoretic possibility of leaving the patient with a first degree block following fast pathway ablation. Therefore, it is our practice to attempt slow pathway ablation unless the refractory period of the fast pathway is inadequate for the patient's physical needs. We revert to fast pathway ablation under that circumstance or if a slow pathway modification can't be performed.

• **Accessory Pathway Ablation:** Typical anatomic locations of accessory pathways are along the tricuspid or mitral annuli, with a preponderance of left-sided pathways. For left-sided pathways, techniques for catheter manipulation include retrograde ablation on the ventricular side of the annulus, and transseptal approach with placement of the

ablation catheter above the mitral annulus. Similarly, right-sided pathways can be approached primarily from above or below the tricuspid annulus. A small percentage of pathways are accessible only from within the coronary sinus. Since early reports, where fairly modest success rates were achieved, accessory pathway ablation is now performed with an expected success rate of greater than 90%. Recurrence rate for accessory pathways is between 6% and 12% and varies with anatomic location.

In our laboratory, mapping for accessory pathway localization is performed both in an anterograde and retrograde fashion; it is our approach to ablate all accessory pathways at the atrial insertion point. We routinely systemically anticoagulate during ablation of left-sided pathways after transseptal access has been achieved. The activated clotting time is followed and maintained at around 220 seconds. Selective patients are anticoagulated for right-sided ablations. Complications of radiofrequency ablation of accessory pathways are reported in around 4% of patients. Complications vary with the approach utilized.

• **Atrial Tachycardia:** At this time, several other arrhythmias are manageable by catheter ablation. Specifically, atrial tachycardia has been demonstrated in our laboratory and by others to be amenable to catheter ablation; our particular technique for mapping involves determination of a paced activation sequence. Occasionally, rather dramatic improvement in ventricular function is observed following successful intervention in persistent ectopic tachycardias. While this is more true in a pediatric population, it has been our experience to see dramatic improvements even in the adult population.

• **Atrial Fibrillation:** Distinct clinical improvement following catheter ablation of the AV node for chronic drug refractory or intolerant patients with atrial fibrillation is often seen. Early experience with AV node ablation using radiofrequency energy was characterized by only modest success rates of around 50%-60%. Again owing to improved technology, the success rate for AV node ablation now approaches 100%. Complete interruption of AV node conduction mandated permanent pacer implantation. To avoid this, experimental work is being done by several investigators in attempting AV node modification for rate control in atrial fibrillation. Attempts at direct catheter ablation of atrial fibrillation are being made, but are experimental at this point. These efforts simulate barriers to atrial fibrillation seen in the Maze surgical procedure devised by James Cox.

• **Atrial Flutter:** Recently, the results with atrial flutter ablation have been encouraging. Once again, for the performance of ablation in atrial flutter, mapping is valuable. There is debate as to the appropriate target in atrial flutter; however, the region surrounding the area of slow conduction in or near the triangle of Koch, bordered by the tricuspid valve and the inferior vena cava, appears to be a site where high success rates can be achieved.

• **Ventricular Tachycardia:** Management of ventricular arrhythmias by radiofrequency catheter ablation is somewhat limited, owing to the small size of lesion created by the radiofrequency energy application. However, for certain forms of monomorphic non-ischemic ventricular tachycardia, success rates are quite acceptable. Other forms of ventricular tachycardia can be ablated or markedly modified. This was first demonstrated with D.C. ablation, but also is true of well-mapped tachycardias using radiofrequency generators.

Patients with incessant tachycardia unresponsive to therapeutic pharmacological techniques should be strongly considered for ablation.

In summary, at this time, radiofrequency catheter ablation is considered to be by many the procedure of choice for symptomatic patients with WPW syndrome. It is our practice to recommend that patients with AV node reentry undergo at least some attempt at medical management prior to committing to performance of AV node modification, this owing to the real, albeit low, risk of development of complete heart block. Referral for ablation of other patient populations typically occurs after multiple drug failures.

In these patients, dramatic improvement in the quality of life can be expected. The future direction of ablation will involve the development of alternate energy sources, alternate catheter types and further refinements of our current technologies. The success of ablative therapeutic techniques is the latest addition to the techniques available in the electrophysiological laboratory. The principles developed in the past continue to be available to elucidate the diagnosis and direct therapy for the patient with arrhythmia. Many of these principles are of major help to the clinician interpreting clinical tracings. Careful interpretation and bedside maneuvers should limit the need for the invasive laboratory but also are the foundation for an efficient informative electrophysiological procedure.

Selected Reading

1. ACC-AHA Task Force Report: Guidelines for clinical intracardiac electrophysiological and catheter ablation procedures. *JACC* 1995; 26:555-573; *Circ* 1995; 92:673-691.
2. Aronson AL: Evaluation of surface EKG findings as prodromata of type II complete heart block. *Circ* 48:122, 1973.
3. Borggrefe M, Budde T, Martinez-Rubio A, et al: Radiofrequency catheter ablation for drug-refractory supraventricular tachycardia. (Abstract) *Circ* 1988; 78:II-305.
4. Breithardt G, Seipel L, Loogen F: Sinus node recovery time and calculated sinoatrial conduction time in normal subjects and patients with sinus node dysfunction. *Circ* 56:43-50, 1977.
5. Calkins H: Radiofrequency catheter ablation of accessory pathways: Is the efficacy and difficulty of the procedure related to accessory pathway location. *JACC* 1991; 19:270A.
6. Calkins H, Sousa J, El-Atassi R, et al: Diagnosis and cure of the Wolff-Parkinson-White Syndrome or paroxysmal supraventricular tachycardias during a single electrophysiologic test. *Ibid*:1612-1618.
7. Cohen A, Fletcher RD, Wish M, Miller F, Cohen R, DelNegro A: "Non-invasive electrophysiology using standard permanent pacemakers in patients with spontaneous ventricular tachycardia or fibrillation." *AJC* 59:564-567, 1987.
8. Damato AN, Lau SH, Helfant RH: Study of atrioventricular conduction in man using electrode catheter recordings of His bundle activity. *Circ* 39:287-296, 1969.
9. Damato AN, Lav SH, Helfant RH et al: Study of the atrioventricular conduction in man using electrode catheter

recordings of His bundle activity. *Circ* 39: 287-296, 1969.

10. Dhingra RC, Amat-y-Leon F, Wyndham C et al: Clinical significance of prolonged sinoatrial conduction time. *Circ* 55:8-14, 1977.

11. Dhingra RC, Deves P, WU D et al: Syncope in patients with chronic bifascicular block. *Ann Int Med* 81:302, 1974.

12. Dhingra RC, Deves P, Wu D et al: Prospective observations in patients with chronic bundle branch block and marked H-V prolongation. *Circ* 53:600, 1976.

13. Dhingra RC, Rosen KM, Rahimtoola SH: Normal conduction intervals and responses in sixty-one patients using His bundle recording and atrial pacing. *Chest*, 64:55, 1973

14. Durrer D, VanDam R, Freud GE et al: Total excitation of the isolated human heart. *Circ* 41:899-912, 1970.

15. Feld GK, Fleck RP, Chen PS, et al: Radiofrequency catheter ablation for the treatment of human type I atrial flutter. Identification of a critical zone in the reentrant circuit by endocardial mapping techniques. *Circ* 1992; 86(4):1233-1240.

16. Fletcher RD, Cohen A, Del Negro A: *Noninvasive Electrophysiological Studies Using Implanted Pacemakers in Modern Cardiac Pacing*, ed. S. Serge Barold, MD. Mount Kisco NY: Futura Publishing Co., 1985.

17. Gallagher JJ, Damato AN: *Cardiac Catheterization and Angiography,* p 220. Philadelphia: Lea and Gebiger, 1974.

18. Gallagher JJ, Gilbert M, Svenson RH et al: Wolff-Parkinson-White Syndrome. *Circ* 51:767, 1975.

19. Goldreyer BN, Kahl FR, Manchester JH et al: Analysis of the HV interval-conduction velocity within the human bundle of His. *Circ* 48:170, 1973.

20. Haines DE, Watson DD, Verow AF: Electrode radius predicts lesion radius during radiofrequency energy heating. Validation of a proposed thermodynamic model. *Circ Res* 1990; 67:124-129.

21. Haines DE: Determinants of lesion size during radiofrequency catheter ablation: the role of electrode-tissue contact pressure and duration of energy delivery. *J. Cardiovasc Electrophys* 1991; 2:509-51.

22. Haissaguerre M: Elimination of atrioventricular nodal reentrant tachycardia using discrete slow potentials to guide application of radiofrequency energy. *Circ* 1992; 85:2162.

23. Huang SKS, Bharati S, Graham AR, et al: Chronic incomplete atrioventricular block induced by radiofrequency catheter ablation. *Circ* 1989; 80:951-961.

24. Josephson ME, Caracta AR, Ricciutti MA et al: Electrophysiologic properties of procainamide. *AJC* 33: 596, 1974.

25. Kuck KH, Schluter M, Geiger M, et al: Radiofrequency current catheter ablation of accessory atrioventricular pathways. *Lancet* 1991; 337:1557-1561.

26. Langberg JJ, Calkins H, Kim YN, et al: Recurrence of conduction in accessory atrioventricular connections after initially successful radiofrequency catheter ablation. *JACC* 1992; 19:1588-1592.

27. Langberg JJ, Chin MC, Rosenqvist M, et al: Catheter ablation of the atrioventricular junction with radiofrequency energy. *Circ* 1989; 80:1527-1535.

28. Lee MA, Morady F, Kadish, A, et al: Catheter modification of the atrioventricular junction with radiofrequency energy for control of atrioventricular nodal reentry tachycardia. *Circ* 1991; 83:827-835.

29. Lee ICI, Wellens HJ, Schurlenburg RM et al: Mechanism and significance of widened QRS complexes during complete atrioventricular block in acute inferior myocardial infarction. *Circ* 47:765-775, 1974.

30. Lesh MD, Van Hare GF, Schamp DJ, et al: Curative percutaneous catheter ablation using radiofrequency energy for accessory pathways in all locations: results in 100 consecutive patients. *JACC* 1992; 19:1303-1309.

31. Lopez-Merino V, Sanchis J, Chorro FJ, et al: Induction of partial alterations in atrioventricular conduction in dogs by percutaneous emission of high-frequency currents. *Am Heart J* 1988; 115:1214-1221.

32. Mandel, WJ, Hayakawa H, Allen HN et al: Assessment of sinus node function in patients with sick sinus syndrome. *Circ* 46:761, 1972.

33. Marcus FI, Blouin LT, Wharton K, et al: Electrophysiological and pathological assessment of chronic first degree atrioventricular block caused by closed-chest catheter ablation with radiofrequency energy in dogs. (Abstract) *JACC* 1987; 9(2):95A.

34. Myerburg RJ, Nilsson K, Castellanos AJ et al: *Cardiac Arrhythmias.* New York: Grune and Stratton, 1973.

35. Narula OS: *His Bundle Electrocardiography and Clinical Electrophysiology,* p. 86. Philadelphia: F. A. Davis Co., 1975.

36. Narula OS: Retrograde pre-excitation. Comparison of antegrade and retrograde conduction intervals in man. *Circ* 50:1129, 1974.

37. Narula OS, Cohen LS, Samet P et al: Localization of A-V conduction defects in man by recordings of the His bundle electrogram. *AJC* 25: 228-237, 1970.

38. Narula OS, Samet P, Javier RP: Significance of the sinus node recovery time. *Circ* 45:140, 1972.

39. Rios J C, Sarin R K, Pooya M et al: The various patterns of aberrant intraventricular conduction in induced premature atrial beats. *AJC* 23:134, 1969.

40. Rosenbaum MB, Elizari MV, Lazzari JO: *Los Hemibloqueros.* Buenos Aires, Pardos, 1968.

41. Scheinman MM, Morady F, Hess DS, et al: Catheter-induced ablation of the atrioventricular junction to control refractory supraventricular arrhythmias. *JAMA* 1982; 248:851-856.

42. Scheinman MM, Peters RW, Modin G et al: Value of intranodal conduction time in patients with chronic bundle branch block. *Circ* 56:240, 1977.

43. Scherlag BJ, Lau SH, Helfant RH, et al: Catheter technique for recording His bundle activity in man. *Circ* 39:13, 1969.

44. Schiulenburg RM, Durrer D: The value of unipolar His bundle recording. *Circ* 52:11-136, 1975.

45. Sellers TD, Campbell RWF, Bashore TM et al: Effects of procainamide and quinidine sulfate in the Wolff-Parkinson-White syndrome. *Circ* 55:15, 1977.

46. Sokolow M and Perloff DB: The clinical pharmacology and use of quinidine in heart disease. *Prog Cardiovasc Dis* 3:316, 1961.

47. Strauss HC, Saroff AL, Bigger JT Jr et al: Premature atrial stimulation as a key to understanding of sinoatrial conduction in man. Presentation of data and critical review of the literature. *Circ* 47: 86, 1973.

48. Swartz J, Tracy C, Fletcher R, et al: A comparative study of direct current and radiofrequency atrial endocardial ablation of accessory pathways. (Abstract) *JACC* 1991; 17:109A.

49. Swisdale N, Wang X, Bekeman K, et al: Factors associated with recurrence of accessory pathway conduction after radiofrequency catheter ablation. *PACE* 1991; 14:2042-2048.

50. Tracy CM, Swartz JF, Fletcher RD, et al: Radiofrequency catheter ablation of ectopic atrial tachycardia using paced activation sequence mapping. *JACC* 1993; 21(4):910-917.

51. Vera Z, Mason DT, Fletcher RD et al: Prolonged His-Q interval in chronic bifasicular block. Relation to impending complete heart block. *Circ* 53:46, 1976.

52. Wellens H J, Schulenburg, R N, Durrer D: Electrical stimulation of the heart in patients with ventricular tachycardia. *Circ* 46:216-226, 1972

53. Wit AL, Weiss MB, Berkowitz WK et al: Patterns of atrioventricular conduction in the human heart. *Circ* 27:345, 1970.

PART II

NORMAL AND ABNORMAL STRUCTURE AND CIRCULATORY FUNCTION

CHAPTER 22

Clinical Anatomy
of the Heart

Bruce F. Waller, M.D.

The heart is situated in the middle mediastinum with its "long-axis" oriented from the left upper abdominal quadrant to the right shoulder. The heart has a base formed by the atria and great arteries and an apex which is formed by the junction of the ventricles and ventricular septum. The sternum and costal cartilages of the third, fourth and fifth ribs overlie the heart anteriorly; about two-thirds of the heart is left of the midline. The heart rests upon the diaphragm and is tilted forward and to the left so that the apex is anterior to the rest of the heart. The normal apex impulse can be palpated in the fourth or fifth intercostal space near the midclavicular line.

The weight and size of the heart vary considerably depending on age, sex, body length, epicardial fat and general nutrition. The average human adult heart weighs approximately 325 ± 75 gm in men and 275 ± 75 gm in women. The borders of the normal cardiac silhouette in a frontal view are formed by the following structures: the top of the cardiac silhouette is formed by the transverse and ascending aorta. The upper right margin is delineated by the superior vena cava. The right atrium provides the remaining right lateral cardiac border. Most of the inferior border is composed of right ventricle. The apex and the lower left lateral cardiac border consist of the left ventricle. The left atrial appendage perches atop the left ventricle and to the side of the pulmonary artery, interjecting on the cardiac border between the left ventricle and pulmonary outflow tract. The pulmonary outflow area forms the rest of the upper left border.

External Features

The atria are separated from the ventricles externally by the coronary sulcus (atrioventricular sulcus), which circles the heart between the atria and ventricles (Figure 1). The right coronary artery, after leaving the aorta, travels in this sulcus between the right atrium and right ventricle until it descends on the posterior surface of the heart. Similarly, the left circumflex artery is found in the coronary sulcus between the left atrium and left ventricle until the artery ramifies posteriorly. Externally, the two ventricles are delineated by interventricular sulci, which descend from the coronary sulcus toward the apex; epicardial fat often obscures these landmarks (Figure 1). The anterior interventricular sulcus contains the left anterior descending coronary artery and courses over the muscular ventricular septum between the right and left ventricles to the apex. It then turns around the apex and continues in the posterior interventricular sulcus on the diaphragmatic surface of the heart. The posterior interventricular sulcus is the pathway for the posterior descending coronary artery, which is usually the terminal branch of the right coronary artery or, less frequently, of the left circumflex artery (Figure 1). The two atria may be delineated externally by a groove on the posterior surface between the right pulmonary veins and the venae cavae. The crux of the heart refers to the area on the posterior-basal surface where the coronary sulcus meets the posterior interventricular sulcus (Figure 1). Internally at this junction, the atrial septum joins the ventricular septum. The coronary artery that crosses this area makes a sharp inward turn at the crux and provides a small artery to the nearby atrioventricular node. The area of the heart below the crux is referred to as the diaphragmatic, or inferior, surface of the heart. A transverse section through the heart is extremely

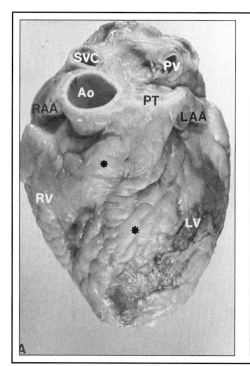

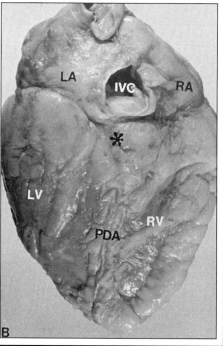

Figure 1. External views of the heart. (A) Anterior surface showing epicardial fat* which obscures the interventricular sulci containing the left anterior descending artery. Ao = aorta; LAA = left atrial appendage; LV = left ventricle; PT = pulmonary trunk; PV = pulmonary vein; RAA = right atrial appendage; RV = right ventricle; SVC = superior vena cava. (B) Posterior surface of heart showing location of posterior descending artery (PDA), crux of the heart (*), and inferior vena cava (IVC). LA = left atrium; RA = right atrium. *(From Waller and Schlant, 38)*

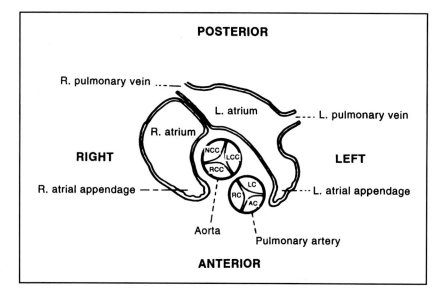

Figure 2. Schematic transverse section through the heart at approximately the level of the second intercostal space. The relation between the left and right atria and the interatrial septum is illustrated. The relative positions of the aortic and pulmonary valves and their cusps are shown. AC = anterior cusp; RC = right cusp; LC = left cusp of the pulmonary valve; LCC = left coronary cusp; RCC = right coronary cusp; NCC = noncoronary cusp of the aortic valve. *(From Waller and Schlant, 38)*

helpful in demonstrating the relations of the cardiac chambers (Figures 2, 3, 4).

The ventricular and atrial septa are aligned obliquely 45° to the left of the midline with the planes of the septa directed approximately from right scapula to left nipple. The entire right side of the heart is to the right of this plane, placing most of the right atrium anterior to the left atrium and most of the right ventricle anterior to the left ventricle.

Fibrous Skeleton

A fibrous tissue framework affords a firm anchor for the attachments of the atrial and ventricular musculature as well as the valvular tissue (Figures 5, 6). At the center of the heart the central fibrous body (right fibrous trigone) fuses together the medial aspect of the mitral and tricuspid valve and the aortic roots. The left fibrous trigone is formed by compact bundles of connective tissue that course from the central fibrous body to the left, posterior inferiorly and anteriorly. Continuations of fibroelastic tissue from the central fibrous body (right fibrous trigone) and the left fibrous trigone partially encircle the mitral and tricuspid valves. These rings of tissue are the mitral and tricuspid annuli, which serve as attachments for the mitral and tricuspid valves as well as for the atrial and

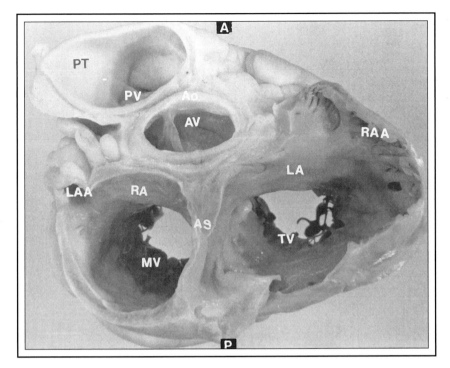

Figure 3. Transverse section through base of heart showing relationship of various chambers and great vessels. A = anterior; Ao = aorta; AS = atrial septum; AV = aortic valve; LA = left atrium; LAA = left atrial appendage; MV = mitral valve; RA = right atrium, RAA = right atrial appendage; P = posterior; PT = pulmonary trunk; PV = pulmonic valve; TV = tricuspid valve. *(From Waller and Schlant, 38)*

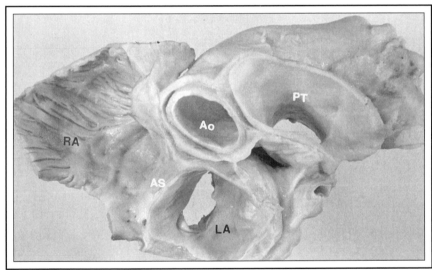

Figure 4. Basal view of heart showing relationship of great vessels and atria. The left atrium (LA) has a smooth endocardium while the right atrium (RA) is trabeculated. The aorta (Ao) is posterior to the pulmonary trunk (PT) but anterior to the atrial septum (AS). *(From Waller and Schlant, 38)*

ventricular muscle. In general, the fibrous skeleton is less well-developed around the tricuspid valve. A triple scalloped line of heavy collagenous tissue extends anteriorly from the left and right fibrous trigones to provide a three-pointed crown-like skeletal support for the aortic root and cusps. A substantial ligament of tissue, the conus ligament, passes from the right side of the aortic root to a similar arrangement of scalloped tissue that surrounds the pulmonic root.

An important extension of the fibrous skeleton, the membranous ventricular septum, extends inferiorly and anteriorly from the central fibrous body (right fibrous trigone). This membranous septum is located at the summit of the muscular ventricular septum, where it provides support for the right coronary and noncoronary aortic cusps (Figure 1). A portion of the membranous ventricular septum extends slightly above the tricuspid valve, forming a small portion of the medial wall of the right atrium. The bundle of His penetrates the central fibrous body and travels along the inferior margin of the membranous portion of the ventricular septum. At the crest of the muscular septum, about the level of junction of the right coronary and posterior (noncoronary) aortic cusps, the His bundle separates into a left bundle branch and a right bundle branch. The left bundle subsequently subdivides into multiple branches that fan out as they spread to the left ventricle.

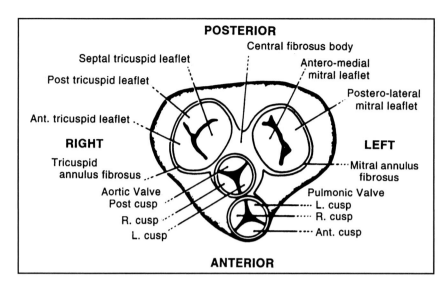

Figure 5. Schematic anterosuperior view of the heart with the atria removed. The components of the fibrous skeleton and the orientation of the leaflets of each valve are shown. *(From Waller and Schlant, 38)*

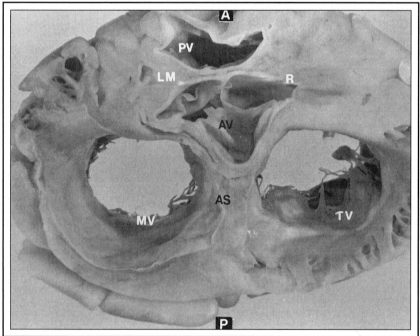

Figure 6. Cross-sectional view of heart showing aortic valve (AV), pulmonary trunk (PT), origin of the right (R) and left main (LM) coronary arteries, tricuspid (TV) and mitral (MV) valves, and the atrial septum (AS). A = anterior; P = posterior. *(From Waller and Schlant, 38)*

Cardiac Chambers

Right Atrium

Venous blood returns to the heart via the superior and inferior venae cavae into the right atrium, where it is stored during right ventricular systole. During ventricular diastole, blood flows from the right atrium into the right ventricle (Figures 1,3,6,8-10). The right atrium forms the right lateral cardiac border and is above, behind, and to the right of the right ventricle (Figures 3,6). Most of the right atrium is to the right and anterior to the left atrium (Figures 3,6). Anteromedially, the right atrial appendage protrudes from the right atrium and overlaps the aortic root (Figure 1). On the posterior external surface of the right atrium a ridge,

the sulcus terminalis (or terminal groove), extends vertically from the superior to the inferior vena cava. This corresponds to an internal muscular bundle, the crista terminalis, which runs along the edge of the entrance to the right atrial appendage to the front of the orifice of the superior vena cava and then to the right side of the inferior vena cava (Figures 8 to 10). The sinus node is usually located at the lateral margin of the junction of the superior vena cava with the right atrium and the atrial appendage, beneath or near the sulcus terminalis (terminal groove; Figure 1). The inner surface of the posterior and medial (septal) walls of the right atrium is smooth, while the surfaces of the lateral wall and of the right atrial appendage are composed of parallel muscle bundles, the pectinate

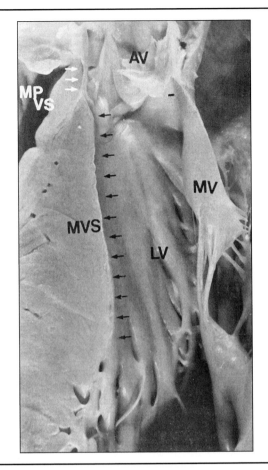

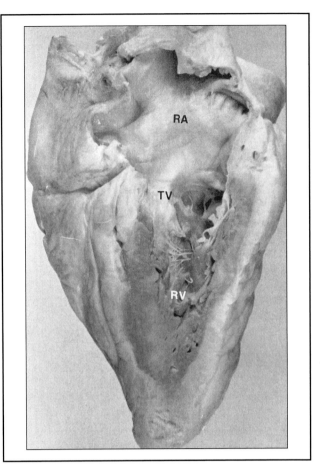

Figure 7. Specimen showing the muscular ventricular septum (MVS) (black arrows) and membranous portion of the ventricular septum (MPVS) (white arrows). LV = left ventricle; MV = mitral valve. *(From Waller and Schlant, 38)*

Figure 8. Long axis view of right side of heart showing right ventricle (RV), right atrium (RA), tricuspid valve (TV). The RV walls are heavily trabeculated. *(From Waller and Schlant, 38)*

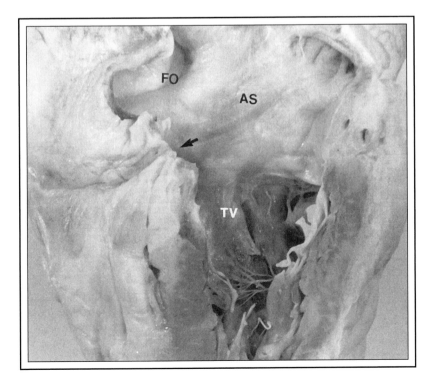

Figure 9. Closeup of right atrium showing atrial septum (AS), foramen ovale (FO), entrance to orifice of coronary sinus (arrow), and tricuspid valve (TV). *(From Waller and Schlant, 38)*

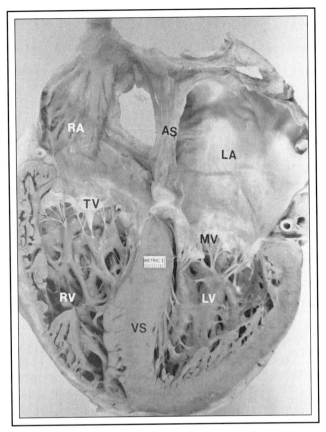

Figure 10. Four chamber view of heart showing morphologic differences between the 4 chambers. The right atrium (RA) is more trabeculated than the left (LA), and the right ventricle (RV) is more heavily and coarsely trabeculated compared to the left ventricle (LV). AS = atrial septum; MV = mitral valve; TV = tricuspid valve; VS = ventricular septum. *(From Waller and Schlant, 38)*

landmark during transseptal catheterization of the left side of the heart. The proximal right coronary artery is in the immediate vicinity as it enters the coronary sulcus. The proximity of the aortic root to the right atrium permits an aneurysm of the sinus of Valsalva to rupture into the right atrium. The atrial septum (Figures 2, 3, 6, 8-10) is found in the posteroinferior portion of the medial wall of the right atrium and extends obliquely forward from right to left. Near the center of the atrial septum there is a shallow depression, the fossa ovalis, which often has a prominent fold, or limbus, anteriorly. The ostium of the coronary sinus is located between the inferior vena cava and the tricuspid valve (Figures 8 to 10). The orifice of the coronary sinus is guarded by a rudimentary flap of tissue, the Thebesian valve. The atrioventricular (AV) node is anterior and medial to the coronary sinus, just above the septal leaflet of the tricuspid valve. The sinus and atrioventricular nodes, as well as the entire conducting pathways, are not grossly visible.

Right Ventricle

The right ventricle receives venous blood from the right atrium during ventricular diastole and propels blood into the pulmonary circulation during

muscles (Figures 8 to 10). The right atrial wall measures almost 2mm in thickness. The superior and inferior venae cavae enter the right atrium posteriorly and medially at its superior and inferior aspects.

The orifice of the superior vena cava usually has no valve; the orifice of the inferior vena cava is flanked anteriorly by an inconstant, rudimentary valve, the eustachian valve, formed by a crescentic fold. The caval orifices may vary in shape and diameter depending upon the phase of respiration, the cardiac cycle, and the contraction or relaxation of surrounding muscular bands. Variation in the orifice may play some role in promoting venous return or preventing atrial reflux.

The medial wall of the right atrium includes the atrial septum and is also important because of its proximity to several structures (Figures 6, 8-10). Anteriorly, the posterior (noncoronary) cusp and the right coronary cusp of the aortic root lean against the medial right atrium, forming a normal slight bulge known as the torus aorticus, which is a useful

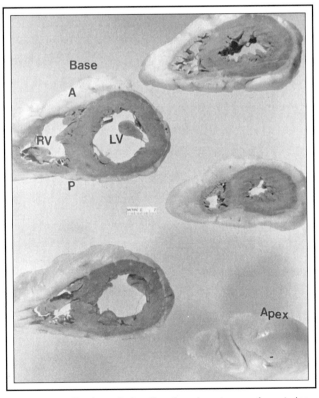

Figure 11. Family of ventricular slices from base to apex. A = anterior; LV = left ventricle; RV = right ventricle; P = posterior; VS = ventricular septum; The LV cavity is more "circular" shaped compared to the more "triangular" shaped RV cavity. *(From Waller and Schlant, 38)*

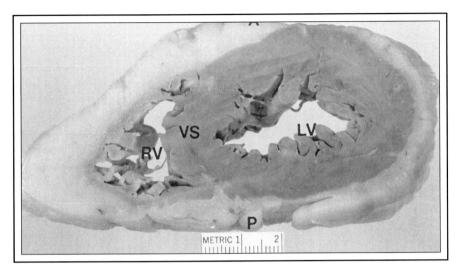

Figure 12. Closeup of ventricular slice seen in Figure 12. This view corresponds to the short-axis echocardiographic views of the ventricular cavities. A = anterior; LV = left ventricle; RV = right ventricle; VS = ventricular septum. *(From Waller and Schlant, 38)*

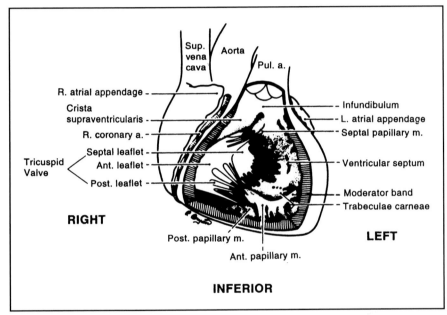

Figure 13. Schematic representation of a frontal view of the heart. The anterior right ventricular wall has been removed to demonstrate the orientation of the tricuspid leaflets and the papillary muscles. The anterior papillary muscle is sectioned. The trabeculated inflow portion of the right ventricle is contrasted with the smooth infundibular (outflow) area. *(From Waller and Schlant, 38)*

ventricular systole (Figures 8 to 13). The right ventricle is normally the most anterior cardiac chamber, lying directly beneath the sternum (Figure 11). Enlargement or hyperactivity of the right ventricle may often be detected by palpation of the sternum or the lower left sternal border. The right ventricle is partially below, in front of, and medial to the right atrium, but anterior and to the right of the left ventricle. Most of the entire inferior border of the frontal roentgenogram view of the heart consists of the right ventricle. The striking difference in configuration between the two ventricles is illustrated by a transverse section (Figures 11, 12). The left ventricular chamber is an ellipsoidal sphere surrounded by relatively thick (8mm to 15mm at autopsy) musculature, well suited to ejecting blood against the high resistance of the systemic vessels. The right ventricle, which normally contracts against very low resistance, has a crescent-shaped chamber and a thin outer wall, measuring 4mm to 5 mm in thickness. The anterior right ventricular wall curves over the ventricular septum, which normally bulges into the right ventricular cavity. Although the ventricular septum forms the medial wall of both ventricles, it seems to contribute predominantly to left ventricle function in normal subjects. The anterior and inferior walls of the right ventricular cavity are lined by muscle bundles, the trabeculae carneae, which often form ridges along the inner surface of the wall or cross from one wall to the other (Figures 8 to 13). A rather constant muscle, the moderator band, crosses from the lower ventricular septum to the anterior wall, where it joins the anterior papillary muscle (Figures 8 to 10). The right bundle branch, after traveling through the muscular ventricular septum, courses through the moderator muscle to the endocardium of the right ventricle.

Functionally, the right ventricle can be partitioned into an inflow tract, an outflow tract, and an apical trabecular component. The trabecular muscles in the apex of the right ventricle are much more coarse than those in the left ventricle. The inflow tract, consisting of the tricuspid valve and the trabecular muscles of the anterior and inferior walls, directs entering blood anteriorly, inferiorly, and to the left at an angle of 60° to the outflow tract (Figure 8). The smooth-walled outflow tract, also referred to as the infundibulum, forms the superior portion of the right ventricle. It is separated from the inflow tract by a thick muscle, the crista supraventricularis, which arches from the anterolateral wall over the anterior leaflet of the tricuspid valve to the septal (medial) wall, where it joins other constrictor bands of muscle that encircle the outflow tract (Figures 8 to 13). Blood entering the infundibulum is ejected superiorly and posteriorly into the pulmonary trunk.

Left Atrium

The left atrium receives blood from the pulmonary veins and serves as the reservoir during left ventricular systole, and as a conduit during left ventricular filling. In addition, left atrial contraction provides a significant increment of blood to the left ventricle, stretching the ventricle and priming it for ventricular ejection. This is sometimes referred to as the "atrial kick" or atrial component of ventricular filling. The left atrium is located superiorly, in the midline, and posterior to the other cardiac chambers (Figures 2, 3, 6, 10, 14). As a consequence of this posterior position, the left atrium is not normally seen in the frontal roentgenogram. The esophagus abuts directly upon its posterior surface, while the aortic root impinges upon its anterior wall. The right atrium is located to the right and anterior (Figure 2). The left ventricle is to the left, anterior, and inferior. The posterior position of the left atrium makes it impossible to palpate externally unless it is massively dilated. With severe mitral regurgitation, however, expansion of the left atrium from the regurgitation and the ejection recoil of the anteriorly located ventricles may force the heart anteriorly, producing a late systolic sternal lift. The left atrium usually enlarges posteriorly and laterally in mitral stenosis or regurgitation, occasionally even reaching the right or left lateral chest. The wall of the left atrium is 3mm, slightly thicker than that of the right atrium. Two pulmonary veins enter posterolaterally on each side, conveying oxygenated blood

from the lungs. Though there are no true valves at the junction of the pulmonary veins and the left atrium, sleeves of atrial muscle extend from the left atrial wall around the pulmonary veins for 1 or 2 cm and may exert a partial sphincter-like influence, tending to lessen reflux during atrial systole or mitral regurgitation (Figures 10, 14).

The endocardium of the left atrium is smooth and slightly opaque (Figures 10, 14). Pectinate muscles are present only in the left atrial appendage, which projects from the anterolateral left atrium, alongside the pulmonary artery. The atrial septum is smooth but may contain a central shallow area, corresponding to the fossa ovalis.

Left Ventricle

The left ventricle receives blood from the left atrium during ventricular diastole and ejects blood into the systemic arterial circulation during ventricular systole (Figures 10 to 12, 14). The left ventricle is roughly bullet-shaped with the blunt tip directed anteriorly, inferiorly, and to the left, where it contributes, with the lower ventricular septum, to the apex of the heart. Although the left ventricle forms the lower left lateral cardiac border in the frontal roentgenogram, the major portion of its

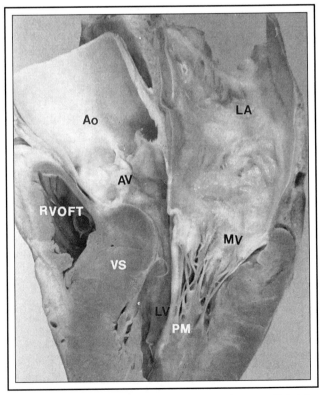

Figure 14. Long axis view of left side of heart showing aorta (Ao), left atrium (LA), left ventricle (LV), mitral valve (MV), papillary muscle (PM) of mitral valve, aortic valve (AV) and right ventricular outflow tract (RVOFT). *(From Waller and Schlant, 38)*

518

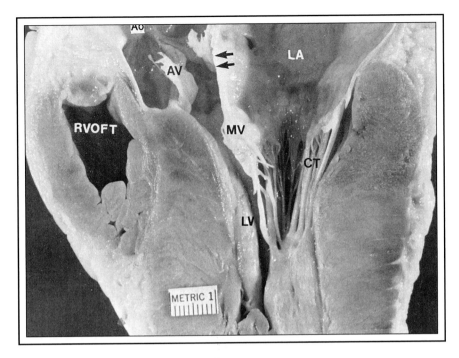

Figure 15. Long axis view of left ventricle showing continuity of aortic (AV) and mitral (MV) valves (arrows), and chordae tendineae (CT) of MV. Ao = aorta; LA = left atrium; LV = left ventricle; RVOFT = right ventricular outflow tract. *(From Waller and Schlant, 38)*

external surface is posterolateral. The left ventricle is posterior and to the left of the right ventricle and inferior, anterior, and to the left of the left atrium. The left ventricular chamber is approximately an ellipsoidal sphere, surrounded by thick muscular walls measuring 8 mm to 15 mm, or approximately two to three times the thickness of the right ventricular wall. The tip of the left ventricular apex is often thin, sometimes measuring 2 mm or less. The medial wall of the left ventricle is the ventricular septum, which is shared with the right ventricle (Figures 1, 10, 12, 14). The septum, which is roughly triangular in shape with the base of the triangle at the level of the aortic cusps, is entirely muscular except for the small membranous septum, located superiorly just below the right coronary and the posterior coronary cusps (Figures 7, 10, 14). The upper third of the septum is smooth endocardium. The remaining two-thirds of the septum and the remaining ventricular walls are ridged by interlacing muscles, the trabeculae carneae. The ventricular wall exclusive of the septum is often referred to as the free wall of the left ventricle.

The anteromedial leaflet of the mitral valve, which is the larger and more mobile of the two mitral leaflets, extends from the top of the posteromedial septum across the ventricular cavity to the anterolateral ventricular wall and separates the left ventricular cavity into an inflow and an outflow tract (Figures 14, 15). The funnel-shaped inflow tract, which is formed by the mitral annulus and by both mitral leaflets and their chordae tendineae,

directs the entering atrial blood inferiorly, anteriorly, and to the left (Figures 14,15). The outflow tract, surrounded by the inferior surface of the anteromedial mitral leaflet, the ventricular septum, and the left ventricular free wall, orients the blood flow from left ventricular apex to the right and superiorly at an angle of 90° to the inflow tract. With the onset of ventricular systole, both mitral leaflets are propelled together and upward, converting the entire left ventricle into an expulsion chamber. The apical portion of the left ventricle is characterized by fine trabeculations.

Cardiac Valves

The heart contains four cardiac valves: two semilunar and two atrioventricular. The two semilunar valves, aortic and pulmonic, guard the outlet orifice of their respective left and right ventricle. The two atrioventricular (AV) valves, mitral and tricuspid, guard the inlet orifice of their respective left and right ventricle. The four cardiac valves are surrounded by fibrous tissue forming partial or complete "rings" (valve annulus). These fibrous rings join to form the fibrous skeleton of the heart, to which also are attached atrial and ventricular myocardium. The area between the septal leaflet of the tricuspid valve, the anterior leaflet of the mitral valve, and the posterior or noncoronary cusp of the aortic valve forms one part of the central fibrous body. The remaining portion is made up of fibrous tissue connecting the left aortic cusp and the anterior leaflet of the mitral valve.

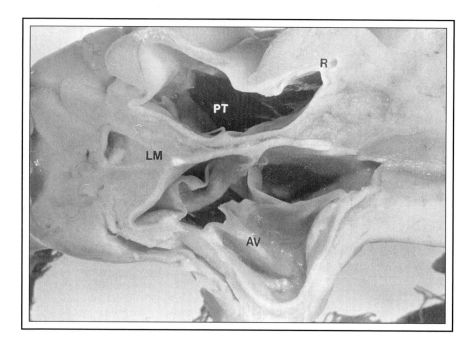

Figure 16. Short axis view of 3-cuspid aortic valve (AV) and pulmonary trunk (PT). L = left main coronary ostium; R = right coronary ostium. *(From Waller and Schlant, 38)*

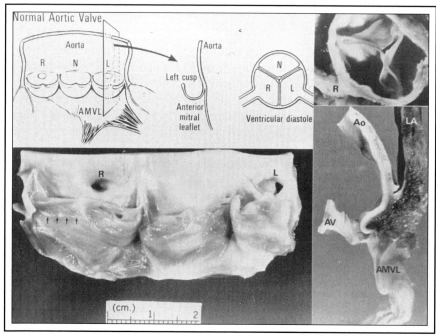

Figure 17. Morphology of the normal aortic valve. AMVL, anterior mitral valve leaflet; Ao = aorta; AV = aortic valve; LV = left main; N = noncoronary cusp; LA = left atrium; R = right; RC = right coronary artery. Arrows point to line of closure. Portion of aortic cusp above the line of closure is called the lunula. *(From Waller and Schlant, 38)*

Histologic Structure

Each cardiac valve has a central collagenous core, the fibrosa, which is continuous with the collagen of the cardiac skeleton and of the chordae tendineae. Both sides of the fibrosa are covered by loose fibroelastic tissue, usually containing mucopolysaccharides, and the entire valve is covered by endothelium. The endothelium and connective tissue of the AV valves are continuous with atrial and ventricular endocardium, and of the semilunar valves, with the aortic and pulmonary intima. Gross and Kugel have proposed that the loose connective tissue on the atrial aspect of the AV valves be termed the atrialis, on the ventricular surface of all four valves the ventricularis, and on the aortic or pulmonary side of the semilunar valves the arterialis. Smooth and striated cardiac muscle may extend onto the proximal one third of the atrialis in the AV valves and often contains blood vessels. The distal two thirds of the normal AV valve and all the semilunar valve is avascular.

Semilunar Valves

The semilunar aortic and pulmonary valves are similar in configuration, except the aortic cusps are slightly thicker. They are situated at the summit of

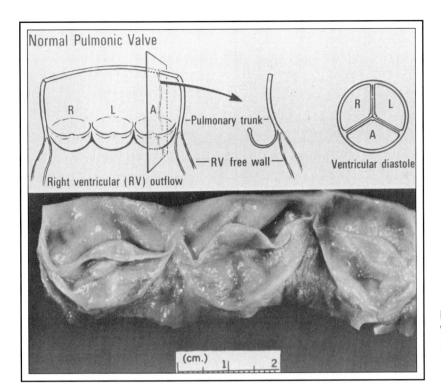

Figure 18. Morphology of the normal pulmonic valve. A = anterior; L = left; R = right. *(From Waller and Schlant, 38)*

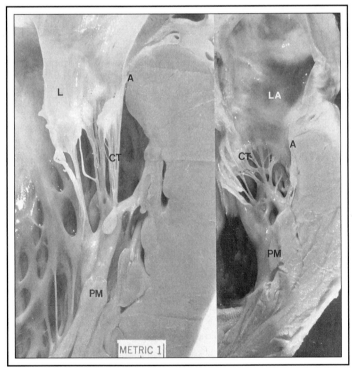

Figure 19. Mitral valve apparatus. (Left): chordae tendineae (CT); leaflet (L); annulus (A); papillary muscle (PM); (Right): left atrium (LA). Note the interchordal connections (arrows) and chordal connections from both anterior and posterior mitral leaflets to the posteromedial papillary muscle (right). *(From Waller and Schlant, 38)*

the outflow tract of their corresponding ventricle, the pulmonary valve being anterior, superior, and slightly to the left of the aortic valve (Figures 3, 5 to 7, 13 to 18). Each valve is composed of the three fibrous cusps. The pulmonary valve differs from the aortic valve by having no annulus or discrete fibrous ring. The U-shaped convex lower edges of each cusp are attached to and suspended from the root of the aorta or pulmonary artery, with the upper free valve edges projecting into the lumen. The cusps, which are often slightly unequal in width, circle the inside of the vessel root. Each semilunar valve consists of three equal-sized or nearly equal-sized semicircular cusps. Each cusp is attached by its semicircular border to the wall of the aorta or pulmonary trunk. The small space

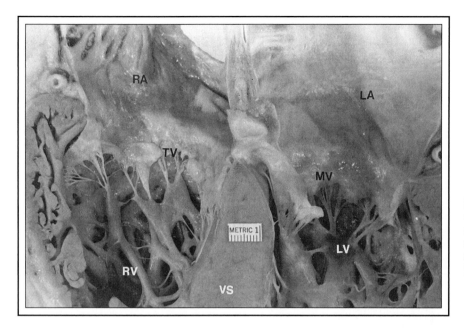

Figure 20. Four chamber view showing mitral (MV) and tricuspid (TV) valves. The annulus of the tricuspid valve is more spiral than the annulus of the mitral valve (MV). LA = left atrium; LV = left ventricle; RA = right atrium; RV = right ventricle; VS = ventricular septum. *(From Waller and Schlant, 38)*

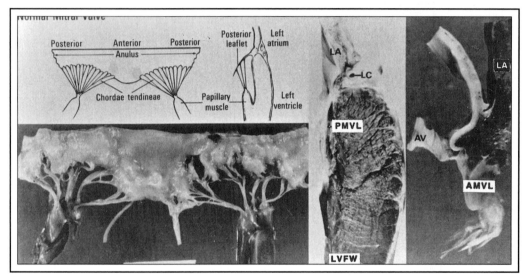

Figure 21. Morphology of the normal mitral valve. AMVL = anterior mitral valve leaflet; Ao = aorta; AV = aortic valve; LA = left atrium; LC = left circumflex coronary artery; LVFW = left ventricular free wall; PL = posterior leaflet. *(From Waller and Schlant, 38)*

between attachments of adjacent cusps is called a commissure.

Each semilunar valve has three commissures. The three commissures lie equally spaced around the aorta or pulmonary trunk, and the circumference connecting these points has been termed the sinotubular junction which is described as the portion of the great vessel separating the sinuses of Valsalva from the adjacent tubular portion of the great artery. In the aorta a distinctive circumferential "hump" or line marks this junction, originally described by Leonardo da Vinci as the "supra-aortic ridge." Each of the ventricular surfaces of the semilunar cusps has a small nodule (much more prominent on the aortic valve [noduli Arantii]) in the center of the free edge marking the contact sites of closure (Figures 17, 18). Behind each cusp the ves-

sel wall bulges outward, forming a pouch-like dilatation known as the sinus of Valsalva. The free edge of each cusp is concave, with a nodular interruption at the center of the cusp, the nodulus Arantii. The portion of the cusp adjacent to the rim is not as thick and may normally contain small perforations. During ventricular systole, the cusps are passively thrust upward away from the center of the aortic lumen. During ventricular diastole, the cusps fall passively into the lumen of the vessel as they support the column of blood above. The noduli Arantii meet in the center and contribute to the support of the leaflets. The geometry of the cusps and the strong fibrous tissue support provide excellent approximations of the leaflets and prevent regurgitation of blood. The anatomy of the two AV valves is considerably more complex than the

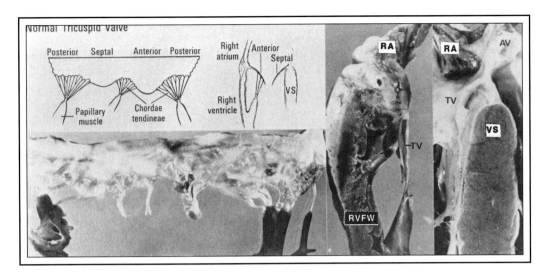

Figure 22. Morphology of the normal tricuspid valve. AV = aortic valve; RA = right atrium; RV = right ventricular free wall; TV = tricuspid valve; VS = ventricular septum. *(From Waller and Schlant, 38)*

anatomy of the semilunar valves (Figures 5, 6, 8, 10, 14, 19 to 22). Both AV valves consist of leaflets (two mitral and three tricuspid), chordae tendineae, papillary muscles (two or three, respectively), and valve annuli. The leaflets are demarcated by commissures located along the valve annular attachment. The anterior leaflet of each of the AV valves is the largest and is roughly semicircular in shape. The posterior mitral leaflet and the posterior and septal tricuspid leaflets have shorter annulus to free edge distances but longer basal attachments, compared to the respective anterior leaflet. Complex chordal structures arise from papillary muscles or directly from ventricular myocardium and insert onto the free edge and several millimeters from the margin on the ventricular surface. The annular structure of the mitral valve primarily surrounds the posterior leaflet, while the anterior leaflet does not have a true annulus but is continuous with the wall of ascending aorta, aortic valve, and membranous ventricular septum. The annulus of the tricuspid is nearly circumferential, is larger than the mitral annulus, and lies at a lower level (more apical) than the mitral annulus. On the atrial surface of the AV valves, 0.5cm to 1 cm from the free edge, is a line of nodular thickening (more prominent on the mitral valve), marking the contact points of closure.

Specific Valve Structure

• Aortic Valve

General: The normal tricuspid aortic valve (Figures 16, 17) is a symmetric structure in which the orifice of the fully opened valve is central and the cusps are easily mobile and retract to the aortic commissures. When the valve is closed, all three cusps meet and overlap equally. The circumferen-

tial distances between each of the three commissures and the depth of the aortic valve sinus (from sinotubular junction to base of sinus) in a normally formed valve are similar (Figure 17). Each of the ventricular surfaces of the aortic cusps has a small nodule in the center of the free edge which marks the closure contact site. A small rim of valve tissue above this nodule, known as the lunula, overlaps the neighboring cusp and serves as a supporting strut. Fenestrations of the lunula are quite common but are of no functional consequence. Fenestrations of the aortic valve lunula increase with age. The sinotubular junction, the aortic sinuses of Valsalva, the valve cusps and commissures, and the junction of aortic valve with the ventricular septum and anterior mitral valve leaflet make up the aortic valve complex. The narrowest circumference is at the lowermost portion of this complex at the junction with the ventricular septum. This circumference (diameter), referred to as the aortic ring, is measured by surgeons to determine the size of an aortic prosthetic valve. Pathologists at necropsy, on the other hand, measure the circumference (8 cm to 10 cm) at the sinotubular junction, which more closely corresponds to the measurements made by the echocardiographers during life.

The three aortic valve cusps have been termed the left, right, and noncoronary (posterior) cusps, with each of the left and right sinuses of Valsalva giving rise to the left and right main epicardial coronary artery, respectively. Knowledge of the adjacent anatomical structures or chambers of the aortic valve is important in determining potential sites of left-to-right shunting. Rupture of the right and noncoronary sinuses of Valsalva may communicate with right-sided chambers (right ventricular outflow tract, right atrium), while rupture of the left sinus of Valsalva generally communicates with left-sided chambers (left atrium or left ventricular outflow tract). Portions of the left and noncoronary cusp are continuous with the anterior leaflet of mitral valve.

Anatomical Variation: The normal tricuspid aortic valve is a symmetric structure composed of three equal-sized cusps. Detailed measurements of commissural diameters and cuspal depth show that some tricuspid aortic valves have marked variation in these measurements. The circumference between one set of commissures may be longer or shorter than in the remaining two sets of commissures, one sinus of Valsalva may be deeper or shallower than the remaining two sinuses, or the combination of these variables may occur in the same aortic valve. These variations in cusp size result in asymmetric lines of closure and may result in accelerated 'wear and tear' (aging) of the valve structure. These congenitally malformed tricuspid valves may be the basis for some of the isolated aortic valve stenoses seen in patients over age 65.

Age-Related Changes: The normal cuspal markings become more prominent with age. The central cuspal nodules thicken and enlarge and the bases of the sinuses of Valsalva typically contain calcific deposits. The body of the aortic valve cusps also thickens, while the cusp lunula often thins and develops fenestrations. Commissures characteristically remain open with normal aging changes and the sinuses of Valsalva dilate with increasing age.

• **Pulmonic Valve**

General: Like the aortic valve, the normal tricuspid aortic valve is a symmetric structure (Figures 6, 18) in which the orifice of the fully opened valve is central and the cusps are easily mobile and retract to the pulmonary trunk attachments. The circumferential distances between each of the three commissures and the depth of the pulmonary valve sinus in a normally formed valve are similar. With the exception of adjacent anatomical connections and coronary ostia, the normal pulmonic and aortic valves are identical in design. The lines of cusp apposition and the central nodules are less prominent in pulmonic valves than in aortic valves, as might be expected from the lower right-sided ventricular pressures. With age, fenestrations of the cusp lunulae appear but, as in the aortic valve, have no functional significance. The three pulmonic valve cusps are named in relation to the aortic cusps - right, left and anterior. The pulmonic valve annulus is about 1.5 cm above the level of the aortic valve annulus, but its circumference is similar (7 cm to 9 cm). The pulmonic valve is discontinuous with the tricuspid valve by muscular structures of the right ventricular outflow tract.

Anatomical Variation: As with the aortic valve, detailed measurements of commissural diameters and cuspal depth reveal variations. The long-term functional significance of these congenitally abnormal tricuspid pulmonic valves with asymmetric closure lines differs from that of the aortic valve in that acquired "senile" (old age) pulmonic stenosis does not occur. This difference presumably is due to the difference in right- and left-sided ventricular systolic pressures.

Age-Related Changes: With increasing age, the pulmonic valve cusps thicken slightly, but far less in comparison to the age-related fibrous thickening seen in aging aortic valves. Calcific deposits in the base of the pulmonic valve sinuses were not observed in 40 hearts from patients aged 90 years to 103 years.

• **Mitral Valve**

General: The mitral valve is much more complex than the semilunar valves. The mitral valve consists of six major anatomical components (Figures 5, 6, 14, 15, 19 to 21): posterior left atrial wall, annulus, leaflets, chordae tendineae, papillary muscles, and left ventricular free wall. Alterations of one, more than one, or all of these components can cause mitral valve dysfunction. The mitral valve annulus forms a major part of the basal attachment of the posterior leaflet. This bundle of fibrous tissue separates left ventricular from left atrial myocardium and is located posterior to the posterior mitral leaflet. The anterior leaflet does not have a true annulus but is continuous with the wall of ascending aorta, aortic valve and membranous ventricular septum. The valve measurement used by surgeons ("mitral ring"), or that obtained by pathologists at autopsy, is not really a measurement of the mitral annulus but of the mitral valve circumference. The circumference of the normal mitral valve ranges from 8 cm to 10.5 cm (mean, 9.4 cm). Unlike the other three cardiac valves, which each have three leaflets or cusps, the mitral valve consists of only two leaflets. The anterior leaflet has a much longer base to margin of closure width (2.3 cm) than the posterior leaflet (1.2 cm), but the circumference (6 cm) of the posterior leaflet (annular attachment) is about twice that of the anterior leaflet (3 cm). Whereas the base to margin widths and circumferences of each mitral leaflet are different, the surface area of each leaflet is similar. The total surface area of both leaflets is about two and one-half times that of the orifice area calculated using the mitral valve circumference. The leaflets are connected to each other at junctions called commissures. In contradistinction to the semilunar commissures, which represent "spaces" between cusps, the commissures of the AV valves are "junctions" of continuous leaflet tissue.

The chordae tendineae of the mitral valve consist of primary, secondary and tertiary chordae which subdivide as they extend from papillary muscles to leaflets (Figures 19 to 21). Some chordae tendineae from each papillary muscle attach to both anterior and posterior mitral leaflets. The spaces between the multiple chordal subdivisions function as secondary orifices between the left atrium and left ventricle. The two left ventricular papillary muscles are termed anterolateral and posteromedial. The anterolateral papillary muscle is usually larger than the posteromedial. The major blood supply of the anterolateral muscle is the left anterior descending coronary artery, while the right coronary artery supplies the posteromedial muscle. The left circumflex artery supplies blood to both papillary muscles. The apices of papillary muscles appear to be sensitive indicators of myocardial hypoxia, since blood supply to the papillary muscle must travel the full thickness of the left ventricular free wall and then retrogradely up the longer axis of the papillary muscle body.

Anatomical Variations: The posterior leaflet of the mitral valve shows considerable variation in its subdivision into one to three scallops -lateral, middle and medial. Virtually all posterior leaflets (96%) are tri-scalloped, with the middle scallop being the largest. The width of the middle scallop is about 1.3 cm, compared to about 1.0 cm for the lateral and medial scallops. Variation in number, width and circumference of the posterior leaflet scallops, however, constitutes the major anatomical variation of the mitral valve. Rare congenital variations of mitral leaflets and chordae include abnormal supernumerary orifices of the mitral valve (bridging leaflet tissue or actual duplication) and aberrant chordae tendineae from atrial septum to mitral valve leaflets. Some hearts have "muscular chords" representing direct insertion of papillary muscles into leaflet edges.

Age-Related Changes: Expected age-related changes of the mitral valve include focal areas of leaflet fibrous thickening, lipid deposits over the ventricular surface of the anterior mitral leaflet, progressive prominence of the lines of closure and calcification of the mitral valve annulus. Since the left ventricular cavity size decreases with increasing age, the mitral valve annulus also decreases with age. This latter change promotes further leaflet contact and increases leaflet fibrous changes. This change in ventricular cavity also cre-ates ventriculo-leaflet area disproportion, so the segments of normal leaflet prolapse into the left atrium.

• **Tricuspid Valve**

General: The tricuspid valve, like the mitral valve, is a complex structure made up of six major anatomical components: right atrial wall, annulus, three leaflets, chordae tendineae, papillary muscles and right ventricular free wall. The three leaflets are termed anterior, posterior, and septal (Figures 5, 6, 8 to 10, 13, 22). The anterior leaflet is usually the largest, with a width of 2.2 cm. The septal leaflet and posterior leaflet measure about 1.5 cm and 2.0 cm in width, respectively. The tricuspid annulus is a nearly circular fibrous structure, much less prominent than the mitral valve annulus but slightly larger in circumference (10 cm to 12.5 cm). The posterior leaflet makes up the largest portion of the annulus (7.5 cm), followed by the anterior (3.7 cm) and septal (3.6 cm) leaflets. The septal leaflet has a characteristic fold or indentation where its annulus passes from the posterior ventricular free wall to the membranous septum (Figure 22). The chordae tendineae of the tricuspid valve are made up of five types: fan-shaped, rough zone, basal, free edge and deep (Figure 22). Of these, the free edge and deep chordae are unique to the tricuspid valve. The chordae arise from a single large anterior papillary muscle, double or multiple septal papillary muscles, and several small posterior papillary muscles. The papillary muscles are attached to the corresponding walls of the right ventricle.

Anatomical Variations: The posterior leaflet of the tricuspid valve shows considerable variation in its subdivision into one to three scallops. The scallops are produced by small clefts marked by fan-shaped chordae. Rare congenital tricuspid valve anomalies include supernumerary orifices created by bridging leaflet tissue or actual valve duplication.

Age-Related Changes: With increasing age, the tricuspid valve leaflet margins of closure become more prominent, and the leaflet acquires focal areas of fibrous thickening. Leaflet or annular calcification are rarely seen unless there is an abnormal calcium balance or the patient has inborn metabolic abnormalities.

Papillary Muscles

The papillary muscles of both ventricles are located below the commissures of the atrioventricular valves. These muscles project from the trabeculae carneae and may be single, bifid, or occasionally

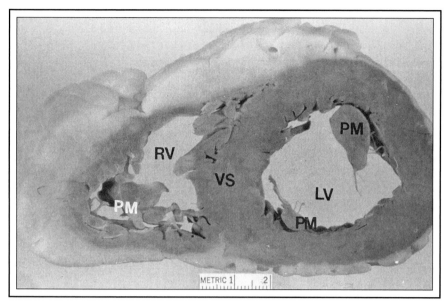

Figure 23. Short axis view of ventricles showing papillary muscles of mitral valve (PM - black) and tricuspid valve (PM - white). LV = left ventricle; RV = right ventricle; VS = ventricular septum. *(From Waller and Schlant, 38)*

a row of muscles arising from the ventricular wall. In the left ventricle the two groups of papillary muscles, located below the anterolateral and posteromedial commissures, arise from the junction of the apical and middle third of the ventricular wall (Figures 7, 8, 9, 10, 14, 15, 19, 20, 23). In the right ventricle there are usually three papillary muscles (Figures 9, 10). The largest is the anterior papillary muscle, which is found below the commissure between the anterior and posterior leaflets, originating from the moderator band as well as from the anterolateral ventricular wall. The posterior papillary muscle lies beneath the junction of the posterior and septal leaflets. A small septal papillary muscle, originating from the wall of the infundibulum, tethers the anterior and septal leaflets high against the infundibular wall. At times this muscle is virtually absent, and the chordae tendineae arise from a small tendinous connection to the infundibulum. The septal leaflet of the tricuspid valve usually has extensive attachments to the ventricular septum. The papillary muscles, because of their relatively parallel alignment to the ventricular wall and their chordal attachments to two adjacent valve leaflets, pull the leaflets of the mitral valve and tricuspid valve together and downward at the onset of isovolumic ventricular contraction.

Chordae Tendineae

Strong cords of fibrous tissue, the chordae tendineae, spring from the tip of each papillary muscle (Figures 7, 10, 14, 15, 19, 20). They often subdivide and interconnect before they attach to the two leaflets directly above. The chordae may attach directly into a fibrous band running along the free edge of the valves, or they may become

incorporated into the ventricular surface of the leaflet a few millimeters back from the edge. Additional chordae run directly from the ventricular wall into the undersurface of the posterolateral leaflet of the left ventricle and the septal and posterior leaflets of the right ventricle. The chordae tendineae, by their attachments to most of the free valvular border and by their numerous cross connections, allow the valve leaflets to balloon upward and against each other and evenly distribute the forces of ventricular systole. Dysfunction or rupture of a papillary muscle or rupture of a chorda tendinea may undermine the support of one or more valve leaflets, producing regurgitation.

Endocardium

Endocardium endothelium appears to share many, if not all, of the many functions of vascular endothelium described below. A newly found agent from endocardial endothelial cells that prolongs myocardial contraction has been provisionally referred to as "endocardin." The prolongation of contraction by endocardin can be overridden by stimulation of endothelium-derived relaxing factor (EDRF), which shortens the duration of contraction.

Pericardium

The heart is enclosed by the pericardium, the two surfaces of which can be visualized by considering the heart as a fist that is plunged into a large balloon or serous pericardium (Figures 24). The surface of the balloon in intimate contact with the fist is analogous to the visceral pericardium or epicardium. This surface encases the heart, extending several centimeters onto each of the great vessels.

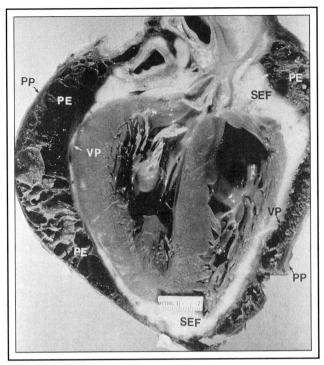

Figure 24. Fibrous pericardial effusion (PE) helps to delineate the 2 normal layers of the pericardial sac – visceral pericardium (VP) and parietal pericardium (PP). Subepicardial fat (SEF) is located just beneath the visceral layer of pericardium. *(From Waller and Schlant, 38)*

It is then reflected back, as is the outer surface of the balloon, to form the parietal pericardium, which is fused to the fibrous pericardium to form the fibrous layer. The two pericardial surfaces are lined by smooth, glistening serous tissue and are separated by a thin layer of lubricating fluid, which allows the heart to move freely within the parietal pericardium. The parietal pericardium is attached by ligaments to the manubrium, the xiphoid process, the vertebral column and the diaphragm. There is normally about 10 ml to 50 ml of thin, clear pericardial fluid, which moistens the contracting surfaces of the visceral and parietal pericardium. Four recesses are frequently present in images or examination of the pericardial space: the superior sinus, the transverse sinus, the postcaval recess and the oblique sinus.

Tomographic Views of the Normal Heart: Basis for Various Cardiac Imaging Techniques

During the last several years, dramatic developments have taken place in the diagnosis of cardiovascular disorders in the area of cardiac imaging techniques. From a previous era of imaging by silhouettes (chest roentgenography, fluoroscopy, angiocardiography), we have emerged into an era of imaging by tomographic scanning (echocardiography, radionuclide tomography, computed tomography [CT], magnetic resonance [MRI]). An understanding of tomographic anatomy is the foundation for proper use and interpretation of these new imaging modalities.

Position of the Heart and Tomographic Axis

New tomographic imaging techniques result in various depictions of the heart that have similarities and differences. The major similarity in the techniques is the planar method of cardiac sectioning. The major difference in these various tomographic techniques is the axis of sectioning relative to the position of the heart in the thorax. Two-dimensional echocardiographic imaging cuts the heart in transverse and longitudinal planes perpendicular and parallel to the heart itself (Figure 9, 25 to 28). The heart serves as the axis of tomographic sectioning. The cavities and chamber walls are sectioned perpendicular and/or parallel to their respective axis. In contrast, CT and MRI imaging cut the thorax in transverse and longitudinal planes. The body serves as the axis of tomographic sectioning. The heart sits in an oblique position relative to the thorax: the atria are located posteriorly and only slightly superiorly; the cardiac apex directed leftward, anteriorly and somewhat inferiorly; and the atrial and ventricular septae and atrioventricular valves are directed anteriorly and somewhat inferiorly. Thus, the right atrium is a right lateral chamber, the left atrium is a midline posterior chamber, the right ventricle is an anterior chamber, and the left ventricle is a posterior chamber.

Sectioning the heart in tomographic planes using the thorax as the axis of reference necessarily results in "distortions" of cardiac cavities, valve structures, and thickness of chamber walls. Oblique sectioning of the cavities and chamber walls may not provide precise anatomic correlates but produce truncated or inflated measurements. Technical changes in CT and MRI presently under development will permit tomographic cardiac sectioning using the heart as the axis of reference. In contrast to imaging modalities using the thorax as the axis of sectioning, echocardiography uses the heart as the axis of sectioning. Thus, precise anatomic correlates can be made in terms of measurements of wall thickness and chamber sizes. Debate among pathologists and anatomists concerning the "proper anatomic orientation and "display" of tomographic cardiac images centers around the principle of reference axis. Arguments that depiction of the heart in an echocardiographic four-chamber view ("valentine shape") is "unconventional" and "nonanatomic" are based upon tomographic imaging that uses the

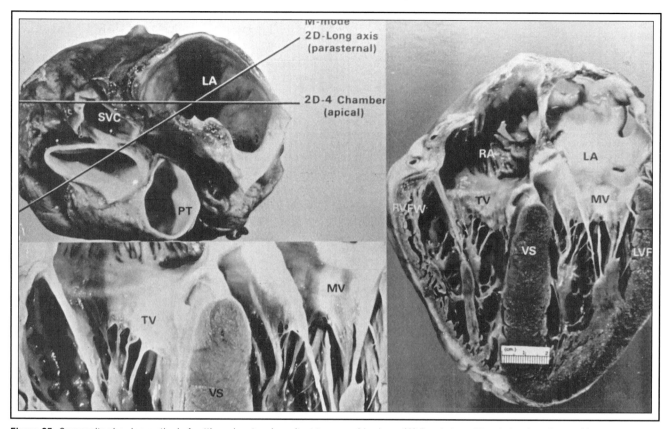

Figure 25. Composite showing method of cutting a heart and resultant tomographic views. **(A)** Basal view of heart showing planes of base-apex sectioning in order to obtain two-dimensional long-axis and two-dimensional, four-chamber echocardiographic views. The parasternal long-axis view is also used to correlate images obtained from M-mode echocardiography. **(B)** Closeup of four-chamber view showing atrioventricular valves (tricuspid [TV], mitral valve [MV]). The annulus of the TV is located more apically than the MV annulus. VS = ventricular septum. **(C)** Four-chamber view of heart. LA = left atrium; LVFW = left ventricular free wall; RA = right atrium; RVFW = right ventricular free wall. *(From Waller and Schlant, 38)*

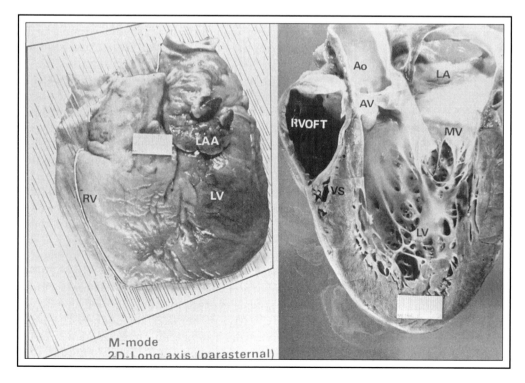

Figure 26. Tomographic sectioning of the heart from base to apex along the planar lines shown in Figure 2 produces views which correlate with echocardiographic parasternal long-axis images. Ao = aorta; AV = aortic valve; LA = left atrium; LAA = left atrial appendage; LV = left ventricle; MV = mitral valve; RV = right ventricle; RVOFT = right ventricular outflow tract; VS = ventricular septum. *(From Waller and Schlant, 38)*

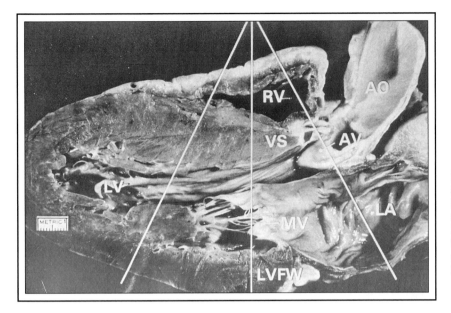

Figure 27. M-mode echocardiographic view showing "ice-pick" views of selected areas of the heart. One view displays the right ventricle (RV), aortic valve (AV), and portions of aorta (Ao), and left atrium (LA). Another more apical view shows the RV, ventricular septum (VS), left ventricular cavity (LV), and left ventricular free wall (LVFW). MV = mitral valve. *(From Waller and Schlant, 38)*

body as the reference axis. However, when one uses the heart as the reference axis, the echocardiographic four-chamber view is quite conventional and anatomic.

The Heart as the Reference Axis

• Short-Axis Method

The short-axis method of sectioning the heart also has been referred to as the "bread loaf" or "ventricular slice" method (Figures 3, 4, 6, 11, 12, 29). The technique involves transverse sectioning of the right and left ventricles at about 1 cm intervals from apex to base perpendicular to the axis of the atrial and ventricular septum. Near the base of the heart (about the level of chordae tendineae-papillary muscle junction), the transverse sections may skip to the level of the semilunar valves and atria (Figures 11, 12, 29). The resulting sections produce a "family of slices" from apex to base (Figures 11, 12). These slices are orientated with the anterior surface on the top and the posterior surface on the bottom. The short-axis method allows clinical morphologic correlation of wall and cavity dimensions and cross-sectional analysis of the cardiac valves. It is the method of choice in cases of atherosclerotic coronary heart disease in which recent and remote myocardial infarcts are likely, in cases of neoplastic infiltration in which location of metastatic implants are possible, and in cases of aortic and mitral valve disease in which assessment of valve structure and valve function (stenotic purely regurgitant) is necessary. This method of sectioning the heart also allows classification of myocardial infarcts into location and size: anterior, posterior, septal and/or lateral; basal, midventricular, apical or base-to-

apex; transmural or nontransmural (subendocardial, subepicardial). Another use of the short-axis view of the aortic valve and adjacent anatomic structures is recognition of the right and left main coronary arteries (Figures 3, 4, 6). The bifurcation of the left main into left anterior descending and left circumflex arteries and proximal portions of these main arteries can be identified with two-dimensional echocardiography. Anomalous origin of the right and left coronary ostia can also be recognized occasionally.

• Two-Chamber Method

The two-chamber method involves sectioning the heart through the inflow tract of the left ventricle and inflow and a portion of outflow tracts of the right ventricle. The plane of left ventricular sectioning is through the left ventricle and left atrium in an anteroposterior fashion and extending from base to apex. The two-chamber left ventricular plane discloses views of left atrium, anterior (septal), and posterior (mural) portions of the mitral valve leaflets, left ventricular cavity, and views of the anterior, apical, and posterior walls of the left ventricle. This view currently is used in assessment of the left ventricle in patients with atherosclerotic coronary heart disease. It provides another plane of sectioning for classification of left ventricular damage. A parallel cut on the right side of the heart discloses a similar view of the right ventricular inflow (right atrium, tricuspid valve, right ventricular body), but also discloses a portion of the right ventricular outflow tract. Although this particular tomographic view has been used less commonly in echocardiography, it would appear to be ideal in assessing right ventricular wall damage, intracavi-

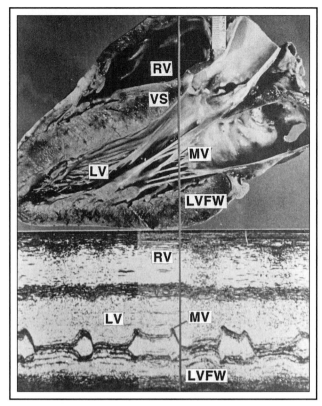

Figure 28. Parasternal long-axis view of heart with correlating M-mode echocardiogram. The "ice-pick" view through the midportion of the heart shows the right ventricle (RV) outflow tract, the ventricular septum (VS), left ventricular (LV) cavity, mitral valve (MV), and left ventricular free wall (LFVW). Systolic measurements on M mode echocardiogram correspond to measurements on the formalin-fixed heart. *(From Waller and Schlant, 38)*

tary masses and right ventricular outflow tract obstruction.

• Four-Chamber Method

The four-chamber method involves sectioning the heart from base to apex in a right-to-left plane along the acute margins of right and left ventricles and corresponding walls of the atria (Figures 10, 20, 25). In the bisected specimen, portions of the tricuspid valve (posterior and septal leaflet), mitral valve (primarily posterior leaflet), atrioventricular valve annuli, chordae tendineae, papillary muscles and each of the four cardiac chambers are visualized. In this view, it is readily apparent that the tricuspid valve annulus is located more apical than the mitral valve annulus. This anatomic finding is useful in identification of the right ventricle in complex congenital heart disease. Once the ventricle is identified, the atrioventricular valve follows concordantly. The corollary is also true in that if the atrioventricular valve can be morphologically identified, the ventricle follows concordantly (that is, recognition of the tricuspid valve as the apical most

atrioventricular valve also identifies the morphologic right ventricle). The four-chamber view is useful in cardiomyopathies for measurement of all four chambers, wall thickness and for identification of cavitary thrombus or tumor.

• Long-Axis Method

The long-axis method of cutting or imaging the heart produces a unique left ventricular inflow/outflow tract view (Figures 8, 9, 14, 15, 26, 27, 30, 31). The left ventricular long-axis view is obtained by sectioning the heart in an anterolateral plane from base to apex. In this longitudinal plane, evaluation of the aortic and mitral valves, proximal portion of the ascending aorta (sinus portion and proximal tubular portion), left ventricular outflow, left ventricular and atrial walls and chamber is possible. Also, a portion of right ventricular outflow tract just apical to the pulmonic valve is viewed on the left ventricular long-axis plane. The right-sided parallel longitudinal section views right atrium, tricuspid valve and body of the right ventricle. The left ventricular long-axis view is on the "standard" two-dimensional echocardiographic views of the

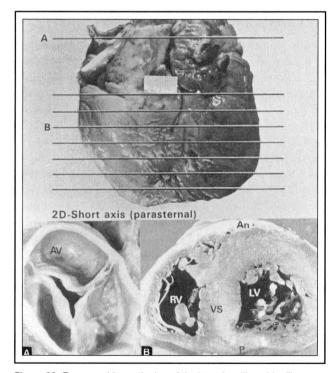

Figure 29. Tomographic sectioning of the heart in a "bread loaf" fashion produces a series of short-axis views of the left ventricle (LV) from apex to base. This "family of ventricular slices" is seen in Figure 8. Section B in the left hand photograph corresponds to a basal view of the ventricles (B) showing right ventricle (RV) and LV, anterior (An) and posterior (P) surfaces of the heart, and the ventricular septum (VS). A very basal view of the heart (line A) produces a view of the aortic valve (AV)(A). *(From Waller and Schlant, 38)*

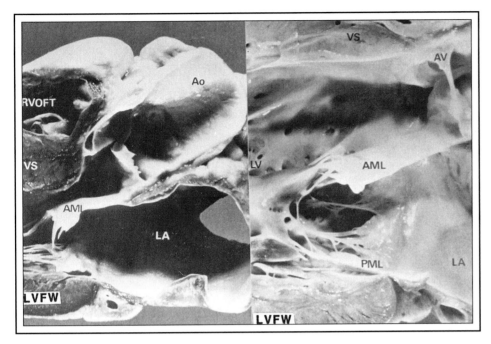

heart and thus is used for coronary, valvular and myocardial heart disease. The long-axis left ventricular section also corresponds to the traditional M-mode echocardiographic image with "ice pick" views of the aorta and left atrium, left ventricular outflow tract and mitral valve, and proximal portion of the ventricular septum, left ventricular cavity and left ventricular free wall. Anatomically, the left ventricular free wall imaged in this plane represents the lateral left ventricular free wall.

The Body (Thorax) as the Reference Axis

Tomographic sections of the heart obtained by use of the body as the reference axis result in cardiac images that differ from those described earlier. Three standard anatomic planes are generally used in computed tomography and magnetic resonance:

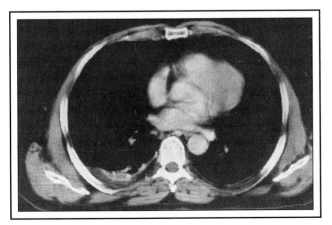

Figure 31. Transverse section of the heart from a computed tomography scan. The perpendicular cut of the thorax creates oblique cuts of the heart. *(From Waller and Schlant, 38)*

transverse (horizontal), frontal (coronal) and parasagittal (paramedian)(Figures 31, 32). Corresponding anatomic cardiac sections produced by these tomographic planes have been well illustrated in several anatomic atlases.

• Transverse (Horizontal) Method

Transverse tomographic planes of the thorax produce sections of the heart with truncated or expanded views of chambers and walls because of the oblique position of the heart within the thorax (Figures 31, 32). Some of the transverse views appear similar to the echocardiographic short-axis views. Transverse sectioning at the level of the great vessels provides an anatomic display of the pulmonary trunk and its bifurcation into the right and left main pulmonary arteries and an adjacent cross section of the ascending aorta. Transverse sections taken of the heart "from the head to the feet" produce a family of oblique cross sections. One horizontal view produces a foreshortened four-chamber view which, when viewed from the left, appears as a two-chamber echocardiographic cut and when viewed from the right appears as a truncated view of right ventricular inflow and an inflated view of the right atrium. Horizontal planes are useful in evaluation of patients with coronary and pericardial heart disease and in patients with diseases of the great vessels (dissection, aneurysm, mediastinal masses).

• Frontal (Coronal) Method

Frontal tomographic planes of the body (thorax) produce the least familiar cardiac images compared

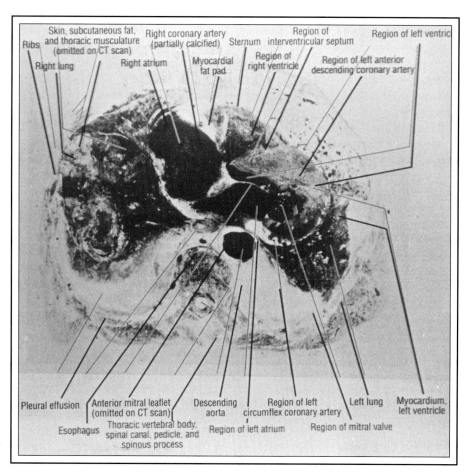

Skin, subcutaneous fat, and thoracic musculature (omitted on CT scan)
Ribs
Right lung
Right atrium
Right coronary artery (partially calcified)
Myocardial fat pad
Sternum
Region of right ventricle
Region of interventricular septum
Region of left anterior descending coronary artery
Region of left ventric

Pleural effusion
Esophagus
Anterior mitral leaflet (omitted on CT scan)
Thoracic vertebral body, spinal canal, pedicle, and spinous process
Descending aorta
Region of left atrium
Region of left circumflex coronary artery
Region of mitral valve
Left lung
Myocardium, left ventricle

Figure 32. Transverse section of a human cadaver thorax. Note the perpendicular cut through the thorax produces truncated and expanded views of various cardiac structures. The anterior left ventricular wall is much thicker than the posterior wall due to the oblique cardiac section. The anterior mitral leaflet appears closer to the right atrium than to the left atrium in this cut. *(From Gambarelli, et al 12)*

with echocardiographic images. Sectioning the thorax from the anterior to posterior (sternum to spine) results in cardiac sections which, at any one time, contain portions of left and right ventricles, aorta and pulmonary trunks, and left and right atria. These cardiac sections also cut the heart obliquely, preventing adequate assessment of chamber size and wall thickness or thinness. This method does provide excellent views of the right ventricular outflow tract, pulmonary trunk and pulmonary trunk bifurcation that are not available in the previously described tomographic cardiac sections. Also, the frontal plane is useful in evaluation of the aortopulmonary window and the vena cavae.

• Parasagittal (Paramedian) Method

Parasagittal tomographic planes of the body (thorax) produce another set of generally unfamiliar views of the heart. Planes of sectioning cut the heart in right to left fashion from shoulder to shoulder. Thus, the right sided structures (vena cavae, right atrium, right ventricle) are viewed last. Some sections resemble the echocardiographic two-chamber views of the right and left sides. This method also cuts chambers and vessels in an oblique fash-

ion that precludes adequate assessment of chamber size and wall thickness in most images. This method is excellent in anatomic evaluation of the aortic aneurysm, dissection and coarctation. In addition to conventional transverse, coronal and sagittal imaging, oblique imaging planes are possible with magnetic resonance. Oblique planes permit cuts of the heart along its long and short axes. The resultant cuts are analogous to the angiographic right and left anterior oblique views. The newest of the cardiac imaging modalities (MRI, cine CT, positron emission tomography) provide depiction of cardiac anatomy with the limitations mentioned above, but also provide an excellent technique for characterization of myocardial tissue. Distinguishing ischemic and scarred myocardium, tumor and fat infiltration and intracavitary tumor versus thrombus are useful morphologic data that cannot be assessed using present echocardiographic modalities.

• Scintigraphic Thallium Imaging

Scintigraphic thallium testing is a popular technique used in conjunction with exercise testing. Present methods of sectioning the heart produce images that closely resemble two-dimensional

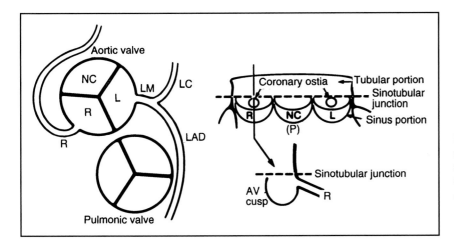

Figure 33. Diagram showing normal aortic origin and epicardial distribution of four major coronary arteries: left anterior descending (LAD), left circumflex (LC), left main (LM), and right (R). AV = aortic valve; NC = noncoronary; P = posterior. *(From Waller and Schlant, 38)*

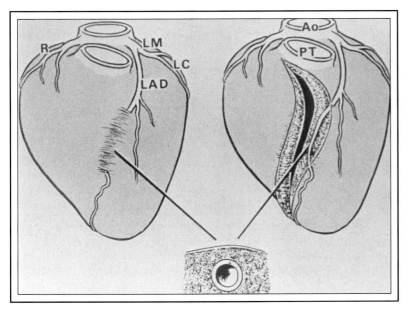

Figure 34. Diagram and photomicrograph showing tunneled epicardial coronary artery. (Left) Middle portion of left anterior descending coronary artery (LAD) lies within ventricular myocardium. Ao = aorta; LC = left circumflex; LM = left main; PT = pulmonary trunk; R = right. (Magnification x 100) *(From Waller and Schlant, 38)*

echocardiographic views, yet are variants of the oblique and sagittal planes. The similarity of these images to that of the echocardiographic views results from using the heart primarily as the axis for imaging.

The Epicardial Coronary Arteries

The epicardial coronary artery system consists of the left and right coronary arteries, which normally arise from ostia located in the left and right sinuses of Valsalva, respectively (Figure 33). In about 50% of humans a "third coronary artery" (conus artery) arises from a separate ostium in the right sinus. Additional smaller ostia may be found in the right sinus, which give rise to multiple right ventricular branches.

Up to five separate coronary ostia have been described. The left main (LM) coronary artery ranges in length from 1mm to 25mm in length before bifurcating into the left anterior descending

(LAD) and left circumflex (LC) branches. The LAD coronary artery measures from 10cm to 13cm in length, whereas the usual nondominant LC artery measures about 6cm to 8cm in length. The dominant right coronary artery (RCA) is about 12cm to 14cm in length before giving rise to the posterior descending artery (PDA). The luminal diameters of the major coronary arteries in adults range as follows: LM 2.0mm to 5.5mm (mean 4mm), LAD 2.0mm to 5.0mm (mean 3.6mm), LC 1.5mm to 5.5mm (mean 3.0mm) and right 1.5mm to 5.5mm (mean 3.2mm). Although the LAD and LC arteries generally taper in diameter as each extends from the left main bifurcation, the RCA maintains a fairly constant diameter until just before the origin of its posterior descending branch. The subepicardial coronary arteries run on the surface of the heart embedded in various amounts of subepicardial fat. Portions of the epicardial coronary arteries may dip into the myocardium ("mural artery" or

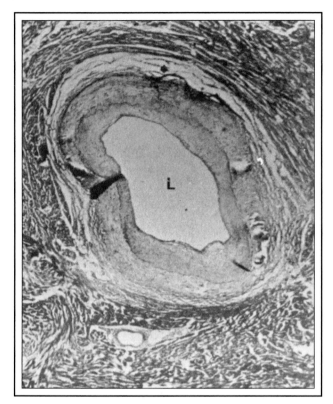

Figure 35. Tunneled left anterior descending coronary artery. The artery is surrounded by myocardium (Myo). L = lumen. *(From Waller and Schlant, 38)*

"tunneled artery") and be covered for a variable length (1 to several mm) by ventricular muscle ("myocardial bridge"; Figures 34 to 36). Tunneled epicardial coronary arteries probably represent a normal variant being recognized in up to 86% of vessels.

Branches of the Major Epicardial Arteries

The branches (Figure 33) of the LAD artery, in their usual order of origin, are the first diagonal, the first septal perforator, right ventricular branches (not always seen in normal hearts), other septal perforators and other diagonal branches. There may be two to six diagonal arteries, including the first diagonal, which may originate separately from the LM trunk. These diagonal branches course laterally over the free wall of the left ventricle in the angle between the LAD and the LC. There are also three to five septal branches, which leave the LAD artery at a right angle and plunge deeply into the ventricular septum. The branches of the LC are variable but may include the sinus node artery (40% to 50%), the left atrial circumflex branch, the anterolateral marginal, the distal circumflex, one or more posterolateral marginals and the PDA (10% to 15%). The anterolateral marginal, which is usually the largest branch, is directed

along the anterolateral wall towards the apex. The branches of the RCA include the conus artery (which may originate from a separate ostia in the right coronary sinus in 40 to 50% of hearts) to the right ventricular outflow area, the artery to the sinus node (50% to 60%), several anterior right ventricular branches, right atrial branches, the acute marginal branch, the artery to the AV node and proximal bundle branches, the PDA and terminal branches to the left ventricle and left atrium. When the sinus node artery originates from the RCA, it runs along the anterior right atrium to the superior vena cava, which it encircles in a clockwise or counterclockwise direction before it penetrates the sinus node. In 40% to 50% of hearts, the sinus node artery originates from the proximal LC and crosses behind the aorta and in front of the left atrium to reach the superior vena cava.

Coronary Ostia

The left and right coronary ostia arise normally within the sinus of Valsalva or at the junction of the sinus and tubular portions of aorta (sinotubular junction; Figures 33, 34). This ostial location allows maximal coronary filling during ventricular diastole. Occasionally, the right or left coronary ostium arises 1 cm or more above the sinotubular junction. This ostial dislocation has been termed high takeoff coronary artery. The record position for a high takeoff coronary artery is 2.5 cm above the sinotubular junction. In addition to the normal variants of a separate conus ostium or several right ventricular branch ostia, certain congenital coronary artery anomalies give rise to a reduced number (single coronary artery), increased number (separate origin of either the LAD, LC, or both) or altered shapes (acute angle takeoff, slit-like) of the coronary ostia.

Coronary Artery Distribution and Myocardial Supply

In the current era of reperfusion therapy for evolving acute myocardial infarction, it has become popular to "infarct artery" of the ventricular myocardium at risk. These phrases indicate that there is a well established relation between a given epicardial coronary artery and its myocardial supply. Although general statements can be made about the coronary distribution, the amount of myocardium supplied by a vessel is variable and is affected by collateral vessels, congenital variations, and other factors. Figure 36 shows a scheme whereby certain areas on various views of the two-dimensional echocardiogram can provide a reasonable prediction of the coronary artery perfusion pattern. Generally, the basal half of the ventricular

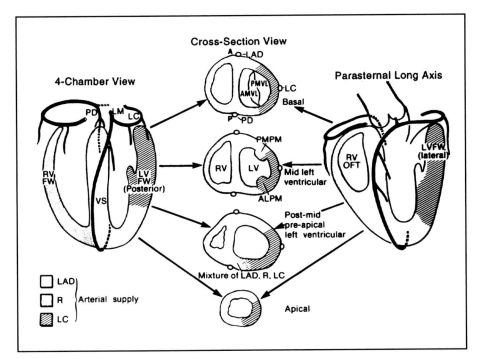

Figure 36. Diagram showing myocardial perfusion patterns of major epicardial coronary arteries as viewed from three tomographic cuts: four-chamber view, cross-sectional view, and parasternal long-axis. A = Anterior; ALPM = anterolateral papillary muscle; LC = left circumflex; LAD = left anterior descending; LM = left main; LV = left ventricle; LVFW = left ventricular free wall; P = posterior; PMPM = posteromedial papillary muscle; RV = right ventricle; RVFW = right ventricular free wall; RVOFT = right ventricular outflow tract. *(Modified from H Feigenbaum: Echocardiography. Philadelphia, Lea & Febiger, 1986: 462)*

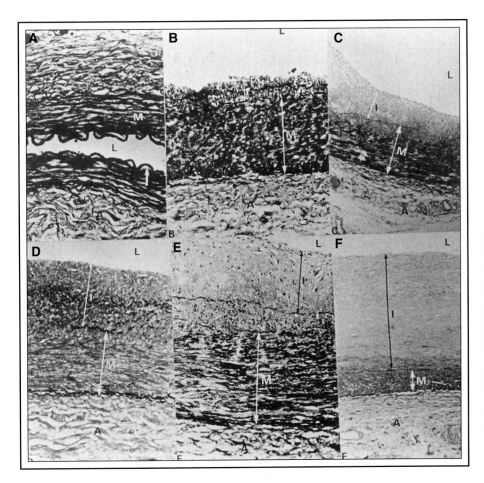

Figure 37. Composite of histologic sections of wall of various epicardial coronary arteries. **(A)** One-day-old artery showing underdeveloped intima, wavey internal elastic membrane (arrow), and well-developed media (M). **(B)** Teenage coronary artery showing further development of intima and media. **(C to F)** Diseased epicardial coronary arteries showing varying degrees of intimal thickening by atherosclerotic plaque, fragmented or disrupted internal elastic membrane, and thinning of media. A = Adventitia; L = coronary lumen. *(From Waller and Schlant, 38)*

535

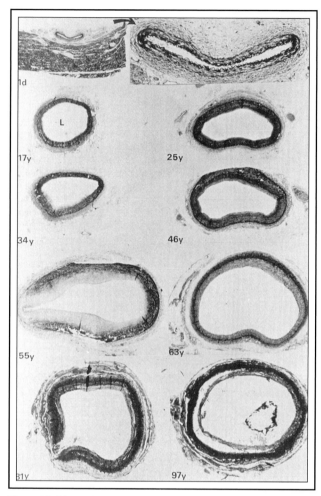

Figure 38. Photomicrographs of left anterior descending coronary artery from nine patients spanning nine decades of life. All arteries (except top right) are photographed at same magnification (x 10). With advancing age, luminal diameter and cross-sectional area increase, intima thickens, and media thins. All arteries are from patients dying of noncardiac disease. D = day; y = year. *(From Waller and Schlant, 38)*

cardiac apex for variable lengths along the posterior left ventricle. At present it is believed that the LAD and its branches nourish the apical wall of the left ventricle, most of the right and left bundle branches and the anterolateral papillary muscle of the left ventricle. When the PDA is provided by the circumflex artery, the entire septum is vascularized by the left coronary system. The LAD can also provide collateral circulation to the anterior right ventricle via the circle of Vieussens, to the posterior ventricular septum by the septal perforations, and to the PDA from the distal LAD or a diagonal branch.

Aging Changes of the Epicardial Coronary Arteries

The epicardial coronary arteries normally undergo significant changes between the fetal state and old age (Figures 37, 38). In fetal coronary arteries the intima is not well developed, consisting of a thin layer of elongated endothelial cells in close contact with the internal elastic membrane. The internal elastic membrane appears as a continuous tube (Figure 38). The media in fetal coronary arteries is well developed consisting of a layer of circular smooth muscle cells and fine elastic fibers (Figure 38). The adventitia is less well developed and consists of a thin layer of connective tissue. Changes in various layers begin after birth and consist of splitting and fragmenting of the internal elastic membrane, proliferation of fibroblasts and an increase in ground substance in the subendothelium. The medial smooth muscles alter their shape and position presumably as a result of a reaction to hemodynamic changes after birth. In the next several months smooth muscles appear between the split internal elastic membrane and form the "musculoelastic layer" between the intima and media. Intimal "cushions" of fibroblasts and elastic fibers occur focally along the intima. The external elastic membrane forms by 6 months. By one year, the intima contains a collection of subendothelial collagen and elastic fibers and a musculoelastic layer that eventually is incorporated into the mature media. In normal human coronary arteries, the amount of smooth muscle and fibroelastic tissue in the intima is a function of age. The intima progressively thickens, so that by late adolescence it is as thick as the media; after adolescence the intima becomes thicker than the media. In middle age the intima may become diseased and markedly thickened by atherosclerotic plaque. The underlying media thins and loses smooth muscle cells. The internal elastic membrane becomes fragmented, duplicates or focally disappears. Degenerative changes such as

septum and the anterior left ventricular free wall is perfused by the LAD coronary artery. A dominant right coronary artery perfuses anterior, lateral, and posterior right ventricular myocardium. The posterior coronary artery (most commonly arising from the RCA) supplies blood to the apical half of the ventricular septum and posterior left ventricular free wall. The LC coronary artery usually perfuses the lateral wall of the left ventricle (defined as that portion of ventricular myocardium located between anterolateral and posteromedial papillary muscles). Unappreciated areas of coronary perfusion include the basal ventricular septum and left ventricular apex. The basal-most portion of the ventricular septum is usually perfused by branches of the posterior descending artery (Figure 3). The apical third of the posterior left ventricle may be predominantly perfused by the LAD artery as it wraps around the

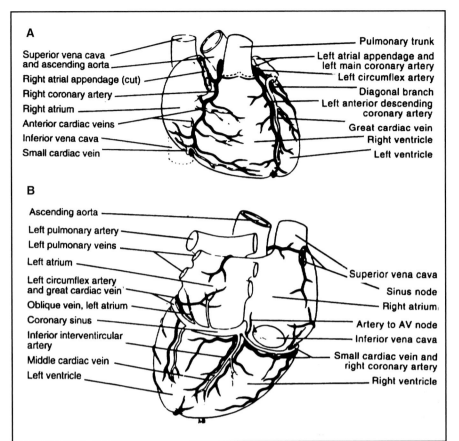

Figure 39. Diagram illustrating the principal arteries and veins **(A)** on the anterior surface of the heart and **(B)** on the posterior and inferior surfaces of the heart. Part of the right atrial appendage has been resected to show the proximal right coronary artery. In (B) the heart is shown more vertically oriented to expose the inferior surface. *(From Walmsley R, Watson H: Clinical Anatomy of the Heart. New York, Churchill Livingstone, 1978 with permission.)*

calcium deposition take place in the intima (atherosclerotic plaque) but calcific deposits rarely involve the media (Monckeberg's medial sclerosis). In old age the coronary arteries become tortuous, the luminal diameter increases, the media thins and calcific deposits increase.

The Coronary Veins

An extensive intercommunicating network of veins provides venous drainage for the coronary circulation. Three venous drainage systems can be considered: the coronary sinus and its tributaries, the anterior right ventricular veins, and the Thebesian veins (Figure 39). The coronary sinus, located in the posterior AV groove near the crux of the heart, receives venous blood from the great, middle, and small cardiac veins, the posterior veins of the left ventricle, and the left atrial oblique vein (of Marshall). The coronary sinus predominantly drains blood from the left ventricle. The anterior interventricular vein lies in the anterior interventricular sulcus, parallel to the left anterior descending coronary artery. It ascends to near the bifurcation of the left main coronary artery and then turns leftward to circle posteriorly under the left atrium in the left atrioventricular sulcus, where it is referred to as the great cardiac vein. Along its pos-

terior course, the great cardiac vein receives venous blood from large marginal and posterior left ventricular branches and then becomes the coronary sinus near the posterior margin of the left atrium. The posterior interventricular vein (middle cardiac vein) arises near the posterior aspect of the cardiac apex and ascends in the posterior interventricular sulcus next to the posterior descending coronary artery and drains either into the right atrium directly or into the coronary sinus just before it empties into the right atrium. The oblique vein of Marshall runs along the posterior left atrium and joins the great cardiac vein at the point where the latter becomes the coronary sinus. The coronary sinus extends 2cm to 3cm within the posterior atrioventricular groove before it opens into the infero-posterior-medial aspect of the right atrium, between the orifice of the inferior vena cava and the septal tricuspid leaflet. A crescent shaped, rudimentary valve, the Thebesian valve, can be seen at its entrance. The total distance from the bifurcation of the left coronary artery to the Thebesian valve is about 9 cm. About 85% of the coronary venous blood, including the drainage from the ventricular septum, the left ventricle, both atria, and some of the right ventricle, is carried by this elaborate system of veins. It is important to note that studies

537

involving catheterization of the coronary sinus often require placing the tip of a catheter in the coronary sinus beyond the entrance of the posterior interventricular vein or other major veins draining the posterior left ventricle.

There are two to four anterior cardiac veins that originate in and drain the anterior right ventricular wall, travel superiorly to cross the right atrioventricular sulcus, and enter either directly into the right atrium anteriorly or into a collecting vein at the base of the right atrium. The small cardiac vein, which receives some branches from the right ventricle and the right atrium, winds around the right side of the heart in the atrioventricular sulcus and terminates either in the coronary sinus or the right atrium. The Thebesian veins are tiny venous outlets draining directly into the cardiac chambers primarily into the right atrium and right ventricle.

Selected Reading

1. Anderson RH, Becker AE: *Cardiac Anatomy.* Gower Medical Publishing, London, 1980.
2. Brock RC: The surgical and pathologic anatomy of the mitral valve. *BHJ* 14:489-513, 1952.
3. Carter BL, Morehead J, Wolpert SM, Hammerschlag SB, Griffiths HJ, Kahn PC: *Cross-sectional Anatomy, Computed Tomography and Ultrasound Correlation.* New York, Appleton Century Crofts 1–60, 1977.
4. Cascos AS, Rabago P, Sokolowski M: Duplication of the tricuspid valve. *BHJ* 29:943-946, 1967.
5. Choe YH, Im JG, Park JH, Ho MC, Kim CW: The anatomy of the pericardial space: A study in cadavers and patients. *AJR* 149:693-698, 1987.
6. Clark JA: An x-ray microscopic study of the blood supply to the valves of the human heart. *BHJ* 27:420-423, 1965.
7. Duran CMG, Gunning AJ: The vascularization of the heart valves: A comparative study. *Cardiovasc Res* 3:290-296, 1968.
8. Edwards BS, Edwards WD, Bambara JF, et al: Anomalies of the left atrium and mitral valve: Cords, flaps and duplication of valves. *Arch Path Lab Med* 107:29-33, 1983.
9. Edwards WD: Applied anatomy of the heart. In: Brandenburg RO, Fuster V, Giuliani ER, et al (eds): *Cardiology: Fundamentals and Practice.* Chicago, Year Book Medical Publisher 47-112, 1987.
10. Elfenbein B, Paplanus SH: Duplication of the mitral and tricuspid valves. *Arch Path* 85:675-680, 1968.
11. Estes EH Jr, Dalton FM, Entman ML, Dixon HB, Hackel DB: The anatomy and blood supply of the papillary muscles of the left ventricle. *AHJ* 71:356-362, 1966.
12. Gambarelli J, Guerinel G, Chevrot L, Matteri M: Computerized Axial Tomography. An anatomic atlas of serial sections of the human body. Berlin, Springer-Verlag 1-41, 1977.
13. Gross L, Kugel MA: Topographical anatomy and histology of the valves in the human heart. *AJP* 7:445-476, 1981.
14. Higgins CB: Overview of MR of the heart. *Am J Radiol* 146:907-914, 1986.
15. Higgins CB, Carlsson E, Lipton MJ: *CT of the Heart and Great Vessels.* Mount Kisco, NY, Futura 1-48, 1983.
16. Janes RD, Brandys JC, Hopkins DA, Johnstone DE, Murphy DA, Armour JA: Anatomy of human extrinsic cardiac nerves and ganglia. *AJC* 57:299-309, 1986.
17. Kennedy JW, Baxley WA, Figley MM, Dodge HT, Blackmon

JR: Quantitative angiocardiography: The normal left ventricle in man. *Circ* 34:272-278, 1966.
18. Lev M, Bharati S: The fibrous skeleton of the heart. In: Hurst JW (ed): *Update IV: The Heart.* New York, McGraw-Hill 7-14, 1982.
19. Mitchell GAG: *Cardiovascular Innervation.* Baltimore, Williams & Wilkins, 1956.
20. Merklin RJ: Position and orientation of the heart valves. *An Anat* 125:375-380, 1969.
21. Nazarian GK, Julsrud PR, Ehman RL, Edwards WD: Correlation between MRI of the heart and cardiac anatomy. *Mayo Clin Proc* 62:573-583, 1987.
22. Prakash R: Determination of right ventricular wall thickness in systole and diastole: echocardiographic and necropsy correlation in 32 patients. *BHJ* 40:1257-1261, 1978.
23. Randall WC (ed): *Nervous Control of Cardiovascular Function.* New York, Oxford University Press, 1984.
24. Ranganathan N, Lam JHC, Wigle ED, Silver MD: Morphology of the human mitral valve: II. The valve leaflets. *Circ* 41:459-467, 1970.
25. Roberts WC, Perloff JK: Mitral valve disease: A clinicopathologic survey of the conditions causing the mitral valve to function abnormally. *Ann Intern Med* 77:939-975, 1972.
26. Roberts WC, Waller BF: Effect of chronic hypercalcemia on the heart: An analysis of 18 necropsy patients. *AJC* 71:371-384, 1981.
27. Roberts WC: The structure of the aortic valve in clinically isolated aortic stenosis—an autopsy study of 162 patients over 15 years of age. *Circ* 42:91-97, 1970.
28. Roberts WC: Morphologic features of the normal and abnormal mitral valve. *AJC* 51:1005-1028, 1983.
29. Rosenquist GC, Sweeney LJ: The membranous ventricular septum in the normal heart. *Johns Hopkins Med* 135:9-16, 1974.
30. Scholz DG, Kitzman DW, Hagan PT, Ilstrup DM, Edwards WD: Age-related changes in normal human hearts during the first 10 decades of life. Part I (growth): A quantitative anatomic study of 200 specimens from subjects from birth to 19 years old. *Mayo Clin Proc* 63:126-136, 1988.
31. Sweeney LF, Rosenquist GC: The normal anatomy of the atrial septum in the human heart. *AHJ* 98:194-199, 1979.
32. Titus JL: Normal anatomy of the human cardiac conduction system. *Mayo Clin Proc* 48:24-30, 1973.
33. Vollebergh FE, Becker AE: Minor congenital variations of cusp size in tricuspid aortic valves: Possible link with isolated aortic stenosis. *BHJ* 39:1006-1011, 1977.
34. Waller BF, Taliercio CP, Slack JD et al: Tomographic views of normal and abnormal hearts: Anatomic basis for various cardiac imaging techniques. Part 1. *Clin Cardiol* 13:804-812, 1990.
35. Waller BF, Taliercio CP, Slack JD et al: Tomographic views of normal and abnormal hearts: Anatomic basis for various cardiac imaging techniques. Part 2. *Clin Cardiol* 13:877-884, 1990.
36. Waller BF: Morphologic aspects of valvular heart disease: Part 1. *Curr Prob Cardiol* IX:13-26, 1985.
37. Waller BF, Morrow AG, Maron BJ, DelNegro AA, et al: Etiology of clinically isolated, severe, chronic pure mitral regurgitation: Analysis of 97 patients over 30 years of age having mitral valve replacement. *AHJ* 104:276-288, 1982.
38. Waller BF, Schlant RC: *Anatomy of the Heart.* (In), *Hurst's The Heart,* Schlant RC, Alexander RW (eds), 18th Ed., McGraw Hill, pp 59-111, 1994.
39. Wilcox BR, Anderson RH: *Surgical Anatomy of the Heart.* New York, Raven, 1985.
40. Zimmerman J: Functional and surgical anatomy of the aortic valve. *J Med Sci* 5:862-868, 1969.

CHAPTER 23

Physiology of the Heart and Vascular System: Basic Concepts and Clinical Applications

Hanjörg Just, M.D.

Advances in the diagnosis and treatment of cardiovascular disease is firmly rooted in an understanding of basic cardiovascular physiology. A command of the physiology of the heart and vascular system allows appropriate interpretation of such clinical phenomena as gallop-rhythm, precordial motion, and variation in venous and arterial pulsations. As a detailed description of the physiologic underpinnings of Dr. W. Proctor Harvey's masterly clinical teachings would fill too large a volume; three selected fields of physiology which serve as examples of the application of basic physiologic concepts to the practice of clinical medicine will be discussed:

1. Contractile geometry and quantitative morphology of the heart.

2. Excitation contraction coupling: The link between structure and function.

3. The vascular system: Determinants of cardiac performance and cardiovascular risk.

General Considerations

The heart and the vascular system circulate approximately 5 liters of blood at rest, during exercise, with varying body positions, and over a wide range of disease states and stressful situations with a remarkable degree of stability of pressure and flow. The heart transforms venous return, which is continuous, into pulsatile arterial blood flow. The right heart fills at 1mmHg pressure and perfuses pulmonary circulation at a mean pressure of 10 mmHg. The left heart propels 5 liters to 15 liters of blood per minute through the systemic circulation,

whereby the windkessel function of the aorta and resonance phenomena in the arterial system allow for pulsatile flow throughout the body.

Flow distribution is regulated through interplay of multiple local, regional, and systemic mechanisms such as autoregulation in the sympathetic nervous system. Conductivity and patency of the blood vessels and regional and/or systemic flow and flow reserve are largely maintained by function of the vascular endothelium. This monolayer cell system releases nitric oxide in response to shear stress from flowing blood at the cell surface and thereby regulates smooth muscle tone.

Return of venous blood to the heart occurs through the largely superficial subcutaneous systemic veins. Propulsion of blood, by a certain vis a tergo, is mainly through the pumping action of working skeletal muscle and more centrally by respiratory motion and pressure change in the abdominal and thoracic cavity. Transformation of continuous into pulsatile blood flow requires rhythm and the coordination of venous return, performance of the heart (atrium, ventricles, heart valves), and input impedance of the arterial system. Interplay of these components can be observed clinically at bedside; venous return can be inferred by inspection of the jugular venous pulse and pressure, and pulse wave velocity by palpation of the carotid and peripheral arterial pulses. The performance of the system therefore, can be deduced from indirect indicators. The well-known Wiggers' scheme represents the clinically relevant phenomena in a simple way (Figure 1).

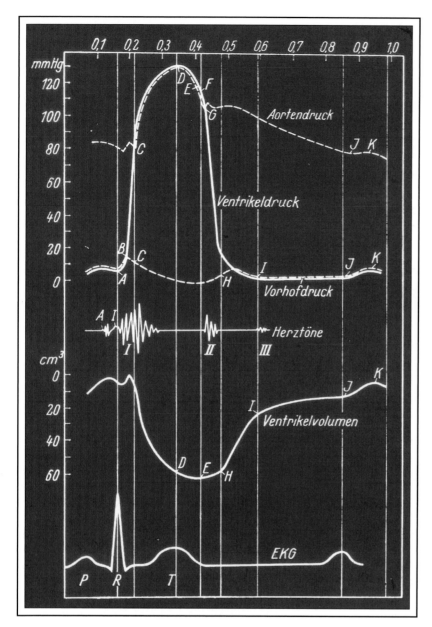

Figure 1. Modified Wiggers Scheme of cardiac dynamics. Ventricular pressure and volume change are given together with atrial and arterial pressure pulse with the ECG (bottom) as time reference. Phonocardiographic indication of the heart sounds (middle) gives valve opening and closure for timing of systole and diastole. This original recording represents the events as measured in the left heart. The same holds for the right heart. Here, however, systole is slightly longer, pulmonary valve closure (P2) follows A2 with inspiration. The dependence of right heart events on respiration is much more pronounced than those of the left heart, and they are quite opposite: As right heart filling increases and therefore systole prolongs, left heart filling is reduced due to retention of blood in the expanding lungs. This effect is barely noticeable. However, increased left ventricular filling with expiration may well exceed a diseased left ventricle's capacity and give rise to a gallop rhythm. Quite the opposite is seen in the right heart: Here inspiratory overfilling will give rise to an inspiratory protodiastolic gallop. These examples may show the tremendous capacity of auscultation in the recognition and differentiation of right and left heart events and/or disease.

CARDIAC PEARL

If not already being done, we should develop the habit of drawing or sketching the various heart sounds and murmurs that we hear when examining our patients (Fig. A). Include it as part of the patient's record on both the office and hospital charts. If done, this invariably increases the accuracy of our auscultation because if we have to sketch what we are hearing, we obviously have to pay strict attention to the various components of the heart cycle. Note should be made of the intensity and splitting of the first heart sound and whether or not it varies in intensity; also, the features of the second sound- its intensity and type of splitting, normal or abnormally widely split ("fixed"). Sketch the murmur as to what part of systole and/or diastole it occurs, as well as any ejection sounds, systolic clicks, gallops, pericardial knocks and normal physiologic third sounds that are heard. If a continuous murmur is present, where in systole or diastole is it loudest? Does it "envelop" the second sound, as is typical of patent ductus arteriosus? I have yet to find a physician or student who sketches what he is hearing who does not greatly improve his expertise in clinical auscultation of the cardiovascular system. Making this a continuing lifelong habit will also result in continued progressive improvement over the years.

W. Proctor Harvey, M.D.

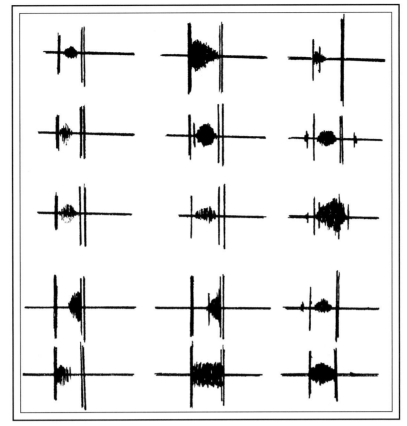

Fig A: Sketches of various murmurs and heart sounds. Top 3, left to right: (1) Note that systolic murmur is short in midsystole with normal aortic and pulmonic components of second heart sound, consistent with innocent murmur. (2) Note holosystolic murmur decreasing in the latter part of systole. This configuration of murmur is seen in acute mitral valve insufficiency, such as with ruptured chorda tendineae. (3) Note ejection sound and short systolic murmur in early systole, plus accentuated, closely split second heart sound, consistent with pulmonary hypertension as with Eisenmenger's ventricular septal defect. Line 2: (1) Early to mid systolic murmur with vibratory component, consistent with innocent murmur (Still's). (2) Note ejection sound following first sound with diamond-shaped murmur and wide splitting of second heart sound that may be present with milder degrees of pulmonic stenosis or atrial septal defect. Ejection sound more likely with valvular pulmonic stenosis. (3) Crescendo-decrescendo systolic murmur, not holosystolic; however, atrial (S_4) and ventricular (S_3) diastolic gallops present, consistent with mitral systolic murmur heard with congestive cardiomyopathy or coronary artery disease with papillary muscle dysfunction and cardiac decompensation. Line 3: (1) Longer, somewhat vibratory crescendo-decrescendo systolic murmur with wider splitting of second heart sound. If second heart sound became single with expiration, atrial septal defect is less likely and if remainder of cardiovascular evaluation is normal, then it is consistent with innocent murmur. (2) Midsystolic murmur, wide splitting of second heart sound that was "fixed"; atrial septal defect. (3) Prolonged diamond-shaped or "kite-shaped" systolic murmur masking the aortic component of second sound with delayed pulmonic component, atrial sound present in presystole, ejection sound present. Typical of valvular pulmonic stenosis of increasing severity. Line 4: (1) Late apical systolic murmur. Prolapsing mitral valve leaflet (systolic click-murmur syndrome, Barlow's syndrome). (2) Systolic click-late apical systolic murmur. Prolapsing mitral leaflet syndrome. (3) Midsystolic murmur, not holosystolic, atrial sound in presystole, consistent with mitral systolic murmur of cardiomyopathy or ischemic heart disease. Bottom line: Early crescendo-decrescendo systolic murmur ending at midsystole, consistent with innocent murmur; or can be seen with small ventricular septal defect, often closing. (2) Holosystolic murmur consistent with mitral insufficiency, ventricular septal defect. (3) Holosystolic murmur peaking in midsystole, also consistent with mitral insufficiency, tricuspid insufficiency, ventricular septal defect. An acute mitral insufficiency may take this configuration where there is a decrease in the murmur in the latter part of systole (in this latter case, atrial and ventricular diastolic gallops are frequent, and the second heart sound may be accentuated).

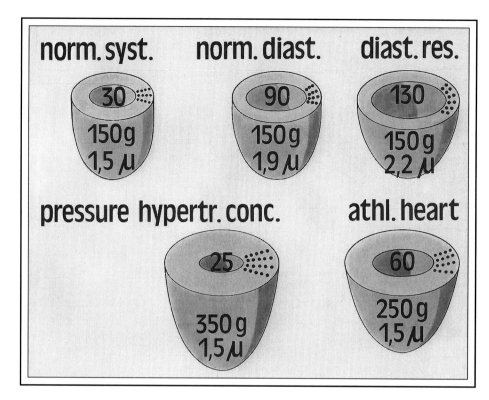

Figure 2A. Left ventricular volumes, muscle mass and sarcomere lengths in normal and well adapted hearts with either pressure or volume overload. It can be seen that from systole to diastole sarcomere length increases and the number of muscle fibers on the ventricular wall cross section decreases due to elongation *and* slippage or rearrangement of the fibers. Diastolic dilational reserve allows for a maximal LV-volume of 130ml and the maximal sarcomere length of 2.2μm at a 40% reduction of fibers on the cross section. Concentric hypertrophy due to pressure overload occurs at small ventricular volumes, keeping stress small and shortening distance high. The number of cells increases only in extreme cases, for the most part a gain in fiber volume due to increased contractile protein, mitochondria and nuclei is seen. In volume overload, or the athlete's heart, increase in size and muscle mass is entirely harmonic. The ability of the fibers to "slip" is augmented. *(modified from Linzbach)*

Adaptation of performance to demand is effected through a cascade of short and long-acting mechanisms:

1. *Frank-Straub-Starling Mechanism:* Increased diastolic filling of the heart, leading to "stretching" of muscle fibers, increases force of contraction of the subsequent beat. Contractile machinery of the myocyte responds to stretch with an increase in calcium sensitivity of contractile proteins. With lesser filling, contractile performance is reduced (Figure 3).

2. *Force/Frequency Relationship (Bowditch-Treppe Phenomenon):* The heart increases force of contraction with increasing heart rate. Increasing heart rate, under the majority of conditions, occurs as a result of increasing sympathetic tone. The force of contraction of both the atria and the ventricles is augmented and atrio-ventricular conduction time is shortened. With higher heart rates, atrial contribution to ventricular performance increases. In addition, myocardial contraction increases intrinsically with increasing heart rate. This mechanism, however, may be altered under diseased conditions.

3. Sympathetic tone with local (myocardial) release of catecholamines, as well as increased systemic levels of circulating catecholamines increases heart rate, atrial, and ventricular force of contraction and shortens atrial-ventricular conduction.

4. Myocardial performance seems to be strongly influenced by release of stimulatory substances from the endocardium and from the vascular endothelium within the myocardium. The nature of the substances has not yet been fully clarified.

Adaptation of the heart to load invokes adaptive mechanisms at a local (myocardial) as well as a systemic level (sympathetic nervous system, renin angiotensin system, atrial natriuretic peptide and others). Adaptations occur on a functional and morphological level. Heart size, muscle mass, and myocardial function are within wide ranges able to adapt. In the following discussion, our current knowledge of the functional anatomy of the myocardium shall be described.

Contractile Geometry and Quantitative Morphology of the Heart

Structure and Function

Muscle mass and chamber size of the heart are closely correlated to blood volume and level of blood pressure. The growing heart undergoes only one wave of mitosis between the first and fourth years of life, while total myocytes double. Thereafter, harmonic growth occurs and the number of cells remains constant within a wide range of adaptations up to the so-called "critical heart weight" of 500 grams. Growth occurs through gain in length and width of individual myocytes. The number of cells remains constant on the cross section of the myocardium at a defined point in time during the cardiac cycle (Figure 2A/B). Mechanisms of harmonic growth are only incompletely understood.

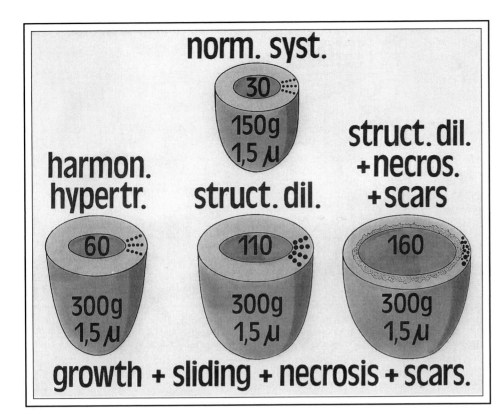

Figure 2B. Under pathologic conditions overload leads to structural dilatation in the first place. Note, that sarcomere length does not increase, fiber slippage past each other allows for the necessary volume increase. Only with extreme dilatation and wall tension increase, as well as with structural damage to the myocardial syncytium, connective tissue contents rises. Fiber sliding is impaired or entirely lost. But never is sarcomere overstretching seen. Instead hyperplasia sets in. *(modified from Linzbach)*

Several growth-stimulating mechanisms have, however, been identified. With "mechanical stretch" for example, intramyocyte protein synthesis is activated within minutes. This mechanism may relate to physiologic protein turnover and constant renewal of all cell structures, may be responsible for the adaptation to load. Clearly load-dependent is the growth-stimulating influence of sympathetic nervous tone, of systemically and locally released catecholamines (noradrenalin and adrenalin). A powerful growth stimulus arises from the renin-angiotensin system, the activation of which brings about a phenotype change, as the heart adapts to augmented volume and/or pressure load. This system seems to be responsible for individual blood pressure level, heart size, and muscle mass, as well as vascular structure and propensity to develop arteriosclerosis.

Myocardial Fiber Size and Orientation

Myocardial fibers are not randomly arranged, but follow a strict system of orientation maintained throughout systole and diastole, and within a wide range of adaptation. The orientation changes from an oblique course in the superficial layers to a more circular, angular course in the middle layers to a longitudinal course in the inner layers of the myocardium. There are no fascia separating the layers, which are more or less a continuum supplying the right and left ventricle.

It is believed that this three-layer orientation of the myocardial fibers allows for mitral and tricuspid valve closure through early activation of the inner longitudinal fibers. This leads to a shortening of the long axis with descent of valve leaflets towards the apex. Contraction of the ringlike layers of the inner part of the myocardium and the outer oblique fibers follows, leading to ejection of blood through circumferential chamber shrinkage. Upon relaxation the reverse occurs. Elastic forces of the myocytes and myocardial connective tissue contributes to active opening of the chamber. This process is aided by the maximally-filled atria at height of systole, which tend to pull the valve leaflets toward themselves, thereby translocating atrial blood into ventricular chambers. The more circular-oriented fibers are dominant in the ventricular walls. The ratio from circumferential to more longitudinally-oriented fibers is approximately 10:1. In the left ventricular free wall, approximately 55% of all fibers are circumferential. Circumferential fibers have an angle of 0 degrees to 22 degrees, the longitudinal ones 67 degrees to 90 degrees. Occasionally, myocardial fibers follow the course of coronary vessels.

Coronary vasculature, in length and width, is closely correlated to muscle mass. As the myocardium grows, the coronary vessels follow. Each muscle fiber is bordered by four capillaries. As fiber size increases, the capillary/muscle fiber ratio

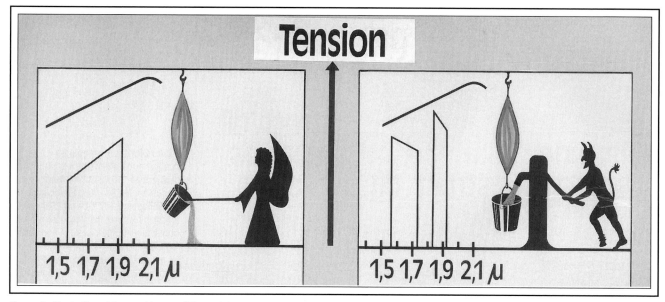

Figure 3. Illustration of the working conditions of the normal (left) and the structurally dilated and scarred heart (right), as seen by A. Linzbach. On top the Frank-Straub-Starling curve is given as it relates to sarcomere length. In the normal heart chamber geometry and fiber rearrangement during contraction allow for a decreasing load as contraction progresses – "as if an angel helped the working heart at a time when the greatest effort is needed". The dilated and scarred heart with larger chamber dimensions and interspersed connective tissue contracts under unfavourable conditions: The working element has to produce more force at lesser distance of shortening due to chamber geometry (law of LaPlace) *and* meets with series elastic elements, *and* cannot rearrange fibers for more efficient shortening: "as if the devil increased the load to the contractile element which is already disabled". The sarcomere may operate at lengths at which forceful contraction may no longer be possible.

remains constant. This means that the perfusion distance increases. With increases of myocardial muscle mass beyond the critical heart weight, the number of capillaries increases and adaptive growth of epicardial coronary arteries begins to lag behind. With systole and diastole, no significant changes in orientation of muscle fibers occur. However, the number of fibers on the myocardial cross-section changes with systole and diastole: with diastolic relaxation, the number of fibers decreases, whereas with systole the converse is true. The intramyocardial rearrangement allows remarkable changes in chamber size without stretching of the individual myocyte. The framework of the myocardial syncytium allows a reduction of the number of fibers by 30% to 40% during physiologic variation in chamber size. This mechanism of slippage is only possible if the myocardial syncytium and reticular fibers of myocardial connective tissue are intact.

The capacity of the myocardium to dilate in response to filling is, under normal circumstances, not utilized to its full extent. A limitation to overfilling is provided by intramyocardial connective tissue and the pericardial sac. The intramyocardial connective tissue consists of an interlace network of type 1 collagen, connected to the fibrous structures of the epicardium and the endocardium. The collagen fibers are predominantly oriented in parallel to the muscle fibers. In dilated hearts these fibers are stretched, whereas in normal ones they take an undulating course.

Sarcomere Length and Chamber Filling

The Frank-Straub-Starling law postulates that the myocytes with increasing chamber filling show increasing stretch, thereby producing a stronger contraction of the following systole. Indeed, the sarcomere length correlates directly with ventricular circumference. Normal sarcomeres contract or relax by 15% to 20% from 2.1 μm to 1.7 μm or vice versa (Figure 2A/B).

Beyond the 2.1 μm length, the Frank-Straub-Starling mechanism comes into play. The longest sarcomeres measure about 2.24 μm; limits then, of the Frank-Straub-Starling mechanism are relatively narrow. In fact, sarcomere lengths are identical within very narrow ranges, with all sizes of ventricular dilatation. The so-called "descending limb" of the Frank-Straub-Starling curve can't be related to true overstretching of the sarcomere. Nevertheless, within a wide range of adaptation to load, the Frank-Straub-Starling mechanism seems to be operative as an important principle of regulation of cardiac performance.

Structure and Dynamics of the Myocyte

The myocardium, constant in cell number throughout life, represents a syncytium. The cyto-

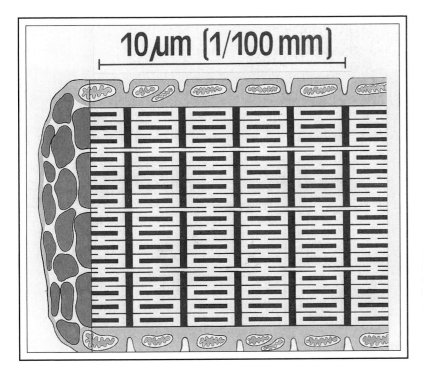

Figure 4. This schematic drawing gives the dimensions of the contractile myocyte with its actin- and myosin- filaments as they overlap and interconnect at the Z-bands. Mitochondria are found at the outer perimeter of the cell.

plasmic membrane, the sarcolemma, is a complex double layer lipid film containing multiple proteins (Figure 4); the inner surface is connected to the cytoskeleton. The sarcolemma appears stretched out during relaxation and shows protuberant structures with contraction at the level of the Z-membranes. With sarcomere length beyond 1.83 µm, sarcolemma is stretched. With shorter lengths, the sarcomere becomes "wavy". The resting length therefore, must be around 1.83 µm to 1.9 µm. Also, stretching of the sarcolemma seems to exert a powerful growth stimulus.

Upon electronmicroscopic examination, a complex inner structure of the myocyte is revealed. The membranous structures of the sarcoplasmic reticulum are worthy of mention (Figures 4, 5). Here the processes of electromechanic coupling take place and it's here where most proteins responsible for calcium homeostasis are located.

The nuclei of the myocytes change their size with contraction and relaxation, as can be seen from changes in configuration of the nuclear membrane. Likewise, the mitochondria, abundantly present in myocardial cells change their configuration with contraction and relaxation. They are always located directly adjacent to the contractile proteins.

The contractile apparatus consists of the actin and myosin filaments, which slide against each other, developing contraction through configuration changes of actomyosin heads. Actin filaments are approximately 1.0 µm, the myosin filaments approximately 1.6 µm in length. The force devel-

oped depends on degree of overlap of the actin and myosin filaments. Maximal overlap is seen between 2.0 µm and 2.25 µm sarcomere length, corresponding to normal diastolic relaxed state.

With cell growth during hypertrophy, length and size of the myocytes increases. This is achieved through an increase in number myofilaments and through addition of sarcomeres. The number of cell nuclei may increase (polyploidy), as does the number and size of the mitochondria. With structural alterations of the myocardium, the connective tissue contents increases and may reach up to 50% of the myocardial mass. When hypertrophy in excess of the "critical heart weight" hyperplasia occurs (number of myocytes increases; Figure 2A/B). At the same time, a loss of slippage of the myocardial fiber sets in. This leads to unfavorable conditions for the individual myocyte. As a consequence of the Law of LaPlace, at larger chamber size, without slippage of the contracting fiber, the distance of shortening decreases, whereas the force of contraction increases (work = force x distance). This initiates a vicious cycle, leading to inevitable deterioration (Figure 3). The process of hypertrophy and dilatation under load or overload conditions or as a result of myocardial damage or disease leads to cellular and subcellular adaptations. This change in myocardial phenotype brings about characteristic functional consequences. In hypertrophy the process of relaxation may be impaired, cell nutrition may be inadequate with resultant ischemia without coronary artery disease. Electric phenom-

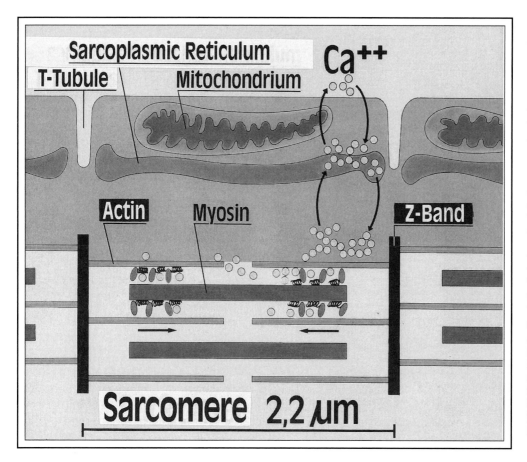

Figure 5. The cartoon depicts the sarcomere and the sarcoplasmic reticulum. Calcium (Ca++) is stored in the sarcoplasmic reticulum (SR). Upon entrance of calcium through the I-type channels of the sarcolemma, SR-Ca++-stores are emptied into the cytosol. Calcium release from the mitochondria is probably of minor importance. The contractile element, consisting of the actin and myosin filaments sliding past each other upon contact of calcium ions with the attached tropinin-tropomyosin-complex, releases the calcium after contraction. The free cytosolic calcium is then reabsorbed into the SR. The necessary enzyme, the sarcoplasmatic reticulum-ATPase, together with the regulatory protein phospholamban is responsible. Prompt removal of calcium allows for the necessary quick relaxation. Under diseased conditions, e.g. in heart failure this mechanism may be impaired (see text).

ena of the myocardium may be altered with subsequent electrical instability and occurrence of sudden cardiac death. In the state of heart failure the myocardial phenotype change may have far reaching functional consequences, which apply to therapeutic management of this systemic disorder. Specific alterations of calcium homeostasis may lead to both decreased performance and reduced electrical stability or a high propensity to develop ventricular arrhythmias, eventually culminating in sudden cardiac death. The myocardial phenotype change may best be indicated by the expression of atrial natriuretic peptide in the ventricular myocardium, whereas this peptide is normally only produced in atrial myocardial cells. This aspect of myocardial phenotype change is highly characteristic and can be used prognostically.

Myocardial Phenotype Changes in Heart Failure and their Consequences

Congestive heart failure is in most instances the result of chronic pressure and/or volume overload. This may result from valvular heart disease, and arterial or pulmonary arterial hypertension. Likewise, heart failure may result from loss of myocardial tissue (myocardial infarction) or from structural defects of a more diffuse nature

(myocarditis). As the myocardium fails to fulfill the body's demand for blood supply at a sufficient pressure level at rest and during exercise, a series of compensatory mechanisms comes into play, which activates neurohumoral systems and induces systemic changes of far-reaching consequences in the peripheral circulation, as well as in parenchyma of different organs. For purposes of this chapter, only myocardial adaptation to the state of heart failure will be considered.

The myocardial phenotype change in heart failure results from stimulation to growth from increased fiber stretch (ventricular dilatation) and simultaneous activation of the sympathetic and the renin-angiotensin systems. During the past few years, some of the mechanical stimuli, hormones, and growth factors have been identified, inducing quantitative and qualitative modulation of myocardial gene expression. In general, hypertrophy involves expression of "immediate early genes" and "late responsive genes", the latter including cardiac specific genes. Among the "immediate early genes" "proto-oncogenes" such as c-myc, y-fos. c-jun are involved, the messenger RNA of which may be increased as early as several minutes after onset of stretch. In addition, one receptor stimulation may result in a selective upregulation of mRNA including "immediate early genes" and "late responsive genes". A moderate degree of hypertrophy is also seen with stimulation of the beta-adrenergic receptor, typically at rest, later down-regulated in the state of heart failure. More recently it has been shown that angiotensin I- and II-receptor activation induces expression of "immediate early genes". The angiotensin II-mediated induction of gene expression closely resembles the program observed, when mechanical stress is applied to myocytes. Enhanced myocardial mRNA expression for angiotensin and the angiotensin-converting enzyme has been observed in several models of cardiac hypertrophy, especially in human hearts with end stages of ischemic or dilated cardiomyopathy. In addition to myocyte hypertrophy and phenotype change, fibroblast hyperplasia with development of interstitial fibrosis seems to be mediated by the renin-angiotensin system, namely through elevation of circulating aldosterone.

Contractile Proteins in Heart Failure

The central element of myocardial force development or shortening is the cross-bridge cycle, when the myosin cross-bridge head attaches to the actin filament, rotates, and develops force while shortening through sliding of the thin filaments past each other. Thereafter it detaches from the actin filament and starts another cycle. Changes in the number of the cross-bridges activated or of the individual cross-bridge cycle may exert profound effects on the contractile performance of the myocardium. The total number of cross-bridges available for activation may in heart failure be reduced due to replacement of contractile proteins by connective tissue. This applies to ischemic cardiomyopathy as well as to hypertrophic, hypertensive heart disease and dilated cardiomyopathy. Therefore, the percentage of contractile proteins in relation to total myocardial mass may be reduced by 20% or more in the state of heart failure, notwithstanding the fact that structural alterations, as described above, hamper contractile performance independent of the total amount of contractile protein present. Recently, it has been demonstrated that the decrease of contractile protein content is of minor importance relative to the effects of altered contractile geometry and of myocardial structure.

Regarding characteristics of the individual cross-bridge cycle, profound alterations have been observed in several models of myocardial hypertrophy. In these studies, reduced activity of myosin ATPase or myofibrillar ATPase, maximum shortening velocity and increased economy of asymmetric force development have been observed. The latter has been interpreted in terms of prolonged attachment time of the cross-bridges and to a reduced cross bridge cycling rate. Changes within the cross-bridge behavior have been attributed to changes in the myosin isoform from V_1 to V_3. The V_1-isoform consists of alpha-myosin-heavy chain and the V_3-isoform of the beta-myosin-heavy chain. In the hypertrophied and failing human heart, however, such isoform shifts have not been observed so far. Normal human ventricular myocardium primarily consists of the myosin isoform V_3 (beta-myosin-heavy chain). Since no shift in the myosin heavy chain-isoforms is observed in the human myocardium, alterations of cross-bridge behavior may be due to changes in the light chains or in thin filament regulatory systems. Alterations in the behavior of the individual cross-bridge cycle, observed in the hypertrophied and failing myocardium, may have two different, important consequences with respect to contractile function: on one hand, prolonged cross bridge attachment, as seen in hypertrophy and failure, may be advantageous from an energy economy point of view. A greater force/time integral is produced per unit of high energy phosphate hydrolysis. On the other hand, prolonged cross-bridge attachment may result in reduced rate of relaxation and in reduced shortening velocity and therefore cause diastolic dysfunction and prevent the myocardium from increasing power output.

Excitation Contraction Coupling: The Link Between Structure and Function

Recent studies with isolated human myocardium have suggested that excitation contraction coupling processes may be of major importance in development of contractile dysfunction in hypertrophy and heart failure. Excitation contraction coupling comprises all processes of calcium homeostasis and calcium-related activation of contractile proteins (Figure 5). Calcium enters the cells through the L-type, voltage-gated, sarcolemmal calcium channel. Then a larger amount of calcium is released from the sarcoplasmic reticulum through the ryanodine-sensitive calcium release channel. The calcium released into the cytosol subsequently binds to the regulatory protein troponin C, thus enabling the actin-myosin interaction. After contraction, calcium is removed from the cytosol mainly by the sarcoplasmic reticulum ATPase. To a lesser extent calcium is removed through the sarcolemmal sodium calcium exchanger, and to an even lesser extent by a sarcolemmal calcium ATPase. During the last few years, considerable work has been performed in analyzing function of various components of excitation contraction coupling in the human heart. Regarding the L-type sarcolemmal calcium channel, recent experiments indicate that mRNA expression of the dihydropyridine receptor is reduced in hearts with dilated or ischemic cardiomyopathy. The sarcoplasmic reticulum calcium release channel and the ryanodine receptor shows reduced mRNA expression. It has been observed in various types of hypertrophy and heart failure. Alteration of gating properties of this channel is seen in dilated cardiomyopathy.

With regard to the sarcoplasmic reticulum calcium ATPase, several studies have demonstrated that expression of dysprotein is reduced at the level of mRNA and protein in failing human myocardium irrespective of course of hypertrophy or failure. Accordingly, a reduced sarcoplasmic reticulum calcium reuptake is seen.

Activity of the sarcoplasmic reticulum calcium ATPase is controlled by the regulatory protein phospholamban. No data have been presented regarding the phospholamban protein in the failing human heart. However, recent mRNA measurement indicates that phospholamban expression may be decreased in parallel with the sarcoplasmic reticulum calcium ATPase. Current evidence indicates that the myocardial phenotype change in hypertrophy and failure involves significant changes of calcium homeostasis, mainly due to a reduced calcium reuptake into the sarcoplasmic reticulum. In this instance, increased amounts of cytosolic calcium may be expected to interfere with diastolic relaxation. This may indeed be the case. However, more recent evidence has been presented that in parallel to reduced calcium reuptake, capacity into the sarcolemmal sodium calcium exchanger is upregulated both in messenger RNA, protein, and function. This observation could easily explain the normal cytosolic calcium levels in the presence of reduced sarcoplasmic reticulum calcium reuptake. The consequence would, however, be that total intracellular calcium is lost to the extracellular space and therefore not available for the next contractile cycle. Here, a major source for the contractile efficiency of the failing human myocardium may be explained.

As a matter of fact, a recent observation on the functional behavior of the failing myocardium supports this hypothesis, allowing insight into therapeutic consequences. In the normal heart, contractile performance increases with heart rate (Bowditch-Treppe Phenomenon). In experiments with calcium-sensitive photoproteins it has been demonstrated that the rate-dependent increase in force of contraction is mediated by an increase in cytosolic calcium. In congestive heart failure, in contrast, the positive force/frequency relationship is flattened or reversed, meaning that with increasing heart rate contractile performance decreases. Optimal performance of the failing myocardium may be seen at heart rates between 30 per minute and 40 per minute. This reversal of the Bowditch-Treppe Phenomenon may easily be explained by a decreased sarcoplasmic reticulum calcium reuptake mechanism in conjunction with an increased expression and activity of the sarcolemmal sodium calcium exchanger. In addition, the subsequent increase in intracellular sodium ions (2 sodium ions are exchanged for 1 calcium ion) will inevitably lead to electrophysiologic consequences in terms of increased tendency to develop after depolarizations and electrical instability of the membranes. It may well be that here an explanation for the increased propensity of the failing myocardium towards ectopic arrhythmias may be found.

Yet other factors may be involved in alteration of calcium homeostasis in the phenotypically-altered failing human myocardium. For example, the role of the mitochondria has not been fully elucidated. In addition, different intracellular calcium binding proteins, such as troponin C or calmodulin, have not fully been investigated.

It seems clear, however, that even in view of reduced available cytosolic calcium, the contractile performance may be well preserved. This may relate to the operation of the Frank-Straub-Starling mechanism. It has been demonstrated that that stretch of the myocyte, as discussed above, alters sensitivity of the contractile proteins towards calcium, thereby allowing higher force of contraction at an unchanged calcium level. In summary, myocardial phenotype changes in hypertrophy and heart failure involve mainly calcium homeostasis and contribute to a major extent to the functional disturbances in heart failure. An outstanding phenomenon in this regard seems to be the inverted force/frequency relationship in the failing human myocardium.

The Vascular System: Endothelial Function and Vascular Risk

The function of the heart cannot be understood without knowledge of the venous and the arterial vascular system. Not only does venomotor tone regulate distribution of blood volume and ventricular filling, but the arterial system through the input impedance of the aorta exerts a major influence upon ventricular performance (the interplay of the neurohumoral systems with the heart and the circulation) that accounts for stability of the system and allows for optimal performance.

The extraordinary impact of arteriosclerosis has focused our interest on this generalized arterial disease, often linked with risk factors such as hypertension, diabetes, smoking, and obesity. Only in recent years has the central role of the endothelium in the regulation of regional and systemic blood flow and of blood pressure been recognized. Even more recently has been the observation that the renin angiotensin system in its vascular, specifically endothelial, representation may be a major risk factor in itself. Since the function of the endothelium is of central importance and the renin angiotensin system the major control mechanism of blood pressure, as well as myocardial mass and vascular compliance, and therefore of myocardial and vascular phenotype, some new observations highlighting the central role of this system will be presented.

Clinical observations demonstrate an enhanced risk for myocardial infarction in patients with sustained activation of the local and/or the systemic renin angiotensin system. For example, a high renin sodium profile or enhanced expression of angiotensin-converting enzyme indicates a high risk of developing coronary disease. Chronic blockade of the system by angiotensin-converting enzyme inhibition in patients with moderate heart failure reduces rate of myocardial infarction and reinfarction. Preliminary experimental evidence suggests that these clinical observations may be based upon an effect of the renin-angiotensin system on the endothelial release of nitric oxide. Nitric oxide (NO) in itself is potentially antiatherogenic, inhibits platelet aggregation, as well as transendothelial migration of lipoproteins, monocytes, and leucocytes. Therefore, activation of the renin angiotensin system may be pro-atherogenic. In animals with experimental or genetic hypertension, vasodilation mediated by release of endothelium-dependent (EDRF) relaxing factor is attenuated both in conductance and resistance arteries. This attenuated vasodilator capacity results mainly from a depressed capacity of the endothelium to produce nitric oxide. This phenomenon has been observed in many models of hypertension. In some of the models it may be related to a downregulation of the endothelial nitric oxide synthase (type 3).

Besides this downregulation of the main nitric oxide producing enzyme other factors may contribute to reduced nitric oxide production, for example, alterations in signal transduction of EDRF releasing receptors, enhanced diffusion distances for endothelial NO due to vascular remodeling in hypertension or increased breakdown of released nitric oxide due to enhanced local formation of free oxygen radicals. While all these mechanisms might be involved to various degrees, the downregulation of the NO synthase seems to be of central importance. Reversal of experimental hypertension restores reduced capacity to produce nitric oxide. Treatment with ACE-inhibitors leads to an improvement in NO production and of endothelial-dependent vasodilation. In rats with hypertension due to suprarenal coarctation of the aorta, chronic treatment with ACE-inhibition normalizes the depressed and/or mediated dilation without lowering elevated mean arterial pressure. Here, a pressure-independent mechanism of endothelial protection is demonstrated. In various models of renal or genetic hypertension the upregulated ACE expression is associated with downregulated expression of endothelial NO synthase and of endothelial NO production. Without normalizing the elevated blood pressure, chronic low-dose ACE inhibitor treatment normalizes the elevated local ACE activity, thereby upregulating depressed expression of endothelial NO production. Therefore, an inverse relationship between local vascular ACE activity and endothelial NO production can be demonstrated and related to the expression of the endothelial nitric oxide synthase of the type 3.

Interestingly, lowering local vascular ACE activity through ACE inhibition in animals on long-term atherogenic diet also enhances the depressed endothelium dependent relaxation in these animals. Hyperlipidemia in itself seems to possess the capacity to suppress endothelial NO production. Endothelial nitric oxide can inhibit several steps in the atherogenic process:

1. NO is an inhibitor of lipid oxidation, acting by radical scavenging, reducing oxidative modification of LDL.

2. NO is a potent inhibitor of platelet activation and aggregation.

3. NO exerts an inhibitory effect on monocyte adhesion to the endothelium and on transendothelial migration of monocytes.

4. NO attenuates accumulation of activated neutrophils in ischemic vascular beds.

5. NO attenuates vascular smooth muscle proliferation and can be considered a potent antiproliferate factor.

With these clearly antiarteriosclerotic effects of nitric oxide in mind, the reduced capacity to produce nitric oxide of the vascular endothelium in hypertension, diabetes, smoking, and in states of activated renin angiotensin system lends itself to an hypothesis linking disturbed endothelial function to premature development of arteriosclerosis.

The role of altered local bradykinin availability has not yet been clarified. Evidence has been presented whereby local bradykinin availability could be the mechanism by which a high local ACE activity downregulates NO synthase expression. Alterations of endothelial NO expression by bradykinin have only been demonstrated in cultured endothelial cells. Therefore, the question of the participation of bradykinin in this process remains open. It is likewise open for discussion that endothelial NO deficiency plays a permissive role in atherosclerosis development, or is a major and primary factor in atherogenesis. In the case of primarily altered, that is, increased activity of the renin angiotensin system with subsequent downregulation of endothelial NO synthase, a primary atherogenic role may be seen. On the other hand, antiatherosclerotic properties of a well-developed endothelial NO producing and releasing capacity may be conceivable and a therapeutic goal worth pursuing.

Selected Reading

1. Drexler H, Zeiher AM, Bassenge E, Just H: Endothelial mechanisms of vasomotor control. *Bas Res Card* (Supp) V86, 2, Steinkopff, Verlag Darmstadt, Springer-Verlag, New York 1991.
2. Hasenfuss G, Holubarsch C, Just H, Alpert NP: Cellular and molecular alterations in the failing human heart. *Bas Res Card* V87, 1, Steinkopff Verlag Darmstadt, Springer-Verlag, New York 1989.
3. Holtz J, Drexler H, Just H: Cardiac adaptation in heart failure. risks due to phenotype changes. *Bas Res Card* Steinkopff Verlag Darmstadt, Springer-Verlag, New York 1992.
4. Jacob R, Just H, Holubarsch C: Cardiac energetics. Basic mechanisms and clinical implications, *Bas Res Card* 82, 2, Steinkopff Verlag Darmstadt, Springer-Verlag, New York 1987.
5. Just H, Drexler H, Hasenfuss G: Pathophysiology and treatment of congestive heart failure. *Card* 84 (Supp) 2: 99-107, 1994.
6. Just H, Drexler H, Zelis R: Regional blood flow in congestive heart failure AJC suppl 8, V62, *York Medical Journal*, Cahners 1988.
7. Just H, Holubarsch C, Scholz H: Inotropic stimulation and myocardial energetics. *Bas Res Card* V84 1 Steinkopff Verlag, Darmstadt; Springer-Verlag, New York 1989.
8. Just H, Hort W, Zeiher AW: Arteriosclerosis: new insights into pathogenetic mechanisms and prevention. *Bas Res Card* V89, 2, Steinkopff Verlag, Darmstadt; Springer-Verlag, New York 1992.
9. Reindell H, Keul E, Doll E: *Heart Failure. Pathophysiological and Clinical Aspects*. G. Thieme Verlag, Stuttgart 1968.
10. Zeiher AM, Schachinger V, Saurbier B, Just H: Assessment of endothelial modulation of coronary vasomotor tone: insights into a fundamental functional disturbance in vascular biology of atherosclerosis. *Bas Res Card.* 89 (Supp) 1: 115-128, 1994.

CHAPTER 24

Pathophysiologic Mechanisms of Heart Disease: Clinical Correlations

Albert A. Del Negro, M.D.

An understanding of normal cardiovascular physiology is fundamental to understanding the pathophysiology of the changes that accompany heart disease. Such a thorough understanding assists in the proper differential diagnosis of the patient with cardiovascular disease and aids in the selection of therapy. The following is a discussion of normal cardiovascular physiology and the pathologic changes encountered in selected cardiovascular disease states. Where appropriate, this chapter will highlight clinical and laboratory findings when they amplify understanding of the physiology of the cardiovascular system.

Cardiovascular Hemodynamics

Normal Intracardiac Pressures

A graphic portrayal of pressure curves in the great vessels and the cardiac chambers illustrates the time and pressure relationships of the cardiac cycle (Figure 1). Ordinarily, right atrial and right ventricular intracardiac pressure is considerably lower than left atrial and left ventricular pressure. Normal right atrial pressure averages from 1 mmHg to 8 mmHg. During right ventricular diastole, there is no pressure gradient between right atrium and right ventricle, but as systole begins and the right ventricle contracts raising right ventricular pressure above atrial pressure, the tricuspid valve closes. The right ventricular pressure continues to rise throughout systole reaching a peak pressure of approximately 15 mmHg to 30 mmHg. Opening of the pulmonary valve occurs when the rising right ventricular pressure reaches the pul-

monary artery diastolic pressure. Main pulmonary artery pressure in peak systole is also 15 mmHg to 30 mmHg, and pulmonary artery diastolic pressure averages 4 mm Hg to 12 mmHg. The normal pulmonary vascular bed is very low in resistance; hence, there is no difference between pulmonary artery diastolic pressure and mean left atrial pressure under normal conditions. For this reason, in the absence of intrinsic pulmonary hypertension, left atrial pressure defines pulmonary artery diastolic pressure and plays a major role in the determination of pulmonary resistance.

Mean left atrial pressure can be determined by direct left atrial catheterization or by a measurement of the pulmonary capillary wedge pressure by occluding a pulmonary artery segment with a balloon-tipped catheter (Swan-Ganz catheter) which permits measurement of down-stream pressure across the low resistance pulmonary capillary bed. Like pulmonary artery diastolic pressure, pulmonary capillary pressure ranges from 4 mmHg to 12 mmHg. Left ventricular mean diastolic pressure is the same as left atrial mean pressure, averaging 4 mmHg to 12 mmHg. The contribution of atrial systole to ventricular filling "tops off" the pressure in the left ventricle and the degree to which this end-diastolic pressure rises with atrial systole is a measure of the distensibility or compliance of the left ventricle. Normal left ventricular end-diastolic pressure does not exceed 12 mmHg.

Onset of left ventricular systole raises the left ventricular pressure above left atrial pressure and closes the mitral valve just before closure of the tricuspid valve. Left ventricular peak systolic pres-

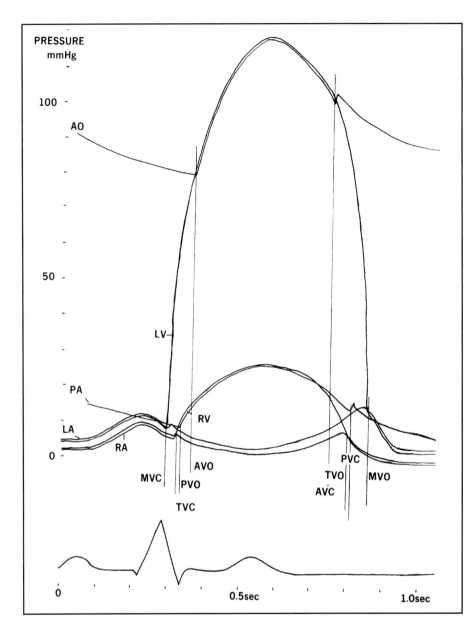

Figure 1. Schematic illustration of the normal cardiac cycle. (MVC = mitral valve closure; TVC = tricuspid valve closure; PVO = pulmonic valve opening; AVO = aortic valve opening; AVC = aortic valve closure; PVC = pulmonic valve closure; TVO = tricuspid valve opening; MVO = mitral valve opening; AO = aorta; PA = pulmonary artery; LA = left atrium; RA = right atrium; LV = left ventricle; RV = right ventricle.) *(From Del Negro AA, 7)*

sure normally is 100 mmHg to 120 mmHg. Aortic valve opening occurs when the rising left ventricular pressure exceeds aortic diastolic pressure. Central aortic and peripheral arterial blood pressure is also in the range of 100 mmHg to 120 mmHg at peak systolic pressure with diastolic pressure falling to 70 mmHg to 80 mmHg diastolic pressure. Mean central aortic pressure averages approximately 70 mmHg to 100 mmHg.

The cardiac output varies with patient size and, in the normal adult, averages approximately 4 liters to 5 liters per minute. The cardiac index is an expression of cardiac output normalized for body size and weight and is computed by dividing the body surface area, derived from height-weight normograms, into the cardiac output. If the average body surface area is approximately 2 m², then a

cardiac output of 5 liters per minute means that individual has a cardiac index of 2.5 liters per minute per square meter of body surface. A resting cardiac output of 0.8 liters per minute may be quite appropriate for an infant and allows calculation of a normal cardiac index of 2.7 liters per minute per square meter if the body surface area is 0.3 meters squared. Likewise, a cardiac output of 7 liters per minute may be normal for a large individual with a body surface area of 2.5 square meters. Normal cardiac index is 2.8 to 4.2 liters per minute per square meter.

Calculation of Resistance

Resistance in the pulmonary and systemic circulations is expressed in Wood units or in dynes/sec/cm⁻⁵. The total systemic resistance is calculated by

552

dividing the mean arterial blood pressure by the cardiac output (Table 1). A normal mean arterial blood pressure of 90 mmHg with a cardiac output of 5 liters per minute yields a total systemic resistance of 18 Wood units. To convert this to dynes sec cm^{-5}, the number of Wood units is multiplied by 80. The total systemic resistance calculated in this hypothetical case is therefore 1,240 dynes sec cm^{-5}. Normal total systemic resistance is 770 to 1500 dynes sec cm^{-5}.

Since the ultimate destination of blood leaving the left ventricle is the right atrium after passing through the systemic circulation, the right atrial mean pressure contributes some small quantity to systemic pressure and the calculation of systemic resistance. Ordinarily, this contribution is insignificant but subtracting mean right atrial pressure from mean arterial pressure prior to dividing by cardiac output removes its influence on systemic pressure and permits the calculation of systemic vascular resistance. Total pulmonary resistance is calculated by dividing the mean pulmonary artery pressure by the cardiac output. If we measure a normal pulmonary artery mean pressure of 15 mm Hg and divide that by a cardiac output of 5 liters per minute, we arrive at a total pulmonary resistance of 3 Wood units or 240 dynes sec cm^{-5}. However, if we subtract the contribution of the left atrial pressure to pulmonary artery pressure, a significantly lower calculation of pulmonary vascular resistance is achieved. Subtracting a normal mean left atrial pressure of 12 mmHg from the mean pulmonary artery pressure of 15 yields a difference of only 3 mmHg. Dividing this by a 5-liter-per-minute cardiac output yields a pulmonary vascular resistance of 0.6 Wood units or 48 dynes sec cm^{-5}.

Normal pulmonary vascular resistance is considerably lower than systemic vascular resistance and, in fact, pulmonary vasculature has an enormous reserve and capability for an increase in its capacitance. In addition, significant pulmonary hypertension may exist without an increase in pulmonary vascular resistance. This occurs in left ventricular failure with a left atrial mean pressure as high as 18 mmHg. In such a patient in whom the pulmonary artery pressure may be 40/18 with a mean pulmonary artery pressure of 26 mmHg, pulmonary artery pressures are elevated. However, if one subtracts the contribution of the mean left atrial pressure of 18 mmHg from the mean pulmonary artery pressure of 26 mmHg and divides that difference by a cardiac output of 4 liters per minute, we calculate a pulmonary vascular resistance of only 2 Wood units or 160 dynes sec cm^{-5}. Pulmonary vascular resistance is normal although total pulmonary

TABLE 1	
Physiologic Calculations	
CALCULATIONS	**NORMAL VALUES**
Cardiac Index = $\dfrac{\text{Cardiac Output}}{\text{Body Surface Area}}$	2.8 to 4.2 liters/min/m^2
Total Systemic Resistance = $\dfrac{\text{Mean Arterial Pressure}}{\text{Cardiac Output}}$	10 to 20 Wood Units (770 to 1500 dynes sec cm^{-5})
Systemic Vascular Resistance = $\dfrac{\text{Mean Arterial Pressure minus Mean Right Atrial Pressure}}{\text{Cardiac Output}}$	10 to 20 Wood Units (770 to 1500 dynes sec cm^{-5})
Total Pulmonary Resistance = $\dfrac{\text{Mean Pulmonary Arterial Pressure}}{\text{Cardiac Output}}$	1.3 to 3.8 Wood Units (100 to 300 dynes sec cm^{-5})
Pulmonary Vascular Resistance = $\dfrac{\text{Mean Pulmonary Arterial Pressure minus Mean Left Atrial Pressure}}{\text{Cardiac Output}}$	0.25 to 1.5 Wood Units (20 to 120 dynes sec cm^{-5})

resistance is elevated in this case because of an elevation of left atrial mean pressure secondary to left ventricular failure.

Conversely, the patient with pulmonary hypertension due to chronic recurrent pulmonary emboli or to chronic obstructive pulmonary disease with hypoxia may have a normal mean left atrial pressure but an elevated pulmonary artery mean pressure. If such a patient has a mean pulmonary artery pressure of 26 mmHg but only a mean left atrial pressure of 6 mmHg, then the assumption of a cardiac output of 4 liters per minute allows us to calculate a pulmonary vascular resistance of 5 Wood units (400 dynes sec cm^{-5}) which is above the upper limit of normal. Patients may maintain similar blood pressures over a relatively wide range of cardiac outputs. Changes in peripheral vascular resistance permit this maintenance of a narrow range of blood pressure despite a widely varying systemic flow. For instance, in a patient with a mean arterial pressure of 90 mmHg whose cardiac output is only 3 liters per minute, the blood pressure is maintained by a twofold increase in peripheral vascular resistance over normal. Congestive heart failure is characterized by such a low cardiac output and high peripheral vascular resistance leading to little or no change in measured peripheral arterial blood pressure. In an opposite fashion, increases in peripheral capacitance or reductions in peripheral vascular resistance may be able to accommodate large increases in cardiac output without change in blood pressure. For example, the patient with hyperthyroidism may have a cardiac output that is two or three times normal. This may occur with little change in measured peripheral arterial pressure because of a concomitant decrease in peripheral vascular resistance.

The Frank-Starling Curve

Two parameters of left ventricular performance can assess its function. The first is the cardiac output or stroke volume. The second is the mean left ventricular diastolic pressure (also the same as mean pulmonary capillary wedge pressure). By controlling all other external factors, such as afterload peripheral resistance and blood pressure, stroke volume and cardiac output will increase if one is able to increase diastolic filling. Conversely, reduced left ventricular filling will result in a drop in stroke volume and cardiac output. Varying the left ventricular diastolic pressure and thereafter measuring the cardiac output enables us to describe a left ventricular function curve or Frank-Starling curve (Figure 2).

The left ventricle can operate on any number of such curves, which vary according to performance. A failing left ventricle shifts to a curve at a lower level, resulting in a lower stroke volume and cardiac output for a given mean diastolic pressure or volume. Increasing mean diastolic pressure or volume in the normal left ventricle would ordinarily raise stroke volume, but because the Frank-Starling curve of congestive heart failure is relatively flat, increases in mean diastolic volume and pressure cause little augmentation of stroke volume. Improving performance of the failing left ventricle will cause a shift to a higher, more normal curve. One can achieve this by increasing the inotropic state of the myocardium with the addition of cardiotonic agents such as digitalis or sympathomimetic amines. Exercise alone, which increases circulating catecholamines, shifts the curve in a normal subject to a higher and steeper one where there is a greater stroke volume and cardiac output for the same left ventricular mean diastolic volume and pressure. Fundamental changes in the myocardium can suddenly result in a rise in left ventricular mean diastolic pressure without a change in diastolic volume. Myocardial ischemia results in such a change and is usually associated with a drop in cardiac output without a change in diastolic left ventricular volume. This is the case because ischemia causes a reduction in myocardial diastolic relaxation or loss of left ventricular diastolic compliance. Even though mean left ventricular diastolic pressure is elevated acutely, left ventricular diastolic volume is unchanged and stroke volume and cardiac output fall to some degree because ischemia impairs contractility by a shift to a flatter Frank-Starling curve. This fall may be reversed by relief of ischemia, which restores the pressure-volume relationship in the left ventricle to normal and improves systolic performance, thus restoring cardiac output to control levels.

Valvular Heart Disease

Aortic Stenosis

• Pathophysiology

Severe aortic stenosis imposes a heavy burden on a left ventricle by causing it to generate systolic pressures far in excess of those usually demanded of that chamber. The response of the left ventricle is to hypertrophy initially without associated dilatation. Oxygen consumption is thus increased by two mechanisms. The first is the increased work of contracting in order to generate higher-than-normal systolic pressures to overcome the obstructed aortic valve. The second is the increased left ventricular muscle mass, which occurs as a compensatory response. Even though there may be no associated coronary artery disease, a disparity may exist between the oxygen supply available to the myocardium through the coronary arteries and the oxygen demand imposed by the hypertrophied left ventricle pumping against an obstructive aortic valve. This is especially the case under conditions of exertion which exaggerates the disparity between oxygen supply and demand. This oxygen imbalance explains the syndrome of angina pectoris associated with this lesion. Commonly the angina is mistaken for that of coronary artery disease where no important coronary disease exists and where the diagnosis of severe aortic stenosis has been overlooked. More confusing is the fact that the angina of aortic stenosis may be treated successfully with many of the same therapeutic modalities useful in the treatment of angina due to coronary artery disease. It is typical for the angina to be relieved by the use of nitroglycerin, for instance, although beta blockers would be expected to worsen the syndrome and perhaps to precipitate congestive failure.

It is well appreciated that angina is a frequent symptom in patients having aortic valve stenosis. About 50% of the patients with angina pectoris have significant coronary artery disease. Aortic valve replacement gives relief of angina in the patients whose coronary arteriograms are normal. When coronary bypass is performed in addition to aortic valve replacement in those patients having coronary arterial disease, the surgical mortality is higher and relief of angina pectoris less predictable. The suggestion that coronary arteriography be performed on all patients over the age 40 in whom surgery is being considered for aortic stenosis makes good sense.

W. Proctor Harvey, M.D.

Congestive heart failure is a critically important finding in the presence of severe aortic stenosis. The primary diagnosis of critical aortic stenosis may be overlooked because, in the presence of congestive heart failure with a reduced cardiac output, the flow across the aortic valve is greatly diminished thereby rendering a smaller transaortic valve gradient and a much softer murmur than would be anticipated in severe aortic stenosis. Additionally, in congestive heart failure due to aortic stenosis the clinical picture is so dominated by dyspnea and the physical findings of gallop rhythm, mitral and tricuspid regurgitation, and elevated venous pressure, that the diagnosis of severe aortic stenosis is easily overlooked. Because calcification of the aortic valve is associated with congestive failure due to severe aortic stenosis, all patients with heart failure and an ejection murmur, however soft, should undergo fluoroscopy to look for the presence of aortic valve

calcium. If calcium is noted in the aortic valve the diagnosis is severe aortic stenosis until proven otherwise. The emphasis on echocardiography as a screening tool in cases of congestive failure also is an aid to the diagnosis.

Etiology of congestive heart failure in aortic stenosis is not well understood but it is presumed to be due to the chronic high systolic pressure that is imposed on left ventricular performance. Even in circumstances where heart failure is quite refractory and left ventricular performance is quite compromised, it may be lifesaving to perform aortic valve replacement. The most ominous symptom of aortic stenosis is syncope or presyncope. In the young patient this may be the first sign of severe aortic stenosis. The significance of this symptom is that it may portend sudden death. In elderly patients, syncope and sudden death are less common than angina pectoris or congestive heart failure, but they are equally feared as symptoms.

The etiology of syncope is a marked reduction in cardiac output, leading to hypoperfusion of the central nervous system and unconsciousness. This usually occurs under conditions of exercise, because of increased peripheral capacitance as skeletal muscle vasculature dilates resulting in reduced peripheral vascular resistance. In the normal individual the increased capacitance can easily be filled by an increase in cardiac output. However, the patient with severe aortic stenosis cannot augment his cardiac output to a level sufficient to fill the increased volume of the vascular bed, and if the increased capacitance is not met by rising cardiac output, blood pressure will fall. The central nervous system and the heart may be underperfused. This will lead to a reduction in coronary blood flow and a compromise of left ventricular performance at a time when

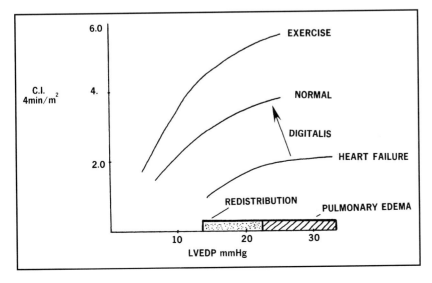

Figure 2. Schematic illustration of a series of Frank-Starling curves relating cardiac index (CI) to left ventricular end-diastolic pressure (LVEDP). The curve describing the failing left ventricle shows that for the same diastolic pressure there is a much lower cardiac index when compared to normal. Use of cardiotonic agents such as digitalis may restore the curve toward normal. Radiographically evident pulmonary redistribution and edema correlate with elevated LVEDP as noted. *(From Del Negro AA, 7)*

supranormal left ventricular performance is demanded. The resultant ischemia may lead to ventricular irritability producing ventricular tachycardia and ventricular fibrillation which is, of course, a fatal arrhythmia. This is understood to be the mechanism of syncope and sudden death in patients with severe aortic stenosis.

• Clinical Findings

History: Many patients present with asymptomatic murmurs. Other patients may come to medical attention because of chest pain, congestive heart failure, or syncope. Most patients under the age of 20 are asymptomatic, but in this age group, when severe aortic stenosis appears, symptoms consist of both presyncope and syncope. Congestive heart failure and chest pain are rare in this age group. Syncope may be the prelude to sudden death, and this symptom should be the signal to start a full evaluation.

Physical Exam: In the young individual with mild aortic stenosis, the only important physical finding may be that of an ejection murmur at the base of the heart radiating to the carotid arteries. Young patients should have an ejection sound to accompany this murmur. The pulse contour should feel normal unless the aortic stenosis is severe. The classical finding of the pulsus parvus and pulsus tardus in severe aortic stenosis is more typical of patients in the age group of 40 years to 60 years. In this circumstance, the ejection sound is usually absent because the valve is so severely stenosed that sudden doming of leaflets at the beginning of systole, which is responsible for the ejection sound, cannot occur. Usually by this point the valve architecture has become so deformed that the murmur of aortic incompetence is also present.

Another sign of severe aortic stenosis is the loss of the aortic component of the second heart sound. In such circumstances one hears only a single second heart sound irrespective of the phase of respiration. Again, this is because of the lack of mobility of the leaflets, which prevents them from closing briskly at the end of systole, thereby preventing them from generating any aortic closure sound. As mentioned above, occasionally a patient will present with far-advanced left ventricular failure. In this circumstance, with cardiac output markedly reduced, flow across the aortic valve is likewise diminished. Consequently, the transvalvular gradient and the intensity of the murmur will be less than expected for a case of severe aortic stenosis. In addition, findings of congestive heart failure, including mitral regurgitation, gallop rhythm, evidence for pulmonary hypertension, and even right heart failure with tricuspid regurgitation, pulsatile hepatomegaly and ascites, may so dominate the clinical picture that auscultation misses a soft aortic stenosis ejection murmur.

CARDIAC PEARL

It is surprising to find, at times, how advanced congestive heart failure can alter heart murmurs. A patient personally evaluated had severe calcific aortic stenosis (necropsy). He had, at one stage during his life, a loud, harsh grade V aortic systolic murmur associated with a palpable thrill. Advanced heart failure ensued and the murmur and thrill disappeared. At that time, one physician, examining the patient for the first time and not being aware of his previous findings on physical examination, brought up the possibility of constrictive pericarditis, since many of the patient's physical findings were related to the right side of the heart.

W. Proctor Harvey, M.D.

• Laboratory Findings

Electrocardiogram: The electrocardiogram typically shows normal sinus rhythm. In the younger patient without severe aortic stenosis the electrocardiogram may be entirely normal. However, a clue to advancing severity of aortic stenosis may be provided in the asymptomatic patient who is less than 20 years of age and in whom new S-T and T wave changes are found that suggest left ventricular strain. The finding of increased left ventricular voltage is not a reliable sign of severe aortic stenosis in the young patient because it is not uncommon to have increased left ventricular forces in the normal person of less than 20 years. In patients older than 40 years, severe aortic stenosis is usually accompanied by signs of left ventricular hypertrophy consisting of increased left ventricular voltages in the precordial leads, S-T and T changes, and left atrial enlargement. As mentioned earlier, it is typical to have normal sinus rhythm on the electrocardiogram in patients with significant aortic stenosis. However, if the rhythm is atrial fibrillation, this may be a clue to the coexisting presence of mitral stenosis in the patient whose etiology of aortic stenosis is rheumatic heart disease.

CARDIAC PEARL

It is worthy of reemphasis that patients with a rheumatic etiology of aortic valve stenosis frequently have associated mitral valve involvement. When only the aortic valve is involved and the stenosis has been thought to be on a rheumatic basis it is much more likely that it will be on a congenital basis. Another clinical finding (cardiac pearl) that has stood the test of time is that if a patient has what appears to be evidence of only aortic valve disease, such as aortic stenosis, and atrial fibrillation is present, there probably is a 90% chance that there is concomitant mitral valve involvement, thereby affording another clue as to the presence of associated mitral valve disease. It is a known clinical point that patients with isolated aortic valve disease, either stenosis or insufficiency or both generally are in normal sinus rhythm.

W. Proctor Harvey, M.D.

Echocardiogram: The echocardiogram in severe aortic stenosis usually shows left ventricular hypertrophy. This is a more sensitive index of left ventricular hypertrophy than the electrocardiogram. In the patient with congenital aortic stenosis due to a bicuspid aortic valve the M-mode echocardiogram of the aortic valve may show an eccentric closure point. In severe aortic stenosis a diminished aortic valve opening may be documented on echocardiogram. As the aortic valve becomes more heavily calcified one will see increased density of echoes reflected back from the region of the aortic valve. Doppler examination is accurate in estimation of the gradient across the aortic valve as well as calculation of the valve area. Doppler studies may also identify coexisting aortic insufficiency. Finally, for patients who have had severe left ventricular decompensation due to aortic stenosis or coexisting coronary artery disease, a dilated and poorly contracting, although hypertrophied, left ventricle may be seen.

Cardiac Catheterization: Cardiac catheterization has as its goal the documentation of the severity of aortic stenosis, the documentation of the status of the coronary arteries, and the estimation of left ventricular performance as measured by ejection fraction. In addition, other valvular abnormalities such as coexisting mitral stenosis or insufficiency may be documented and their severity quantitated precisely. Simultaneous measurement of left ventricular and peripheral arterial pressure is essential for the documentation of the severity of aortic stenosis.

It is important to obtain an accurate measurement of cardiac output when documenting the transaortic valve gradient in order to estimate the aortic valve area. This yields a more accurate determination of the severity of aortic stenosis than the

measurement of the gradient alone because low cardiac output states may be associated with very low gradients, even in the face of severe aortic stenosis. The valve area calculated using the Gorlin formula takes into account not only the gradient but also the cardiac output. This formula provides an accurate estimation of the valve area over a wide range of cardiac outputs and valve gradients. Since the advent of Doppler evaluation, the measurement of gradients and the calculation of aortic valve area by cardiac catheterization is of less critical importance. This relegates the role of cardiac catheterization to the diagnosis of coexistent coronary artery disease. Cardiac catheterization thus should include coronary arteriography, especially in the elderly patient who may also present with angina pectoris.

Although some dispute exists about the safety of left ventriculography in severe aortic stenosis, it is a safe procedure when properly performed. The large volumes of contrast material that may induce peripheral vasodilatation have the potential to precipitate a drop in peripheral vascular resistance, which may compromise blood pressure. This risk can be minimized by utilizing smaller quantities of contrast material and by paying adequate attention to the state of hydration prior to left ventriculography.

The diagnosis of severe aortic stenosis is justified by the finding of a significantly reduced aortic valve area of less than one square centimeter. With children, it is more appropriate to calculate an aortic valve index, which normalizes the valve area for the body surface area. Valve area index, however, is less relied upon as a guide to the severity of aortic stenosis than the valve area in adults. In children it is also less commonly used because the valve gradient alone is a sensitive index of the severity of aortic stenosis. This is the case because congestive heart failure with a low stroke volume is exceedingly rare in the congenital aortic stenosis patient less than 20 years of age.

Aortic Insufficiency

• Pathophysiology

Significant aortic insufficiency imposes a volume load on the left ventricle. If half of each stroke volume of the left ventricle regurgitates back into that chamber, then the heart pumps 2 liters for every liter that it sends to the body. In a patient with a 50% regurgitant fraction, the heart must pump 10 L/min in order to maintain a normal forward cardiac output. This is the essential problem with aortic insufficiency, which over a period of years causes

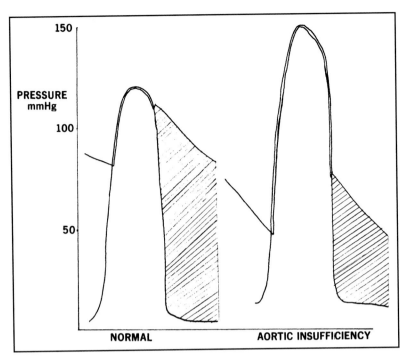

Figure 3. Schematic illustration of normal left ventricular and aortic pressure curves (left) and pressure curves seen in severe aortic insufficiency (right). The shaded areas represent the transmyocardial perfusion pressure, which is reduced in aortic insufficiency. A further reduction in this gradient occurs as left ventricular failure produces a rise in left ventricular diastolic pressure. This reduced perfusion pressure diminishes oxygen delivery in the face of increased demand and is the mechanism for angina pectoris in isolated severe aortic insufficiency. *(From Del Negro AA, 7)*

a diminution in left ventricular systolic function because of the chronically overtaxed cardiac systolic performance. Unfortunately, repair of the aortic insufficiency after developing left ventricular failure does not always improve left ventricular performance. This is because the diminution in systolic function by chronic aortic insufficiency may not be reversible if surgery is delayed beyond certain ill-defined end-points. A cardinal hallmark of aortic insufficiency is left ventricular dilatation. If the cardiac output normally is 5 L/minute and aortic insufficiency causes a 50% regurgitant fraction, compensatory dilation of the left ventricle occurs to maintain cardiac output in the normal range because half of each stroke volume regurgitates into the left ventricle. Analysis of the diastolic function of the left ventricle in patients with aortic insufficiency shows that left ventricular mean diastolic pressure remains in the normal range over a very wide range of left ventricular diastolic volume. This relationship defines a compliant left ventricular diastolic state. This is fortunately the case in patients with chronic aortic insufficiency because if it were not possible to maintain normal diastolic pressures with large diastolic volumes, then prompt elevation of left ventricular diastolic pressure would occur producing the clinical picture of congestive heart failure.

Patients with chronic aortic insufficiency and dilated left ventricles have a high oxygen demand imposed on the coronary bed because of increased left ventricular diameter as well increased left ventricular muscle mass. These factors increase wall tension and elevated oxygen demand. In addition, the higher-than-normal stroke volume also obligates higher oxygen demand. Consequently, patients with limitation of coronary blood flow due to coronary artery disease are especially prone to left ventricular ischemia and angina pectoris. Even in the patient with normal coronary arteries, the ability of the coronary blood flow to rise may be insufficient to meet the increased oxygen demand of the myocardium. Failure to increase oxygen delivery to meet demand may not be due to any intrinsic abnormality of the coronary arteries, but is unique to hemodynamics of aortic insufficiency. The normal patient has a diastolic arterial pressure of 80 mmHg. Because coronary blood flow occurs mainly during diastole, the pressure gradient between the diastolic arterial pressure and the left ventricular diastolic pressure will determine the transmyocardial perfusion pressure, which in the normal individual ranges close to 70 mmHg (Figure 3). This wide pressure gradient facilitates coronary blood flow and delivery of oxygen to the myocardium. In the patient with chronic aortic insufficiency, the diastolic arterial pressure may be as low as 40 mm Hg. Even if the left ventricular diastolic pressure is normal at 10 mmHg to 12 mmHg, the transmyocardial perfusion pressure will approximate only 30 mmHg. This narrow transmyocardial perfusion pressure compromises coronary blood flow in chronic aortic insufficiency and creates a state of relative cardiac ischemia.

The patient who develops left ventricular failure with severe chronic aortic sufficiency is worse off.

The chronic state of aortic insufficiency results in an elevation of left ventricular diastolic pressure as left ventricular performance declines further narrowing the transmyocardial perfusion pressure. In such a patient, delivery of oxygen-rich blood to the myocardium will diminish which may further deteriorate diastolic left ventricular function and lead to a further decline in systolic function. Given an understanding of this physiology, it is not difficult to understand why the patient with chronic aortic insufficiency may develop angina pectoris even in the absence of coronary artery disease. Aortic insufficiency can occur abruptly, such as in a patient with acute bacterial endocarditis which destroys a previously normal aortic valve, or a dissecting aortic aneurysm which causes insufficiency of the valve because of loss of the support for the sinuses of Valsalva. A sudden massive leak of the aortic valve induced by these clinical circumstances leaves the left ventricle totally unprepared to accept the large diastolic volumes imposed by acute insufficiency. The result is that the left ventricular diastolic pressure rises abruptly. This is reflected back to the left atrium and into the pulmonary capillary bed, and prompt pulmonary edema occurs. In addition, left ventricular dilatation cannot occur quickly enough to accommodate the severe and sudden incompetence of the aortic valve; therefore, heart size usually is normal early in the course of acute aortic insufficiency in the face of a normal or near-normal left ventricular dimension.

Another factor that makes acute aortic insufficiency especially dangerous is that there is compromise of diastolic filling of the left ventricle from the left atrium. This is the case not only because of the high left ventricular diastolic pressures due to poor left ventricular compliance but also because as regurgitation occurs, the rising left ventricular diastolic pressure may quickly exceed the mean left atrial pressure well before diastole is finished. This will prematurely close the mitral valve before complete left atrial emptying has occurred.

CARDIAC PEARL

The faint grade 1 or 3 aortic diastolic murmur of a congenital bicuspid aortic valve is frequently overlooked. Infective endocarditis following simple dental extractions, cleaning, or filling may affect the valve, damage it and produce wide-open severe aortic regurgitation requiring valve replacement.

This emphasizes the need for early surgical treatment for acute severe aortic insufficiency, such as may result from infective endocarditis. Worthy of emphasis is that the

physician may be misled by the fact that the diastolic blood pressure might not be as low as is the usual pressure in chronic severe aortic insufficiency, where the diastolic blood pressure may be 40, 30, with sounds heard down to 0. However, in some cases of the acute type, the blood pressure may be in the range such as 116/76 mmHg, thereby misleading the physician into thinking that it is not severe. Another clue is the fact that the 1st heard sound may be faint. A premature closure of mitral valve can occur, at times prominent or even loud, and can be misinterpreted as either the 1st or 2nd heart sound. It is an extra sound resulting from this premature closure of the mitral valve, occurring when the left ventricular end-diastolic pressure exceeds the left atrial and pulmonary capillary pressure.

It is important to recognize this acute, severe aortic insufficiency and to move quickly for surgical replacement, which can be lifesaving; delay, on the other hand, may be lethal.

W. Proctor Harvey, M.D.

• Clinical Findings

History: Early in aortic insufficiency no symptoms occur because degree of insufficiency is mild. Even after aortic insufficiency quantitatively increases and cardiomegaly occurs, there still may be no symptoms. The patient with chronic aortic insufficiency comes to medical attention usually with development of one of three symptoms. The first is congestive heart failure. This is quite an ominous sign in aortic insufficiency and implies that gradual loss of diastolic compliance of the left ventricle has occurred, which is most typically due to chronic volume overload. This is especially dangerous because it is usually accompanied by diminution in systolic function that may not be recoverable even if aortic valve placement is performed. A second major symptom is fatigue, which is due to the drop in forward cardiac output caused by the diminution in systolic function. Fatigue and symptoms of congestive heart failure almost always coexist in severe aortic insufficiency; a third important symptom is that of angina pectoris, which occurs for the reasons mentioned above.

CARDIAC PEARL

Patients with severe aortic regurgitation may have chest pain localized to the substernal area that can be so severe as to simulate acute myocardial infarction.

I remember a West Virginia mountaineer

who had severe, advanced aortic regurgitation. His bedroom was heated by a wood stove and on awakening in the morning, as he started the fire in the wood stove to heat up the cold bedroom, he would have onset of severe substernal precordial pain. He claimed he would set fire to an entire set of book matches and inhale the heat. This would relieve his chest pain. No electrocardiographic evidence of myocardial infarction could be found.

W. Proctor Harvey, M.D.

Patients with acute aortic insufficiency most typically present with acute pulmonary edema. The suddenness of the aortic insufficiency leaves the left ventricle unable to accept the large volume load as noted above, and left ventricular diastolic pressure rises precipitously producing the clinical picture of pulmonary edema with a relatively normal heart size initially. Infective endocarditis as the cause of aortic insufficiency may evade diagnosis at first. Commonly, if aortic insufficiency is mild initially, it is easily overlooked and fever is not connected with valvular infection. In such circumstances the initial diagnosis may be fever of unknown origin until positive blood cultures prompt the clinician to initiate a more careful cardiac examination. Aortic valve endocarditis due to an aggressive organism can lead to rapid destruction of the aortic valve and the clinical picture of acute severe aortic regurgitation with severe left ventricular failure. A less aggressive organism causing endocarditis and aortic sufficiency may produce mild chronic aortic insufficiency initially.

Numerous complications may befall the patient with ineffective endocarditis as a cause of aortic insufficiency. Vegetations on the aortic valve may become dislodged and cause septic systemic emboli. Regurgitation into the cavity of the left ventricle along the anterior mitral leaflet or chordal tendineae of the mitral valve may extend the infection to the mitral valve, causing perforation of the anterior leaflet and severe mitral insufficiency. Extension of the infection into the aortic annulus can result in ring abscess which may precipitate heart block because the atrioventricular conduction system lies subjacent to the aortic valve. Finally, rapid progressive left ventricular failure may occur. As with aortic stenosis, patients who have chronic, mild aortic insufficiency should begin antibiotic prophylaxis before dental procedures or other nonsterile procedures likely to cause bacteremia.

Physical Exam: The classical blood pressure finding in aortic insufficiency is a wide pulse pressure. The characteristic arterial pulse in pure aortic insufficiency is the bisferiens or twin-peaked pulse. Numerous bedside physical findings of aortic insufficiency have been described over the years. Some of these signs are Quincke's pulses, water-hammer pulse, and Duroziez's sign. These signs are of passing clinical importance because they are not present in all cases of aortic insufficiency nor are they an index of the severity of aortic insufficiency or of the need for operation. Jugular venous pulse evaluation usually is unremarkable unless there is such severe left ventricular failure that pulmonary hypertension and right ventricular failure occur as well. Auscultation of the heart may show a soft first heart sound and a normally split second heart sound. In pure aortic regurgitation or aortic regurgitation associated with mild aortic stenosis an ejection sound will be heard. There is almost always a systolic ejection murmur, due to the increased flow across the aortic valve or to associated valvular aortic stenosis. The high-pitched blowing diastolic murmur heard along the left sternal border diagnostic of aortic insufficiency is best heard with the patient leaning forward in forced expiration. The diaphragm of the stethoscope should be applied with firm pressure. Radiation of the diastolic murmur may give a clue to etiology of the aortic regurgitation; valvular aortic regurgitation generates a murmur that is best heard along the left sternal border. Aortic regurgitation that is due to dilatation of the aortic root, as in Marfan's Syndrome or aortic dissection, generates a murmur that radiates to the right of the sternum rather than to the left.

• Laboratory Findings

Electrocardiogram: In significant aortic regurgitation, left ventricular hypertrophy, usually associated with S-T and T-wave changes and left atrial enlargement, is the rule. Unless there is associated mitral stenosis, a patient's rhythm usually is normal. Echocardiogram will document dilatation of the heart as well as presence of left ventricular hypertrophy. A universal finding in significant aortic insufficiency is diastolic fluttering of the anterior mitral valve leaflet. This occurs because in diastole the left ventricle fills simultaneously by way of the left atrium and the aortic root. The anterior mitral leaflet is the structure that divides these two pathways of left ventricular filling and flutters during diastole as it is caught in the streams filling the ventricle from each aspect. A dilated aortic root can be documented on echocardiogram, and left atrial enlargement may also be noted as a reflection of left ventricular failure. Premature mitral valve closure is found in acute severe aortic insufficiency.

560

Echocardiogram: The echocardiogram is a sensitive tool to aid clinicians in deciding the proper time for surgery. A left ventricular end-systolic dimension of 5.5 cm or greater reflects left ventricular dilation as well as diminished left ventricular systolic effort. Associated with this finding is a poor outcome following aortic valve replacement. In these patients, left ventricular hypertrophy fails to regress and continued evidence of left ventricular dysfunction persists despite relief of aortic insufficiency by aortic valve replacement. Hence, many clinicians use this finding is a sensitive marker of the need for aortic valve replacement. Thus, the cardiac output and stroke volume are usually in the normal range so that one may rely on the measurement of valve gradient alone to estimate severity of aortic stenosis.

Mitral Stenosis

• Pathophysiology

In mitral stenosis due to rheumatic heart disease, early symptoms are absent. It is interesting to note that in acute rheumatic fever mitral stenosis does not exist, although mitral valve insufficiency is present. As the initial valve lesion heals, leaving a scarred valve, the wear and tear on the valve over time produces progressive stenosis and fusion of the commissures occurs. Furthermore, shortening and fusion of the chordae tendineae also may contribute to obstruction.

Obstruction at the mitral valve obstructs emptying of the left atrium and elevates the left atrial pressure. The pressure rise is reflected across the pulmonary vascular bed and raises the pulmonary artery pressure. In the mitral stenosis patient at rest, however, the mean left atrial pressure may be only 13 mmHg to 14 mmHg or slightly above the upper limit of normal in this early stage of the disease. This will have little impact on pulmonary artery pressure which may be normal under the circumstances.

Patients with more severe obstruction at the mitral valve level have mean left atrial pressures ranging from 18 mmHg to 20 mmHg. This means that the pulmonary artery diastolic pressure is at least 20 mmHg and, as a reflection of the obstruction at the mitral valve level, pulmonary artery systolic pressure also is elevated in the range of 45 mmHg. Pulmonary artery mean pressure will be measured at approximately 25 mmHg in such a patient. This is considered moderate pulmonary hypertension, but because there is no difference between pulmonary artery diastolic pressure and left atrial mean pressure, pulmonary vascular resistance is entirely normal. If one calculates the pulmonary vascular resistance in such a circumstance in a patient with a cardiac output to five liters per minute, one measures a resistance of only one Wood unit, or within normal limits. The pulmonary hypertension in such a circumstance is passive because it is entirely due to elevation of left atrial pressure. Among initial therapies for heart failure in mitral stenosis are diuretics and digitalis. Unless the rhythm is atrial fibrillation with rapid ventricular response, digitalis in this setting is of little value because left ventricular function in mitral stenosis is usually normal and the "heart failure" is not due to left ventricular factors.

It is instead due to high pressure in the left atrium secondary to mitral valve obstruction. Diuresis achieves one important end in such a circumstance by reducing the intravascular volume which in turn reduces the cardiac output. As the cardiac output falls and flow across the mitral valve is reduced, left atrial pressure will fall and pulmonary vascular congestion will improve.

In clinically significant mitral stenosis, two factors will elevate left atrial pressure. One is volume overload which results in a normal or near-normal cardiac output. If the mitral stenosis is severe enough, normal flows across the mitral valve will obligate a high left atrial pressure and create the clinical picture of pulmonary vascular congestion and heart failure. Interestingly, another factor is heart rate. As heart rate increases, it does so mainly at the expense of a shortened diastolic filling time since systolic ejection time is relatively fixed over a wide range of heart rates. That results in a shortened diastolic filling time as heart rate increases. This leaves the atrium less time per cardiac cycle to empty completely. The result is a high left atrial residual volume at the end of each diastole, which, added to the incoming blood from the pulmonary veins, elevates the left atrial pressure.

This is why it is not surprising for a patient with significant mitral stenosis who has no evidence of heart failure in normal sinus rhythm at rest to develop signs of pulmonary edema associated with the onset of paroxysmal atrial fibrillation and a rapid ventricular response. The use of betablockers or verapamil and diltiazem to slow the ventricular response is helpful in this circumstance because they slow the ventricular response, producing a lengthening of the diastolic filling period and permitting more complete atrial emptying during each cardiac cycle. In the past, digitalis was the drug of choice for the treatment of the rapid ventricular response to atrial fibrillation, but it may be relatively ineffective in this situation when used alone.

The patient with mitral stenosis will pass through four distinct stages in the course of rheumatic heart disease. These stages correspond to significantly different clinical patterns. The first is the asymptomatic stage, in which there is minimal mitral valve obstruction early in the disease. This results in little if any elevation of left atrial pressure and little or no pulmonary hypertension. The second stage is associated with more progressive mitral valve obstruction. As mitral stenosis worsens, left atrial pressure elevates even in the resting state and the response to exercise with an increased heart rate is even further elevation of left atrial pressure. This results in a high pulmonary venous pressure and consequently a high pulmonary capillary wedge pressure. Passive pulmonary hypertension develops and, because pulmonary compliance is reduced by the high pulmonary venous pressure, the work of breathing is increased and dyspnea becomes an important clinical symptom. The next stage is associated with the development of active pulmonary hypertension. After exposure to a high left atrial pressure for many years, the intima of the pulmonary arterioles thicken and the muscular media hypertrophy. Pulmonary hypertension develops with increased pulmonary vascular resistance in response to chronically elevated left atrial pressure. In this circumstance, pulmonary artery diastolic pressure is higher than left atrial pressure, which nonetheless is still elevated. Until this point there has been no compromise of cardiac output, and dyspnea continues to be an important symptom.

The next phase in the course of the patient with mitral stenosis is the development of right heart failure because of chronic pulmonary hypertension, which is now severe. This phase is dominated clinically by signs of right heart failure associated with tricuspid regurgitation, a high right atrial pressure, signs of hepatic congestion, ascites, and peripheral edema. Cardiac output is reduced in these circumstance because of the right heart failure; hence, flow across all the valves of the heart, including the stenosed mitral valve, is reduced. Paradoxically, dyspnea no longer becomes a problem but is replaced by fatigue as the dominant clinical symptom. It's important for the clinician to recognize that this is a sign of advanced mitral stenosis and is due to a reduction in the cardiac output. Patients should not be permitted to progress to the last stage of mitral stenosis. The operation for replacement of the mitral valve in such a circumstance is associated with a higher mortality rate, and there may be the need for additional surgery to treat the significant tricuspid insufficiency that has occurred as a consequence of right heart failure.

• Clinical Findings

History: As indicated above, the history in patients with mitral stenosis early in its course may be unimpressive. In fact, only approximately 50% of the patients who have rheumatic mitral valve stenosis know that they have suffered an episode of rheumatic fever. As mitral valve obstruction becomes more severe with progressive valve scarring, dyspnea and later active pulmonary hypertension and right heart failure dominate the scene. Arrhythmias are common in mitral stenosis. The most common arrhythmia, of course, is atrial fibrillation and this is associated with a significant incidence of systemic embolization. With obstruction at the mitral valve level, atrial fibrillation results in loss of active atrial contraction, resulting in marked stasis of blood in the left atrium contributing to potential for atrial appendage thrombosis. It is from such thrombi that small clots may embolize to the systemic circulation and cause important end-organ deficits. For this reason it's important to treat the patient with mitral stenosis who has atrial fibrillation with anticoagulants. Incidence of emboli seems to be the highest in the first year after the onset of atrial fibrillation, although it is associated generally with advanced degrees of mitral valve obstruction. Nevertheless, lifelong anticoagulation after the onset of atrial fibrillation is recommended.

CARDIAC PEARL

A history of rheumatic fever or symptoms of same should be specifically asked about; fortunately today, in most sections of the United States, the incidence of rheumatic heart disease has declined greatly and it would be a very uncommon cause of a murmur. A "cardiac pearl"- if there is a history of rheumatic fever, there is a 50% chance of having a rheumatic heart; another "pearl"- only one-half of patients having rheumatic mitral stenosis have a history of rheumatic fever.

This "50% rule" is an easy way to remember both of these observations.

There is a so-called rheumatic triad- rheumatic fever, mitral stenosis, atrial fibrillation. When two of these are present, the other will also be evident or probably will be forthcoming.

For example, if a patient has mitral stenosis and a history of rheumatic fever, even though there is normal sinus rhythm at the time of your examination, it is likely that atrial fibrillation will develop in the future.

W. Proctor Harvey, M.D.

Physical Exam: A common finding in significant mitral stenosis is the irregularly irregular pulse. This is due to atrial fibrillation. The examination of the chest may show rales if there is significant pulmonary venous congestion. The jugular venous pulse may be normal in early stages but in late stages will be elevated and have a contour consistent with tricuspid regurgitation. Palpation of the precordium will demonstrate a palpable second heart sound due to pulmonary hypertension and also will show a left parasternal lift in early systole that is consistent with right ventricular hypertrophy. Cardiac auscultation will demonstrate a loud first heart sound and a normally split second heart sound with an increased pulmonary closure sound. The opening snap associated with mitral stenosis is best heard at the cardiac apex or along the left sternal border. Its proximity to the aortic component of the second heart sound is predictive of left atrial pressure and correlates well with severity of mitral stenosis. A short interval between the aortic component of the second heart sound and the opening snap indicates a severe case of mitral stenosis; diastolic rumble of mitral stenosis is best heard at the cardiac apex, and in severe cases of mitral stenosis will last the duration of diastole. In later stages of mitral stenosis, mitral insufficiency accompanies the murmur of mitral stenosis because the valve apparatus becomes so scarred and fixed that it is incapable of competent closure. In patients with advanced mitral stenosis, right-sided heart failure dominates the clinical picture. The lungs may be free of rales, but one may note the elevated venous pressure and tricuspid regurgitation, both by presence of the murmur along the left sternal border that increases with inspirations and by a pulsatile and engorged liver. In such a circumstance ascites and significant peripheral edema also are present.

• Laboratory Findings

Electrocardiogram: The electrocardiogram in advanced mitral stenosis usually shows atrial fibrillation. If normal sinus rhythm is present, one should be able to note presence of left atrial enlargement. Varying degrees of right ventricular hypertrophy may be seen on the electrocardiogram, ranging from mild right axis deviation and shallow S waves in lead V_1, to overt evidence of right ventricular hypertrophy with monophasic tall R waves in V_1. Rarely is there associated evidence for left ventricular hypertrophy unless there is coexistent aortic stenosis or severe mitral insufficiency.

Echocardiogram: The echocardiogram is vitally important in assessment of mitral stenosis. Not only can the size of the left atrium be measured directly noninvasively, but the orifice area of the mitral valve can be calculated with the Doppler technique. If a good-quality echo can be obtained, calculation of the mitral valve area by 2-D echo should correlate closely with that derived from cardiac catheterization. Presence of tricuspid regurgitation permits the estimation of the peak systolic pulmonary artery pressure.

Cardiac Catheterization: All patients expected to require mitral valve replacement should undergo cardiac catheterization. The diagnostic goals of catheterization are to document the severity of mitral stenosis, to assess degree of pulmonary hypertension, evaluate presence or absence of mitral regurgitation that may contribute to the gradient; to assess left ventricular systolic function, evaluate other possible valve pathology such as associated aortic stenosis or aortic insufficiency, and assess status of the coronary arteries. Using a formula derived by Gorlin and Gorlin, one may calculate the mitral valve area with accuracy in mitral stenosis. This formula, similar to that for aortic stenosis, but using a different constant, takes into account mean valve gradient, cardiac output, and diastolic filling period to calculate valve area. Mitral valve areas of 1.2 cm^2 or less indicate clinically important mitral stenosis and the need for mitral valve replacement. Valve areas of greater than 1.2 cm^2 generally are not associated with clinically important symptoms and hence are evocative of mild stenosis only. The importance of preoperative cardiac catheterization is paramount. Some patients with mild mitral stenosis will have important congestive symptoms not due to mitral stenosis but instead due to associated left ventricular dysfunction. Clinically, dyspnea of severe left ventricular failure and that of advanced mitral stenosis are indistinguishable, whereas a carefully done catheterization will be able to differentiate between these two problems and avoid unwarranted surgery in the latter case.

Pericardial Disease

Important physiologic states associated with pericardial disease are those of cardiac tamponade and chronic constrictive pericarditis. There are numerous causes of cardiac tamponade, including acute viral pericarditis with significant accumulation of pericardial fluid, uremic pericarditis, and pericarditis associated with metastatic disease to the pericardium. In children especially, bacterial infection of the pericardium may lead to cardiac tamponade. Chronic constrictive pericarditis is a late sequelum, usually of acute pericarditis, which

563

may have been occult in presentation. The over-whelming majority of patients with chronic constrictive pericarditis probably had an episode of acute viral pericarditis at some time. Tuberculous pericarditis is a less common cause of chronic constriction in the modern era than it was in the pre-antibiotic era.

Cardiac Tamponade

• Physiology

Cardiac tamponade exists when significant compression of the heart by fluid contained within a tensely distended pericardial sac, compromises ventricular filling. Impairment of diastolic filling of both ventricles occurs as intrapericardial pressure rises and this in turn leads to a reduction in stroke volume, cardiac output, and blood pressure. In its extreme form cardiac tamponade is life-threatening, and death will occur unless pericardial compression is relieved.

A spectrum of pericardial tamponade exists. Minimal compression of the heart by a significant pericardial effusion with little drop in cardiac output may occur. If left unchecked, the gradually rising intrapericardial pressure will impede diastolic filling and lead to a progressive decline in cardiac output with concomitant hypotension. Cardiac tamponade may occur acutely because of a penetrating chest wound that causes acute hemopericardium. In such cases, as little as 100 mL to 150 mL of blood can lead to sudden death. Pericardial effusion that accumulates over a prolonged period of time, however, gradually distends the pericardium and will not lead to hemodynamic embarrassment until volumes of fluid as large as a liter or more accumulate.

• Clinical Findings

Several signs enable the clinician to diagnose a significant pericardial effusion that produces hemodynamic embarrassment. The first sign is pulsus paradoxus (or pardoxicus). Ordinarily, inspiration increases venous return to the right heart. Pulmonary vascular capacitance also increases with inspiration. As a result, pulmonary venous return to the left atrium declines slightly with inspiration. Thus, a slight reduction in left heart filling with inspiration is normal. This results in an inspiratory fall in stroke volume, which may be associated with a slight drop in systolic pressure of from 3 mmHg to 5 mmHg in the normally respiring patient. Pulsus paradoxus is an exaggeration of this normal pattern. The patient with cardiac tamponade on quiet inspiration will drop systolic blood pressure by 10 mmHg or greater.

The mechanism of pulsus paradoxus is well-established; it's due to the normal increase in right heart return that occurs during inspiration. In presence of a tense pericardial sac with its fluid distributing pressure equally to the right and left sides of the heart, the increased right heart filling occurs at the expense of left ventricular volume return. Echocardiographic studies document a marked diminution in diastolic dimension of the left ventricle in patients with cardiac tamponade during inspiration. The proper method of determining pulsus paradoxus is to inflate blood pressure cuff higher than peak systolic pressure and then slowly deflate it until the Korotkoff sounds are heard first in end-expiration. The pressure is noted and the blood pressure cuff is further deflated until Korotkoff sounds are heard at peak inspiration and peak expiration. The difference in pressure when Korotkoff sounds are first noted in inspiration and when they are heard through both phases of respiration should be less than 10 mm Hg. If greater than this, pulsus paradoxus is present. Patients should exert no greater than a normal inspiratory effort. Pulsus paradoxus can be present in a variety of other conditions including hyperventilation in normal individuals. It's also present in congestive heart failure and chronic obstruction pulmonary disease in which patients make greater-than-normal efforts to respire.

CARDIAC PEARL

The term "paradoxical pulse" is really a misnomer because when it is clinically apparent, it is really only an exaggeration of the normal pulse. The decrease in amplitude of the pulse coincident with inspiration is an important sign of pericardial tamponade, and may be a sign of restrictive cardiomyopathy, or chronic pulmonary disease such as emphysema or asthma.

Pulsus paradoxus can be present with constrictive pericarditis, but it is more likely to occur with cardiac tamponade.

W. Proctor Harvey, M.D.

Another clinical finding that corroborates diagnosis of cardiac tamponade is an elevated jugular venous pressure; compressing pericardial fluid is responsible for this elevated pressure. The configuration of the jugular venous contour is also suggestive of cardiac tamponade when it shows a preserved X descent but an absent Y descent. This is an important distinction between tamponade and constrictive pericarditis, the latter associated with an exaggerated X and Y descent in the jugular venous pulse. Cardiac auscultation may be of little value in cardiac tamponade except to demonstrate distant heart sounds or perhaps a pericardial friction rub.

• Laboratory Findings

Numerous laboratory aids are helpful in diagnosis of cardiac tamponade. The first is the electrocardiogram, which may show a reduced voltage or universal electrical alternans in which all elements of the EKG including P, QRS and T waves alternate in vector. The latter finding is virtually diagnostic for cardiac tamponade. The mechanism of electrical alternans is an alternating pendulum motion of the heart in the pericardial sac, swinging on its pedicle. A chest x-ray will generally show a markedly enlarged cardiac silhouette with pulmonary vascular congestion in cases where compressing effusion accumulates gradually. Echocardiogram is helpful in positively identifying the presence of a large effusion and diastolic collapse of the right atrium. If diagnosis of tamponade can be made before the patient develops a critically compromised hemodynamic state, then one should proceed to a right heart catheterization to verify diagnosis. Findings on cardiac catheterization reflect the understanding of the physiology of tamponade since there should be no difference between right atrial pressure and pulmonary capillary wedge pressure. In fact, all diastolic pressures in the heart will be the same because they are determined by the intrapericardiac pressure and not by independent factors. Furthermore, in the performance of a pericardiocentesis, there should be no difference between pericardial pressure and right atrial pressure, again reflecting the fact that intrapericardiac pressure defines the diastolic filling of all chambers of the heart. Normally, intrapericardiac pressure is the same as intrapleural pressure and drops during inspiration.

• Treatment

Expertise in the aspiration of fluid from the pericardium is of prime importance in treating pericardial tamponade. Several approaches exist, but pericardiocentesis should not be performed without a unipolar electrocardiographic monitor attached to the pericardiocentesis needle. Such monitoring allows detection of the moment at which the myocardium is touched by the finding of current of injury. One should obviously avoid further advancement of the pericardiocentesis needle if this occurs. Such advancement may result in laceration of a coronary artery or of the right ventricle or right atrium, with obvious disastrous consequences. The state of cardiac tamponade is relieved immediately

on withdrawal of no more than 20 mL to 30 mL of fluid. It is this critical volume that reduces intrapericardiac pressure significantly and allows greater diastolic filling of both ventricles. This in turn results in a higher stroke volume and a restoration of blood pressure toward normal.

While preparing for pericardiocentesis, several supportive measures can assist in stabilizing the patient. Paradoxically, although patients appear to be fluid-overloaded with elevated venous pressure on physical examination and pulmonary vascular congestion on roentgenogram, administration of additional volume can somewhat overcome the effect of a compressing pericardial effusion and result in increased diastolic filling and increased stroke volume and blood pressure. In addition, use of isoproterenol and dopamine may improve cardiac emptying and thereby increase stroke volume and blood pressure. Operative excision of the interior portion of the pericardium not only permits drainage of fluid but also provides the opportunity for cytologic examination and bacteriologic culture of a specimen of tissue. This may be hazardous in the hemodynamically compromised patient, however, and removal of even small amounts of fluid by pericardiocentesis can stabilize the patient and permit a more elective operative approach.

Constrictive Pericarditis

• Physiology and Clinical Findings

Presence of constrictive pericarditis is suggested by the findings of an elevated venous pressure, the failure of right atrial pressure to fall on inspiration, the presence of ascites and edema, the absence of cardiac murmurs, and the presence of a loud early-diastolic sound known as the pericardial knock sound. In contrast to the patient with cardiac tamponade, the venous pressure shows a prominent X and Y descent; failure of the venous pressure to fall with inspiration is known as Kussmaul's sign. This helps to distinguish constrictive pericarditis from cardiac tamponade, in which Kussmaul's sign is absent.

CARDIAC PEARL

A clinical cardiac pearl that has stood the test of time concerning the clinical diagnosis of constrictive pericarditis is the combination of a pericardial knock sound and distention of the jugular venous pulse. When a patient is examined and a sound is heard in early diastole about the timing of the opening snap, two main possibilities arise; of course, the most

565

common is an opening snap of mitral stenosis. When the patient is turned to the left lateral position, the point of maximum impulse of the left ventricle (which may be in a very localized spot- the size of a quarter or a half dollar) is found and the bell of the stethoscope is placed very lightly over this area, the characteristic rumble of mitral stenosis, if present, will be heard, thereby establishing the diagnosis. However, if no rumble is heard despite this maneuver and carefully listening over this localized area, the physician should carefully double-check the jugular veins if he has not done so already. If elevation of pressure in the jugular veins is present, the extra diastolic heart sound may not be an opening snap, but a pericardial knock sound. An immediate clue as to the diagnosis of constrictive pericarditis is thereby afforded by this combination of findings.

W. Proctor Harvey, M.D.

Filling of the ventricles and the state of compliance of both the right and left ventricles is determined by the thickened and fibrotic pericardium that surrounds the heart. Often systolic function is not impaired and overall heart size may be normal. In mild cases of pericardial constriction, there may be little or no elevation of right-sided pressure, especially if there has been vigorous diuresis of a previously edematous patient. Because the process extends to both ventricles, and because transpiration continues to augment right heart return, pulsus paradoxus is present in constrictive pericarditis in up to 30% of cases.

• Laboratory Findings

Laboratory aids in the diagnosis of constrictive pericarditis include the chest roentgenogram, which may show an overall normal size cardiac silhouette but with a rim of calcium around it if the disease process is very long-standing. The electrocardiogram may show atrial fibrillation because the pericardial process may cause irritation of the atrial epicardium leading to this rhythm disturbance. Furthermore, chronically elevated atrial pressures also are a stimulus to atrial fibrillation, seen in slightly less than 50% of such patients. The echocardiogram is helpful in that it may show an increased echodensity of the pericardium. In most cases, the echocardiogram demonstrates normal systolic effort of the heart and a failure of gradual diastolic expansion of the posterior wall of the left ventricle. This finding is reversible following surgery but it is not specific for constrictive pericarditis; it is also present in cardiomyopathy such

as that related to amyloidosis or to other entities in which there is extensive ventricular scarring.

Cardiac catheterization should be performed to confirm the diagnosis of pericardial constriction because myopathic states of the myocardium may provide an identical picture clinically. Cardiac catheterization should verify an equalization of diastolic pressures on both the right and left sides of the heart. Caution is advised on interpretation of the data if the pressures are low and unequal because excessive diuresis can result in this finding. In circumstances in which the diagnosis of constriction is suspected but not verified because of excessive diuresis, administration of a liter of saline over a short period of time will quickly cause equalization of pressures confirming the presence of a constrictive process.

When the finding of identical pressures in diastole may be due to a myopathic process rather than to constrictive pericarditis, exercise on the catheterization table can differentiate between constrictive pericarditis and restrictive cardiomyopathy. If cardiomyopathy is the explanation for the clinical picture, there will be a rise in both right and left ventricular diastolic pressures with a proportionately higher rise in left ventricular diastolic pressure. This does not occur in constrictive pericarditis because both diastolic pressures rise together and show no tendency to separate with exercise. Peak systolic pulmonary pressure in constrictive pericarditis is rarely greater than 50 mmHg. When the clinical picture is due to cardiomyopathy, the peak pulmonary artery systolic pressure commonly is greater than 50 mmHg. Much has been written about the so-called square root sign, the unique configuration of the right ventricular pressure contour in constrictive pericarditis. This also may be found in cases of cardiomyopathy with a restrictive picture, however.

• Treatment

The diagnosis of constrictive pericarditis often is not verified until operative removal of the pericardium. Even postoperatively the diagnosis may not be verified until some time after surgery when right atrial and left atrial pressures begin to fall toward normal. Once the diagnosis is made with a reasonable certainty, operative intervention is recommended even in mild cases because rapid progression total severe constrictive picture may occur. Furthermore, early surgery is recommended because of the easy removal the pericardium compared to later when there has been time to permit intense calcification of the pericardium and growth of calcium into the epicardial surface of the myocardium making surgical removal much more difficult and hazardous.

Cardiomyopathy

Pathophysiology

Cardiomyopathy is cardiac dysfunction that is due to a primary disorder of the cardiac muscle. Cardiomyopathy can be divided into two types. The first is dilated cardiomyopathy which is characterized by low cardiac output and signs of congestive heart failure, including pulmonary congestion and peripheral edema. The second is hypertrophic cardiomyopathy characterized by greater-than-normal systolic function of the heart and marked decrease in left ventricular diastolic compliance. Consequently, dyspnea is a dominant symptom in association with pulmonary congestion in both forms, but dilatation of the heart in hypertrophic cardiomyopathy is a late event in the course of the disease. Hypertrophic cardiomyopathy may be either obstructive, in which there is disproportionate thickening of the left ventricular septum compared to the posterior free wall of the left ventricle, or concentric, in which there is symmetric thickening of the left venticular wall.

Dilated Cardiomyopathy

There are numerous causes of dilated cardiomyopathy. Some of the more common include idiopathic, viral, alcoholic, toxic (such as due to therapy with Adriamycin) and familial. In this syndrome angina is usually absent and the findings of low cardiac output and pulmonary congestion dominate the clinical picture. Dilated cardiomyopathy affects both the right and left ventricles, but usually signs of left ventricular dysfunction are preeminent. It is in this group of patients that therapy with afterload reduction is most beneficial, especially in the face of a high left ventricular diastolic pressure and a high mean left atrial pressure. Such patients also may have mitral regurgitation because the mitral valve and chordae tendineae require an intact, functioning left ventricular free wall and normally contracting papillary muscles for proper function. Mitral regurgitation thus is an extremely common finding in patients with cardiomyopathy in which there is marked left ventricular dilation and marked reduction in the vigor of contraction throughout all muscular elements of the heart. Treatment of patients who have mitral regurgitation with vasodilators significantly reduces the degree of regurgitation and contributes to the improvement in hemodynamics.

The selection of vasodilator depends on the clinical situation. If signs of low output are dominant without a great deal of pulmonary congestion, then pure afterload reducing agents (such as hydralazine, prazosin and more recently the ACE inhibitors) are not only helpful for the treatment of low output in dilated cardiomyopathy, but they also may prolong life for the cardiomyopathy patient. Use of these agents reduces the impedance to left ventricular ejection and can significantly reduce the degree of associated mitral regurgitation. Administering a preload-reducing agent like nitroglycerine to such a patient in whom left ventricular diastolic pressure may be relatively normal results in a reduction in filling of the left ventricle and concurrent reduction in stroke volume and cardiac output. One should forego use of such agents in this case since significant reductions in stroke volume and cardiac output may occur.

However, if pulmonary congestion is severe and left ventricular diastolic pressure and left atrial mean pressure are greatly elevated, then vasodilator therapy with agents that reduce both afterload and preload (such as nitrate therapy or a combination of nitrates and hydralazine) may be the most effective mode of therapy along with diuretics.

Hypertrophic Cardiomyopathy

Because of high left ventricular diastolic pressure due to reduced left ventricular compliance in hypertrophic cardiomyopathy, dyspnea is an extremely common symptom in this clinical syndrome. Although vasodilating agents are safe for patients with dilated cardiomyopathy, they are harmful for patients with hypertrophic cardiomyopathy. Vasodilating agents tend to make the left ventricular cavity, which is reduced in size in this syndrome, even smaller. This may compromise stroke volume and lead to a marked drop in cardiac output to symptomatic levels. Therapy should instead aim at increasing diastolic compliance and promoting left ventricular diastolic relaxation. Beta-adrenergic blockers and the calcium channel blocker verapamil best achieve this result, the latter able to increase diastolic compliance in patients with hypertrophic cardiomyopathy. Whereas cardiotonic agents such as digitalis may be helpful in dilated cardiomyopathy, they are harmful to the patient with hypertrophic cardiomyopathy because they tend to reduce compliance further. This intensifies the symptoms of chest pain and dyspnea.

Left Ventricular Failure

The fundamental abnormality in congestive heart failure in most cases is a diminution in systolic function. This commonly occurs in coronary artery disease because of repeated episodes of myocardial necrosis that diminish the mass of myocardium available for systolic work. Chronic ischemia may compromise vigor of contractility and contribute to a decline in systolic function. This results in a reduced systolic stroke volume and ultimately a reduced cardiac output. The Frank-Starling curve (Figure 2), which relates the cardiac output to the left ventricular diastolic volume or pressure, significantly changes shape in the heart failure patient compared to normal. In left ventricular failure, this curve is shifted downward and to the right so that for the same diastolic volume or pressure there is a lower stroke volume or cardiac output. The challenge in congestive heart failure is to restore the curve to its original normal shape; this is achieved by addition of sympathetic influences or by use of cardiotonic agents. Furthermore, reducing aortic impedance against which the left ventricle works will increase left ventricular emptying, stroke volume, and cardiac output if left ventricular filling remains unchanged.

Compensatory Mechanisms

Numerous secondary changes occur in response to the initial drop in stroke volume and cardiac output in order to maintain intact cardiovascular physiology. The first is an increase in sympathetic tone. Although this can result in an increase in contractility, it also results in an increase in peripheral resistance so that, in the face of a drop in cardiac output, blood pressure remains unchanged. The increase in sympathetic tone results in an increase in venous tone, which augments venous return to the heart and raises left ventricular diastolic volume and pressure. This will be an ineffective measure to improve cardiac output if the Frank-Starling curve is flat over a wide range of diastolic pressures, a curve that defines congestive heart failure. The increased sympathetic drive also increases heart rate; this is an adaptation to increase cardiac output in the face of a diminished stroke volume.

Laboratory evaluation of left ventricular performance demonstrates how these mechanisms operate. One parameter of left ventricular function is the ejection fraction. If the left ventricle starts with a normal diastolic volume of 100 mL of blood and performs with a normal ejection fraction of 60%, stroke volume is 60 mL. If the ejection fraction falls to 40% because of declining systolic performance, it will reduce cardiac output. The reflex increase in sympathetic tone in part overcomes this drop by increasing the heart rate and contractility, but car-

diac dilation occurs to compensate for this drop in stroke volume. In such a hypothetical circumstance (an increase in diastolic volume from 100 mL to 150 mL through the compensatory mechanism of left ventricular dilatation) a reduced ejection fraction of 40% will still produce the normal 60-mL stroke volume.

Consequences of Compensatory Factors

Several important consequences of these compensatory mechanisms occur. As venous return to the heart increases and cardiac dilation occurs, left ventricular diastolic pressure becomes elevated. This causes an increased left atrial pressure which raises the pulmonary venous pressure and results in pulmonary vascular congestion. Dyspnea becomes a significant symptom when the pulmonary capillary wedge pressure rises to the range of 18 mmHg to 20 mmHg. Oxygenation is not compromised in this circumstance, but the high pulmonary venous pressure makes the lungs less compliant and increases the work of breathing. This increased work of breathing is perceived by the patient as dyspnea. At this level of pulmonary venous pressure, pulmonary venous congestion should be obvious on the chest x-ray. As pulmonary venous pressure rises to 20 mmHg to 25 mmHg, the plasma oncotic pressure is exceeded and fluid moves across the vascular bed into the interstitium creating interstitial pulmonary edema. The most extreme circumstance of pulmonary edema exists when the pulmonary venous pressure is 30 mmHg to 35 mmHg. At this level there is massive fluid extrusion into the interstitium and alveolar spaces.

The findings in the right heart depend on the time course of the development of left ventricular failure. Sudden massive left ventricular failure due to ruptured chordae tendineae of the mitral valve and sudden severe mitral regurgitation will cause pulmonary edema with little change in left ventricular heart size and no sign of right heart failure. Right-sided filling pressures that can easily be estimated at the bedside are no reflection of the state of the left side in an acute myocardial infarction. This is because the right sided findings may lag behind the onset of acute left ventricular failure by 8 hours to 12 hours. Consequently, it is important to assess acute changes in left ventricular performance in acute myocardial infarction by performing right heart catheterization to evaluate pulmonary capillary wedge pressure. On the other hand, insidious onset of left ventricular failure due to chronic ischemic heart disease that has a time course of weeks to months results in chronic high left atrial pressures, longstanding pulmonary hypertension,

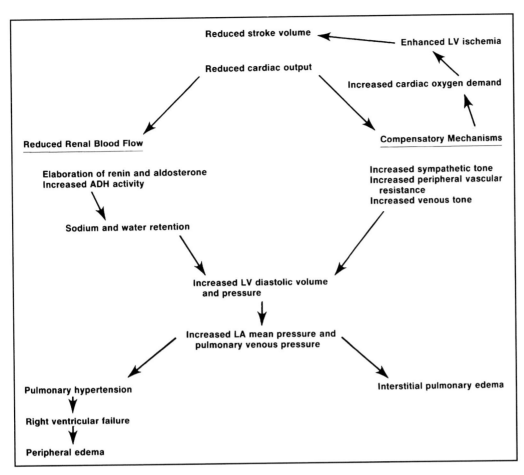

Figure 4. Left ventricular failure. (LV = left ventricle; LA = left atrium; ADH = antidiuretic hormone.) *(From Del Negro AA, 7)*

and eventual right heart failure with evidence of high central venous pressure, congestive hepatomegaly, and peripheral edema.

Several important renal factors contribute to chronic left ventricular failure (Figure 4). The first is the reduced renal blood flow. The kidney misinterprets this reduction in renal blood flow to mean that there is an inadequate circulating blood volume. Indeed, any reduction in renal blood flow results in this response whether it is due to lowered cardiac output because of hypovolemia or congestive heart failure. Renal factors therefore attempt to increase blood volume by retaining sodium by activating the renin-angiotensin II system to reduce sodium excretion. In addition, the kidney elaborates an antidiuretic hormone in an attempt to increase free water retention.

All of these compensatory mechanisms operate to the detriment of the patient with congestive heart failure. An increase in peripheral vascular resistance leads to an increased afterload and an increase in oxygen demand. If the etiology of heart failure is ischemic heart disease, the increased oxygen demand may cause further deterioration in left ventricular performance. Retention of sodium and water by the kidney as well as increases in venous

tone will raise left ventricular diastolic pressure and volume. Although raising the diastolic pressure and volume will increase the stroke volume and cardiac output in an individual operating on a normal Starling curve, it may have little effect in increasing cardiac output in the individual with congestive heart failure who is on a relatively flat Starling curve. Instead of augmenting cardiac output, increases in diastolic volume and pressure will aggravate the clinical picture by further raising left atrial pressure.

Therapy

Therapy for congestive heart failure is aimed not only at improving systolic performance of the heart but also at reducing deleterious effects of the compensatory mechanism. Improving the muscular function of the heart is the least efficacious way of dealing with congestive heart failure, because the drug most commonly used, digitalis, is a relatively weak cardiotonic agent. It is for this reason that other measures are more effective in treating heart failure. These include dietary sodium and fluid restriction, and use of diuretics to promote a negative salt and water balance. This aims at the treatment of fluid overload which causes pulmonary congestion and peripheral edema. One may be able to reduce the elevated peripheral vascular resistance by the use of vasodilating agents such as hydralazine. These drugs selectively reduce the afterload against which the heart must push. This usually results in an increased stroke volume and an increased cardiac output, which counterbalances the reduced peripheral vascular resistance, resulting in little change in blood pressure. ACE inhibitors have a unique role in treatment of congestive heart failure, as they may actually prolong the life of the patient with advanced congestive heart failure by augmenting stroke volume and increasing cardiac output. This therapy should not be combined with excessive diuresis since a significant drop in cardiac output and blood pressure may result. Drugs such as nitroglycerin and isosorbide dinitrate may have a mixed effect; they promote a reduction in peripheral vascular resistance by their effect on arteriolar vasodilation, but they also reduce venous return to the heart by causing venodilation. The latter effect reduces pulmonary congestion and causes a decrease in the left atrial pressure. Often a balanced effect in preload and afterload is desirable so that one may be able to combine ACE inhibitors with nitrates and obtain an effect that is greater than with either agent alone.

Other Forms of Congestive Heart Failure

Heart Failure as an Ischemic Equivalent

The state of myocardial perfusion influences left ventricular compliance in the patient with ischemic heart disease. Compared to the normal situation in which there is no oxygen supply-demand imbalance, the ischemic myocardium becomes stiff in diastole. In short, it loses properties of elasticity because of an inability to relax which is induced by the ischemic state. This reduced compliance means that for the same diastolic volume as in the normal circumstance, diastolic left ventricle pressure is elevated. Left atrial pressure also becomes elevated, and this is reflected into the pulmonary bed. Pulmonary venous pressures as high as 20 mmHg to 25 mmHg are not unusual in this circumstance, and the pattern of interstitial pulmonary edema may be noted on chest x-ray. Nitroglycerine achieves two beneficial effects in this circumstance: the first effect is to reduce venous return and hence reduce diastolic pressure and relieve pulmonary congestion. It does this at the cost of a reduced stroke volume, however, and a fall in blood pressure will accompany this. The fall in blood pressure is also due to some afterload reduction, a primary effect of the drug. The result is that the myocardium works

against a lower afterload, which reduces oxygen consumption, restoring oxygen supply-demand ratio to a normal range, relieving the ischemia, and thereafter restoring left ventricular diastolic compliance and pressure to normal. Of course, nitroglycerine may cause coronary artery dilation and improve oxygenation of ischemic areas as well.

The duration of ischemia and congestion in this circumstance is so short that the brief time course does not permit associated right ventricular failure to occur. In many patients a painless episode of sudden dyspnea is due to ischemia and is the equivalent of angina pectoris. Often the patient with angina pectoris will complain of shortness of breath in association with chest pain; pathophysiology of this state is identical to that of the patient with painless ischemia.

High-Output Congestive Heart Failure

High-output congestive heart failure is less understood than that associated with poor myocardial performance. The patient with high-output congestive heart failure has a greater-than-normal cardiac output. Some of the clinical situations that are associated with this syndrome are chronic anemia, thyrotoxicosis, and arteriovenous fistulae. All of these lead to an increase in the demand for cardiac output. Initially this increased demand is easily met, but the longevity of the demand over a period of months to years ultimately leads to a decompensation of systolic and diastolic functions of the left ventricle. This may in turn lead to cardiac dilation and full-blown right- and left-sided congestive heart failure. The treatment obviously is correction of the underlying cause for high-output failure, but the common therapies for standard congestive heart failure are also appropriate.

CARDIAC PEARL

A soldier was admitted to Walter Reed Army Hospital with classic signs of advanced cardiac decompensation. However, at first, no specific etiology could be determined. His diagnosis was that of dilated cardiomyopathy. Careful auscultation over the back paid off when listening over a scar over the lower spine and detecting a continuous loud murmur. The scar was the result of a previous lumbar disc operation. An arteriovenous fistula had been created at surgery, which resulted in his heart failure. Following surgical correction of this fistula, his heart returned to normal, another example of a curable type of heart disease.

W. Proctor Harvey, M.D.

570

Selected Reading

1. Acar J, Ducimetier P, Cadihac M et al: Prognosis of surgically-treated chronic aortic valve disease: predictive indicators of early postoperative risk and long-term survival, based on 439 cases. *J Thor Card Surg* 82:114, 1981.

2. Adelman AG, Wigle ED, Felderhof CH, et al: Current concepts of primary cardiomyopathy. *Card Med* 2:495, 1977

3. Barry WH, Brooker JZ, Alderman EL et al: Changes in diastolic stiffness and tone of the left ventricle during angina pectoris. *Circ* 49:255, 1974.

4. Braunwald E, Lambrew CT, Rockof SD et al: Idiopathic hypertrophic subaortic stenosis. *Circ* 29/30 (Suppl IV), 1964.

5. Braunwald E, Sonnenblick EH, Ross J Jr: Mechanisms of cardiac contractions: in Braunwald E (ed): *Heart Disease: A Textbook of Cardiovascular Medicine;* WB Saunders, Philadelphia 1992.

6. Bush CA, Stang JW, Wooley CF, Kilman JW: Occult constrictive pericardial disease: diagnosis by rapid volume expansion and correlation by pericardiectomy. *Circ* 56:924, 1977.

7. Del Negro AA: In: *Cardiac Imaging in Infants, Children, and Adults.* Elliott LP (ed); JB Lippincott Company, 1991.

8. Fowler NO: *Cardiac Diagnosis and Treatment,* 3rd ed. New York, Harper & Row, 981, 1981.

9. Fowler NO: Physiology of cardiac tamponade and pulsus paradoxus: Physiological, circulatory and pharmacologic responses in cardiac tamponade. *Mod Con Card Dis* 47; 115, 1978.

10. Fowler NO: The significance of echocardiographic-Doppler studies in cardiac tamponade. *JACC* 11:1081, 1988.

11. Franciosa JA, Cohn JN: Immediate effects of hydralazine in patients with left ventricular failure. *Circ* 59:1085, 1979.

12. Goodwin JF: Congestive and hypertrophic cardiomyopathies. A decade of study. *Lancet* 1:731, 1970.

13. Gorlin R, Gorlin G: Hydraulic formula for calculation of area of stenotic mitral valve, other cardiac valves and central circulatory shunts. *AHJ* 41:1-29, 1951

14. Graettinger JS, Parsons RL, Campbell JA: A correlation of clinical and hemodynamic studies in patients with mild and severe anemia with and without congestive heart failure. *Ann Int Med* 58: 617, 1963

15. Grossman W, Baim DS (eds): *Cardiac Catheterization, Angiography, and Intervention* 5th ed; Baltimore, Williams & Wilkins, 1995.

16. Henry WL, Bonow R, Borer JS et al: Observations of the optimum time for operative intervention for aortic regurgitation. *Circ* 61:471-483, 1980.

17. Huxley RL, Gaffney A, Corbett JR et al: Early detection of left ventricular dysfunction in chronic aortic regurgitation as assessed by contrast angiography, echocardiography, and rest and exercise scintigraphy. *AJC* 51:1542-1550, 1980.

18. Kirkorian G, Hancock EW: Pericardiocentesis. *AJM* 65:808, 1978.

19. Laurent F, De Vernejoul F, Galery JJ, Brun P: Echocardiography in the evaluation of constrictive pericarditis. *Arch Mal C* 73:85, 1980.

20. Littman D, Spodick DH: Total electrical alternans in pericardial disease. *Circ* 17:912, 1958

21. Lorell BH, Braunwald E: Pericardial disease. In Braunwald E (ed) *Heart Disease: A Textbook of Cardiovascular Medicine.* WB Saunders, Philadelphia 1992.

22. Parker JO, Di Giorgi S, West RO: A hemodynamic study of acute coronary insufficiency precipitated by exercise: observations on the effect of nitroglycerine. *AJC* 17: 470, 1966.

23. Reddy PS, Curtiss EI, O'Toole JD, Shaver JA. Cardiac tamponade: hemodynamic observations. *Circ* 58:265, 1978.

24. Ross J, Braunwald E: Aortic stenosis. *Circ* 38 (Suppl) 5:61, 1968.

25. Rowe JC, Bland EF, Sprague HB, White PD: The course of mitral stenosis without surgery: Ten and twenty year perspectives. *Ann Int Med* 52:741 1960.

26. Selzer A, Cohn KE: Natural history of mitral stenosis: a review. *Circ* 45:878-890, 1972.

27. Shabetai R, Fowler NO, Guntheroth WG: The hemodynamics of cardiac tamponade and constrictive pericarditis. *AJC* 26: 480, 1970.

28. Wigle ED, Felderhof CH, Silver MD, Adelman AG: Hypertrophic cardiomyopathy: characterization of 26 patients without functional limitation. *AJC* 41:803, 1978

29. Ziady GM, Oakley CM, Raphael MJ, Goodwin JF: Primary restrictive cardiomyopathy. *BHJ* 37:556, 1975.

CHAPTER 25

Clinical Approach to Heart Failure

David L. Pearle, M.D. and Robert DiBianco, M.D.

Congestive Heart Failure (CHF), or simply, Heart Failure (HF) is a clinical syndrome characterized by abnormalities of systolic and diastolic ventricular function and neurohormonal regulation. Although no universally accepted definition exists, the syndrome is associated with effort intolerance, salt and water retention, dyspnea at rest and with exertion, reduced longevity. It is complicated by an increased frequency of arrhythmias, end-organ dysfunction, intracardiac thrombosis and embolic phenomena. This definition as proposed by Drs. Jay N Cohn, Milton Packer and others emphasizes current concepts of pathophysiology and the lessons learned from large scale, placebo-controlled, therapeutic trials.

The classic circulatory model of "backward" and "forward" heart failure remains valid and useful. This model considers the pathophysiologic state in which an abnormality of cardiac function results in the failure of the heart to pump blood at a rate commensurate with the needs of the metabolizing tissues (forward failure), or to do so only at elevated filling pressures in the right or left ventricles (backward failure). With "forward failure", a reduced exercise tolerance results from inadequate oxygen delivery to exercising muscle; with "backward failure", exercise limitation is explained by increased left ventricular filling and pulmonary venous pressures causing dyspnea.

Implicit to both definitions are abnormalities of ventricular function during systole or diastole. Abnormalities of systolic function resulting in a diminished ventricular ejection fraction with an inadequate stroke volume of blood pumped from the ventricle is the classic concept of forward heart

failure. Backward heart failure may be considered to result from abnormalities of ventricular relaxation (diastolic dysfunction) that result in abnormally high ventricular filling pressures, often without associated abnormalities of contractility (Table 1). The distinction between systolic and diastolic dysfunction is clinically important because therapy

---

TABLE 1

Myocardial Causes of Systolic and Diastolic Heart Failure

SYSTOLIC

- Coronary artery disease (ischemic heart disease)
- Dilated cardiomyopathy of unknown cause (Idiopathic)
- Dilated cardiomyopathy of known cause:
  - Familial
  - Viral
  - Parasitic
  - Chronic pressure or volume overload
  - Drugs (adriamycin, alcohol, cyclophosphamide, doxorubicin, disopyramide, flecainide)
  - Metabolic (hypocalcemia, hypophosphatemia)
  - Sickle cell anemia

DIASTOLIC

- Hypertrophic cardiomyopathy
- Restrictive cardiomyopathy (example, endocardial fibroelastosis)
- Infiltrative cardiomyopathy (amyloid, sarcoid, hemochromatosis, glycogen storage disease)
- Ventricular hypertrophy in response to chronic pressure overload
  - Hypertension
  - Aortic Stenosis or other outflow tract obstruction
  - Pulmonary hypertension

TABLE 2

Non-Myocardial Causes of Circulatory Failure

A. Cardiac
  Valvular stenosis or regurgitation
  Congenital malformations
  Supraventricular and ventricular arrhythmias

B. Pericardial
  Constrictive pericarditis
  Tamponade

C. Non-Cardiac
  Renal failure
  High output states
    Thyrotoxicosis
    Anemia
    AV fistula
    Pregnancy
    Thiamine deficiency

---

is different for these two abnormalities. However, in most patients with heart failure, both types of ventricular dysfunction coexist, especially in heart failure resulting from coronary atherosclerosis.

Since the syndrome of heart failure may not be "congestive", that is, associated with pulmonary (interstitial or alveolar) or systemic edema, the abbreviation "CHF" is often represented as Clinical or Chronic heart failure rather than "Congestive". More recently, the term "Heart Failure" is increasingly preferred.

The syndrome of "circulatory failure" resulting in signs and symptoms of heart failure can exist without either systolic or diastolic ventricular dysfunction. Nonmyocardial causes of circulatory failure are listed in Table 2. Patients with signs and symptoms of heart failure require appropriate evaluation to exclude the presence of correctable valvular, pericardial and noncardiovascular conditions which may be a cause of circulatory failure without ventricular dysfunction. It is clinically important to identify these conditions because their treatment and prognosis differ markedly from that of patients with heart failure secondary to ventricular dysfunction.

Background

Heart failure is a problem of already immense significance that is growing dramatically in incidence and prevalence. This clinical syndrome afflicts nearly 1% to 2% of the entire U.S. population and represents the most common cause for hospitalization of patients over age 65. Unlike the incidence and mortality of most cardiovascular dis-

orders, which have decreased in the U.S. over the past 20 years, the incidence, prevalence and mortality of heart failure are rising and will probably continue to increase for the forseeable future as more patients survive acute myocardial infarction and the population becomes more aged. Some U.S. statistics that provide perspective of the problem are as follows:

• **Incidence:** Each year 3 cases of heart failure develop for each 1,000 persons under age 65. This is increased to greater than 10 cases per 1,000 in those over age 65 years.

• **Prevalence:** Heart failure afflicts 1% of all persons under age 50 and more than 10% of those over age 80.

The prevalence of heart failure approximately doubles for each decade of life.

There are approximately 4 million doctor visits, 500,000 hospitalizations and 5 million hospital days annually for heart failure in the U.S. Hospitalizations for heart failure more than doubled between 1975 and 1985, predominantly as a result of heart failure in patients over age 55 years.

• **Mortality:** Approximately 35% of patients die within 1 year of establishing the diagnosis with even higher mortalities observed for increased severity of heart failure. The 6-year mortality rate ranges from 67% for women to 82% for men; death rates are 4 to 8 times greater than in general age-matched populations. Mortality rates are age-specific with 200 times as many deaths at age 75 as at age 35. Mortality rates are race-specific with blacks having approximately 20% higher mortality compared to age-matched whites beyond the age of 65 years.

• **Racial Variation:** In blacks, the higher prevalence and greater severity of hypertension contributes to an increased incidence and prevalence of heart failure; in whites ischemic heart disease is more commonly the underlying cause of heart failure.

• **Trends:** Increased incidence and prevalence of heart failure reflects multiple trends including an improved survival of patients with angina, hypertension and acute myocardial infarction, better reporting and recognition of heart failure and the progressive aging of the population. This trend has continued despite the marked decrease in mortality rates from coronary heart disease and hypertension, the recognized major risk factors for heart failure. Coronary heart disease confers a fourfold increase in the risk of developing heart failure; hypertension triples the risk. Hypertension and coronary heart disease are the predominant causes of heart failure in Westernized society accounting for 80% of all cases.

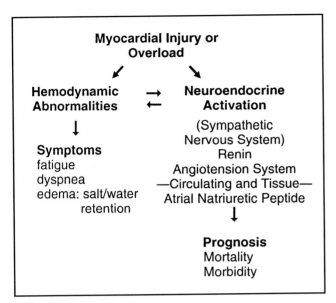

Figure 1. Pathophysiology of heart failure

Contents of figure:

Myocardial Injury or Overload

Hemodynamic Abnormalities → ← **Neuroendocrine Activation**

Symptoms
fatigue
dyspnea
edema: salt/water
retention

(Sympathetic Nervous System)
Renin
Angiotension System
—Circulating and Tissue—
Atrial Natriuretic Peptide

Prognosis
Mortality
Morbidity

Pathophysiology

Heart failure is characterized by a complex series of pathophysiologic changes involving cardiac structure and performance, the peripheral circulation, neuroendocrine perturbations and alterations in mutiple organ systems. Some of the physiologic abnormalities are primary while others are compensatory, with the relative roles of each component and their complex interactions incompletely understood. The pathophysiology of heart failure may be artificially divided into hemodynamic and neuroendocrine paradigms for discussion purposes (Figure 1).

• **Hemodynamic Paradigm:** Cardiac contractility is depressed in most patients with heart failure. This may be the result of an absolute loss of myocardial fibers secondary to necrosis, reduced myocardial blood flow and ischemic dysfunction or a by-product of myocardial hypertrophy stimulated by a pressure or volume overload which decreases systolic contractile function and diastolic compliance. Multiple altered biochemical mechanisms may result in impaired contractility and contribute in a primary or secondary manner to the syndrome of heart failure. These diverse abnormalities are only partly elucidated.

Changes in ventricular diastolic compliance, that is, a rise in ventricular filling pressure disproportionate to changes in left ventricular volume, can occur as a result of both passive and active processes. Passive processes include an increase in muscle stiffness due to growth of both myocardial fibers and collagen among other remodeling changes. Active processes include abnormalities of the energy-dependent relaxation process of early diastole, a process that begins in the earliest, preclinical phase of heart failure in most patients. Abnormalities of systolic and diastolic dysfunction coexist in most patients; although diastolic dysfunction, which usually precedes systolic dyfunction, may exist in more-or-less pure (or predominant) form. In addition to these cardiac structural and functional abnormalities, the syndrome of heart failure involves interactions of preload, aortic impedance and neurohormonal activation.

• **Neuroendocrine Paradigm:** When cardiac performance cannot meet the metabolic and circulatory needs of the body, heart failure is present. No matter what the cause of ventricular dysfunction, neuroendocrine "compensatory" mechanisms are triggered to maintain cardiac output and blood pressure. Although vasoconstrictor and vasodilator systems are simultaneously activated, vasoconstrictive systems predominate and become detrimental by producing an excessive systemic vascular resistance (Figure 1). The vasoconstrictor systems are the sympathetic nervous system (SNS) and renin-angiotensin and aldosterone system (RAAS).

Increased SNS activity as represented by increased plasma levels of norepinephrine is present in heart failure and provides prognostic value since norepinephrine levels correlate directly with disease severity and mortality. Both beta- and alpha-adrenergic receptors are activated. The beta-adrenoreceptor responses cause a faster heart rate and stronger force of myocardial contraction, which augment cardiac output. Enhanced alpha-adrenoreceptor activity yields arterial vasoconstriction (increased afterload that augments peripheral perfusion pressures) and venoconstriction (increased preload that increases ventricular filling and is positively inotropic). The detrimental effects of SNS stimulation include down-regulation of beta-adrenergic receptors, a possible direct toxic effect on the myocardium, alterations of regional distribution of blood flow, increased arrhythmias and most importantly reduced survival. The mechanisms by which increased SNS activity decreases survival in heart failure remain incompletely understood.

Activation of the RAAS in heart failure provides prognostic value since the levels of activation correlate with disease severity and mortality. Activation of the RAAS augments systemic vascular resistance and compromises cardiac output. Release of the enzyme renin triggers the transformation of angiotensinogen to the inactive precursor, angiotensin I. Angiotensin-converting enzyme (ACE) then converts angiotensin I into the extremely potent circulating and locally active vasoconstrictor angiotensin II. Afterload is increased via direct systemic vasoconstriction caused by angiotensin II. Preload is increased through the stimulation of aldosterone secretion, which causes sodium and water retention, stimulation of thirst (centrally via the hypothalamus) and increased water reabsorption by the kidneys leading to an expanded blood volume and reduced serum sodium concentration in severe heart failure. The RAAS is predominantly activated through interactions with the SNS and reduced renal perfusion. Other neurohormonal systems altered in heart failure include arginine vasopressin (antidiuretic hormone), atrial naturetic factor, endothelial derived relaxant factor, endothelin, prostaglandins and others.

Increases in preload and cardiac contractility from these compensatory mechanisms increase cardiac output. Excessive peripheral vasoconstriction and reduced cardiac output trigger fluid retention directly through renal and indirectly through RAAS-mediated mechanisms. Elevated right and left ventricular filling pressures produce systemic (dependent) edema, increased lung water and respiratory work. As reductions in cardiac output occur, additional increments in vasoconstrictor hormones are engendered, resulting in a progressive cycle of compromised cardiac performance, metabolic disturbances and symptoms of low output (fatigue), and congestion (dyspnea and edema).

Clinical Diagnosis of Heart Failure

The clinical evaluation of the patient with heart failure (Table 3) must address several important issues:

• Is ventricular dysfunction present and if so, what is the cause?

• Is the clinical syndrome associated with systolic dysfunction, diastolic dysfunction or both?

• Does the patient have causes for circulatory failure independent of ventricular dysfunction?

• Are there identifiable factors precipitating or exacerbating the syndrome that can be modified (especially underlying ischemic heart disease)?

• What is the prognosis for the patient under evaluation?

The "five-finger approach" of Dr. W. Proctor Harvey remains relevant for clinical assessment of the patient suspected of having heart failure and is a succinct way to focus skills, teach, and gain information crucial to answering the above questions needed for patient management (Figure 2). The history, physical examination, electrocardiogram, chest x-ray and special laboratory tests (noninvasive and invasive) are all important in addressing these issues. One could argue that the first four "fingers" combined with an echocardiogram (as the

TABLE 3
Descriptors of the Clinical "Diagnosis" of Heart Failure

History:	Dyspnea on exertion or at rest
	Fatigue
	Weight gain
Physical:	Sinus tachycardia, pulsus alternans
	Elevated jugular venous pressure
	Pulmonary rales
	Cardiomegaly, atrial gallop (fourth heart sound)
	Ventricular gallop (third heart sound)
	Hepatomegaly
	Peripheral (dependent) edema
Chest X-ray:	Increased pulmonary vascularity
	Pleural effusion
	Cardiac silhouette enlargement
Electrocardiogram:	Left atrial overload pattern
	Ventricular hypertrophy or possibly prior myocardial infarction
Echocardiogram:	Enlarged left atrium
	Systolic failure
	Enlarged left ventricular chamber size
	Variable left ventricular wall thickness
	Poor contractility (low ejection fraction)
	Diastolic failure
	Normal left ventricular chamber size
	Increased left ventricular wall thickness
	Normal or increased contractility (normal or increased ejection fraction)

first "special lab test") provide the essential information needed to evaluate and manage the patient with heart failure.

History

Manifestations of heart failure are generally most prominent and easily detectable in the history. The patient experiences fatigue and dyspnea on exertion, which in its severest form progresses to breathlessness and profound fatigue even at rest. Some patients, because of an insidious onset of symptoms, attribute the lack of stamina to "growing old" or "being out of shape". Symptoms of heart failure almost always reflect important abnormalities in ventricular function; it is recognized however that ventricular dysfunction correlates poorly with symptoms and only modestly with survival within the subgroup of patients with heart failure. The poor correlation between symptoms and ventricular dysfunction may be in part explained by the importance of neurohormonal responses and peripheral vascular compensation that is still poorly understood.

Dyspnea is present early in the course of heart failure, initially occurring only with severe exertion and emotional stress. Later in the natural history

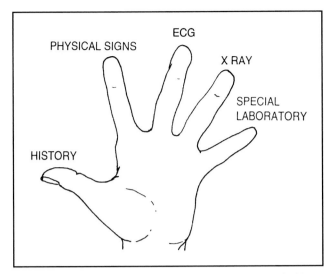

Figure 2. The 5-finger approach to clinical diagnosis as described by W. Proctor Harvey, M.D.

of the disease, dyspnea occurs with mild exertion and finally at rest as heart failure progresses. Dyspnea may also occur when the patient is recumbent and be reported as orthopnea, paroxysmal nocturnal dyspnea or trepopnea (positional dyspnea such as that which occurs when lying in the left lateral decubitus position). As heart failure progresses, ventricular filling pressures rise (especially the left atrial and pulmonary venous pressures), interstitial pulmonary pressure increases and peribronchiolar edema and airway resistance increase resulting in decreased pulmonary compliance and increased work of breathing. A nocturnal cough and rarely hemoptysis mark the appearance of alveolar edema as severe heart failure develops.

Fatigue is an easily elicited complaint of patients in heart failure and results from multiple causes, including a reduced cardiac output with impaired delivery of oxygen to the tissues, increased work of breathing limiting energy expenditures for other organ (muscle) functions, and probably reduced rest associated with sleep disturbances from orthopnea, paroxysmal nocturnal dyspnea, and nocturia, which are so commonly reported by patients with heart failure.

Edema that is bilateral, dependent and typically associated with a weight gain secondary to salt and water retention is a common finding in heart failure. Systemic edema results from elevations of right ventricular end-diastolic pressure and right atrial mean pressure and hydrostatic effects on capillaries leading to reduced reabsorption.

Other symptoms commonly seen in heart failure include right upper quadrant discomfort (attributed to hepatic venous engorgement), loss of appetite,

and in later stages of the syndrome ascites and cachexia. Nocturia (reflecting an improvement in sodium excretion probably resulting from improved renal blood flow while the patient is at supine rest) can occur in heart failure as can unexplained weight gain secondary to salt and water retention.

Symptoms are often described in semiquantitative terms using a single estimation of the limitation the symptoms pose for the patient. The measure of "functional class" most commonly used for heart failure patients is the New York Heart Association Functional Classification (Table 4). This classification system though highly subjective, offers a "short-hand" for description of disease severity. It is compromised especially by variability in what different observers see as "normal" activity. However, despite these limitations, large studies demonstrate that the NYHA Functional Classification system, applied to patients with left ventricular dysfunction, identifies distinct risk groups. Patients with mild to moderate symptoms (NYHA Class II-III) have an annual mortality of 10% to 25%, while patients with severe symptoms (NYHA Class IV) suffer an annual mortality approaching 60%. A more objective classification system based on maximum oxygen consumption determined by exercise testing has been described by Weber and is a valuable research tool.

Physical Exam

Systemic disorders possibly causing or aggravating heart failure must be evaluated as part of a general medical examination. The cardiovascular physical examination in suspected heart failure can yield valuable diagnostic and prognostic information; although studies assessing the correlation between specific physical findings felt to be characteristic of heart failure and the presence of actual heart failure are low in specificity and sensitivity. The general appearance of the patient with heart failure may display "anxiety" and "fear" especially

TABLE 4
NYHA Functional Classification

Class I.	No limitation to exercise tolerance or symptoms on usual activities of daily living
Class II.	Mild limitation of exercise tolerance with provocation of symptoms by ordinary exertion
Class III.	Moderate limitation of exercise tolerance with symptom provocation by less than ordinary exertion.
Class IV.	Severe limitation of exercise tolerance with symptoms at rest.

when heart failure is severe or acutely decompensated. There may be associated tachypnea, diaphoresis and cold extremities (with cyanosis in severe cases). Vital signs reveal sinus tachycardia (at times with pulsus alternans) and inconsistent changes in systolic and diastolic blood pressure; although hypertension as a primary problem or secondary to elevated catecholamines may be seen. Elevation of venous pressure (most easily assessed from the internal jugular pulse) and an abnormal response to abdominal compression (positive hepatojugular reflux) are typical as are pulmonary rales with pleural effusions. A laterally displaced and sustained cardiac apex beat with an atrial and ventricular gallop (S_4 and S_3 respectively) is often identifiable as is hepatomegaly and peripheral (dependent) edema.

CARDIAC PEARL

The faint ventricular gallop that has the better prognosis is the one which is detected as an early sign of congestive heart failure and which disappears after treatment. As a rule, such treatment needs to be continued. A ventricular diastolic gallop is frequently associated with a slight pulsus alternans. On the other hand, the finding of a definite pulsus alternans is almost always associated with a ventricular diastolic gallop. Both these findings indicate a failing myocardium, and too little attention has been paid to them in the past. In addition, alternation of the intensity of heart sounds and/or murmurs is frequent when a ventricular diastolic gallop and pulsus alternans are present. Nearly all these findings are clues indicating some degree of cardiac decompensation (Fig. A).

W. Proctor Harvey, M.D.

The "congested state" of the patient with heart failure has a typical appearance despite different cardiac etiologies. The "congested state" from heart failure must be differentiated from that associated with renal failure, hepatic failure and that which may accompany severe obesity or chronic lung disease. The symptom complex and physical signs of

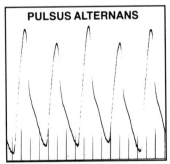

PULSUS ALTERNANS

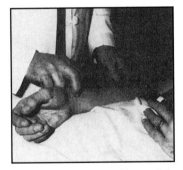

Fig A: Ventricular diastolic gallop is frequently associated with a pulsus alternans, alternation of the second sound and alternation of murmurs. The prognosis of patients with these clinical findings is not a good one.

Pulsus alternans detected by careful palpation of radial pulse.

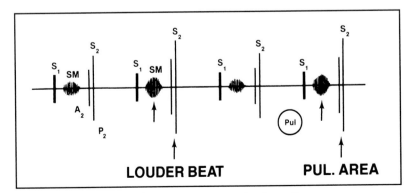

LOUDER BEAT   **PUL. AREA**

Note alternation of intensity (↑) of both second sound and systolic murmur every other beat. This man with coronary heart disease had advanced heart failure.

578

heart failure are also accompanied by abnormalities of the clinical laboratory (especially the chest x-ray, electrocardiogram and echocardiogram).

Chest X-ray

Confirmatory evidence of cardiomegaly associated with elevated pulmonary venous pressures is available from the typical pattern of interstitial and or alveolar pulmonary edema on the chest x-ray, accompanied by signs of left atrial enlargement. The sensitivity and specificity of these findings is poor for the diagnosis of heart failure or specific hemodynamic abnormalities. More severe forms of heart disease are associated with increased interstitial markings, peribronchiolar edema or "cuffing" and thickening of the interlobular spaces manifested by so-called Kerley B lines, often associated with pleural effusions.

CARDIAC PEARL

Hydrothorax can be a complication of advanced congestive heart failure. It is not seen as frequently now as it was in the past due to better present day medical treatment. Hydrothorax accompanying heart failure may be bilateral, but in my experience is more commonly present in the right thorax. This is probably best explained by simple gravity and the fact that these patients are more likely to lie and sleep on their right side than their left. Patients having enlarged hearts, often with an arrhythmia, such as atrial fibrillation, are conscious of their heart action when lying on their left side; therefore most prefer to sleep on their right side and/or back.

When a left hydrothorax is present in a patient with heart disease, rule out the possibility of an etiology rather than heart failure.

W. Proctor Harvey, M.D.

Electrocardiogram

An electrocardiogram may indicate an atrial overload pattern, ventricular hypertrophy, ventricular conduction delay, or evidence of prior myocardial infarction. Each increases likelihood of underlying cardiac disease, although neither the presence of electrocardiographic abnormalities nor their absence prove or disprove diagnosis of heart failure.

Echocardiogram

The most informative non-invasive test for patients suspected of having heart failure is the 2-D echocardiogram. Although initially understood and used exclusively by the cardiologist, the utility of this technique, its ease of application, specificity for defining cardiac structure, widespread availability and acceptable cost has promoted its use today to the generalist. The "echo" will confirm that heart failure is present. This is most easily identified by evidence of increased left atrial size, since this thin walled chamber is an excellent manometer of chronic left ventricular filling pressure. The left atrium is virtually always increased in size in chronic left ventricular failure. Although the left atrium is at times increased in size because of mitral regurgitation that has not yet progressed to heart failure, the diagnosis of heart failure must be placed in serious doubt without left atrial enlargement.

Since the appropriate drug treatment of heart failure depends on the type of ventricular function abnormality present, it is necessary in all patients to determine whether there is a failure of contractility (systolic failure) or relaxation (diastolic failure; Table 1). The echo provides the best and most easily applied discriminator between patients with "systolic" and "diastolic" heart failure (Figure 3). The echocardiogram elucidates cardiac structure and thus identifies valvular or pericardial problems.

Value of information obtained from the echocardiogram cannot be overemphasized in the clinical management of the heart failure patient. The benefit more than compensates for the time, effort and cost in obtaining this test. It is strongly recommended that the physician have this information early in the evaluation of all such patients.

T A B L E   5
Special Cardiac Laboratory Tests

1. **Biochemical and metabolic measurements**
2. **Arrhythmia detection through**
   - monitoring or recording
   - correlation of symptoms with (or without) arrhythmia
   - provocation during electrophysiologic testing
3. **Exercise testing with or without metabolic measurements**
   - submaximal
   - maximal
4. **Nuclear imaging to determine**
   - myocardial perfusion
   - ventricular function
   - myocardial metabolism
   - myocardial cell integrity (Gallium, Antimyosin antibody scanning)
5. **Cardiac catheterization with hemodynamic definition**
6. **Coronary and left ventricular angiography**
7. **Myocardial biopsy**

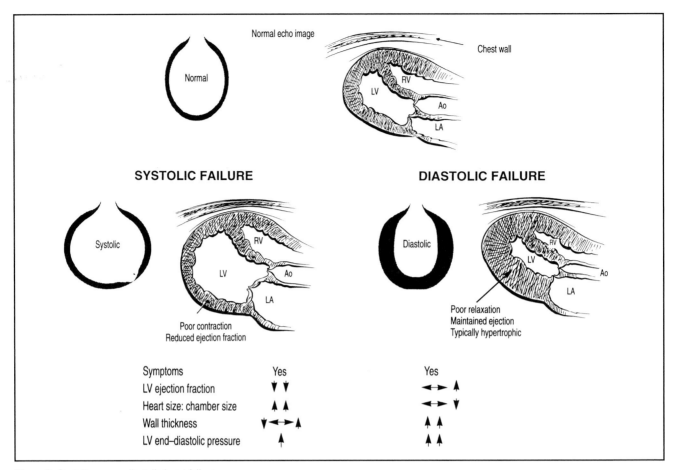

Figure 3. Systolic versus diastolic heart failure

Special laboratory or "fifth finger" techniques provide useful and at times critical information necessary for optimal patient assessment and care (Table 5). Cardiac catheterization will identify right and left heart pressures, cardiac output, pulmonary and systemic circulatory resistances, valvular gradients, and calculations of valve areas and presence of abnormal communications or shunts. This is a valuable technique for defining the significance of pericardial restriction or constriction, assisting in determination of systolic versus diastolic dysfunction, and intracavitary gradients such as seen with hypertrophic cardiomyopathy. Left ventriculography can aid in the assessment of chamber size, regional and global contractility and structural valvular abnormalities and incompetence, especially of the mitral valve. Presence of segmental left ventricular dysfunction suggests ischemic heart disease, whereas the finding of global dysfunction is characteristic of a viral, toxic or immunologic etiology to the cardiomyopathy. Assessment of coronary anatomy is the most common indication for invasive cardiac testing today and is used to define the most common etiology of heart failure, namely, coronary artery disease.

Endomyocardial biopsy has a low diagnostic yield for myocarditis and is widely used to detect rejection following cardiac transplantation. In addition, the implications of a positive biopsy are controversial with regard to therapy. Perhaps future diagnostic capabilities including genetic analysis and techniques to evaluate specific cellular abnormalities may increase the value of this technique.

Causes of Heart Failure

Heart failure can be produced by a variety of structural causes according to whether the predominant mechanism results in direct myocardial damage, from ventricular overload or from compromised cardiac filling. "Pure" forms of some disorders may produce systolic *or* diastolic dysfunction, although most patients with congestive heart failure demonstrate a combination of these disorders.

CARDIAC PEARL

**Listen with the stethoscope over areas other than the precordial heart areas.
Be sure to listen over every scar.**

TABLE 6
Precipitating Causes of Heart Failure

- Dietary indiscretion (especially sodium)
- Failure to comply with medication prescriptions
- Myocardial ischemia
- Tachy- or Brady-arrhythmias (especially atrial fibrillation)
- Drugs (depress cardiac function; may produce excessive vasoconstriction or salt and water retention).
  Anti-inflammatory (Non-Steroidal Anti-Inflammatory Drugs)
  Anti-arrhythmic drugs (disopyramide, flecainide, verapamil)
  Calcium channel blocking agents or
  Beta-adrenergic blocking agents
- Anemia
- Sepsis (usually secondary to pulmonary or urinary cause)
- Metabolic deficiencies (nutritional such as hypophosphatemia)
- Compromised renal function
- Hyper- and Hypo-thyroidism

A soldier was admitted to Walter Reed Army Hospital with classic sign of advanced cardiac decompensation. However, at first, no specific etiology could be determined. His diagnosis was that of dilated cardiomyopathy. Careful auscultation over the back paid off when listening over a scar over the lower spine and detecting a continuous loud murmur. The scar was the result of a previous lumbar disc operation. An arteriovenous fistula had been created at surgery, which resulted in his heart failure. Following surgical correction of this fistula, his heart returned to normal- another example of a curable type of heart disease.

W. Proctor Harvey, M.D.

Circulatory Failure Without Myocardial Dysfunction

Signs and symptoms of congestive heart failure can be produced by non-cardiac conditions in the presence of normal systolic and diastolic function. Table 2 lists the major non-cardiac causes of circulatory failure. It should be recognized that each of these conditions may exacerbate mild underlying heart failure secondary to ventricular dysfunction.

Precipitating Causes of Heart Failure

Factors, at times unrelated to the fundamental etiology of heart failure, may play a role in precipitating or exacerbating a clinical event. Recognition and treatment of these factors may contribute importantly to preventing the event or mitigating symptoms and sequelae even in the face of progres-

sion of the underlying disease. Some of these important determinants are listed in Table 6.

CARDIAC PEARL

A patient with heart disease may have no evidence of cardiac decompensation, but acute pulmonary edema can occur with the change from normal sinus rhythm to atrial fibrillation. In some patients, this also may be the first indication of underlying heart disease.

W. Proctor Harvey, M.D.

Natural History

The natural history of patients with heart failure generally involves a period of asymptomatic ventricular dysfunction of variable duration followed by a relentless and progressive increase in symptoms from the time of their appearance until death. Throughout the course of this there is a high risk of "unexpected" mortality referred to as sudden cardiac death. Although many factors tend to identify the patient at risk for early mortality (Table 7) virtually none are helpful in the individual patient and few are powerful enough to discriminate between groups of patients segregated by individual descriptors.

- **Etiology:** There is probably a higher mortality rate for patients with heart failure secondary to coronary artery disease than non-ischemic cardiomyopathy; this is especially true in the first year following myocardial infarction and probably less so after 1 year. Active inflammatory disease with biopsy evidence of antibody to heart antigen may be a poor prognostic sign.

- **Symptoms:** The severity of symptoms as estimated by the New York Heart Association Functional Class correlates with an increased annual mortality (Figure 4).

TABLE 7
Predictors of Increased Mortality in Heart Failure

- Etiology
- Symptoms
- Ventricular dysfunction
- Hemodynamic disturbances
- Neurohormone disturbances
- Complications
  Arrhythmia frequency
  Thrombosis/Embolism

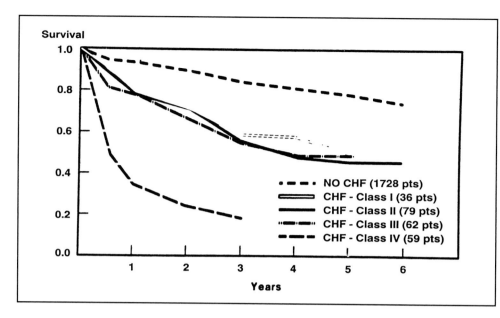

Figure 4. Survival probabilities in 236 patients with congestive heart failure according to NYHA functional classification compared to 1728 patients with no history of congestive heart failure.

• **Ventricular Dysfunction:** Most of the common descriptors of left ventricular function have been shown to correlate inversely with survival when the entire spectrum of ventricular function is assessed, that is, from extremely poor ventricular function in patients with heart failure up to and including asymptomatic normal subjects. Within subsets, with particularly narrow limits, these correlations often lose statistical significance. Some indices often displaying a correlation with survival are left ventricular ejection fraction and stroke work index. Reduced right ventricular systolic function defined as either a low RV ejection fraction or RV chamber enlargement, has also been shown to predict an increased mortality.

• **Exercise Capacity:** Exercise capacity as a measure of ventricular performance, including maximum oxygen consumption or the capacity for continued exercise at a submaximal workload correlates inversely with mortality. It has been suggested that measurements of submaximal exercise such as prolonged walking may correlate better with symptoms reported during activities of daily living and overall survival as compared to peak performance estimated by maximal exercise capacity and oxygen consumption. Maximum exercise capacity and the 6-minute walk test that assesses exercise against a submaximal workload correlate with relative risk of mortality and are suggested to better subdivide patients according to functional impairments and prognosis than the NYHA functional classification.

• **Hemodynamic Disturbances:** Left ventricular end-diastolic pressure and volume correlate inversely with survival whereas the cardiac index correlates directly.

• **Neurohormone Disturbances:** Neuroendocrine abnormalities including high plasma renin activity, high plasma norepinephrine and epinephrine levels and electrolyte imbalances, especially reduced serum sodium concentration, are predictive of increased mortality.

Complications

• **Ventricular arrhythmias** in the form of frequent premature ventricular contractions of multiform variety or in pairs complicates the clinical profile of greater than 80% of patients with heart failure. Approximately half of patients with more severe degrees of heart failure have nonsustained ventricular tachycardia, a presumptive contributor to greater than 50% of sudden cardiac deaths. Whether the frequency of arrhythmia is related to structural or hemodynamic factors, electrolyte or neurohormonal disturbances or drug treatments is unclear. It has been suggested that an independent relationship of ventricular arrhythmia to mortality exists; however, the failure of antiarrhythmic drug treatment to alter prognosis counters this hypothesis. It may be that ventricular ectopic activity predominantly reflects the extent of other structural and functional disturbances, a hypothesis supported by its direct correlation with severity of ventricular dysfunction.

• **Thrombosis and embolic phenomena** are frequently found in post mortem studies of patients dying with heart failure. They appear to be more frequent in patients with atrial fibrillation and represent a continuing threat to survival. Studies to date have not provided clear evidence of worsened survival when these problems are clinically identified; but, this may be the result of limited sample

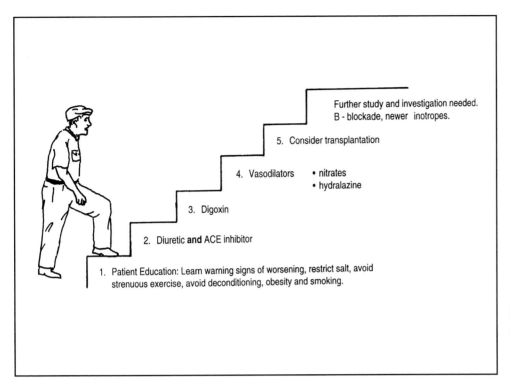

5. Consider transplantation

Further study and investigation needed.
B - blockade, newer inotropes.

4. Vasodilators
• nitrates
• hydralazine

3. Digoxin

2. Diuretic **and** ACE inhibitor

1. Patient Education: Learn warning signs of worsening, restrict salt, avoid strenuous exercise, avoid deconditioning, obesity and smoking.

Figure 5. Pharmacologic approach to treatment of heart failure secondary to systolic dysfunction.

sizes and extent of follow-up and the difficulty of identifying these problems pre-mortem.

Therapeutic Concepts and Correlations

• **Preventing Heart Failure (Table 8):** Risk factors for developing heart failure include the standard risk factors for coronary heart disease such as age, hypertension, elevated cholesterol, glucose intolerance (especially overt diabetes), cigarette smoking, electrocardiographic evidence of left ventricular hypertrophy, and obesity. Coronary heart disease confers a fourfold increase in the risk of developing heart failure; hypertension triples the risk. Supporting the importance of risk factors is the observation that while only about 10% of non-diabetic individuals can be identified as high risk by risk factor analysis, these individuals comprise 40% of those who will develop heart failure. The role of controlling risk factors is important and must be emphasized, especially in the presence of diabetes. Many of the predisposing factors (hypertension, hyperlipidemia, and hyperglycemia, smoking, and obesity) can be modified and would be expected to have favorable effects on the atherosclerotic process, thereby reducing incidence and severity of coronary heart disease and its complications including heart failure.

Some risk factors for heart failure actually represent the expression of impaired cardiac function, which appears early in the natural history of the syndrome; these include increased heart rate and heart size, a reduced left ventricular ejection fraction, a reduced vital capacity and T-wave abnormalities on the ECG. It is known that patients with these findings demonstrate an increased incidence of overt heart failure, hospitalization for heart failure, and a worsened mortality.

Heart failure, a frequent complication of myocardial infarction, often begins in the early post-MI period and shows a progressive and continued incidence, with the result that it is the most likely underlying etiology of heart failure detected late. The newest approach to reducing incidence of heart failure post-MI is to initiate ACE inhibitor therapy after myocardial infarction to limit ventricular damage (or remodeling) and thereby reduce subsequent risk of heart failure. During the acute phase of a myocardial infarction, it is beneficial to reestablish coronary perfusion with thrombolytic treatments and control hypertension, wall stress, and ischemia. Following an MI, beta blockade, aspirin, and ACE inhibition has been associated with reductions in recurrent MI, total mortality, cardiovascular mortality, occurrence of severe heart failure, and hospitalization for heart failure.

Treatment of heart failure is rarely directed at the cause of the disease, which is usually irreversible unless a nonmyocardial factor or precipitating condition (Tables 2 and 6) can be identified and corrected. The goals of treatment in patients with heart failure are to make them feel better and live longer. Current therapies have been demon-

---

TABLE 8

Prevention of Heart Failure

Primary Prevention: Control risk factors for CHD, especially hypertension, the major causes of heart failure:

- Systolic blood pressure
- Total cholesterol (and LDL-cholesterol)
- Glucose intolerance and diabetes mellitus
- Cigarette smoking
- Obesity and sedentary lifestyle

Secondary Prevention:

Post myocardial infarction

- Control ischemia (thrombolysis, beta blocker, aspirin)
- Control remodeling (nitrates, ACE inhibition)

---

strated to reduce symptoms, improve quality of life as demonstrated by subjective assessment, improve exercise tolerance, reduce hospitalizations and lengthen survival. However, most patients with heart failure remain significantly limited by their disease and life expectancy remains severely curtailed. Despite recent progress, treatment for heart failure remains one of the frontiers of medicine.

Nonpharmacologic Treatment of Heart Failure

A discussion of the management of heart failure should begin with the role of nonpharmacologic treatments such as *patient education* directed toward the disorder itself, compliance with dietary restrictions of sodium, exercise recommendations, and advice on when to seek additional medical attention.

CARDIAC PEARL

Dietary restriction of sodium: This is one of the most important aspects of treatment; it is also one of the most neglected.

Think how often we see patients with heart disease and failure who are taking an appropriate drug or drugs but do not restrict the sodium intake in their diet. Too often the patient is allowed to eat what he or she wants, thinking that a good diuretic will take care of it. It is particularly important for patients having more advanced degrees of cardiac decompensation to restrict their sodium intake. I still find this to be the most common need for "tightening" and improving their symptoms. Many patients are told to "cut down on the salt" but no specific dietary education and counseling is given. Many patients say that they are on sodium restriction, but questioning them about what they eat for each meal quickly identifies no significant

restriction. In addition, when discussing diet with some of our clinic patients, they may be aware of the need to eat less salty foods, but unfortunately, because of their low income, they have to eat more of the higher sodium content foods such as processed meats and canned soup; however, these patients can still be advised which foods in particular to avoid.

Sodium restriction is number one in treatment of more advanced degrees of cardiac decompensation. Despite the use of drugs, benefit to the patient may not occur unless there is rigid sodium restriction.

Of course, with mild cardiac decompensation, more moderate restriction of salt in the diet may suffice (not adding extra salt to food when eating, or only adding a small amount to make it "tasty").

A cardiac pearl to know that a patient is adhering to his low sodium diet is when he says, "The food is too salty when I eat in restaurants or away from home." I have heard this unsolicited statement from many patients.

W. Proctor Harvey, M.D.

Commonly, a lack of understanding of heart failure and the effects of noncompliance, coupled with denial mechanisms, is pivotal in contributing to the clinical deterioration and the recurrent need for urgent medical care and repeated hospitalizations. Nonmyocardial causes and precipitating factors for heart failure should be identified and treated; restiction of sodium intake and avoiding excess weight are prudent recommendations. Obese patients should lose weight and smokers should discontinue cigarettes. Moderate sodium restriction is indicated, even if diuretics can control overt sodium retention so that lower and safer doses can be used. Although patients should be discouraged from severe physical exertion that provokes ischemic symptoms or hemodynamic instability, and periods of bed rest may be indicated for acute decompensation, careful and moderate physical training has been demonstrated to improve symptoms and exercise capacity in patients with all degrees of heart failure. Noncompliance with medications, dietary indiscretion, inadequate discharge planning or follow-up, failed social support systems and delay in seeking medical attention are major factors contributing to hospitalizations for decompensated heart failure. These facts underscore the importance of education of the patient and family. Patients with marked ventricular dysfunction are at risk for systemic and pulmonay emboli (especially if atrial fibrillation is present) and the use of anticoagulants and anti-platelet agents should be considered in the absence of contraindications.

Patients having chronic cardiac decompensation are more likely to have thrombophlebitis, and in turn pulmonary emboli; this may explain why medical treatment is not working. Searching for this possible complication and treatment with anticoagulants can then result in good control of the patient's heart failure.

W. Proctor Harvey, M.D.

Pharmacologic Treatment of Heart Failure

Treatment of heart failure has been most successful using a polypharmaceutical approach referred to as "triple therapy": diuretics, angiotensin converting enzyme inhibitors, and a digitalis glycoside (almost exclusively digoxin in the U.S.). This represents the standard of care for patients with heart failure and poor systolic function. Additional vasodilators including nitrates and/or hydralazine may also be used as adjunctive treatment (Figure 5). Treatments with beta adrenergic blockers have also shown success in selected cases but remain unapproved by the FDA, as do all other therapies, at the date of this publication. Heart transplantation is the only accepted and FDA approved surgical procedure for treatment of heart failure although other less complicated procedures continue to be evaluated. The substantial benefit resulting from transplantation with respect to symptom relief and the unrivaled improvement in survival since the advent of cyclosporin A into immunosuppression protocols using azothioprine and prednisone explain the growth of this complex intervention. The major limitation of expanded use of this modality of treatment continues to be the availability of donor hearts.

• ACE Inhibitors

ACE inhibitors have been demonstrated to improve symptoms, reduce hospitalizations, and prolong survival in patients with impaired LV systolic function independent of symptom status. Because of their unmatched benefits in improving survival, ACE inhibitors represent the foundation of therapy for heart failure secondary to poor systolic function. Originally tested because of their vasodilator activity, the efficacy of these weak indirect vasodilators, in contrast to the lack of efficacy of more potent vasodilators such as minoxidil, suggest that other and perhaps more important mechanisms of ACE inhibitor actions account for their benefits. As the potential adverse role of neurohor-monal activation has been recognized, the activity of ACE inhibitors as neurohormonal antagonists has been postulated as their major action. ACE inhibitors have been demonstrated to reduce ventricular enlargement, mortality and acute ischemic events in survivors of myocardial infarction. The secondary prevention of recurrent myocardial infarction suggests beneficial effects on coronary arteries by mechanisms not yet defined.

Benefits of ACE inhibitors are not dependent on concomitant therapy with digoxin which some clinicians omit in more mildly symptomatic patients with systolic failure, and should be omitted in all patients with "pure" diastolic heart failure where contractility is not impaired. Studies confirm that ACE inhibition is effective in improving hemodynamics, reducing symptoms and extending exercise tolerance beyond that achieved with diuretic and digitalis alone. Moreover, with ACE inhibitor treatment, hospitalizations are less frequent, electrolyte balance favors potassium and magnesium conservation, and mortality is less frequent. The improvements in symptoms and exercise capacity with ACE inhibitors generally are of greater magnitude and more predictable than seen with conventional vasodilators.

The principal adverse effects of ACE inhibitors are systemic hypotension, functional renal insufficiency, hyperkalemia, cough and angioneurotic edema. The lower side effect profile of ACE inhibitors compared to agents such as hydralazine and minoxidil also provides an additional incentive for use. First-dose hypotension is an increased risk for patients with severe heart failure, activated renin angiotensin systems, hyponatremia or hypovolemia. Patients may be protected from this adverse reaction by repleting intravascular volume prior to ACE inhibitor initiation (reducing diuretic or liberalizing fluids), using small doses to initiate ACE inhibitor therapy and choosing patients with dilated left ventricles that are mechanically unrestricted in filling or emptying. Cough appears to be the most clinically apparent and bothersome side effect necessitating ACE inhibitor discontinuation. The cough is generally nonproductive (irritative) and thought to be mediated by kinins. It is seen in 5% to 20% of patients and results in discontinuation of treatment in approximately 1% to 5% of patients.

• Digitalis Glycoside (Digoxin)

After 200 years of use, and considerable controversy over efficacy, digoxin has been confirmed as effective treatment for reducing symptoms of heart failure. Digoxin exerts salutary hemodynamic effects, increases ejection fraction, improves exercise tolerance, and reduces need for hospitalization. It is beneficial in patients with atrial tachyarrhythmias or sinus rhythm and in patients already using ACE inhibitors. Digoxin controls the ventricular response in patients with chronic atrial tachyarrhythmias such as atrial fibrillation and flutter, an accepted and recognized early benefit of its use.

Digoxin is commonly believed to exert its effects by increasing cardiac contractility as a consequence of inhibition of cellular membrane sodium potassium ATPase. Additonal data support that digoxin reduces sympathetic nervous outflow, improves disturbed baroreceptor function and reduces RAAS activity. Digoxin provides incremental benefits in patients already on ACE inhibitors.

• **Diuretics**

One of the earliest manifestations of heart failure is retention of sodium and water with the development of pulmonary congestion and peripheral edema. Diuretics combined with dietary sodium restriction can restore sodium balance and reduce signs and symptoms of fluid overload. Diuretics are the most commonly prescribed agents for management of heart failure, a fact most assuredly resulting from their prompt and reliable action in controlling salt and water retention. Diuretics exert their beneficial effects much faster than either digoxin or ACE inhibitors, which may take weeks or even months to achieve full therapeutic benefits. Although diuretics produce favorable effects in heart failure secondary to either systolic or diastolic dysfunction, symptoms of heart failure progress in patients treated only with diuretics. This may be explained by diuretic-induced activation of neurohormonal mechanisms, producing further inappropriate vasoconstriction.

CARDIAC PEARL

"I go to bed tired. I get up tired." I have heard patients say this for many years. This is the chronic fatigue that is a prominent symptom of chronic heart failure. It is to be expected and often can be helped by a general "tightening" of the patient's medical management.

The basic treatment for congestive heart failure is as follows:
1. Dietary restriction of sodium
2. Diuretics
3. ACE inhibitors
4. Digitalis
5. Vasodilators
6. Control of arrhythmias, if possible

7. Restriction of unnecessary physical activities
8. Search for "reversible" or "curable" causes of heart failure (cardiac surgery, pulmonary emboli, infections, drug toxicity)
9. Patient education

Diuretics are a fundamental mainstay in treating heart failure. We now have many effective diuretic agents that vary in potency.

The intermittent use of diuretics is effective for mild to moderate decompensation. Some patients need a diuretic only once or twice a week rather than daily.

Diuretics may be more effective on the days when there is less physical activity and more rest takes place.

I have seen many patients who have little or no diuretic response during the busy weekdays, but on a quiet restful Sunday have a prompt significant response to their diuretic tablet of that day.

Of course, with more advanced degrees of heart failure, the stronger diuretics are needed and necessary. Combinations of diuretics, two or even three, can be effective in these patients whereas only one is not.

Hypokalemia (potassium depletion) may be a complication of diuretic therapy. Symptoms of fatigue, weakness and general malaise are clues to suspect this side effect of diuretic therapy and to prevent and treat with supplemental potassium (usually potassium chloride). Serum potassium levels should be checked at intervals to maintain the proper normal level.

It is important to remember that, while many hypokalemic patients complain of weakness and fatigue, others will be asymptomatic. Also, remember that potassium loss can occur with diarrhea and the excessive use of laxatives.

Patients should be advised to eat more of the foods having a higher potassium content.

A word of caution: In patients with coronary artery disease who have already had a myocardial infarction and are taking digitalis and diuretics, low serum potassium can precipitate ventricular arrhythmias, including tachycardia, fibrillation, and death. Monitoring serum potassium at intervals is a precautionary measure. Also, this should be done with elderly patients and alcoholics, because poor nutrition (poor appetite and decreased food intake) depletes potassium; also, they may be taking diuretics.

W. Proctor Harvey, M.D.

Although recognized to have adverse metabolic effects including electrolyte (Na^+, K^+, Mg^{++}, Cl^-) depletion with associated alkalosis, they are generally well tolerated. It is often necessary to provide potassium and magnesium supplementation to control excessive loss of these electrolytes with chronic diuretic use. In the patient with heart failure, it is important to avoid excessive depletion of intravascular volume, which can produce hypotension, further depressing cardiac output and exacerbating orthostatic symptoms common in heart failure patients.

Loop diuretics such as furosemide, bumetanide, and torsemide have emerged as the preferred agents for heart failure over thiazides and potassium-sparing diuretics. The latter have the disadvantage of more limited sodium excretion and loss of efficacy in patients with even moderate renal insufficiency. Resistance to diuretics can be overcome by combining loop and thiazide diuretics (especially furosemide and metalozone), using intravenous loop diuretics or adding drugs that increase renal blood flow such as low dose dopamine.

• Direct-Acting Vasodilators

Recognition of the important role of inappropriate peripheral vasoconstriction in chronic heart failure by Dr. Jay Cohn and others resulted in clinical trials of vasodilators in heart failure. While arterial dilators such as hydralazine produced short-term hemodynamic benefits, beneficial effects long-term are not sustained. More potent arterial dilators such as minoxidil have also been ineffective.

The combination of nitrates and hydralazine was the first pharmacologic intervention to demonstrate improved survival in patients with moderately severe heart failure. This combination also improved symptoms, hemodynamics, and ejection fraction. In a direct comparison to ACE inhibitor (enalapril) in the Second Veterans Admninstration Heart Failure Trial (VeHFT II), nitrates and hydralazine proved superior for improving exercise tolerance. The combination of nitrates and hydralazine however, was less successful than ACE inhibitor treatment with enalapril for improving survival. Furthermore, the combination of hydralazine and nitrate was not well tolerated with 40% of patients having to discontinue one or both drugs because of side effects.

The isosorbide-dinitrate combination remains an alternative in patients unable to tolerate ACE inhibitors and may be helpful as adjunctive treatment in those patients whose clinical improvement is unsatisfactory with ACE inhibitors, though the latter is an unproven hypothesis. It may be particularly effective in patients with mitral or aortic regurgitation.

Calcium channel blocking agents are effective arterial vasodilators and have been confirmed in most short-term studies using parenteral administration in patients with chronic heart failure to produce hemodynamic benefit. However, the first generation calcium channel blockers (nifedipine, diltiazem, and verapamil) have not exerted beneficial long-term effects. These drugs can cause short-term adverse reactions and may increase the long-term frequency of episodes of heart failure and mortality. The lack of efficacy of these agents has been attributed to their intrinsic negative inotropic activity and stimulation of the RAAS and SNS.

Second generation calcium channel blocking agents (amlodipine, felodipine) have been demonstrated to be effective arterial vasodilators and enhance baroreceptor responsivity but without the activation of neurohormonal systems. Whether the favorable preliminary effects of these agents in heart failure will be confirmed by large well-controlled trials is not yet known.

• Positive Inotropic Agents

Use of agents to stimulate contractility would seem to be a rational approach to therapy of heart failure if depressed contractility is considered the primary mechanism of reduced cardiac output. Yet, despite the discovery of many agents proven to be positively inotropic through different mechanisms of action (with the exception of digoxin) there are none available for treatment of chronic heart failure in the U.S. For the short-term treatment of heart failure, the only positive inotropic agents approved for use are intravenous catecholamines and phosphodiesterase inhibitors.

Beta-adrenergic receptor agonists are the mainstay of therapy for acute heart failure producing short-term hemodynamic improvements. Unfortunately, these short-term benefits produced with intravenous use have not been demonstrated chronically. Tolerance, with loss of drug action, increased heart rate and arrhythmia, and higher sudden death rates have compromised many of these agents and precluded their clinical long-term oral use.

The cardiovascular selective phosphodiesterase inhibitors amrinone and milrinone are alternative inotropic and vasodilator agents for the short-term intravenous management of cardiac decompensation. Similar to beta-adrenergic receptor agonists these drugs increase cardiac output while simultaneously reducing ventricular filling pressures. They do so without acting through the beta receptor and hence are not associated with development of tolerance mediated by receptor down-regulation. Oral use of these agents has been limited both by unacceptable side-effects and by decreased survival. The placebo-controlled Prospective Randomized Milrinone Survival Evaluation (PROMISE) in patients with chronic heart failure on digoxin, diuretic, and ACE inhibitor found a 28% increased mortality associated with oral milrinone use.

Newer agents with multiple pharmacologic actions, only some of which are known, continue to be tested in patients with heart failure. Vesnarinone, an oral inotropic agent acting by inhibition of potassium currents, increasing intracellular sodium through opening of sodium channels and mild phosphodiesterase activity has been associated with a favorable effect on survival and is presently under clinical investigation and appears promising for clinical use. Pimobendan, a cardiovascular selective phosphodiesterase inhibitor, remains under study having demonstrated beneficial effects on exercise capacity and symptoms.

• Beta-Adrenergic Receptor Antagonists

Beta receptor blocking drugs can have adverse effects on cardiac contractility and heart rate with resultant decreases in cardiac output and exacerbation of heart failure. Use of beta blockers for the treatment of heart failure has therefore been skeptically viewed by many clinicians and although these agents are still considered investigational, several well-designed studies have confirmed beneficial effects. Beta blockade has been shown to improve ventricular function (myocardial contractility and relaxation) in patients with dilated cardiomyopathy. Beta receptor blockade up-regulates the beta adrenergic receptor making these receptors more responsive to graded doses of beta agonists. In addition, beta blockers can favorably alter baroreceptor mediated increases in sympathetic discharge hence reducing neurohormonal activation. Relatively small trials with metoprolol, bucindolol and carvedilol have shown beta blockade to be well tolerated when introduced at small dosages that are gradually titrated upward. Treatment has been associated with increased exercise capacity, increased LV ejection fractions and improved indices of systolic and diastolic function which develops very slowly over weeks to months of treatment. Large scale survival trials are in progress. Combined alpha and beta blockade (carvedilol, bucindolol) is attractive in that peripheral vasoconstriction may be reduced for added afterload reduction. A large-scale study of these agents is underway in patients with heart failure. Currently, the FDA has not approved beta blockade for the treatment of heart failure.

• Adjunctive Agents

Antiarrhythmic agents are of controversial value in patients with heart failure. The high frequency of both supraventricular and ventricular arrhythmia in patients with asymptomatic left ventricular dysfunction and symptomatic heart failure and the high incidence of sudden cardiac death (presumably of arrhythmic origin) in these patients has prompted evaluation of antiarrhythmic agents of all types. To date, there have been no decisive studies that show benefit in patients with heart failure as a result of antiarrhythmic treatment. Amiodarone is currently being investigated in several large clinical trials and has generated some enthusiasm based on favorable results from small studies. However, a heart failure patient is at increased risk for adverse hemodynamic effects and proarrhythmic events. Both of these inherent risks of antiarrhythmic drugs increase directly as heart failure worsens. Use of agents to suppress arrhythmia, therefore, in patients with heart failure is not currently recommended, and the expected benefits of drug versus device treatment of arrhythmia must be individualized.

Anticoagulants are generally used to prevent embolic stroke in patients with heart failure. The exact incidence of intracavitary thrombus in heart failure is unknown; however it is generally agreed that the incidence of embolic stroke rises with increasing disability from heart failure and the presence of chronic atrial fibrillation or a large segmental dyskinetic area (left ventricular aneurysm). These agents should be considered in patients at high risk for embolic events.

Cardiac Transplantation

Reduced survival of patients with advanced degrees of heart failure can be improved by cardiac transplantation, an option that presently is limited by availability of suitable donor hearts. In general, candidates for transplantation should be in heart failure with moderately-severe-to-severe functional limitation (New York Heart Association Functional Class III-IV), have a poor prognosis with comprehensive medical treatment or available surgical options, be free of pulmonary hypertension or systemic diseases that can jeopardize the transplanted heart, and be free of drug dependencies or emotional or social limitations that would compromise follow-up involving complex medical regimens. The age range has been extended upward since the early introduction of this technique when it was limited to patients under age 50 years and is dependent, in part, on the general medical health of the recipient. Older potential recipients are considered only if they lack pulmonary hypertension, peripheral vascular disease, neurological disease, malignancy, renal disease and mental illness. As surgical and immunosuppressive techniques have improved, especially since the introduction of cyclosporine, the risks of transplantation have been reduced as outcomes have improved.

Therapy of Acute Heart Failure

Patients with acute heart failure have many of the pathophysiologic and clinical manifestations of those with chronic heart failure, except that their pulmonary congestion and peripheral hypoperfusion are severe enough to be immediately life-threatening. The first goal of treatment is immediate hemodynamic and clinical stabilization, so that the cause for the acute decompensation or exacerbation of chronic heart failure can be identified and treated. Some pharmacologic agents, especially adrenergic drugs and phosphodiesterase inhibitors, which are deleterious when used chronically, are valuable for the short-term management of acute heart failure.

Pulmonary congestion presenting as acute pulmonary edema can be caused by non-cardiac conditions such as high altitude stress, narcotic overdose or alveolar-capillary membrane injury which may require specific cause-related therapy. In these instances pulmonary capillary wedge pressure is normal; however when the etiology is heart failure, the primary hemodynamic abnormality is a marked increase in pulmonary venous pressure.

Adequate oxygenation must be maintained either by increasing the concentration of inspired oxygen, positive end-expiratory pressure or assisted or controlled ventilation. Morphine sulfate remains not only a time-honored drug but one that is also highly effective as an arterial and venodilator yielding a prompt shift of blood volume from the central circulation yielding a reduction in pulmonary venous pressure. Morphine sulfate accomplishes these actions through antagonism of the vasoconstrictive effects of the sympathetic nervous system, acting as a neurohormonal antagonist.

Intravenous administration of a loop diuretic can elicit a prompt diuresis, reducing intravascular volume and consequently pulmonary venous pressure. These agents, furosemide, bumetanide, torsemide, may produce beneficial vasodilatory actions in addition to their diuretic effects, possibly resulting from intrarenal prostaglandin release. To achieve an effective diuresis, it is often necessary to use combination diuretic therapy, the addition of dopamine in dopaminergic agonist (renal arterial vasculature dilating) dosages in patients with severely compromised renal function.

Direct acting vasodilators such as nitroglycerin and nitroprusside are highly effective in the treatment of pulmonary edema acting through combined arterial and venous dilatation. Nitroglycerin may be administered cutaneously, orally, sublingually or intravenously. Sublingual use is simple to use and offers early onset of action that can provide prompt relief in less severe syndromes. Intravenous use can allow careful titration of drug effect and high bioavailability although at the expense of continuous monitoring of drug effect. Although both agents act through combined arterial and venous vasodilatation at high dose, nitroprusside is more potent as an arterial dilator and is generally preferred for patients with severe peripheral vasoconstriction, hypertension, or regurgitant valvular disease. Nitroglycerin is preferred treatment for patients with underlying ischemic heart disease.

The pulmonary "congestion" of acute heart failure is associated with variable degrees of "forward" failure presenting as peripheral hypoperfusion with cardiogenic shock as the most severe manifestation. Positive inotropic agents, many of which have significant vasodilating properties, are effective acutely in treating pulmonary congestion and peripheral hypoperfusion.

Sympathomimetic drugs vary in their degree of alpha-1 and alpha-2, beta-1 and beta-2 adrenergic agonist activity yielding different profiles with respect to myocardial contractility, peripheral vasoconstriction or dilatation and acceleration of heart rate. Many of these effects are dose-dependent.

Dopamine demonstrates unique dose-dependent activities including renal-mesenteric dilating action at low doses, increased cardiac contractility and heart rate at moderate dosages and augmented peripheral vascular resistance at high doses. It is generally selected at low doses to augment renal perfusion and diuresis in patients with compromised cardiac output. It can be used in profound states of hypotension to support arterial blood pressure temporarily until correction of primary hemodynamic problems allows its withdrawal. In moderate dosages, dopamine can be used to temporarily augment cardiac output; however, it is associated with increased heart rate, atrial and ventricular arrhythmias, peripheral (alpha-adrenergic receptor mediated) venous and arterial vasoconstriction and rebound withdrawal reductions in cardiac output compromising it's overall value. Improvements in cardiac output are often more directly attributable to increases in heart rate than stroke volume and have been associated with a reduction in arterial oxygen tension as increases in pulomary capillary wedge pressure and central circulation blood volume result from reduced venous capacitance (venoconstriction).

Intravenous dobutamine is preferred to moderate dose dopamine for the short-term management of acute heart failure. It stimulates beta-1, beta-2, and has less alpha-1 receptor agonist activity than dopamine. It exerts positive inotropic effects with an increase in cardiac output resulting primarily from increases in stroke volume with modest effects on heart rate and blood pressure. Pulmonary capillary wedge pressure is reduced as cardiac output is improved. This agent has the most favorable hemodynamic profile for the short-term support of heart failure. As with the use of any catecholamine however, patients should be continuously assessed for tachyphylaxis (tolerance), increased arrhythmia, provocation of ischemia and unacceptable elevations of heart rate and blood pressure. Other catecholamines including isoproterenol, with predominant beta adrenergic agonism, epinephrine and norepinephrine with combined alpha and beta agonism, and phenylephrine with isolated alpha agonism can be used to correct observed derangements of hemodynamics in selected patients with heart failure.

Phosphodiesterase inhibitors such as amrinone and milrinone are effective inotropic and vasodilator agents ("inolators") for the short-term intravenous management of heart failure. These agents are associated with dose-dependent increases in cardiac output and decreases in pulmonary capillary wedge and right atrial pressures. Because these agents do not act through adrenergic receptor agonism they can be used in situations where there is tolerance or blockade of the adrenergic receptors. In addition, phosphodiesterase inhibitors can be combined with catecholamine support of the failing ventricle for enhanced contractility and reductions in peripheral resistance. Lower doses of both agents may be used chronically without the development of tolerance.

Cardiogenic shock is the most severe manifestation of acute heart failure. It is characterized by both pulmonary congestion and severe systemic hypoperfusion. Blood pressure and cardiac index are low (usually < 90 mmHg or 100 mmHg below previous hypertensive levels of arterial blood pressure with cardiac indices of <2.2 L/minute/m^2). The clinical syndrome of cardiogenic shock is defined by reductions in cardiac output severe enough to compromise blood flow to vital organs (brain, heart and kidneys). Clinical manifestations include hypotension, cutaneous vasoconstriction (skin hypoperfusion), lactic acidosis (skeletal muscle hypoperfusion), mental obtundation (cerebral hypoperfusion) oliguria and generalized weakness.

Therapy for cardiogenic shock involves general and specific measures that must be instituted aggressively for an optimal outcome. A Swan-Ganz pulmonary artery catheter is usually placed to assure wedge pressure is kept between 15 mmHg-20 mmHg. It should be emphasized that the treatment of acute heart failure is designed to stabilize the patient and prevent imminent deterioration or demise. Pharmacologic treatments consisting of inotropic and pressor treatments are used to maintain tissue perfusion. Intraaortic counterpulsation or left ventricular assist devices may be required when pharmacologic treatments prove inadequate or to allow needed diagnostic or therapeutic procedures.

In cases in which an identifiable and remedial problem is not defined and corrected the prognosis is extremely poor; therefore simultaneous with treatment must be attempts to identify and treat the causes or contributing factors to heart failure such as myocardial infarction, complications of acute myocardial infarction including ventricular septal defect, ruptured papillary muscle or extensive ventricular aneurysm or pseudoaneurysm. Precipitating factors such as sustained brady- or tachy-arrhythmias, ischemia, sepsis, respiratory failure, volume overload or renal failure must be identified and corrected as indicated.

Treatment of Diastolic Heart Failure

Clinical studies of patients with diastolic heart failure are presently inadequate to direct the physician in the routine management of these patients. It is generally accepted that all guidelines for prevention of hypertension and coronary heart disease apply to these patients and that any contributions secondary to pericardial disease be eliminated. Justification for pharmacologic treatment is anecdotal in general and not based on results from large controlled randomized trials. Hypertension should be controlled since this is a strong stimulus to left ventricular hypertrophy and can be modified successfully. Reductions in hypertrophy would be expected to reduce relaxation abnormalities and improve diastolic function. The antihypertensive use of ACE inhibitors, calcium channel blockers, selective alpha-1 inhibitors and beta blockers are acceptable.

One must avoid excessive heart rate lowering with antihypertensive agents such as verapamil, diltiazem and beta blockers since in the occasional patient, this may compromise cardiac output and be poorly tolerated. Diuretics should be used to control pulmonary and systemic congestion without depleting intravascular volume excessively. Monitoring serum blood urea nitrogen (BUN) and creatinine may be helpful, generally avoiding prere-

590

nal azotemia defined as a BUN/creatinine ratio of greater than 20/1.0. Digoxin should be avoided unless its use is mandated by the presence of a supraventricular tachyarrhythmia with a rapid ventricular response that is unresponsive to other treatments (verapamil, diltiazem or beta blocker). Control of ischemia is important since relaxation, an active metabolic process, is worsened during ischemia. The usual inability of the hypertrophied and stiff ventricle with diastolic heart failure to increase cardiac output in response to peripheral vasodilatation makes the use of direct-acting vasodilators such as hydralazine and high dose nitrates problematic. Arterial vasodilatation accompanying the use of these agents may be associated with hypotension.

Our understanding of the pathophysiology of heart failure has advanced from the solely hemodynamic to a combined neuroendocrine and hemodynamic emphasis, largely because of results from major studies using ACE inhibitors and other therapeutic agents. Clearly, there is more to learn about the genetics in relation to the biology of heart failure and the interactions among different neurohormonal systems. As we observe, learn and review, we must keep in mind the major importance of heart failure as a growing clinical problem. Certain goals seem reasonable as we attempt to prevent, control and regress heart failure.

Heart Failure: Future Goals

Heart failure goals include prevention, by controlling risk factors such as hypertension, coronary artery disease, and left ventricular systolic dysfunction; early identification of those with risk of asymptomatic left ventricular systolic dysfunction and treating them before heart failure arises; routine clinical characterization of those with heart failure by objective testing for optimal care; diagnostic and prognostic information (by determination of LV ejection fraction) is required at least once for all heart failure patients; pathogenic information to elucidate qualitative and quantitative changes in myocardial function including gene expression, with hypertrophy and progression to myocardial systolic dysfunction, leading to genetic targets for treatment; early treatment of systolic heart failure (presymptomatic phase) and later when apparent; effective treatment of diastolic heart failure; identification of particular types and mechanisms of heart failure to supply effective treatment; and resolution, with the goal to improve quality of life and increase survival of heart failure patients with non-pharmacologic guidelines and pharmacologic therapy.

Selected Reading

Definitions
1. Gaasch WH: Diagnosis and treatment of heart failure based on left ventricular systolic or diastolic dysfunction. *JAMA* 1994; 271:1276-80.
2. Marantz PR, Alderman MH, Tobin JN: Diagnostic heterogeneity in clinical trials for congestive heart failure. *Ann Intern Med* 1988; 109:55-61.
3. Rapaport E: Congestive heart failure:diagnosis and principles of treatment. In: *Drug Treatment of Heart Failure*, [Editor JN Cohn], Chapter 6, 1988 pages 127-46.

Background
1. Ho KKL, Pinsky JL, Kannel WB, Levy D: The epidemiology of heart failure: The Framingham Study. *JACC* 1993; 22 [Suppl A]:6A-13A.
2. Morbidity and mortality weekly report from the Centers for Disease Control and Prevention. Mortality from congestive heart failure -United States, 1980-1990. *JAMA* 1994; 271:813-4.
3. Schocken DD, Arrieta MI, Leaverton PE, Ross EA: Prevalence and mortality rate of congestive heart failure in the U.S. *JACC* 1992;20:301-6.

Pathophysiology
1. Atlas SA, Cody RJ, Laragh JH. *Atrial natriuretic peptide in heart failure.* In *Heart Disease* [Editor E. Braunwald], Fourth edition Update No. 2, 1992, pages 19-30.
2. Dzau VJ, Packer M, Lilly LS, et al: Prostaglandins in severe congestive heart failure. *NEJM* 1984; 310:347-52.
3. Francis GS,Benedict C, Johnstone DE, et al: Comparison of neuroendocrine activation in patients with left ventricular dysfunction with and without congestive heart failure. A substudy of the studies of left ventricular dysfunction (SOLVD).*Circ* 1990; 82:1724-30.
4. Myers J, Froelicher VF: Hemodynamic determinants of exercise capacity in chronic heart failure. *Ann Intern Med* 1991; 115:377-86.
5. Poole-Wilson PA: Relation of pathophysiologic mechanisms to outcome in heart failure. *JACC* 1993;22 [Suppl A]:22A-9A.
6. Schrier RW: Pathogenesis of sodium and water retention in high-output and low-outout cardiac failure, nephrotic syndrome, cirrhosis and pregnancy. *NEJM* 1988; 319;1065-72 and 1127-34.
7. Zelis R, Flaim SF: Alterations in vasomotor tone in congestive heart failure. *Prog Cardiovasc Dis* 1982; 24:437-59.

Clinical Approach (Making the Diagnosis of Heart Failure)
1. Braunwald E: *Clinical Manifestations of Heart Failure.* In *Heart Disease,* Chapter 16 [Editor E Braunwald], Philadelphia, WB Saunders Co, 1988, p 471-84.
2. Srebro J and Karliner JS: Congestive heart failure. *Curr Probl Cardiol* 1986; 23:1.
3. Stevenson LW, Perloff JK: The limited reliability of physical signs for estimating hemodynamics in chronic heart failure. *JAMA* 1989;10:884.

Causes of Heart Failure
1. Abelmann WH and Lorell BH: The challenge of cardiomyopathy. *JACC* 1989; 13:1219-39.
2. Johnson RA, Palacios I: Dilated cardiomyopathies of the adult. *NEJM* 1982; 307:1051-8, and 1119-26.

Precipitating Causes of Heart Failure
1. Monane M, Bohn RL, Gurwitz JH, et al: Noncompliance with congestive heart failure therapy in the elderly. *Arch Intern Med* 1994; 154:433-437.

Natural History

1. Erikson H, Svardsudd K, Larsson B et al: Risk factors for heart failure in the general population: The study of men born 1913. EHJ 1989; 10:647-56.

Predictors of Increased Mortality

1. Cohn JN, Levine TB, Olivari MT et al: Plasma norepinephrine as a guide to prognosis in patients with chronic congestive heart failure. *NEJM* 1984; 311:819.
2. Criteria Committee, New York Heart Association, Inc. Diseases of the Heart and Blood Vessels. Nomenclature and criteria for diagnosis. 9th Edition Boston, Little Brown, p 254.
3. Lee WH, Packer M. Prognostic importance of serum sodium concentration and its modification by converting-enzyme inhibition in patients with severe chronic heart failure. *Circ* 1986; 73:257.
4. Packer M: Sudden unexpected death in patients with congestive heart failure: a second frontier. *Circ* 1985; 72:681.

Therapeutic Concepts and Correlations

1. Hoffman RM, Psaty BM, Kronmal RA: Modifiable risk factors for incident heart failure in the coronary artery surgery study. *Arch Intern Med* 1994; 154:417-23.
2. Multicenter Diltiazem Post-Infarction Research Group: The effect of diltiazem on mortality and reinfarction after myocardial infarction. *NEJM* 1988; 319:385.
3. Pfeffer MA, Braunwald E, Moye L for the SAVE Investigators: Effect of captopril on mortality and morbidity in patients with left ventricular dysfunction after myocardial infarction. Results of the Survival and Left Ventricular Enlargement Trial. *NEJM* 1992; 327:669-77.
4. The Acute Infarction Ramipril Efficacy (AIRE) Study Investigators: Effect of ramipril on mortality and morbidity of survivors of acute myocardial infarction with clinical evidence of heart failure. *Lancet* 1993; 342:821-8.
5. The SOLVD Investigators: Effect of enalapril on mortality and the development of heart failure in asymptomatic patients with left ventricular dysfunction. *NEJM* 1992; 327:685-91.

Treatment of Chronic Heart Failure

1. Packer M: How should we judge the efficacy of drug therapy in patients with chronic congestive heart failure? The insights of six blind men. *JACC* 1987; 9:433.

General Measures

1. Coats AJS, Adamopoulous S, Meyer TE, et al: Effects of physical training in chronic heart failure. *Lancet* 1990; 335:63-66.

Pharmacologic Treatment of Heart Failure

1. Packer M: Therapeutic options in management of chronic heart failure. *Circ* 1989; 79:198-204.

Ace Inhibitors

1. The Captopril Digoxin Multicenter Research Group. Comparative effects of captopril and digoxin in patients with mild to moderate heart failure. *JAMA* 1988; 259:539.
2. Captopril Multicenter Research Group: A placebo-controlled trial of captopril in refractory chronic congestive heart failure. *JACC* 1983; 2:755.
3. Cohn JN, Johnson G, Ziesche S, et al: A comparison of enalapril with hydralazine-isosorbide dinitrate in the treatment of congestive heart failure. *NEJM* 1991; 325:303-310.
4. The CONSENSUS Trial Study Group: Effects of enalapril on survival in severe congestive heart failure. Results of the Cooperative North Scandinavian Enalapril Survival Study (CONSENSUS) *NEJM* 1987; 316:1429.
5. Dzau VJ, Hollenberg NK: Renal response to captopril in

severe heart failure. Role of furosemide in natriuresis and reversal of hyponatremia. *Ann Intern Med* 1984; 100:777.
6. Pflugfelder PW, Baird MG, Tonkon MJ, et al: Clinical consequences of angiotensin-converting enzyme inhibitor withdrawal in chronic heart failure: a double-blind, placebo-controlled study of quinapril. *JACC* 1994.
7. The SOLVD Investigators: Effect of enalapril on survival in patients with reduced left ventricular ejection fraction and congestive heart failure. *NEJM* 1991; 325:293.

Digitalis Glycoside (Digoxin)

1. Georghiade M, Hall V, Lakier JB, Goldstein: Comparative hemodynamic and neurohormonal effects of intravenous captopril and digoxin and their combinations in patients with severe heart failure. *JACC* 1989; 13:134-142.
2. Gheorghiade M, Ferguson D. Digoxin-A neurohormonal modulator in heart failure. *Circ* 1991; 84:2181-2186.
3. Guyatt GH, Sullivan MJ, Fallen EL, et al: A controlled trial of digoxin in congestive heart failure. *AJC* 1988; 61:371-375.
4. Packer M, Georghiade M, Young JB et al for the RADIANCE Study. Withdrawal of digoxin from patients with chronic heart failure treated with angiotensin-converting enzyme inhibitors. *NEJM* 1993; 329:1-7.
5. Sullivan M, Atwood JE, Myers J, et al: Increased exercise capacity after digoxin administration in patients with heart failure. *JACC* 1989; 13:1138-1143.
6. Uretsky BF, Young JB, Shahidi FE, et al on behalf of the PROVED Investigative Group: Randomized study assessing the effect of digoxin withdrawal in patients with mild to moderate chronic heart failure: Results of the PROVED Trial. *JACC* 1993; 22:955-62.

Diuretics

1. Anand IS, Veall N, Kalra GS, et al: Treatment of heart failure with diuretics: body compartments, renal function and plasma hormaones. *EHJ* 1989; 10:445-450.
2. Cody RJ, Covit AB, Schaer GL et al. Sodium and water balance in chronic congestive heart failure. *J Clin Invest* 1986; 77:1441-1452.

Direct-Acting Vasodilators

1. Cohn JN, Archibald DG, Ziesche S, et al: Effect of vasodilator therapy on mortality in chronic congestive heart failure. Results of a Veterans Administration cooperative study (V-HeFT). *NEJM* 1986; 314:1547-1552.

Positive Inotropic Agents

1. DiBianco R, Shabetai R, Silverman BD, et al: Oral amrinone for the treatment of chronic congestive heart failure. Results of a multicenter, randomized double-blind and placebo-controlled study. *JACC* 1984; 4:855.
2. DiBianco R, Shabetai R, Kostuk W, et al: A comparison of oral milrinone, digoxin, and their combination in the treatment of patients with chronic heart failure. *NEJM* 1989; 320:677.
3. Feldman A, Bristow M, Parmley W and the Vesnarinone Study Group: Effect of vesnarinone on morbidity and mortality in patients with heart failure. *NEJM* 1993; 329:149-155.
4. Packer M, Carver MD, Rodeneffer RJ, et al: Effect of oral milrinone on mortality in severe chronic heart failure. *NEJM* 1991; 325:1468-1475.

Beta-Adrenergic Receptor Antagonists

1. Domanski MJ and Eichhorn EJ. Beta blockade in congestive heart failure-The need for a definitive study. *AJC* 1994; 73:597-599.
2. Eichhorn EJ. The paradox of beta-adrenergic blockade for the management of congestive heart failure. *AJM* 1992; 92:527-538.

Adjunctive Agents
1. Chakko CS, Gheorghiade M: Ventricular arrhythmias in severe heart failure. Incidence, significance and effectiveness of antiarrhythmic therapy. *AHJ* 1985;109:497.

Transplantation
1. Copeland J: Cardiac transplantation. *Curr Probl Card* 1988; 13:1-224.
2. Hill AB, Chiu RCJ: Dynamic cardiomyoplasty for the treatment of heart failure. *Clin Cardiol* 1989; 12:681-8.
3. 24th Bethesda Conference: Cardiac Transplantation. *JACC* 1993; 22:1-64 .

Treatment of Diastolic Heart Failure
1. Bonow RD, Udelson JE: Left ventricular diastolic dysfunction as a cause of congestive heart failure. *Ann Intern Med* 1992; 117:502-510.
2. DiBianco R: Changing syndrome of heart failure. *J Hyper* 1994; 12: 573-584.
3. Grossman W: Diastolic dysfunction in congestive heart failure. *NEJM* 1991; 325:1557-1564.

The Agency for Healthcare Policy and Research (AHCPR) has recently issued Clinical Practice Guidelines on managing patients with left ventricular systolic dysfunction. A summary of the Guidelines, excerpted from the AHCPR's Quick Reference Guide for Clinicians, follows.

Clinical Practice Guidelines

Heart Failure: Management of Patients with Left Ventricular Systolic Dysfunction

Purpose and Scope

Heart failure is a clinical syndrome or condition characterized by signs and symptoms of intravascular and interstitial volume overload, including shortness of breath, rales, and edema or manifestations of inadequate tissue perfusion, such as fatigue or poor exercise tolerance.

Heart failure is a major public health problem. The National Heart, Lung, and Blood Institute estimates that more than 2 million Americans have heart failure and that about 400,000 new cases of heart failure are diagnosed each year. Heart failure claims the lives of more than 200,000 people in the United States annually. Almost 1 million hospitalizations occur each year for patients with this condition, at an estimated cost of more than $7 billion. Total treatment costs for heart failure, including physician visits, drugs, and nursing home stays, were more than $10 billion in 1990.

This Quick Reference Guide for Clinicians provides recommendations concerning outpatient evaluation and care of patients with heart failure due to left ventricular systolic dysfunction, the most common cause of heart failure. It does not address management of patients with heart failure occur-

ring despite normal ventricular systolic performance or due to surgically correctable valvular disease. This Guide is intended for use by a broad range of healthcare practitioners, including family physicians, physician assistants, nurse practitioners, internists, cardiologists, cardiac surgeons, and clinical nurse specialists. Consultation is advised when patients remain symptomatic despite appropriate care, or experience significant adverse effects, or when invasive management is contemplated.

The most significant recommendations in the Clinical Practice Guideline are described here in an abbreviated form. Readers should refer to the official text of the Clinical Practice Guidelines for supporting discussion, citations, and levels of evidence for each recommendation.

Highlights of Patient Management

Initial Evaluation

All patients who complain of paroxysmal nocturnal dyspnea, orthopnea, or new onset of dyspnea on exertion should undergo evaluation for heart failure unless history and physical examination clearly indicate a noncardiac cause for their symptoms, such as pulmonary disease.

Although the physical examination can provide important information about the etiology of patients' symptoms and appropriate initial treatment, physical signs are not highly sensitive for detecting heart failure. Therefore, patients with symptoms highly suggestive of heart failure should undergo echocardiography radionuclide ventriculography to measure left ventricular ejection fraction if physical signs of heart failure are absent. Patients with less specific symptoms (such as fatigue or edema of the lower extremities) should only undergo such testing when physical or radiographic signs of heart failure are present.

Conversely, many physical findings of heart failure are not highly specific. Elevated jugular venous pressure and a third heart sound are the most specific findings and are virtually diagnostic in patients with compatible symptoms. Pulmonary rales or peripheral edema are relatively nonspecific findings, however. Presence of these signs does not require measurement of left ventricular ejection fraction if other symptoms, signs, and radiographic findings of heart failure (such as cardiomegaly and pulmonary vascular congestion) are absent or if they can be attributed to other causes. Table 1 summarizes tests that should be performed to evaluate patients with new-onset signs or symptoms of heart failure for underlying causes.

A variety of conditions can mimic or provoke

TABLE 1

Echocardiography and Radionuclide Ventriculography Compared in Evaluation of Left Ventricular Performance

Test	Advantages	Disadvantages
Echocardiogram	Permits concomitant assessment of valvular disease, left ventricular hypertrophy and left atrial size Less expensive than radionuclide ventriculography in most areas Able to detect pericardial effusion and ventricular thrombus More generally available	Difficult to perform in patients with lung disease Usually only semiquantitative estimate of ejection fraction provided Technically inadequate in up to 18 percent of patients under optimal circumstances
Radionuclide ventriculogram	More precise and reliable measurement of ejection fraction Better assessment of right ventricular function	Requires venipuncture and radiation exposure Limited assessment of valvular heart disease and left ventricular hypertrophy

---

heart failure, including pulmonary disease, myocardial infarction, arrhythmias, anemia, renal failure, nephrotic syndrome, and thyroid disease. These conditions should be considered in every patient with suspected heart failure of new onset. The guidelines do not address management of those with these conditions.

Hospital Management

The presence or suspicion of heart failure and any of the following findings usually indicates a need for hospitalization:

1. Clinical or electrocardiographic evidence of acute myocardial ischemia.

2. Pulmonary edema or severe respiratory distress.

3. Oxygen saturation below 90% (not due to pulmonary disease).

4. Severe complicating medical illness (e.g., pneumonia).

5. Anasarca.

6. Symptomatic hypotension or syncope.

7. Heart failure refractory to outpatient therapy.

8. Inadequate social support for safe out-patient management.

Occasionally, patients with one of the above findings may be managed at home or in an assisted living or nursing home setting if the clinician believes it is safe to do so and adequate follow-up can be arranged. Heart failure is one of the most common causes for recurrent admission to hospitals, and many of these admissions may be avoidable. Readmission rates as high as 57% within 90 days have been reported in patients over the age of 70 years. Proper discharge planning is essential to prevent those unnecessary readmission. Patients with heart failure should be discharged from the hospital only under the following circumstances:

1. Symptoms of heart failure have been adequately controlled.

2. All reversible causes of morbidity have been treated or stabilized.

3. Patients and caregivers have been educated about medication, diet, activity, exercise, and symptoms of worsening heart failure.

4. Adequate outpatient support and follow-up care have been arranged.

Patients hospitalized for heart failure should be seen or contacted within one week of discharge to make sure they are stable in the outpatient setting and to check their understanding of and compliance with the treatment plan. This guideline does not address management strategies specific to the hospital setting (such as invasive hemodynamic monitoring and intravenous dobutamine).

Clinical Volume Overload

During initial evaluation, the clinician should determine if the patient manifests symptoms or signs of volume overload. Symptoms and signs of volume overload include orthopnea, paroxysmal nocturnal dyspnea, dyspnea on exertion, pulmonary rales, a third heart sound, jugular venous distention, hepatic engorgement, ascites, peripheral edema, pulmonary vascular congestion, or pulmonary edema on chest radiograph.

Patients suspected of having heart failure with signs of significant volume overload should be started immediately on a diuretic. Patients with mild volume overload can be managed adequately with thiazide diuretics, while those with more severe volume overload should be given a loop diuretic. Patients with severe volume overload may require intravenous loop diuretics and/or hospitalization. See Table 2 for agents and dosing.

TABLE 2
Medications Commonly Used for Heart Failure

Drug	Initial dosage	Target dosage	Recommended maximum dosage	Major adverse reactions
Thiazide diuretics Hydrochlorothiazide	25 mg every day	As needed	50 mg every day	Postural hypotension, hypokalemia, hyperglycemia, hyperuricemia, rash; rare severe reactions include pancreatitis, bone marrow suppression and anaphylaxis
Chlorthalidone	25 mg every day	As needed	50 mg every day	Same as above
Loop diuretics		As needed	240 mg twice daily	Same as thiazide diuretics
Furosemide	10 to 40 mg every day	As needed	10 mg every day	Same as above
Bumetanide	0.5–1.0 mg every day	As needed	200 mg twice daily	Same as above
Ethacrynic acid	50 mg every day			
Thiazide-related diuretic Metolazone	2.5 mg*	As needed	10 mg every day	Same as thiazide diuretics
Potassium-sparing diuretics Spironolactone	25 mg every day	As needed	100 mg twice daily	Hyperkalemia, especially if administered with ACE inhibitor; rash; gynecomastia (spironolactone only)
Triamterene	50 mg every day	As needed	100 mg twice daily	Same as above
Amiloride	5 mg every day	As needed	40 mg every day	Same as above
ACE inhibitors Enalapril	2.5 mg twice daily	10 mg twice daily	20 mg twice daily	Hypotension, hyperkalemia, renal insufficiency, cough, skin rash, angioedema, neutropenia
Captopril	6.25 to 12.5 mg three times daily	50 mg three times daily	100 mg three times daily	Same as above
Lisinopril	5 mg every day	20 mg every day	40 mg every day	Same as above
Quinapril	5 mg twice daily	20 mg twice daily	20 mg twice daily	Same as above
Digoxin	0.125 mg every day	As needed	As needed	Cardiotoxicity, confusion, nausea, dizziness, tachycardia, lupus-like syndrome
Hydralazine	10 to 25 mg three times daily	75 mg three times daily	100 mg three times daily	Headache, nausea, dizziness, tachycardia, lupus-like syndrome
Isosorbide dinitrate	10 mg three times daily	40 mg three times daily	80 mg three times daily	Headache, hypotension, flushing

ACE = angiotensin converting enzyme
*—Given as a single test dose initially.

Left Ventricular Function

Measurement of left ventricular performance is a critical step in the evaluation and management of almost all patients with suspected or clinically apparent heart failure. Combined use of history, physical examination, chest radiography, and electrocardiography does not appear to be reliable in determining whether a patient's symptoms and physical findings are due to dilated cardiomyopathy, left ventricular diastolic dysfunction, valvular heart disease, or a noncardiac etiology. Therefore, echocardiography or radionuclide ventriculography can substantially improve diagnosed accuracy.

Patients with suspected heart failure should undergo echocardiography or radionuclide ventriculography to measure left ventricular ejection fraction (if information about ventricular function is unavailable from previous tests). Most patients with signs and symptoms of heart failure are found to have ejection fractions of less than 40%. Patients with ejection fractions of 40% or greater may still have heart failure on the basis of valvular disease or stiffness of the ventricular wall (diastolic dysfunction). The recommendations in this Quick Reference Guide for Clinicians are designed for patients with heart failure due to left ventricular systolic dysfunction (ejection fractions of less than 35% to 40%).

Screening for arrhythmias, as with ambulatory electrocardiographic (Holter) recording, is not warranted as part of patient evaluations with heart failure. Patients with a history of syncope or near-syncope should be referred immediately to a cardiologist with expertise in arrhythmias.

General Counseling

Patients with heart failure should be informed about their diagnosis, including prognosis, symptoms of worsening heart failure, and what to do if these symptoms occur. Information should also be provided concerning the benefits of regular activity, dietary restrictions, necessary medications, and the importance of compliance. It is vital that patients understand their disease and be involved in developing a planned cure. In addition, family members and their caregivers should be included in counseling and decision-making.

• **Activity:** Regular exercise such as walking or cycling should be encouraged for all patients with stable heart failure. Even short periods of bed rest result in reduced exercise tolerance and aerobic capacity, muscular atrophy, and weakness. Recent studies show that patients with heart failure can exercise safely, and regular exercise may improve functional status and decrease symptoms. An explanation of the importance of exercise can help prevent patients from becoming afraid to perform daily activities that might provoke shortness of breath. Patients should be advised to stay as active as possible. Evidence is insufficient to recommend routine use of formal rehabilitation programs for patients with heart failure, although patients who are anxious about exercising on their own or who are dyspneic at a low work level may benefit from such programs.

• **Diet:** Sodium should be restricted to as close to 2 grams per day as possible and in no cases should exceed 3 grams daily. Alcohol use is discouraged. Patients who drink alcohol should be advised to consume no more than one drink per day (one glass of beer or wine, or one mixed drink or cocktail containing no more than 1 oz of alcohol). Patients with heart failure should be advised to avoid excessive fluid intake. However, fluid restriction is not advisable unless patients develop hyponatremia. Patients should be advised to keep a diary of their daily weights and to advise the clinician if a weight gain of 3 lb to 5 lb or more occurs within a week or since the previous visit with the clinician.

• **Medications:** Medications are prescribed for patients with heart failure for two basic reasons:

1. To reduce mortality (angiotensin converting enzyme [ACE] inhibitors, isosorbide dinitrate/hydralazine).

2. To reduce symptoms and improve functional status (ACE inhibitors, diuretics, digoxin). Patients should be provided with complete and accurate information concerning medications they are taking, including the reasons the medications are being prescribed, dosing requirements, and possible side effects.

• **Compliance:** Because noncompliance is a major cause of morbidity and unnecessary hospital admissions for heart failure, educational programs or support groups can be helpful in the care of patients with heart failure. Noncompliance may reduce life expectancy (for example, if patients are not taking beneficial medications) and is also a major cause of hospitalizations. Practitioners should be aware of the problem of noncompliance and its causes and should discuss the importance of compliance at follow-up visits while assisting patients in removing barriers to compliance (such as cost, side effects, or complexity of medical regimens).

• **Prognosis:** Patients with heart failure must understand the serious implications of this diagnosis, including a five-year mortality rate approaching 50% in some studies. Patients should be encouraged to complete advance directives regarding their health care preferences. Patients, families, and caregivers must be provided with accurate information to make decisions and plans for the future, while maintaining hope and emphasizing that good quality of life is still possible.

Initial Pharmacologic Management

Table 2 summarizes the usual dosing and potential adverse effects of the pharmacologic agents commonly used to treat patients with heart failure.

• **Diuretics:** Diuretics are extremely useful for reducing symptoms of volume overload, including orthopnea and paroxysmal nocturnal dyspnea. Diuretics should be started immediately when patients present with symptoms or signs of volume overload. Although initiation of diuretics is important in these patients, it is also important to avoid overdiuresis before starting ACE inhibitors. Volume depletion may lead to hypotension or renal insufficiency when ACE inhibitors are started or when doses of these agents are increased to full therapeutic levels. After the ACE inhibitor is increased to full therapeutic levels, additional diuretic therapy may be necessary to optimize the patient's status.

• **ACE Inhibitors:** Because of their beneficial effects on mortality risk and functional status, ACE inhibitors should be prescribed for all patients with left ventricular systolic dysfunction unless specific contraindications exist such as a history of intolerance or adverse reactions to these agents, a serum potassium level greater than 5.5 mmol per L, or symptomatic hypotension. Patients with contraindications to ACE inhibitors and patients with intolerance to these agents should be given isosorbide dinitrate/hydralazine. ACE inhibitors may be considered as sole therapy in patients who present with fatigue or with mild dyspnea on exertion and who do not have any signs or symptoms of volume overload. Diuretics should be added if symptoms persist in these patients despite treatment with ACE inhibitors or if volume overload develops at a later time.

• **Digoxin:** Digoxin increases the force of ventricular contraction in patients with left ventricular systolic dysfunction. Although physical functioning and symptoms may improve with digoxin, its effect on mortality is unknown. Digoxin should be initiated along with ACE inhibitors and diuretics in patients with severe heart failure. Patients with mild to moderate heart failure will often become asymptomatic with optimal doses of ACE inhibitors and diuretics; these patients do not require digoxin. Digoxin should be added to the therapeutic regimen of those patients whose symptoms persist despite optimal doses of ACE inhibitors and diuretics. Digoxin dosing and precautions are discussed in the Guidelines.

• **Anticoagulation:** Routine anticoagulation is not recommended. Patients with a history of systemic or pulmonary embolism or recent atrial fibrillation should receive anticoagulation therapy until a prothrombin time ratio of 1.2 to 1.8 times each individual control time is reached (International Normalization Ratio of 2.0 to 3.0). Although there has never been a controlled trial of anticoagulation for patients with heart failure, the risks of routine treatment, including intracranial or gastrointestinal hemorrhage, do not appear warranted given the relatively low incidence of significant thromboembolic events in this population.

Revascularization

Coronary artery disease is currently the most common cause of heart failure in the United States, and some patients may benefit from revascularization. In particular, patients with viable myocardium subserved by substantially stenotic vessels may reasonably be expected to obtain longevity benefits and,

perhaps, improved quality of life if the stenosis is successfully relieved. On the other hand, revascularization entails significant morbidity and mortality. Before studies are initiated to determine if patients are candidates for revascularization (i.e., have viable myocardium subserved by stenotic arteries), it is important to first determine if any conditions exist that may preclude intervention or could raise risk of revascularization above any potential benefit. These may include the following situations:

1. Patient would not consider surgery or is unable to give informed consent.

2. Severe comorbid diseases, especially renal failure, pulmonary disease, or cerebrovascular disease (such as severe stroke).

3. Very low ejection fraction (for example, less than 20%).

4. Patients with illnesses that indicate a projected life expectancy less than or equal to one year. These include advanced cancer, severe lung or liver disease, chronic renal disease, advanced diabetes mellitus, and advanced collagen vascular disease.

5. Technical factors, including previous myocardial revascularization or other cardiac procedure, history of chest irradiation, and diffuse distal coronary artery atherosclerosis.

Patients without contraindication to revascularization should be advised of the possibility of revascularization, including its potential benefits and harms. Three parameters are important:

1. Likelihood of surgically correctable lesions.

2. Expected benefits of revascularization.

3. Expected risks and potential harms of revascularization.

These parameters vary depending on several factors, including whether clinical evidence of myocardial ischemia is present and the patient's general health. Counseling should be based on patients' individual characteristics, particularly on an assessment of patients' risk factors for coronary artery disease. Patients can be classified into three major subgroups:

1. Those who have neither angina nor a history of myocardial infarction.

2. Patients without significant angina (angina that limits exercise or occurs frequently at rest) but who have a history of myocardial infarction.

3. Patients with significant angina pectoris.

• **No Angina and No Myocardial Infarction:** The likelihood of coronary disease in patients who have heart failure without angina or history of myocardial infarction varies depending on patient risk factors such as age, sex, smoking history, hyperlipidemia, hypertension, family history of premature coronary artery disease, and diabetes.

Patients should be counseled concerning expected benefits and risks of evaluation for ischemia, including the fact that there is no evidence from controlled trials to show that revascularization benefits heart failure patients in the absence of angina. It is unclear whether patients without a history of myocardial infarction or significant angina should be routinely evaluated for ischemia. The decision about whether to perform physiologic tests for ischemia or coronary angiography should be based on a consideration of patients' risk factors for coronary artery disease and the likelihood of alternative etiologies (for example, alcoholic cardiomyopathy).

• **No Angina and History of Myocardial Infarction:** Available evidence suggests that as many as half of all patients who have myocardial infarction have clinically important myocardial ischemia in areas supplied by other coronary arteries. There are no data, however, to show that revascularization of these areas is beneficial, in terms of increased life expectancy or enhanced quality of life, in the absence of angina. Nevertheless, patients with large areas of ischemia may possibly benefit from revascularization. Patients without angina but with a history of myocardial infarction should undergo a physiologic test for ischemia and should undergo cardiac catheterization if ischemic regions are detected. This strategy will fail to detect a small number of patients with false-negative physiologic tests. However, in view of the lack of evidence that these patients benefit from surgery, together with a consideration of the morbidity, mortality, and cost of catheterizing all patients in this group, this drawback is considered relatively minor. Although there are a number of acceptable physiologic tests for ischemia, the most widely available and accepted procedure for determining presence of ischemic myocardium is myocardial perfusion scintigraphy, such as thallium scanning, with post-stress, redistribution and rest reinjection imaging.

• **Angina:** Potential benefit of revascularization is clearest and probably greatest in those with severe or limiting angina or angina-equivalent (such as recurrent acute episodes of pulmonary edema despite appropriate medical management). Available evidence suggests that about 75% of heart failure patients with significant concomitant angina have operable disease. Although the three randomized trials of coronary artery bypass graft (CAB) surgery excluded patients with heart failure or severe left ventricular dysfunction, several cohort studies and registries suggest that those with angina and impaired left ventricular function have improved functional status and survival if they undergo bypass surgery.

Patients with heart failure without contraindications to revascularization and who have exercise-limiting angina, angina that occurs frequently at rest, or recurrent episodes of acute pulmonary edema, should be advised to undergo coronary artery angiography as the initial test for significant coronary lesions. Some patients may need physiologic testing for ischemia to interpret significance of the findings from coronary artery angiography.

• **Counseling and Decision:** Based on results of physiologic testing and/or cardiac catheterization, the physician should give the patient a refined estimate of risks and benefits of revascularization. The patient can then decide if he or she desires revascularization. No data are available that address the question of how much ischemia should be present to justify the risk of revascularization for a chance of improvement in survival. In general, patients with severely depressed ejection fractions (less than 20%) should undergo revascularization only if large areas of ischemia are detected. Patients with less severely depressed ejection fractions may be willing to risk surgery for more modest-sized ischemic areas. The lack of data in this area makes it difficult to justify revascularization for small ischemic areas, except when severe angina is present.

• **Continue Medical Management:** If a patient is not a candidate for revascularization, studies show insufficient evidence of reversible ischemia, or surgery has been performed but the patient still has residual left ventricular dysfunction, then medical therapy should be continued. As stated previously, an assessment of compliance is recommended at each visit. Use of a home health nurse or visiting nurse may be helpful for this purpose.

• **Revascularize:** Coronary artery bypass grafting is the only revascularization procedure shown to prolong life in patients with angina and left ventricular dysfunction. The effect of coronary artery angioplasty on survival of heart failure patients has not been studied, nor are the risks of angioplasty in heart failure patients known. The choice between CAB and angioplasty will depend on numerous considerations, including multiple technical factors (for example, coronary anatomy), relative risk of the two procedures in individual patients, and patient preferences.

Follow-Up

Careful history and physical examination should be the main guide to determining outcomes and directing therapy. A thorough history should include questions regarding physical functioning, mental health, sleep disturbance, sexual function, cognitive function, and ability to perform usual work and social activities. On follow-up visits, patients should be asked about presence of orthopnea, paroxysmal nocturnal dyspnea, edema, and dyspnea on exertion. It is important to remember that patients are likely to experience changes in symptoms before there is evidence of deterioration on physical examination. Patients should be encouraged to keep a daily weight report and to bring that with them when visiting their practitioner. Patients should be instructed to call if they experience an unexplained weight gain greater than 3 lb to 5 lb since their last clinical evaluation. Family members or caregivers can often contribute important additional information about the patient's status and compliance when asked similar questions. In some cases, it may be desirable to interview family members or caregivers apart from a patient in order to validate the patient's report. If discrepancies do occur, additional measures should be instituted for clarification. In addition to questions about symptoms and activities, providers should ask about other aspects of patients' health-related quality of life, including sleep, sexual function, mental health, appetite, or social activities. A worsening in any of these parameters may indicate the need to adjust therapy. To ensure optimal care for heart failure, the provider must view the disease in the context of the patient's life and see how the patient is coping with the disease. Consultation with psychologists, health educators, and clinical specialists may be necessary to deal with problems such as depression, trouble adhering to complicated dietary or medical regimens, or poor functional status.

The Heart Failure Guideline Panel recommends against use of other tests such as echocardiography or exercise testing for monitoring the response of heart failure treatment. No data exist to suggest that the monitoring of these endpoints contributes information beyond that obtained by a careful history and physical exam. However, repeat testing may be useful in patients with a new heart murmur, a new myocardial infarction, or sudden deterioration despite compliance with medications. Repeat testing as part of evaluation for transplantation may also be necessary.

Additional Pharmacologic Management

If patients remain symptomatic on a combination of a diuretic, an ACE inhibitor and digoxin, they should be seen at least once by a cardiologist. Patients with persistent volume overload despite initial medical management may require more aggressive administration of the current diuretic (e.g., intravenous administration), more potent diuretics, or a combination of diuretics (Table 2).

Patients with persistent dyspnea after optimal doses of diuretics, ACE inhibitors, and digoxin should be given a trial of hydralazine and/or nitrates. The addition of a vasodilator to an ACE inhibitor may relieve symptoms. Direct vasodilators may be particularly helpful in patients with hypertension or evidence of severe mitral regurgitation. Even patients with blood pressure in the usual normal range benefit by reducing their blood pressure with direct vasodilators. Alternatively, if a patient primarily has symptoms of pulmonary congestion or has a low systolic blood pressure, nitrates are preferred over arterial vasodilators.

Some evidence shows that gradual incremental therapy with low-dose beta blockers may produce long-term improvements in symptoms and in natural history in patients with heart failure. However, because beta blockers may also cause acute deterioration in patients with heart failure, this form of treatment should be considered experimental at this time.

Heart Transplantation

Consideration should be given to cardiac transplantation in patients with severe limitation and/or repeated hospitalization because of heart failure, despite aggressive medical therapy, and in whom revascularization is not likely to convey benefit. Patients with severe symptoms should be referred to a cardiologist to ensure that medical therapy is optimized prior to referral for possible transplantation. Practitioners should refer to existing documents concerning heart transplantation for further information on criteria for patient selection.

Patients with poor systolic function whose symptoms are controlled with optimal medical management need not be referred for transplantation. Where appropriate, patients with severe symptoms uncontrolled by optimal medical management who are unable to obtain a heart transplant should be informed of the availability of experimental treatment protocols for which they may be eligible (such as new drugs or mechanical assist devices).

Prevention in Patients with Left Ventricular Systolic Dysfunction

Asymptomatic patients found to have moderately or severely reduced left ventricular systolic function (ejection fraction less than 40%) should be treated with an ACE inhibitor to reduce the chance of developing clinical heart failure.

Probably the largest number of such patients

will be those who have recently sustained a myocardial infarction. For this reason, ejection fraction should be determined in most patients following a myocardial infarction unless they are at low risk for significant systolic dysfunction, i.e., unless they meet all of the following criteria:

1. No previous myocardial infarction.

2. Inferior infarction.

3. Relatively small increase in cardiac enzymes (less than two to four times normal).

4. No Q waves develop on electrocardiogram.

5. Uncomplicated clinical course (no arrhythmia or hypotension).

Other asymptomatic patients without infarctions may be found to have reduced ejection fraction on evaluation of heart murmurs or cardiomegaly. These patients should also be treated with ACE inhibitors.

The clinical practice guidelines were developed by an interdisciplinary, non-federal panel comprising healthcare professionals and consumer representatives. Panel members were Marvin A. Konstam, MD, co-chair; Kathleen Dracup, D N Sc, Rn, co-chair; Michael B. Bottorff, Pharm D; Neil H Brooks, MD; Robert A Dacey, MD; Sandra B Dunbar, DSn, RN; Anne B. Jackson, MA, RN; Mariell Jessup, MD; Jerry C. Johnson, MD; Robert H. Jones, MD; Robert J. Luchi, MD; Barry M. Massie, MD; Bertram Pitt, MD; Eric A. Rose, MD; Lewis J. Rubin, MD; Richard F. Wright, MD. Konstam M, Dracup K, Baker D et al: Heart failure: evaluation and care of patients with left ventricular systolic dysfunction. Clinical Practice Guidelines No. 11. AHCPR publication No. 94-0612. Rockville, Md. Agency for Healthcare Policy and Research, Public Health Service, US Dept of Health and Human Services, June 1994.

Selected Reading

1. Alderman EL, Fisher LD, Litwin P, Kaiser GC et al: Results of coronary artery surgery in patients with poor left ventricular function (CASS) *Circ* 1963; 68:785-95.

2. Amsdorf MF, Bump TE: Management of arrhythmias in heart failure. *Card Clin* 1989; 7 145-69.

3. Bounous EP, Mark DB, Pollock ET, et al: Surgical survival benefits for coronary disease patients with left ventricular dysfunction. *Circ* 1988; 78 (3 pt 2):1151-1157.

4. Chakko S, Woska D, Martinez H et al: Clinical, radiographic, and hemodynamic correlations in chronic congestive heart failure: conflicting results may lead to inappropriate care. *AJM*; 1991:90:353-359.

5. Christakis GT, Ivanov J, Weisel RD et al: The changing pattern of coronary bypass surgery. *Circ* 1989; 80(3 Pt 1).

6. Coats AJ, Adamopoulous S, Meyer TE, Conway J, Sleight P: Effects of physical training in chronic heart failure. *Lancet* 1990; 335:63-66.

7. Cody RI: Management of refractory congestive heart failure. *AJC.* 1992; 69; 141G-9G.

8. Cohn JN, Archibald DG, Ziesche S et al: Effect of vasodilator therapy on mortality in chronic CHF. Results of Veterans Administration Cooperative Study. *NEJM* 1986; 314: 7-52.

9. Cohn JN, Johnson G, Ziesche S, Cobb F, et al: Comparison of enalapril with hydralazine-isosorbide dinitrate in treatment of chronic CHF. *NEJM* 1991; 325: 303-310.

10. Dougherty AH, Naccarelli GV, Gray EL et al: Congestive heart failure with normal systolic function. *AJC* 1984; 54: 778-782.

11. Dracup K, Walden JA, Stevenson LW, Brecht ML: Quality of life in patients with advanced heart failure. *Heart Lung Transplant* 1992; 11(2 Ft 1):273-279.

12. Dubach P, Froelicher VF: Cardiac rehabilitation for heart failure patients. *Card* 1989;76:368-373.

13. Effect of enalapril on mortality and the development of heart failure in asymptomatic patients with reduced left ventricular ejection fractions. The SOLVD Investigators. *NEJM* 1992; 327:685-691 [Published erratum] *NEJM* 1992; 327:1768.

14. Effect of enalapril on mortality in severe CHF. Results of the Cooperative North Scandinavian Enalapril Survival Study (CONSENSUS). The CONSENSUS Trial Study Group. *NEJM* 1987; 316:1429-1435.

15. Effect of enalapril on survival in patients with reduced left ventricular ejection fractions and CHF. The SOLVD Investigators. *NEJM* 1991; 325:293-302.

16. Falk RH: A plea for a clinical trial of anticoagulation in dilated cardiomyopathy (Editorial). *AJC* 1990; 65:14-15.

17. Fleg JL, Hinton PC, Lakatta EG, Marcus FL, et al: Physician utilization of laboratory procedures to monitor outpatients with CHF. *Arch Int Med* 1989; 149:393-396.

18. Ghali JK, Kadakia S, Cooper RS, Liso YL: Precipitating factors leading to decompensation of heart failure. Trials among urban blacks. *Arch Int Med* 1988; 148:201-306.

19. Ghali JK, Kadakia S, Cooper RS, Liso YL: Bedside diagnosing of preserved vs impaired left ventricular systolic function in heart failure. *AJC* 1991; 67: 1002-1006.

20. Hannan EL, Kilburn H Jr, O'Donnell F, et al: Adult open heart surgery in New York State. Analysis of risk factors and hospital mortality rates. *JAMA* 1990; 264: 2768-2774.

21. Hartzler GO, Rutherford BD, McConahay DR, Johnson WL: High-risk percutaneous transluminal coronary angioplasty. *AJC* 1988; 61: 33G-37G.

22. Jaeschke R, Oxman AD, Guyatt GH: Do congestive heart failure patients in sinus rhythm benefit from dioxin therapy? A systematic overview and analysis. *AJM* 1990.88:279-286.

23. Kannel WB: Epidemiological aspects of heart failure. *Card Clin* 1989:7:1-9.

24. Kotler TS, Diamond GA: Exercise thallium-201 scintigraphy in the diagnosis and prognosis of coronary artery disease. *Ann Int Med* 1990:113: 684-702.

25. Marantz PR, Tobin JN, Steingart RM, Budner N, et al: Relationship between left ventricular systolic function and CHF diagnosed by clinical criteria. *Circ* 1988;77:607-612.

26. Molgaard H, Kristenson BO, Baandrup U: Importance of abstention from alcohol in alcoholic heart disease. *Int J Card* 1990; 26: 373-375.

27. On bedrest in heart failure. *Lancet* 1990; 336: 75-76.

28. Perlman LV, Isenberg EL, Donovan L, Fleming DS: Public health nurses and prevention of recurrence of CHF. *Geriatrics* 1969; 24:82-89.

29. Pfeifer MA, Braunwald E, Moye LA, Basta L et al: Effect of captopril on mortality and morbidity in patients with left ventricular dysfunction after myocardial infarction.Results of the survival and ventricular enlargement trial. The SAVE Investigators. *NEJM* 1992; 327:669-677.

30. Preliminary report: Effect of encainide and flecainide on mortality in a randomized trial of arrhythmia suppression after myocardial infarction. The Cardiac Arrhythmia Suppression Trial (CAST) Investigators. *NEJM* 1989; 321: 406-417.

31. Vinson JM, Rich MW, Sperry JC, Shah AS, McNamara T: Early readmission of elderly patients with CHF. *J Am Ger Soc* 1990:1290-1295.

CHAPTER 26

Clinical Approach to the Patient in Shock

Joseph R. McClellan, M.D.

Acute circulatory collapse, or shock, occurs in an array of conditions that ultimately lead to inadequate oxygen delivery to the organs, tissues, and cells. Shock results from a variety of pathophysiological alterations with different etiologies and clinical manifestations. Rapid treatment is vital to prevent mortality in this condition. Clinical recognition of shock depends on a high index of suspicion and an understanding of the pathophysiology of initial signs and symptoms. Bedside diagnosis is required to initiate early, appropriate therapy and to decide which procedures and interventions are necessary for further diagnosis and treatment.

The unifying concept for all types of shock is that the syndrome results from inadequate oxygen transport to the organs. Systemic oxygen transport (DO_2) must match oxygen consumption (VO_2) and shock results from an increase in demand for oxygen or the inability to maintain normal oxygen supply. When oxygen transport is inadequate to meet cellular requirements, anaerobic metabolism ensues and the generation of high energy phosphate compounds is impaired. With cellular hypoxia the mitochondrial oxygenation of glucose through the Krebs citric acid cycle is inhibited and ATP is produced only by anaerobic glycolysis in cytoplasm. Anaerobic metabolism cannot proceed beyond the conversion of pyruvate to lactate and generates less than 10% of ATP produced by aerobic metabolism. Lactic acid accumulates and blood lactate levels reflect the cumulative cellular oxygen deficit that develops. Ultimately cell death occurs.

Oxygen consumption varies substantially in shock states. A number of factors including hormonal status, breathing, fever, and physical activity can increase oxygen consumption. Frequently, early in shock, VO_2 rises and oxygen delivery must also be increased concomitantly. As shock progresses, VO_2 may decrease and tissue survival will depend on anaerobic metabolism. Optimizing oxygen delivery is necessary for the initial therapy of shock states and forms the basis for the principles of management. Oxygen delivery depends on oxygen carrying capacity (the hemoglobin), oxygenation (percent hemoglobin saturation) and the blood flow or cardiac output. Fundamental causes of shock results in reduction of one or all of these determinants of oxygen delivery. When arterial blood flow diminishes, the initial compensatory mechanism is an increase in tissue oxygen extraction with a corresponding reduction in the venous oxygen saturation. As the level of oxygen delivery further decreases, oxygen extraction increases maximally, anaerobic metabolism ensues and the VO_2 will no longer increase. A fixed or declining VO_2 in association with elevated lactic acid production identifies a patient subgroup with a high mortality rate.

Hemodynamic Derangements in Shock

Peripheral Resistance

Adequate organ perfusion requires the maintenance of a sufficient flow of oxygenated blood. The arterial pressure is the force which maintains the blood flow and is directly dependent on stroke volume (cardiac output) and peripheral resistance. This driving force, which is the pressure difference between two vascular beds, determines the amount of flow that occurs. The pressure difference that develops when blood passes through a tube occurs because of energy loss and the peripheral resistance is defined as the reduction in pressure that occurs per unit flow. Resistance increases when there is a decrease in cross-sectional area and is inversely proportional to the fourth power of the radius of the tube. An increase in the length of the tube or in the viscosity of the fluid also raises systemic vascular resistance. Arterioles primarily control peripheral resistance and the distribution of the blood flow to and within an organ, and are modulated by a variety of influences which alter their diameter.

The autonomic nervous system and the modulation of its activity by the arterial baroreceptors, myocardial receptors, and chemoreceptors control the peripheral resistance. These receptors input to the medullary vasomotor centers that regulate release of catecholamines from the adrenal medulla and sympathetic nerves. Variable responses in multiple vascular beds occur which determine the amount of flow to the various organ systems. Reduction in blood pressure is sensed by the baroreceptors and produces a decrease in afferent inhibitory impulses to the vasomotor center. This results in increased sympathetic outflow with preferential vasoconstriction in the skeletal muscle and splanchnic vascular beds but only minimal change in the cerebral and coronary circulation.

These vascular beds also have the capacity for local autoregulation and can maintain adequate blood flow over a wide range of arterial pressures. Autoregulation occurs in the cerebral, coronary and renal circulation and protects these organs when systemic hypotension occurs. A variety of other humoral factors also influence the peripheral circulation including a number of vasoactive mediators which are released in response to endotoxins. Intense peripheral vasodilation with an associated loss of autoregulation produces maldistribution of blood flow in the microcirculation, which can ultimately lead to cellular injury and organ failure.

Cardiac Output

Central to the maintenance of an effective circulation is myocardial pump function. Cardiac performance is dependent on intrinsic cardiac properties which include contractility, relaxation, diastolic stiffness, and heart rate as well as extrinsic properties which are the preload or venous return, afterload, primarily determined by peripheral resistance, and the pericardium. Preload may be inadequate because of a reduction in the circulating blood volume. This is a common cause of shock and results from a variety of conditions including hem-

orrhage or excessive fluid loss. Preload is also dependent on the total capacity of the venous bed which can be rapidly altered. Catecholamines and vasopressin may diminish venous capacity and help to augment venous return while other vasoactive mediators can produce venodilation and decreased venous return. Effective preload may also be reduced in pericardial tamponade or restriction and other cardiac conditions which are characterized by abnormal diastolic compliance.

Afterload is the resistance to ejection of blood from the ventricle and impedance of outflow is determined by the characteristics of the vascular tree. The afterload can be approximated from the arterial blood pressure and left ventricular wall stress which is largely determined by the left ventricular cavity size as well as intracavitary pressure. Cardiac function depends on anatomic integrity of the pump as well as cardiac contractility. Toxins, acute inflammatory conditions, acute valvular insufficiency or obstruction, left to right shunts and cardiac dysrhythmias may all lead to severe reductions in cardiac output. Cardiogenic shock most commonly occurs because of an acute myocardial infarction with loss of a substantial amount of cardiac muscle mass. Frequently, multiple hemodynamic abnormalities occur simultaneously in shock which are related both to the control of the peripheral vasculature and the cardiac output. However, the predominant derangement leads to the clinical classification of shock states (Figure 1).

Clinical Classification

• **Hypovolemic:** In hypovolemic shock the fundamental abnormality is inadequate circulating volume to maintain effective cardiac output. The loss of intravascular volume is most frequently due to hemorrhage or dehydration and is commonly seen with trauma, surgery, severe vomiting or diarrhea or loss of skin integrity due to burns or bullous dermatologic diseases. During early phases of hypovolemia, inadequate venous return and stroke volume are compensated by increased sympathetic tone mediated by the baroreceptor reflex. As hypovolemia progresses, hypotension and organ hypoperfusion develops.

• **Distributive:** Sepsis is the model for distributive shock, although other conditions including systemic anaphylaxis or autonomic blockade can produce a similar state. Estimates are that a million patients per year develop bacteremia and approximately one half progress to frank shock with a mortality between 40% and 60%. Septic shock produces acute alterations in the distribution of blood, which occur because of abnormalities in vascular reactiv-

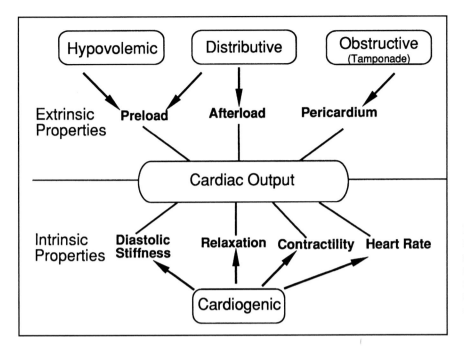

Figure 1. Clinical Classification of Shock. Cardiac output is controlled by both intrinsic and extrinsic properties. The four major categories of shock, hypovolemic, distributive, obstructive, and cardiogenic are determined by their major hemodynamic derangement.

ity. In most forms of shock the central abnormality is a reduction in the stroke volume and overall cardiac output. In the initial phase of sepsis, the primary alteration is arterial vasodilation with reduction in peripheral vascular resistance and increased cardiac output. Diffuse arterial vasodilation is related to the effects of endotoxins, exotoxins and cytokines. Cytokines are released by macrophages and lymphocytes in response to circulating endotoxins.

The cytokines include tumor necrosis factor, which produces vasodilatation and hypotension and renal, pulmonary and endothelial damage, as well as interleukin 1, which activates T-cells and interleukin 2 which causes fever and hypotension. Multiple other mediators are released including kinins, histamines, prostaglandins, lipid A, ß-endorphins and leukotrines with variable effects, and produce constriction or dilatation of arterial and post-capillary venules. Vasodilatation may be mediated on a cellular level by the release of nitric oxide. These alterations in the microcirculation, accompanied by loss of normal autoregulation, lead to regional imbalances of blood flow. The net result is that some vascular beds receive inadequate flow while in others there may be arteriovenous shunting with cellular and tissue hypoxia. Other mechanisms responsible for the hemodynamic abnormalities include increased vascular permeability as well as venous dilatation and blood pooling with a reduction in effective circulating blood volume. Depression of myocardial function also occurs in septic shock. Initially, there is a decrease in diastolic function, followed by impaired systolic func-

tion of both the right and left ventricle. Acute respiratory failure and associated acute pulmonary hypertension may contribute to the right ventricular dysfunction. Both water and lipid-soluble circulating myocardial depressant factors have been implicated in this myocardial dysfunction. If the syndrome resolves, myocardial function will gradually improve.

Distributive shock, with sepsis as a model, is quite complex with features of hypovolemic and cardiogenic shock. The complicated nature of this hemodynamic syndrome often requires multiple interventions for successful resolution, however, the mortality in septic shock remains high in spite of improved antibiotic therapy and greater understanding of the pathophysiology. Death usually results from multiple organ failure and the mortality increases to 80% when three organ systems are affected.

• **Obstructive Shock:** In obstructive shock, the primary mechanism is an impairment of the venous return to the right or left ventricle. The obstruction may occur in the venous system, pulmonary artery or pericardium and the net result is inadequate stroke volume and cardiac output. This form of shock is exemplified by pericardial tamponade in which the underlying mechanism is limitation of ventricular filling during diastole. The pericardium contributes to the circulation by assisting in control of the hydrostatic forces of the heart, the prevention of acute ventricular dilatation, and the maintenance of the diastolic interrelationships of the ventricles. The normal pericardium is a relatively stiff, non-compliant sac, and intrapericardial pressure

603

TABLE 1
Mortality in Acute Myocardial Infarction

	CLASSIFICATIONS				
	CLINICAL[1]		HEMODYNAMIC[2]		
CLASS	PHYSICAL EXAM	MORTALITY (%)	CARDIAC OUTPUT (L/min/m²)	PCW (mmHg)	MORTALITY %
I	NORMAL	8	> 2.2	< 18	3
II	RALES <50% S₃	30	> 2.2	> 18	9
III	RALES >50% Pulmonary edema	44	< 2.2	< 18	23
IV	SHOCK	> 80	< 2.2	> 18	51

[1] Killip, T. III: Treatment of myocardial infarction in a coronary care unit: A two year experience with 250 patients. AJC 20:457, 1967.
[2] Forrester, J.S.: Medical therapy of acute myocardial infarction by application of hemodynamic subsets. NEJM 295: 1356, 1976.

will rise rapidly if fluid is added. Therefore, if fluid accumulates quickly in the pericardium, for example, with acute hemorrhage after cardiac perforation, intrapericardial pressure rises rapidly. Diseases of the pericardium, including malignancy and connective tissue disease, are usually associated with a slower rate of accumulation of fluid. During this more gradual increase in pericardial fluid the compliance of the pericardial sac increases and pressure rises slowly. However, the limits of pericardial stretch will be reached and then the intrapericardial pressure will also begin to rise rapidly.

As intrapericardial pressure rises, the transmural pressure gradient between the pericardial sac and right atrium and ventricle decreases which leads to a reduction in venous return with a resultant fall in stroke volume. Initial compensatory mechanisms include an increase in sympathetic tone with tachycardia and increased peripheral resistance. Hypertension may even occur early in the course of tamponade. Peripheral venoconstriction also increases the venous pressure and central blood volume. As tamponade progresses, compensatory mechanisms are inadequate to maintain perfusion and shock ensues. Tamponade also alters the pattern of venous return and cardiac chamber filling. Ejection fraction is usually increased and at end-systole the total intracardiac volume is low with a concomitant decrease in intra-pericardial and right atrial pressure. The low intracardiac pressures initially enhance venous return. In early diastole, the intracardiac volume and pressure in the pericardium rapidly rises which impedes further diastolic filling of the right atrium. Echocardiography may demonstrate collapse of the right atrium in diastole, which is an early but non-specific sign of tamponade physiology. Acute pulmonary embolism is another form of obstructive shock. With acute obstruction of the pulmonary artery there is a reduction in the effective cross-sectional area of the pulmonary vasculature. This may lead to sudden, severe pulmonary hypertension, right ventricular pressure overload and decompensation and a reduced stroke volume. A fall in right-sided stroke volume results in reduced venous return to the left heart and impaired systemic cardiac output. These changes can occur quite abruptly with profound hypotension and rapid death.

• **Cardiogenic Shock:** The fundamental defect in cardiogenic shock is an inadequate cardiac output which results from an abnormality in intrinsic myocardial function or an acute anatomical derangement in cardiac structure. Cardiogenic shock usually occurs when contractile function is lost due to a reduction in myocardial mass, most commonly from an acute myocardial infarction. Autopsy studies have shown that a 40% loss of functioning myocardium is present in patients with fatal cardiogenic shock. Historically, approximately 15% of patients with an acute myocardial infarction developed shock, usually between the first and sixth hospital day. Since the introduction of thrombolytic therapy the occurrence of shock has decreased to approximately 7% but mortality has remained essentially unchanged and ranges between 60% and 90%. Acute coronary angioplasty has been recently demonstrated to produce a substantial improvement in outcome. Both clinical assessment and hemodynamic classification have been valuable in risk stratification and prediction of mortality in patients with an acute infarct (Table 1).

Acute coronary obstruction initiates a cascade of events. Interruption of blood flow produces cell death with a loss of contractile mass and a fall in stroke volume and arterial pressure. Reduction in coronary perfusion pressure leads to progressive myocardial cellular ischemia and death with a further reduction in myocardial contractile ability. When a critical mass of functioning myocardium is lost, irreversible shock ensues. Abnormalities in diastolic function also occur and contribute to the pathophysiology. Acute ischemia and infarction produce a decrease in myocardial compliance. The ventricle becomes "stiff" with an elevation in intracardiac pressures, pulmonary vascular congestion and reduced left ventricular filling and stroke volume.

Hypotension during a myocardial infarction can also occur because of a reduction in venous return. Forrester defined four hemodynamic subsets, based on measured cardiac output and level of pulmonary capillary wedge pressure, that occur in patients with an acute infarct. Most important is the recognition that shock may occur because of absolute or relative hypovolemia. Marked increases in vagal tone are frequently observed, especially early in the course of an MI, with intense venodilitation and bradycardia. The increase in venous capacitance leads to a reduction in preload and stroke volume. These patients often need massive volume infusions to restore adequate cardiac output. Heart failure from any cause including restrictive and congestive cardiomyopathies and valvular or ischemic disease can ultimately lead to a profound reduction in cardiac output and circulatory failure. Cardiac dysrhythmias can also cause acute circulatory collapse.

Diagnosis of Shock

Because of the wide-ranging etiologies, shock can occur in a variety of settings. In hospitalized patients, shock most frequently is encountered in association with sepsis, in the post-operative period, or during the course of an acute myocardial infarction. Constant vigilance of high risk patients must be maintained for early detection. The development of hypotension is the classic sign of circulatory collapse. However, this may be a late occurrence in the course of shock because a variety of compensatory mechanisms can maintain systemic blood pressure in spite of other severe circulatory derangements.

General Appearance

The patient with shock often exhibits only nonspecific signs reflective of organ hypoperfusion. One of the early symptoms is an alteration in sensorium with agitation or confusion which may be the initial manifestation of circulatory failure, especially in the elderly. Patients with sepsis may first exhibit hyperventilation with an associated metabolic alkalosis which can precede the development of fever (or hypothermia), chills or frank rigors. Other clinical signs are often specific to the particular etiology and pathophysiology. However, central to all shock states is the recognition of a decrease in cardiac output and tissue perfusion. Reduction in stroke volume will lead to intense vasoconstriction especially to the skin and skeletal muscle and produce cool, clammy, and often mottled extremities. In sepsis there will be an increase in cardiac output with intense peripheral vasodilation and maintenance of perfusion to the skin. This "warm" shock phase is transient but may be quite intense and associated with a very high cardiac output. The development of the classic signs of shock such as hypotension, oliguria, obtundation, and metabolic acidosis often do not occur until the late stages of shock. Initial compensatory mechanisms including peripheral vasoconstriction and tachycardia help maintain systemic blood pressure and cardiac output. Hypotension does not ensue until these mechanisms are no longer able to compensate for the decrease in stroke volume. When hypotension begins, subsequent decrease in blood pressure can be very rapidly progressive. Metabolic acidosis may precede frank hypotension but also reflects severe tissue hypoperfusion and anaerobic metabolism and signifies a late stage of shock.

Physical Examination

The environment of the intensive care unit can provide formidable challenges to the physician attempting to perform a careful physical examination. Critical care units are often crowded and noisy and patients frequently have numerous lines and tubes, for example jugular venous catheters, that may obscure important physical findings. Invariably, it seems, ECG monitoring leads are placed directly over the left ventricular impulse and interfere with palpation and auscultation. Heart sounds and murmurs are obscured by a mechanical ventilator. Unfortunately, these kinds of difficulties often lead to neglect and deemphasis of the physical examination and the loss of potentially important information. Special efforts and a little extra time are often needed to ensure adequate assessment with techniques such as assisting respiration with a bag device, instead of a mechanical ventilator, during the physical examination.

• **Vital Signs:** The careful monitoring of vital signs is of utmost importance in the early detection of shock. The first clue of incipient circulatory fail-

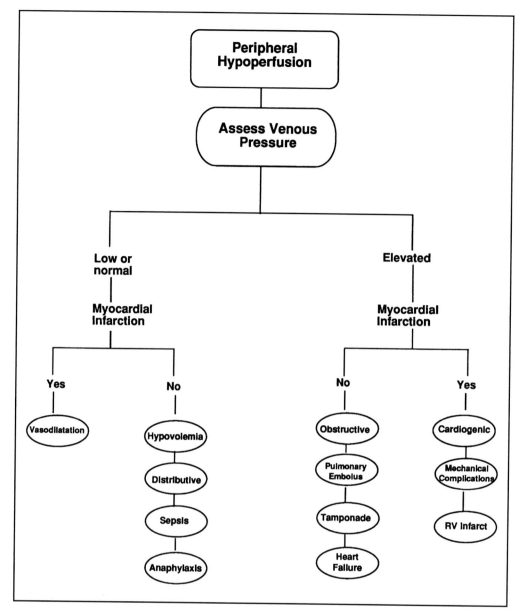

Figure 2. Initial clinical approach to the patient in shock.

ure is often an "unexplained" tachycardia as a result of increased sympathetic tone. Additionally, "unexplained" tachypnea may be the initial clue to sepsis, however, hypotension is frequently the first recognized sign of shock. A mean arterial pressure of 60 mmHg is usually required to maintain organ perfusion but below this level tissue oxygen delivery is usually inadequate. Diastolic pressure may be disproportionately low and reflects vasodilatation and rapid run-off into the periphery as well as hypovolemia. Perfusion of the coronary circulation is significantly dependent on the diastolic pressure and may be impaired at low levels.

• **Jugular Venous Pressure and Pulse:** After the initial recognition of hypoperfusion, the proper and accurate assessment of the jugular venous pressure (JVP) and waveform is critical for diagno-

sis and administration of rapid and effective therapy. The JVP can provide the first clue to the etiology of the shock state (Figure 2). Technique and accuracy of the bedside estimate of venous pressure has been described. When confronted with a patient with early shock, the initial clinical assessment begins with two questions: is the peripheral perfusion adequate? Second, is venous pressure low, normal, or increased? If initial venous pressure is low and peripheral perfusion is inadequate, it is likely that absolute or relative hypovolemia is of major importance in the circulatory pathophysiology. Patients with an acute myocardial infarction may present with an intense increase in vagal tone with bradycardia, marked venodilation and peripheral pooling of blood with reduced venous return. Although left-sided pressures may be normal or increased, venous pressure will be low and these patients will also improve with volume administration. Presence of an acute infarct is confirmed by the typical clinical symptoms, other physical signs, and characteristic changes on the electrocardiogram. The vast majority of patients without prior cardiac disease or an MI with low venous pressure will have hypovolemic or distributive shock.

If peripheral perfusion is inadequate and the jugular venous pressure is normal or elevated the assessment becomes more complex. Intense increases in sympathetic tone can produce venous as well as arterial vasoconstriction with maintenance of a normal venous pressure in the presence of hypovolemia. Patients with severe generalized cardiac dysfunction of any etiology, such as congestive cardiomyopathy, will have an elevated venous pressure. Obstructive forms of shock will also present with increased venous pressure. After an acute pulmonary embolus there may be severe right ventricular pressure overload and failure with increased right atrial pressure and a prominent A-wave. In addition there may be associated significant tricuspid regurgitation and a large regurgitant V-wave. Cardiac tamponade is also characterized by elevated venous pressure.

Kussmaul's sign (increase in venous pressure with inspiration) is seen most frequently with constrictive pericarditis but can be present in the effusive-constrictive type of pericardial effusion as well as with a right ventricular infarct. Cardiac tamponade alters the pattern of cardiac filling, but an increase in the jugular venous pressure does not occur in cardiac tamponade until a significant increase in intra-pericardial pressure is present. In early diastole, during the rapid passive filling of the right and left ventricle, intra-pericardial pressure rises. The increase in intra-pericardial pressure is transmitted to the right atrium and reduces the transmural right atrial pressure gradient leading to a decrease in venous return. There is also a characteristic alteration in venous wave form with a more prominent x-descent. After right ventricular systole the relatively empty right ventricle fills quickly creating a rapid fall in pressure and a prominent x-descent. Right atrial pressure then rises with venous return and intra-pericardial pressure also increases. Because of the constricting effect of the pericardial effusion and high intra-pericardial pressure, the right atrial pressure remains high and the y-descent is blunted. Elevation of venous pressure is the most frequently recognized sign in the patients with cardiac tamponade. As noted, Kussmaul's sign does not occur with tamponade but is a sign of constrictive pericarditis which does not usually present with shock or circulatory collapse. Patients with constrictive pericarditis will characteristically have both a prominent x- and y-descent.

Approximately 50% of patients with inferior myocardial infarctions will have associated right ventricular involvement, although it is clinically recognized less often. Acute right ventricular ischemia or infarction will reduce systolic function and may also decrease right ventricular compliance. The most important clinical feature is elevation of the venous pressure, usually greater than 7 mmHg to 8 mmHg. Kussmaul's sign may also be observed. In spite of the elevated right atrial pressure, left heart filling may be reduced leading to inadequate cardiac output and peripheral perfusion. Volume infusion is critically important in restoring cardiac output in this situation. Analysis of the jugular venous pressure and wave form is also valuable in identifying other causes of acute cardiac decompensation, including congenital disorders and valvular heart disease, and are discussed in other chapters.

Another important value of bedside analysis of the venous pressure is the observation of responses to acute volume administration. Many shock states are characterized by absolute or relative hypovolemia and initial therapy with volume infusion is vital in the management of these patients. An initial volume bolus can be given while awaiting further detailed hemodynamic information. The assessment of the response to fluid therapy should include careful observation of the venous pressure as well as monitoring of the arterial blood pressure and clinical signs of organ perfusion. Analysis of the jugular venous wave form may also be of assistance in the bedside diagnosis of cardiac dysrhythmias, especially in distinguishing between supraventricular and ventricular tachycardia.

Right heart pressure information observed in the jugular venous pressure is useful as a guide to initial therapy but may be misleading in some settings and often not optimal for the continued management of the patient with shock. However, it does assist in deciding whether hemodynamic monitoring and other diagnostic modalities are required. The recognition of increased venous pressure creates a differential diagnosis which includes left ventricular failure, cardiac tamponade or restriction, right ventricular infarction or acute right ventricular failure from pulmonary hypertension. Other clues from the physical examination can often be observed which will assist in the diagnosis (Table 2).

• **Arterial Pulse and Pressure:** The characteristic pulse in shock is rapid with a decreased volume. Occasionally, especially in the early stage of

	PHYSICAL FINDINGS	CONFIRMATORY/DIAGNOSTIC TEST
RV INFARCT	JVP - Y > X Descent Kussmaul's sign Pulsus paradoxus Right sided S_3 Tricuspid regurgitation Absent RV lift	Chest X-Ray - absence of CHF ECG - Inferior MI - ST elevation in right-sided leads V_3R, V_4R Echo - RV dilation Wall motion abnormality
PULMONARY EMBOLISM	JVP - increased A-wave and V-wave RV Lift P_2, delayed with expiratory splitting Right sided S_3 Tricuspid regurgitation	Chest X-Ray - pulmonary artery "cutoff," dilatation ECG - S, Q_3; S_1, S_2, S_3 Echo - RV clot, pulmonary hypertension RV dysfunction
PERICARDIAL TAMPONADE	JVP - prominent x-descent and blunted y-descent Pulsus paradoxus S_3 absent S_1 and S_2 decreased intensity	Chest X-Ray - globular heart, loss of hilar vessels ECG - electrical alternans Echo - effusion, diastolic atrial collapse
CHF-LV FAILURE	Pulsus alternans S_3 gallop MR, TR Pulmonary crackles	Chest X-Ray - cardiomegaly, venous redistribution Echo - LV size and global function, valvular abnormalities

TABLE 2
Peripheral Hypoperfusion with Elevated Venous Pressure

sepsis with vasodilation, there may be sensed an adequate or increased stroke volume with a low diastolic pressure and a well-preserved, brisk upstroke in the arterial pulse contour. In this situation, the blood pressure appears to be "adequate". The sensation of the pulse is the force perceived at the fingertips and is dependent on the pulse pressure and not the absolute level of systolic pressure. Obviously, there is no substitution for the direct measurement of arterial pressure, however, a rapid bedside estimate of arterial pressure can be made by direct graded compression of the brachial artery while palpating the radial artery. If arterial wall is stiff, more pressure may be needed to occlude the vessel which may again produce a false sense of adequate blood pressure. A mean arterial pressure of 60 mmHg is usually necessary to maintain effective organ perfusion, and diastolic pressure is important in maintenance of adequate coronary artery perfusion. Marked reductions in diastolic pressure may lead to worsening myocardial ischemia, especially with co-existent coronary artery disease. With hypovolemia, inadequate cardiac output is compensated by an increase in heart rate. Initially, this may be measured only during postural changes, and the early detection of shock can be improved if arterial blood pressure and pulse are obtained in the supine and standing positions. Both the systolic and diastolic pressure will further decrease as the patient develops a progressive reduction in stroke volume.

Another important clue to the early recognition of shock, as well as the etiology, is measurement of the pulsus paradoxus. During normal respiration the arterial blood pressure decreases during inspiration less than 8 mmHg to 10 mmHg and usually in the 2 mmHg to 4 mmHg range. An exaggeration of this normal respiratory variation is characteristically recorded in cardiac tamponade. Cyclic changes in intrathoracic pressure during normal respiration are transmitted to the pericardial space and substantially alter the filling characteristics in both the right and left ventricle. During inspiration and the generation of negative intrathoracic pressure, there is pooling of blood in the pulmonary venous circulation and a decrease in the venous return to the left heart. Concomitantly, venous return is increased to the right heart. These changes are magnified in many other conditions. An increase in pulsus parodoxus can be seen with hypovolemia, asthma or airway obstructions from any cause, and acute pulmonary embolus. In hypovolemia, the effects of the already reduced preload are magnified during normal respiration. Alterations in intrathoracic pressure, such as an increase in negative intrathoracic pressure induced by airway obstruction, will magnify the effects of normal inspiration and produce a larger pulsus paradoxus. Acute obstruction of the pulmonary arterial bed by a pulmonary embolus produces a series of effects including a reduction in pulmonary blood volume and left heart venous return. In addition, acute bronchospasm and airway obstruction can occur with further reduction of negative intrathoracic pressure and a larger paradoxical pulse.

Pericardial tamponade is the classic cause of pulsus paradoxus. When intrapericardial pressure rises, transmural diastolic pressure will decrease with reduction in venous return and stroke volume. During inspiration, there will be a decrease in intrapericardial pressure and right atrial pressure. Venous return to the right ventricle will increase and the right ventricular dimension normally enlarges. If the right ventricle is restrained from dilating outward by the pericardial effusion, the ventricular septum will be "shifted" and distended into the left ventricle. This "septal shift" will alter the compliance of the left ventricle and the increased ventricular diastolic pressure will further inhibit venous return, exaggerating the normal respiratory effects and increasing the measured amount of pulsus paradoxus.

When pulsus paradoxus is observed in hypotensive patients, for whatever reason, absolute or relative hypovolemia is playing a role in the pathophysiology and initial therapy should almost always include volume administration. The rapid infusion of volume in cardiac tamponade will increase venous return at the expense of elevated intracardiac pressures but can partially restore stroke volume and be life-saving. Similarly, with pulmonary hypertension or an acute right ventricular infarct, right-sided pressures will rise with the administration of volume, and peripheral edema may result. However, the increase in venous return and intracardiac diastolic volume is often necessary to restore adequate cardiac output. Other information usually obtained by careful analysis of the pulse contour may be obscured by the shock state because of the associated low stroke volume. Often the characteristic pulses usually observed, for example, with chronic aortic insufficiency, will not be detected on physical examination.

• **Cardiac Examination:** When severe peripheral hypoperfusion is recognized, the initial focus of the cardiac examination is to discern whether or not acute cardiac decompensation is the primary cause of the circulatory collapse. Physical examination will be most useful in the differential diagnosis of patients with an elevated venous pressure. The recognition of pulmonary crackles and increased venous pressure assist in the diagnosis. On cardiac examination, the hallmark finding of left ventricular decompensation remains the presence of an S_3 gallop. With hypovolemic shock and early distributive shock with low venous pressure, cardiac examination will be normal except for the presence of a

tachycardia. With cardiac tamponade, the percussed cardiac heart border may fall distinctly outside the palpable left ventricular impulse. The first and second heart sounds may be of diminished intensity but the second heart sound will be normally split. Absence of a third heart sound in association with marked cardiomegaly and jugular venous pressure elevation may be an important clue to the presence of a significant pericardial effusion. Palpation in acute pulmonary hypertension may detect a prominent subxiphoid right ventricular lift. After an acute pulmonary embolus, at least 30% of the pulmonary vascular bed must be obstructed before pulmonary hypertension develops. The mean pulmonary artery pressure is usually under 40 mmHg unless there is pre-existing lung disease or chronic elevation of pulmonary artery pressure. The pulmonic component of the second heart sound is increased in intensity. Right ventricular electrical-mechanical systole is prolonged with a resultant prolongation in the A_2 - P_2 interval and persistent expiratory splitting may also be detected. Recognition of a right-sided S_3 gallop which characteristically will increase in intensity during inspiration is a useful sign of right ventricular decompensation. A right ventricular infarct may be suspected when a right-sided S_3 occurs without associated evidence of pulmonary hypertension. Typically, a right ventricular infarct does not produce a prominent right ventricular lift and is almost invariably associated with an acute inferior or posterior myocardial infarction.

Recognition of the causes of circulatory collapse during the course of an acute myocardial infarction also requires careful clinical evaluation. After an acute myocardial infarction, an S_4 is almost always audible in patients with sinus rhythm and an S_3 occurs in patients with significant left ventricular dysfunction. Acute mechanical complications including mitral regurgitation and ventricular septal rupture are also first detected by cardiac examination. Disruption of the mitral valve apparatus may occur at any level and the extent and severity of mitral regurgitation will determine the clinical picture observed. With sudden elevation of left atrial and pulmonary venous pressure, significant pulmonary hypertension often develops with a loud and delayed P_2. The murmur of acute mitral regurgitation may be holosystolic but frequently is decrescendo and can end long before the second heart sound. This occurs because of a marked elevation in left atrial pressure and reduction in the gradient between the left ventricle and left atrium in mid-systole. The regurgitant jet of acute mitral regurgitation is frequently directed toward the atrial septum producing a murmur which radiates predominately to the base and even into the neck. This murmur can be confused with aortic stenosis and bedside maneuvers can assist in distinguishing the origin of the murmur. For example, the murmur of acute mitral regurgitation will increase in intensity with handgrip while the murmur of aortic stenosis will be diminished. After acute rupture of the ventricular septum, the usual finding is a holosystolic murmur at the third and fourth left intercostal space which radiates across the chest from left to right and is often associated with a palpable thrill. It can be confused with acute mitral regurgitation, and both murmurs respond similarly to bedside maneuvers, especially ones that decrease afterload.

Acute aortic regurgitation also can provide challenges in clinical diagnosis. As discussed, the pulses may not be characteristic and the left ventricular impulse may be normal in size and not displaced on palpation. Left ventricular end-diastolic pressure may also rise abruptly in mid-diastole, leading to early closure of the mitral valve and marked elevation in pulmonary venous and arterial pressure. The first heart sound may be diminished and the pulmonic component of the second heart sound may be both increased in intensity and delayed. Rapid rise in the left ventricular end-diastolic pressure produces a reduction in the amount of regurgitation in mid-diastole and the diastolic murmur may be quite short and soft.

CARDIAC PEARL

Pertinent clinical findings of a patient who has the onset of an acute aortic regurgitation: An early closure of the mitral valve may be present, producing a sound that is readily heard, particularly if one searches for it; the first heart sound is often faint; and the diastolic blood pressure may be in the 60s or upper 50s rather than in the lower 50s, 40s, and upper 30s as is usually present with chronic severe aortic regurgitation. This audible sound in diastole that is associated with the early closure of the mitral valve lends solid support to the valvular origin as the genesis of the first heart sound.

W. Proctor Harvey, M.D.

Acute aortic and mitral regurgitation from other causes, most commonly bacterial endocarditis, will also provide similar potentially confusing findings on examination. In addition, the severity of chronic valvular disease may be difficult to recognize in the patients with acute circulatory collapse with low

flow states. For example, in aortic stenosis the pulse characteristics could be obscured and attributed to the low stroke volume and the murmur will be softer. Complex situations occur when hypotension from whatever cause complicates pre-existing cardiac disease and other diagnostic modalities are often valuable in understanding the cause of the circulatory collapse and the associated clinical picture.

In summary, the integrated clinical assessment including evaluation of venous and arterial pulses and cardiac examination provide important clues to the differential diagnosis of circulatory collapse (Table 2). After the physical exam is performed strategies for initial treatment and further diagnostic evaluation can be reasonably formulated.

Noninvasive Assessment

• **Laboratory:** A variety of biochemical abnormalities are recognized in shock but are often nonspecific. Arterial blood gases will often demonstrate an initial respiratory alkalosis, especially with sepsis. As tissue hypoxia progresses a metabolic acidosis will develop. Arterial hypoxemia is commonly observed and is multi-factorial in origin, but primarily related to worsening ventilation-perfusion matching with a definable increase in intrapulmonic shunt flow. As tissue hypoxemia progresses, metabolic acidosis will develop. Serum lactate levels measured from arterial or mixed venous samples will rise and are important predictors of survival, i.e., as the lactate level increases the observed mortality also rises. Improved tissue perfusion is also reflected by decreasing lactate levels. Hyperglycemia is common early due to increased catecholamines, glucagon, and cortisol. Later hypoglycemia will be observed with a decrease in gluconeogenesis and depletion of hepatic glycogen stores. Leukocytosis is frequently seen and early white cell forms including bands and metamyelocytes are released in response to bone marrow hypoxia. With sepsis, neutropenia occurs in a small number of patients and is also associated with a high mortality. Thrombocytopenia may occur as a part of generalized intravascular aggregation of all blood cell components and also can be an accompaniment of disseminated intravascular coagulation.

Other laboratory abnormalities reflect widespread organ damage, e.g., generalized elevation in liver aminotransferases and lactic dehydrogenase. Rising serum urea nitrogen and creatinine with a low urine osmolality (<350 mOSM) and high urine sodium excretion (> 40 mEq/L) are found with acute renal failure.

• **Electrocardiogram:** The initial surface electrocardiogram provides important clues to the etiology of acute circulatory collapse. Also, constant cardiac monitoring should be employed in the hypotensive patient to observe for the development of a cardiac dysrhythmia. A variety of alterations occurring during the course of shock including elevated catecholamines, electrolyte imbalance, and acidosis, as well as vasoactive drugs used in treatment, may precipitate the development of cardiac dysrhythmias.

The ECG assists in the initial determination of whether or not an intrinsic myocardial abnormality is present. Acute myocardial infarction can be demonstrated from the initial electrocardiogram in 60% of patients. The hallmark is the presence of upwardly curving S-T segment elevation. The presence of S-T segment depression in both anterior and inferior infarcts is generally a reciprocal change but is related to the size and the extent of the infarct. Extensive S-T segment depression is associated with a higher short and long term mortality when compared to patients without S-T depression. A scoring system based on the amplitudes and duration of the resultant Q- and R-waves can be employed to predict the extent of left ventricular dysfunction as well as the short term prognosis. The occurrence of S-T segment elevation and loss of R-wave in right sided leads (V_3R and V_4R) in association with an acute inferior or posterior infarct are sensitive indicators of a right ventricular infarction but do not predict the severity of right ventricular failure.

Distributive shock with sepsis as well as hypovolemic shock produce only non-specific ECG changes. Pericardial tamponade may be characterized by low voltage and electrical alternans due to the swinging motion of the heart within the pericardial effusion. Other signs of pericarditis, including PR segment depression and ST elevation are frequently detected. In constrictive pericarditis, low voltage may also be present but electrical alternans is not characteristically seen. After an acute pulmonary embolus, the most common ECG changes are the occurrence of non-specific S-T segment depression and T-wave flattening. The classic changes of an S wave in lead I and a Q wave in lead III or the S_1, S_2, S_3 pattern are less common. The ECG may also suggest acute right ventricular pressure or volume overload with a pattern of hypertrophy, right axis deviation and right atrial enlargement. Electrocardiograms are also useful in the recognition of electrolyte abnormalities. An acute metabolic acidosis and associated hyperkalemia can be recognized by the presence of tall symmetrical T-waves and prolongation of conduction both in the atrium and the ventricle. Other clues to a cardiac etiology of shock includes evidence of chamber hypertrophy or enlargement which, for example, may suggest chronic valvular heart disease.

• **Chest X-Ray:** Initial value of chest x-ray in the acutely hypotensive patient is to assess cardiac size and pulmonary vascularity which assists in the initial differential diagnosis and treatment. The chest x-ray findings are integrated with the entire clinical picture and are extremely accurate in predicting elevated pulmonary venous pressure in congestive heart failure. Marked increases in left atrial and pulmonary venous pressure are reflected in the typical findings of cephalization of blood flow with increased venous return from the apices, peribronchial cuffing, increased interstitial markings and frank alveolar filling initially in the perihilar area. The acute respiratory distress syndrome (ARDS) is a frequent consequence of prolonged hypoperfusion, especially in association with sepsis. In ARDS, there is a loss of integrity of the alveolar capillary membrane leading to extravasation of fluid into the alveolar space at lower levels of venous pressure. The radiographic appearance may be difficult to distinguish from congestive heart failure and the important clues are the presence of cardiomegaly, apical venous redistribution and pleural effusions.

Cardiomegaly suggests a cardiac etiology for the shock; however, heart disease is common and multiple conditions may exist simultaneously, becoming an important confounder for accurate diagnosis. For example, the patient with aortic stenosis who develops acute gastrointestinal hemorrhage from colonic AV malformations may have cardiomegaly but low filling pressures. In addition, in this situation, shock can be rapidly progressive because of the decreased compliance of the hypertrophied left ventricle. Bedside examination and the recognition of low venous pressure in a patient with cardiomegaly may be the initial clue to the diagnosis. Often, however, hemodynamic monitoring is necessary to further evaluate these complex situations.

An array of other radiographic findings may assist in diagnosis. With a large pericardial effusion, the heart appears globular with loss of the distinctive borders and outline of the hilar vessels. Acute right heart enlargement can be recognized by reduction in the retrosternal airspace on the lateral view. After an acute pulmonary embolus, there may be an enlargement of the proximal pulmonary arteries with an abrupt "cutoff" or narrowing of a central pulmonary artery. Aortic abnormalities including dissection are usually readily visible on the plain chest x-ray.

The chest x-ray can also be useful in the diagnosis of mechanical complications during acute myocardial infarction. With acute mitral regurgitation, there is a sudden and marked elevation of left atrial and pulmonary venous pressure leading to the rapid development of the typical x-ray appearance of acute pulmonary edema. Ventricular septal rupture will increase pulmonary blood flow but will not raise left atrial pressure acutely and pulmonary edema occurs later as a consequence of progressive left ventricular dysfunction. Correlation of x-ray findings in patients who develop acute systolic murmurs may be the key to establishing the diagnosis. Patients with right ventricular infarction and shock will also have normal pulmonary vascularity.

• **Echocardiogram:** Echocardiographic information can be quickly and accurately obtained in the hypotensive patient and complement the clinical examination. Esophageal echocardiography is also being increasingly employed in the evaluation of the acute cardiac emergency. Transesophageal

echo is safely and easily performed at the bedside in critically ill patients providing excellent images and is of most importance when transthoracic views are suboptimal. A major value of echo is to assess myocardial performance and discern if there is a cardiac cause for the hemodynamic changes. Global left ventricular dysfunction and segmental wall motion abnormalities can be recognized and assist in confirming the diagnosis. Severity of left ventricular dysfunction can be quantified and right ventricular size and function can also be assessed. Doppler flow velocities are used to measure cardiac output and flow across valves and within cardiac chambers. Echocardiographic information also complements the measurements of intracardiac pressure. Starling's law relates the end-diastolic volume, but not necessarily the end-diastolic pressure, to stroke volume. Pressure information is easier to obtain and is frequently substituted for volume determinations. However, the measured pressure is a function of the compliance of the chamber, as well

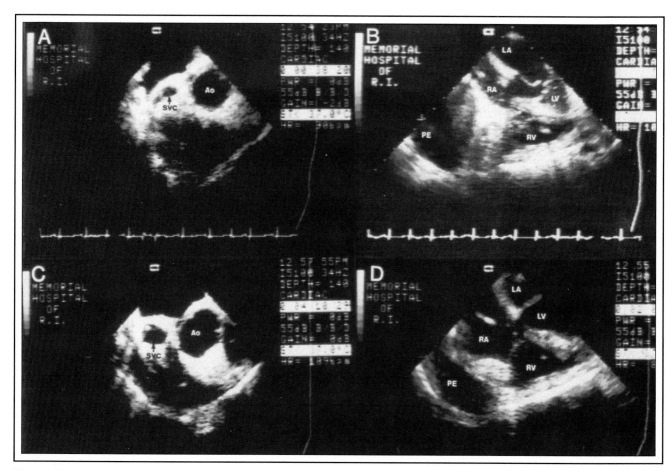

Figure 3. Transesophageal views of short axes (Panel A and C) and four chamber (Channel B and D) in a patient with purulent pericarditis and tamponade. Panels A and B show compression of the lumen of the superior vena cavas (SVC) and right atrial (RA) and right ventricular (RV) chambers by the pericardial effusion (PE). Panels C and D demonstrate an increase in the size of the right heart chambers after pericardiocentesis. AO= aorta; LA= left atrium; LV = Left ventricle. *(With permission from Golub, R.J.: Usefulness of transesophageal echocardiography in the surgical drainage of a loculated purulent pericardial effusion. AHJ 126: 724, 1993.)*

as the volume, and echocardiography can be used to assess pressure and volume relationships. Echocardiography is also valuable in establishing the diagnosis and assisting with the treatment of the patient in shock. Pericardial effusion was one of the first conditions recognized on echo and is diagnosed by the presence of an echo free space around the left ventricle. Evidence of tamponade pathophysiology includes collapse of the right atrium and ventricle during diastole as well as a decrease in vena cava size (Figure 3). Analysis of changes in Doppler flow patterns can also be utilized to detect the hemodynamic consequences of cardiac tamponade. During inspiration Doppler analysis demonstrates a reduction in early mitral inflow while during expiration, there will be a decrease in tricuspid inflow. These changes can be predicted from the dynamic pathophysiology of cardiac tamponade previously reviewed. Echocardiography can also be used to guide pericardiocentesis and the intrapericardial placement of drainage catheters.

Bedside echo also has a role in detection of an acute pulmonary embolus. First, the right atrial or ventricular clot may be directly visualized. Additionally, the consequences of acute pulmonary hypertension are visualized with right ventricular enlargement and reduced systolic function as well as right atrial enlargement. Pulmonary artery pressure is estimated from velocity of the regurgitant jet of tricuspid insufficiency combined with the clinical assessment of right atrial pressure. The consequences of the mechanical complications of myocardial infarction can also be imaged. The presence of a new wall motion abnormality may assist in the early detection of an acute infarct and the extent of the observed left ventricular dysfunction can be used to predict early complications including the likelihood that congestive heart failure or shock will develop. Papillary muscle and chordal rupture can be directly visualized and the severity of mitral regurgitation is estimated from the size of the regurgitant jet on color flow analysis. Free wall rupture with resultant pseudoaneurysm or pericardial effusion can also be directly visualized. Evaluation of the right ventricular size and function can confirm the diagnosis of an associated right ventricular infarct. Also, a combination of color flow and direct imaging may detect the presence of ventricular septal defects and confirm the location and size of multiple defects. Other potential cardiac causes of shock including severe aortic stenosis, hypertrophic obstructive cardiomyopathy and aortic dissection can be recognized by echocardiography. During sepsis, left ventricular dysfunction frequently develops and the extent and sever-

ity of depression of myocardial function can be followed.

Clearly, rapid bedside transthoracic or transesophageal echo can be extremely valuable in the care of the patient with acute hemodynamic collapse (Table 3). Elements of the history and physical examination remain extremely important, however, in deciding when an immediate echo will be of the most value.

• **Nuclear Techniques:** *Radionuclide Angiography (RNA)* – Bedside radionuclide angiography can be performed on patients with shock to assess both left and right heart function. Left ventricular ejection fraction is an excellent prognostic indicator of outcome in patients with acute myocardial infarction. The mechanical complications of an infarct, including left ventricular aneurysm formation, mitral regurgitation and ventricular septal defects can also be detected utilizing volume and shunt flow analyses of the right and left ventricles. Global measurements of left ventricular function are based on changes in counts in the cardiac blood pool and, in general, are more accurate than similar information obtained from echocardiography. However, the echocardiogram often allows for improved analysis of segmental wall motion, and has important logistic advantages including ease in bringing equipment to the bedside with less complicated and faster completion of studies. Echo-

---

T A B L E   3

Echocardiogram in Shock

ASSESS MYOCARDIAL PERFORMANCE

Regional abnormalities
Global function

PERICARDIAL EFFUSION / TAMPONADE

Demonstrate effusion
Doppler flow patterns
Diastolic collapse of atria and ventricles
Assist pericardiocentesis / drainage

PULMONARY EMBOLUS

RV size and function
Pulmonary hypertension
Atrial or ventricular clot

ACUTE MYOCARDIAL INFARCTION - COMPLICATIONS

RV Infarct
Aneurysm / pseudoaneurysm
Acute mitral regurgitation
Ventricular septal defect

cardiography may also be superior for sequential analysis and observing the effects of interventions in regional and global wall motion.

Myocardial Perfusion Imaging – The primary application of perfusion imaging is detection of the presence, size and location of defects which result from abnormal myocardial blood flow. Perfusion images can be obtained in critically ill patients and are most useful during the course of acute myocardial infarction. Myocardial viability can often be assessed accurately with rest and redistribution thallium images. Documentation of viable myocardium can predict the potential for improvement with coronary interventions. Infarct size can also be readily determined using SPECT imaging. The use of Technetium-99 sestamibi, which only minimally redistributes, has been valuable in observing the response to thrombolytic therapy as well as predicting the extent and severity of left ventricular dysfunction.

Hemodynamic Monitoring

Since introduction of the flow directed balloon flotation catheters in 1970, bedside hemodynamic monitoring has been extensively employed in the management of critically ill patients. Unfortunately, many questions remain regarding the proper use and relative value of these techniques. Pulmonary artery catheterization has significant risks including the development of local complications such as hemorrhage, pneumothorax, and ventricular arrhythmias (Table 4). Other complications which are related to long-term placement of the catheter include pulmonary infarction, pulmonary artery rupture or perforation, sepsis, thrombus formation and rarely endocarditis. Significant reductions in mortality in acute myocardial infarction have been achieved with systemic thrombolytic therapy which provides a strong impetus to avoid invasive cardiac monitoring and reduce the potential for serious hemorrhage. The complication rate of right heart catheterization may also be reduced if the duration of indwelling catheter time is shortened. Catheters are often most valuable to confirm the diagnosis and observe the response to an acute intervention.

There is no clear documentation that hemodynamic monitoring improves the outcome in patients with acute myocardial infarction or other critical illnesses. The Worcester Heart Attack study group analyzed the use and outcomes of pulmonary artery catheterization in 3,263 patients with an acute MI. They could not demonstrate any beneficial effects on survival either during the in-hospital phase or on long-term follow-up. A similar analysis was performed in 19 ICUs in major medical centers which

TABLE 4
Complications of Hemodynamic Monitoring
PULMONARY ARTERY CATHETERS
Local Placement 　Hemorrhage 　Pneumothorax 　Ventricular arrhythmias **Long-Term Placement** 　Pulmonary infarction 　Pulmonary artery rupture/perforation 　Sepsis 　Thrombosis 　Catheter knotting 　Endocarditis
ARTERIAL CATHETERS
Thrombosis/arterial occlusion Local infection and sepsis Nerve compression Arterial embolization
URINARY CATHETERS
Hemorrhage Local infection/sepsis

had a significant variability in the frequency of use of pulmonary artery catheters. No evidence of reduced mortality with hemodynamic monitoring was recorded, and in fact, the unit with the lowest catheter utilization had the lowest severity-weighted mortality. These studies suggest the potential for improved outcomes in critically ill patients with more judicious applications of invasive monitoring, and reaffirm the necessity for careful clinical evaluation.

In patients with an acute myocardial infarction, the clinical assessment of hemodynamic subsets is quite accurate. Also, clinical evaluation is excellent in predicting prognosis (Table 1). Forrester found that clinical criteria accurately predicted the hemodynamic state with an overall 83% accuracy in 200 patients studied. The major limitation of clinical assessment was the recognition of reduced cardiac output. However, the combination of clinical and x-ray criteria identified the presence of pulmonary congestion in 68 of 70 patients with hemodynamic subset IV (peripheral hypoperfusion with pulmonary edema) (Table 1). Clinical and radiographic assessment has not proven to be as valuable in patients with multiple organ failure, especially with associated alterations in pulmonary capillary permeability. However, many patients who present with hypotension, especially patients with uncomplicated hypovolemia, can be diagnosed and managed quite well without invasive hemodynamic monitoring.

Pulmonary Artery Catheterization

Pulmonary artery catheterization is useful to confirm the cause of shock and to assess the initial response to therapy. It is often possible to perform a diagnostic right heart catheterization procedure, obtain confirmatory hemodynamic information, and then remove the catheter. The data obtained during bedside catheterization include intracardiac pressures in the right heart chambers and the pulmonary artery as well as balloon occlusion pressure which reflects pulmonary venous and left atrial pressure. Proper measurements require careful positioning of well-maintained and frequently calibrated transducers. Oxygen saturations measured from the vena cava and right heart chambers are used to detect an intra-cardiac shunt and also to calculate cardiac output. The mixed venous oxygen saturation obtained in the pulmonary artery is necessary to determine cardiac output by the Fick principle (Table 5). Currently available catheter systems have an available fiberoptic system for continuous monitoring of the mixed venous oxygen saturation. Thermodilution cardiac outputs can also be directly obtained from catheters with thermistors which can recognize changes in temperature.

In the complex environment of the critical care unit, bedside pressure measurements must be carefully analyzed, especially in patients on mechanical ventilation with end-expiratory pressure. The important intravascular pressure is the transmural pressure which equals the measured vascular pressure minus the pleural pressure. If pleural pressure is increased, for example, by the application of end-expiratory pressure, measured intravascular pressure may also increase while transmural pressure and cardiac output decrease. This effect of end-expiratory pressure on transmural pressure is not linear and varies with many factors including the compliance of the lung. Direct measurement of pleural pressure, for example, with esophageal balloon occlusion, can assist in accurate measurements but may be cumbersome, potentially uncomfortable and is performed infrequently. Patients on mechanical ventilation or with obstructive airways disease may also have wide swings of measured vascular pressures throughout the respiratory cycle. Improved accuracy in pressure determinations can be obtained by simultaneous analysis of tracings of respiratory and pressure waveforms and standardizing the measurement of pressures at end-expiration (with no respiratory airflow).

Cardiac output is measured by thermodilution techniques using an injectate into the right atrium with a known temperature and thermistor at the tip of the catheter to detect the change in temperature. This technique requires thorough mixing of the injectate in the right ventricle to accurately calculate the stroke volume. The indicator must be injected in the right atrium and the thermistor should be positioned in the main pulmonary artery. At least three samples should be obtained and averaged. Cardiac output can also be estimated by using the Fick Principle. Simply stated, the amount of blood flow through an organ can be determined if a substance is removed or added to the circulation. In this case, oxygen is the substance removed. The flow or cardiac output is obtained by calculating the volume of blood required to transport the oxygen removed from the air over time. Cardiac output equals the oxygen consumption (VO_2) divided by the difference in oxygen content between the pulmonary venous and arterial blood (the AVO_2 difference). Oxygen content equals the hemoglobin x 1.34 (ml of oxygen carried per gram of hemoglobin) x the percent saturation. Oxygen consumption can be directly measured by collection and analysis of expired air. This is often difficult and impractical to perform at the bedside in patients who are critically ill. Oxygen consumption is often then assumed to be $140cc/m^2$. However, wide variations in oxygen consumption occur in critically ill patients, which introduce important errors into this "assumed" cardiac output calculation. An alternative is continuous monitoring of the mixed venous oxygen saturation which reflects the global integrity of the cardiopulmonary unit and will decrease if either arterial oxygen saturation or cardiac output decreases. If arterial oxygen saturation is maintained, a fall in venous saturation usually reflects a reduction in cardiac output or an increase in oxygen consumption without a concomitant rise in cardiac output. Mixed venous oxygen may also be elevated if the blood bypasses the vascular bed capable of extracting oxygen; i.e., it is shunted around the capillary bed. In this situation, there is a normal or high mixed venous oxygen saturation while tissue perfusion is inadequate and is frequently observed during sepsis.

After right heart pressures and cardiac output are determined, an appropriate hemodynamic classification can be constructed. The principal information utilized are the cardiac index and balloon occlusion or pulmonary capillary wedge pressure. In general, a cardiac index of 2.2 $L/min/m^2$ is required to maintain adequate tissue perfusion and defines the lower limit of acceptable cardiac output.

Adequate cardiac output must be related to peripheral demand and in some forms of shock, for example sepsis, it must be much higher to maintain effective organ perfusion. Normal right heart pressures in mmHg are: right atrial 2-8, pulmonary artery 15-30 / 5-12, with a mean of 9-16, and pulmonary capillary wedge of 5-12. When the alveolar-capillary membrane is intact and intravascular osmotic pressure is normal, extravasation of fluid into the pulmonary interstitial space occurs at a pressure of 18 mmHg. This number is then frequently used as an upper limit for optimal filling pressure. Other useful data which assists in the understanding of the pathophysiology includes oxygen saturations from the vena cava and right heart chambers and the calculations of A-VO$_2$ difference and systemic and pulmonary vascular resistance (Table 5).

Hemodynamic profiles are used to classify the shock state. Low right atrial or balloon occlusion pressure confirms that relative or absolute hypovolemia is present and defines hypovolemic shock. In distributive shock from sepsis or anaphylaxis, there is arterial and venous vasodilatation with decreased systemic vascular resistance, increased cardiac output and peripheral pooling of blood with low cardiac filling pressures. As septic shock progresses left ventricular dysfunction develops, myocardial contractility is depressed and cardiac output falls in spite of normal or elevated preload.

Equalization (within 5 mmHg) of right atrial, right ventricular end-diastolic, pulmonary artery diastolic and balloon occlusion pressures is the characteristic finding in pericardial tamponade. Similar equalization of pressures also may occur in restrictive cardiomyopathy and other diagnostic modalities including the chest x-ray, echocardiogram, or cardiac magnetic resonance images can be valuable in distinguishing between these conditions. After an acute pulmonary embolus or right ventricular infarction, the pulmonary artery and right heart pressures will be elevated while the wedge pressure remains low or normal. Four hemodynamic subsets have been modeled in patients with an acute myocardial infarction (Table 2). Cardiogenic shock is characterized by a cardiac index less than 2.2 L/min/m^2 when the pulmonary capillary wedge pressure is greater than 18 mmHg. Occasionally a patient with an MI will have low filling pressures and low cardiac output recognized by hemodynamic monitoring (as well as the physical exam).

CARDIAC PEARL

This emphasizes to me the great improvement in diagnosis and treatment of shock that has occurred- and quite rapidly- due to our ability to obtain accurate observations in our laboratories and to correlate them with the clinical picture. Only a few decades ago, procedures now common in the hemodynamics laboratory would have been considered too hazardous to the patient. Today, hemodynamic monitoring via the Swan-Ganz catheter is accepted as "routine" in coronary care units. Not too long ago, the thought of a catheter introduced into the heart of a patient with an acute myocardial infarction would have caused physicians to "shudder", thinking of the danger to the patient. Of course, now it is known that this is a very safe procedure, and the information derived from its use can be life saving.

W. Proctor Harvey, M.D.

Arterial Cannulation

Arterial pressure monitoring is often necessary for the care of the unstable, hypotensive patient when accurate blood pressure measurements can be difficult to acquire with a sphygmomanometer or Doppler technique. An arterial pressure catheter also facilitates obtaining multiple arterial blood gases and blood samples. The preferred site of cannulation is the radial artery. Prior to insertion, an Allen Test (alternate occlusion of the ulnar and radial arteries) to assess the collateral flow in the palmar arch should be performed. In patients with

---

TABLE 5
Hemodynamic Monitoring - Useful Calculations

(A) FLOW
Oxygen content = Hgb x 1.34 (mL O$_2$/gm Hgb) x % saturation
AVO$_2$ Difference = Arterial oxygen content – mixed venous oxygen content
Cardiac output (CO) = $\dfrac{\text{Oxygen consumption (VO}_2)}{\text{AVO}_2 \text{ Difference}}$

(B) RESISTANCE
Systemic vascular resistance (SVR) = $\dfrac{\text{Mean aortic pressure – Mean RA pressure}}{\text{Systemic blood flow (CO)}}$
Total pulmonary resistance = $\dfrac{\text{Mean PA pressure}}{\text{Pulmonary blood flow}}$
Pulmonary vascular resistance (PVR) = $\dfrac{\text{Mean PA pressure – Mean LA pressure}}{\text{Pulmonary blood flow}}$

RA = Right atrial
PA = Pulmonary artery
LA = Left atrial

severe hypotension and peripheral vasoconstriction, the femoral artery can usually be rapidly cannulated and is often an excellent alternative for initial monitoring. Arterial catheters also have the potential for serious complications including thrombosis, local infection and sepsis, hemorrhage, nerve compression syndromes and arterial embolization. Prior to cannulation, one should carefully consider the indications. The time the catheter is left indwelling should be limited to the period which is absolutely necessary for the optimum care of the patient. In general, the risk of complications increase over time and strong consideration should be given to removing this catheter after four days.

Urinary Catheters

Acute reduction in renal blood flow leads to oliguria and the hourly quantification of urinary output, which reflects renal blood flow and is indicative of perfusion to other organs, is often of value in the management of patients with severe hypotension. The minimal adequate urine output is 0.5 cc /kg/hour. Again, however, this information is not obtained without serious risks. Urinary tract infections are the most frequent nosocomial infection in hospitalized patients and are related to the frequency and duration of indwelling catheter use (most commonly employed in the ICU). The consequences of sepsis may be severe with the mortality of catheter-associated bacteremia reported to be 10% to 30% Duration of catheterization is extremely important in the development of infection and bacteriuria occurs in approximately 5% to 10% of patients per day of indwelling catheter use. Careful clinical examination with assessment of vital signs, mental status and the peripheral circulation can frequently be effective in assessing organ perfusion. Collection of excreted urine and daily weights can often be substituted for direct hourly measurement of urine output, especially after the patient has stabilized.

Principles of Management

Management of patients with shock can be divided into two phases. The initial phase begins when first confronted with a patient with hypotension who requires a clinical decision regarding immediate treatment. The first goal is to reestablish effective organ perfusion and quickly restore mean atrial pressure to at least 60 mmHg. Treatment modalities available to achieve this goal are; (1) rapid volume administration to provide adequate filling of the right and left ventricle, (2) an ionotropic agent to augment cardiac contractility, (3) an arterial vasoconstrictor to restore effective perfusion pressure, and (4) a combination of these interventions. Each approach has potential dangers. Volume administration in the patient with cardiogenic shock may produce worsening pulmonary edema. Ionotropic and vasoconstrictor agents increase heart rate, peripheral resistance and cardiac contractility which can result in higher myocardial oxygen requirements and the potential for worsening myocardial damage in patients with an acute myocardial infarction. However, extremely low levels of arterial pressure and myocardial hypoperfusion also cause infarct extension.

During this initial phase of treatment, therapy must often be administered without the luxury of detailed hemodynamic information. In the vast majority of patients, rapid volume administration should be part of the initial therapy. Elevation of the legs produces an immediate increase in central blood volume. Assessment of the level of venous pressure, combined with chest and cardiac examination, frequently will identify the patient with cardiogenic shock and elevated filling pressures. Severe reductions in arterial perfusion pressure may require rapid correction with an arterial vasoconstrictor even if hypovolemia is present. Vasoconstrictors can be quickly withdrawn as volume is restored. Other immediate therapy includes supplemental oxygen and analgesics. Hypoxemia and intrapulmonic shunting is a frequent accompaniment of shock and oxygen administration can protect against arterial desaturation and further impairment of oxygen delivery. Patients are often apprehensive or in pain and analgesics should be administered. Relief of discomfort can decrease sympathetic outflow and may also reduce cardiac and peripheral oxygen requirements. Systemic acidosis depresses cardiac function, predisposes to cardiac dysrhythmias and alters responsiveness to vasoactive drugs. The pH should be restored if it is less than 7.3. Cardiac dysrhythmias require immediate treatment. Wide-complex tachycardias of ventricular origin are frequently misdiagnosed as supraventricular and the administration of verapamil or beta blockers often leads to worsening hypotension. Prompt DC countershock is an effective strategy in the management of both supraventricular and ventricular tachyarrhythmias with hypotension, especially when complicating an acute myocardial infarction. Bradyarrhythmias usually respond to atropine and external or temporary wire pacing.

Simultaneously with initial treatment, clinical assessment will assist with prioritizing the other diagnostic information that needs to be obtained. Evaluation should include an electrocardiogram, chest x-ray, and laboratory studies including arterial blood gases, chemistries including renal and hepatic function, glucose, electrolytes, a complete blood count, coagulation profile and serum lactate. If cardiac tamponade is likely, an echocardiogram is useful to confirm the diagnosis and assist with pericardiocentesis. In patients with a known pericardial effusion, immediate unguided pericardiocentesis may be necessary and life-saving. When hemodynamic monitoring is required for further diagnosis and management, care should be taken to continually observe the condition of the patient when inserting the pulmonary artery catheter or other monitoring devices.

The second phase of management begins after acute stabilization. Attention focuses on utilizing the information available to address the cause of the circulatory derangements and developing a strategy to correct the underlying problem as well as maintaining the most effective hemodynamic management. Subsequent therapy can be assessed by the effects on cardiac output, oxygen delivery and oxygen consumption, as well as indices of tissue perfusion including mixed venous oxygen, arterial lactate and systemic acidosis.

Hypovolemic Shock

Simple hypovolemic shock may respond rapidly to volume restoration and a major focus of management is the search for the cause of fluid or blood loss. The goal of therapy is to maximize oxygen transport by increasing preload, restoring stroke volume and ensuring adequate oxygen carrying capacity. In general, volume loss from acute hemorrhage should be replaced with red blood cells to maintain a hematocrit of at least 30, especially if active bleeding continues. Controversy continues regarding which type of fluids should be administered. Crystalloid fluids contain NaCl as the major constituent while colloids contain larger, osmotically active particles which are more likely to remain in the intravascular space. Crystalloids can freely diffuse into the interstitium, hence larger volumes are required for effective resuscitation, and peripheral edema is more common. However, both fluids are effective in restoring intravascular volume and no convincing differences in outcomes related to the choice of fluid have been demonstrated. Volume infusion can be administered in a "bolus" fashion with an initial amount between 500cc and 2 L to 3 L depending on assessed severity of volume depletion, with clinical and hemodynamic evaluation after each infusion. Restoration of adequate mean blood pressure, resolution of resting tachycardia, and postural changes in blood pressure and pulse rate, as well as improved peripheral perfusion, indicate adequate volume replacement has been accomplished.

Distributive Shock

The next phase in the treatment of sepsis begins with a search for the underlying cause and prompt administration of effective antibiotics, which significantly improves survival. Gram negative organisms are a frequent cause of septic shock and initial therapy should include at least two bacteriocidal agents providing appropriate coverage for the likely pathogens. Cultures should be obtained promptly and antibiotics should be administered as quickly as possible. Controlling the source of the infection by interventions such as prompt surgical drainage of an abscess or excision of a necrotic focus is often necessary. High dose systemic glucocorticoids do not improve outcome. Immunotherapy including monoclonal antibodies to endotoxin appears to increase early survival in sepsis but this result has not been substantiated with further evaluation. Prompt restoration of adequate tissue perfusion is of utmost importance in prevention of multiple organ failure.

Hemodynamic management of the septic shock patient usually requires invasive monitoring. The goals of therapy are to maximize systemic oxygen transport by assuring adequate circulating blood volume and cardiac output. Fluids are given until balloon occlusion pressure approaches 18 mmHg while measuring cardiac output, urine output, mixed venous oxygen, lactate and clinical indicators of organ perfusion. Occasionally, massive amounts of fluid are required to accomplish this aim and may result in extensive peripheral edema. If systemic blood pressure remains low, ionotropic agents and vasoconstrictors are added to restore adequate perfusion pressure. Vasoconstrictors may be detrimental because they produce further reduction in flow to some vascular beds with worsening tissue perfusion. Alternatively, when adequate circulating volume and perfusion pressure are restored, vasodilators such as nitroprusside may be valuable in restoring perfusion to vascular beds and reversing acidosis. Nitroprusside can produce peripheral vasodilation in intensely constricted vascular beds with restoration of effective tissue oxygenation. Ionotropic agents and augmentation of cardiac output may be useful even when initial measured cardiac output is normal or high but inadequate to restore effective tissue oxygenation.

Frequently, dobutamine is the initial vasoactive agent employed after adequate perfusion pressure is restored with volume administration. Dobutamine increases cardiac output in the range of 30% to 80% and does not cause significant arterial vasoconstriction. Peripheral resistance usually falls because of a reflex inhibition in sympathetic tone by the baroreceptors resulting from the increased stroke volume. Dopamine may also be an effective initial therapy. High dose dopamine causes vasoconstriction and restoration of perfusion pressure, while lower doses increase renal blood flow. A combination of vasoactive agents are often employed to capitalize on their combined effects and therapy is tailored to the hemodynamic conditions. For example, low dose dopamine and dobutamine may be synergistic in increasing cardiac output and restoring renal blood flow. Controversy exists regarding the extent of further treatment. Shoemaker has suggested that interventions should be maximized in an attempt to optimize oxygen delivery and incremental therapy should be given as long as oxygen delivery, oxygen consumption, and cardiac output are increased. This approach is based on the evaluation of hemodynamics in survivors of postoperative shock. Hemodynamic profiles in patients who survive demonstrate an early increase in cardiac output, oxygen consumption and delivery while non-survivors have normal or reduced outputs and oxygen uptake. Patients who do not survive also present with larger arterial-alveolar oxygen gradients and more intrapulmonic shunting of blood flow.

Obstructive Shock

Initial treatment of pericardial tamponade should be volume infusion. This will often generate enough stroke volume to maintain adequate cardiac output until definitive therapy is completed. The alternatives for subsequent therapy include: pericardiocentesis, subxiphoid pericardial drainage or a formal pericardiectomy. Pericardiocentesis should be performed, when possible, with hemodynamic monitoring and fluoroscopy and is often ideally accomplished in the cardiac catheterization laboratory. Echocardiography can assist with the guidance of needles and catheters and may improve overall success and outcomes. Pericardiocentesis has a significant risk, including lacerations of the heart, coronary arteries or other intrathoracic structures. A subxiphoid pericardiotomy is a useful alternative. This procedure can be performed under local anesthesia with direct visualization and placement of an intracardiac drainage catheter. Another major cause of obstructive shock is an acute pulmonary embolus. Alternatives for therapy in patients with severe hemodynamic compromise include the use of thrombolytic agents and direct embolectomy. Thrombolytic therapy has the important advantages of rapid administration as well as the avoidance of surgical trauma. Mortality in acute pulmonary embolus with circulatory collapse remains high and there are no definitive studies documenting improved outcome with either modality.

Cardiogenic Shock

The approach to cardiogenic shock has been reviewed in the chapter on acute myocardial infarction. In spite of hemodynamic monitoring, intraaortic balloon pumps and a wide array of vasoactive agents, overall mortality from cardiogenic shock remains high. Direct restoration of blood flow, within 24 hours, with acute percutaneous transluminal coronary angioplasty appears to hold the most promise for improved in-hospital and long-term survival. Surgical therapy for mechanical complications is often urgently required but the mortality with acute ventricular septal rupture as well as acute severe mitral regurgitation remains high.

Conclusion

Acute circulatory collapse is the result of a complex array of disorders with variable pathophysiology and presenting signs and symptoms. The mortality in many conditions is quite high but can be improved by rapid recognition of the shock state and prompt administration of effective therapy with reversal of the underlying cause. Careful clinical assessment and skills in physical diagnosis are of the utmost importance in the early recognition and treatment of acute circulatory collapse. Hemodynamic monitoring and other noninvasive modalities can complement the clinical assessment and are also important in the proper care of these patients. Improved treatment strategies are needed to reduce mortality especially for cardiogenic and septic shock.

Selected Reading

Hemodynamics

1. Abboud FM: Reflex control of the peripheral circulation. *Prog Card Dis* 18: 371, 1976.
2. Astiz ME: Peripheral vascular tone in sepsis. *Chest* 99: 1072, 1991.
3. Bland RD: Hemodynamic and oxygen transport patterns in surviving and non-surviving post-operative patients. *Crit Care Med* 13:85, 1985.
4. Braunwald E: Regulation of the circulation. *NEJM* 290: 1420, 1974.
5. Gilbert JC: Determinants of left ventricular filling and of the diastolic pressure volume relation. *Circ Res* 64: 827, 1989.
6. Grossman W: Diastolic properties of the left ventricle. *Ann Intern Med* 84: 316, 1976.
7. Harezi RC: Diastolic function of the heart in clinical cardiology. *Arch Int Med* 148: 99, 1988.

8. Hess OM: The role of the pericardium in interactions between the cardiac chambers. *AHJ* 106: 1377, 1983.

9. Hinshaw LB: *Fundamental Mechanisms of Shock.* New York, Plenum Press, 1972.

10. Katz AM: Regulation of myocardial contractility 1958-1983. *JACC* 1:126, 1983.

11. Lefer AM: *Molecular and Cellular Aspects of Shock and Trauma.* Liss Inc, New York, 1983.

12. Rackow EC: Cellular oxygen metabolism during sepsis and shock: the relationship of oxygen consumption to oxygen delivery. *JAMA* 259: 1989, 1988.

13. Rackow EC: Pathophysiology and treatment of septic shock. *JAMA* 266: 548, 1991.

14. Ross J: Afterload mismatch and preload reserve: A conceptual framework for the analysis of ventricular function. *Prog Card Dis* 18: 255, 1976.

15. Ross J: Cardiac function and myocardial contractility: A perspective. *JACC* 1: 52, 1983.

16. Shoemaker WC: Circulatory mechanisms of shock and their mediators. *Crit Care Med* 15: 787, 1987.

17. Weil MH: Experimental and clinical studies in lactate and pyruvate as indicators of the severity of circulatory shock. *Circ* 41: 989, 1970.

Clinical Classification

18. Forrester JS: Medical therapy of acute myocardial infarction by application of hemodynamic subsets. *NEJM* 295: 1356, 1976.

19. Fowler NO: Cardiac tamponade: A comparison of right versus left heart compression. *JACC* 12: 187, 1988.

20. Hands ME: The in-hospital development of cardiogenic shock after myocardial infarction: Incidence, predictors of occurrence, outcome and prognostic factors. *JACC* 14: 40, 1989.

21. Killip T, III: Treatment of myocardial infarction in a coronary care unit: A two year experience with 250 patients. *AJC* 20: 457, 1967.

22. Knause W: Prognosis in acute organ-system failure. *Ann Surg* 202: 685, 1985.

23. Page DL: Myocardial changes associated with clinical shock. *NEJM* 285: 133, 1971.

24. Parker M: Septic shock. *JAMA* 250: 3324, 1983.

25. Parrillo JE: A circulatory myocardial depressant substance in humans with septic shock. *J Clin Invest* 76: 1539, 1985.

26. Parker MM: Profound but reversible myocardial depression in patients with septic shock. *Ann Int Med* 100: 483, 1984.

27. Pasternak RC and Braunwald E: Acute myocardial infarction: in Isselbacher KJ, Braunwald E, Wilson JD et al, eds.; *Harrison's Principles of Internal Medicine.* 13th Edition, New York, McGraw Hill 1994.

28. Shabetai R: Pericardial and cardiac pressure. *Circ* 77: 1, 1988.

Clinical Diagnosis

29. Antman E: Demonstration of the mechanism by which mitral regurgitation mimics aortic stenosis. *AJC* 42:1044, 1978.

30. Bell WR: Clinical features of submassive and massive pulmonary emboli. *AJM* 52: 355, 1977.

31. Cintron GB: Bedside recognition, incidence and clinical course of right ventricular infarction. *AJC* 47: 224, 1981.

32. Cohen SI: Pulsus paradoxus and Kussmaul's sign in acute pulmonary embolism. *AJC* 44: 378, 1979.

33. Cohn JN: Blood pressure measurement in shock: Mechanism of inaccuracy in ascultatory and palpatory methods. *JAMA* 199:118 1967.

34. Dell'Italia L: Physical examination for exclusion of hemodynamically important right ventricular infarction. *Ann Inter Med* 99: 608, 1983.

35. Harvey WP: Bedside diagnosis of arrhythmias. *Prog Card Dis* 8: 419, 1966.

36. Kreger BE: Gram negative bacteremia IV: Re-evaluation of clinical features and treatment in 612 patients. *Am J Med* 68: 344, 1980.

37. Logue RB: Second heart sound in pulmonary embolism and pulmonary hypertension. *JACC* 78: 38, 1966.

38. Lorell B: Right ventricular infarction: Clinical diagnosis and differentiation from cardiac tamponade and pericardial constriction. *AJC* 43: 465, 1979.

39. McIntyre KM: Determinants of cardiovascular responses to pulmonary embolism, in *Pulmonary Thromboembolism.* ed Osner KM. Yearbook Medical, Chicago, 1973, p. 144.

40. Morgenroth J: Acute severe aortic regurgitation: pathophysiology, clinical recognition, and management. *Ann Int Med* 87: 223, 1977.

41. Perloff JK: Auscultatory and phonographic manifestations of pure mitral regurgitation. *Prog Card Dis* 5:172, 1962.

42. Ronan JA: Clinical diagnosis of acute severe mitral insufficiency. *AJC* 27: 284, 1971.

43. Shabetai R: Hemodynamics of cardiac tamponade and constrictive pericarditis. *AJC* 70: 480, 1970.

44. Shabetai R: Pulsus paradoxus. *J Clin In* 44: 1882, 1965.

45. Shaver JA: Sound pressure correlates of the second heart sound: an intracardiac sound study. *Circ* 53: 997, 1976.

Noninvasive Assessment

46. Bates ER: Limitations of thrombolytic therapy for acute myocardial infarction complicated by congestive heart failure and cardiogenic shock. *JACC* 18: 1077, 1991.

47. Bounous EP: Prognostic value of the simplified selvester QRS score in patients with coronary artery disease. *JACC* 11: 35, 1988.

48. Fisch C: Electrocardiography and Vectorcardiography in: Braunwald E: *Heart Disease* WB Saunders 1992.

49. Gacioch AV: Cardiogenic shock complicating acute myocardial infarction: The use of coronary angioplasty and the integration of the new support devices into patient management. *JACC* 19: 654, 1992.

50. Gibbons RJ: Features of tomographic 99m-Tc-hexakis-2-methoxy-2 methylpropyl isontrile imaging for assessment of myocardial area at risk and the effect of treatment in acute myocardial infarction. *Circ* 80:1277, 1989.

51. Gore JM: Community wide assessment of use of pulmonary artery catheters in patients with AMI. *Chest* 92: 721, 1987.

52. Harrison MR: Usefulness of color Doppler flow imaging to distinguish ventricular septal defect from acute mitral regurgitation complicating myocardial infarction. *AJC* 64: 697, 1989.

53. Helmecke F: 2-D echocardiography and Doppler color flow mapping in the diagnosis and prognosis of ventricular septal rupture. *Circ* 81: 1775, 1990.

54. Hlastky MA: Prognostic significance of precordial ST segment depression during inferior acute myocardial infarction. *AJC* 55: 325, 1985.

55. Kasper W: Echocardiographic findings in patients with proved pulmonary embolus. *AHJ* 112: 1284, 1986.

56. Lee L: Percutaneous transluminal coronary angioplasty improves survival in acute myocardial infarction complicated by cardiogenic shock. *Circ* 78: 1345, 1988.

57. Levine MJ: Implications of echocardiographically assisted diagnosis of pericardial tamponade in contemporary medical patients. *JACC* 17: 59, 1991.

58. Lopez-Sendon J: Electrocardiographic findings in acute right ventricular infarction: Sensitivity and specificity of electrocardiographic alterations in right precordial leads V_4R, V_3R, V_1 and V_3. *JACC* 6: 1273, 1985.
59. Milne EN: The radiologic distinction of cardiogenic and noncardiogenic edema. *Am J Radiol* 144: 879, 1985.
60. Stein PD: The electrocardiogram in acute pulmonary embolism. *Prog Cardiovasc Dis* 17: 247, 1975.
61. Swan HJC: Catheterization of the heart in man with the use of flow directed balloon tipped catheters. *NEJM* 283: 447, 1970.
62. Usher BW: Electrical alternans: Mechanisms in pericardial effusion. *AHJ* 83: 459, 1972.

Hemodynamic Monitoring

63. Forrester JS: Correlative classification of clinical and hemodynamic function after acute myocardial infarction. *AJC* 39: 137, 1977.
64. Gore JM: A community wide assessment of the use of pulmonary artery catheters in patients with acute myocardial infarction. *Chest* 92: 721, 1987.
65. Knaus WA: An evaluation of outcome from intensive care in major medical centers. *Ann Intern Med* 104: 410, 1986.
66. Swan HJC: Catheterization of the heart in man with the use of flow directed balloon tipped catheters. *NEJM* 283: 447, 1970.

Therapy

67. Bates ER: Limitations of thrombolytic therapy for acute myocardial infarction complicated by congestive heart failure and cardiogenic shock. *JACC* 18: 1077, 1991.
68. Bone R: Methylprednisolone in severe sepsis study group: A controlled trial of high dose methylprednisolone in treatment of severe septic shock. *NEJM* 317: 653, 1987.
69. Callahan JA: Pericardiocentesis assisted by two-dimensional echocardiography. *J Thorac Cardiovasc Surg* 85: 877, 1983.
70. Gacioch, AV: Cardiogenic shock complicating acute myocardial infarction: The use of coronary angioplasty and the integration of the new support devices into patient management. *JACC* 19: 654, 1992.
71. Golub RJ: Usefulness of transesophageal Doppler echocardiography in the surgical drainage of a loculated purulent pericardial effusion. *AHJ* 126:724, 1993.
72. Lee L: Percutaneous transluminal coronary angioplasty improves survival in acute myocardial infarction complicated by cardiogenic shock. *Circ* 78: 1345, 1988.
73. Mitchell JP: Tissue plasminogen activation for pulmonary embolism resulting in shock: Two case reports and discussion of the literature. *AJM* 90:255, 1991.
74. Rackow EC: Fluid resuscitation in circulatory shock: comparison of the cardiorespiratory effects of albumin, hetastarch, and saline solutions in patients with hypovolemia and septic shock. *Crit Care Med* 11:839, 1983.
75. Shoemaker WC: Therapy of shock based on pathophysiology, monitoring and outcome prediction. *J Crit Care*, 1987.
76. Ziegler EJ: Treatment of gram-negative bacteremia and septic shock with HA-1A human monoclonal antibody against endotoxin. *NEJM* 324: 429, 1991.

PART III

Clinical Electrophysiology: Cardiac Arrhythmias and Conduction Disturbances

CHAPTER 27

Clinical Recognition
and Management of
Cardiac Arrhythmias

Bernard D. Kosowsky, M.D.

The latter half of the 20th century has seen dramatic advances in technologies related to cardiac arrhythmias. Sophisticated diagnostic and therapeutic techniques have altered the management of most rhythm disturbances. Unfortunately, there appears to have been a concomitant regression in the clinical skills of electrocardiographic rhythm interpretation, related to the increased complexity of clinical situations due to the survival of sicker patients, the availability of more effective monitoring techniques, and the use of potent medications and complicated devices. Furthermore, arrhythmia management is often removed from the clinical arena to the electrophysiologic laboratory, thus depriving the bedside clinician the opportunity to deal with, and learn about, cardiac arrhythmias.

The great cardiologists of the early 20th century were able to masterfully diagnose and describe most known arrhythmias, primarily using their powers of clinical observation. Wenckebach described his form of heart block before the invention of the electrocardiogram. Sir Thomas Lewis documented a large variety of ventricular and supraventricular arrhythmias based upon pulse wave analyses and auscultation. Much of their efforts were of limited clinical value as the treatments available to them consisted of bedrest, digitalis, and, occasionally, bromides. In contrast, there now exists a panoply of medications and interventions available for managing rhythm disorders. Yet, the improper diagnosis of an arrhythmia can result in serious or even fatal consequences, such as when verapamil is administered for rapid ventricular tachycardia. A coming together of enhanced clinical

diagnostic acumen with advanced knowledge of mechanisms and therapy should be the goal of the modern practitioner caring for the patient with cardiac arrhythmias.

Normally, regularly-spaced cardiac impulses arise in the sinus node, high in the right atrium. The signal is transmitted via specialized conduction pathways to the atrioventricular (AV) node, while at the same time spreading throughout the two atria causing atrial depolarization. The impulse is delayed within the AV node due to decremental conduction and emerges into the His bundle. From there, the right and left bundle branches of the Purkinje system distribute the impulse to the two ventricles in a uniform fashion. Alterations in this pattern of impulse formation and conduction, or deviations in rate or rhythmicity of the beats, are termed "arrhythmias". Although the word "dysrhythmia" may be technically more appropriate, the term arrhythmia is widely accepted in common usage.

There have been many attempts, unfortunately generally unsuccessful, to classify cardiac rhythm disorders. Arrhythmias have been categorized by their mechanism, rate, site, and clinical relevance. However, no uniform simple classification has emerged to aid the clinical practitioner.

Arrhythmias can be divided into those related to abnormal impulse formation and those due to abnormal conduction. The sinus node can be the origin of an arrhythmia when the rate is inappropriate or irregular. Traditionally, normal sinus rhythm is the term used for sinus rates between 60 and 100 beats per minute, although a range of 50 to

90 might be more appropriate for an adult at rest. A faster rate in infants, or in adults with sympathetic nervous system stimulation, may be called sinus tachycardia but, in fact, may not be abnormal. Sinus bradycardia can be seen in healthy individuals during sleep and in those superbly conditioned. Irregularities of sinus rhythm can range from respiratory sinus arrhythmia (acceleration with inspiration) and nonrespiratory sinus arrhythmia, to pathological sinus pauses and sinus arrest.

Cardiac impulses originating from other than the sinus node are termed "ectopic". These may arise elsewhere in the atria or anywhere along the His-Purkinje system in the AV junctional area or the ventricles. The mechanism can be enhanced normal automaticity, abnormal automaticity, or afterdepolarizations either early or delayed. Clinically indistinguishable may be impulses generated from re-entrant circuits, especially when these entail small loops at the terminal Purkinje-muscle bundle junction. These abnormal impulses are, in fact, a result of an abnormal conduction pattern in which unidirectional block predisposes to a circus movement resulting in repetitive firing in the atrium or ventricle. Larger re-entrant circuits account for AV nodal re-entrant tachycardia and tachyarrhythmias associated with the Wolff-Parkinson-White (WPW) syndrome.

Abnormalities in conduction can occur at any site within the heart. An impulse may fail to exit the sinus node due to block at the sino-atrial junction. This may occur sporadically or follow a pattern as in Wenckebach type I block. Rarely, block occurs within the specialized atrial conduction tissue, with the resultant failure to deliver the sinus impulse to the AV node or the left atrium. In the latter case, there may be independent beating of the two atria or parasystole. In severe hyperkalemia, there can be reasonably normal conduction from the sinus to the AV node, but the atrial tissue may not be depolarizable. This results in "normal sinus rhythm" but without discernible P-waves or atrial function.

The AV node is the most common site at which an abnormality in conduction causes a rhythm disturbance. Conduction blocks range from a minor prolongation in transmission time, to complete block with resultant asystole. PR interval prolongation is termed first degree AV block. In second degree block, some beats are conducted while others are blocked. The pattern of conducted and blocked beats may be fixed or variable, and the occurrence of block may be appropriate or pathologic. In the presence of a marked supraventricular tachycardia such as atrial flutter or fibrillation, AV block is necessary to preserve cardiac function. When the ratio of supraventricular beats to conducted beats is less than 2:1, the conduction pattern may be categorized as Mobitz type I (Wenckebach) or Mobitz type II. A total interruption of AV conduction is termed third degree block. Block within the intraventricular conduction system, or fascicles, may only cause a distorted pattern of impulse transmission with a wide QRS complex, unless all fascicles are blocked, in which case complete heart block, either intermittent or stable, will ensue. It is evident that categorizing arrhythmias by their mechanism can result in ambiguities, whereby conduction abnormalities present as enhanced activity, such as re-entrant tachycardias, and accelerated stimulation can produce high degrees of conduction block.

The clinician is confronted with the problem of a patient with the symptoms suggestive of a rhythm disturbance, or with a documented arrhythmia that requires analysis. Aside from making a diagnosis, he must determine if the arrhythmia is simple and benign or potentially dangerous. The rhythm may suggest the presence of some underlying problem such as a disease process or a drug reaction. Although at times interventions are necessary to aid in the elucidation of an arrhythmia, generally careful analysis can identify the correct diagnosis and allow for its appropriate management. Even the most seemingly complex rhythm patterns can be unraveled if approached in a systematic fashion.

Clinical History

A carefully-obtained history can augment one's ability to decipher an arrhythmia. The presence of an underlying disease can serve as a clue to define the nature of a rhythm disorder. A wide complex tachycardia is more likely to be ventricular in origin in a patient with known coronary artery disease and previous myocardial infarction, whereas a similar appearing rhythm in a patient with advanced pulmonary disease or thyrotoxicosis is more prone to be supraventricular.

A history of WPW is invaluable in trying to interpret a wide complex tachycardia. Congenital heart disease is commonly accompanied by rhythm disturbances, and atrial fibrillation is seen in adults with atrial septal defect and in lesions which produce an enlarged left atrium. Atrial fibrillation often complicates the surgical repair of transposition of the great arteries; a significant proportion of patients with Ebstein's Anomaly will also have WPW and its associated arrhythmias. Abnormalities that result in ventricular overload or strain are more likely to result in ventricular arrhythmias. Patients with

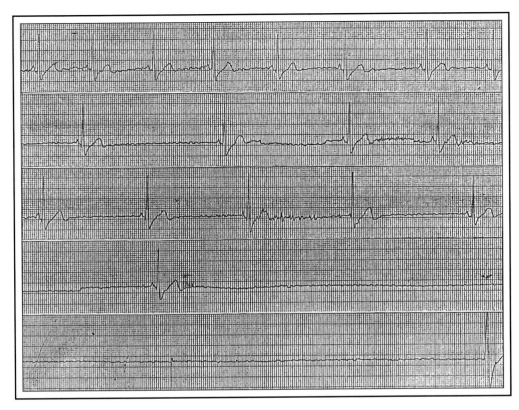

Figure 1. Continuous monitor recording from a 54-year-old woman during a venipuncture. Patient had history of syncope during blood drawing.

Lyme disease or Chagas disease may present with conduction disturbances or heart block.

A propensity for specific arrhythmias may be inherited. Long Q-T interval syndromes with and without deafness, and ventricular dysplasia can occur in families and result in ventricular tachycardia, and WPW and its associated arrhythmias may also be familial.

Information about the patient such as presence of fever, anemia, or postoperative state, differentiates sinus tachycardia from other entities, with atrial fibrillation often complicating postoperative pulmonary or cardiac surgery.

Many drugs affect cardiac rhythm. Digitalis toxicity produces a variety of disorders including atrial, junctional, and ventricular tachycardia with and without AV block. Frequent premature ventricular beats are often the first manifestation of digitalis excess. Class IA and IC anti-arrhythmic drugs can promote ventricular arrhythmias, with rapid ventricular tachycardia of the torsade de Pointes variety occurring especially in the setting of Q-T prolongation. Psychotropic drugs of the tricyclic class can provoke ventricular tachyarrhythmias, whereas lithium use is associated with a variety of bradyarrhythmias and conduction disorders. Hyperkalemia can be associated with apparent sinus arrest and can also result in bona fide cardiac arrest. Beta agonists and theophylline medications can provoke a variety of supraventricular arrhyth-

mias, especially in patients with advanced pulmonary disease.

Circumstances and symptoms related to an arrhythmia may have diagnostic significance; for example, provocation with caffeine or alcohol suggests a supraventricular origin to a tachycardia. Certain provocative circumstances could suggest vagotonia rather than anatomic disease as the cause for bradyarrhythmia or conduction disturbances (Figure 1). A gradual onset of tachycardia is more likely to be seen with sinus tachycardia or enhanced automoticity, whereas sudden onset and cessation are seen with re-entrant disorders.

Symptoms during an attack can be helpful in elucidating the nature of the arrhythmia. In general, atrial tachyarrhythmias are better tolerated than ventricular ones, although it is not uncommon for patients with ventricular tachycardia to tolerate very rapid rates, even in the presence of compromised ventricular function (Figure 2).

CARDIAC PEARL

Paroxysmal Atrial Tachycardia: Some patients can have a very rapid ventricular rate of 180 or so and have no symptoms. Others may become dizzy and are immediately aware of the abrupt change in rhythm.

Called to mind are two patients, one a teenage young lady, the star of her basketball

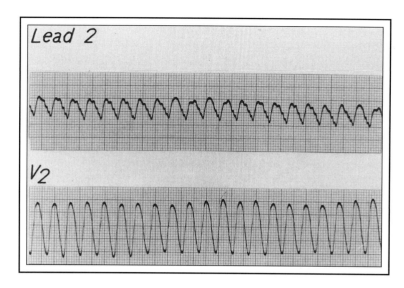

Lead 2

V2

Figure 2. Recordings from a 43-year-old man with a history of two prior myocardial infarctions and known left ventricular dysfunction. The patient developed palpitations while unloading a truck and presented with a blood pressure of 110/60 with no other symptoms other than slight diaphoresis. A diagnosis of ventricular tachycardia was confirmed by intra-atrial electrogram.

team, who had no heart disease except episodes of paroxysmal atrial tachycardia. Usually she could play competitive basketball without any difficulty, but when this tachycardia occurred she would have to stop. Her tachycardia was well controlled by beta blockers.

Another patient was a lineman for a National Football League team. Occasionally he would have sudden onset of rapid tachycardia and would become dizzy; at that point he would take himself out of the game.

Other patients, however, can have the rapid heart rate of paroxysmal atrial tachycardia without any significant symptoms even during the arrhythmia.

W. Proctor Harvey, M.D.

A sensation of rapid pulsation in the neck often accompanies AV nodal re-entrant tachycardia. This is caused by atrial contractions against a closed tricuspid valve. Intermittent pulsations are experienced in the presence of ventricular tachycardia with AV dissociation, however, a regular pulsation can be experienced when there is a 1:1 retrograde conduction.

Syncope is more likely to occur with ventricular tachycardias, since supraventricular arrhythmias rarely produce the extremely rapid rates required for sudden loss of consciousness, although atrial flutter with 1:1 conduction and atrial fibrillation in WPW must also be considered. A blackout spell, which is a transient loss of vision, can occur with paroxysmal ventricular or atrial tachyarrhythmias. Inadequate perfusion of the retinal arteries requires less of a fall in cerebral perfusion pressure, and therefore will occur in circumstances of less profound hemodynamic compromise. Polyuria is not an uncommon symptom with tachycardia,

lasting 20 minutes or more. This may be more often noted with supraventricular arrhythmias but is not specific.

CARDIAC PEARL

More common than realized is the fact that patients having rapid tachycardia (such as paroxysmal atrial tachycardia) may have profuse diuresis associated with it.

I had not been aware of this until the late Paul Wood of London made this observation on some of his patients. One patient prone to episodes of paroxysmal tachycardia had such an urgency for urination with the onset of tachycardia that she would have to stop to urinate while traveling on a bus from her home to the city. She would excrete a voluminous amount of urine. I have also seen this with rapid atrial fibrillation, although it is not nearly as common as with paroxysmal atrial tachycardia.

It would seem logical to explain this interesting phenomenon as due to the atrial natriuretic factor.

After the late Dr. Paul Wood first called to our attention that polyuria occurred in some patients who had paroxysmal tachycardia, our observations have certainly confirmed this interesting fact. Unless the patient is specifically questioned concerning polyuria associated with tachycardia, the patient usually does not mention it. The diuresis may be quite profuse in some. This is a good example of how "we find what we look for." There are two parts of this axiom, however, in that in order to find what we are looking for, we must know what we are looking for. A short time ago I evaluated a patient who has had serious, almost incapacitating bradycardia-tachycardia syndrome. With his tachycardia, he described his diuresis as an incredible "profound" diuresis. He has had a cardiac pacemaker implanted, which should take care of the problem.

W. Proctor Harvey, M.D.

When a paroxysmal tachycardia is not documentable, the patient can be asked to tap out the rhythm as it was perceived. The rate and regularity may be valuable clues to a tentative diagnosis. In addition, the patient should be questioned about maneuvers that might have been successful in terminating the tachycardia.

CARDIAC PEARL

Paroxysmal Atrial Tachycardia: The history is that of a sudden onset and cessation of a tachycardia. Rapid, regular ventricular rates of 180 to 200 or above are classic for paroxysmal atrial tachycardia. Carotid sinus pressure, if correctly applied, can, in most patients, result in reversion to normal sinus rhythm.

Self-Reversion of Paroxysmal Atrial Tachycardia- Many patients have learned ways to stop their own paroxysmal atrial tachycardia:

1. Straining, as with a bowel movement.

2. Placing their hands in ice water and then straining.

3. Lying on their stomachs with their head hanging over the edge of the bed and then straining.

4. Some patients will stick their finger down their throat to produce gagging, which is sometimes effective.

5. Some patients have learned that getting into a bathtub of cold water can revert the tachycardia.

W. Proctor Harvey, M.D.

Physical Examination

Careful physical examination can help in the diagnosis of arrhythmia where the ECG might be ambiguous. At times, rhythm disturbances can be diagnosed on the basis of physical examination alone. Heart rate and rhythmicity are readily ascertainable. It is best to examine the apical pulse, as there may be a pulse deficit in the peripheral pulse, especially in atrial fibrillation and early premature beats. The measurement of the blood pressure can be helpful in determining the nature of a paroxysmal bradycardia. In vagotonic states, both the blood pressure and pulse rate are low, whereas other bradycardias often display an exaggerated pulse pressure.

The jugular venous pulse may signal atrial activity that might be obscured on the ECG. In atrial flutter with block, small deflections in the venous pulse will be seen at a multiple of the carotid pulsation. Giant or cannon "A" waves are seen during AV dissociation, such as ventricular tachycardia, complete heart block, and blocked premature atrial beats. An "A" wave preceding a premature pulse denotes a premature atrial beat and a long interval between the "A" and "C-V" waves suggests the presence of first degree AV block. It should be recalled that Wenckebach identified his phenomenon by observing the venous and carotid pulsations.

The intensity of the first heart sound (S_1) may be affected by, and vary with, the PR interval. A soft regular S_1 is heard with first degree heart block. In AV dissociation there is a seemingly random variation in the intensity of S_1. In Wenckebach block one may hear a progressive diminution in the intensity of S_1 followed by a pause and then a loud first sound. There are times when an early premature beat will close the AV valves but not fully open the semilunar valves. In this case, one can hear an S_1 but a diminished or absent S_2, which might in fact sound like an S_3 but occurring only in beats followed by pauses.

CARDIAC PEARL

A changing intensity of the first heart sound is best illustrated by complete heart block where there is a frequent changing of the P-R relationship. The presence of a slow ventricular rate, generally around 40, plus a changing intensity of the first heart sound, producing the classical "bruit de canon" (sudden loud booming first heart sounds with the shorter P-R intervals), plus the frequent detection by auscultation of atrial sounds generally permits a bedside diagnosis of complete heart block.

Another example of a changing intensity of the first sound may be heard with ventricular tachycardia. It is particularly important to listen specifically for this. In a patient having paroxysmal tachycardia, the presence of multiple sounds plus the lack of slowing of the rate from carotid sinus pressure leads to the quick suspicion of ventricular tachycardia, and, after electrocardiographic documentation, more prompt treatment for this urgent type of tachycardia.

W. Proctor Harvey, M.D.

A paradoxically split second sound is heard in beats that have an altered ventricular depolarization of the left bundle branch type. This can be

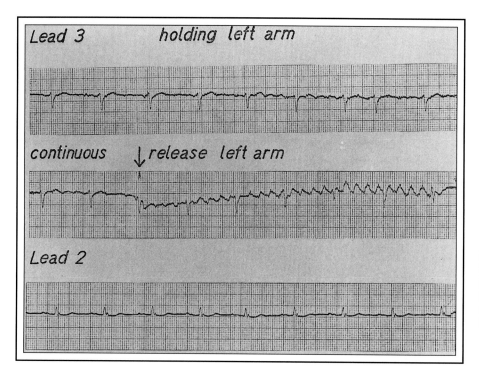

Figure 3. The effect of left arm tremor on the electrocardiogram. Lead 2 (bottom), and Lead 3 with the left arm restrained reveal normal sinus rhythm. When the left arm is released, a pattern similar to atrial flutter is evident.

noted in right ventricular premature beats, right ventricular pacing, and cases of idioventricular rhythm and ventricular tachycardia.

A fourth heart sound can accompany a premature atrial beat even though the P wave on the ECG may be obscured. An S_4 of variable timing and intensity can be appreciated in AV dissociation. Blocked PACs may result in a summation-type gallop heard on beats preceding long pauses.

Rhythm Documentation

Proper identification of rhythm disturbances is facilitated by utilizing appropriate materials and tools. The basic information generally is contained on an electrocardiographic recording. Most diagnostic electrocardiograms are recorded or mounted such that only a few seconds of information is available for review. This greatly compromises the ability to analyze other than the most obvious arrhythmias. Monitor strips are generally longer recordings from usually a single lead. Unfortunately, the lead recorded may have been chosen to provide the largest or most upright QRS complex in order to satisfy the sensing requirements of the monitor's rate detector. That particular lead often is not optimal for identifying P waves nor for best distinguishing differences in QRS morphology. Changing the lead being recorded, or moving the location of the electrodes to unconventional sites, may facilitate the rhythm analysis. Multichannel recordings of simultaneous leads help identify ambiguous deflections.

Simultaneous leads provide the most accurate determination of the AV conduction time. There has been much dispute regarding the "best" lead in which to measure the PR interval. The PR interval is defined as the time between the initial P-wave deflection to the initial portion of the QRS complex. An isoelectric segment of the P or QRS complex in a particular lead could falsely shorten or lengthen the PR interval. This can be overcome by measuring the interval between the very first P-wave deflection on one of simultaneously recorded leads to the initial QRS deflection on the same or other leads.

Choosing the proper portion of rhythm strip to analyze can be crucial. Generally, the most valuable information is at the very onset of an arrhythmia, and, at times, at its termination. Very long strips of a monotonous tachycardia are much less valuable than a short strip on which is recorded minor alterations in the pattern such as an extra beat or pauses.

Heart rate measurement is facilitated by use of a special "rate stick" usually provided on a ruler. The rate is determined by lining up the location of an impulse 2 or 3 intervals from the original beat and reading the rate from the rule. This is quite adequate for heart rates below 100 beats per minute. However, at rapid rates the accuracy of this method is very unsatisfactory. This can be corrected by counting a multiple of the prescribed beats and then multiplying the result accordingly. Thus, one can count twelve instead of three beats, and if this

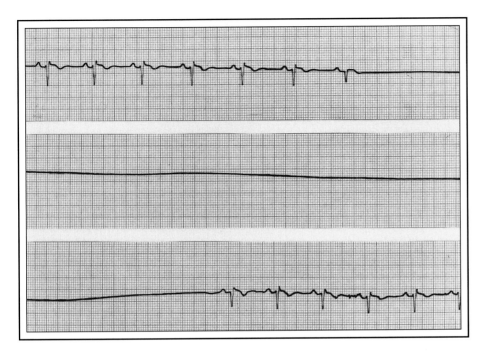

Figure 4. Holter monitor recording from a patient with a history of syncope. The apparent asystole is artifact. Note the loss of the U wave in the last beat on the upper strip.

then corresponds to a rate of 45 on the rule, the true heart rate will be 180. Similarly, counting "boxes" is reasonable at slow heart rates, but at rapid rates the observational error could cause a major discrepancy. Regularity and rhythmicity are most easily judged by use of a caliper. These should be stiff enough to maintain a constant interval but loose enough to readily allow change.

It is important to be alert to artifactual information on ECG recordings. Extraneous signals may result from patient motion or tremor, or from stray electrical signals (Figure 3). Problems with paper drive speed, or tape malfunction in memory devices such as Holter recordings, can mimic serious rhythm disturbances. Poor electrode contact or device malfunction can produce signal loss and mimic asystole (Figure 4). Careful attention to the morphology of the tracing may give a clue to such problems since physiologic signals rarely produce abrupt deflections or perfectly straight lines.

Categories of Arrhythmia

In clinical practice, one is presented with the recording of an arrhythmia which calls for a diagnosis and management plan. The pattern may deviate from normal in site of origin, conduction pattern, rhythmicity, or rate. Thus arrhythmias can be categorized as ectopic, abnormally conducted, erratic, tachycardic, or bradycardic. It is important to recognize that not all arrhythmias are pathologic. Some rhythm disturbances are in fact solutions to less apparent rhythm disorders, and the management needs to be addressed to the true problem, not the heart's attempt to resolve it.

Ectopic

In normal circumstances, the dominant pacemaker is in the sinus node. However, the beat can originate in a variety of different locations and yet retain normal rate and rhythmicity often without any adverse hemodynamic consequences. An ectopic atrial focus is identified by abnormal appearing P-waves. Unlike normal sinus rhythm, wherein the P-wave vector is downward and to the left, an ectopic focus often produces inverted P waves in the inferior limb leads. The P-wave morphology may vary from beat to beat without major changes in P intervals. This has been termed "wandering atrial pacemaker", although, in fact, this might represent alterations in intra-atrial conduction pathways rather than variations in pacemaker site.

Initial focus for cardiac stimulation can also arise in the AV nodal area or the ventricles, producing junctional or idioventricular rhythms, respectively. In assessing an ectopic rhythm, whether atrial, nodal, or ventricular, one must consider the status of the sinus node. If sinus node activity is inadequate or absent, the ectopic rhythm may not be a problem but in fact a solution. This is especially true for atrial and junctional escape rhythms. A ventricular escape rhythm would imply an inadequacy of both atrial and junctional pacemakers or atrioventricular block.

Escape atrial rhythms replace the sinus node as the dominant pacemaker, and therefore normal P waves are not present. Ectopic foci in the junctional or ventricular tissues may conduct to and depolarize the atrium and sinus node producing inverted

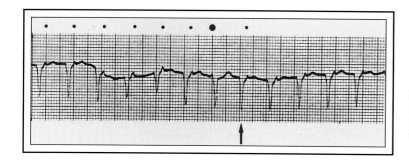

Figure 5. Atrial tachycardia at a rate of 140 beats per minute with a long PR interval. The 7th P wave (large dot) is premature as is the 8th QRS complex (arrow). The 7th P-wave which precedes the 7th QRS conducts to the 8th QRS.

or retrograde P waves. In the absence of such conduction, the ventricles can beat independently from the atria, which is termed "A-V dissociation". In this situation, there is a regular atrial rhythm at a rate different from the ventricular rate without one interfering with the other. Rarely, there may be dissociation between or within the atria themselves. Electrical pacing is an artificial means of producing an ectopic focus within the ventricles or atria.

Conduction Abnormalities

Abnormal conduction patterns can exist in the presence of a normal rate and rhythm. Although technically these should not be considered arrhythmias, such conditions often are part of a spectrum of disorders which do cause rhythm disturbances. Prolonged but preserved conduction between the atria and ventricles is termed "first degree AV block" and is manifested by a prolongation of the PR interval. The conventional upper limit of normal for the PR interval is 0.20 seconds, although there may be minor adjustments for age and heart rate. PR prolongation with intact conduction can, on rare occasions, be as long as one second. With an unusually long PR interval, the P-wave may be in front of the QRS complex preceding the beat it is conducting to (Figure 5). This phenomenon is also likely to occur during atrial pacing at a rapid rate. AV conduction time is sensitive to autonomic tone and to the interval from the previously conducted beat (RP interval). It can also be affected by

ischemia and a variety of pharmacologic agents. Rapid regular atrial rates may result in a regular pattern of second degree AV block such as 2:1 or 4:1, preserving a normal ventricular rate and rhythmicity. In this circumstance, the problem is the atrial tachyarrhythmia, whereas the conduction block protects the ventricles from an excessive rate of firing. In the absence of autonomic stimulation, the AV node should be able to conduct 1:1 up to a rate of approximately 150 beats per minute.

AV conduction time may be shorter than normal (<0.12 sec.) in the presence of accelerated conduction via bypass tracts such as in the Wolff-Parkinson-White and the Lown-Ganong-Levine (LGL) syndromes. These are noteworthy for their associated tachyarrhythmias and are recognized by presence of a short PR interval with (WPW) or without (LGL) a delta wave (Figure 6).

Asymmetric intraventricular conduction delay distorts the normal appearance of the QRS complex. Patterns of left or right bundle branch block, left anterior or posterior hemiblock, nonspecific intraventricular conduction delay, and combinations thereof, do not themselves alter cardiac rhythm, but may be associated with or progress to higher levels of AV block.

Electrical alternans is characterized by rhythmic variation in the amplitude of various components of the electrocardiogram. Most often it is the QRS complex that is affected, although the P, T, and U waves may be individually or commonly involved.

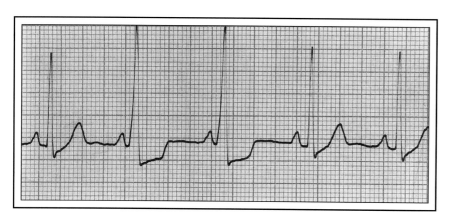

Figure 6. Monitor recording from a patient with intermittent Wolff-Parkinson-White Syndrome. The second and third beats display short PR intervals with delta waves with no change in the atrial rhythm.

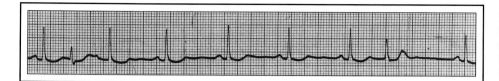

Figure 7. A Lead 2 recording displaying two premature ventricular beats. The first PVB is interpolated between two normal sinus beats, the second is associated with a compensatory pause.

The most frequently noted pattern is 2:1 alternation, whereby every other beat is taller. Electrical alternans is not uncommon in tachycardias such as AV reciprocating tachycardia with retrograde conduction along an accessory pathway, and may also be seen in rapid ventricular tachycardia. Electrical alternans at more normal heart rates is seen with large pericardial effusions.

Erratic Rhythms

The simplest deviation from normal rhythmicity is the occurrence of a single premature beat that occurs prior to the next scheduled sinus beat. An ectopic impulse can arise in the atrium (PAC), ventricle (PVC), or less commonly in the AV node-junctional area (PJC). Such a beat generally supercedes the next normally scheduled beat, although occasionally a premature depolarization can be interpolated between two normal beats (Figure 7). The effect of a premature beat on the underlying sinus rhythmicity depends on whether the sinus node is depolarized by the ectopic impulse. Generally, an impulse arising in the ventricle will have more difficulty reaching the sinus node before its next scheduled depolarization, either because of retrograde conduction block or simply due to the fact that the sinus fires before the time it takes for a relatively late premature beat to traverse the distance from the ventricle to the high right atrium. In such a case, the underlying sinus rhythm is not disturbed and the subsequent P-wave and its associated QRS are on schedule. The interval between the P-wave of the beat preceding the PVC and the one following it will equal two P-P intervals, and

the pause following the PVC will be longer than the normal interval by the amount that the premature interval was shorter. This "compensatory pause" is seen in the majority of PVCs. Since a PVC depolarizes the ventricle in an abnormal fashion, the resultant QRS will be wider and of a different configuration from the normally conducted beats. More commonly, the beat is monophasic or diphasic in lead V_1, and, if notched, the R wave is larger than the R'.

Atrial premature beats are more likely to reach and depolarize the sinus node before its next scheduled firing. The reset sinus node will then produce the next P-wave before a full compensatory pause. Occasionally, the reset sinus node will not immediately resume its previous rhythmicity and the pause can exceed that which would be normally expected. Generally, a PAC can be recognized by a premature, different looking P-wave preceding an earlier appearing normally configured QRS. At times, the P-wave is obscured by the preceding T-wave or by a flattened morphology. A relatively early PAC may find the AV node partially refractory, resulting in a prolonged PR interval. PACs, therefore, usually display a normal or prolonged interval. Since the major portion of the PR interval is related to AV conduction, and intra-atrial conduction is via specialized tracts from the sinus to AV nodes, PACs arising "lower" in the atrium will not necessarily be associated with a shorter PR interval.

An early PAC may find the ventricular conduction system not fully repolarized, resulting in aberrated ventricular conduction (Figure 8). This is more likely to occur in the right ventricular His-

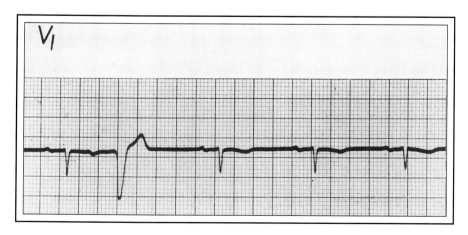

Figure 8. Lead V_1 recording of a premature atrial beat with aberrant ventricular conduction. Note the distortion of the T wave preceding the abnormal beat and the similarity of the initial portion of the QRS complex of the premature beat to the normal beats.

633

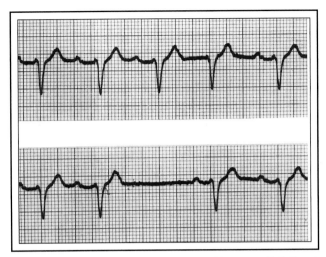

Figure 9. Lead 2 rhythm strip from a 50-year-old woman with "skipped beats." The 4th QRS in the upper strip is premature and is preceded by a slightly distorted T-wave containing a premature atrial beat with a long PR interval. The pause in the lower strip is caused by a premature atrial beat in the T-wave of the second complex which fails to conduct.

a T-wave, giving the impression that there is a sinus pause, transient sinus arrest, or sinus exit block. Blocked PACs are far more common than any of these entities, and careful examination of the T-wave at the beginning of an abruptly lengthened R-R interval will often reveal a subtle distortion, denoting a superimposed P-wave (Figure 9). Blocked PACs in a bigeminal pattern simulate sinus bradycardia.

A premature beat originating in the AV node-junctional region will display a normal QRS morphology, but without an antecedent conducted P-wave. When there is depolarization of the atrium as well as the ventricle from the junctional focus, a P-wave may be seen just in front of or beyond the QRS deflection. The P-wave morphology generally reflects retrograde conduction and is inverted in the inferior leads. Although a very early PJC could find the His-Purkinje system partially refractory and therefore conduct aberrantly, it is unwise to invoke the diagnosis of "junctional with aberrancy" unless one can independently confirm the presence of junctional beats.

Premature beats occurring in a row, from any source, can appear as couplets or triplets. It is a matter of semantics as to when one begins to call such an event a paroxysm of tachycardia, with definitions ranging from three to six or more beats.

More complex erratic beating is seen in a variety of arrhythmias. The irregular rhythm may in fact be chaotic, but very often follows a pattern, albeit subtle, which greatly facilitates the diagnosis. Truly chaotic beating at normal heart rates is seen in controlled atrial fibrillation and chaotic atrial rhythm. The latter is often seen in patients with pulmonary disease and is characterized by seemingly random variations in P-wave rate and morphology, often accompanied by varying PR intervals (Figure 10). The term "sick sinus syndrome" includes many supraventricular disorders often consisting of brief paroxysms of extra beats and pauses in no apparent pattern (Figure 11).

The pattern of an irregular heart rhythm may be

Purkinje system, resulting in a right bundle branch block type pattern. In such a case, the initial QRS deflection will be similar to that of normal beats, and the pattern in lead V_1 is more likely to be rSR'. However, aberration can occur elsewhere in the ventricles and total reliance on the QRS morphology is not advised. Aberration occurs more readily when the premature beat is early, and follows a beat with a long R-R interval (Ashman's phenomenon). Clearly, the most definitive means of diagnosing a PAC is by identifying a premature P-wave. Aberrrantly conducted beats in atrial fibrillation are difficult to diagnose definitively, and one must rely on the pattern of short after long as well as the QRS morphology. One can seriously challenge the diagnosis of Ashman's phenomenon if an earlier beat after a longer pause conducts normally in an adjacent sequence.

When a premature P-wave occurs very early in the cycle, it may find the AV node and/or the His-Purkinje system refractory, resulting in a blocked PAC. The early blocked P-wave is often obscured by

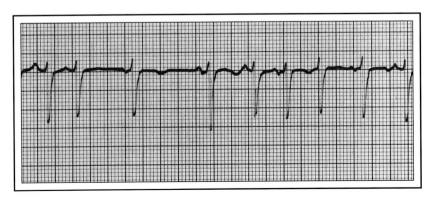

Figure 10. Chaotic atrial rhythm or multi-focal atrial tachycardia characterized by varying P-wave morphologies and PR intervals.

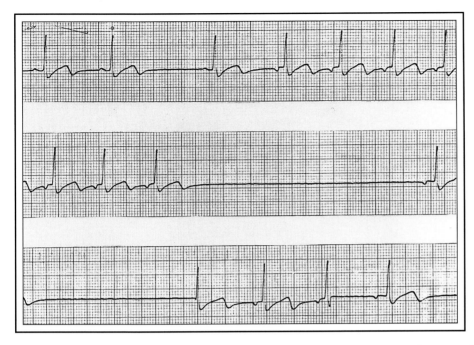

Figure 11. Continuous monitor recording from a 44-year-old truck driver with syncope.

obvious, or may only be discernible after careful examination and measurement. At times, the presence of a pattern can be assumed by the occurrence of a repeated sequence of beats, even if the nature of the pattern is unknown.

The sinus node may display a fluctuation in its firing rate resulting in a sinus arrhythmia. In respiratory sinus arrhythmia the rate quickens upon inspiration and slows on expiration. This pattern can be identified on long rhythm strips where the frequency of peaks and valleys of heart rate corresponds to the patient's respiratory rate. Sinus arrhythmia is common in young people, is presumed to be due to fluctuations in vagal tone, and is of no clinical significance. Similar heart rate variations occur less commonly independent of the breathing pattern.

Alternation in autonomic tone also causes ventriculo-phasic sinus arrhythmia. This is evident in cases of 2:1 heart block in which the P-P interval which encompasses a QRS complex is different from the P-P interval without a QRS complex within it (Figure 12). Depending upon where in the cycle the QRS falls, the P-P interval surrounding it may be shorter or longer than the other interval. Stimulation of baroreceptors by the arterial pulsation in the alternating intervals produces a phasic effect on the rate of sinus firing.

Simple ectopic beats can occur in patterns such that they follow every normal beat or every second, third, or more beat resulting in bigeminy, trigeminy, quadrigeminy, etc. The premature beats may be atrial or ventricular and less commonly junctional. The coupling interval to the previous normal beat is generally fixed, and the mechanism is thought to be either re-entry or afterdepolarization. When the premature bigeminal beat falls early in the cycle, the resulting contraction may be too weak to be felt as a peripheral pulse. Thus, when there is a full compensatory pause, the peripheral pulse can be half the apical pulse. Occasionally, the patterned premature beats may occur as couplets (Figure 13).

Ventricular bigeminy occurs in a variety of cardiac disorders, including digitalis toxicity, ischemia, and heart failure. This rhythm can also be chronic, and, in fact, the pattern of alternating long and short intervals predisposes to self-perpetuation as postulated by Langendorf and Pick as their "law of bigeminy". Once established, the rhythm may persist and is generally benign in that it does not degenerate to more dangerous rhythms. However, when a ventricular bigeminal rhythm first begins, the second PVC of the cycle, although it has the same coupling interval as the first PVC, will now be

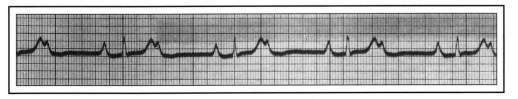

Figure 12. Rhythm strip demonstrating normal sinus rhythm with 2:1 A-V block. The PP intervals encompassing a QRS complex are shorter than the PP intervals without a QRS complex.

635

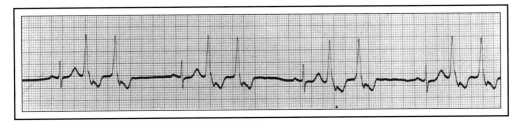

Figure 13. Lead 2 strip from an 80-year-old man who presented with a slow pulse. Coupled premature ventricular beats follow each normal beat.

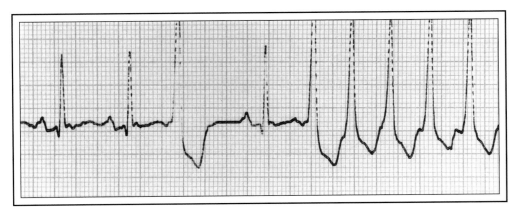

Figure 14. Monitor rhythm strip revealing ventricular tachycardia commencing with the second cycle of a bigeminal rhythm. The coupling intervals of the two cycles are equal.

following a beat whose antecedent R-R interval is longer and whose repolarization is therefore delayed. This is more likely to induce a sustained arrhythmia such as ventricular tachycardia or fibrillation (Figure 14).

Although it is usually not necessary to treat bigeminy, therapy is indicated when there is an inappropriately slow pulse rate, unacceptable symptomatic palpitations, or when more dangerous rhythms are provoked, especially in the presence of ischemia as in the early course of an acute myocardial infarction. Antiarrhythmic therapy with type I drugs is effective. An increase in the underlying heart rate brought about by atrial pacing may alter the conditions enough to abolish a re-entrant pathway. Unlike the pattern where the premature beat is linked to the previous normal beat, impulses can arise from an ectopic focus and fire independently of the underlying rhythm. This situation, known as parasystole, is relatively uncommon since the abnormal focus must be protected or isolated from the normal conduction system and thus not depolarized by the faster underlying rhythm.

There is no relationship between the beats from the two sources; therefore, the coupling intervals vary. When both rhythms are regular, each can be marched out separately. Since the tissue may be refractory after a depolarization, not every beat of each rhythm will be manifest, but the interval between beats from each focus will have a common denominator. Characteristically, when the two wave forms appear simultaneously, a fusion beat will occur whose morphology will be some combination of the two beats (Figure 15). Parasystole is more

commonly seen in the ventricles, while atrial parasystole is more rare and less likely to be noticed even when present. Parasystole can occur when separate foci arise in the right and left atria.

Despite the fact that in parasystole "premature" beats occur at different points in the cardiac cycle including the late repolarization phase, provocation of sustained tachyarrhythmia is uncommon. If treatment is required, one must employ techniques that reduce automaticity such as the use of type I anti-arrhythmic drugs.

When the upper and lower chambers of the heart beat independently, it is termed AV dissociation. In this situation, as with parasystole, the foci must be protected from each other, usually by antegrade and retrograde AV conduction block. AV dissociation is not a specific diagnosis, but rather a description of a phenomenon brought about by an abnormality of rhythm formation or conduction. An accelerated ventricular or junctional focus may beat faster than the underlying sinus rate. If this rhythm fails to conduct retrogradely and depolarize the atria, the sinus node will beat independently at a slower rate, and the two rhythms will march through each other in a dissociated fashion.

Alternatively, in the presence of complete heart block, the atria will generally beat faster than an independent ventricular or junctional escape focus with no meaningful relationship between the two. The management of AV dissociation is related to the underlying ectopic rhythm or heart block, not the presence of AV dissociation per se.

In complete AV dissociation, a beat from one chamber never affects the rhythm in the other

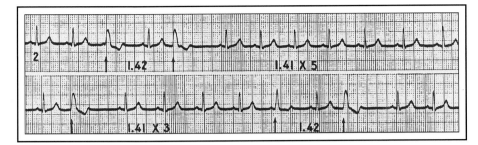

Figure 15. Continuous Lead 2 rhythm strip demonstrating normal sinus rhythm at a rate of approximately 75 (R–R=0.8 sec) with independent idioventricular beats at a cycle length, or multiple, of 1.41 sec. The seventh QRS complex on the lower strip is a fusion beat.
(Courtesy William P. Nelson, MD)

chamber, and the ventricular rate is generally regular. However, it is possible to have the atria and ventricles beating independently with some degree of conduction preserved. In this situation, an occasional impulse can be transmitted from the atrium to the ventricle, producing a depolarization which is earlier than the next scheduled ventricular beat, thus interfering with the otherwise regular rhythm. This phenomenon is called AV dissociation with interference or interference dissociation. A characteristic pattern of this would be a regular idioventricular or junctional rhythm with periodic early beats. The early beats will invariably be preceded by P-waves with a normal or somewhat prolonged PR interval. The PR intervals may vary depending on where in the cycle the P-wave falls (Figure 16). One may need to see several such beats in a long continuous strip to be convinced that this is a bona fide pattern. The implications and management of interference dissociation are similar to that of standard AV dissociation except for the knowledge that complete heart block is not present.

A special situation in which the recognition of interference dissociation is important is in the patient with underlying 2:1 block. It is not uncommon for such a patient to display an escape junctional or ventricular rhythm at a rate faster than one-half the sinus rate. Superficially, one will then see a regular atrial rate faster than a different regular ventricular rate, suggesting the presence of complete heart block. However, the occurrence of occasional early ventricular beats preceded by reasonably timed P waves, indicates the preservation of some AV conduction. This condition is no worse than the underlying 2:1 block and demonstrates the presence of an adequate escape mechanism, which is very different from the implications of documenting complete heart block.

Second degree heart block of less than a 2:1 ratio produces some of the most classic patterns of cardiac arrhythmias. The pattern of the blocked beats depends on the site of the conduction abnormality. AV nodal tissue displays the characteristic of decremental conduction, whereby the impulse can be delayed to a variable degree, at times quite considerable, and yet maintains the ability to conduct. Conduction within, and especially below, the His bundle is much more of an all or none phenomenon. The usual conduction patterns that are generated from block above and below the His bundle are termed Mobitz I (Wenckebach) and Mobitz II block.

Mobitz I Block

The hallmark of Wenckebach block is a progressive prolongation of the PR interval, culminating in a blocked atrial beat associated with a pause in the ventricular rhythm. The pause is terminated by a conducted beat with the shortest PR interval of the cycle which, in turn, serves as the first beat of the next sequence (Figure 17). The number of atrial beats in a cycle may vary from three to more than 20. In the classic form, the PR interval lengthens progressively with each successive beat of the cycle. However, the increment by which the PR interval prolongs decreases with each beat. This results in a minor shortening of the R-R interval of successive beats (Figure 18). It is important to recognize that the PR intervals may progressively lengthen by an increasing or variable increment resulting in no clear pattern of R-R intervals without vitiating the diagnosis of Wenckebach block.

The pattern of Wenckebach block can be recognized by the progressive prolongation of PR intervals leading to a blocked beat and a pause. In fact, the periodicity of grouped beats followed by a pause of less than 2 R-R intervals may be so characteris-

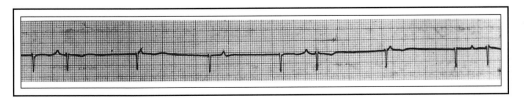

Figure 16. Lead 1 recording from a 52-year-old woman with sinus bradycardia at a rate of 39 and a junctional escape rhythm at a rate of 45. P-waves that fall outside the refractory periods are able to conduct.

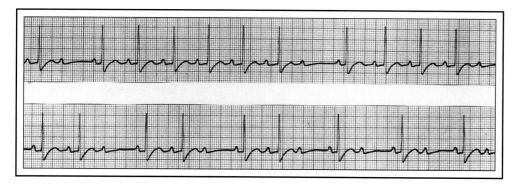

Figure 17. Continuous monitor strip from a 49-year-old woman with an acute inferior myocardial infarction. There is normal sinus rhythm with minor prolongation of PR intervals and dropped beats, progressing to 2:1 A-V block.

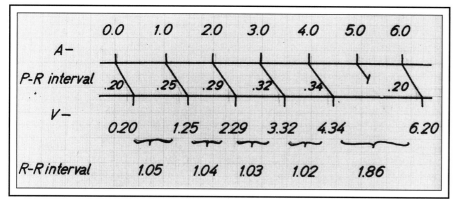

Figure 18. Ladder diagram of typical Wenckebach periodicity. Intervals are in seconds. A = atrium, V = ventricle.

tic as to suggest the diagnosis even in the absence of visible P-waves. When there is variation in the number of beats in each complete cycle, one will see, for example, groups of three, four, five, and six QRS complexes which are not completely regular, followed by pauses, with longer pauses occurring in those cycles with fewer beats. Assuming the presence of a regular atrial rate, and that the first PR interval of each of the cycles will be similar, the time interval from the beginning of one cycle to the next will contain n + 1 P-waves, where n is the number of QRS complexes in the sequence. By measuring accurately the duration of several different cycles and dividing each by its appropriate n + 1, one will find a common result which represents the P-P, or initiating stimulus-to-stimulus interval. Although this exercise is unnecessary when P-waves are evident, it will allow one to entertain the diagnosis of Wenckebach block in an otherwise obscure rhythm (Figure 19) and in the presence of atrial fibrillation with junctional rhythm.

In this latter situation, a seemingly benign pat-tern of irregular ventricular beats with atrial fibrillation may in fact represent digitalis toxicity with junctional tachycardia and atrioventricular block of a Mobitz I variety. Similarly, a characteristic pattern of P-waves occurring in groups separated by pauses can represent sino-atrial Wenckebach block (Figure 20). Finally, Wenckebach periodicity of QRS complexes can be identified in situations in which there are many more P-waves than QRS complexes. AV block can occur at more than one level in the conduction system such that there is 2:1 block at a higher level with Wenckebach block at a lower level, with each pause containing three successively dropped P-waves. This phenomenon occurs commonly during the transition from atrial flutter with 2:1 to atrial flutter with 4:1 block (Figure 21). The appearance of this Wenckebach periodicity in the presence of 2:1 block should not be considered a new problem, but rather part of the process of correcting the rapid rate response. More complex patterns can occur when there is Wenckebach block at the upper level or both levels of multilevel block.

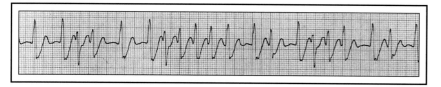

Figure 19. Monitor lead displaying a rhythm which superficially appears chaotic with varying QRS morphologies. Careful analysis reveals the rhythm to be atrial tachycardia with periods of 7 to 6, 5 to 4, 4 to 3, and 3 to 2 Wenckebach as well as 2:1 block. QRS complexes that occur at a rapid rate are of a different morphology from those following longer pauses.

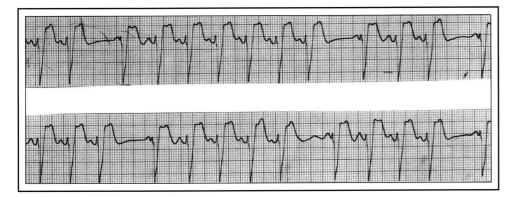

Mobitz II Block

Since conduction at or below the His bundle tends to be all or none, there is no opportunity for significant variations to occur in the PR interval. Conducted beats will display their particular PR interval, whereas nonconducted beats will be blocked completely. The resultant pattern is a series of regularly conducted beats followed by a pause which, assuming a regular atrial rate, is twice or a larger multiple of the P-P interval.

Mobitz II block occurs most commonly in the fascicles of the bundle branch system. Intermittent block in the His bundle, in the anatomically very short common bundle or simultaneous intermittent block in the already divided branches is less likely. Most often there is preexisting disease in one bundle branch in which case block in the contralateral bundle will result in a completely blocked beat, or a series of block beats. Characteristically, therefore,

the QRS complex of the conducted beat is wide and often displays a right or left bundle branch block pattern (Figure 22). Conversely, in Mobitz I block the QRS configuration is usually normal, although it is possible to have an intraventricular conduction defect independent of the AV nodal disorder.

When conduction block is localized to the AV node, an escape focus can arise in the junctional or high ventricular areas providing a relatively reliable and rapid ventricular rhythm. AV nodal block may be only a transient phenomenon secondary to ischemia such as in an acute inferior wall myocardial infarction, drug usage, or related to temporary alterations in vagal tone.

Conduction block below the His bundle is often associated with extensive Purkinje system disease. The duration of block and the reliability and rate of any escape mechanism is less favorable than that of AV nodal block and Mobitz II block cannot be attributed to alterations in autonomic tone. Mobitz I block can often be managed conservatively and can respond to vagolytic therapy such as atropine. Mobitz II block generally signals the need for pacemaker therapy since the problem is often chronic and the likelihood of complete heart block and prolonged asystole is great. Atropine is not indicated in Mobitz II block, and, in fact, speeding of the sinus node by a vagolytic drug can result in a greater compromise of intraventricular conduction with resultant worsening of the heart block.

Tachycardic Rhythms

A heart rate greater than 100 beats per minute is considered tachycardia. The site of origin of the tachycardia may be supraventricular or ventricular.

Supraventricular Tachycardia

In sinus tachycardia, the sinus node drives the heart at a rapid rate in response to physiologic or pathologic stimuli. Rapid heart rates are appropriate in infants and in adults during exercise or emotional stress. Sinus tachycardia is observed in association with a multitude of circumstances such as

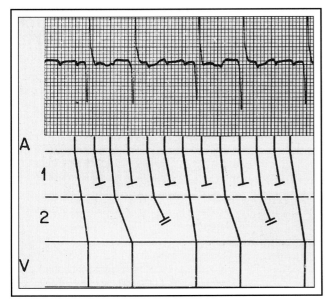

Figure 21. Ladder diagram depicting atrial flutter with two levels of block in the A-V conduction system. There is 2:1 block at the upper level and 3:2 Wenckebach at the lower level resulting in grouped beating. *(Courtesy American Heart Association)*

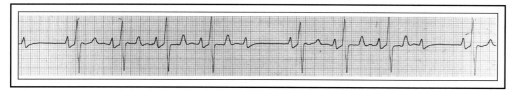

Figure 22. Monitor lead displaying normal sinus rhythm with occasional blocked beats not preceded by PR prolongation. The QRS duration is 0.12 seconds.

fever, hypotension, anemia, congestive heart failure, and thyrotoxicosis as well as in response to a variety of pharmacological agents. The range of heart rate in sinus tachycardia is quite great. In infants and during extreme stress, the heart rate may exceed 200 beats per minute. More commonly, rates of up to 150 beats per minute are noted. The tachycardia develops and recedes gradually rather than with an abrupt change in rate. Sinus tachycardia is characterized by a normal appearing P wave, with a normal PR interval when compared to a baseline electrocardiogram.

At times the P-wave may in fact be somewhat more pronounced and distinct, reflecting a more rapid and well coordinated atrial depolarization. Although under certain circumstances a rapid atrial rate can cause a slowing of AV conduction, the autonomic stimulation which accounts for the sinus tachycardia will also enhance AV conduction and thus preserve the normal PR relationship. Unless the patient is known to have underlying atrial or AV nodal disease, one should not diagnose sinus tachycardia if one does not see distinct, well conducted P-waves before each QRS complex. Slowing of the heart rate will be achieved by correcting or controlling the factors that are provoking the tachycardia. The sinus node's pacemaker function can be usurped by a rapid ectopic atrial focus. Ectopic atrial tachycardia is a characteristic of digitalis toxicity, and is also seen with advanced pulmonary disease. The P-wave morphology is different from the underlying sinus rhythm, and the PR interval is often longer since the atrial rate is fast while AV conduction is not being facilitated. In digitalis toxicity, the atrial tachycardia is commonly associated with second degree AV block in a Wenckebach or 2:1 pattern. This rhythm can occur in paroxysms. The rate may accelerate during its

first few beats, then continue in a nearly regular fashion. In patients with pulmonary disease, the P-wave morphology may vary from beat to beat often with differing PR intervals. This is called multifocal atrial tachycardia.

Rate of the atrial tachycardia related to digitalis excess will vary directly with the degree of toxicity. Reversal of the process by the use of specific antibodies, supplemental potassium, phenytoin or discontinuation of the drug will result in progressive slowing of the ectopic rate culminating in the re-emergence of sinus rhythm. Ectopic rhythms associated with pulmonary disease respond poorly to medications and require correction of the underlying disease process.

A very common form of supraventricular tachycardia is called "PAT" or paroxysmal atrial tachycardia, although in reality it is most often due to re-entry within the AV node. In this situation, there exist two conduction pathways; one with the property of slower conduction and a shorter refractory period (alpha) and the other which conducts more rapidly with a longer refractory period (beta). An early premature atrial beat can descend the alpha pathway, enter the beta pathway at a point lower in the junction and then conduct retrogradely to the atria, establishing a re-entrant circuit. Characteristically, the PR interval is long and the RP interval so short that the P-wave is obscured by the QRS complex (Figure 23). A re-entrant circuit in the opposite direction, in which antegrade conduction is via the faster pathway, is uncommon. In this situation, the P-wave is clearly identifiable and the PR interval is normal or somewhat prolonged. Although there is a P-wave preceding each QRS complex, in reality the P-wave does not actually conduct to the ventricle but rather both chambers are activated by impulses emerging from the re-

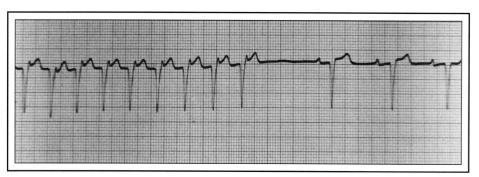

Figure 23. Rhythm strip of A-V nodal re-entrant tachycardia with carotid sinus massage (black bar). During the tachycardia the P wave is seen to distort the terminal portion of the QRS complex.

entrant circuit in the AV junction. Impulses emerging from the His bundle generally will activate the ventricles in a normal fashion. However, it is not uncommon to have rate related aberrated conduction producing a wide QRS complex tachycardia.

A different form of re-entrant tachycardia is seen in the Wolff-Parkinson-White syndrome. A rapidly conducting accessory pathway, generally with a longer refractory period, bypasses the AV node and enters the ventricle directly. In normal sinus rhythm the impulse will traverse both the accessory pathway and the AV node producing the characteristic short PR interval and delta wave. A premature atrial beat may find the accessory pathway refractory and thus conduct via the AV node exclusively. Beyond the AV node the impulse can enter the accessory pathway and return rapidly to the atrium, establishing a re-entrant circuit. In the absence of an underlying intraventricular conduction defect or rate related aberrancy, the QRS morphology will be normal, without a delta wave. Less commonly, the antegrade pathway will be via the bypass tract resulting in a wide complex tachycardia, often similar in morphology to the abnormal QRS of the baseline WPW.

CARDIAC PEARL

One would think that a patient having the Wolff-Parkinson-White syndrome with a short P-R interval would have a loud first heart sound; however, it is usually of normal intensity.

The shortening of the P-R interval is at the expense of the wide QRS, so the total time from the onset of the P-wave to the end of the QRS is about normal. The right ventricle is stimulated early and the left ventricle response is on time.

A historical note concerning the Wolff-Parkinson-White Syndrome (a short P-R interval, wide QRS and episodes of a supraventricular tachycardia).

Dr. Louis Wolff of Boston and Sir John Parkinson of London had apparently independently observed these patients. Dr. Paul Dudley White of Boston was instrumental in putting the records of these patients together and arranging for their publication. The syndrome was, therefore, reported in the medical literature introducing what became known as the Wolff-Parkinson-White Syndrome. Drs. White and Wolff, being in the same city, knew each other. Dr. White also knew Dr. Parkinson but Dr. Wolff did not. It was not until following the Second World Congress of Cardiology held in 1950 (Washington, D.C.) that Dr. White introduced Dr. Wolff to Dr. Parkinson.

W. Proctor Harvey, M.D.

There are several other variants of re-entrant tachycardias in patients with pre-excitation. There may be multiple accessory pathways in which case the rate will be more rapid and the QRS wide. A bypass tract that can only conduct retrogradely will allow re-entrant tachycardias, but will never display the characteristic short PR and delta wave either during normal sinus rhythm or tachycardia (concealed WPW). Typical AV nodal re-entry can occur in patients with an incidental partial bypass via Mahaim fibers resulting in a wide complex tachycardia. Precise delineation of these mechanisms generally require electrophysiologic study with mapping.

A re-entrant circuit can arise in the atrium and include the sinus node. The resultant P wave will be similar in morphology to that of sinus rhythm and the PR interval will tend to be somewhat prolonged. Unlike sinus tachycardia, this rhythm will start and stop abruptly.

Re-entrant supraventricular tachycardias are generally short-lived and self-terminating. The rate of PAT is usually approximately 150 bpm and does not cause hemodynamic compromise. With more rapid rates, such as may be seen with WPW, or in the setting of underlying heart disease, the tachycardia may be tolerated poorly and require prompt treatment. Blocking of one of the pathways by means of vagotonic stimulation may be achieved by

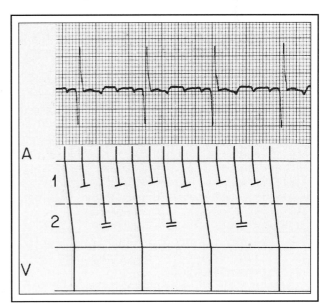

Figure 24. Ladder diagram of same patient as Figure 21, after digitalis therapy. 4:1 A-V block can be considered to have resulted from progression of block at the lower level to 2:1.
(Courtesy American Heart Association)

641

interventions such as carotid sinus massage, Valsalva maneuver, or provocation of a diving reflex (Figure 23). These may be successfully initiated by the patient or medical personnel.

CARDIAC PEARL

Carotid sinus stimulation (or pressure) is still a very useful maneuver that can be performed in the office or at the bedside. The technique of performing carotid sinus pressure is shown in Figures A and B.

The physician's stethoscope is placed over the precordium to monitor any change in rhythm. (One does not have to hold the stethoscope.) The patient's head is positioned over the physician's left arm. The head is turned to the left and the carotid artery is palpated at the angle of the right jaw. This is where the carotid sinus is located. Press this area with your index and middle finger (some physicians prefer to use their thumb) and feel for the carotid pulsation. Stop the pressure immediately if a response is obtained. If available, the electrocardiogram should be recording the procedure. Remember not to use prolonged carotid sinus stimulation, since serious consequences can occur, such as prolonged cardiac systole, and even death. Instead press over the carotid sinus for 3 to 5 seconds, then let up for 5 to 10 seconds. Repeat this several times.

It is necessary to apply sufficient pressure that it will usually cause some discomfort to the patient.

When carotid sinus pressure is not effective, it usually means that the exact spot of the carotid arterial pulsation at the angle of the jaw has not been located.

If the patient has a rapid tachycardia, slowing of the ventricular rate with carotid sinus pressure rules out the most serious arrhythmias that of ventricular tachycardia.

Precautions- Do not use carotid sinus pressure in a patient who has known cerebral vascular disease. The temporary cessation of blood flow resulting from the carotid sinus pressure can decrease cerebral blood flow to the point of causing convulsions and even a stroke. Personally observed was a patient who had convulsions following carotid sinus pressure; fortunately this did not result in any permanent damage.

Do not use simultaneous carotid sinus pressure over both right and left sides of the neck.

Even though pressure over the eyeballs has been used and advocated as vagus nerve stimulation in the past, don't use it. Serious injury to the eye can and has resulted.

Carotid sinus hypersensitivity has been noted in some patients with advanced aortic stenosis.

Hypersensitive carotid sinuses do exist, but are not common. However, such a possibility should be ruled out to avoid serious complications such as asystole and ventricular arrhythmias that can result from carotid sinus pressure.

Make sure there is no abnormality of the carotid arteries, as might be signalled by the finding of significant bruits over either of the carotids. History of previous transient ischemic attack (TIA) or stroke also would contraindicate carotid artery stimulation. If there is no significant change in carotid pulsation or presence of a bruit, place the stetho-

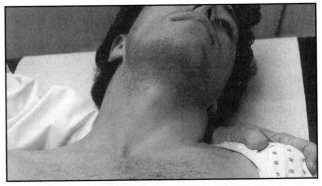

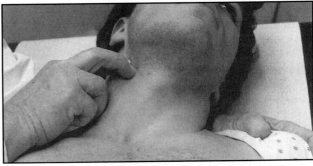

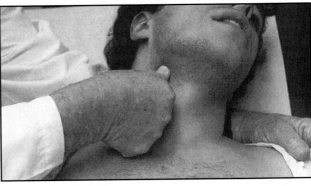

Fig A: Carotid Sinus Pressure - Remove the pillow and position the patient's head over your left arm (top). Locate the carotid artery pulsation just under the angle of the right jaw. Exert pressure with the index and middle fingers or thumb. Listen with your stethoscope resting over the precordium (no hand is necessary to hold the stethoscope in place).

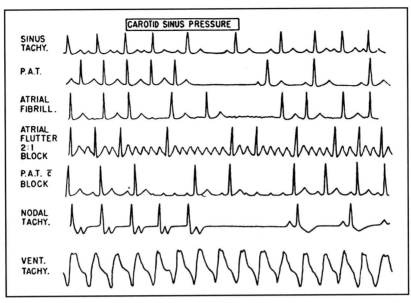

Fig B: Composite Artist's Sketch of Effect of Carotid Sinus Pressure on Various Tachycardias. First strip: Note gradual slowing and gradual return to former rate with normal sinus tachycardia. Second strip: Paroxysmal atrial tachycardia (PAT) abruptly stopped, followed by regular rhythm. Third strip: Atrial fibrillation. Rate originally irregular and rapid. Immediate slowing with irregular return to former rhythm. Fourth strip: Note prompt slowing with irregular "jerky" return to original 2:1 flutter. The atria remain undisturbed. Fifth strip: Carotid pressure produces slowing with return to former rate. Note atrial waves easily identified slowing. Sixth strip: Abrupt reversion from nodal rhythm to normal (like paroxysmal atrial tachycardia). Seventh strip: No effect whatsoever on ventricular tachycardia.

scope over the chest to monitor any change in the rhythm. (The stethoscope can be positioned so that both hands are free); then while listening with the stethoscope, very gently touch the area for carotid sinus stimulation to make sure it is not a hypersensitive carotid sinus.

W. Proctor Harvey, M.D.

Acute pharmacologic intervention with intravenous verapamil or adenosine is highly effective, while intravenous digoxin therapy acts more slowly. In an urgent situation, direct current cardioversion can immediately restore sinus rhythm. Long-term preventive treatment can be achieved by the use of digitalis, verapamil, and/or beta blockers.

The presence of wide complex tachycardia or suspicion of WPW complicates therapy. Since verapamil will not benefit ventricular tachycardia and can seriously worsen already compromised left ventricular function, one must be certain that one is dealing with supraventricular tachycardia with aberrated conduction before utilizing this drug. If in doubt, DC cardioversion can be effective in terminating the tachycardia whether it be supraventricular or ventricular. Both verapamil and digitalis can enhance conduction through an accessory pathway, which could be very dangerous when WPW is associated with atrial flutter or fibrillation.

Patients with re-entrant supraventricular tachycardia refractory to simple therapy, or WPW in which there is a threat of atrial flutter/fibrillation with a dangerously rapid ventricular response, should undergo electrophysiologic testing to assess drug responsiveness and the susceptibility to extremely rapid ventricular rates. When indicated, catheter or surgical ablation of one or more conduction tracts has proven to be a highly effective and safe form of treatment.

Atrial flutter is thought to result from a re-entrant mechanism within the atria. Since the pathway does not include more slowly conducting tissues, the circuit time is shorter and the resultant rate faster than AV or sinus nodal re-entrant tachycardias. The flutter rate can range from the low 200s to above 400 beats per minute, although a rate of 300 is a common finding. Typically, the flutter waves produce a sawtoothed pattern on the electrocardiographic baseline, especially in the inferior leads. Slow rates, bordering on those seen in atrial tachycardias, are found in patients with large, diseased atria and in the presence of Type IA antiarrhythmic drugs. Atrial flutter at very rapid rates may look and behave more like atrial fibrillation. This rhythm is often somewhat irregular with variations in morphology of the flutter waves and the rhythm cannot be overdriven by rapid atrial pacing.

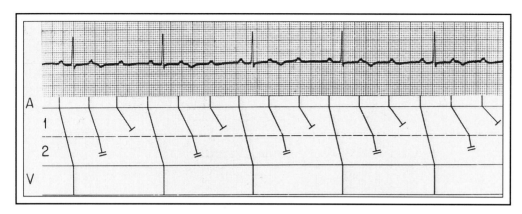

Figure 25. Ladder diagram depicting 3:1 block consisting of Wenckebach at an upper level and 2:1 block at a lower level in the conduction system. *(Courtesy American Heart Association)*

The ventricles are protected from the rapid atrial rate by physiologic block within the AV node. The most common conduction ratios are 2:1 and 4:1 block, depending on such factors as the flutter rate, the status of the AV node, autonomic tone, and the use of pharmacologic agents. In these circumstances, the interval between a QRS complex and the preceding flutter wave is constant, although one cannot necessarily identify which flutter wave is the one which conducts. In fact, since atrial flutter is a continuous wave coursing through the atria, a flutter to R interval does not represent a true conduction time. Other conduction ratios are generally irregular and do not display a fixed relationship between the flutter and R waves. In these conditions, there usually is block at more than one level of the AV conduction system. Often, one can discern Wenckebach periodicity due to 2:1 block at a high level and Mobitz I block at a lower level (Figure 21). Four to one block generally is the result of 2:1 block at two separate levels (Figure 24). Three to one block with a fixed flutter to R interval is rare, and usually results from 3:2 Wenckebach at an upper level with a 2:1 block below it (Figure 25). A rapid ventricular response due to 1:1 conduction can occur when the flutter rate is relatively slow and when AV conduction is facilitated by an abnormal pathway or enhanced conductivity such as in infants or with exaggerated autonomic tone.

The diagnosis of atrial flutter may be most difficult when the conduction ratio is 2:1. In this circumstance, one flutter wave may be "buried" within the QRS complex, while the other one may be obscured by a T-wave. When the ventricular rate is approximately 150 beats per minute this rhythm can be confused with AV nodal re-entrant tachycardia if one does not recognize either of the flutter waves, or with an ectopic or atypical paroxysmal atrial tachycardia if one does identify an atrial depolarization before each QRS. Carotid sinus stimulation or other vagal maneuvers can transiently increase the AV block and unmask the rapid flutter waves (Figure 26).

CARDIAC PEARL

Atrial Flutter: A patient with an untreated atrial flutter having a tachycardia usually has a 2:1 block.

A woman about 30 years of age had returned to her home in the midwest for a holiday; while there she had the onset of a rapid tachycardia and was taken to the emergency room of a local hospital; a drug was administered which caused successful reversion to normal sinus rhythm. On returning home she was referred to me for evaluation. Her description of the tachycardia was corroborated by her watching my moving hands over my chest simulating a very rapid rate of regular rhythm; she said, "Yes, it was just like that." This indicated paroxysmal atrial tachycardia. She then showed me the electrocardio-

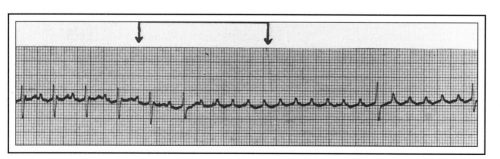

Figure 26. Lead II recording in a patient with atrial flutter with 2:1 block. Right carotid sinus massage (bar between arrows) increases the degree of block and unmasks flutter waves.

gram that had been taken during her tachycardia (which I had been unaware she had possession of)- the computer readout stated that it was atrial flutter. The ventricular rate was 214. A patient on no medication and who had atrial flutter would be 2:1 block; therefore the atrial rate would be 428.

Atrial flutter is usually between 250 and 350 beats per minute; 428 is too fast for the usual flutter; 214 is consistent with paroxysmal atrial tachycardia. The computer readout was incorrect. This emphasizes that even though most computer interpretations are correct, the "human" electrocardiographer should review the tracings.

Untreated flutter is generally 2:1 block. It may simulate paroxysmal atrial tachycardia. With carotid sinus stimulation, an abrupt slowing may take place, but there is a so-called "jerky" return to the previous rate.

This is due to the temporary change of the 2:1 block to higher grades of block such as 4:1, 3:1, and so forth and then back to the original regular 2:1 block. Carotid sinus pressure does not cause reversion of the tachycardia to normal sinus rhythm. However, carotid sinus stimulation can cause paroxysmal atrial tachycardia to revert to normal sinus rhythm.

W. Proctor Harvey, M.D.

Atrial flutter may occur in paroxysms lasting from only a few beats to hours and days, or may be chronic, especially in patients with advanced cardiac disease. Persistent atrial flutter may be difficult to manage since the AV conduction ratio often changes by a multiple of 2, producing marked swings in heart rate with or without provocation. A variety of drugs can be used in an attempt to control the ventricular rate. Digitalis, the calcium channel inhibitors verapamil and diltiazem, and beta blockers all slow conduction through the AV node. However, despite relatively large doses and multiple agents, the conduction ratio may remain at 2:1.

Because of these difficulties, often the best therapeutic strategy is to get the patient out of atrial flutter. If spontaneous conversion to normal sinus rhythm does not occur within two to three days, low

energy cardioversion may be employed with a high degree of success. Atrial thrombus is not likely to form during relatively short periods of flutter and thus anticoagulation is not necessary. Type IA and IC anti-arrhythmic agents are effective in converting acute atrial flutter to sinus rhythm. However, these must be used with caution since they act by first slowing the atrial flutter rate. Thus, a rapid flutter rate of 300 bpm with 2:1 AV block can be converted to a slower flutter rate of 200-220 bpm in which case 1:1 conduction may ensue with clinical deterioration caused by the excessive ventricular response. This can be avoided by the prior use of drugs to slow AV conduction, such as digitalis or verapamil.

It is not uncommon for atrial flutter to convert spontaneously to the more easily controllable atrial fibrillation. Conversion to atrial fibrillation is facilitated by digitalis therapy, and is generally preceded by a progressive increase in the flutter rate. If normal sinus rhythm cannot be achieved or maintained, atrial fibrillation may be the rhythm of choice. Fibrillation can be induced by very low energy cardioversion or atrial pacing using single or trains of rapid stimuli. A high level of digitalization will help prevent the rhythm from reverting to flutter.

Atrial fibrillation is the most commonly occurring supraventricular tachycardia. Atrial depolarization is totally discoordinated in the presence of multiple and varying re-entrant circuits, resulting in the loss of any effective atrial contraction. The AV node is presented with an enormously large number of impulses, only some of which are transmitted to the ventricle. The interplay of AV nodal repolarization and multiple levels of concealed conduction and block result in a random pattern of beats emerging from the bundle of His. In the absence of underlying AV nodal disease, the ventricular rate is generally rapid, especially with the acute onset of the arrhythmia. Clinical problems relate to the hemodynamic effect of losing the atrial kick, to an excessively rapid ventricular rate, and/or to the uncomfortable sensation caused by the irregular heartbeat.

Most often atrial stretch contributes to the occurrence of fibrillation. This is seen in a variety of

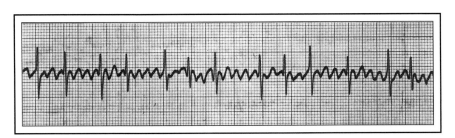

Figure 27. Lead 2 recording of atrial fibrillation displaying a course baseline and an irregular ventricular rhythm.

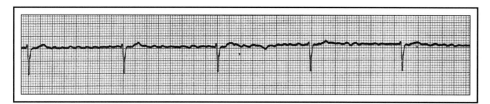

Figure 28. Lead 3 recording of atrial fibrillation with a regular junctional rhythm at a rate of 37 beats per minute.

clinical circumstances in which atrial pressure or volume is increased. Atrial fibrillation commonly complicates mitral valve disease, and occurs later and less frequently in the course of aortic valve disease. A large proportion of patients with atrial fibrillation have enlarged atria resulting from long standing hypertension. Congestive heart failure from any cause can lead to atrial fibrillation. This arrhythmia is also associated with ischemic heart disease and is not uncommon during acute myocardial infarction or in the late stages of ischemic cardiomyopathy. However, it is not likely for atrial fibrillation to be the first or only manifestation of coronary artery disease since the vascular supply to the atria is from the proximal portions of the coronary arteries, and interruption of this blood supply would almost certainly be associated with more manifest problems elsewhere in the heart. Atrial fibrillation may appear late in the course of an atrial septal defect resulting in clinical deterioration.

Atrial fibrillation may result from mechanical irritation of the atria as in pericarditis and following cardiac or pulmonary surgery, or may be precipitated by excesses of alcohol, caffeine, thyroid hormone, or autonomic stimuli. When no underlying cause can be identified, it is termed lone atrial fibrillation.

Atrial fibrillation is characterized by a coarse baseline on the electrocardiogram reflecting chaotic atrial activation. The deflections may be large and at times mimic P-waves or flutter waves but without a true pattern (Figure 27). In long-standing disease with fibrotic atria the deflections may be quite small and approach the appearance of a flat line. The ventricular rhythm is erratic and fails to fit any pattern. At more rapid rates, the rhythms superficially may appear regular but it does not hold up to careful measurement. It is possible to have fibrillating atria with an independent regular ventricular rhythm such as from an escape junctional or ventricular focus in the presence of high degree AV block (Figure 28), or a more rapid ventricular focus such as in junctional or ventricular tachycardia.

In the absence of an underlying ventricular conduction disturbance, the QRS complexes in atrial fibrillation will be normal. The presence of occasional wide complex abnormal beats can represent premature ventricular contractions or merely aberrated conduction of a supraventricular impulse. Since in this situation it is impossible to identify a premature atrial depolarization, one must rely on the long followed by short sequence as well as characteristics of the QRS morphology such as an rSR' in lead V_1, in order to support a presumption of Ashman's phenomenon. At times it may be impossible to diagnose definitively a particular beat, in which case it may be safer to assume that the beat is ventricular in origin.

Atrial fibrillation may be paroxysmal lasting for only a few seconds up to hours and days. Once it is established for many days, it will tend to continue chronically, unless it was caused by a reversible disorder which has been corrected. Management of this arrhythmia relates to control of the ventricular rate, conversion and prevention, and avoidance of complications.

Heart rate control can be accomplished by drugs that block AV conduction such as digitalis, the calcium channel blockers verapamil and diltiazem, and beta blockers. All can be used intravenously for acute management and orally for long-term control. Although these medications are reasonably effective in controlling the resting ventricular rate, they usually do not adequately limit the heart rate during sympathetic stimulation such as during exercise or at the time of the acute onset of a paroxysm. The combined use of digitalis and verapamil often provides the most effective rate control.

Type IA and IC antiarrhythmic drugs are effective at modest doses in reducing the recurrence of paroxysmal atrial fibrillation. Considerably larger doses are needed to convert fibrillation to sinus rhythm, especially once the arrhythmia has become established. Because of the high risk of toxicity from the medications, it is preferable to utilize DC cardioversion except for situations in which the fibrillation is short lived or the underlying provocative factor is resolved. Favorable results have been reported with the use of amiodarone, propafenone, and sotalol, but none are yet approved for use in the United States for atrial fibrillation. Patients with atrial fibrillation are often treated with digitalis and it had long been thought that this drug is instrumental in reverting the rhythm back to normal. Recent studies demonstrate no benefit of digitalis in converting atrial fibrillation to normal sinus rhythm and, in some circumstances, the drug may potentiate the arrhythmia.

Aside from the hemodynamic consequences of atrial fibrillation, there is a risk of clot formation in the poorly contracting atria with resultant peripheral emboli. This risk is present in both chronic and paroxysmal atrial fibrillation and may be especially prevalent upon the resumption of normal sinus rhythm and the return of atrial contraction. It is therefore advisable to anticoagulate a patient for approximately three weeks prior to attempting conversion either electrically or with drugs. Anticoagulation of chronic atrial fibrillation is recommended especially in the presence of atrial enlargement, heart failure, valvular disease, or a history of emboli. Long-term anticoagulation is generally not required in patients with lone atrial fibrillation and the absence of structural disease.

In situations in which atrial fibrillation cannot be controlled by standard means, ablation of the AV node with the insertion of a ventricular pacemaker may be necessary. In patients with WPW and paroxysmal atrial fibrillation, ablation of the bypass tract(s) is necessary to prevent potentially fatal arrhythmias. The recent development of surgical procedures which interrupt atrial pathways provides a novel means of reestablishing more normal atrial function. These procedures are reserved for refractory cases which also require atrio-ventricular synchrony.

CARDIAC PEARL

Atrial Fibrillation: The unexplained onset of atrial fibrillation in a patient who is 50 years of age or older may be a clue to the presence of underlying coronary artery disease. However, this is not necessarily true, since other conditions can cause this.

One example was President Bush's atrial fibrillation, which apparently was triggered by hyperthyroidism. His hyperthyroidism was treated and in turn the atrial fibrillation has apparently been controlled.

There is still a place for the medical treatment of paroxysmal atrial fibrillation. Too often the first step in management is to have electroconversion, whereas if antiarrhythmic drugs are given under supervision this can be accomplished medically.

It is best to have the patient under supervision in the hospital when attempting conversion to normal sinus rhythm, either with medication or electroconversion.

When it is not possible to control atrial fibrillation after trying several antiarrhythmic

drugs, it may be best for both physician and patient to "accept" and live with a chronic atrial fibrillation with a ventricular range in the 60s and 70s.

A patient with heart disease may have no evidence of cardiac decompensation, but acute pulmonary edema can occur with the change from normal sinus rhythm to atrial fibrillation. This also may be the first indication of underlying heart disease in some patients.

W. Proctor Harvey, M.D.

Ventricular Tachycardia

Ventricular tachycardia (VT) is a series of beats originating in the ventricles at a rate greater than 100 per minute. The arrhythmia may be paroxysmal or sustained, and may be as short as three beats or incessant. This rhythm is of major clinical significance since it often is associated with hemodynamic compromise and can degenerate into fatal ventricular fibrillation (VF). The mechanism is generally thought to be due to re-entrant circuits at a micro or macro level. The rhythm can be precipitated by an early cycle PVC which interrupts the previous T-wave (R on T phenomenon), but more often begins with a late cycle premature beat.

Ventricular tachycardia can occur in the absence of any underlying cardiac disease, but most often is a manifestation of some structural or metabolic abnormality. A common cause for VT is ischemic heart disease. Ventricular tachycardia may occur at the very onset of an acute myocardial infarction and its degeneration to ventricular fibrillation is the likely cause of most sudden cardiac deaths. The risk of VT remains high during the first 24 hours of an MI, but generally it can be effectively treated or prevented by judicious use of intravenous lidocaine, without subsequent problems. Ventricular tachycardia occurring later in the course of an MI, or in association with myocardial scarring, is more likely to be recurrent and troublesome. Brief runs of nonsustained VT may be tolerated without requiring treatment. However, longer runs may pose difficult management problems. Ventricular tachycardia does not commonly occur during episodes of classic angina, but can complicate major ischemic events such as seen with Prinzmetal's angina or extreme physical exertion.

Ventricular tachycardia may accompany a variety of other disorders of the ventricle such as cardiomyopathy, valvular heart disease, especially mitral regurgitation, right ventricular dysplasia, and congenital heart disease. Digitalis at toxic levels, psychotropic drugs, and anti-arrhythmic agents may be proarrhythmic for VT. Torsade de

Pointes occurs in the setting of a long QT interval which may be related to bradycardia, anti-arrhythmic drugs, or a congenital predisposition.

Ventricular tachycardia is characterized by wide complex QRS's in a regular or slightly irregular pattern. The rate may speed progressively and then stabilize, or may degenerate into a more chaotic pattern or even ventricular fibrillation. The diagnosis is made with certainty when one can identify independent atrial activity with P-waves marching through the rhythm. When P-waves cannot be identified, or when P-waves occur following each QRS, the rhythm must be differentiated from a supraventricular tachycardia with aberrancy. When in doubt, it is generally best to assume that a wide complex tachycardia is ventricular in origin.

CARDIAC PEARL

For a number of years we have been impressed with the clinical observation that ventricular tachycardia frequently sounds quite different from other tachycardias. On careful analysis, it became apparent that the additional sounds in ventricular tachycardia were a major reason for this auscultatory peculiarity. These sounds are apparently produced by wide splitting of the first and second heart sounds plus gallop sounds. Because of the widening of the QRS complex there is a wide splitting of the first and second heart sounds; a ventricular gallop is usually present as is also an atrial gallop sound. In addition, in some patients a sound in systole may be heard in addition to those already mentioned. As a result, multiple sounds may be heard, and when in combination with a changing intensity of the first heart sound and a slightly irregular ventricular rate, the characteristic auscultatory findings of ventricular tachycardia are present. These features, in addition to the lack of response to carotid sinus pressure, can result in prompt recognition of this serious arrhythmia. Most, although not all, patients with ventricular tachycardia show these auscultatory findings. Production of these multiple sounds is probably related to a number of factors: the degree of widening of the QRS complex, duration of the ventricular tachycardia, lack of cardiac reserve, and the degree of cardiac decompensation.

W. Proctor Harvey, M.D.

Careful analysis of the QRS morphology can provide valuable clues to the proper diagnosis. In a majority of cases, aberrantly conducted beats will display an rSR' pattern in lead V_1 and a QRS in V_6,

with a right bundle-branch-block-like pattern. Conversely, ventricular tachycardia is more likely to have a left bundle-branch-block-like pattern with a monophasic R or qR morphology in V_1. Other patterns that suggest VT are equiphasic QR or RS complexes in V_1 or rS and QS complexes in V_1 with slurred initial portions. Upright QRS complexes in all precordial leads are almost always due to VT rather than aberrancy. QRS durations of greater than 0.14 seconds and a frontal plane axis more negative than -30° strongly favor ventricular tachycardia (Figure 29). Examination of the onset of the arrhythmia may show an initial PVC or a brief run of a clear cut supraventricular tachycardia preceding the wide complex tachycardia, which may suggest the nature of the subsequent arrhythmia.

The rate of ventricular tachycardia ranges from 100 to approximately 250 beats per minute. Still faster rates produce a pattern which appears saw toothed and which obscures the definition of the QRS and T-waves. This pattern is called ventricular flutter and is ominous because of its adverse hemodynamic consequences and its propensity to lead to ventricular fibrillation.

Torsade de Pointes denotes a form of rapid polymorphic VT in which the QRS axis shifts back and forth. The complexes gradually change from upright to inverted and back again in this rhythm which is almost always associated with a long QT interval in the underlying beats. The rhythm can arise from the use of anti-arrhythmic drugs such as those in Class IA and IC as well as amiodarone and sotalol. It is often precipitated by a sudden slowing of heart rate as might occur with a compensatory pause following a premature beat. Discontinuation of the offending agent and establishment of a faster heart rate can help restore a normal rhythm. Intravenous magnesium sulphate has been used to reverse drug induced torsade. In bidirectional VT, which can complicate advanced digitalis toxicity, there is beat to beat alternation in the polarity of the QRS complex.

Termination of acute episodes of ventricular tachycardia can be achieved pharmacologically by use of intravenous lidocaine. Other drugs including bretylium and Class IA and IC agents may be effective. In the presence of hemodynamic compromise, prompt electrical conversion is indicated. A brisk blow to the precordium, or chest thump, can halt ventricular tachycardia. On rare occasions this maneuver can instead precipitate ventricular fibrillation (Figure 30). Synchronized DC cardioversion is appropriate when the QRS complex is discrete and able to trigger a properly timed discharge. In this situation, a single low energy shock may be

648

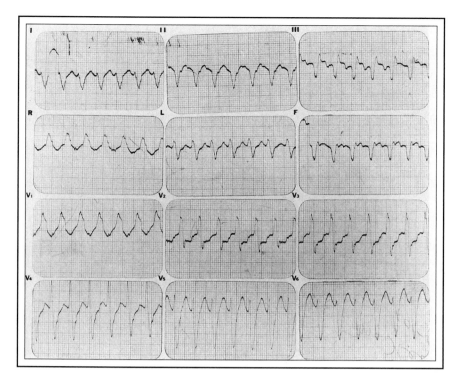

Figure 29. Twelve lead electrocardiogram of ventricular tachycardia. Note the abnormal axis and wide QRS complexes.

effective. In polymorphic VT or ventricular flutter synchronization may not be feasible, or triggering may erroneously occur on the T-wave. It is therefore advisable to use unsynchronized defibrillation at high energy to avoid provocation of VF. Stabilization of the rhythm will usually require correction of underlying problems and at least temporary treatment with anti-arrhythmic agents.

The long-term management of a patient with documented paroxysmal tachycardia is challenging. The outlook varies from the benign prognosis for nonsustained VT in the setting of a structurally normal heart to the high risk of recurrence for the untreated patient who has been resuscitated from sudden cardiac death.

Nonsustained VT lasting less than 30 seconds and without hemodynamic compromise occasionally occurs in otherwise healthy patients and generally does not warrant therapy. Similar rhythms in patients with known ischemic disease, compromised left ventricular function (ejection fraction less than 35%), or late potentials on signal averaged ECGs may be markers for potentially more dangerous or fatal arrhythmias. If sustained monomorphic VT cannot be induced by exercise or electrophysiological studies (EPS), the prognosis is generally good and anti-arrhythmic therapy is not indicated. Patients in whom sustained VT can be induced and those whose primary problems are paroxysmal sustained VT, tend to do better if they can be treated with a drug that has proven to be effective on serial EPS. Unfortunately, none of the

anti-arrhythmic drugs currently available is terribly effective, and most carry substantial risks of provoking arrhythmias and other side effects. Recent studies have demonstrated the efficacy of sotalol and amiodarone as first line agents—but not without risk.

The disappointing results of anti-arrhythmic drug therapy has fostered major advances in the electrical treatment of VT. Overdrive pacing with brief trains of rapid stimulation have long been known to be an effective means of terminating VT. Unfortunately, this intervention can at times provoke a more rapid tachycardia or VF, and therefore it was not safe to utilize in an unsupervised fashion. The development of reliable implantable defibrillators has now allowed the employment of extremely sophisticated devices which can be programmed to first attempt overdrive pacing, and, if necessary, low or high energy defibrillation. These devices are often used in conjunction with drug therapy.

Surgical or catheter ablation of critical foci or conduction pathways are also employed in the management of serious ventricular arrhythmias. This strategy is especially valuable in the minority of cases in which there is bundle branch re-entry or VT originating in the right ventricular outflow tract. Ablation of VT originating within or at the borders of aneurysms or ischemic areas is less successful but can be curative.

Untreated ventricular fibrillation is almost universally fatal although on rare occasions one can

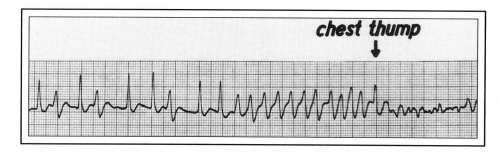

Figure 30. Lead 2 recording from a 65-year-old man four days following an acute myocardial infarction. A chest thump delivered in an attempt to terminate rapid ventricular tachycardia resulted in degeneration to ventricular fibrillation.

see brief runs of VF which terminate spontaneously. VF is manifested by a wavy electrocardiographic baseline without discrete QRS complexes. The morphology may vary from relatively large deflections similar to ventricular flutter or torsade to a near flat line with minor undulations. The only effective therapy is electrical defibrillation, which may only be possible in conjunction with the correction of underlying problems such as hypoxia and electrolyte or metabolic disturbances. Use of anti-arrhythmic agents and catecholamines may facilitate defibrillation. Patients who survive VF in the early stages of an acute MI have a good prognosis. VF occurring in the absence of an acute provocation is associated with a high risk of reccurrence. EPS are often not helpful in these cases and an implantable defibrillator with or without drug therapy is generally warranted.

Bradycardic Rhythms

Bradycardia is an inadequate ventricular rate which almost always implies a slowing of the sinus node or an A-V conduction disorder. Occasionally, frequent blocked PAC's, especially when in a bigeminal pattern, can result in symptomatic ventricular bradycardia. The sinus node is richly innervated via the autonomic nervous system. Increased vagal tone and resultant sinus slowing is caused by a large variety of physiological and pathologic conditions. The heart rate in a normal person at rest may dip below 50 or 60 beats per minute, especially during sleep and in one who is physically well conditioned. Increased vagal tone associated with vomiting, fright, and other psychological stimuli can cause profound sinus slowing. When acute atrial slowing is accompanied by the appearance of A-V block, it is almost certainly due to vagotonia.

Sinus bradycardia occurs in association with hypothyroidism, hypothermia, increased intracranial pressure, and may accompany an acute viral illness. This rhythm is common in the early stages of an otherwise uncomplicated acute inferior wall myocardial infarction. The mechanism is thought to be vagal stimulation induced by a reflex from the posterior left ventricular wall as well as possible compromised blood flow to the sinus node.

Severe hypoxia is a potent stimulus of vagal tone. It is not uncommon for a patient to have marked sinus slowing when presenting in profound cardio-pulmonary distress. In this situation it is far more likely that hypoxia caused sinus bradycardia, than that a primary sinus node disorder produced cardio-pulmonary collapse.

Idiopathic sinus bradycardia is an uncommon phenomenon and may be part of the spectrum of the sick sinus syndrome which also includes frequent sinus pauses and sinus arrest. Rarely sino-atrial or sinus exit block can reduce the number of impulses delivered to the A-V node. A variety of pharmacological agents produce sinus bradycardia as a side effect. The list includes diltiazem, lithium, beta blockers, reserpine, digitalis, and nitroglycerin. Unfortunately, no available drug can be relied upon to therapeutically slow a fast heart rate.

CARDIAC PEARL

Slow Ventricular Rate: If on examining a patient you note normal sinus rhythm with a slow ventricular rate such as in the 50s or 60s, think of two things: One, the patient is in good physical training and has developed a slow rate from vagal tone; or two, that the patient might be on a beta blocker.

For instance, one might examine a person aged 55 or so, and find that he has a healthy slow ventricular rate. You might say, "Are you in any athletic or physical conditioning program such as swimming, playing tennis, or jogging at this time?" And he says, "No." "Are you on a beta blocker?" Again, the answer is "no." then you might ask, "Were you ever active in athletics?" and the patient may answer, "Oh yes, I used to run the mile when I was on the track team in college;" or mention previous participation in some other sport. It is interesting that the vagal tone that is responsible for this development of a slow rate in athletic training when a person was younger, may still persist at a later age in some patients.

W. Proctor Harvey, M.D.

Sinus bradycardia is characterized by normal P-waves and QRS complexes at a slow rate. There may be an associated prolongation of PR interval or a higher degree of A-V block. Sinus bradycardia can be inferred when there is a slow escape rhythm originating in the atrium or junction which takes over the pacemaker function.

Most often sinus bradycardia requires no treatment. In the symptomatic patient elimination of provocative stimuli and the temporary use of intravenous atropine can reverse the vagotonic state. Chronotropic catecholamines can be administered intravenously in emergencies and atrial and/or ventricular pacing is indicated for longer term therapy.

Ventricular bradycardia can be caused by an interruption in the conduction of beats from the atrium. Most commonly, block occurs within the A-V node or the ventricular fascicles. Second degree A-V block may cause bradycardia depending on the atrial rate and the extent of the block. Persistent second degree block at normal atrial rates generally denotes advanced conduction system disease. In 2:1 block due to A-V nodal disease the QRS complex is usually narrow, and the rhythm may have been preceded by Wenckebach type (Mobitz I) block. When the conduction disturbance is within the ventricles, the QRS complex generally is wide with a right or left bundle branch block pattern.

The ventricular rate in complete heart block will depend on the site of the escape focus. A-V nodal block is usually associated with a junctional rhythm at a rate of 40 to 50 beats per minute and a narrow QRS complex. Block due to fascicular disease requires an escape focus lower in the ventricle, which will tend to be slower and less reliable. Periods of prolonged asystole are more likely to complicate a wide complex escape rhythm, resulting in syncope.

CARDIAC PEARL

A slow ventricular heart rate plus a changing intensity of the first heart sound indicates complete heart block.

In complete heart block, wherein the atrial rate is independent of the ventricular rate, there are multiple opportunities for a change in the relation of the P-wave to the QRS complex. Therefore, when the P is close to the first heart sound, it may be loud. On the other hand, when it is not close and the P-R interval is prolonged and at a distance away from the first heart sound, the sound may be faint. This results in a changing intensity of the first heart sound; at intervals, when the P-R interval is short, an abrupt loud first sound (the "bruit de canon" or "cannon shot") occurs which is an auscultatory finding diagnostic of complete heart block.

Of course, if the ventricular rate is slow, about 40 beats per minute, an early to midsystolic murmur is usually present and in addition, atrial sounds may be heard in diastole, if searched for.

The diagnosis of complete heart block can be suspected by paying attention to the jugular venous pulsations in the neck and by observing a slow regular heart rate (approximately 40 beats per minute). If a sudden "cannon wave" occurs, it indicates that atrial contraction is occurring simultaneously with ventricular contraction. This is common with complete heart block.

If one placed a ping pong ball over the right supraclavicular fossa, the cannon wave might well knock it off.

It is a misconception that in complete heart block the loud first heart sound (the so-called "bruit de canon" or cannon shot) occurs at the same time as the cannon wave in the jugular venous pulse. This is incorrect.

The loud auscultatory sound has no relation to the cannon wave of the jugular venous pulse. However, they may occur simultaneously if the P-R interval is short enough to produce a loud first sound, and the next P-wave (atrial contraction) occurs with ventricular systole.

Complete heart block (in addition to causing a change in intensity of the first sound, atrial sounds heard in diastole, and the visual "cannon waves" in the neck) can also cause faint arterial pulsations which relate to atrial contraction. This represents a seldom recognized physical finding.

Palpation of the radial, brachial, carotid or femoral arterial pulses can identify a pulsation that is coincident with the atrial contraction of diastole. It is interesting that this is a faint but definite arterial pulsation, indicating that the atrial contraction is producing a wave traversing the left ventricle and aortic valve in order to be palpated at the arterial pulse.

W. Proctor Harvey, M.D.

Complete heart block is characterized by a slow regular ventricular rhythm which is independent of any atrial depolarizations. Ventricular escape foci, especially in acquired heart disease, tend to be unreliable. Unprovoked pauses can cause prolonged asystole and resultant Stokes-Adams syncope. For this reason, pacemaker therapy is warranted in patients with complete heart block especially in the presence of a slow ventricular escape focus or any history of syncope.

651

Selected Reading

1. Akhtar M.: Clinical spectrum of ventricular tachycardia. *Circ* 82:1561, 1990.

2. Akhtar M, Shanasa M, Jazayeri M. et al.: Wide QRS complex tachycardia. Reappraisal of a common clinical problem. *Ann. Intern. Med.* 109:905, 1988.

3. Albers GW, Sherman DG, Gress DR, et al: Stroke prevention in nonvalvular atrial fibrillation: a review of prospective randomized trials. *Ann. Neurol.* 30:511, 1991.

4. Castellanos A, Myerburg RJ: The wide electrophysiologic spectrum of tachycardias having R-P intervals longer than the P-R intervals. *PACE* 10:1382, 1987.

5. Chakko S, Kessler KM: Recognition and management of cardiac arrhythmias. *Curr Prob Card.* V20:53-120, 1995.

6. Cox JL, Boineau JP, Schuessler RB, et al. Successful surgical treatment of atrial fibrillation: Review and clinical update *JAMA.* 266:1976, 1991.

7. El-Sherif N, Craelius W, Boutjdir M.: Early afterdepolarizations and arrhythmogensis. *J. Cardiovasc. Electrophysiol.* 1:145, 1990.

8. Falk RH, Podrid PJ: *Atrial Fibrillation: Mechanisms and Management.* Raven Press, New York 1992.

9. Fazekas T, Scherlag BJ, Vos M. et al: Magnesium and the heart: antiarrhythmic therapy with magnesium. *Clin. Cardiol.* 16:768, 1993.

10. Ferrer MI: *The Sick Sinus Syndrome,* Futura, Mt. Kisco, 1974.

11. Fisch C: *Electrocardiography of Arrhythmias,* Lea & Febiger, Phila. 1990.

12. Grogin HR, Scheinman M: Evaluation and management of patients with polymorphic ventricular tachycardia. *Cardiol. Clinics.* 11:39, 1993.

13. Jackman WM, Friday KJ, Clark M, et al.: The long QT syndromes: a critical review, new clinical observations and unifying hypothesis. *Prog. Cardiovasc. Dis.* 31:115, 1988.

14. Josephson ME, Horowitz LN, Waxman HL, et al: Sustained ventricular tachycardia: Role of the 12-lead electrocardiogram in localizing site of origin. *Circ* 64:257, 1981.

15. Josephson ME, Wellens HJJ: Differential diagnosis of supraventricular tachycardia. *Cardiol. Clinics.* 8:411, 1990.

16. Josephson ME, Wellens HJJ: *Tachycardias: Mechanisms, Diagnosis, Treatment.* Lea & Febiger. Phila. 1984.

17. Kosowsky BD, Latif P, Radoff A: Multilevel atroventricular block. *Circ* 54:914, 1976.

18. Kutalek SP: The genetics of cardiac arrhythmias. *Cardio* (Supplement) April:25, 1993.

19. Langendorf R, Pick A, Winternitz M: Mechanism of intermittent ventricular bigeminy. I. Appearance of ectopic beats dependent upon length of the ventricular cycle, the "rule of bigeminy". *Circ* 11:422, 1955.

20. Lewis T: *Clinical Disorders of the Heart Beat,* Paul B. Hoeber, New York 1921.

21. Marcus FI, Fontaine GH, Guiraudon G, et al: Right ventricular dysplasia: A report of 24 adult cases. *Circ* 65:384, 1982.

22. Marriott HJL, Sandler IA: Criteria, old and new, for differentiating between ectopic ventricular beats and aberrant ventricular conduction in the presence of atrial fibrillation. *Prog. Cardiovasc. Dis* 9:18, 1966.

23. Martin D, Mendelsohn ME, John RM et al: *Atrial Fibrillation.* Blackwell Scientific, Boston 1994.

24. Rosen MR, Janse MJ, Wit AL: *Cardiac Electrophysiology: A Textbook.* Futura, Mt. Kisco 1990.

25. Sager PT, Bhandari AK: Wide complex tachycardias. *Cardiol. Clinics.* 9:595, 1991.

26. Shine KI, Kastor JA, Yurchak PM: Multifocal atrial tachycardia. *NEJM* 279:344, 1968.

27. Stewart RB, Bardy GH, Greene LH: Wide complex tachycardia: Misdiagnosis and outcome after emergent therapy. *Ann. Intern. Med.* 104:766, 1986.

28. Surawicz B, Fisch C: Cardiac alternans: Diverse mechanisms and clinical manifestations. *JACC* 20:483, 1992.

29. Welebit V, Podrid P, Lown B, et al: Aggravation and provocation of ventricular arrhythmia by antiarrhythmic drugs. *Circ* 65:886, 1982.

30. Waldo AL, Henthorn RW, Plumb VJ: *Atrial flutter: Recent observations in man,* in Josephson ME, Wellens HJJ (eds): *Tachycardias: Mechanisms, Diagnosis, Treatment,* Lea & Febiger, Phila. 1984, p. 113.

31. Wathen MS, Klein GJ, Yee R, et al: Classification and terminology of supraventricular tachycardia. *Cardiol. Clinics.* 11:109, 1993.

32. Wellens HJJ, Bar FW, Lie KI. The value of electrocardiogram in the differential diagnosis of a tachycardia with a widened QRS complex. *Am. J. Med.* 64:27, 1978.

33. Wenckebach KF: Zur analyse des unregelmassigen pulses. *Z. Klin. Med.* 37:975, 1899.

34. Winters SL, Stewart D, Gomes JA.: Signal averaging of the surface QRS complex predicts inducibility of ventricular tachycardia in patients with syncope of unknown origin: A prospective study. *JACC* 10:775, 1987.

35. Wyse DG: Pharmacologic therapy in patients with ventricular tachyarrhythmias. *Cardiol. Clinics.* 11:65, 1993.

36. Zipes DP, Jalife J: *Cardiac Electrophysiology from Cell to Bedside.* W.B. Saunders Co., Phila. 1995.

CHAPTER 28

Clinical Approach to the Patient with Palpitations

Cynthia M. Tracy, M.D.

An uncomfortable awareness of the heartbeat is a common complaint. Palpitations may be related to severe cardiac rhythm disturbances or may be entirely benign. The clinician, by careful evaluation, is frequently able to categorize patients as having either benign or malignant arrhythmias without extensive invasive testing. In the evaluation of the patient with palpitations there are essentially three questions which must be answered:
1) What is it the patient is feeling?
2) What kind of a heart is it occurring in?
3) What if anything needs to be done about it?

Evaluation of Palpitations: A Stepwise Approach

History

The initial step in evaluating the patient with palpitations is a detailed history. Typically, the patient will seek evaluation after cessation of the acute symptom. However, information regarding the chronicity of symptoms is often diagnostically helpful.

Patients with reentrant forms of arrhythmia will have noted symptoms over a period of several years. Often, there will be a gradual increase in the symptomatology as the patient ages. This may well be related to an increased frequency of PACs and PVCs which act as triggers for reentrant tachyarrhythmias.

CARDIAC PEARL

Paroxysmal Atrial Tachycardia may be transient, lasting only a few seconds or min-

TABLE   1
Atrial Fibrillation – Associated Conditions and Causes

I.   **Aging**

II.   **Congenital heart disease:**
  Ebstein's anomaly
  atrial septal defect
  primary degenerative disease of the conduction system
  hypertrophic cardiomyopathy

III.   **Acquired:**
  A. postoperative repair of congenital lesions-
      atrial septal defect repair
      mustard procedure
      tetralogy of Fallot
  B. coronary artery disease
  C. coronary artery bypass surgery
  D. hypertensive heart disease
  E. infiltrative lesions
  F. mitral stenosis or regurgitation

IV.   **Toxic:**
  drugs
  alcohol

utes, or it may persist for hours, days, and in some cases even longer.

Atrial tachycardia is more commonly present in individuals having no other evidence of heart disease than in those having underlying organic heart disease. Some have only one attack, others have infrequent attacks at intervals of months to years, and still others have more frequent recurrences varying from every few hours to every several weeks. It appears to be more prevalent in a nervous, tense individual, who can generally give a good description of his tachycardia. As a rule, it is of sudden onset unrelated to any particular event, although in some individuals it appears to be related to emotional upsets, sudden physical exertion, or a certain motion of the body. Palpitation is generally noted and the patient can often specifically identify his tachycardia after watching the physician's hand as he imitates the rapid, regular motion over his own precordium. The patient often describes this rapid regular rhythm as a "fluttering" or a "pounding". Symptoms include nervousness, weakness, apprehension, dizziness, and rarely syncope. Surprisingly, some are unaware that tachycardia has been present. The patient whose heart is otherwise healthy usually tolerates this paroxysm of tachycardia without any particular difficulty, and in fact, many continue on in their work or other activities. Characteristically, the attack ceases abruptly and generally no residual myocardial damage is evident, either on electrocardiogram or clinical evaluation. (At times, however, nonspecific S-T and T-wave changes may be noted on the electrocardiogram, which can persist for days. These are designated as post-tachycardia myocardial changes, and in the absence of other evidence may have no special significance.) In patients with heart disease the paroxysm of atrial tachycardia may be attended by significant symptoms, as is also true of any other type of rapid heart action. The patient with known heart disease may be seriously incapacitated by uncontrolled tachycardia, particularly if it lasts for hours or days, rather than minutes. Cardiac decompensation, angina, or even myocardial infarction may occur in a susceptible diseased heart. In some, blood pressure drops, the pulse pressure becomes quite narrow, thereby predisposing to thrombosis of the peripheral vessels. Severe chest pain coincident with a rapid rate may be noted in patients with coronary disease; occasionally this type of pain, characteristic of coronary insufficiency, may be first noted during such a paroxysm. A few patients with severe aortic insufficiency have been personally observed having paroxysmal atrial tachycardia. It generally goes badly with them; precordial chest pain is frequent and the abnormally forceful beat of the heart associated with the leak of the aortic valve greatly accentuates the peripheral atrial signs of aortic insufficiency, thereby causing great annoyance as well as the possibility of discomfort and/or cardiac decompensation. Fortunately, this type of tachycardia is not common in these patients.

Occasionally, a patient with paroxysmal atrial tachycardia presents a history of precipitating events such as emotional upset, undue nervousness, fatigue, indigestion, alcohol (particularly in excess), or in combination with a gallbladder attack. If possible, the physician should observe the patient during the episode of paroxysmal tachycardia and document this on the electrocardiogram. In this way he can arrive at an accurate diagnosis, making sure that there is not confusion with other tachycardias.

W. Proctor Harvey, M.D.

Atrial fibrillation is the most common arrhythmia in the elderly, with the incidence increasing with age. The patient often presents shortly after the onset of symptoms. While the incidence at age 25 to 35 is only 2 to 3 per 1,000, by the ages 62 to 90, this has increased to 50 to 90 per 1,000. Detailed historic information may provide clues to the etiology of the atrial fibrillation (Table 1).

Patients presenting with ventricular arrhythmias face a varied prognosis; again, historic information may provide initial information regarding etiology of the ventricular arrhythmia, and help differentiate between benign ventricular arrhythmias and more malignant forms. As noted above, simple PVCs are present commonly in the general population (35% to 50%) and their prevalence increases with age. Their pathologic significance varies tremendously with underlying heart diseases, and historic clues can help differentiate benign from malignant PVCs (Table 2).

CARDIAC PEARL

Some women complain of palpitation due to extrasystoles only when pregnant, and particularly during the last trimester. Without other evidence of heart disease, they are benign, generally disappearing following delivery, and the patient can be reassured about them. It is also a matter of interest that supraventricular tachycardias such as paroxysmal atrial tachycardia or paroxysmal atrial fibrillation also may occur in some women only during pregnancy.

Benign arrhythmias during pregnancy may be misinterpreted as evidence of heart disease. Particularly in the last two trimesters of pregnancy the patient may note cardiac irregularities of which she had been unaware before; she may describe these as skipped beats, turning over of the heart, a momentary pressure in the neck, extra beats, etc. These usually represent premature beats, generally of ventricular origin. In addition, the patient

TABLE 2

Ventricular Arrhythmias: Evaluation and Classification

CLINICAL FEATURES	STATUS	CARDIAC EVALUATION	CLASSIFICATION
Asymptomatic or palpitations	Structurally normal	History, physical, ECG, Holter, TTM, +/– ETT, +/– echocardiogram	Benign
Asymptomatic or palpitations	Structural heart disease	History, physical, ECG, Holter or TTM, ETT, echocardiogram, +/– cardiac cath, +/– electrophysiologic testing	Potentially malignant
Symptoms of altered cardiac output-syncope, cardiac arrest, sustained VT	With or without structural heart disease	History, physical, ECG, Holter or TTM, ETT, echocardiogram, cardiac cath, electrophysiologic testing	Malignant

may be more aware of the normal heart beat since the ventricular rate is increased with the more active circulation associated with increased cardiac output. At times, some patients note tachycardias such as paroxysmal atrial tachycardia or paroxysmal atrial fibrillation. Paroxysmal atrial tachycardia appears more frequently than fibrillation. These tachycardias may not be evident when the patient is not pregnant. On the other hand, the patient may have had rare episodes of paroxysmal atrial tachycardia that become more frequent during the pregnancy. As a rule, the cardiac arrhythmias are not serious when there is no other evidence of heart disease, and the patient can be reassured concerning them. Control of the arrhythmias generally presents no problem, but in a few patients specific antiarrhythmic drugs may be required for control.

W. Proctor Harvey, M.D.

Additional information provided by the initial detailed history includes exacerbating or precipitating factors. Not infrequently, patients present with palpitations at times of changes in their life circumstances. The patient with increased stress may be more prone to the development of all forms of arrhythmias. However, peculiar exposures to chemical toxins such as alcohol, drugs and caffeine must be elicited from the history.

CARDIAC PEARL

Alcohol in smaller amounts, such as several cocktails or glasses of wine, can "trigger" (or precipitate) arrhythmias in the patient who has underlying heart disease. This occurs much more frequently than is generally realized; premature beats and atrial fibrillation can occur causing uncomfortable symptoms in a patient. At times, atrial fibrillation with a rapid ventricular rate produces cardiac decompensation- even pulmonary edema. If a careful history elicits a recurrent arrhythmia such as atrial fibrillation following even small amounts of alcohol ingestion, it is wise to advise our patient to refrain from its use. However, some patients do not heed such advice and have the recurrent problem. Fortunately, however, the majority follow the advice of no alcohol.

Alcohol, usually in larger amounts, or "binges" can produce arrhythmias such as atrial fibrillation in a perfectly normal heart. I recall seeing a young sailor at a teaching conference in a naval hospital, who after a weekend "binge" had atrial fibrillation which required hospitalization; the electrocardiogram documented atrial fibrillation. After reversion to normal sinus rhythm, the "P" waves in the limb leads and in lead V1 indicated left atrial enlargement; these were transient changes. In addition, transient left atrial enlargement was also demonstrated on the heart x-rays.

From a clinical point of view, it is probable that ingestion of a large amount of alcohol in a patient with heart disease (such as coronary artery disease or cardiomyopathy) can "trigger" a ventricular arrhythmia causing sudden death.

W. Proctor Harvey, M.D.

Although uncommon, familial forms of arrhythmias exist and a family history of similar symptoms and sudden death should be sought. Hereditary conditions include hypertrophic cardiomyopathy and the Wolff-Parkinson-White syndrome.

Symptomatology

PACs and PVCs are the most common form of arrhythmia for which the patient seeks medical attention. Frequently, it is impossible on an historic basis to distinguish between these two conditions. Often, the patient is aware of the post-extra systolic beat owing to the prolonged diastolic filling time, and they may describe a sensation of the heart stopping. This is also particularly true of the patient presenting with tachy/brady or sick sinus syndrome.

While the patient may be aware of the tachycardia, it is more frequently the bradyarrhythmia which causes the alarming symptom (Figure 1).

CARDIAC PEARL

The detection of extrasystoles may forewarn the physician of impending arrhythmias. For example, atrial extrasystoles occurring with mitral stenosis may lead one to suspect that atrial fibrillation may develop in the near future. In addition, if a patient has had attacks of paroxysmal rapid heart action and the physician has not observed the episode, the finding of atrial extrasystoles between these episodes would make him suspect that his tachycardia was supraventricular in type. On the other hand, if ventricular extrasystoles were heard the physician might deduce that it was more likely of ventricular origin, such as would be exemplified by a patient with known coronary artery disease having had a recent previous tachycardia and now has multiple ventricular extrasystoles. In addition, the patient with frequent ventricular extrasystoles during the course of an acute myocardial infarction might serve as a warning of a subsequent ventricular arrhythmia.

W. Proctor Harvey, M.D.

A useful tool in differentiating palpitations can be elicited by having the patient "tap" out the arrhythmia with their hand. AV reentrant or AV nodal reentrant tachycardia is typically of abrupt onset, rapid and regular. The patient often notes an abrupt cessation as well, although sinus tachycardia may follow longer episodes of SVT and the offset may be more difficult for the patient to distinguish. Typically, the patient taps out the rapid regular rhythm. Alternatively, atrial fibrillation is frequently tapped out as a rapid, irregular beat.

CARDIAC PEARL

A cardiac pearl to aid in the office or bedside evaluation of a patient's complaint of palpitation of the heart: what is palpitation to one patient is not to another, who may describe other sensations or personal interpretations. The use of one's hand over the precordium can be useful and diagnostic (Fig. A). The hand is moved for the patient to observe, up and down at a regular rate similar to the heartbeat. A quick beat, followed by a pause, simulates the premature beat. More than one quick motion, two or three or more, can thus be simulated. Bigeminal or trigeminal rhythm is also easily reproduced. The patient may indicate that the palpitation was not one of these but that the heartbeat was faster. Then the hand can move with a more vigorous and regular motion, with the physician stating at the time that this feeling is what may occur if someone has a temporary fright or near accident while driving the car; the heart normally speeds up with a normal sinus tachycardia.

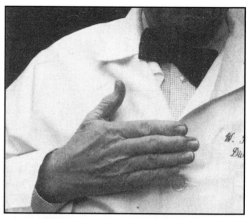

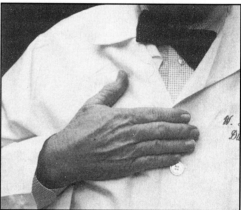

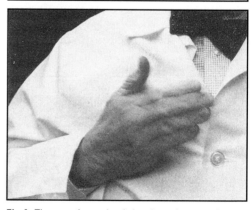

Fig A: The use of examiner's hand moving over the precordium to stimulate the patient's arrhythmia (palpitation). Top panel, Fingers off the chest wall. Middle panel, Fingers touching chest wall. Lower panel, Hand moving rapidly up and down, simulating various tachycardias.

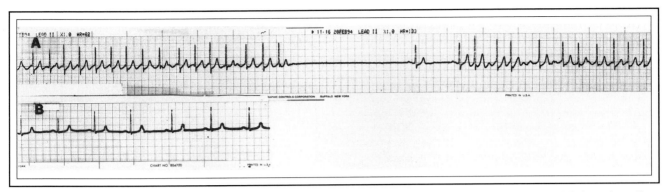

Figure 1. A 75-year-old patient presented to the emergency room with complaints of near syncope. Minimal symptoms occurred during tachycardia and symptoms of near syncope correlated with pauses **(A)**. Minutes later, sinus rhythm resumed **(B)**. This patient with sick sinus syndrome received a dual chamber pacer and a beta blocker.

The patient may then say, "It was faster." Now the physician should move the hand faster and ask the patient to identify the motion as a fast irregular or regular one. It is interesting that the patient frequently can immediately and correctly identify the irregular motion of atrial fibrillation or the regular motion of paroxysmal atrial tachycardia.

W. Proctor Harvey, M.D.

Associated symptomatology may help determine etiology of palpitations. Historically, patients with A-V reentrant tachycardia will often complain of a full sensation in the throat which occurs during the tachycardia and is related to the simultaneous contraction of the atrium in the ventricle. Patients with A-V nodal reentrant tachycardia also are prone to pre-syncope or syncope during their episodes of tachycardia; this is due to decreased cardiac output, owing to decreased ventricular filling due to the loss of A-V synchrony (Figure 2). With A-V reentrant tachycardia, the retrograde atrial activation and atrial contraction occurs distant enough from ventricular filling and often cardiac output is maintained.

The physician should question the patient regarding additional symptoms which may point to associated illnesses. Patients presenting with histories of structural heart disease or myocardial infarction are at greater risk for more malignant forms of arrhythmia and further evaluation, based on the history, is required. Patients with anxiety disorders frequently complain of palpitations and the physician should frankly question the patient as to their emotional response to symptoms and their emotional status at the time of palpitations.

CARDIAC PEARL

Premature Contractions (Extrasystoles) can arise from any part of the heart, the atrium, A-V node, and ventricle. Extrasystoles alone in the absence of other evidence of heart disease should not be looked upon as indicating underlying organic heart disease since they are frequently found in patients with normal hearts. On the other hand, they are also commonly associated with all forms of heart disease. The total cardiovascular evaluation, including a complete, careful history, physical examination, x-ray and laboratory tests, is essential in deciding whether or not extrasystoles are benign. It is most important to understand their significance because they may be causing undue anxiety in a patient. Extrasystoles may or may not produce symptoms. In some, they are first noted on a routine physical examination and the patient is completely unaware of them. In others, they are quite aware of this heart irregularity which is quite bothersome to them, and often causes apprehension. As a rule, individuals who have a thin chest and are of a more nervous temperament are more likely to be aware of the irregularity of the heart. The sensation of extrasystoles of the heart is described in various ways, such as "my heart skipped," "a wave comes over me," a "fullness of the throat," "my heart turned over," a "fluttering in the heart," "choking in the throat," "shortness of breath," etc. Occasionally, there is a momentary pain with the irregularity, and on rare occasions the patient's body may actually have a momentary tremor after extrasystole. They generally occur when the heart rate is slow, often when the patient is resting, or about to fall asleep at bedtime. With exercise such as walking, or other ways in which the heart rate is speeded up, these benign extrasystoles are likely to disappear. Ventricular extrasystoles are the most common of all arrhythmias and frequently occur without any evidence of heart disease. One may ask a large group of physicians in an audience when this topic is being discussed as to how many have had extrasystoles, and approximately two-thirds will answer in the affirmative. I have noted extrasystoles occasionally, and the following observations have been made: they seem to be related to the combination of fatigue and emotional tension. At other times, a hearty meal with a subsequent gaseous abdominal distension appears to be related to extrasystoles. If they are frequent they are bothersome, and it is possible to identify each one. It is therefore easy to understand why patients who complain of extrasystoles often want some type of therapy to eliminate them. My first awareness of these extrasystoles occurred more than 40 years ago, several hours before delivering a paper at a medical society meeting: being pressed for time the evening meal was skipped. Suddenly I was aware of a wave-like sensation that arose from the lower anterior chest region to the throat producing a feeling of regurgitation and a mild pressure. This was followed immediately by a sinking feeling and a "thump" in the chest. It was apparent that extrasystoles were present, and on auscultation it was noted that an extrasystole was present every third or fourth beat. These continued until the beginning of the lecture that evening, and then promptly disappeared. Since this time, usually on occasions associated particularly with fatigue, unusual tension, and/or a hearty meal, extrasystoles may recur temporarily- lasting a few minutes to an hour or so. This personal experience has been helpful in evaluating and reassuring patients who are having similar symptoms. The patient is generally comforted when no evidence of heart disease is found, and he is told that his physician also has had similar experiences.

W. Proctor Harvey, M.D.

Physical Examination

Other than atrial fibrillation, the luxury of examination during a symptomatic episode is rarely afforded to the physician. Nevertheless, to the astute clinician, clues are available as to the etiology of arrhythmia if present during the exam. Remarkably, the diagnosis of type I second degree heart block was first made on physical exam by Wenckebach, in 1899, by analysis of venous pulsations. Typical findings are often present in the patient with atrial fibrillation and apparent even before auscultation. Oscillation in the venous pulsation is noted in the neck. Classically, the irregularly irregular rhythm and variability of the first heart sound are diagnostic for atrial fibrillation.

Similarly, flutter waves may be noted in the venous pulsations of the patient in atrial flutter. Cannon A-waves can be seen in patients with AV dissociation related to ventricular tachycardia or those in com-

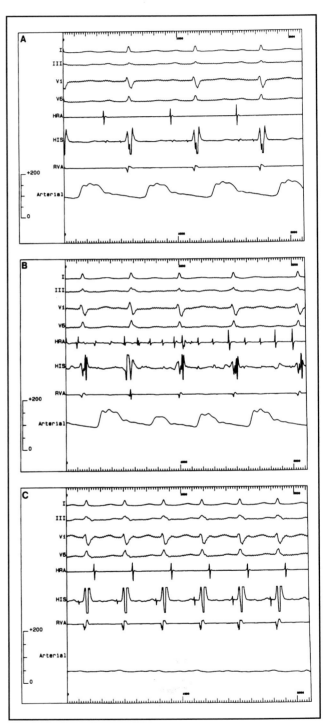

Figure 2. This 64-year-old patient presented with syncope. In the electrophysiology laboratory, mild hypertension was present during sinus rhythm **(A)**. During atrial fibrillation, the blood pressure was reasonably maintained **(B)**. With induction of AV nodal reentrant tachycardia, marked hypotension occurred **(C)**. The patient underwent AV nodal modification which eliminated AV nodal reentry and alleviated symptoms.

TABLE 3
Medical Conditions Associated with Cardiac Arrhythmias

I. ENDOCRINOPATHIES

- Acromegaly – PVCs, conduction delays
- Hyperthyroidism – atrial fibrillation, PSVT, flutter, heart block, sinus tachycardia
- Hypothyroidism – bradycardia, PVCs
- Adrenal Insufficiency – sinus bradycardia, conduction delays
- Pheochromocytoma – sinus tachycardia, SVT

II. NEUROLOGIC DISORDERS

- Progressive Muscular Dystrophies (including Duchennes) – sinus tachycardia, sinus node dysfunction, atrial arrhythmias
- Myotonic Muscular Dystrophy – PACs, sinus bradycardia, atrial flutter, atrial fibrillation, ventricular tachycardia, conduction delay
- Acute Cerebral Accidents – sinus bradycardia, sinus tachycardia, atrial arrhythmias (PACs, fib, flutter, SVT), ventricular arrhythmias (PVCs, VT, V-fib)

III. INFECTIOUS DISEASES

- Endocarditis – atrial and ventricular arrhythmias and conduction disease
- Chagas' disease – conduction disease, ventricular arrhythmia (PVCs, VT), sinus bradycardia, atrial fibrillation

IV. RHEUMATOLOGIC DISORDERS

- Ankylosing Spondylitis – conduction delays
- Reiter's Disease – conduction delays
- Rheumatoid Arthritis – 1st degree AV block, conduction delays, atrial fibrillation, PACs and PVCs
- Systemic Lupus Erythematosus – AV and SA node disease
- Progressive Systemic Sclerosis – conduction delays
- Hurler Syndrome – conduction delays
- Sarcoidosis – conduction delays, heart block, atrial arrhythmias, ventricular arrhythmias

V. NEOPLASTIC DISEASE

- Pericardial involvement – atrial fibrillation, AV block, tachyarrhythmias
- Cardiac Amyloidosis – atrial flutter and fibrillation, AV block
- Radiation therapy – conduction delays

VI. LUNG DISEASE

- COPD/Respiratory Failure – PSVT, atrial flutter, multifocal atrial tachycardia, junctional tachycardia, AV dissociation, PVCs, VT, VF

plete heart block. In AV nodal reentrant tachycardia, the atrium may contract at a time when the tricuspid valve is closed and result in prominent A-waves.

A host of medical illnesses can present with cardiac arrhythmias. The physician should examine the patient closely for processes associated with cardiac arrhythmias which can be detected by physical exam (Table 3) or elicited by patient history.

Similarly, structural abnormalities of the heart can provide the setting for cardiac arrhythmias and palpitations. Structural heart disease, such as valvular lesions, hypertrophic or dilated cardiomyopathy, can often be detected on physical examination. The patient with mitral valve prolapse is more likely to exhibit PACs and PVCs, and the typical click or murmur is frequently readily apparent.

Additional associated diseases such as hypertension and hypertensive heart disease can often be detected in patients presenting with arrhythmias. Rarely, however, auscultation alone will help distinguish one form of arrhythmia from another.

Diagnostic Tools

Electrocardiogram

A baseline 12-lead electrocardiogram performed during an asymptomatic period is normal more often than not. However, specific abnormalities associated with arrhythmias can sometimes be observed. Careful evaluation of the electrocardiogram can reveal Wolff-Parkinson-White syndrome, a persistent juvenile AV node, and signs of conduction system disease. First degree AV block and bifascicular block in a patient complaining of severe palpitations or pre-syncope may point to intermittently worsened conduction disease. Atrial fibrillation or flutter are readily determined if present on the 12-lead electrocardiogram.

Additional clinical information relevant to the evaluation of the patient with palpitations is available by 12-lead electrocardiography, including evidence for old myocardial infarction or ischemia. Also, signs of left ventricular hypertrophy and repolarization abnormality can point towards hypertensive heart disease and non-compliant myocardial chambers. ST segment changes and voltage criteria for hypertrophy may be present in patients with hypertrophic cardiomyopathy. The QT interval should be evaluated carefully for prolongation.

Ambulatory Electrocardiographic Monitoring

To further the evaluation of the patient presenting with complaints of palpitations, it is necessary to correlate rhythm disturbances with symptomatology. For this purpose, 24-hour ambulatory monitoring may be quite valuable. This is particularly true if the palpitations are easily precipitated or occur frequently. In preparation for the ambulatory monitoring, the patient should be instructed to keep a complete diary of activities and symptoms during the 24-hour period. A variety of systems are commercially available for analysis of 24-hour recordings. It is important for the laboratory evaluating the recorded data to pay particular attention to the onset and offset of any tachyarrhythmia detected. These data may give important information as to the mechanism of the tachyarrhythmia.

CARDIAC PEARL

It is evident that ambulatory ECG monitoring should be performed more often in evaluating patients who have transient neurologic symptoms, particularly those who have some underlying problem with the heart. Recently, I personally observed a patient with documented prolapse of the mitral valve who had a syncopal episode; she was subsequently clinically observed to have an arrhythmia that might have explained the syncopal episode.

W. Proctor Harvey, M.D.

A limitation with ambulatory monitoring is the spontaneous variability of cardiac arrhythmias. Recent multicenter studies have demonstrated the utility of repeated ambulatory monitorings in the management of patients with even malignant ventricular arrhythmias. However, because of the spontaneous variability of cardiac arrhythmias, a significant percentage of ectopy suppression must be demonstrated between 24-hour recordings in order to demonstrate efficacy of an intervention. For the elucidation of palpitations, the spontaneous variability of cardiac arrhythmias presents a serious problem with the exclusive use of 24-hour ambulatory monitoring. A single, 24-hour ambulatory electrocardiogram frequently fails to provide a direct recording of the symptomatic arrhythmia. Nevertheless, markers such as PACs or PVCs can be quantified during the 24-hour period and may be of use in determining the etiology of the patient's symptoms.

Heart Rate Variability

In addition to 24-hour recording of heart rate and rhythm, it is possible to utilize the tapes to assess the autonomic tone. Recent data indicate that the autonomic nervous system plays an important role in the pathogenesis of cardiac arrests. Interplay between sympathetic and parasympathetic nervous systems, and their influence on the heart can be detected by analysis of heart rate variability. Heart rate variability is a technique whereby small beat-to-beat variations are analyzed in time and frequency domains.

These algorithms have been shown to be estimates of autonomic tone and are applied to 24-hour ambulatory electrocardiographic recordings. Analysis of the variation in the R-R intervals in our laboratory is performed with a Marquette series 8000 Holter system. Spectral and non-spectral analyses are performed.

Spectral analysis uses a mathematical function (Fast Fourier transform) to separate the R-R intervals into characteristic frequencies. Alterations in parasympathetic tone result in rapid changes in heart rate and are primarily reflected in the high frequency component of spectral analysis. Conversely, sympathetically mediated oscillations occur less rapidly and are reflected primarily in the low frequency component. Parasympathetic influences are reflected to some degree in this low frequency component as well.

Non-spectral or time domain parameters can be used to analyze sympathetic and parasympathetic influences. These parameters and their predominant determinants are:
• *Mean RR* - mean coupling interval between all normal beats.
• *SDANN* - standard deviation for all normal-normal beat coupling intervals within a 5-minute

period. This is a measure of short term heart rate variance and reflects sympathetic as well as parasympathetic influences.

• *SD* - mean of all 5-minute standard deviations of RR's (sympathetic and parasympathetic).
• *pNN50* - percentage of beats that are greater than 50 msec different computed from triplets of normal beats (parasympathetic).
• *rMS* - root mean square of the difference of successive beats computed from triplets of normal beats (parasympathetic). Studies have demonstrated that the risk of malignant ventricular arrhythmias is increased by increased sympathetic efferent activity or by withdrawal of vagal efferent activity. Thus, a finding of decreased heart rate variability on 24-hour ambulatory monitoring may suggest an increased risk for ventricular fibrillation.

Transtelephonic Monitoring

For patients whose palpitations (particularly those owing to paroxysmal arrhythmias such as AVNRT or AVRT) occur sporadically, the development of the small event ECG recorders has greatly improved the ability of the clinician to determine the etiology of the symptoms. There are essentially two kinds of recorders. For patients who experience fleeting episodes of tachycardia or palpitations, a device with a memory loop can be very useful. This device when activated by the patient will store in memory up to 1 minute of data prior to patient device activation. The information stored on tape can be then transmitted via telephone to the receiving station. Alternatively, patients who experience palpitations which are of longer duration can be provided with a simple event recorder which the patient applies at the time of their symptomatic palpitations. These stored data are then transmitted via telephone to the receiving station.

Evaluation for Underlying Heart Disease

As previously stated, palpitations may be relegated to a benign or a malignant category. Palpitations in patients presenting with structurally normal hearts, other than for the Wolff-Parkinson-White syndrome, rarely are prognostically important. It is, therefore, important to rule out structural heart disease and to assess the underlying milieu in which the palpitations are occurring.

Echocardiography

Echocardiography, particularly for patients presenting with symptomatic PVCs, can be extremely helpful. Particular attention should be paid to wall motion, valve integrity, and evidence for structural heart disease such as hypertrophic cardiomyopathy, dilated cardiomyopathy, or mitral valve prolapse. For the patient with symptomatic PVCs or non-sustained ventricular tachycardia, evidence for prior myocardial infarction must be sought.

CARDIAC PEARL

If one has a patient in their 20s or 30s who complains of palpitation that could be due to frequent premature beats or episodes of paroxysmal atrial tachycardia or paroxysmal atrial fibrillation, be sure to consider the possibility of mitral valve prolapse.

This appears to be more common in women than men (although, of course, it does occur in men). Also, some women with mitral valve prolapse have such palpitations only when they are pregnant. Though mitral valve prolapse can occur in children, teenagers and older patients, consider the possibility of mitral valve prolapse especially in the young adults just described.

Various arrhythmias can occur with mitral valve prolapse. The most frequent are benign premature ventricular contractions. Many patients are unaware or are not bothered by them. No treatment (except reassurance) is usually necessary.

W. Proctor Harvey, M.D.

Exercise Treadmill Testing

The exercise treadmill test is also a useful tool in the evaluation of palpitations. This test can be utilized for a number of purposes, and particularly for patients with ventricular arrhythmias, information regarding ischemic status of the patient can be obtained. Further, for patients presenting with palpitations who have underlying conduction system disease, some assessment as to the conduction system reserve can be obtained by observing the PR interval and heart rate response to exercise (Figure 3).

For other conditions such as WPW syndrome, the stress test may give some limited information as to the anterograde conduction properties of the accessory pathway. However, the stress test provides no information regarding retrograde accessory pathway conduction.

Exercise treadmill testing even in the asymptomatic population may result in the induction of some form of arrhythmia. Atrial or junctional premature complexes can occur with exercise in asymptomatic people; more sustained arrhythmias such as AVNRT or AVRT can sometimes be precipi-

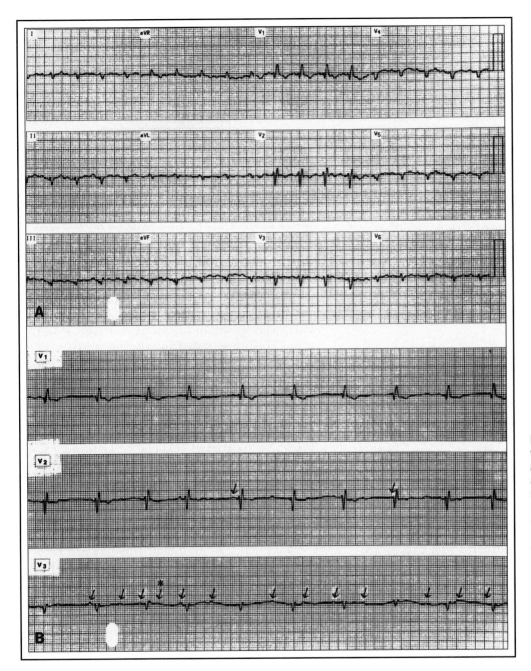

Figure 3. This 27-year-old transplant recipient with advanced atherosclerosis was admitted with complaints of syncope. A right bundle branch block was present at rest **(A)** prior to exercise. Approximately two minutes into exercise, high grade A-V block occurred associated with light headedness. P waves are indicated by arrows. Notice at * the appearance of an early P wave likely arising from his native atrium.

tated by exercise treadmill testing in patients who have history of such arrhythmias. When this occurs, observations regarding onset and termination of tachycardia and P-wave location may prove useful in determining mechanism of the cardiac arrhythmia.

Isolated premature ventricular contractions occur in a sizeable number of normal people undergoing treadmill testing. Their occurrence is more frequent in patients who present with underlying heart disease. In the ongoing management of a patient who has presented with documented ventricular arrhythmias, exercise treadmill testing can be of great utility. The induction of sustained ven-

tricular arrhythmia during exercise testing is rare. However, non-sustained VT as a hallmark for more sustained arrhythmias is occasionally reproducibly induced on treadmill testing.

In fact, 10% to 15% of patients with a history of sustained ventricular tachycardia can be induced by exercise treadmill testing. In this instance, repeat stress testing as an adjunct to ambulatory ECG monitoring may be of utility in the management of such patients undergoing drug treatment.

It should be emphasized that in people with structurally normal hearts and exercise induced ventricular arrhythmia, there are no negative prognostic implications. Conversely, patients with

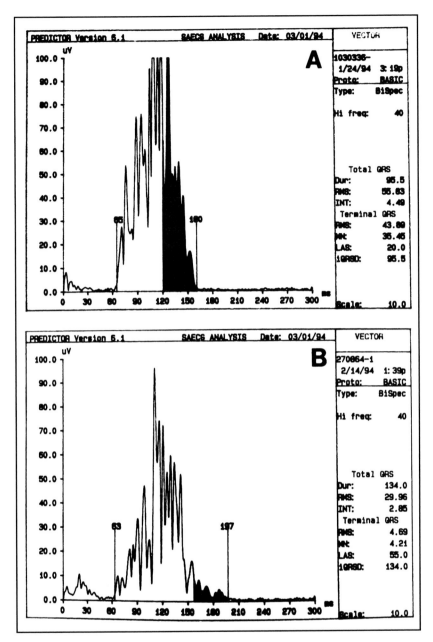

Figure 4. (A) is representative of a normal signal averaged electrocardiogram. The QRS duration is < 110 msec; the root mean square (RMS) of the terminal 40 msec of the complex is > 25 microvolts and low amplitude signals (LAS) are present for less than 35 msec. Conversely, in panel B is pictured a signal averaged electrocardiogram which is abnormal by all three parameters.

dilated cardiomyopathy or ischemic cardiomyopathy, particularly post-infarction patients, may be higher risks for sudden death if repetitive ventricular arrhythmias are found on exercise treadmill testing.

Another important use of exercise treadmill testing is in the management of patients with palpitations related to atrial fibrillation. Repeat exercise tests can be used to determine the adequacy of heart rate response control with medication.

Signal Averaged Electrocardiography

Risk stratification is required for the patient whose palpitations have been related to ventricular arrhythmias. Further evaluation is required in order to determine the need for invasive investigation and the necessity of treatment. The signal-averaged electrocardiogram is a tool useful for determining prognostic significance of ventricular arrhythmias. This computer based technique was first described in 1978; it has allowed the detection of microvolt level signals in the electrocardiogram. These low amplitude, high frequency signals are not normally seen in the surface electrocardiogram. Abnormalities detected by signal averaging appear to correlate with slower, fragmented passage of electrical activity through diseased myocardium. The signal averaged ECG has been utilized in the evaluation of several patient groups, including post-infarction patients.

In this population, signal average along with Holter monitoring and ejection fraction determination are useful in evaluating prognosis; in patients with non-sustained ventricular tachycardia or suspicion of ventricular tachycardia, the signal average can be of use in determining and predicting the inducibility at the time of an electrophysiologic test.

The signal average recording is performed during sinus rhythm, using standard bipolar orthogonal X, Y, and Z leads. It requires from 250 to 1000 wave forms averaged to achieve a noise level of less than .4 microvolts. The wave forms are then amplified, digitized and averaged. They are filtered with a bi-directional filter, using a high band pass frequency of 40Hz. The X, Y and Z leads are then combined into a vector magnitude to give the filtered QRS complex. The onset and offset of the QRS complex are determined by a computer algorithm.

Analysis of the filtered QRS includes: 1) Filtered QRS duration (in milliseconds); 2) Root mean square (RMS) voltage of the terminal 40 milliseconds at the QRS complex (in microvolts); and 3) Duration (in milliseconds) of low amplitude signals (LAS) less than 40 microvolts in the terminal QRS.

For analysis purposes, late potentials are considered present if the filtered QRS duration is greater than 110 milliseconds, the root mean square (RMS) of the terminal 40 milliseconds is less than 25 microvolts and low amplitude signals are present for ≥ 35 milliseconds (Figure 4). While predictive value of the signal average varies with patient populations, for the patient presenting with sustained and inducible ventricular tachycardia following a myocardial infarction, the signal average has been found to be abnormal in 79% to 92% of cases. This contrasts strikingly with a positive signal average rate of 0% to 2% in healthy volunteers. The signal average can be viewed as one potential tool in the evaluation of the symptomatic patient presenting with palpitations. Clearly, it will be of greater utility to perform a signal average in the patient in whom myocardial infarction has occurred and who is suspected to be at high risk for ventricular arrhythmias.

Electrophysiologic Testing

Electrophysiologic testing is rarely useful in the diagnosis of simple palpitations. Patients who present with episodic non-sustained symptoms are best diagnosed by the above-described procedures. Invasive electrophysiologic testing is rarely indicated for patients with structurally normal hearts other than for those with tachycardia related to AV nodal reentry or AV reentry. The electrophysiologic test is rarely of utility in assessing the sinus node in those patients who present with sinus tachycar-

dia. It is of some utility in assessing conduction system disease, although the exercise treadmill test, ambulatory ECG monitor and/or event recorder may well determine the presence of significant conduction system disease.

For patients in whom supraventricular tachycardia has been identified or in whom the symptom is suggestive of a reentrant tachycardia, electrophysiologic testing can provide useful diagnostic information as well as open the possibility of definitive treatment by catheter ablation.

For the patient with documented ventricular arrhythmia, electrophysiologic testing should be considered in certain subgroups. Low grade ventricular ectopy in the patient with a structurally normal heart does not present a significant negative prognostic indicator and these patients should not undergo electrophysiologic testing. Isolated PVCs even in patients with known structural heart disease rarely require electrophysiologic testing. Individuals presenting with non-sustained ventricular tachycardia who are symptomatic and have structural heart disease should undergo further testing. For the post-myocardial infarction patient with non-sustained ventricular tachycardia and symptoms of palpitations, risk stratification likely will include electrophysiologic testing.

Treatment of Palpitations

Benign PACs and PVCs

Successful management of the patient presenting with palpitations will depend on the clear understanding of etiology and pathologic significance of the symptom. For patients who present with structurally normal hearts and isolated supraventricular or ventricular premature beats, simple reassurance may be enough to if not eliminate symptoms, at least alleviate the anxiety related to the occurrence of the palpitation. The majority of these patients can be managed in this fashion after they have been reassured as to the benign nature of their symptomatology. It has been my experience that the best approach is to discuss the findings with the patient and to carefully explain that, although they do indeed have some premature complexes, these will not affect prognosis.

CARDIAC PEARL

Probably most people who have an occasional premature beat are not even aware of it. Even those having frequent premature beats may not be conscious of them or may

notice only a portion. I recall being asked, when a young physician, to evaluate a member of the Harvard crew regarding his participation in an upcoming race. He was a well-developed, healthy, strapping athlete, looking the picture of health. He was without symptoms, but on examination I realized why this evaluation was requested. He had many premature ventricular beats (none occurring in short runs of ventricular tachycardia), although with a basic normal sinus rhythm. To my amazement, he was not aware of any of these beats. The remainder of his evaluation was normal. He was told to go ahead and participate in the race, which he did, and he did not have any problems. This patient taught me that a person could be insensitive to an arrhythmia. Of course, many patients do feel irregularity of their heart beat and promptly report to their physician for advice and treatment. Most people who have occasional premature beats do not need medication, only explanation and reassurance. When I have such anxious and worried patients, I tell them about my own premature beats, which I have had for more than 40 years, and relate that I am not worried about these benign beats. Often this reassurance suffices as far as their treatment is concerned.

Patients with more advanced degrees of aortic regurgitation are more likely to be aware of their arrhythmia than persons with no heart disease. Those patients with advanced aortic regurgitation become accustomed to the "bobbing" up and down of their head. When a premature beat occurs that alters the regular prominent pulsations, the patient is immediately aware but tolerates it. However, if atrial fibrillation is present, producing irregular "bobbing", it can be very bothersome to the patient, and he or she will seek help to alleviate this sensation. Cardiac pearl: fortunately, most patients with a single aortic valvular lesion, aortic regurgitation, stenosis, or a combination of stenosis and regurgitation have a normal, regular sinus rhythm.

Another cardiac pearl: if atrial fibrillation is present, suspect the possibility of a concomitant mitral valve lesion.

W. Proctor Harvey, M.D.

For the patient in whom reassurance alone is unsuccessful, a beta blocker either in a continual dose or to be used on a p.r.n. basis, can provide significant amount of symptomatic relief. Very rarely would such an individual be treated with antiarrhythmic drugs.

For the patient in whom the palpitation is primarily related to anxiety or panic attacks, alteration in life stress and psychotherapy are the most useful form of therapy.

Ventricular Ectopy in Patients With Structural Heart Disease

Palpitations which are related to a more pathologic etiology, such as PVCs in the setting of ischemic heart disease, must be managed more aggressively. Paramount in the treatment of such patients is an accurate definition of the ischemic status, ventricular function and, in most cases, coronary anatomy. In the category of patient in whom potentially malignant ventricular arrhythmias have been identified, electrophysiologic testing may be warranted.

Atrial Fibrillation

Management of the patient who presents with palpitations related to atrial fibrillation will depend upon the underlying heart disease; chronic atrial fibrillation in patients presenting with valvular disease clearly places them at an increased risk for stroke. It is often difficult to distinguish the morbidity and mortality faced by patients with atrial fibrillation from the consequences of their underlying heart disease. Nevertheless, atrial fibrillation has been associated in some categories of patients with doubled cardiovascular mortality and death. For the patient with underlying heart disease, stroke prevention is of utmost importance. While some debate exists in the literature, there is good agreement that use of warfarin is relatively safe and effective as stroke prevention. Correction or optimization of underlying heart disease in patients with atrial fibrillation is mandatory.

CARDIAC PEARL

The incidence of stroke associated with atrial fibrillation can be reduced by the use of anticoagulants such as warfarin (Coumadin).

With life expectancy increasing, more patients will have atrial fibrillation; the above pearl will be even more apropos.

It is of interest that several decades ago there was controversy as to whether anticoagulants were indicated for patients having atrial fibrillation.

However, recent analysis showed that patients who have atrial fibrillation will be less prone to thromboembolic events if they are on warfarin (Coumadin). Of course, contraindications to anticoagulant administration should be checked before use of these drugs.

Stroke represents one of the most serious and devastating complications that can occur in cardiovascular disease. Recovery and improvement, if this occurs, is generally slow compared with other diseases. However, if we see some improvement, even though slight, it is a sign that additional improvement is possible, but again not likely to be rapid. Since patients who have suffered a stroke are so depressed and discouraged, they need to know and should be told that improvement can take place, but slowly; if it occurs more quickly, good. It is a bonus.

W. Proctor Harvey, M.D.

For patients presenting with atrial fibrillation without overt heart disease, again, correction of underlying conditions such as hyperthyroidism or removal of toxins such as alcohol, is mandatory. The strategy for management in patients with structurally normal hearts then includes control of heart rate, identification and correction of the precipitating factors, and consideration of cardioversion, and attempts at maintenance of sinus rhythm. We have found that heart rate control in atrial fib-

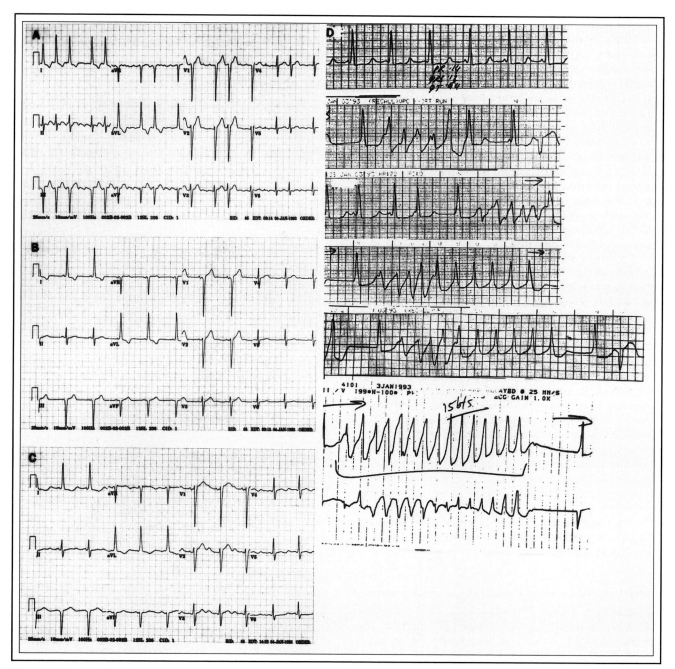

Figure 5. A 79-year-old patient with renal insufficiency was admitted with symptomatic atrial fibrillation **(A)**. Cardioversion was performed **(B)** and therapy with procainamide initiated. Three days later, the patient was noted to have a markedly prolonged QT interval **(C)**. The pronestyl level was therapeutic, but the NAPA level was elevated. Recurrent torsades occurred **(D)**. Procainamide was discontinued.

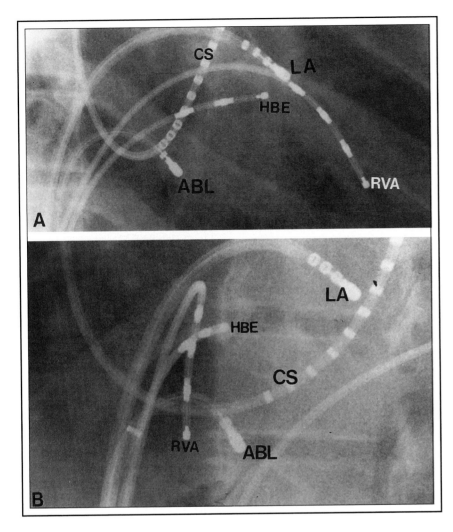

Figure 6. Pictured are right **(A)** and left **(B)** anterior oblique projections of catheter positions during ablation of the right posteroseptal accessory pathway in Figure 7. The ablation was carried out with the large-tipped bipolar catheter positioned just below the coronary sinus os. A second large-tipped catheter was placed in the left atrium via a transseptal approach to facilitate mapping.

rillation is best achieved by the use of calcium channel antagonists such as diltiazem. These provide the best heart rate control during exercise when compared to digoxin or to beta blockers. Nevertheless, digoxin and beta blockers remain important adjuncts in the therapy of patients with atrial fibrillation. Acute management for the symptomatic patient with atrial fibrillation is best achieved with IV diltiazem.

When considering cardioversion for the patient presenting with palpitations related to atrial fibrillation, it is our practice to cardiovert within the first 24 hours of symptom onset. If, however, the patient presents more than 24 hours following onset of symptoms, we will anticoagulate the patient for three to four weeks, achieve rate control and readmit for cardioversion. At that point, the question of long term anti-arrhythmic therapy often arises.

Long term use of primary antiarrhythmics in the management of atrial fibrillation should be reserved for the patient in whom other options have been exhausted. While proarrhythmia is relatively

uncommon in patients with structurally normal hearts; most patients with atrial fibrillation have some structural abnormality. In this population, the risk of precipitation of ventricular arrhythmias through the use of antiarrhythmics is real (Figure 5). In a recent meta-analysis, Coplen et al reported a threefold increase in mortality in patients with atrial fibrillation treated with quinidine as compared to controls.

Catheter Ablation

The development of newer sources of energy delivery and improved catheter technology has increased the applicability of catheter ablation in the management of patients presenting with symptomatic arrhythmias. Radiofrequency energy produces tissue damage by desiccation. Energy at 500 Hz to 750 Hz is delivered to the myocardium in a monopolar fashion through a catheter positioned against the endocardium. This technique when applied in the laboratory is curative in approximately 95% of patients treated for Wolff-Parkinson-White syndrome. Approximately 90% of patients

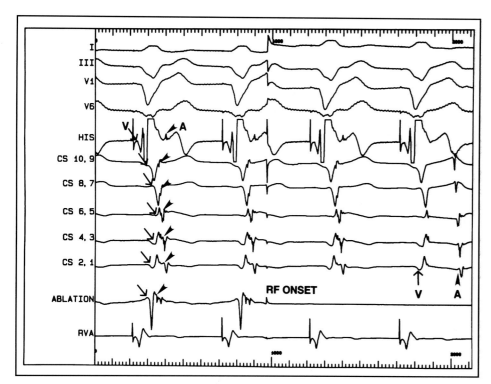

Figure 7. Surface and intracardiac electrocardiograms correspond with catheters in figure 6. Note CS 10, 9, etc., correspond with electrode pairs of the catheter positioned in the coronary sinus. Pair 10, 9 is the most proximal to the coronary sinus and 2, 1 is the most distal. Ventricular deflections, as recorded at each site, are indicated by the arrow; atrial deflections by the arrow head. Retrograde activation is consistent with retrograde posteroseptal accessory pathway conduction. The earliest retrograde atrial activation is recorded on the ablation catheter. Less than one second following the onset of radiofrequency energy application, there is an abrupt alteration in retrograde activation consistent with interruption of accessory pathway conduction.

treated for AV nodal reentrant tachycardia can undergo successful AV node modification without necessitating permanent pacemaker. A 1% to 3% incidence of complete heart block occurs with AV nodal modification. For patients presenting with atrial flutter, approximately a 50% to 90% cure rate can be expected. As mentioned above, for patients who present with atrial fibrillation uncontrollable by medication, AV nodal ablation is often an effective form of treatment and can result in reversal of myocardial depression related either to drug suppression or persistent tachycardia. Likewise, for patients with ectopic atrial tachycardia, approximately a 70% cure rate can be achieved in the laboratory. These patients who are frequently young and otherwise have structurally normal hearts can, therefore, be prevented from developing tachycardia related cardiomyopathy and can avoid the need for long term drug management.

A comprehensive discussion of catheter ablation is beyond the scope of this chapter. However, for all the above conditions, successful ablation is dependent on the accurate localization of the target tissue to be ablated. With multiple reference catheters (Figure 6), it is possible to accurately map the electrical activation sequence within the heart. Energy delivery through the ablation catheter when correctly positioned will result in rapid effect (Figure 7). In our patient population at sites of permanent accessory pathway interruption, the mean time to effect is less than 4 seconds. Typically, following catheter ablation, patients can be discharged the following morning and return to work one or two days later.

Selected Reading

1. Antman EM, et al: Transtelephonic electrocardiographic transmission for management of cardiac arrhythmias. *AJC* 1986;58:1021.
2. Bjerregaard, P: Premature beats in healthy subjects 40-79 years of age. *Eur Heart J* 1982;3:493.
3. Borggrefe M, Hindricks G, Haverkamp W, Budde T, Breithardt G: *Radiofrequency ablation. In:* Zipes DP, Jalife J, eds. *Cardiac electrophysiology — from cell to bedside.* Philadelphia: W.B. Saunders 1990;997-04.
4. The Boston Area Anticoagulation Trial for Atrial Fibrillation Investigators. The effect of low-dose warfarin on the risk of stroke in patients with non-rheumatic atrial fibrillation. *NEJM* 1990;323:1505-11.
5. Boudoulas H, Kligfield P, Wolley CF: *Mitral valve prolapse: sudden death. In:* Boudoulas H, Wooley CF, eds. Mitral valve prolapse and the mitral valve prolapse syndrome. Mount Kisco, NY: Futura 1988.
6. Braunwald E: *Heart Disease: A Textbook of Cardiovascular Medicine.* Vol 2, 3rd Ed. Philadelphia: W.B. Saunders 1992.
7. Brodsky M, et al: Arrhythmias documented by 24-hour continuous ambulatory electrocardiographic monitoring in 50 male medical students without apparent heart disease. *AJC* 1977;39:390.
8. Coplen SE, Antman FM, Berlin JA, Hewitt P, Chalmers TC: Efficacy and safety of quinidine therapy for maintenance of sinus rhythm after cardioversion. *Circ* 1990;82:1106-16.
9. Engle TR, Luck JC: Effect of whiskey on atrial vulnerability and holiday heart. *JACC* 1983;1:816-18.
10. Fagerberg B, Lindstedt G, Stromblad SO, et al: Thyrotoxic atrial fibrillation: An under diagnosed or over diagnosed condition? *Clin Card* 1990;36:620-27.

11. Falk RH: Flecainide induced ventricular tachycardia and fibrillation in patients treated for atrial fibrillation. *Ann Intern Med* 1989;111:107-11.

12. Fananapazir L, Tracy CM, Leon MB, et al: Electrophysiologic abnormalities in patients with hypertrophic cardiomyopathy: A consecutive analysis in 155 patients. *Circ* 1989; 80:1259-68.

13. Feinberg WM, Seeger JF, Carmody RF, Anderson DC, Hart RG, Pearce LA: Epidemiologic features of asymptomatic cerebral infarction in patients with nonvalvular atrial fibrillation. *Arch Intern Med* 1990;150:2340-44.

14. Fleg, JL and Kennedy HL: Cardiac arrhythmias in a healthy elderly population: Detection by 24-hour ambulatory electrocardiography. *Chest* 1982;81:302.

15. Hinkle, LE, Carver ST, Stevens, M: The frequency of asymptomatic disturbances of cardiac rhythm and conduction in middle-aged men. *AJC* 1969;24:629.

16. Kadish AH, Morady F: *Torsades de pointes. In:* Zipes DP, Jalife J, eds. *Cardiac electrophysiology—from cell to bedside.* Philadelphia: W.B. Saunders 1990;605-10.

17. Kannel WB, Wolf PA: *Epidemiology of Atrial Fibrillation. In:* Falk RH, Podrid PJ, eds. *Atrial Fibrillation: Mechanisms and Management.* New York: Raven Press 1992;81-92.

18. Kennedy HL: Long-term electrocardiographic recordings. In: Zipes DP, Rowlands DJ, eds. *Progress in Cardiology.* Philadelphia: Lea and Febiger:1988;237-56.

19. Kennedy HL, et al: Long-term follow-up of asymptomatic healthy subjects with frequent and complex ventricular ectopy. *NEJM* 1985;312:193.

20. Kleiger RE, et al: Decreased heart rate variability and its association with increased mortality after acute myocardial infarction. *AJC* 1987;59:256.

21. Klein RC, Machell C: Use of electrophysiologic testing in patients with nonsustained ventricular tachycardia: Prognostic and therapeutic implications. *JACC* 1989;14:155-61.

22. Kuchar DL, Thorburn CW, Sammel NL: Prediction of serious arrhythmic events after myocardial infarction: Signal-averaged electrocardiogram, Holter monitoring and radionuclide ventriculography. *JACC* 1987;9:531-38.

23. Leather RA, Kerr CR: *Atrial Fibrillation in the Absence of Overt Cardiac Disease. In:* Falk RH, Podrid PJ, ed. *Atrial Fibrillation: Mechanisms and Management.* New York: Raven Press 1992;93-108.

24. Mancini GBJ, Goldgerger AL: Cardioversion of atrial fibrillation: consideration of embolization, anticoagulation, prophylactic pacemaker and longterm success. *AHJ* 1982;104:617-21.

25. Morganroth J, Horowitz LN: Antiarrhythmic drug therapy 1988: For whom, how and where? *AJC* 1988;62:461-65.

26. Morganroth J, et al: Limitations of routine long-term electrocardiographic monitoring to assess ventricular ectopy frequency. *Circ* 1980;61:690.

27. Paul T, Guccione P, Garson A Jr: Relation of syncope in young patients with Wolff-Parkinson-White syndrome to rapid ventricular response during atrial fibrillation. *AJC* 1990;65:318-21.

28. Petersen P, Boysen G, Godtfredsen J, Andersen B: Placebo-controlled, randomised trial of warfarin and aspirin for prevention of thromboembolic complications in chronic atrial fibrillation: the Copenhagen AFASAK study. *Lancet* 1989;1:175-79.

29. Petersen P, Kastrup J, Helweg-Larsen S, Boysen G, Godtfredsen J: Risk factors for thromboembolic complications in chronic atrial fibrillation. The Copenhagen AFASK Study. *Arch Intern Med* 1990;150:819-21.

30. Platia E: *Management of Cardiac Arrhythmias: The Non-pharmacologic Approach.* Philadelphia: J.B. Lippincott 1987.

31. Podrid PJ, Falk RH: *Management of Atrial Fibrillation—An Overview. In:* Falk RH, Podrid PJ, ed. *Atrial Fibrillation: Mechanisms and Management.* New York: Raven Press 1992;389-11.

32. Ruffy R, Roman-Smith P, Barbey JT: Palpitations: evaluation and management. In: Zipes DP, Rowlands DJ, eds. *Progress in Cardiology.* Philadelphia: Lea and Febiger: 1988;131-38.

33. Ruskin JN: The Cardiac Arrhythmia Suppression Trial (CAST). *NEJM* 1989;321:386-87.

34. Savage DD, Garrison RJ, Castelli WP et al. Prevalence of saturated (annular) calcium and its correlates in a general population-based sample: the Framingham study. *AJC* 1983;57:1375-78.

35. Scheinman MM, Morady F, Hess DS, Gonzalez R: Catheter induced ablation of the atrioventricular junction to control refractory supraventricular arrhythmias. *JAMA* 1982; 248:851-55.

36. Segal BJ: *Diagnostic Techniques. History and Physical Examination of Patients with Arrhythmia. In:* Horowitz LN, ed. *Current Management of Arrhythmias.* Philadelphia: B.C. Decker 1991;17-43.

37. Simson MB: *Signal-averaged electrocardiography: Methods and clinical applications. In:* Braunwald E, ed. Heart disease update. Philadelphia: W.B. Saunders 1989:145.

38. Sobotka PA, et al: Arrhythmias documented by 24-hour continuous ambulatory electrocardiographic monitoring in young women without apparent heart disease. *AJC* 1981; 101:753.

39. Solomon AJ, Tracy CM: The signal-averaged electrocardiogram in predicting coronary artery disease. *AHJ,* Vol 122(5); 1991:1334-39.

40. Stroke Prevention in Atrial Fibrillation Study Group Investigators. Preliminary report of the stroke prevention in atrial fibrillation study. *NEJM* 1990;322:863-68.

41. Swartz, JF, Tracy CM, Fletcher RD: Radiofrequency endocardial catheter ablation of accessory atrioventricular pathway atrial insertion sites. *Circ,* Vol 87 (2);1993:487-99.

42. Tracy CM, Swartz JF, Fletcher RD, Hoops HG, Solomon AJ, Karasik PE, Mukherjee D: Radiofrequency catheter ablation of ectopic atrial tachycardia using paced activation sequence mapping. *JACC* Vol 21 (4);1993:910-17.

43. Veltri EP, Platia EV, Griffin LSC, Reid PR: Programmed electrical stimulation and long-term follow-up in asymptomatic, non-sustained ventricular tachycardia. *AJC* 1985; 56:309-14.

44. Zeldis SM, Levine BJ, Michelson EL, Morganroth J: Cardiovascular complaints: Correlation with cardiac arrhythmias on 24-hour electrocardiographic monitoring. *Chest* 1980; 78:456.

669

CHAPTER 29

Syncope and Sudden Death: Diagnosis and Treatment

Albert A. Del Negro, M.D., and Ross D. Fletcher, M.D.

The essential dilemma in the diagnosis and treatment of syncope is that the same symptom, loss of consciousness, has many etiologies of widely differing clinical implications. On the one hand, cardiac arrest and death is not usually part of the syndrome in the patient with syncope due to sick sinus syndrome, which is generally not a life-threatening condition. On the other hand, paroxysmal non-sustained ventricular tachycardia may portend sudden death and have precisely the same presenting symptoms as the more benign condition. This is the case because the common denominator of syncope is a reduction in blood pressure resulting in altered cerebral perfusion and function to the point of near or complete loss of consciousness. It is a dangerous pitfall in the clinical evaluation of patients with syncope or presyncope to believe that this symptom has a benign etiology, when in fact its cause may be life-threatening.

Fortunately, a careful and complete clinical evaluation which considers any and all etiologies will save the clinician from this pitfall. Such an evaluation necessarily begins with a detailed history and includes physical examination, electrocardiogram, chest x-ray, laboratory, and where indicated, other special procedures. When the clinician follows such a course, he or she rarely mistakes a benign for a malignant cause. Proper and successful therapy, then, proceeds from such an orderly approach to patient evaluation.

CARDIAC PEARL

Syncope generally connotes an abnormality of either the cardiovascular or cerebrovascular systems. However, syncope (defined as nontraumatic loss of consciousness) is found in 6%-20% of presumably healthy individuals. It is therefore apparent that it occurs much more commonly than generally realized.

Syncope and/or dizziness can be a frightening experience to our patients, the cause of which needs analysis and treatment including prevention, if possible.

A history of dizziness, near syncope, or syncope immediately suggests the possibility of arrhythmia which can occur in the absence of other cardiac pathology, or be a sign of heart conditions such as aortic stenosis, hypertrophic cardiomyopathy, and myocarditis.

W. Proctor Harvey, M.D.

Diagnosis of Syncope

A carefully-obtained history offers important clues to the proper etiologic diagnosis of syncope. The reports of observers may detail antecedent chest pain or complaints of palpitations. Syncope after prolonged upright posture is a common history in the vasodepressor syndrome of neuro-cardiogenic syncope (Figure 1). Loss of consciousness at rest suggests a sudden arrhythmia, while exertional syncope may be the first clue to significant valvular heart disease or ischemic heart disease. A prior history of coronary artery disease, myocardial infarction or congestive heart failure of any etiology should lead the clinician to suspect a lethal ventricular arrhythmia. Knowledge of an antecedent arrhythmia or a history of conduction system disease is of obvious importance and calls arrhythmia to mind as an etiology, and drug history is important to review with patients. Administration of pharmacologic agents such as digitalis or beta blockers may evoke profound bradycardia episodes

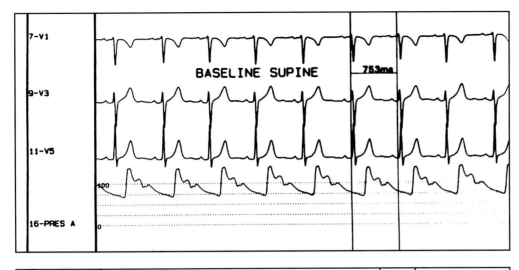

Figure 1A. Baseline supine heart rate and blood pressure in a patient with recurrent syncope of neurocardiogenic origin.

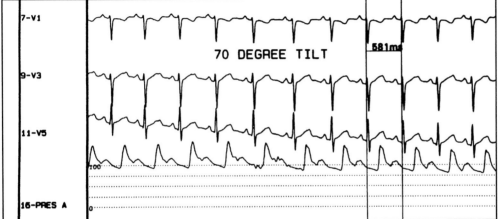

Figure 1B. 70 degree upright tilt after 10 minutes. Heart rate is faster than 100/min and blood pressure averages 150/85 mmHg.

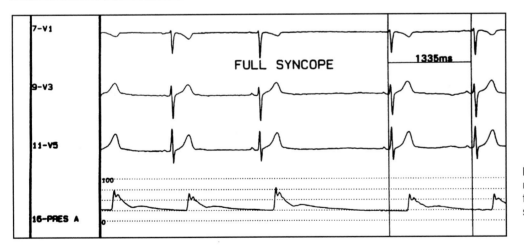

Figure 1C. After 22 minutes of upright posture, blood pressure falls to 70/25 mmHg and full syncope occurs.

which present as syncope. Notable also is the class of pharmacologic agents such as nitrates or calcium channel blockers known to produce vasodilatation, which aggravate vasodepressor syncope. In evaluation of syncope, a history of other family members with seizures, syncope, or sudden death suggests familial prolonged QT interval syndrome. In such patients, polymorphous non-sustained ventricular tachycardia is the alarming cause of loss of con-

sciousness. The length of the syncopal episode (seconds to hours) may give clues to etiology. Cardiac arrhythmias, neuro-cardiac syncope and the exertional pre-syncope/syncope associated with severe valvular aortic stenosis is usually short-lived. The duration of the history (days to years) is valuable in assessment of patients with atrio-ventricular nodal reentry tachycardia or reentrant arrhythmias due to an accessory pathway in the Wolff-Parkinson-

White syndrome who may have a life-long or at least a year long history.

Seizure activity and incontinence of bowel or bladder associated with syncope are worrisome symptoms and suggest profound and life-threatening arrhythmias as etiology. Facial or head trauma incurred in a syncopal fall likewise is of concern since these findings occur with profound hypotension often associated with potentially lethal ventricular arrhythmias. If chest pain precedes the onset of syncope caused by a lethal ventricular arrhythmia, such as sustained ventricular tachycardia or ventricular fibrillation aborted by cardiac resuscitation, the clinician must suspect active and provocable cardiac ischemia first. The treatment of such underlying ischemia must precede consideration of the arrhythmia per se.

Finally, although syncope patients often receive a detailed neurologic evaluation including costly and time-consuming laboratory examinations, a primary neurologic disorder as a cause of syncope is much less common than a primary cardiovascular disorder. Much valuable time is wasted searching for a disorder which does not exist, and after being cleared by neurologic evaluation, the cardiologist is finally consulted. One can avoid this mistake by realizing the unlikelihood of a neurologic disorder and focusing one's clinical tools to obtain an accurate history.

Categories of Syncope

Syncope From Primary Hemodynamic Disturbances

Postural Hypotension

• **Clinical Presentation:** Postural hypotension usually results in near-loss of consciousness. In this syndrome, hypotension results from the change in position from sitting or lying to upright. Near-loss of consciousness is usually transient and resolves as hemodynamics readjust to the posture change. In fact, every individual has a postural drop in blood pressure to some extent, but symptomatic patients have an exaggerated fall in pressure to the extent that cerebral perfusion is compromised. Complete loss of consciousness is possible, but most such patients have varying degrees of pre-syncope with posture change and learn to moderate symptoms by slowing posture changes.

• **Mechanism:** A contracted blood volume is the principal cause of postural hypotension. Compensatory vasoconstrictor reflexes may operate appropriately, but are unable fully to compensate. Over diuresis, excessive fluid loss from perspira-

tion or diarrhea without sufficient volume replacement, or even gastrointestinal hemorrhage, are common clinical scenarios for postural hypotension. Drug therapy with nitrates, alpha constrictor antagonists, and beta adrenergic blockers also cause this response. The ganglionic blocker bretylium most profoundly causes postural hypotension by depleting the nerve ending of norepinephrine so that there can be absolutely no vasoconstrictor compensation to posture change. Prolonged bed rest results in deconditioning of the normal reflex vasoconstrictor responses so that postural hypotension occurs when the patient is mobilized out of bed.

CARDIAC PEARL

Micturition syncope can occur when a man is urinating. A man may awaken from sleep and, still sleepy, goes to the bathroom to urinate. Postural hypotension develops, contributing to it might be some vagal stimulation coincident with straining with urination, and syncope results. The occurrence of this in women would be unusual, since they are sitting while urinating.

W. Proctor Harvey, M.D.

Postural hypotension complicates diseases associated with peripheral neuropathy. The peripheral neuropathy associated with diabetes mellitus results in loss of appropriate vasoconstrictor responses upon the change from lying to upright position, and peripheral neuropathy of chronic renal insufficiency produces similar responses. Finally, in the neurologic syndrome of absent reflexes (Shy-Dragher syndrome) there is no reflex vasoconstriction, and no reflex increase in heart rate when changing position from lying to upright posture. The result is profound hypotension and pre-syncope or syncope.

• **Diagnosis:** A history of pre-syncope arising from lying or sitting positions suggests diagnosis of postural hypotension. History also commonly elicits use of anti-hypertensive drugs or diuretics which worsen the syndrome. Caution should be exercised to consider the possibility of Addison's disease (prior history of tuberculosis) or Sheehan's syndrome (pituitary infarction peripartum). The chronic dialysis patient is a common victim of this syndrome; the problem in such patients may be so profound as to require saline infusions to bolster blood volume post dialysis even at the cost of fluid overload and clearcut congestive heart failure. The simplest test for this syndrome is the comparison measurement of blood pressure in the supine position and after

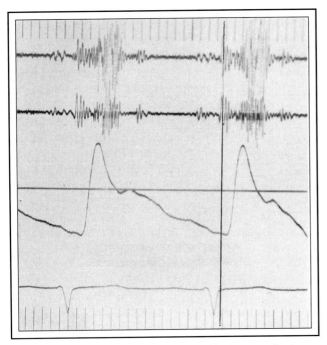

Figure 2. Phonocardiogram and indirect carotid artery recording in a patient with obstructive hypertrophic cardiomyopathy given amyl nitrite to inhale. The first heart sound is preceded by a loud atrial sound (fourth heart sound) and there is a "spike and dome" appearance to the carotid pulse contour.

standing for two minutes: a fall of greater than 10mmHg in systolic pressure after two minutes of upright posture confirms the diagnosis. Patients with postural hypotension should also have an endocrine evaluation to exclude Addison's disease and diabetes. A thorough physical examination should exclude valvular heart disease and obstructive hypertrophic cardiomyopathy, although exertionally-related syncope and pre-syncope are more common presenting symptoms of these conditions (Figures 2, 3). Finally, a renal evaluation will exclude a salt-losing nephropathy which may present as postural hypotension.

- **Treatment:** Several measures can mitigate symptoms associated with postural hypotension. Initially, one should counsel the patient to a arise from lying to sitting slowly and to wait some seconds before standing, allowing whatever compensation possible to occur. Where possible, one should avoid drugs that cause vasodilatation such as nitrates and ACE inhibitors. Therapy with beta-blocking agents is generally undesirable in pure postural hypotension, and centrally active alpha constrictor antagonists are also undesirable. After these measures, use of a support leotard will reduce severity of the syndrome by enhancing venous return. Use of mineralocorticoids such as fludrocortisone acetate will enhance vasoconstriction and improve symptoms.

CARDIAC PEARL

Recently I was asked to see a patient who had two syncopal episodes within the past three months. The possibility of mitral valve prolapse had been considered even though no physician had detected a systolic click (or clicks) and/or a late apical systolic murmur. On evaluation of the patient, he had no evidence of mitral valve prolapse. His history, however, revealed that hypertension had been detected several months before, for which a diuretic had been prescribed. I asked him when he last felt dizzy. He replied, "When I got up from my chair in the waiting room to come in the office." His blood pressure was then taken and it was 140/90 sitting and promptly fell to 98/50 on standing. This postural hypotensive effect was documented several times after this.

He was taking twice to three times the usual dose of the diuretic used to control his hypertension which presumably resulted in hypotension and syncope. His symptoms

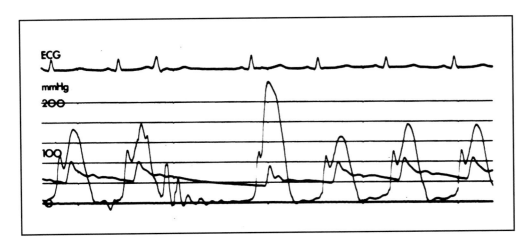

Figure 3. Simultaneous brachial artery and left ventricular pressure recordings in a patient with obstructive hypertrophic cardiomyopathy. After the premature ventricular contraction, there is diminution of the pulse pressure on the next sinus beat (Brockenbrough response) unique to this entity.

started after taking the diuretic. Adjustment of his antihypertensive medication was the obvious answer to treat his symptoms of dizziness and syncope.

W. Proctor Harvey, M.D.

Vasodepressor Syncope

• **Clinical Presentation:** This recently more clearly categorized syndrome has several alternate names including neuro-cardiogenic syncope and vaso-vagal syncope. Typically, syncope occurs following prolonged upright posture. Often, there is a long antecedent history of such symptoms, and the syndrome is sometimes associated with cardiac bradyarrhythmias which aggravate the primary hemodynamic disturbance. In its purest form, however, there is no contributing bradycardia.

• **Mechanism:** Patients subject to this develop inappropriate venodilatation in response to prolonged upright posture. This results in reduced stroke volume and cardiac output and blood pressure. Although a significant bradycardia does not occur with this response in the classic case, notably lacking is reflex tachycardia. Instead, further venodilatation occurs which worsens hypotension; eventually syncope results from hypotension and cerebral hypoperfusion. Although venodilatation is the initiating physiologic event, there is an absence of the usual compensatory mechanisms such as vasoconstriction.

• **Diagnosis:** The presenting symptom of syncope following prolonged standing suggests diagnosis of vasodepressor syncope. Reproduction of symptoms with measurement of blood pressure in the course of a tilt test is the definitive way to make the diagnosis. There are several protocols for the performance of a tilt test, and the procedure can be shortened by administration of isoproterenol to provoke a positive response if upright (60 degrees to 80 degrees) tilt does not. Although a significant bradyarrhythmia is not present in the pure form of vasodepressor syncope, profound bradycardia may coexist with the vasodepressor component. Thus, evaluation of one with this suspected diagnosis should include a Holter monitor or an event recorder for the patient with only infrequent symptoms.

• **Treatment:** Curiously, beta blockers are the drugs of choice. Often, the addition of a scopolamine patch will complement beta blockade. A repeat tilt test on therapy will assess treatment efficacy; when a significant bradyarrhythmia complicates the syndrome, permanent pacing is also indicated. The pacing modality of choice is dual chamber rate responsive pacing since single cham-

ber ventricular pacing will aggravate the hypotensive response and because sinus node dysfunction usually is present in such patients. One may achieve further support of blood pressure with the use of fludrocortisone, and alpha adrenergic vasoconstrictors are under study at present for therapy of vasodepressor syncope. Patients should avoid vasodilator therapy and the use of a support leotard may enhance pharmacologic therapy in resistant cases.

Although symptomatic orthostatic hypotension is an uncommon problem in clinical practice, the physician may have a very tough nut to crack to effectively control it. The use of dual chamber pacing has been beneficial.

W. Proctor Harvey, M.D.

Primary Pulmonary Hypertension

• **Clinical Presentation:** Exertional dyspnea and syncope are the most typical presentations for primary pulmonary hypertension. More often occurring in females under age 40, cough, progressive dyspnea and even hemoptysis are prominent symptoms. Palpitations due to atrial fibrillation are common. Time course is usually short, and most patients die within one year of the onset of clinical congestive heart failure that ultimately occurs.

A cardiac pearl concerning syncope in a young person (teenage, 20s, 30s) and most likely a female- be sure to consider and look for primary pulmonary hypertension.

W. Proctor Harvey, M.D.

• **Mechanism:** Progressive obstruction of the pulmonary vascular bed is the cause of the symptoms due to primary pulmonary hypertension. The resulting hypoxia is exacerbated by intra-pulmonary arterio-venous shunting, which worsens with exertion. The pulmonary vascular obstruction places a fixed upper limit on the cardiac output. Exercise increases this demand which cannot be met and hypotension and vascular collapse necessarily occur. This is the cause of syncope in this syndrome.

• **Diagnosis:** Progressive dyspnea, cyanosis, hemoptysis, and syncope, especially in young females, should suggest the diagnosis of primary pulmonary hypertension. Physical findings include clubbing of the digits, and the cardiovascular examination lends clues to severity of the syndrome. The jugular venous pulse will demonstrate elevated pressure and if right heart failure is severe enough, there will be the C-V venous contour of tricuspid regurgitation. Precordial examination will show a right ventricular lift proportional to the pulmonary pressure. The pulmonary component of the second heart sound will be accentuated and the murmur of high pressure pulmonary insufficiency may be audible. The murmur of tricuspid insufficiency will be audible, and the abdominal examination will demonstrate pulsatile hepatomegaly in cases with marked right heart decompensation. The prognosis is ominous if these latter findings of right heart failure are present. The electrocardiogram may show right ventricular hypertrophy, right heart strain, or right ventricular conduction delay. Chest x-ray shows reduced pulmonary markings and a prominent right heart silhouette.

Ultimately, the diagnosis of primary pulmonary hypertension is one of exclusion, ruling out first all of the other clinical entities which can produce this constellation of symptoms and clinical findings. A cardiac catheterization is necessary to exclude Eisenmenger's lesions from intracardiac shunts, as well as to exclude pulmonary emboli. The pulmonary arteriogram will show a "pruned" appearance to the pulmonary vasculature.

• **Treatment:** The cardiac catheterization is also the vehicle for therapy. There is no satisfactory therapy for this progressive and ultimately fatal disease, but empiric therapy is aimed at the reduction in pulmonary artery pressure without compromise in cardiac output. With a flow-directed catheter in place in the pulmonary artery, one assesses the effect on pulmonary artery pressure and resistance with various vasodilators from nitrites to ACE inhibitors. No two patients will respond similarly and this fact emphasizes the utility of such an empiric approach. Finally, full dose anticoagulation is a common therapeutic alternative since postmortem examination often demonstrates intra-pulmonary thrombosis, and because right heart failure predisposes to thromboembolism. There is no demonstration, however, that anticoagulation either alters the course of the disease or prolongs life.

Pulmonary Embolism

• **Clinical Presentation:** Sudden syncope and presyncope with exertion along with cough, exertional dyspnea and hemoptysis are the presenting symptoms of pulmonary embolism. Some patients will present with new onset atrial fibrillation and pleuritic chest pain. Often, there is a history of

antecedent leg trauma or prolonged travel that gives a clue to the possibility of lower extremity venous thrombosis. Inactivity, bed rest, and congestive heart failure also predispose to venous thrombosis and are common background clinical features.

Further emphasizing the need to move and exercise the leg muscles when traveling was a physician acquaintance and patient, who drove nonstop from upstate New York to Washington, D.C. and developed thrombophlebitis in the right calf region; a pulmonary embolus occurred requiring emergency hospital admission. He had kept his leg in the same position on the accelerator pedal. He did not have heart disease. Cardiac pearl: "An ounce of prevention." Break up prolonged automobile trips by stopping at intervals, such as every hour, getting out of the car and walking around.

On an airplane, get an aisle seat if possible and get up and walk at intervals. During travel, remember to occasionally wiggle your feet and move your legs at intervals.

W. Proctor Harvey, M.D.

• **Mechanism:** Acute and severe pulmonary embolism may compromise so much of the pulmonary bed that obstruction to pulmonary blood flow results in a low or at least fixed cardiac output. As in the case of primary pulmonary hypertension, exertion, then, is associated with syncope and pre-syncope because of the inability to increase cardiac output in the face of increased demand. Considerable intra-pulmonary shunting occurs, which exacerbates hypoxia (especially with exertion) and this further leads to cardiac dysfunction and a declining cardiac output.

• **Diagnosis:** Acute dyspnea, pleuritic chest pain, and hemoptysis suggest pulmonary embolism. Syncope, when it accompanies this syndrome, is particularly ominous since it implies inadequate cardiac output and hypotension. Acutely, there will be no sign of right heart failure, but the subtle finding of a right sided fourth heart sound may be present. In patients with chronic recurrent pulmonary emboli, pre-syncope is common as is exertional dyspnea and the findings of pulmonary hypertension and right heart failure are usually present. The electrocardiogram will reflect pulmonary hypertension with right axis deviation compared to prior tracings, and acutely the findings of new right axis deviation with T wave inversion in III is typical. The chest x-ray may show nothing acutely, or there may be atelectasis, signs of segmental hypoperfusion, a pleural based wedge-shaped infiltrate or a pleural effusion. Lung ventilation/perfusion scanning will demonstrate a perfusion defect in pulmonary segments ventilated; this strongly establishes diagnosis. In seriously ill individuals, pulmonary angiography with measurement of pressures can assist in the decision to augment anticoagulation therapy with caval interruption.

• **Treatment:** Anticoagulation with heparin is the cornerstone of the initial therapy of pulmonary embolism. This is followed soon after with anticoagulation with warfarin for at least six weeks. For patients who present with syncope, or who are hemodynamically unstable, or who have greater than 50% of pulmonary vasculature compromised by clot, cardiac catheterization with measurement of pressures and selective pulmonary angiography establishes the anatomy and physiology, confirms the diagnosis, and assists in the estimation of the need for inferior vena caval interruption.

Syncope Due To Valvular Heart Disease

Valvular Aortic Stenosis

• **Clinical Presentation:** Syncope is the classic presentation for patients with severe valvular aortic stenosis. Most typically, exertion provokes this symptom and syncope at rest, if it occurs in valvu-

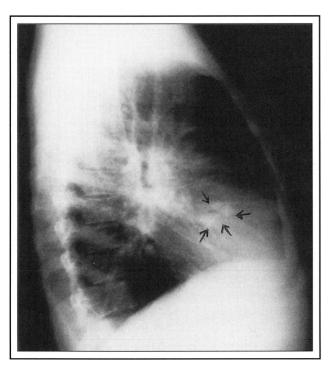

Figure 4. Lateral chest x-ray of a patient with severe calcific aortic stenosis and syncope. The resting aortic valve gradient measured 110 mmHg.

lar aortic stenosis, has another mechanism. Shortness of breath is another cardinal symptom, and exertional chest pain indistinguishable from classic angina pectoris is the third classic symptom of severe aortic stenosis. Interestingly, syncope, although it may occur at any age, is a more common presenting symptom of severe aortic stenosis in patients under 20 years old. The same is true of sudden death, but angina and congestive heart failure are more common presenting findings in patients over the age of 40 years.

• **Mechanism:** The severely stenotic aortic valve places a fixed upper limit to the cardiac output. Any exertional increase in demand for cardiac output cannot be met and hypotension occurs which will cause syncope. Of greater risk is fall in coronary blood flow resulting from hypotension, since the resulting myocardial ischemia will predispose to cardiac arrhythmias. This enhances the probability of ventricular tachycardia and ventricular fibrillation, which is the mechanism of sudden death in severe aortic stenosis.

CARDIAC PEARL

Concerning valvular obstruction, it is logical that the closer the stenotic valve to the brain, the more likelihood of occurrence of dizziness and/or syncope; hence, aortic valve or outflow obstruction is the culprit.
W. Proctor Harvey, M.D.

• **Diagnosis:** A history of a heart murmur in a patient with syncope or aborted sudden death always raises the possibility of severe aortic stenosis. A simple careful physical examination may not only demonstrate an aortic outflow murmur, but the skilled clinician will also be able to estimate severity of the lesion. Findings favoring severity include a slow rising pulse, a precordial thrill, a single second heart sound, the absence of an ejection sound, and a long and late-peaking murmur of aortic stenosis. The electrocardiogram should show left ventricular hypertrophy, and aortic valve calcification may be present on the chest x-ray (Figure 4). Echocardiographic and Doppler estimation of the severity of the stenosis is extremely accurate and cardiac catheterization should document a severely narrowed valve area in addition to evaluating the coronary circulation. This latter diagnostic test is especially important for those severe aortic stenosis patients who present with angina pectoris.

An important pitfall in evaluating aortic stenosis occurs in patients with congestive heart failure.

Such patients have a marked reduction in stroke volume and cardiac output. Intensity of the murmur of aortic stenosis, however, is greatly dependent on flow across the valve. Both flow and systolic ejection time are reduced by heart failure and these factors greatly reduce intensity as well as length of the murmur of severe aortic stenosis leading to clinical underestimation of severity of the lesion. In fact, the findings of congestive heart failure with congested lungs, elevated venous pressure, the murmur of mitral regurgitation due to left ventricular dilatation, gallop rhythm, and congestive hepatomegaly may be so dominant as to obscure aortic stenosis totally. For this reason, severe aortic stenosis should always be in the differential diagnosis of unexplained congestive heart failure.

CARDIAC PEARL

It is surprising to find, at times, how advanced congestive heart failure can alter heart murmurs. A patient personally evaluated had severe calcific aortic stenosis (necropsy). He had, at one stage during his life, a loud, harsh grade V aortic systolic murmur associated with a palpable thrill. Advanced heart failure ensued and the murmur and thrill disappeared. At that time, one physician, examining the patient for the first time and not being aware of his previous findings on physical examination, brought up the possibility of constrictive pericarditis, since many of the patient's physical findings were related to the right side of the heart.

W. Proctor Harvey, M.D.

• **Treatment:** Treatment of severe aortic stenosis is relatively straightforward. Operative replacement of the aortic valve is the only treatment of choice. In patients deemed too ill to withstand cardiopulmonary bypass and operative replacement of the aortic valve, aortic balloon valvuloplasty may at least transiently reduce the gradient. This temporizing measure will permit improvement of clinical status and act as a bridge to operative replacement of the diseased valve.

Mitral Valve Obstruction

• **Clinical Presentation:** As a cause of syncope, mitral valve obstruction, whether due to rheumatic mitral stenosis, congenital parachute mitral valve, or left atrial myxoma, is rare although not uncommon. Exertional syncope may occur, but patients with left atrial myxoma may experience syncope with specific posture changes. Symptoms of patients with left atrial myxoma are especially position-sensitive, and pre-syncope and syncope upon arising from or upon changing position while reclining are typical of this disorder. The overriding symptom of mitral valve obstruction of any etiology, however, is dyspnea since obstruction at the mitral valve level is the root cause of the symptoms. Systemic embolism and new onset atrial fibrillation are also common presenting complaints.

• **Mechanism:** The mechanism of syncope for patients with obstruction at the mitral valve level is that such patients cannot increase their cardiac output with exertion because the obstruction creates a fixed upper limit to left ventricular filling and consequently to stroke volume. As exertion requires a higher cardiac output, that requirement cannot be met and cerebral perfusion falls. For the patient with a left atrial myxoma, simply rolling over in bed can cause the pedunculated tumor to fall into the mitral annulus and obstruct flow sufficiently to cause syncope. The impediment to transmitral flow of any etiology also is the cause of the major symptom common to all forms of mitral valve obstruction: dyspnea. If allowed to progress sufficiently, right heart failure occurs which paradoxically results in relief of dyspnea. The dominant sign of mitral valve obstruction in this situation is that of right-sided heart failure.

• **Diagnosis:** Prior history of rheumatic fever is present in only 50% of patients with rheumatic mitral stenosis. A careful physical examination will uncover the cardinal features of mitral stenosis. A loud first sound is typical, though in advanced calcified rheumatic mitral stenosis, a fixed valve may be incapable of the rapid acceleration and deceleration necessary to generate a loud first sound, as well as an opening snap. The one physical finding common to all etiologies of obstruction at the left atrial-left ventricular level is a diastolic rumble. This finding should lead to an evaluation by echocardiography which will confirm diagnosis and differentiate among the diverse etiologies of obstruction at this level. Cardiac catheterization will establish presence or absence of coronary disease and assist in surgical staging.

• **Treatment:** Operative replacement or repair and balloon mitral valvuloplasty are the two therapeutic alternatives for rheumatic mitral stenosis. Patients of young age who have little calcium in the valve are the best candidates for this latter therapy. For atrial myxoma, after excluding tumors elsewhere in the heart, operative removal of the tumor and its pedicle is the treatment of choice. Often, there is damage to the mitral apparatus, which can only be assessed intraoperatively. Careful evaluation and attempted mitral repair rather than replacement is the more desirable surgical approach in such patients.

In a patient having dizziness or syncope, always consider the possibility of a myxoma of either the left or right atrium. If there are signs of tricuspid stenosis and the patient has syncope, be sure to rule out myxoma of the right atrium which at times obstructs the orifice of the tricuspid valve. Tricuspid valvular stenosis due to rheumatic etiology is much less likely to cause syncope. The same applies to mitral valve stenosis and syncope- always rule out myxoma, as this is more likely the cause than being due to rheumatism.

W. Proctor Harvey, M.D.

Syncope Due to Right Ventricular Outflow Obstruction

• **Clinical Presentation:** Exertion is the most common setting for syncope due to right ventricular outflow obstruction and the most common setting is young patients with pulmonary stenosis. This often will coexist with a ventricular septal defect associated with Tetralogy of Fallot. In such patients, cyanosis from left to right shunting at the ventricular level is usually present, and in infants, crying, irritability, increased cyanosis and syncope form a familiar symptom complex. Occasionally, patients will have isolated severe pulmonary stenosis; many of these will have been patients whose associated ventricular septal defect closed spontaneously, leaving them with isolated right ventricular outflow tract obstruction.

• **Mechanism:** As in other obstructive valve lesions associated with syncope, a fixed stroke volume and cardiac output is present. The demand for an increase in cardiac output which exercise imposes cannot be met, and blood pressure falls resulting in cerebral hypoperfusion and syncope. In patients with Tetralogy of Fallot, exercise or crying results in a fall in systemic peripheral resistance; this increases the right-to-left shunt across the ventricular septal defect, resulting in an increase in peripheral cyanosis. Spasm of the right ventricular infundibulum thereafter occurs and further increases the right-to-left shunt, diminishes pulmonary flow, and causes hypotension and syncope. Squatting to relieve dyspnea with exertion and presyncope is a compensatory maneuver in Tetralogy of Fallot since it increases peripheral resistance thereby reversing some of the increased right to left shunt and improving pulmonary flow.

• **Diagnosis:** Diagnosis of pulmonary stenosis is relatively simple to make since severe cases have the characteristic murmur of best heard in the pulmonary area. The worst cases will have no ejection sound or only a soft ejection sound which decreases in intensity with inspiration. The earlier and softer the ejection sound is on auscultation, the worse the severity of obstruction in valvular pulmonary stenosis. Tetralogy of Fallot patients are easily differentiated from patients with isolated pure valvular pulmonary stenosis in that they usually present in early infancy with cyanosis and the characteristic murmur. The electrocardiogram will demonstrate right ventricular hypertrophy in severe cases, and the chest x-ray will show reduced pulmonary flow, a post stenotic dilatation of the main pulmonary artery segment. Older patients may also show calcification of the pulmonary valve, and echocardiogram will be helpful in evaluation of the overriding of the aorta in Tetralogy patients as well as estimation of presence of a ventricular septal defect. With careful echo imaging, one may evaluate pulmonary atresia with a ventricular septal defect, an important differential diagnosis in cyanotic patients.

In isolated severe pulmonary stenosis, echocardiography is of limited diagnostic value in the estimation of severity, but cardiac catheterization definitively establishes not only severity, but evaluates potential associated anomalies such as presence of a ventricular septal defect or atrial septal defect and defines size of the pulmonary arteries, and presence of associated infundibular stenosis, all of which are important considerations for surgical repair.

• **Treatment:** Therapy for treatment of severe isolated pulmonary stenosis now includes balloon valvuloplasty. This often leaves the patient with some degree of pulmonary valve insufficiency which is clinically not hemodynamically significant since a normal or low pulmonary resistance and pressure usually accompany isolated cases. Patients with Tetralogy of Fallot, of course, will require surgical relief of obstruction along with closure of the ventricular septal defect.

Syncope Due to Cardiac Bradyarrhythmias

Sick Sinus Syndrome

• **Clinical Presentation:** The clinical profile of patients with the sick sinus syndrome is as varied as the several arrhythmias with which such patients will present. Typically, in addition to frank syncope, there is a history of fatigue, multiple episodes of pre-syncope, exercise intolerance, and paroxysms of palpitations. Sudden death as a cardinal symptom is distinctly unusual and although symptoms may be long-standing and progressive, life-threatening loss of consciousness is not considered one of the aspects of this syndrome. Patients with syncope due to this syndrome are typically elderly. Most have associated coronary artery disease only because of the fact that coronary disease is so prevalent in the elderly population. Many have no underlying heart disease, however.

• **Mechanism:** The primary mechanism of syncope in the sick sinus syndrome is an inappropriately slow heart rate to the point that cardiac output is insufficiently low to maintain adequate cerebral perfusion. There are at least four distinct categories of arrhythmic disturbance associated with the sick sinus syndrome. These are persistent symptomatic sinus bradycardia, symptomatic sinus pauses, symptomatic carotid sinus hypersensitivity, and the bradycardia-tachycardia syndrome. The last of these is the most interesting and probably the most common. Often, there is a history of syncope and subsequent hospital monitoring demonstrates paroxysms of atrial arrhythmia, usually atrial fibrillation, followed by reversion to sinus bradycardia at slow rates associated with symptoms. A post-tachycardia pause may last several seconds and be the cause of syncope. Symptoms of pre-syncope or syncope may also occur with tachyarrhythmias, especially if cardiac output is compromised with the tachycardia because of a rapid rate in association with underlying coronary, or valvular heart disease. Identification of the tachycardia in the bradycardia-tachycardia syndrome inevitably leads to therapy to provide protection against future tachycardia occurrences. Virtually all such antiarrhythmic therapies will exacerbate the bradycardia associated with the bradycardia-tachycardia syndrome. This not only reinforces the diagnosis but compounds the treatment and makes pacemaker therapy all the more indicated.

• **Diagnosis:** The necessary component to making the diagnosis is the term "symptomatic". Many patients will have profound sinus bradycardia with heart rates in the 40 beats per minute range. If these patients have no symptoms of syncope or pre-syncope attributable to bradycardia, one cannot rightfully make the diagnosis of sick sinus syndrome however strong the clinical suspicion. Prolonged monitoring is the cornerstone of proper diagnosis. For patients whose symptoms are only intermittent and for whom a 24-hour ambulatory monitor is therefore unlikely to be diagnostic, an event monitor with a patient-activated memory loop is most helpful. Patients can use such a device for prolonged periods of time until symptoms occur. The monitoring physician can receive reports of such patient-activated recording of rhythm within minutes of the clinical event. Many times, the strict criteria for the diagnosis of sick sinus syndrome cannot be fulfilled despite a strong clinical suspicion; for this reason, the guidelines established for the absolute indication for pacemaker therapy in this group of patients include documentation of heart rates below 35 beats per minute and/or pauses equal to or greater than three seconds irrespective of symptoms. These criteria take into consideration the patient with symptoms which are ill-defined but whose demonstrated monitoring reliably confirms generally agreed-upon profoundly slow heart rates which warrant pacemaker therapy.

CARDIAC PEARL

It is evident that ambulatory ECG monitoring should be performed more often in evaluating patients who have transient neurologic symptoms, particularly those who have some underlying problem with the heart. Recently, I personally observed a patient with documented prolapse of the mitral valve who had a syncopal episode; she was subsequently clinically observed to have an arrhythmia that might have explained the syncopal episode.

W. Proctor Harvey, M.D.

Additionally, a treadmill exercise test may assist in deciding in favor of pacemaker therapy in bradycardia patients who do not meet the strict criteria for pacemaker implantation. Such a test, if it demonstrates the failure to adhere to established norms for exercise-related heart rates in the normal elderly population, will lend support to decision to implant a permanent pacemaker. Cardiac electrophysiologic testing may yield less diagnostic information than simple monitoring, but it will be useful for the patient for whom bradycardia has not yet been established as the cause of symptoms of presyncope and syncope. The most valuable tests are the sinus node recovery time (corrected for the resting heart rate) and the sinus node conduction time. A measure of the longest pause associated with carotid sinus stimulation is also valuable, and since there is a frequent association of sinus node disorders with conduction system disease, cardiac electrophysiologic testing also permits evaluation of AV nodal and His-Purkinje conduction times and refractoriness.

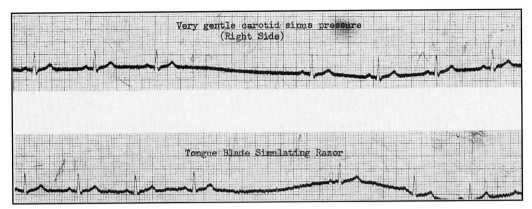

Fig A: Hypersensitive Carotid Sinus - Upper tracing: Prompt slowing with very gentle carotid sinus pressure. Lower tracing: Similar slowing with pressure over same area with a tongue blade.

CARDIAC PEARL

In my experience, a hypersensitive carotid sinus is an uncommon cause of dizziness and syncope, although it certainly does occur. I recall an interesting patient.

A 47-year-old man was evaluated in the office because of a syncopal episode, and the patient's concern that he had heart disease. Pertinent findings from history: While shaving, he stated "everything went blank." He was found lying on the floor by his wife shortly after this. Apparently he remained "unconscious" for one or one and one half minutes. Profuse perspiration was present. He was then hospitalized at Georgetown University Hospital. Carotid arteriogram was normal. He was seen by neurology and neurosurgical consultants. No intracranial or vascular lesion was demonstrated. He was discharged with the final diagnosis of postural hypotension.

Because the patient believed he had heart disease, he was referred for evaluation. There was no previous history of cardiovascular disease. Physical exam was normal except for the following interesting finding: Remembering from the history that the patient's syncopal episode occurred while shaving, gentle carotid sinus pressure was applied on the right side (the same position of the razor blade when syncope occurred). There was prompt slowing. A wooden tongue blade simulating the razor when shaving was applied over the right carotid sinus area, again resulting in abrupt slowing, as shown in Figure A. Diagnosis: Hypersensitive carotid sinus.

This illustrates the importance of a careful detailed history.

Also "handed down" in medical anecdotes folklore is the example of the streetcar conductor who would get dizzy (or faint) only when he turned his trolley, looking in one direction (probably to the right), but not in the opposite direction. This was due to the conductor's high celluloid or starched neck collar that pressed on the carotid sinus thereby producing dizziness or syncope. I was told about this as relating to a conductor of a streetcar in Boston. I suspect the same story was told about a conductor in some of our other cities.

Personally observed is that a patient suffering with significant aortic stenosis may develop a hypersensitive carotid sinus following digitalization; in fact it may be strikingly so.

If there is true hypersensitivity, very gentle carotid sinus pressure is, as a rule, all that is required to produce slowing of the heart beat.

Also of great importance are these words of caution concerning carotid sinus stimulation: It is always wise to place one's stethoscope on the precordium so as to be listening to the heart whenever pressure on the carotid sinus is applied with one's finger, or fingers. In this way, any change in heart rhythm is immediately appreciated and carotid pressure should cease.

Clinically, the right carotid sinus is usually more sensitive than the left.

W. Proctor Harvey, M.D.

• **Treatment:** Treatment of established sick sinus syndrome is permanent pacemaker implantation. Dual chamber rate responsive pacing is the preferred mode of pacing, especially in view of the fact that atrial fibrillation is more common in patients treated with VVI pacing alone. Rate-responsive pacing allows tailoring of the heart rate to physical task and provides a more appropriate heart rate for activity. This is especially valuable in patients with congestive heart failure whose stroke volume is fixed and whose ability to increase cardiac output depends solely on increases in heart rate.

Permanent pacing also assists with the therapy of the associated tachyarrhythmias associated with the sick sinus syndrome since any antiarrhythmic therapy will exacerbate the bradycardia aspect of this entity. The bradycardia support a permanent pacer permits makes it a safe and simple matter to administer antiarrhythmic agents that ordinarily cause bradycardia and exacerbate symptoms associated with this syndrome.

Atrio-Ventricular Block

• **Clinical Presentation:** The hallmark clinical sign of atrio-ventricular block is Stokes-Adams attacks. In these patients, sudden syncope is the typical presentation. Fatigue and dyspnea with new onset congestive heart failure are frequent coexistent features. Some patients will give a history of syncope or presyncope at rest while others will report exertion induced syncope or exercise intolerance. Occasionally, atrio-ventricular block patients suffer sudden death, which if aborted by successful resuscitation confuses the clinical picture. Fortunately, cardiac electrophysiologic study will identify atrio-ventricular block as an important problem and result in appropriate anti-bradycardia therapy.

• **Mechanism:** An inadequately slow heart rate due to atrio-ventricular block causes a clinically significant reduction in cardiac output, blood pressure, and cerebral perfusion. This is the cause of pre-syncope and syncope in this setting. There is a risk of sudden death in this circumstance since profoundly slow heart rates are capable of inducing dangerous tachyarrhythmias in susceptible patients. Such slow heart rates create marked heterogeneity of repolarization of the ventricular myocardium which predisposes to polymorphous ventricular tachycardia and even ventricular fibrillation. The patient with coronary artery disease will become ischemic with profound bradycardia providing a further stimulus for ventricular fibrillation. When such patients suffer ventricular fibrillation and present with aborted sudden death, the clinical evaluation can be skewed away from bradyarrhythmia toward a tachyrhythmia leading to misdiagnosis and mismanagement.

Several disorders produce atrio-ventricular block and the presentation with AV block should initiate an evaluation to consider these possibilities. There are two potential sites for atrio-ventricular block and their evaluation and treatment differ. These categories reflect the locus of block which may reside within the atrio-ventricular node or within the distal His-Purkinje system.

• **A-V Nodal Block:** Considered to be a more benign form of A-V block, A-V nodal block can result from one of several infiltrative myocardial disease. These diseases include sarcoidosis, myxedema, hemochromatosis, and calcification in the area of the atrio-ventricular node due to aortic or mitral annular calcification. Infective endocarditis and Lyme disease are infectious causes, the former especially after endocarditis complicates prior aortic valve replacement. Drugs which may cause atrio-ventricular block include digitalis where tachyarrhythmias due to increased automaticity such as junctional tachycardia and ventricular tachycardia may accompany atrio-ventricular block. Other agents such as beta blockers and calcium channel blockers also may be associated with A-V nodal block. Systemic diseases which cause A-V nodal block include ankylosing spondylitis and Reiter's syndrome. A-V nodal block occurs in approximately a third of patients with acute inferior wall myocardial infarction. Fortunately, recovery to intact A-V conduction is the rule and the bradycardia associated with inferior infarction is usually amenable to pharmacologic treatment with atropine. Myocardial developmental growth of patients with corrected transposition of the great vessels causes anatomic disruption of the atrio-ventricular node and complete heart block occurs in adolescence or early adulthood. Congenital complete heart block probably occurs at the A-V nodal level and is a poorly understood condition in which patients may present in infancy or even in utero. Although such patients usually do not have syncope, congestive heart failure can result from the prolonged associated bradycardia which results in progressive cardiac dilatation to accommodate the slow rate while preserving the cardiac output.

• **His-Purkinje Block:** Heart block in the His-Purkinje system is much more ominous than that within the atrio-ventricular node. A-V nodal patients can rely on junction escape rhythm for heart rate support; this is usually sufficient to prevent full loss of consciousness. Junctional, or His bundle rhythm, responds to sympathetic and parasympathetic influences resulting in sufficiently stable and appropriate rates to forestall presyncope or syncope. This is not true of heart block located within the bundle of His or in the infra-Hisien location. The latter patients default to idio-fascicular or idio-ventricular rhythm to maintain rate. Such rhythms are notoriously unstable and inappropriately slow. For these reasons, syncope, Stokes-Adams attacks and even sudden death are more common in patients with infra-Hisien block than in patients with A-V nodal block. Common clinical settings for infra-Hisien or distal heart block include idiopathic conduction system degeneration, (Lev's

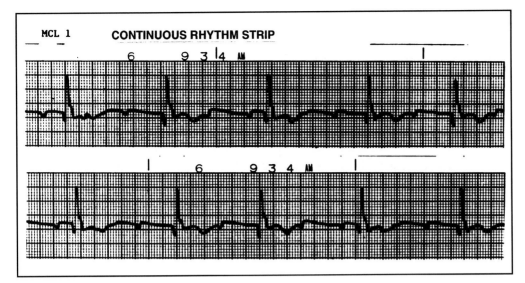

Figure 5. Rhythm strip demonstrating high grade A-V block and intermittent conduction in a patient with severe calcific aortic stenosis and syncope.

disease), valvular aortic stenosis, mitral stenosis, (often with associated annular calcification), and even pure mitral annular calcification. Growth of calcium into the conduction system is responsible for the heart block in these latter circumstances (Figure 5).

When heart block accompanies acute anterior myocardial infarction, syncope and collapse are the usual clinical result. The cause of heart block in this circumstance is necrosis of the interventricular septum and the proximal His-Purkinje system. When this occurs, idiofascicular or idioventricular rhythm is the default cardiac rhythm, and abrupt progression to asystole with cardiac arrest is not uncommon. Patients in this circumstance develop sudden bradycardia which compromises cardiac output and blood pressure frequently resulting in Stokes-Adams attacks. This is unquestionably a clinical situation calling for pacemaker support. Antiarrhythmic agents which impair conduction below the atrioventricular node can precipitate infra-Hisien block. This usually occurs in susceptible individuals with His-Purkinje delay who receive antiarrhythmics such as the Vaughn-Williams class I-A drugs quinidine, procainamide and disopyrimide. The class I-C agent flecainide, a drug with strong sodium channel blocking activity, also may precipitate infra-Hisien block. Antiarrhythmic agents in the class III category, amiodarone and sotalol, can certainly cause infra-Hisien block but also have strong conduction delay effects at the A-V nodal level. Cardiac electrophysiologic study can identify patients with impaired infra-Hisien delay and caution the clinician to avoid antiarrhythmic drugs in these classes.

• **Diagnosis:** Syncope and presyncope occurring in patients with atrio-ventricular conduction delays or bundle branch block on ECG evaluation suggests the diagnosis of intermittent A-V block as the cause of syncope. Contemporary evaluation so quickly jumps ahead to laboratory evaluation that the discovery of a slow pulse during physical examination is hardly noted. Often, A-V block is intermittent or a function of heart rate and the complaints of intermittent pre-syncope are dismissed unless the patient demonstrates the finding for the clinician during physical examination.

CARDIAC PEARL

First Degree Heart Block and Dizziness- A patient having first degree heart block may at times have unexplained dizziness or near syncope. The dizziness may be related to a temporary change from first degree block to 2:1 or complete block.

It is during this change that the symptoms may occur. Dizziness is unlikely to occur when the block is a constant 2:1, first degree, or complete block.

W. Proctor Harvey, M.D.

There is no question, however, that the electrocardiogram is the most important diagnostic tool in the evaluation of syncope due to A-V block. Clues to the diagnosis may simply be the presence of first degree A-V block, the finding of other conduction delays such as left or right bundle branch block, associated hemiblock, or the observation of left bundle delay alternating with right bundle delay. If these are the only objective findings, additional studies are necessary to establish the diagnosis. These may be as simple as exercise during ECG monitoring. A-V block provoked by exercise almost always implies block below the atrio-ventricular

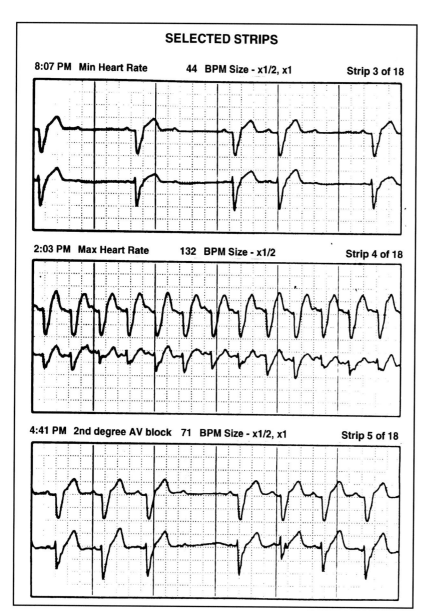

SELECTED STRIPS

8:07 PM   Min Heart Rate   44   BPM Size - x1/2, x1   Strip 3 of 18

2:03 PM   Max Heart Rate   132   BPM Size - x1/2   Strip 4 of 18

4:41 PM   2nd degree AV block   71   BPM Size - x1/2, x1   Strip 5 of 18

Figure 6. Selected rhythm strips in a patient with syncope and Mobitz type II A-V block. The P-R intervals before and after the dropped beats are identical. Note that faster atrial rates actually facilitate conduction in this patient.

node. Exercise unmasks infra-Hisien block because the associated sympathetic surge increases the sinus rate but does not improve conduction in diseased tissue below the A-V node and at least second degree block will occur. This provides an opportunity to secure additional information since the pattern of the second degree block in this circumstance should be Mobitz II, or fixed A-V conduction times before and after the dropped beat. This is diagnostic of infra-Hisien block (Figure 6).

Other studies of syncope patients with suspected syncope due to A-V block include ambulatory, or Holter monitoring. Performed as an outpatient, this is a useful test for the patient with frequent daily symptoms. It is also useful for the patient with intermittent symptoms in order to associate these symptoms with electrocardiographic findings.

Another device, the patient-operated event monitor, permits the patient to activate a continuous memory loop ECG recording which, upon interrogation, "plays back" the ECG for a period before and after the activation. This is especially useful for the patient with infrequent symptoms. Patients with frank syncope, especially those who sustain trauma in the syncopal episode, should be hospitalized for observation and treatment. The resting ECG and monitoring may provide the previously mentioned clues to A-V block as the cause of syncope, but invasive cardiac electrophysiologic study (EPS) will establish the diagnosis with certainty and even assist in the selection of therapy. EPS will provide information about the integrity of A-V conduction by permitting measurement of the PR subintervals, the AV nodal and His-Purkinje conduction times.

Atrial pacing will stress these areas when heart block is not present at rest, permitting full evaluation of the potential for heart block. Furthermore, EPS permits evaluation of additional etiologies of syncope such as ventricular tachycardia.

For cases of AV nodal dysfunction, the finding of an abnormal AV nodal conduction time and refractoriness in the course of EPS with absolutely normal His-Purkinje function does not necessarily prove the association of heart block with syncope. For this reason, the demonstration of heart block with symptoms of syncope and presyncope is vital to making the proper diagnosis. Prolonged monitoring will best provide the information to make the diagnosis. The same cannot be said of His-Purkinje dysfunction, for there are generally agreed-upon absolute limits of normal and abnormal function in this vulnerable area. A-V block below the bundle of His produced by incremental atrial pacing is distinctly abnormal and constitutes an etiologic cause of syncope. Similarly, a conduction time from the His bundle to the ventricle in excess of 100 msec is dangerously prolonged and sufficient to explain the cause of syncope in the absence of other etiologies.

• **Treatment:** Permanent pacing is the treatment of choice for any patient with symptomatic second or third degree heart block not due to some reversible factor. Consequently, withdrawal of these factors is the first step in treatment. Withdrawal of beta-blockers or calcium channel blockers when possible may reverse the A-V block occurring at the AV nodal level. The judicious and intermittent use of intravenous atropine can support the heart rate in the usually temporary A-V block associated with acute inferior myocardial infarction. If atropine does not reverse the A-V block, it will speed the default escape junctional rhythm. Temporary transvenous or even transcutaneous pacing will support the heart rate for resistant cases of A-V block complicating acute inferior infarction. This is especially the treatment of choice if the drug-resistant bradycardia resulting from A-V block encourages bursts of ventricular tachycardia. Most cases of A-V block complicating acute inferior infarction are self-limited and last only hours to days. Some cases, however, are so profound and slowly resolving that permanent pacing is the treatment of choice.

• **Pacing Modalities:** Dual chamber pacing is the mode of choice for patients free of chronic atrial fibrillation. This mode of pacing is increasingly the most widely used, even for patients without complete heart block. The trend toward selection dual chamber pacing reflects the fact that single chamber ventricular pacing provides only minimal support of heart rate to the disadvantage of left ven-

tricular function. Especially in the patient with loss of left ventricular compliance, single chamber ventricular pacing results in a syndrome of dyspnea, fatigue, and symptoms of low cardiac output. Exercise intolerance is also a cardinal feature of this syndrome appropriately named "pacemaker syndrome". The cardiac diseases most associated with loss of left ventricular compliance include coronary artery disease, systemic hypertension, aortic stenosis, and hypertrophic cardiomyopathy. There is also a strong association with a history of prior myocardial infarction. The etiology of this syndrome is the adverse hemodynamics associated with atrio-ventricular dissociation in patients with single chamber ventricular pacing. A-V dissociation results in loss of appropriate pre-systolic stretch thereby reducing stroke volume and cardiac output; dyspnea occurs as a result of simultaneous left ventricular and left atrial systole. Atrial contraction against a closed mitral valve raises pulmonary capillary wedge pressure and, at other times, atrioventricular dissociation results in mitral regurgitation. These circumstances are magnified if the patient with a single chamber ventricular pacemaker has intact ventriculo-atrial conduction. Patients with symptomatic bradyarrhythmias who remain in sinus rhythm have a higher incidence of atrial fibrillation subsequent to single chamber ventricular pacing compared to those treated with dual chamber pacing. The proposed reason for this difference is that left atrial pressure is chronically higher in patients with A-V dissociation, a circumstance avoided by dual chamber pacing. For all of these reasons, dual chamber pacing is now the pacing modality of choice for all patients with underlying sinus whether the pacing indication is sick sinus syndrome or heart block.

Use of rate-responsive pacing provides an additional advantage to pacemaker patients. This is a useful modality of pacing especially since many patients have either sinus node dysfunction or take drugs which inappropriately slow the sinus node. There are several physiologic sensors capable of rate modulation, the first of which was the activity sensor provided by the stimulation of a piezoelectric crystal fixed to the interior of a pacemaker can. Patient motion excites the crystal which emits an electric current proportional to the degree of motion. An algorithm in the pacemaker logic translates this generated current to an increase in heart rate. Other sensors include the accelerometer, also a motion sensing device, temperature, and oxygen saturation, all of which vary with activity. Use of other sensors to provide rate modulation is presently under study, including a QT interval sensor, and a sensor to estimate right ventricular dv/dt. Moreover, combining several sensors together may provide so-called "on line" evaluation of the patient's physiologic state and permit even finer tuning of the rate responsive algorithm.

The patient treated with permanent dual chamber pacing who has drug-refractory paroxysmal atrial fibrillation poses a special challenge to the clinician. Since the atrial lead will sense atrial fibrillatory activity and attempt to pace the ventricle at rapid rates limited only by the upper rate limit of the pacemaker, such patients should be paced dual chamber in the DDIR mode which only paces the atrium at the low activity-indicated-rate of the pacer. There is no atrial sensing in this mode, yet patients will still reap the benefit of rate responsive pacing with atrio-ventricular association if the intrinsic atrial rate in sinus rhythm is below the programmed low rate of the pacemaker or if there is intact or only impaired A-V conduction. Some pacemaker manufacturers address this problem by "mode switching" to VVIR mode when atrial impulses are sensed in the post ventricular atrial refractory period (PVARP), returning to DDDR mode when two consecutive atrial sensed events fall outside the PVARP.

CARDIAC PEARL

There is no question that the use of cardiac pacing in the treatment of selected patients with heart disease has represented one of the most significant advances of the past several decades. We are seeing patients who are comfortable and leading productive lives, who certainly would have died a number of years ago had it not been for cardiac pacemakers.
W. Proctor Harvey, M.D.

Syncope Due To Cardiac Tachyarrhythmias

Ventricular Tachycardia

• **Clinical Presentation:** Presyncope and syncope are the cardinal presenting symptoms of ventricular tachycardia. The patients may complain of palpitations prior to loss of consciousness. The hemodynamic embarrassment may be so severe as to cause seizure activity, which may obscure the proper diagnosis. A frequent presentation is palpitations with a wide QRS tachycardia in a patient with a prior history of coronary artery disease. Finally, many cases of hemodynamically embarrassing ventricular tachycardia present with sudden death, having had ventricular tachycardia

deteriorate to ventricular fibrillation. In this situation, the mechanism of syncope is obvious.

• **Mechanism:** The mechanism of syncope in patients with ventricular tachycardia is hypotension and cerebral hypoperfusion caused by the rapid rate; most patients will have underlying structural heart disease. In this setting, the rapid rate of the tachycardia is even less well-tolerated. The loss of atrial kick caused by the A-V dissociation of even slow ventricular tachycardia compromises stroke volume and cardiac output to the extent that symptomatic hypotension is the rule even if frank syncope does not occur.

• **Diagnosis:** There are several clinical settings where syncope or presyncope is likely related to ventricular tachycardia. Classifying these settings beforehand can aid in the orderly approach to diagnosis. Briefly, these settings are coronary artery disease, dilated non-ischemic cardiomyopathy, hypertrophic cardiomyopathy, and ventricular tachycardia in the absence of structural heart disease. A final category is syncope due to drug induced ventricular tachycardia.

• **Coronary Artery Disease:** The association of coronary artery disease with ventricular tachycardia is so strong that this rhythm disturbance is the most likely diagnosis for the coronary disease patient with syncope. In addition, the diagnosis of first choice in a coronary artery disease patient presenting with a wide QRS tachycardia is ventricular tachycardia. Furthermore, presyncope plus non-sustained ventricular tachycardia (NSVT) is the harbinger of sustained ventricular tachycardia, with risk of sudden death in the setting of coronary artery disease. Bearing the serious consequence of misdiagnosis in mind, it is of obvious importance to recognize this association and to be respectful of the potential for this arrhythmia in this population presenting with syncope or presyncope. Too often, the coronary artery disease patient with presyncope submits to costly and inappropriate neurologic evaluation when the first diagnostic consideration should be a dangerous rhythm disturbance.

When the patient with coronary artery disease presents with presyncope, a vigorous search for ventricular tachycardia should ensue. With prolonged monitoring in hospital, such a patient may demonstrate nonsustained runs of ventricular tachycardia. If ambient ectopy is sparse, prolonged monitoring may be unrevealing and proper diagnosis will require more provocative testing. These include the signal averaged electrocardiogram (SAECG), which may demonstrate delayed low amplitude cardiac electrical activity following the end of the surface QRS. In patients with a recent myocardial infarction, a low ejection fraction, and nonsustained ventricular tachycardia in the post myocardial infarction period, the finding of late potentials has positive predictive association with inducible ventricular tachycardia. Even in the absence of demonstrable late potentials, unexplained syncope in the coronary disease patient should suggest a lethal ventricular arrhythmia. Ultimately, the diagnostic evaluation of unexplained syncope in the coronary artery disease patient includes an evaluation of coronary artery anatomy, cardiac function, and potential for inducible ventricular arrhythmia. Thus, all such patients should undergo cardiac catheterization with left ventricular cineangiography, and invasive cardiac electrophysiologic study (EPS). Nuclear stress testing will provide evidence of inducible ischemia. If present, an ischemic episode may be the cause of the ventricular tachycardia ensuing in a syncopal episode. If inducible ischemia proves to be the cause of ventricular arrhythmia such patients should not undergo EPS until after the treatment of ischemia.

CARDIAC PEARL

Listen over the neck in every patient. A physician in his sixties had several episodes of syncope. He had a history of a previous myocardial infarction. Our first thought was that a ventricular arrhythmia, transient tachycardia, or fibrillation would explain the syncope. Instead, on physical examination a loud continuous murmur was heard over both carotid arteries and each proved to be 90% occluded. Endarterectomy solved this problem. The lesson we learned: Listen over the neck in every patient.

The figure illustrates how valuable information can be quickly obtained by listening over the neck. The bell chest piece should be used in order to make an air seal; this particularly applies to listening over the suprasternal notch (Figures A, B and C).

W. Proctor Harvey, M.D.

• **Dilated Non-ischemic Cardiomyopathy:** The symptom of syncope or presyncope in patients who have no coronary disease, but who have left ventricular dysfunction (such as dilated non-ischemic cardiomyopathy) should again suggest the diagnosis of ventricular tachycardia. Such patients ordinarily first have left ventricular dysfunction defined by noninvasive studies followed by invasive confirmation of normal coronary arteries with cardiac catheterization and coronary angiography. Signal averaged electrocardiography is of little use since it is less sensitive as a marker for ventricular tachycardia in this group. Despite the lower sensitivity of invasive cardiac electrophysiologic study in these patients (only 60% of known ventricular tachycardia patients with non-ischemic dilated cardiomyopathy will have inducible ventricular tachycardia with EPS), such study can be of great assistance in diagnosis and management when positive.

• **Hypertrophic Cardiomyopathy:** Syncope or presyncope in patients with hypertrophic cardiomyopathy requires an aggressive diagnostic approach.

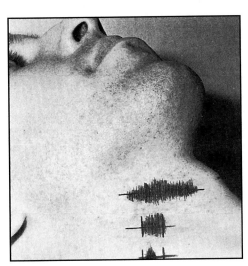

Fig A: Type of murmurs (bruits) heard in the neck, not including innocent venous hum: Top: Continuous murmur of obstruction. Middle: Carotid artery occlusion of mild to moderate degree. Lower: Short early to mid (innocent) systolic murmur heard in supraclavicular fossa bilaterally.

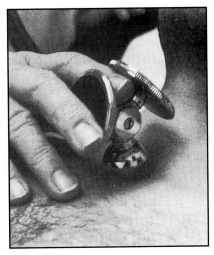

Fig B: Use the bell of the stethoscope to listen over the suprasternal notch.

687

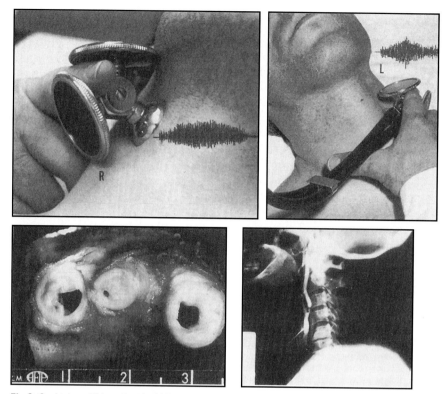

Fig C: Occlusion - This patient had bilateral carotid artery occlusion producing a continuous murmur on both sides. R = right neck, L = left neck. Note pathology of carotid artery occlusive disease and carotid arteriogram demonstrating occlusion.

Irrespective of whether or not obstruction is present in patients with this familial disease, syncope or presyncope is usually due to ventricular tachycardia. Considering that sudden death is common in this group of patients, especially if there is a history of a first degree relative with hypertrophic cardiomyopathy and sudden death, aggressive diagnosis and treatment is necessary. Such patients should have diagnostic cardiac catheterization, extensive arrhythmia monitoring, and invasive EPS. Inducible ventricular tachycardia provides a target for potential drug therapy, but a negative EPS does not rule out the possibility of ventricular tachycardia as a cause of syncope and presyncope.

• **Syncope From Ventricular Tachycardia in Absence of Structural Heart Disease:** Patients without a prior history of coronary artery disease presenting with unexplained syncope will require a similar diagnostic approach with some modifications. Ordinarily, a young patient with syncope or presyncope and a low probability of coronary disease should first undergo exercise testing and evaluation of cardiac function noninvasively. Exercise-induced ventricular tachycardia due to triggered automaticity may be the cause of syncope or presyncope in this group. If this test provokes ventricular tachycardia, the patient should undergo diag-

nostic cardiac catheterization and coronary angiography, possibly with endomyocardial biopsy absolutely to exclude structural heart disease. Although exercise-induced ventricular tachycardia itself may be a target for therapy, invasive EPS provides additional helpful information such as the location of the arrhythmogenic focus and its inducibility by programmed stimulation or burst pacing. In cases of inducible tachycardia, EPS provides an opportunity to assess antitachycardia pacing techniques for the termination of arrhythmia. EPS also provides an opportunity to assess antiarrhythmic drug therapy in the most controlled and safest setting. Such an assessment includes not only administration of antiarrhythmic agents, but testing of drug efficacy against the beta-adrenergic stimulation of isoproterenol.

• **Syncope From Q-T Interval Prolongation-Induced Ventricular Tachycardia:** This usually familial syndrome is the result of unequal cervical sympathetic inputs to the heart, resulting in widely divergent repolarization states throughout the heart. *Torsades de pointes* occurs as a result and patients with this syndrome succumb early in life. The surface ECG may show Q-T interval prolongation, but many patients will have normal resting tracings with Q-T interval prolongation provoked with sympathetic stimulation (exercise, adrenalin) or parasympathetic withdrawal (atropine administration). Syncope or ventricular tachycardia in any young patient without overt heart disease should suggest this diagnosis.

• **Syncope From Drug-Induced Ventricular Tachycardia:** Ventricular tachycardia associated with syncope may be the result of the proarrhythmic effect of drugs administered for treatment of other forms of arrhythmia. A classic circumstance is the patient with atrial fibrillation who is given quinidine in whom *Torsades de pointes* occurs as an idiosyncratic reaction. Virtually all antiarrhythmic agents share the potential for the aggravation of established arrhythmias or the creation of new and more dangerous arrhythmias. The precise incidence of this problem is unknown but several studies estimate the risk at 5% to 25% for the commonly used agents. The potential for proarrhythmia of these drugs makes out-patient, unmonitored administration ill-advised. It is now a standard of care to hospitalize and perform electrocardiographic monitoring for all patients while new antiarrhythmic therapy is initiated.

CARDIAC PEARL

Remember that antiarrhythmic drugs can also be pro-arrhythmic, and ironically produce the same fatal arrhythmia that one is trying to prevent.

Therefore, careful observation and follow-up after initiation of a new antiarrhythmic drug is essential. The possibility of a pro-arrhythmia effect of a drug is not appreciated as well as it should be.

The following is a case in point, which I only learned about recently:

A friend, who is in his late 70's, developed atrial fibrillation. He was anticoagulated as a precaution to prevent emboli coincident or following reversion to normal sinus rhythm. Wisely, he was admitted to the hospital for

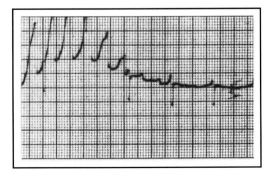

Fig A: Torsades de pointes.

attempt at medical conversion with quinidine before resorting to electroconversion. On quinidine, he is reported to have developed "torsades de pointes" ventricular arrhythmia and cardiac arrest (Figure A). Fortunately he was immediately and successfully resuscitated.

This is a reminder to us that the drug we use to control arrhythmias can also cause them. It is, of course, important that the possibility of this adverse, sometimes very serious, effect be looked for. This is currently apropos, because many newer drugs are being introduced and advocated for treatment of arrhythmias.

W. Proctor Harvey, M.D.

Cardio-active drugs given in toxic amounts also may result in syncope due to ventricular tachycardia. The classic example of this is ventricular tachycardia caused by digitalis intoxication. The hallmarks include the obvious history of administration of digitalis glycosides, and a common setting is the elderly patient with renal impairment whose excretion of digitalis is compromised. Another common setting is concurrent administration of digitalis with other antiarrhythmic agents which interact to raise digitalis levels. These drugs include quinidine, verapamil, cardizem, and amiodarone. The diagnosis of digitalis intoxication rests strongly on the patient's drug history, age and renal status. Electrocardiographic monitoring may detect other classic digitalis toxic arrhythmias besides ventricular tachycardia such as accelerated idioventricular rhythm, complete heart block, junctional tachycardia with A-V dissociation, and atrial tachycardia with block.

Drugs which by themselves may have no primary cardiac electrophysiologic effect may under certain circumstances cause ventricular tachycardia and syncope. Recent reports detailed use of terfenidine in concert with erythromycin, leading to decreased terfenidine excretion, resulting in high serum levels. Life-threatening arrhythmias resulted from the primary effect of extremely high levels of terfenidine on ventricular repolarization causing polymorphous ventricular tachycardia. Other drugs which may cause disturbances of repolarization and lead to ventricular tachycardia and syncope include the phenothiazines, and the tricyclic antidepressants.

• **Treatment:** Treatment of syncope and presyncope due to ventricular tachycardia ranges the gamut, from withdrawal of causative drug therapy to implantation of the internal cardioverter defibrillator. The initial steps in therapy are to withdraw

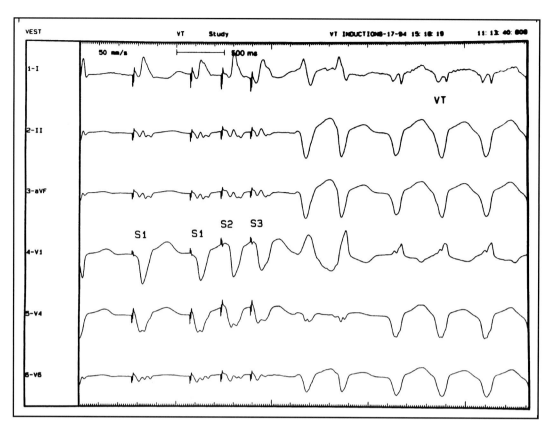

Figure 7. Electrophysiologic induction of monomorphic ventricular tachycardia using programmed stimulation.

reversible factors; thus, in patients with coronary artery disease, relief of ischemia is paramount. For those coronary disease patients whose syncope is mediated by ischemia, anti-ischemic drug therapy, coronary angioplasty or coronary artery bypass surgery should precede cardiac electrophysiologic evaluation since no antiarrhythmic measures will be effective in the face of a variable ischemic milieu. If coronary bypass is performed, the surgeon and electrophysiologist should place epicardial defibrillation patches and assure adequate defibrillation thresholds at the conclusion of bypass surgery in anticipation of the potential need for implantation of an internal cardioverter-defibrillator (ICD). Following recovery from surgery, the cardiac patient should undergo a pre-discharge invasive cardiac electrophysiologic evaluation. With the protection afforded by the surgical relief of ischemia, such a provocative test is safe, associated with negligible mortality. If no arrhythmia is inducible, one concludes that the ventricular tachycardia was ischemia-mediated and no further therapy is warranted. The post coronary bypass induction of ventricular tachycardia at EPS, however, predicts recurrence of VT in the future and one proceeds as in the patient with no reversible causative factor for syncope due to ventricular tachycardia.

In patients whose ventricular tachycardia is not due to reversible factors, the primary step in treatment is to establish a target for therapy. The target most commonly developed is invasively-induced ventricular tachycardia at the time of EPS. Cardiac electrophysiologic study establishes this by the technique of programmed stimulation (Figure 7). Arrhythmia so-induced has the same characteristics as the naturally-occurring arrhythmia with respect to morphology. Induction of ventricular tachycardia during a baseline EPS study in the absence of antiarrhythmic agents is usually a reproducible phenomenon especially in the coronary artery disease group of patients. After treatment with antiarrhythmic drug therapy, the subsequent conversion of a positive EPS (inducible ventricular tachycardia) to a negative test (inability to induce ventricular tachycardia) predicts that drug's efficacy in preventing future episodes if all else remains constant and the patient remains faithful to his drug regimen.

Such a drug challenge may occur in the EPS laboratory at the time of the baseline study. The initial drug usually tested is procainamide, primarily because there is an intravenous preparation of this drug which is safe to administer under these conditions and which can achieve therapeutic levels quickly. If such a challenge prevents induction of VT, treatment with oral procainamide in a dose to achieve therapeutic levels will protect the patient from recurrent ventricular tachycardia. If such a

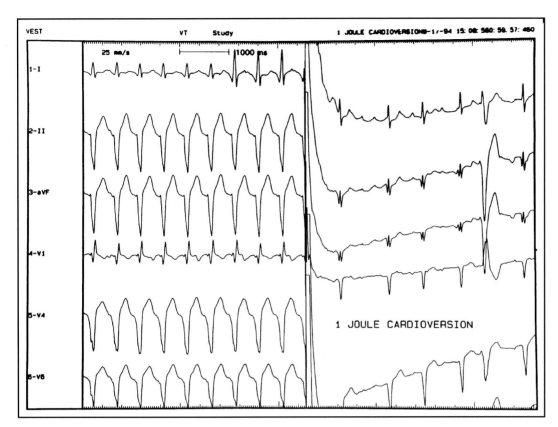

25 mm/s   1000 ms

1-I

2-II

3-aVF

4-V1

5-V4

6-V6

1 JOULE CARDIOVERSION

Figure 8. Cardioversion from ventricular tachycardia using one joule delivered by an implantable cardioverter/defibrillator.

challenge fails to prevent ventricular tachycardia induction, a second drug such as lidocaine or Inderal may be added, again at the initial EPS. If no drug or drug combination succeeds in preventing induction of ventricular tachycardia at the initial trial, the syncope patient with ventricular tachycardia has two choices. These include a trial of other drugs with only an oral preparation (quinidine, propafenone, sotalol, or amiodarone) and retesting after reaching a steady state, or implantation of an internal cardioverter-defibrillator. If the oral drug trial succeeds in preventing induction of ventricular tachycardia, that regimen should be continued in the expectation of at least an 80% chance of protection against recurrent ventricular tachycardia and syncope in the coming year (Figure 8). If the oral drug trial fails to prevent ventricular tachycardia induction on a subsequent EPS, most electrophysiologists would recommend implantation of a defibrillator tailored to the arrhythmia's characteristics and the patient's clinical profile. One would elect this route in the anticipation that failure of drug therapy likely will result in a ventricular tachycardia recurrence rate of approximately 60% in the next 12 months. Therapy is selected for the patient in this empiric manner.

Of largely historic interest now is the surgical removal of the arrhythmogenic focus during cardiopulmonary bypass, often with concomitant coronary or valvular surgery. Successful surgery requires a reliably inducible and stable monomorphic arrhythmia. Intraoperative mapping at normothermia while on cardio-pulmonary bypass identifies the site of the reentrant ventricular arrhythmia. A resection of the subendocardium at this point removes the focus and provides success at arrhythmia control in the majority of patients. This therapy for drug-refractory ventricular tachycardia is little used presently largely because of the high operative mortality compared to defibrillator therapy. In clinical use since the mid 1980s, transcatheter high energy shock ablative therapy for the treatment of drug-refractory ventricular tachycardia remains an option for patients with monomorphic ventricular tachycardia from a single focus. Mapping of the tachycardia in the electrophysiology laboratory establishes the earliest endocardial electrogram which precedes the surface appearance of the QRS and delivery of 200 joules to 300 joules through the mapping catheter to that site follows; the intense electrical field thus generated disrupts cell membranes and will destroy the cells responsible for a critical portion of the reentry circuit necessary for perpetuation of the tachycardia. Success rates depend upon precise mapping and on the fact that only a single tachycardia morphology is present. The procedure is associated with relatively low morbidity and mortality, yet requires considerable sophistication in equipment and expertise. Thus, this technique is not in widespread use today.

Under study at present is the use of radio frequency ablation for treatment of drug refractory ventricular tachycardia due to coronary artery disease. In a fashion similar to high energy shock ablation, intracardiac mapping of the ventricle identifies the site of earliest endocardial activation. Delivery of radiofrequency energy to this site creates thermal injury, raising the tissue temperature to 70 degrees to 100 degrees centigrade and destroying the neighboring tissue. Initial success rates are low and probably relate to the limited area of damage created by this ablative technique. Further research is active in this area because of the relative safety of radio frequency ablative therapy. A subset of patients with syncope and ventricular tachycardia will have no inducible arrhythmia target for therapy. This is rare in the group of patients with coronary artery disease, but it is relatively common for patients with idiopathic dilated cardiomyopathy or hypertrophic cardiomyopathy. In this circumstance, an EPS which cannot reproduce the clinical arrhythmia gives scant comfort and, knowing the recurrence rate of the tachyarrhythmia is at least 20% to 30% over the next 12 months in this population of patients, there can be no expectation that drug therapy will be successful in treatment and protection in the absence of a reproducible target.

Because of the high recurrence rate, patients in this category should receive ICD therapy, for that is the only therapy which will treat expected recurrences. Furthermore, the cost of chronic drug therapy, the high incidence of side effects and drug intolerance, and the degree to which patients lack the ability to comply with drug regimens all conspire to make a pharmacologic approach less desirable than device therapy in general. This puts ICD therapy in a more favorable light as an option for syncope due to ventricular tachycardia in selected patients.

Ventricular Fibrillation

• **Clinical Presentation:** Sudden loss of consciousness with seizure activity, and sudden death is the result of ventricular fibrillation. If left untreated, this arrhythmia uniformly results in mortality. Survival from this arrhythmia depends entirely on successful and timely resuscitation. Some patients will report antecedent palpitations for minutes prior to loss of consciousness which implies the initial rhythm is ventricular tachycardia with little hemodynamic compromise. Most typically, coronary artery disease patients will com-

prise the majority in this group, and acute ischemia is a common presenting clinical setting. Thus, patients will frequently have an antecedent history of angina, myocardial infarction, and congestive heart failure. Additionally, some coronary artery disease patients will present with acute myocardial infarction and subsequently succumb to sudden death from ventricular fibrillation. Another subset of patients with sudden death from ventricular fibrillation will have no overt heart disease. If survival from this arrhythmia occurs, sudden death is by definition "aborted".

• **Mechanism:** Ventricular fibrillation (VF) can occur in the electrically unstable setting of acute ischemia with or without infarction. Ischemia creates great heterogeneity of repolarization in the heart; this then creates a ripe setting for VF. Hemodynamically unstable ventricular tachycardia is another mechanism by which a patient may suffer VF by exacerbating ischemia. As with ventricular tachycardia, VF may be the result of an idiosyncratic response to an antiarrhythmic agent or to other drugs which affect repolarization. Another class of patient susceptible to VF is the patient with the congenital QT prolongation syndrome. In this category of patient, heterogeneity of repolarization is the genesis of VF, often unmasked by adrenergic stress.

• **Diagnosis:** Successful resuscitation implies correct diagnosis of ventricular fibrillation. A family history of premature death and a history of a "seizure" disorder in a young patient may be the only clue to the congenital QT interval syndrome as cause of sudden death. The idiosyncratic antiarrhythmic drug-induced form of VF is the only one which may be self-limited and a drug history is of obvious importance in diagnosis.

• **Treatment:** For the coronary artery disease patient with VF, the most important question is whether or not VF was accompanied by evidence of myocardial infarction. If infarction is the clinical setting for VF, the annual recurrence of VF is only on the order of 2% to 3% and treatment of the underlying coronary artery disease is the correct approach. This includes cardiac catheterization with anti-ischemic drug therapy, coronary artery bypass surgery, or coronary angioplasty. After control of ischemia, cardiac electrophysiologic study will provide a meaningful assessment of the arrhythmia potential of the patient. An EPS that does not induce any arrhythmia in such a circumstance is comforting and no therapy short of that directed toward ischemia is warranted. If a post-ischemia therapy EPS induces ventricular tachycardia, recurrent arrhythmia is likely to occur and the patient will require additional primary anti-arrhythmic therapy. EPS-guided empiric therapy detailed above is the recommended course. Initiation of ventricular fibrillation at the time of an EPS performed in this setting is regrettable and not considered an endpoint upon which clinical decisions should be made. The one exception to this is the patient with residual inducible ischemia following therapy. Since no anti-ischemic regimen can be expected to protect the patient against this confounding variable in the arrhythmia patient, ICD therapy is most appropriate in this circumstance. If there is no myocardial necrosis associated with VF even in the presence of coronary artery disease, the clinician pursues a somewhat different therapeutic approach. First, a work-up of the background of heart disease is appropriate again including cardiac catheterization with coronary angiography and measures of ventricular function and an assessment of inducible ischemia. If there is no inducible ischemia, or if there is no coronary artery disease, ICD therapy is the treatment of choice because of the expected 20% to 30% recurrence rate of ventricular fibrillation in the next year. If inducible ischemia is present and playing a role in the possibility of sudden death, treatment of ischemia should precede any other therapy. Post-ischemia treatment, the clinician should pursue EPS-guided therapy.

Considerations in Selection of Patients for ICD Therapy

Indications

The North American Society of Pacing and Electrophysiology (NASPE), The American Heart Association, and The American College of Cardiology's consensus conference established the generally accepted indications for ICD implantation which are divided into three classes as follows: (Table 1).

Class I: ICD therapy is indicated based upon the consensus.

Class II: ICD therapy is an option but consensus does not exist.

Class III: ICD therapy is generally not justified.

• **Choice of Specific Devices:** Several factors govern the choice of a specific ICD. All implanted devices must have the ability to revert ventricular fibrillation with predictability. This is established at the time of implantation by testing of defibrillation thresholds by the repeated induction of ventricular fibrillation and the application of a defibrillating charge by an external device. The assurance of the ability to defibrillate is necessary even for

---

TABLE 1
Guidelines For ICD Implantation

CLASS I

1. Patients with sustained ventricular tachycardia or ventricular fibrillation in whom EPS cannot be used to predict the efficacy of pharmacologic therapy.
2. Recurrent spontaneous ventricular tachycardia and/or fibrillation despite antiarrhythmic drug therapy.
3. Spontaneous ventricular tachycardia or fibrillation in a patient with drug intolerance or non-compliance.
4. Persistently EPS inducible ventricular arrhythmia despite all other therapies.

CLASS II

1. Syncope of uncertain etiology in a patient with inducible ventricular tachycardia or fibrillation refractory to drug therapy or with therapy limited by inefficacy, intolerance or noncompliance.

CLASS III

1. Sustained ventricular tachycardia or fibrillation in the setting of acute ischemia, infarction, adverse drug effect or other reversible cause.
2. Recurrent syncope of undetermined etiology in a patient with no identifiable or inducible ventricular arrhythmia.
3. Incessant ventricular arrhythmia.
4. Ventricular fibrillation due directly to preexcitation and atrial fibrillation.
5. Medical, surgical, or psychiatric contraindications.

---

the patient with only monomorphic ventricular tachycardia and no history of ventricular fibrillation because of the possibility that either low energy cardioversion or anti-tachycardia pacing will accelerate ventricular tachycardia to ventricular fibrillation. After this requirement is met, other considerations apply.

The patient with only ventricular fibrillation and no other inducible arrhythmia will require a device capable only of defibrillation at a minimum. The patient with inducible ventricular tachycardia capable of reversion to normal rhythm with anti-tachycardia pacing should receive a device capable of both variable energy cardioversion and anti-tachycardia pacing. Third generation defibrillators almost always possess the ability to provide back-up VVI bradycardia pacing (Figure 9). While it is attractive to believe that the ventricular fibrillation patient with severe bradycardia can be adequately treated with a defibrillator with bradycardia pacing, in reality the truly pacemaker-dependent patient does not prosper with VVI pacing alone. Most if not all of the patients in this category have cardiac dysfunction which makes dual chamber pacing a desirable mode, an option not yet available

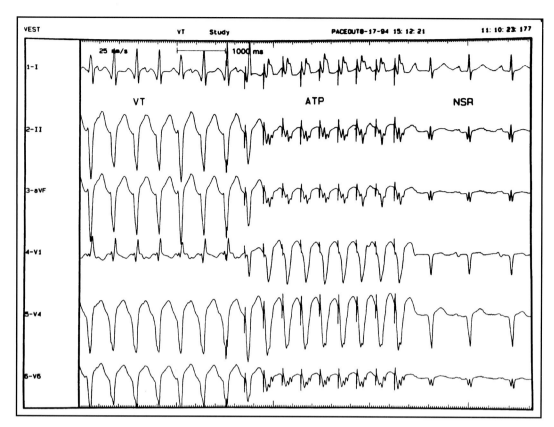

Figure 9. Anti-tachycardia pacing (ATP) delivered by an implantable cardio-verter/defibrillator terminates ventricular tachycardia to sinus rhythm.

in the current generation of defibrillators. Furthermore, most clinicians recognize the superiority of rate-responsive pacing in these patients and this option is also not yet available in the current generation of ICDs. Thus, most patients requiring long-term pacing will be better served by the implantation of a separate dual-chamber, rate-responsive pacemaker in addition to the ICD.

Implantation of a separate pacemaker in a patient with an implanted ICD poses several problems. The pacemaker, whose discharge measures from 2.5 volts to 5.0 volts or greater, may easily be sensed by the ICD whose sense amplifier is set to recognize electrical signals as low as 0.3 mv or less. The ICD may thus sense the pacer output as well as the resulting QRS. Double sensing by the ICD may occur and result in double counting and triggering of an inappropriate ICD discharge. Use of bipolar pacers, the implantation of pacing leads at a site remote from the ICD rate-sensing leads, and careful intra-operative evaluation of the potential of pacemaker-ICD cross-talk will all serve to avoid this adverse interaction.

• **Electrode Configuration:** Originally, implantation of an ICD required the epicardial placement of defibrillating mesh patches by way of a thoracotomy. The accepted mortality for this procedure is approximately 2% since most patients have low ejection fractions and compounding risk

factors, such as congestive heart failure, low cardiac output, and active ischemia. While statistics are not yet clearly available, the risk of the procedure is probably far less with the use of the nonthoracotomy, endocardial defibrillating lead implantation. Operative times are shorter, recovery is more rapid, and discharge from the hospital is more timely than with the thoracotomy approach. With judicious placement of endocardial defibrillating leads and the use of an additional subcutaneous patch where needed to lower defibrillation thresholds, the success rate for conventional monophasic defibrillators approaches 90%. The advent of biphasic shock waveforms has the advantage of lowering the defibrillation threshold by at least 30% to 50% and results in a nearly 100% endocardial implantation success rate. Thus, implantation of an ICD with biphasic waveforms and an endocardial shocking lead(s) is the standard of care for patients requiring ICD therapy, with few exceptions. Furthermore, the nonthoracotomy lead implantation technique should have a much lower morbidity and mortality than heretofore possible with standard thoracotomy techniques for implantation (Figure 10).

• **Drug vs Device Therapy:** Several factors influence the choice of device therapy over drug therapy for ventricular tachycardia, including antiarrhythmic drug intolerance (drug-induced

694

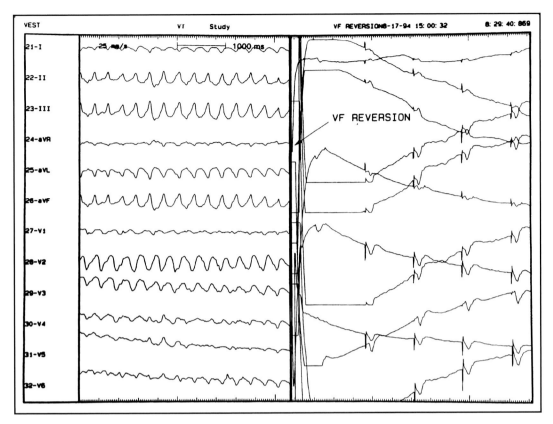

Figure 10. Defibrillation to sinus rhythm occurs using a biphasic 10 joule shock delivered by an implantable cardioverter/defibrillator.

lupus erythematosus or thrombocytopenia, for example), drug refractoriness (the classic indication), an unstable disease substrate (inoperable coronary disease with recurrent ischemia), and patient lack of compliance. When used appropriately with proper programming and follow-up of the device, as well as assiduous management of confounding factors such as congestive heart failure and myocardial ischemia, the patient with a defibrillator will live a relatively unrestricted lifestyle. Many such patients, however, also require associated antiarrhythmic therapy to reduce the frequency of their episodes of ventricular tachycardia. After implantation of an ICD, the addition of antiarrhythmic therapy will require an assessment of the effect of drug therapy upon the rate of the induced tachycardia since virtually all antiarrhythmic therapy will have some such effect requiring reprogramming of the device. Furthermore, antiarrhythmic therapy may elevate the energy requirement for successful defibrillation. It is therefore routine to repeat an EPS after reaching a steady state of antiarrhythmic drug therapy in ICD patients not only to asses the effect of drug therapy on tachycardia rate, but also to verify that defibrillation thresholds have not risen as a drug effect.

Since patients are never static in their clinical profile, the implanted defibrillator should be as versatile and adaptable as possible in order to provide appropriate therapies for the many changing clinical situations. The patient with post-shock symptomatic pauses who has a simple defibrillator without back-up pacing may need an additional pacemaker or a new device with the capacity for bradycardia pacing. The patient whose previously fast VT slows to a rate with the potential for termination by antitachycardia pacing should have that option available without the need for implantation of a new device. Thus, most clinicians recommend ICD therapy with a device sophisticated enough to adapt to the several potential changes in the patient's clinical status.

CARDIAC PEARL

One has to be impressed with the many significant advances that have occurred as well as those that are presently evolving concerning the understanding and management of ventricular arrhythmias and sudden death.

It is obvious that the problem is not a simple one. It is also apparent that a number of serious, often fatal arrhythmias that formerly were untreatable are now being successfully managed.

The amount of research on these arrhythmias is fortunately great and predictably will continue to result in even better management and prevention in the future. The research

and patient application of both drugs plus the advances of treatment by implantable devices, pacemakers and surgery give solid support to the fact that prevention and treatment of ventricular arrhythmias (and of course, sudden death) will be better and better.

W. Proctor Harvey, M.D.

Selected Reading

1. Akhtar M, Jazayeri M, Sra J: Cardiovascular causes of syncope:identifying and controlling trigger mechanisms. *Postgrad Med* 8: (2) 87-94; 1991.

2. Akinboboye OO, Brown EJ Jr, Queirroz R et al: Recurrent pulmonary embolism with second-degree atrioventricular block and near-syncope. *AHJ* 9:126: 731-732; 1993.

3. Crane JK, Shih HT: Syncope and cardiac arrhythmia due to an interaction between itraconazole and terfenadine. *AJM* 10:95 (4) 445-446; 1993.

4. Denniss AR, Ross DL, Richards DA et al: Electrophysiologic studies in patients with unexplained syncope. *Int J Card* 5: 35 (2): 211-217; 1992.

5. Dilsizian V, Bonow RO, Epstein SE et al: Myocardial ischemia detected by thallium scintigraphy is frequently related to cardiac arrest and syncope in young patients with hypertrophic cardiomyopathy. *JACC* 9:22: (3) 805-807; 1993.

6. Gilligan DM, Nihoyannopoulos P, Chan WL et al: Investigation of a hemodynamic basis for syncope in hypertrophic cardiomyopathy. Use of a head-up tilt test. *Circ* 6:85 (9) 2140-2148; 1992.

7. Hopson JR, Rea RF, Kienzle MG: Alterations in reflex function contributing to syncope: orthostatic hypotension, carotid sinus hypersensitivity and drug-induced dysfunction. *Herz* 6:18 (3) 164-175; 1993.

8. Kapoor W: Evaluation and management of the patient with syncope. *JAMA* 11/22: (18) 2553-2560; 1992.

9. Lehman MH, Saksena S: Implantable cardioverter defibrillators in cardiovascular practice: report of the policy conference of the North American Society of Pacing and Electrophysiology. *PACE* 14: 969; 1991.

10. Linzer M, Prystowsky EN, Divine GW et al: Predicting outcomes of electrophysiologic studies of patients with unexplained syncope: preliminary validation of a derived model. *J Gen Int Med* 3: 6 (2): 113-120; 1991.

11. Moazez F, Peter T, Simonson J et al: Syncope of unknown origin: clinical, noninvasive, and electrophysiologic determinants of arrhythmia induction and symptom recurrence during long-term follow-up. *AHJ* 1:121: 81-88; 1991.

12. Sra JS, Anderson AJ, Sheikh AH et al: Unexplained syncope evaluated by electrophysiologic studies and head-up tilt testing. *Ann Int Med* 6/15: 114 (12): 1013-1019; 1991.

13. Sra JS, Jazayeri MR, Avitall B et al: Comparison of cardiac pacing with drug therapy in the treatment of neurocardiogenic (vasovagal) syncope with bradycardia or asystole. *NEJM* 4/15: 328 (15) 1085-1090; 1993.

14. Sra JS, Murthy V, Natale A et al: Circulatory and catecholamine changes during head-up tilt testing of neurocardiogenic (vasovagal) syncope. *AJC* 1: 73 (1) 33-37; 1994.

15. Wilmshurst PT, Willicombe PR, Webb-Peploe MM et al: Effect of aortic valve replacement on syncope in patients with aortic stenosis. *BHJ* 12: 70 (6) 542-543; 1993.

16. Winkle RA, Mead RH, Ruder MA et al: Long-term outcome with the automatic implantable cardioverter-defibrillator. *JACC* 5:13 (6) 1353-1361; 1989.

CHAPTER 30

Sudden Cardiac Death: Noninvasive Risk Stratification with Special Emphasis on Heart Rate Variability

Donald H. Singer, M.D.

Paroxysmal dysrhythmias, principally ventricular tachyarrhythmias, represent the leading cause of sudden death in the western world. In the U.S., such disturbances claim about 400,000 lives annually, usually in the setting of chronic coronary disease. This total represents approximately 50% of all cardiovascular deaths. Death due to this cause, designated "sudden cardiac death" (SCD), usually strikes in the prime of life, frequently without prior warning. In up to 25% of cases, SCD is the first manifestation of severe underlying heart (coronary) disease. Mortality rates for the initial episode of out-of-hospital cardiac arrest are very high. In addition, untreated or empirically-treated survivors of the initial event have a 30%-40% risk of dying during the following year. Economic and social costs are correspondingly high. Early, preferably noninvasive, identification of patients at high risk of SCD for purposes of risk factor modification is a key need.

Risk Factors for Sudden Cardiac Death

Current pathophysiologic models presume that occurrence of SCD represents an interaction between two sets of conditions: 1) an abnormal anatomic substrate and 2) functional disturbances, often transient, which serve to electrically destabilize the myocardium and trigger onset of ventricular tachyarrhythmias and fibrillation. Substrate abnormalities include myocardial scarring associated with coronary artery disease and cardiomyopathies, ventricular hypertrophy, A-V nodal

bypass tracts, and conduction system disease. The occurrence of partially depolarized cells in ischemic and diseased hearts, with resultant localized delays in, and fragmentation of, excitation and conduction, represents still another type of abnormal substrate. Potential triggering events are represented by such conditions as acute ischemic/reperfusion injury, early premature beats (R-on-T phenomenon), abrupt rate increases, electrolyte imbalance, drug toxicity and fluctuations in autonomic balance. Many other examples could be cited.

Numerous investigators have sought to identify reliable predictors of SCD from among these and other pathophysiologic factors. Many have been proposed, but none have proven sufficiently specific or reliable. This probably reflects the fact that development of malignant ventricular dysrhythmias is undoubtedly due to multiple causes. In addition, these factors are nonspecific and may not provide adequate insight into the unique mechanism underlying SCD in any given individual. The most widely cited follow.

Myocardial Damage/Dysfunction

In 1975, Cobb and colleagues pointed out the importance of myocardial damage and ventricular dysfunction manifested respectively by wall motion abnormalities/left ventricular aneurysm and low (< 40%) ejection fraction, as risk factors for SCD. Associations between SCD and the occurrence of multi-vessel obstructive coronary disease also were noted. The predictive utility of these factors with respect to risk of SCD has been reaffirmed many times. Anatomic studies have confirmed that chronic occlusive coronary disease represents the dominant underlying pathology in SCD patients. In one large study, (Perper and colleagues, 1975) stenosis > 75% was found in three or four major vessels in 61% of 169 hearts from SCD patients. In contrast, 24% of specimens had only one or no vessels with stenosis > 75%. Healed myocardial infarction was correspondingly very common in SCD patients, occurring in 40 to > 70% of autopsies (Newman and colleagues, 1982).

Hypertrophic ventricular myocardium also has been identified as an independent risk factor for SCD. Associations between SCD and hypertrophy have been reported for patients with hypertensive and valvular heart disease, hypertrophic cardiomyopathy, pulmonary hypertension, and right ventricular overload states secondary to congenital heart disease. Indeed, some workers have suggested that patients with hypertrophic myocardium are at particular risk of arrhythmic death. However, relationships to left ventricular dysfunction and other factors need to be clarified.

Late Potentials

Development of the signal averaged electrocardiogram, based on techniques similar to those employed for detection at the body surface of His bundle and other specialized cardiac tissue potentials, has focused interest on occurrence of late potentials as a risk factor for ventricular tachycardia and SCD. Late potentials are high frequency, low amplitude (1 to 2 microvolts) deflections which occur immediately following completion of the QRS complex. They are not readily apparent in the standard body surface electrocardiogram because the signal-to-noise ratio of conventional ECG machines does not permit distinctions between late potentials and noise, i.e., electrical activity from non-cardiac sources, such as muscle potentials. Signals are recorded using orthogonal XYZ leads, digitized, averaged, and passed through a bidirectional filter to minimize artifacts. The noise, which is completely random, is largely cancelled out by the averaging of many, usually 250 to 350, QRS complexes. This, together with filtering and other methods of noise reduction, permits detection of even very low amplitude cardiac signals.

Late potentials are thought to reflect impulse spread in regions of delayed and fragmented excitation and conduction in ischemic and diseased myocardium, including particularly the boundary zones about myocardial infarcts. Since such conditions are thought to predispose to reentry, findings of late potentials suggest a propensity to develop ventricular tachyarrhythmias/fibrillation. Although the implications of late potentials are still controversial, their absence appears to be associated with a lower risk of ventricular tachycardia, at least in the post myocardial infarction population and possibly also in patients with non-ischemic cardiomyopathy. Insofar as ventricular fibrillation and SCD are concerned, late potentials appear to be less predictive than for ventricular tachycardia. Correction of the orthogonal leads for the effects of residual noise by visual overreading techniques may improve predictive value. Further clarification is required.

Ventricular Ectopy

Frequency and complexity of ventricular ectopy, usually defined from 24-hour Holter monitoring recordings, also has been identified as an independent risk factor for SCD, particularly in the post-myocardial infarction population. However, there are reports that even complex ventricular ectopy may be more a manifestation of severity of underlying heart disease than an independent risk factor. In contrast to the previously cited risk factors, all of which reflect substrate abnormalities, ventricular ectopy represents a trigger mechanism for SCD.

Overall, sensitivity and specificity of ventricular ectopy appear low. However, predictive value of at least some types of ventricular ectopy, i.e., sustained monomorphic ventricular tachycardia, has been confirmed by programmed ventricular stimulation studies. In addition, although the significance of non-sustained ventricular tachycardias, particularly the polymorphic varieties, requires further clarification, findings in some studies that up to 45% of patients are inducible in response to programmed electrical stimulation underscore the potential predictive utility of Holter findings of this dysrhythmia. Unfortunately, Holter monitoring usually does not allow identification of specific individuals at high risk of SCD. Controversies concerning the effectiveness of the prophylactic use of antiarrhythmic agents in protecting against SCD make for further uncertainties with respect to the predictive utility of ventricular ectopy.

Inducibility

Invasive electrophysiologic studies have provided strong suggestive evidence that SCD survivors at high risk of a second episode are distinguishable on the basis of whether or not they developed sustained runs of rapid ventricular tachycardia and/or fibrillation in response to programmed electrical stimulation of the ventricle ("inducibility"). The key role of electrophysiologic study in evaluation and management of SCD survivors is widely accepted. The method also has been used to distinguish benign from potentially lethal ventricular dysrhythmias, including non-sustained ventricular tachycardias, and to guide antiarrhythmic therapy. However, the inducibility criterion may be of uncertain utility in a number of clinical settings, including recent myocardial infarction and cardiomyopathy.

In addition, the methodology does not provide adequate insights with respect to non-inducible patients, even in SCD survivors. Although most studies suggest that risk of a second episode of ventricular fibrillation is low in non-inducible SCD survivors, contrary findings also have been presented. Indeed, some studies report that up to 35% of non-inducible patients experience a second episode of SCD. Available studies also do not adequately address the question of the fate of non-inducible, non-sustained ventricular tachycardia patients. Finally, invasive electrophysiologic studies are costly and are not entirely risk-free. Despite these caveats, inducibility represents the current "gold standard" for determination of risk of SCD.

Autonomic Dysfunction and SCD

Clinical and Experimental Studies

Fluctuations in autonomic neural activity have been receiving increased attention both with respect to their role in the initiation and perpetuation of ventricular tachyarrhythmias and ventricular fibrillation and their predictive value as a marker of subgroups of patients at high risk of SCD. Experimental and clinical studies dating back many years suggest that the autonomic nervous system, particularly an imbalance between its sympathetic and parasympathetic components, represents an important determinant of the predisposition to ventricular tachycardia and ventricular fibrillation. Lown and Verrier (1976) have shown that sympathetic activity decreases fibrillation threshold and predisposes to ventricular fibrillation. The report by Coumel and associates (1983) of catecholamine dependent ventricular tachycardia/fibrillation represents another case in point, as does the known relationship between the hereditary form of the prolonged QT syndrome and autonomic imbalance. Findings that psychologic and emotional stress can trigger ventricular tachyarrhythmias and SCD are also pertinent. Voodoo death syndromes in primitive cultures probably represent an example in this regard (Cannon, 1957, Burrell, 1963).

Emotions and heart disease represent a real aspect of cardiology that is not often a subject of discussion. Also this topic is not well delineated or appreciated by probably the majority of medical personnel. Certainly, for myself this has been a fascinating subject for over three decades. My interest was initiated by a 29-year-old patient. She had no evidence of heart disease, and had been diagnosed as having a psychoneurosis; psychotherapeutic interviews were recommended in order to give her some insight into her emotional problems. I was a Fellow in Cardiology at that time, and her hospital stay coincided with a project that I was doing on the effect of amyl nitrate on heart sounds. Continual phonocardiographic tracings were recorded before, during, and after inhalation of amyl nitrate. She along with twelve other patients volunteered for the test. She happened to be the last patient, and when it became her turn I noted that she appeared extremely apprehensive. The procedure was then explained in detail in order to reassure her that no pain or harmful effects would occur. She obviously had heard the "pop" sound coinciding with breaking of the amyl nitrate pearl when the preceding patients on the ward were tested, and she was likewise reassured as to the harmlessness of the procedure. She indicated that she fully understood, but her apprehension was very apparent. She carefully watched each step of the procedure. A preliminary examination of the heart revealed no abnormality and her electrocardiogram was normal. Finally the phonocardiograph was connected and a continuous strip on lead two was started. While the tracing was running, the small tin box containing the pearls of amyl nitrate was brought out, and her eyes focused on the box. A pearl was then brought close to her nostrils and her facial expression was one of fear. At that instant, a short burst of rapid beats was heard (and recorded) followed by a return to the original rhythm. I did not break the amyl nitrate pearl. The phonocardiogram showed that a short paroxysm of ventricular tachycardia had taken place. The patient had sensed the change in rhythm and said it was similar to the type of palpitations she had noted in the past. From her history it was inferred that she may have experienced episodes of premature contractions and tachycardia.

This brief run of tachycardia therefore seemed to afford true support to the possibility of the old expression of being "frightened to death," since ventricular tachycardia could of course, lead to a fatal ventricular fibrillation. Our hospital was across the street from Harvard Medical School so I went to the Department of Physiology and asked Dr. Eugene Landis, Professor and Head of the Department, if he knew of any literature concerning death from fright. He stated that Dr. Walter Cannon, his predecessor as Chairman of the Department of Physiology, had indeed written an article on voodoo death. It happened that there was one remaining reprint in the department – which he gave me. This article was entitled: Voodoo Death, *American Anthropologist* 44:169–181, 1942, by Cannon, W.B.

Voodoo death according to Dr. Cannon has been recorded by competent observers. Such a mode of death produced by fright or fear follows the "hexing" of the subject by the "medicine man" or by "black magic." It has been recorded among native tribes of South America, Africa, Australia, New Zealand, and the Pacific Islands. An example of the "voodoo" myths of the ignorant superstitious native is taken from Cannon's fascinating article: a young man on a journey lodged in a friend's house for the night; the friend had prepared for their breakfast wild hen, a food strictly banned by a rule that must be inviolably observed by the immature. The young fellow demanded whether it was indeed a wild hen and when the host answered "no" he ate of it heartily, and proceeded on his way. A few years later when the two met again, the old friend asked the younger man if he would eat a wild hen. He answered that he had been solemnly charged by a wizard not to eat that food. Thereupon the host began to laugh and asked him why he had refused it now after eating it at his table before. On hearing this news his friend immediately began to tremble, so greatly was he possessed by fear, and in less than 24 hours he was dead.

W. Proctor Harvey, M.D.

More pertinent to Western culture is the occurrence of SCD in individuals, many young, without evidence of structural cardiovascular abnormalities. A neural trigger also would seem reasonable in these cases.

CARDIAC PEARL

I have been on the "look out" for various emotional events producing apparent cardiovascular effects. They certainly do occur. To name only a few personally observed: atrial fibrillation occurring with a lie detector test, whereas not occurring with an exercise test;

a man with coronary artery disease and an old myocardial infarct who had numerous attacks of documented ventricular tachycardia. A common cause of such an arrhythmia was a heated argument that the man had with his wife and son. Other emotional effects are multiple premature ventricular contractions in a young healthy member of the Harvard Crew team before a race; they disappeared after the event took place; a young physician had a disturbing bigeminal rhythm occur while waiting to deliver his first paper to a learned medical society, and the arrhythmia disappeared shortly after his talk was underway; another patient who was to receive the first human prosthetic valve would frequently have his normal sinus rhythm change to bigeminy coincident with a discussion of the planned surgical operation on his heart. This patient never had his operation, since he went into fatal ventricular fibrillation on the morning he was being prepared for his operation.

W. Proctor Harvey, M.D.

In contrast, vagal activity increases ventricular fibrillation threshold and appears to protect against malignant ventricular tachyarrhythmias. In conscious dogs with healed myocardial infarction, direct vagal stimulation after onset of acute ischemia prevented ventricular fibrillation (Vanoli and colleagues, 1991). Conversely, atropine enhanced susceptibility to ventricular fibrillation (DeFerrari and colleagues, 1991). Findings that patients with heart disease exhibit defective parasympathetic control mechanisms further support this hypothesis (Eckberg and colleagues, 1971). Findings that cardioactive drugs with strong anti-adrenergic and reflex vagal activity, for example, beta adrenergic blocking agents, appear to protect against SCD, whereas drugs with predominant parasympatholytic actions, for example, standard antiarrhythmic agents, are often pro-arrhythmic, are also pertinent in this regard.

Cellular Electrophysiologic Considerations

Cardiac dysrhythmias represent disturbances in the normal pattern of impulse formation and conduction in the heart. Pro- and antiarrhythmic effects of physiologic and pharmacologic interventions that influence heart rate and rhythm, including the autonomic mediators acetylcholine and the catecholamines, are generally defined in terms of their effects on the cellular electrophysiologic changes which underlie automaticity and conduction. There is an enormous literature; the interested reader is referred to any one or more of the excellent textbooks, monographs, and reviews in the field.

For purposes of this discussion, recall that the heart consists of two general tissue groupings: 1. Ordinary "working" atrial and ventricular myocardial cells, which are responsible for contractile work. Excitation of working myocardium also underlies inscription of the P, QRS, and ST-T waves of the standard body surface electrocardiogram; 2. A chain of specialized tissues, including the sinoatrial and atrioventricular nodes, specialized atrial tissues which link the nodal regions, and ramifications of the His-Purkinje system of the ventricle. The specialized tissues represent residual portions of the embryonal cardiac tube and are responsible for spontaneous impulse formation (automaticity) and for orderly distribution of the cardiac impulse from its point of origin to all portions of the heart.

Normal automaticity results from the ability of the specialized cells to undergo spontaneous diastolic (phase 4) depolarization. If this process lowers diastolic potential to a critical level, the threshold potential, a new regenerative action potential (impulse) ensues. Cells with the fastest rate of phase 4 depolarization, usually S-A nodal cells, function as the pacemaker of the heart; the remainder serve as latent or reserve pacemakers. Normal atrial and ventricular myocardial cells do not have the capability for undergoing phase 4 depolarization and thus do not normally serve a pacemaker function.

Conduction is a complex process resulting from sequential depolarization of contiguous areas of resting membrane by the propagating action potential. The ability to excite adjacent areas of resting membrane and, therefore, to conduct, as well as the rate at which conduction occurs, is dependent on the magnitude of the fast inward sodium current. This, in turn, is dependent on the level of membrane potential at excitation. Conduction velocity is, thus, critically related to the level of membrane potential in the path of impulse spread. Other factors being equal, conduction velocity is maximal in fibers in which the diastolic membrane potential approximates -85 to -95 mV. Reduction in membrane potential is associated with slowing of conduction, significant conduction disturbances generally making their first appearances at membrane potentials <-70 mV. Depolarization to still lower levels results in progressively more marked slowing of conduction, culminating in complete block at -50 mV or below. At such low potential levels, the fast inward sodium current is largely inactivated, and depolarization and conduction become primarily dependent on the slow inward calcium current. Cells in which depolarization is dependent on the

fast and slow inward currents are termed "fast" and "slow" response cells, respectively.

Changes in impulse formation and/or conduction in the sinus and other portions of the specialized tissues underlie changes in sinus rate in response to changing physiologic need, as well as a variety of conduction disturbances and dysrhythmias. Insofar as ventricular dysrhythmias are concerned, these have long been considered to arise in the His-Purkinje system, at least in normal hearts. Ventricular myocardial cells have not been thought to play a major role in normal hearts. In ischemic and diseased hearts, however, there is suggestive evidence that ventricular myocardial cells also may play a major roll (see below).

Since lethal dysrhythmias and SCD usually occur in patients with structural heart disease, as opposed to subjects with normal hearts, electrophysiologic findings in heart muscle from patients with ventricular tachyarrhythmias or from animal models appear pertinent. Specimens of ischemic and diseased human ventricle and experimentally infarcted dog heart differ strikingly from normal (Ten Eick and colleagues, 1976 and Singer and colleagues, 1981) in that they contain large numbers of partially depolarized, slow response type myocardial fibers interspersed among more normally polarized, fast response cells. Excitability and conduction are depressed. Many of the slow response cells exhibit spontaneous diastolic depolarization and beat spontaneously. Early and late afterdepolarization, as well as a multiplicity of oscillations, also occur (abnormal automaticity). These conditions would be expected to predispose to local block, fragmentation of excitation and conduction, and reentry, as well as to dysrhythmias due to multiple mechanisms. The findings provide suggestive evidence that partially depolarized ventricular myocardial cells may contribute importantly to development of ventricular tachyarrhythmias. It follows that interventions which predispose to further depolarization and enhancement of normal and abnormal automaticity would be expected to be pro-arrhythmic. Conversely, normalization of the diastolic potential would exert antiarrhythmic effects.

Catecholamine effects on automaticity and conduction have been studied extensively. In normal heart, these agents principally act to increase the slope of phase 4 depolarization of normally automatic cells throughout the specialized tissues with resultant development of sinus and ectopic tachyarrhythmias. Enhancement of supraventricular automaticity is opposed by reflex vagal activity resulting from catecholamine induced increases in stroke volume and in central aortic and carotid pressures. The vagally mediated depression of phase 4 depolarization decreases the repetition rate of sinus and other supraventricular automatic cells and further facilitates development of ventricular dysrhythmias. At least some cases of stress-related catecholamine dependent ventricular tachycardia may be explicable on this basis. Increases in sympathetic (catecholamine) activity occur locally as well as globally in conjunction with such conditions as non-uniform adrenergic nerve distribution and activation and localized increases in norepinephrine release from ischemia and potassium depolarized adrenergic nerve terminals. Resulting local increases in automaticity further increase electrical inhomogeneity which, in turn, predisposes to fragmentation of excitation and conduction and development of reentrant tachyarrhythmias, including ventricular tachycardia and fibrillation. Such changes probably contribute importantly to ventricular dysrhythmia in ischemia/infarction.

Catecholamine actions on partially depolarized cells may differ strikingly from normal. More specifically, these agents act to hyperpolarize (i.e., make more negative) the diastolic potential of partially depolarized cells, restoring it towards more normal or even normal levels and improving excitability and conduction. This has been attributed to an increase in K^+ conductance of the membrane, with resultant increase in outward K^+ current, possibly the delayed rectifier current, and/or to an increase in activity of the Na^+/K^+ ion exchange pump. The hyperpolarizing action usually is associated with diminution in or abolition of spontaneous diastolic depolarization and spontaneous beating. To the extent that arrhythmia originates in such partially depolarized cells, these actions would be antiarrhythmic. Sometimes, however, hyperpolarization is accompanied by enhancement of automaticity.

In addition, catecholamines, by virtue of their slow inward current enhancing effects, may induce development of abnormal automatic activity in partially depolarized myocardial cells with resultant further slowing and fragmentation of conduction. These actions, together with automaticity enhancing effects on normal Purkinje fibers, are pro-arrhythmic. The association between sympathetic activity and ventricular tachyarrhythmias suggests that the overall effect of catecholamines is, in fact, also pro-arrhythmic.

In contrast, acetylcholine's principal actions on cardiac electrical activity, namely, to decrease phase 4 depolarization of automatic cells and to hyperpolarize partially depolarized cells, are both antiarrhythmic. These effects reflect activation of acetylcholine sensitive potassium channels with resultant increases in outward potassium current. Cardiac cells in all parts of the heart are affected by acetylcholine. However, acetylcholine sensitivity differs for cells in different parts of the heart. The effects are most pronounced on SA nodal cells. Cells in the His-Purkinje system and, to an even greater degree, ventricular muscle cells are much less sensitive. Differences in sensitivity relate to differences in parasympathetic receptor density. Thus, although depressive effects on His-Purkinje automaticity may contribute to protective effect of vagal activity against ventricular tachyarrhythmias and SCD, the role of hyperpolarization is probably much more important, particularly in view of findings in large populations of partially depolarized ischemic and diseased heart muscle.

Findings by Bailey and colleagues (1972) that, in a dog ischemia model, acetylcholine hyperpolarizes partially depolarized Purkinje cells and depresses/abolishes automaticity of such cells, with resultant improvement in excitability and conduction, are pertinent in this regard. There also is evidence that indirect vagal influences play a role, serving to oppose the depolarizing and other pro-arrhythmic effects of increased sympathetic tone. This reflects, at least in part, the action of acetylcholine in decreasing cyclic AMP.

Heart Rate Variability (HRV)

It follows from the foregoing that quantitative indices of autonomic activity have the potential to serve as predictors of risk of SCD and possibly also of risk of mortality due to other causes. This requires clinically utilizable measures of sympathetic and parasympathetic activity. Although direct determination of efferent vagal activity is not yet possible in conscious humans, a number of indirect measures are available. Attention has focused on the spontaneous cyclical changes in heart rate and in hemodynamic parameters, including arterial blood pressure and stroke volume. These have been known since ancient times and have been systematically examined at least since the 18th century. The cyclical change in sinus rate over time is termed heart rate variability or heart period variability.

HRV is attributed to cyclical fluctuations in autonomic tone, virtually disappearing following combined sympathetic and parasympathetic blockade and cardiac transplantation. Early experimental animal studies and time domain HRV studies on man suggested that the spontaneous respiratory fluctuations in sinus rate were mediated solely by efferent vagal activity. More recently, frequency

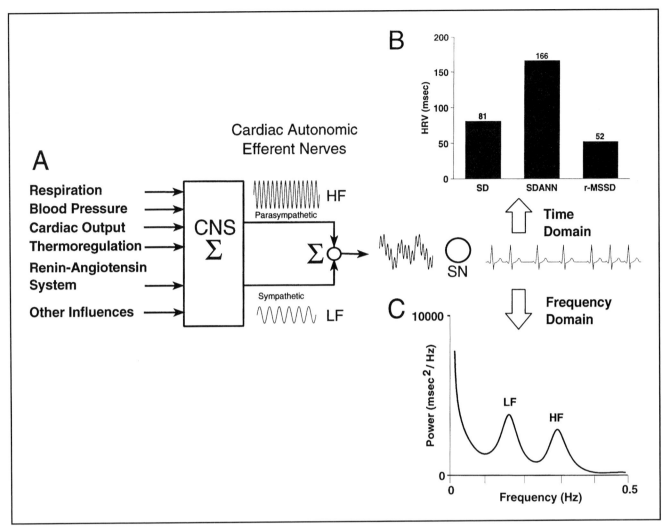

Figure 1. Neuroregulatory influences on sinus rate and rhythm, heart rate variability (HRV), and differences between time and frequency domain analysis of HRV. Neuroregulatory influences (A) are integrated centrally (CNS) and influence the sinus node (SN) via the autonomic nervous system. Time domain HRV analysis (B) reflects overall autonomic activity but does not separate out sympathetic and parasympathetic components. Power spectral analysis (C), on the other hand, can distinguish high-frequency (HF) and low-frequency (LF) components that are thought to reflect parasympathetic and predominantly sympathetic activity, respectively. *(Modified after Ori Z, et al: Cardiology Clinics 10: 1992).*

domain studies have provided strong suggestive evidence that HRV reflects oscillations in sympathetic-parasympathetic balance associated with a variety of factors including respiration, baroreceptor reflexes, vasomotor control, and thermoregulatory processes. Akselrod in his now classic 1982 report confirmed the contribution of these factors and also noted the role of the renin-angiotensin system. Since these early studies there has been increasing recognition of the importance of HRV as an index of autonomic function.

Figure 1 shows a simplified schematic representation of the neuroregulatory influences on sinus rate and rhythm which underlie HRV as well as examples of time and frequency domain analyses. Figure 2 shows graphic depictions of 24-hour HRV determinations, defined in terms of mean heart

rate (Panel A) and a time domain measure (SD measure) Panel B for a normal control and a heart transplant patient. HRV differences between the two subjects are striking using both methods. The virtual disappearance of HRV in the transplant patient reflects the effects of cardiac denervation and underscores the autonomic basis of HRV.

Determinations of baroreflex sensitivity (BRS) also may be used to assess parasympathetic influences on the heart. BRS is expressed by the slope of the regression line correlating the degree of R-R interval prolongation occurring in response to blood pressure increases induced by a pressor agent. The correlation between HRV and baroreflex sensitivity is high but not perfect. This reflects the fact that the two methodologies explore different aspects of the autonomic control of the heart: HRV is a direct

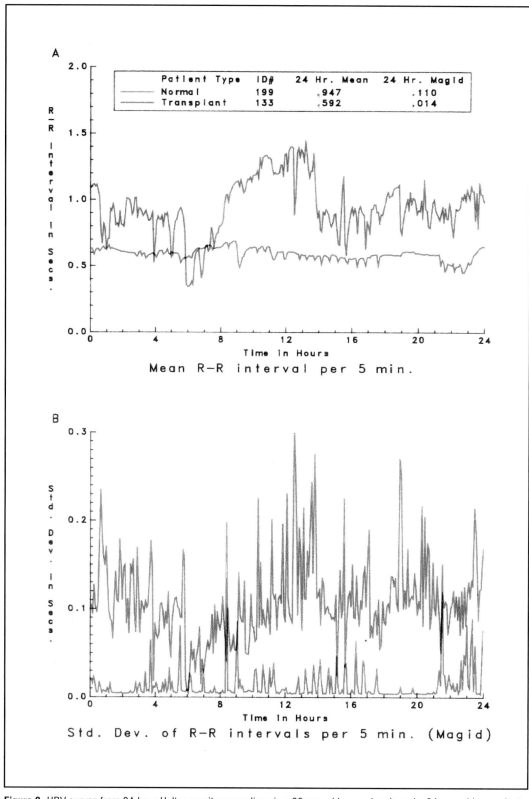

Figure 2. HRV curves from 24-hour Holter monitor recordings in a 30 year old normal male and a 34 year old transplant patient. Time in hours indicates running time of tape. Absolute starting times differ for the two tapes (ID # 199 = 16:15; ID # 133 = 08:00). Panel A shows curves derived by calculating the mean of all normal R-R intervals in successive 5 minute segments. Panel B shows curves for the same two patients obtained by determining the standard deviation of all normal R-R intervals in successive 5 minute segments during the same 24-hour period. Overall 24 hour mean heart rate and HRV determination (SD measure) are indicated in the key. Note the markedly lower HRV of the transplant patient as opposed to the normal control. *(Modified after Singer, D, et al. J Electrocard 88 (Suppl): 1988).*

TABLE 1
Time Domain Heart Rate Variability Measures

MEASURE	UNIT	DESCRIPTION
A. R-R Interval Analysis		
SDNN	Msec	SD* of the mean of all normal** R-R intervals during the total recording period, usually 24 hours***
SDANN	Msec	SD of the means of all normal R-R intervals calculated for successive 5 minute time blocks during the total recording period
SD****	Msec	Mean of the SD of all normal R-R intervals in successive 5 minute time blocks during the total recording period
B. Interval Difference Analysis		
Counts	Beats	Total number of instances per hour in which two consecutive R-R intervals differ by more than 50 msec.
pNN50	Percent	Proportion of the differences between R-R intervals that exceed an arbitrary limit, usually 50 msec, computed over the entire recording period
r-MSSD	Msec	Root mean square of differences between successive R-R intervals over the entire recording period
SDSD	Msec	SD of successive differences between normal R-R intervals over the entire recording period
C. Miscellaneous		
CV	Msec	The coefficient of variation of the SD obtained by dividing the SD value for each 5 minute period by the mean R-R interval for that period and averaging all 5 minute CV values over the total recording period
Day-Night Difference	Msec	The difference between the mean of all normal R-R intervals recorded during the day and during the night

* SD = Standard Deviation
** "Normal" R-R Interval = Interval between two sinus beats without intervening ectopic beats
*** Since most HRV studies are Holter monitor based, the usual recording period is 24 hours
**** The SD measure is also referred to as the SDNN index

Description of time domain HRV measures in current use. Measures are divided into three groupings as shown.

measure of cardiac vagal tone, whereas BRS measures reflex vagal activity. BRS also has been reported to be a sensitive predictor of risk of ventricular tachycardia and SCD in the post-myocardial infarction population.

HRV: Methods of Analysis

There are two major approaches to HRV analysis: time domain analysis and frequency domain analysis:

Time Domain Analysis

Time domain analysis of heart rate (or R-R interval) variability consists of applying simple statistical analytic techniques to an R-R interval series. The R-R interval is used even though true sinus rate is defined by the P-P interval because R-R is more reliably detected and is normally equal to P-P. A number of time domain measures have been proposed. Table 1 lists the principal measures with brief descriptions of each. The measures fall into two general classes.

1} *R-R Interval Analysis:* This approach defines HRV in terms of fluctuations in sinus rate about the mean by determining the standard deviation of an R-R interval series for a given time block, usually five minutes. Subsequent computation of the mean of the standard deviations of all sequential five minute time blocks included in the total recording period allows assessment of HRV changes over prolonged periods, usually 24 hours for Holter monitor based recordings. This measure, designated the standard deviation (SD) measure, is also referred to as the SDNN Index. A variant of this method is to determine the mean of the R-R interval series for each five minute time block and then to calculate the standard deviation of all five minute interval means in the recording (SDANN measure). These measures are broad based and subject to diurnal and other long term trends which affect heart rate.

2} *R-R Interval Difference Analysis:* This class of indices, which measures differences in duration between adjacent R-R intervals, includes the rMSSD measure (the root mean square of successive R-R interval differences) and the PNN50 measure (the proportion of the differences between adjacent R-R intervals that exceed an arbitrary limit, usually 50 msec). In contrast to indices computed from R-R interval measurements, this group of measures is only minimally, if at all, affected by long term trends, and is thought to reflect primarily alterations in parasympathetic activity.

Frequency Domain (Heart Rate Power Spectrum) Analysis

Power spectral analysis decomposes the heart rate signal into its frequency components and quantifies them in terms of their energy content, termed "power". A principal attraction of the method is that, in addition to measuring parasympathetic activity, it provides insights into sympa-

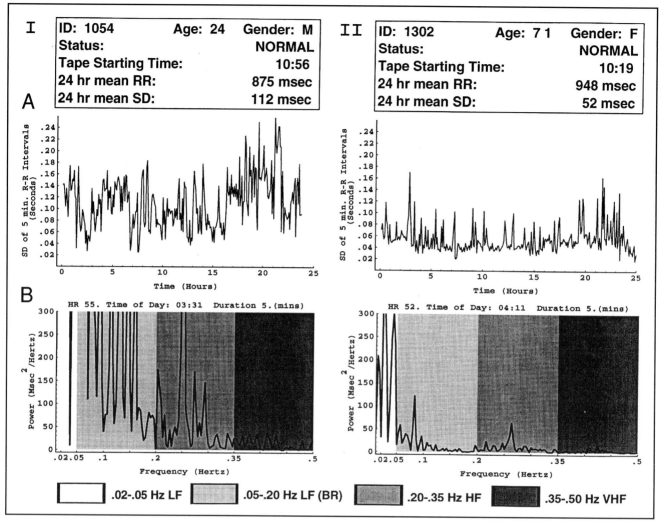

Figure 3. Twenty-four hour time domain HRV curves (SD measure) (IA, IIA) and 5-minute FFT power spectral (IB, IIB) for healthy 24-year-old man (I) and 71-year-old woman (II) subjects to show age-related differences. Patient information and 24-hour mean R-R and HRV values are indicated in the enclosed rectangles. HRV is much greater and fluctuates more markedly over the 24-hour recording period (circadian variation) (IA and IIA) for the younger (IA) as compared with the elderly (IIA) individual. Spectral power also is much higher over the whole frequency range for the younger individual (IB). Note that these high power levels cause peaks of spectral spikes to be cut off in the LF and HF bands. *(Modified after Ori Z et al: Cardiology Clinics 10: 502-503, 1992).*

thetic activation and sympatho-vagal balance, which cannot be determined from time domain analysis. Power spectral analysis also permits the monitoring of HRV changes over very short (2 minutes-5 minutes) time blocks. This, in turn, facilitates assessment of the nature of autonomic changes which precede, and may serve to trigger, acute changes in state, including angina, ventricular tachyarrhythmias and SCD.

Energy distribution in the different frequency components is currently estimated in two major ways: 1. The Fast Fourier Transform (FFT) and 2. Use of a linear model, usually the Auto-Regressive Model. The spectra produced by using the autoregressive model represent a continuum and are smoother in appearance. Figure 1 shows a

schematic representation of records obtained using autoregressive model. However, if the desired information is distributed over a wide frequency range or if the noise level is high, power spectral analysis is a more appropriate choice. All of the power spectral records used in this chapter were obtained using FFT analysis. Figures 3 and 4 show 5-minute and compressed 24-hour FFT power spectral records obtained during ambulatory monitoring of a healthy young subject (Panel A) and a healthy elderly subject (Panel B). Discrete spectral peaks in the HF and LF frequency range are characteristic of the normal condition.

The heart rate power spectrum encompasses at least three major frequency bands ranging from 0.01 to 0.35 Hz. Band boundaries are defined differ-

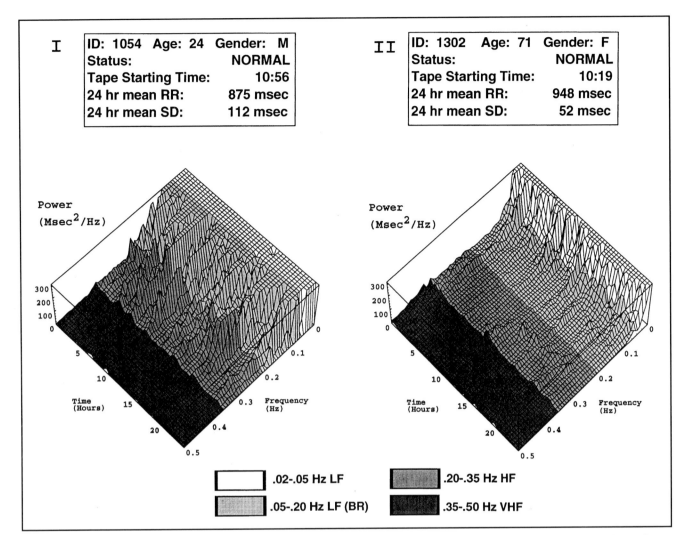

Figure 4. Twenty-four hour FFT power spectra for the same two individuals depicted in Figure 2. Scales are the same for the two traces. Twenty-four hour FFT power records are computed by taking the average of successive 2-minute spectra for each 30-minute period and creating a surface plot at these averages. Again, note the much higher power, including both HF and LF power (particularly the former), exhibited by the younger individual (I) and that the power differential persisted throughout the recording period. Also note the markedly diminished fluctuations in power over the 24 hours (ie, decreased circadian variation) in the elderly individual (II), a finding corresponding to the smaller fluctuations in HRV in Figure 3 (IIA). *(Modified after Ori Z et al: Card Clinics 10: 504-505, 1992).*

ently by different authors. The bands, together with the most commonly employed boundaries are:

1) *High frequency band (HF: 0.2 - 0.35 Hz),* associated with parasympathetic activity. Peak frequency varies with respiration but approximates 0.25 HZ. We have noted still higher frequency components (.35-.50 Hz), which comprise a very high frequency band. This may reflect non-respiration related parasympathetic function.

2) *Low frequency band (LF: 0.04 to 0.2 Hz)* which is ill defined but has been attributed to thermoregulatory processes, peripheral vasomotor activity and the renin-angiotensin system. This band currently encompasses the intermediate frequency Baroreceptor Band (.05-.15 Hz). The LF band is thought to be modulated by both sympathetic and parasym-

pathetic activity, but predominantly by the latter.

3) *Very low frequency band (VLF: 0.01 - 0.04 Hz)* also has been identified and proposed as a marker of sympathetic activity. However, recent pharmacological and physiological testing of sympathetic modulation of HRV power spectrum suggests that VLF power cannot be viewed simply as a measure of sympathetic modulation.

4) *Ultra low frequency band (ULF: 10^{-2} to 10^{-5} Hz).* Kobayashi and Muscha (1982) reported that the heart can fluctuate at even longer periodicities than those comprising the VLF band. The physiologic significance of the ULF band is unknown. However, it is of interest to note that one study reported low ULF power to be the best predictor of risk of SCD.

A number of power determinations are possible:

1) *Total power.* The total area under the power spectral curve.

2) *Power of individual frequency components.* The area under the portion of the curve related to each component.

3) *Normalized or fractional power.* The ratio of the power of the individual components to total power.

4) *LF/HF ratio.* The ratio of LF to HF power is generally considered to be a measure of sympathovagal balance, a conclusion supported by many experimental and clinical studies. As the physiologic basis of the power spectral components, particularly the VLF band, are further clarified, other ratios probably will be found to be more appropriate for the purpose.

Correspondence of Time and Frequency: Domain Measures of HRV

Comparisons between frequency and time domain measures show that the latter correlate with one or more of the power spectral components. Although time domain measures are generally thought to primarily reflect parasympathetic activity, r-MSSD and pNN50 have been reported to be most sensitive in this regard. However, even they are influenced by the sympathetic outflow and possibly by other regulatory mechanisms as well.

Table 2 summarizes the relationships between time and frequency domain measures for normal subjects. Note that total power and the SD measure are virtually equivalent. Other time and frequency domain measures, despite the high degrees of correlation, are not necessarily interchangeable. The high degree of correlation between time domain measures and the power spectrum components suggests that all of the former also are strongly influenced by parasympathetic activity.

Methodologic Caveats

HRV determinations are highly sensitive to methodologic error and artifact. For optimum utility, every effort must be made to ensure omission of intervals containing premature beats and non-conducted P waves or their replacement with interpolated R-R values. Attention also must be paid to data collection methods. If the data are collected on magnetic tape, flutter may be introduced on playback. In a different vein, the fiduciary accuracy of the R wave detection algorithms also must be protected since errors can influence heart rate analysis.

Frequency domain measures are generally much more sensitive to technical artifacts such as timing

TABLE 2 — Correlation Between Time and Frequency Domain Measures				
TIME DOMAIN		**FREQUENCY DOMAIN**		
	Total power*	LF power*	HF power*
SD measure	1.0	0.92	0.90
SDNN	0.87	0.85	0.68
pNN50	0.92	0.81	0.92
r-MSSD	0.94	0.91	0.98

*Correlation coefficients relating time and frequency domain measures. Abbreviations: SD measure = mean of the standard deviations of successive 5 minute R-R intervals over 24 hours; r-MSSD = root-mean-square of the differences of successive R-R intervals; pNN50 = proportion of adjacent R-R intervals > 50 msec different; SDNN = standard deviation of 24-hour R-R intervals *(Modified after Kleiger et al [84]).*

Correlations between the results of time and frequency domain analysis of heart rate variability in healthy subjects. Note high levels of correlation. *(Modified after Ori et al: Cardiology Clinics 10: p 506,1992)*

error due to differences in taping speed or missing data due to ectopic beats than are time domain measures. For optimum reliability and reproducibility, the heart rate signal must meet a number of conditions which are prerequisites for meaningful power spectrum analyses: ideally the signal should be random, stationary, and sufficiently long. Since, in reality, these conditions are not always met or even monitored, power spectral determinations may be subject to unpredictable variations, particularly at lower frequencies.

Renewed interest has recently been evinced in frequencies lower than 0.04 Hz in view of reports that 1) The VLF portion of the spectrum (0.01-0.04 Hz) reflects a purer form of sympathetic activity than the LF band and 2) the VLF and ULF (10^{-2}-10^{-5}) portions of the spectrum, particularly the latter, may represent a predictor of SCD. However, it is important to note that meaningful determinations of VLF and ULF power may be difficult to achieve because decreases in frequency to such low levels are associated with an increasing propensity to violate the rules governing power spectral determinations, violations which diminish reliability despite the most sophisticated preprocessing.

It is also noteworthy that the reliability of power spectral determinations diminishes with decreases in the power of the signal and of the signal-to-noise ratio. This is pertinent with respect to clinical states associated with low HRV, including all-cause mortality and SCD. This occurs because 1) at low signal levels, the relative contribution of noise to the power spectrum is increased; 2) energy from the VLF and ULF bands spreads into the higher frequency ranges, with resultant increases in noise level.

HRV: Clinical Considerations

A burgeoning experimental and clinical literature attests to the growing interest in the contribution of altered autonomic function, defined in terms of HRV, to morbidity and mortality associated with a variety of physiologic and pathophysiologic conditions. Physiologic conditions are represented by normal aging, diurnal variations in cardiovascular function, various vagomimetic and sympathomimetic maneuvers (e.g., mental stress and physical exertion). Pathophysiologic processes include numerous disease states, among them diabetes; *neurogenic syncope;* chronic renal disease; arterial hypertension; coronary and other types of structural heart disease and their major complications, myocardial infarction, congestive heart failure, and cardiac arrhythmias. *An association with rejection of heart transplants also has been postulated.* The *relationship* between low HRV and both all-cause mortality and SCD is of particular interest because of the potential applicability of HRV methodology to considerations of risk stratification. Frequency domain studies have the added potential for providing added insights into the nature of autonomic changes associated with different physiologic and pathophysiologic states.

It is tempting to think that HRV methodology may improve capabilities for early detection of autonomic neuropathies and monitoring progression of disease. The methodology also may lead to more rational therapeutic approaches by facilitating selection of drugs with the ability to correct autonomic imbalances associated with different pathophysiologic states. Utility for follow-up of heart transplant reinnervation and for prediction of rejection also has been suggested.

HRV: A Powerful Predictor of All-Cause Mortality

Numerous studies, using a variety of methodologies, have shown low HRV to be a powerful predictor of all-cause mortality. Early studies made use of relatively simple time domain measures, e.g., the presence or absence of sinus arrhythmia, and measurements of maximum-minimum P-P intervals and computation of the standard deviation of mean sinus P-P intervals in short rhythm strips. Perhaps the earliest description of the relationships between heart rate fluctuations and mortality is contained in a 1965 report on fetal monitoring showing that diminished beat-to-beat variability in heart rate signified fetal distress and a need for rapid delivery. Subsequent reports have confirmed this relationship.

Another early study relating HRV to mortality was that reported by Wolf and colleagues in 1978 for a population of soldiers admitted to an army hospital for acute myocardial infarction. HRV was defined in terms of the presence or absence of sinus arrhythmia in 60 second rhythm strips obtained on admission to the hospital. After controlling for such factors as infarct location and initial sinus rate, they found that patients with acute myocardial infarction who did not exhibit sinus arrhythmia on the initial ECG had a much greater chance of dying during the hospitalization (15.5%) than did those exhibiting sinus arrhythmia (4.1%). Indeed, absence of sinus arrhythmia was the most powerful predictor of mortality in his study.

Masaoka and colleagues (1985) used similarly simple measures to examine the association between HRV, aging and diabetes. Subjects were told to breathe as deeply as possible at a rate of 6 times per minute for one minute and HRV, defined as maximum minus minimum beats per minute, was determined. HRV was found to decrease with aging and the duration and severity of diabetes, being most severe in insulin dependent diabetics with autonomic neuropathy. Insofar as relationships to mortality are concerned, it has been shown that diabetic patients with clinical signs of autonomic neuropathy and abnormal tests of autonomic function (e.g., Valsalva maneuver and handgrip test) have disproportionately high mortality rates relative to similar type patients with normal test results. Relationships between normal aging and mortality are self evident and require no comment.

The advent of Holter monitoring and computer technology have revolutionized HRV analysis by making possible long-term determinations of HRV, usually 24 or 48 hours, and detailed statistical analyses of the data. Kleiger and colleagues (1987) used time domain HRV analysis of 24-hour ambulatory ECG recordings to extend Wolf's observations on the relationships between this parameter and post-myocardial infarction mortality in a group of 850 patients followed for three years after acute infarction. Low HRV (SDNN measure) was found to be a powerful independent predictor of long-term mortality in survivors of myocardial infarction. Similar observations have been reported by others.

Indeed, low HRV may be a more powerful predictor of mortality than such standard determinants as left ventricular ejection fraction, wall motion abnormalities, frequency and complexity of ventricular ectopy, standard ECG indices, exercise capacity, and the signal averaged ECG. Pilot studies by Van Hoogenhuyze and colleagues (1991) showing that mortality in a mixed group of congestive heart failure patients was associated with the lowest

TABLE 3
HRV Values for SCD and Reference Subjects

		SCD GROUPS				REFERENCE GROUPS			
Study	N	Age (years)	SDANN (msec)	SD (msec)	N	Age (years)	SDANN (msec)	SD (msec)	Composition Control
Martin et al (1987)	3	62.7±14	42±17	22±10	20	32±12	154±50	76±14	Healthy young subjects
Magid et al (1985)	20	59±9	55±23	27±15	18	57±10	71±33	44±24	Complex VEA patients*
Van Hoogenhuyze et al. (1991)	10	66±7	54±7	26±5	15	63±14	87±11	40±6	Complex VEA patients**
Rich et al. (1988)	3	54±17	55±31	NA	90	55±9	99±2	NA	Cath/patients without MAE***

All values given are mean ± SD.

SCD = sudden cardiac death; NA = not available; MAE = major arrhythmic event.

* Patients with asymptomatic complex ventricular ectopy (Lown grade III-IVa) in a setting of structural heart disease, who were non-inducible during electrophysiologic study.

** Patients with asymptomatic complex ventricular ectopy (Lown grade IVb) who did not experience major arrhythmic event during follow-up.

*** 94 consecutive patients admitted for cardiac catheterization studies for a variety of disease states who did not experience major arrhythmic event during 1-year follow-up.

Comparison of time domain HRV values (SDANN and SD measures) for SCD and reference subjects. Reference subjects include both healthy young subjects and patients with asymptomatic, complex ventricular ectopy. *(Modified after Van Hoogenhuyze D, et al: J Electrocard 22: p 205, 1989.)*

levels of HRV (SD measure) for the group, underscore its potential utility for risk stratification in the non-coronary as well as coronary population.

The ability of beta-adrenergic blocking agents to protect against the occurrence of SCD following myocardial infarction is pertinent to considerations of the autonomic contribution to SCD and the predictive value of HRV with respect to mortality. These agents, which are among the small handful of cardioactive drugs known to simultaneously depress adrenergic activity and reflexly increase vagal tone, also increase HRV. It is tempting to think that, to the extent that the antiarrhythmic effects of this group of drugs stem from their strong indirect autonomic actions (as opposed to their weak, direct, quinidine-like membrane stabilizing activity), HRV can be used as a simple tool for monitoring therapeutic effectiveness.

It follows from the foregoing that agents which depress parasympathetic activity should be proarrhythmic and should increase risk of SCD. Class IA and Class IC anti-arrhythmic agents represent a case in point. These agents, which include quinidine and procainamide, exhibit strong indirect atropine-like effects and are well known for proarrhythmic activity. Zuanetti and colleagues (1991) compared the autonomic effects of a Class IC agent (flecanide) with those of propafenone and amiodarone on HRV. They found that amiodarone, which generally does not exhibit major pro-arrhythmia, did not modify HRV. In contrast, flecanide and

propafenone, both of which have been shown to increase mortality, decreased HRV (pNN50) significantly, a finding interpreted as reflecting depressive effects on parasympathetic activity. There was no information concerning possible sympathetic effects.

Correlations between HRV and mortality also have been made for a number of non-cardiac disease states, including diabetes and alcoholic neuropathy, both conditions associated with high risk of ventricular tachyarrhythmias and SCD. Early studies by Masaoka (1985) on diabetics have been previously alluded to. Findings by Ewing and colleagues (1980) that diabetics with autonomic neuropathy exhibited a five-year mortality rate (56%) that was three times higher than for patients with normal autonomic function are of particular interest in that of those who died, almost 30% experienced SCD. In addition, there was a surprising absence of coronary artery disease. In a similar vein, Johnson and Robinson (1988) found that depressed vagal activity in chronic alcoholics was associated with an increased risk of mortality, particularly due to cardiovascular causes.

HRV: Sudden Cardiac Death

Time domain studies by Magid and colleagues (1985), Martin and colleagues (1987), Rich and colleagues (1988), and Singer and colleagues (1988) showing that HRV (SD and SDANN measures) was significantly lower in SCD survivors and in patients experiencing SCD during ambulatory monitoring than for non-SCD patients with structural heart disease and normal controls, respectively, support suggestions that this method may be useful in identifying individuals at high risk of sudden death. Table 3 compares HRV for SCD and reference normal and asymptomatic VEA patients from four studies; the fact that HRV was comparable for individuals who experienced SCD during ambulatory monitoring and SCD survivors is important in that it indicates that low levels of HRV in the SCD survivors were not due to physiologic changes associated with the cardiac arrest. Findings of a progressive reduction in HRV, defined in terms of 24-hour mean low and high frequency power, in individuals who died during Holter monitoring are supportive in this regard. However, conflicting evidence also has recently been reported.

To test the hypothesis that HRV could correctly discriminate between inducible and non-inducible SCD survivors, inducible and non-inducible "asymptomatic VEA" patients (patients with complex ventricular ectopy but without syncope or SCD), and normal controls, all subjects were Holter monitored for 24 hours prior to programmed ventricular stimulation and while off antiarrhythmic drugs. A step-wise discriminant analysis controlled for suspected covariates. Univariate analysis showed that inducible and non-inducible patients did not differ with respect to age, sex, mean R-R interval, ejection fraction, cardiac drugs (digitalis or beta blocking agents), and frequency or complexity of ventricular ectopy. HRV of inducible SCD survivors was found to be markedly lower than normal. HRV of inducible SCD survivors also appeared lower than that of non-inducible SCD survivors although differences were not as pronounced.

Inducible asymptomatic VEA patients also were found to exhibit low HRV, thus further underscoring the relationship between HRV, inducibility, and risk of sudden death. HRV of non-inducible asymptomatic VEA patients also was diminished, but differences did not reach statistical significance when compared with normal controls. These findings are supported by studies of Kjellgren and colleagues (1994) of 59 patients referred for routine electrophysiologic study in which the 28 inducible patients exhibited significantly lower HRV than did the 31 non-inducible patients. Combining low HRV (SD measure < 30 msec) and inducibility correctly identified all patients post cardiac arrest who died during a 100 month follow up period.

Figure 5 (Panels A and B) compares HRV (SD measure) of a representative inducible SCD patient, an age-matched non-inducible, asymptomatic, complex ventricular ectopy patient, and a normal control. Similarities between HRV patterns of the SCD-inducible patient and those for the transplant patient (Figure 2) are striking, a finding consistent with marked depression of autonomic function. The SD measure generally provided the best separation from normal. Correlations between low HRV and inducibility of SCD survivors suggest the potential utility of HRV as a predictor of risk of SCD and as a possible screen for programmed ventricular stimulation studies.

Despite the putative importance of sympathetic activity to considerations of SCD, very little power spectral information is available. The paucity of such studies may be due, at least in part, to the fact that time domain determinations are easier to make and also provide excellent correlations with mortality. However, Meyers and colleagues (1986) suggested that power spectral analysis may be even more useful, changes in the HF component providing the best separation between SCD survivors, non-SCD patients with chronic structural heart disease, and normal controls. LF power did not distinguish SCD and non-SCD heart disease patients but was significantly lower in both groups than in normals. In a different vein, it was previously noted that one group of investigators has reported low ULF power, rather than low HF or high LF power, to be the best marker of risk of SCD.

Most studies of the relationship between HRV and SCD have been carried out in the coronary population. However, studies by Fei and colleagues (1994) on seven patients with primary ventricular fibrillation and three cardiomyopathy patients with ventricular fibrillation confirm significantly lower HRV for SCD survivors in non-coronary populations than for healthy age and gender matched controls. Interestingly enough, in this study SCD patients and controls differed significantly with respect to power spectral determinations but not with respect to time domain measures. In addition, hourly HRV analysis showed that minimum observed HRV values were significantly lower in the SCD patients than in the normal controls, whereas maximum hourly HRV remained unchanged, suggesting that this mode of analysis may provide additional information relevant to considerations of risk.

HRV methodology also has been applied to the sudden infant death syndrome (SIDS). Gordon and colleagues (1984) compared the heart rate and respiratory power spectra during quiet sleep of infants who subsequently died from SIDS with those of healthy controls. They found significant enhance-

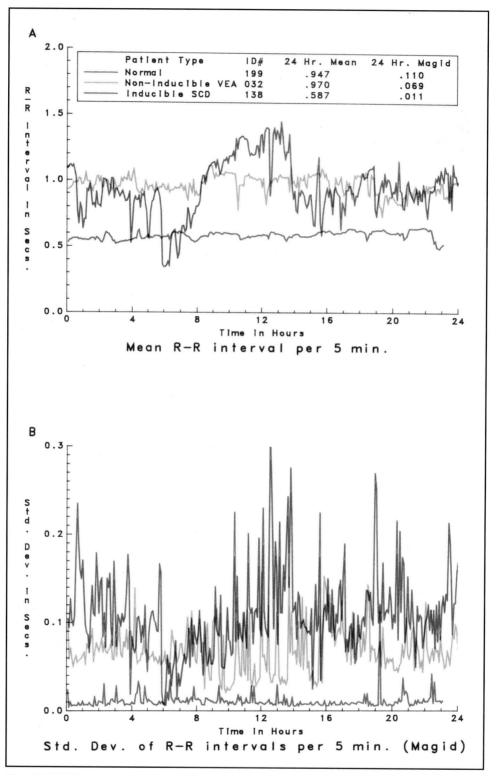

Figure 5. HRV determinations in a 52-year-old inducible male SCD survivor and a 53-year-old noninducible man with "asymptomatic" complex ventricular ectopy, both with coronary disease, and a normal control. Data presentation format is the same as that for Figure 2. The normal control curves were obtained from the same individual as in Figure 2. Time (in hours) indicates running time of tape. Absolute starting times differ for the three tapes (ID #199 = 16:15;ID # 032 = 13:15; ID # 138 = 09:25). Note that HRV (SD measure) of the inducible SCD patient was markedly lower than that of the control. HRV of the inducible SCD patient also appeared somewhat lower than that of the noninducible "asymptomatic" VEA patient. HRV of the latter appeared diminished as compared with control. However, these latter differences did not reach statistical significance. *(Modified after Singer DH et al: J Electrocard (Suppl); S50 1988).*

ment of LF, but not HF, power in the heart rate power spectrum and a widened HF band in the respiratory spectra, in SIDS infants. However, in a second study on a larger population, the same investigators reported that these characteristics did not adequately distinguish SIDS infants from controls. In a subsequent similar type investigation, Kluge et al (1988) found HF power to be significantly lower in the SIDS children than in controls, a finding consistent with parasympathetic withdrawal and comparable with findings in adult SCD cases.

HRV: Aging and Sudden Cardiac Death

Time domain studies have clearly shown that HRV decreases with increasing age, the decline being generally attributed to age related reduction in parasympathetic activity . However, sympathetic activity also declines with age. Figure 6 shows a graphic depiction of the gradual monotonic decline in HRV of 70 normal subjects aged 22 years-81 years. Since, as noted above, development of chronic heart disease per se and SCD also have been associated with declining vagal activity, it is necessary to define areas of HRV overlap between age-matched SCD patients, patients with organic

heart disease but without SCD, and the healthy elderly. Cutoff points to separate these groups need to be established.

Preliminary observations suggest that it may be possible to define cutoff points for time domain measures which separate SCD survivors from non SCD patients with heart disease (sensitivity = 80% and specificity = 66%). However, distinctions between low HRV due to heart disease or high risk of SCD and that due to aging, are more complex. Our own data suggest that SCD patients over age 60 often exhibit substantially lower 24-hour mean HRV (SD measure) than do younger SCD patients. Comparisons between mean 24-hour HRV for a 40-year-old (SD=45 msec) and a 76-year-old (SD=21 msec) individual who experienced SCD during ambulatory monitoring (Figure 7) are illustrative in this regard. However, comparisons with Figure 3 show that HRV for both young and elderly SCD patients were much lower than those for age matched normals. Findings by Odemuyiwa and colleagues (1992) that arrhythmic death is a more common mode of dying and is more reliably predicted by HRV in postinfarct patients younger than 60 years than in those over 60 underscore the influence of aging on HRV.

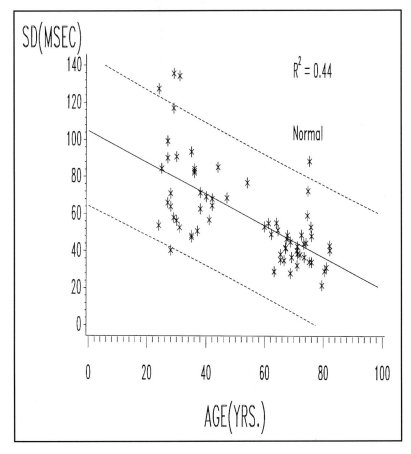

Figure 6. Linear regression line (solid line) with 95% confidence limits (broken lines) and correlation coefficient to show gradual decline in HRV with aging in 70 patients, aged 22 to 81 years. Note the occasional individuals who fall outside the 95% confidence limits. Such "outliers" could detract from the potential utility of HRV analysis for risk stratification and other clinical purposes. *(Modified after Ori Z et al: Card Clinics 10: 507, 1992).*

713

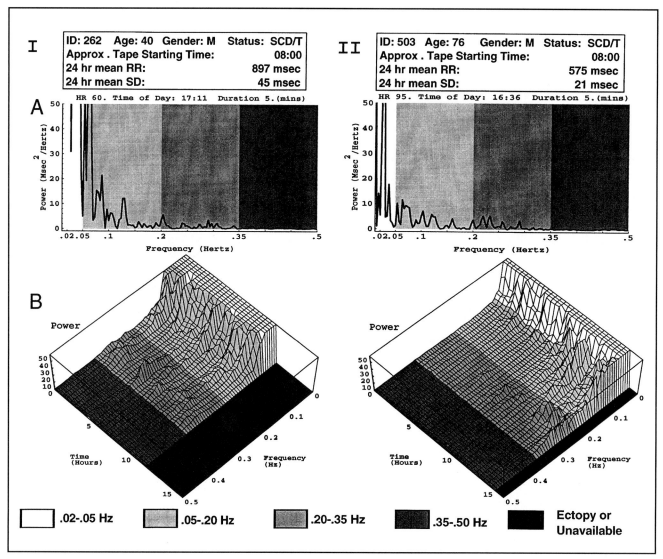

Figure 7. Representative 5-minute (IA, IIA) and 13- and 15-hour (IB, IIB) FFT power spectral traces from 40- and 76-year-old individuals who experienced SCD during ambulatory monitoring (SCD/T). Power is extremely low (note scale) at all frequencies, but particularly in the HF and in the higher ranges of the LF bands, for both individuals. The records in IB appear to show a further gradual decline in the respiratory sinus arrhythmia band (.05-.20 Hz) over time. The baroreceptor component (.20-.35 Hz) of the LF band, on the other hand, appeared to increase somewhat further, particularly during the last 2-3 hours of the recording. In contrast, power in all bands increased somewhat in the records in IIB during the last 2 hours of the recording. Irrespective of these changes, the records are suggestive of sympathetic dominance throughout the monitoring period for both patients. *(Modified after Ori Z et al: Card Clinics 10: 522,523, 1992).*

Observations by Monir and colleagues (1992) concerning differences between cycle length dependence of HRV of normal individuals and patients with symptomatic heart disease, could prove useful in distinguishing low HRV due to aging from that due to disease and risk of SCD. More specifically, it was found that normal individuals of all ages exhibit a linear relationship between cycle length (heart rate) and HRV: HRV increases with increases in cycle length to a maximum at cycle length 1000 msec. In contrast, the strength of the relationship was variably decreased in patients with symptomatic heart disease. In patients with high grade, complex ventricular ectopy and severe congestive failure, the slope of the relationship was markedly depressed and in some individuals was almost flat. The possibility that the relationship may cease to hold in patients with end stage disease and at high risk of SCD needs to be investigated. Our own preliminary observations support the view that the relationship may actually cease to hold in such patients. Larger prospective studies are needed. If further documented, marked depression or disappearance of the cycle length dependence of HRV could represent another indicator of risk of SCD.

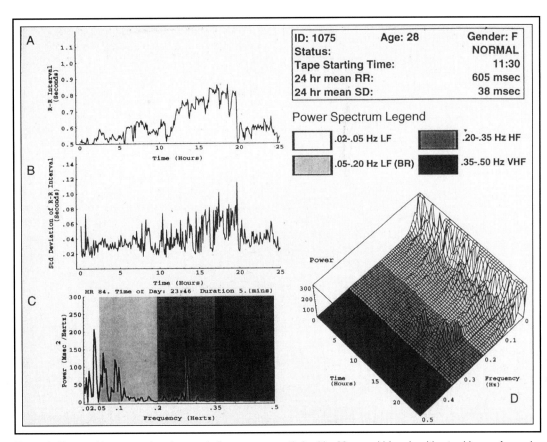

Figure 8. Time and frequency domain records from an apparently healthy 28-year-old female without evidence of organic disease. Physical examination was normal; laboratory data with the exception of HRV also were normal. Mean 24 hour HRV (SD measure) was abnormally low for age (38 msec). Power spectrum analysis revealed reduction in HF and baroreceptor power with transient increases in these parameters occurring in conjunction with periods of lower heart rate. LF power remained high, findings suggestive of sympathetic dominance.

This type of analysis also provides a potential tool for distinguishing "normal outliers," i.e., normal individuals with lower than expected HRV for age, since such individuals, in contrast to those in whom low HRV indicates heart disease and high risk of SCD, should exhibit normal cycle length dependence of HRV. In addition, application of the concept of cycle length dependence of HRV could allow one to distinguish "normal outliers" who exhibit low HRV in relation to high mean heart rates due to transient hypersympathetic states (Figure 8) from patients with pathologic reduction in vagal activity. One additional focus of study would be to compare HF and LF power at comparable cycle lengths in normal individuals and SCD survivors to assess the extent to which these differ.

HRV: Circadian Rhythms and Sudden Cardiac Death

Increased incidence of acute cardiovascular events, including SCD, myocardial infarction, transient myocardial ischemia and arrhythmias, during the early morning hours, particularly in patients with heart disease, suggests a possible relationship to altered circadian fluctuations in autonomic tone.

Studies on normal subjects and patients without organic heart disease have shown that HRV exhibits circadian variation, the lowest values occurring upon awakening in the morning. In a study of 44 patients with coronary disease complicated by myocardial infarction, of whom 22 were SCD survivors, HRV (SD measure) was found to be significantly lower in the SCD group (Huikuri and colleagues, 1992). The 24-hour mean HF spectral area also was lower in the SCD patients. However, the circadian variation in time and frequency domain measures of HRV did not differ between the two groups. Thus, survivors exhibited very low HRV in the morning immediately on awakening, corresponding to the time period with the highest incidence of SCD. These observations support conclusions that alterations in autonomic balance contribute to the increased prevalence of SCD during the morning hours and underscores the potential utility of HRV determinations as a marker of increased risk.

HRV and Sudden Cardiac Death:
Long-Term Predictive Value

Use of low HRV as a predictor of risk of SCD has been most extensively examined with respect to long term survival after myocardial infarction. In general, both experimental and clinical studies indicate that HRV is a powerful long-term predictor of risk of SCD.

Experimental studies by Hull and colleagues (1990) showed that low HRV distinguishes dogs at increased risk of development of SCD in response to exercise and transient ischemia one month post-experimental myocardial infarction (sensitivity: 88%; specificity: 80%). This was confirmed by Algra and colleagues (1993) in a large scale clinical epidemiologic survey of 6,693 consecutive Holter monitored patients followed for periods of up to 2 years showing that individuals with low HRV (SD measure < 25 msec) had an increased risk of SCD independent of other factors. Dougherty and Burr (1992) compared baseline 24 hour HRV determinations for SCD survivors who were alive one year after the event with those from patients who died of a subsequent episode during the follow-period. Baseline HRV was significantly lower in those who died than in survivors. Pilot data (Ahmed and colleagues, 1992) from long-term (to 8 years) follow-up of SCD survivors with mortality as the end point confirm the strong predictive value of low HRV (SD < 30 msec) for recurrence of major arrhythmic events: of seven patients exhibiting two or more major arrhythmic events, five died during the observation period.

Of these, four exhibited very low HRV (SD: < 20 msec). Odemuyiwa and colleagues (1991) found low HRV to be the single best predictor of major arrhythmic events after myocardial infarction, superior to such powerful variables as ventricular ejection fraction, heart rate, late potentials, and frequency and complexity of ectopic beats. Optimum risk stratification was achieved using a combination of HRV with late potentials or ventricular ectopy.

Most studies of the association between low HRV and SCD have been based on determinations from 24-hour Holter monitoring records. Recently, because of considerations of convenience and cost, there has been a surge of interest in HRV determinations from short term records. In a study of 715 patients (Bigger and colleagues, 1993), power spectral measures (VLF, LF, HF, LF/HF) of HRV determined 2 weeks after myocardial infarction proved to be powerful predictors of SCD and all-cause mortality during a 2.5 year follow-up period regardless of whether HRV was determined from short (2 min

to 15 min) or long (24 hr) recordings. Predictive value was even further improved when HRV was used in combination with New York Heart Association functional class criteria.

The combination of HF power and New York Heart Association criteria provided the highest positive predictive accuracy, underscoring the protective effect of parasympathetic activity in this population. A preliminary report (Bigger and colleagues, 1993) to the effect that risk of death following myocardial infarction could be successfully predicted using HRV determinations calculated from 2 minutes-15 minutes electrocardiographic records also is pertinent.

During the past year, we have had the opportunity to examine short term ECG machine based time and frequency domain HRV determinations derived from analysis of 1,027 beats and to make comparisons with conventional Holter based measurements. To date, records from approximately 100 patients have been accumulated. Preliminary evaluation suggests that, in general, HRV determinations appear more or less comparable for the two techniques provided that the mean heart rates for the time blocks studied approximate each other. As might be predicted, comparability was closest when the cycle length distributions in ECG machine and Holter based records were similar. The relationship between mean heart rate and comparability of the HRV determinations using the two methods is being investigated in detail. If confirmed, it would underscore the potential importance of cycle length dependence analysis to short term HRV studies. Reproducibility of short term HRV determinations also is being assessed. The half dozen comparisons made to date suggest that baseline measurements show a high degree of reproducibility one to six months after initial study in the absence of intervening changes in clinical state or mean heart rate.

HRV and Sudden Cardiac Death:
Short-Term Predictive Value

Since substrate conditions thought to predispose to SCD may be present for prolonged time periods prior to the event, the question arises as to the nature of the changes that trigger onset of ventricular fibrillation. Acute alterations in autonomic balance, more specifically, increases in sympathetic and/or decreases in parasympathetic activity with resultant accentuation of sympathetic dominance, represent one possible trigger.

Coumel, in a 1990 report on HRV changes associated with onset of ectopic tachyarrhythmias, concluded that paroxysmal ventricular as well as supraventricular tachyarrhythmias may be triggered by autonomic changes. In support, he showed a case of paroxysmal ventricular tachycardia in which onset of the tachycardia was immediately preceded by changes in heart rate and heart rate oscillations consistent with increased sympathetic activity, and a sympathetic trigger for the tachyarrhythmia. Interestingly, the report also described an example of a paroxysmal supraventricular (atrial fibrillation) tachyarrhythmia, the onset of which was preceded by heart rate changes consistent with an increase in parasympathetic activity. Conclusions concerning the relationships between the onset of ventricular tachyarrhythmias and increases in sympathetic tone are tempered by suggestive evidence that in individuals at highest risk, the degree of sympathetic increase required to trigger the dysrhythmia may be too small to permit ready identification, possibly because of high baseline levels of sympathetic activity.

HRV analysis in patients who experienced SCD during Holter monitoring, particularly changes occurring during the few minutes preceding the terminal event, might be expected to yield important clues. Early observations from our own laboratory were encouraging. Time domain HRV values (SD measure) determined during the five minutes immediately preceding the onset of ventricular fibrillation were compared with those obtained during the preceding five minute period for eleven SCD patients. HRV decreased between the two time periods (p=<.02). Similarities in mean heart rate between the two periods indicated that the decrease in HRV was not a function of change in rate.

Early Holter-based time and frequency domain HRV studies on eight patients with coronary disease who experienced SCD during monitoring (Singer and colleagues, unpublished data) revealed that twenty-four time domain HRV values were very low, i.e., SD <30 msec., in all but the youngest member of the group, a level consistent with that previously reported for SCD patients. HF power also was extremely low. LF power, although much lower than normal, was nevertheless still very much greater than the power in the HF bands. Given the virtual disappearance of HF activity, it seems reasonable to assume that the residual LF power largely reflected non-vagal (sympathetic) activity. To the extent that this holds, the records are indicative of sympathetic dominance throughout the monitoring period. The generally fast sinus rates, which these patients also exhibited, support this interpretation.

Figure 7 shows representative records for the period preceding SCD from 40-year-old (Panel I)

and 76-year-old (Panel II) males with coronary artery disease. Two HF (0.15-.50 Hz) bands and two LF bands (.02 Hz-.20 Hz), putative indices of parasympathetic and sympathetic activity respectively, were measured. Note the virtual disappearance of HF power in both individuals with resultant dominance of LF power. To the extent that the residual LF power reflects non-vagal (sympathetic) activity, the records suggest sympathetic dominance throughout the monitoring period. The generally fast sinus rates are consistent with sympathetic dominance.

Detailed analyses of frequency domain changes in all eight patients of the group during the hour preceding the onset of ventricular fibrillation showed continued LF (sympathetic) dominance. Six of the eight patients also appeared to exhibit an additional surge in LF power just prior to the terminal event, suggesting the possibility of a sympathetic trigger. Figure 9 shows records obtained during the hour preceding the onset of ventricular fibrillation from the same two patients depicted in Figure 7. Note the continuing decline of all power in all components of the power spectrum, particularly HF power, for both patients during the pre-terminal 10 minutes-15 minutes. The last few minutes of the record are characterized by virtually unopposed LF power, highlighting both the sympathetic contribution to the genesis of SCD and the possibility of a sympathetic trigger for the terminal event.

Findings (Huikuri and colleagues, 1993) that time and frequency domain HRV measures were significantly lower prior to the onset of sustained, as compared with non-sustained, ventricular tachyarrhythmias are supportive, as are findings (Yoshida and colleagues, 1992) that the LF/HF ratio increases significantly just prior to the onset of sustained ventricular tachyarrhythmias. Recent reports (Pelliccia and colleagues, 1992) that episodes of ventricular tachycardia were preceded by increases in LF power during the five minutes before the event also deserve mention. Evidence that episodes of ischemia are immediately preceded by increases in indices of sympathetic tone, i.e., increases in heart rate and in low frequency power, also are pertinent in that this condition is frequently associated with ventricular dysrhythmias.

However, as Coumel (1990) has suggested, delineation of specific patterns of autonomic change which serve to trigger lethal ventricular tachyarrhythmias is complex and difficult. For example, two of the eight patients in the group discussed above did not exhibit clear-cut increases in baroreceptor power prior to the onset of ventricular fibril-

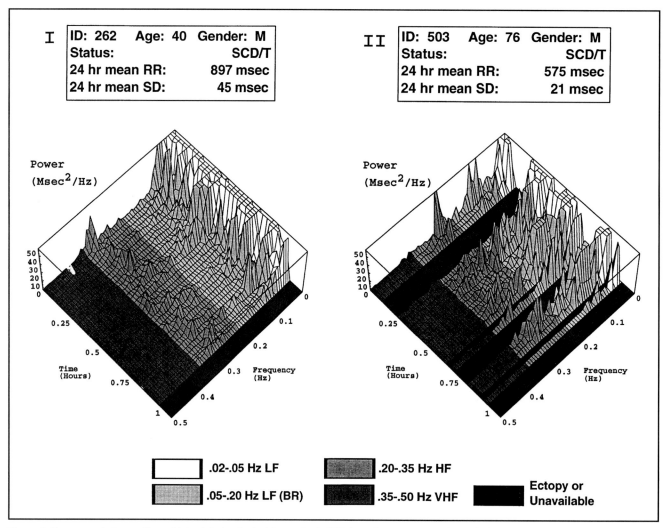

Figure 9. Power spectral recordings obtained during the last hour prior to SCD from the same two patients depicted in Figure 7. The dark bands in Panel II represent periods of time during which meaningful spectral data could not be obtained due to ectopy or other causes. Both records show marked reduction in power at all frequencies. During the 15 minutes prior to SCD, power at all frequency ranges decreased still further. Power in the HF and baroreceptor bands virtually disappeared, leaving LF power virtually unopposed, a finding which could suggest a sympathetic trigger for the terminal dysrhythmia. *(Modified after Ori Z et al: Card Clinics 10: 524,525, 1992).*

lation. Rather, in these individuals, the few minutes just prior to SCD were characterized by small surges in both HF and LF power. In addition, of the six patients who did experience preterminal surges in LF power, two exhibited similar appearing increases in this parameter earlier during the monitoring period. However, these early surges were not associated with ventricular fibrillation. Findings by Vyberal and colleagues (1993) further highlight difficulties in defining the specific pattern of changes which trigger SCD.

This study, in which HRV was evaluated on an hour by hour basis during the monitoring period with special attention to the hour just prior to SCD, did not show consistent patterns of autonomic change of the type which might be expected to trigger ventricular fibrillation. Studies utilizing power

changes in the LF and VLF as indices of sympathetic activity would help clarify the nature of autonomic triggers of ventricular dysrhythmias. In view of reports to the effect that power levels in frequency bands <0.04 Hz, principally the ULF band, may serve as a predictor of risk of SCD, changes in this parameter also deserve study. However, care must be taken to observe the previously described methodologic caveats with respect to analysis of low frequencies. High levels of ectopy which characterize the preterminal period may markedly distort time and frequency domain HRV determinations, particularly the latter. Improved methods for electronically compensating for ectopy and other artifacts are needed.

In addition, high base levels of sympathetic dominance in SCD patients may make it difficult to precisely define additional, possibly small, changes in autonomic activity needed to trigger lethal ventricular tachyarrhythmias, at least using current methods. Use of new and more sophisticated indices of HRV may facilitate a better understanding of patterns of HRV change associated with SCD. Application of "chaos theory" also shows promise.

Combinations of Risk Factors

Combinations of risk factors may be a more potent indicator of risk of SCD than any individual measure. For example, Kuchar and colleagues (1987) and Gomes and colleagues (1987) showed that combination of a late potential and low ejection fraction served to identify subjects at high risk of ventricular tachycardia, ventricular fibrillation, and SCD with a remarkably high degree of sensitivity (80%-100%) and specificity (89%-100%). In addition, Farrel and colleagues (1991) found the combined occurrence of a late potential and low heart rate variability (HRV), a measure of autonomic function to be the best predictor of a major cardiac event after myocardial infarction (sensitivity: 58%, specificity: 93%, positive predictive accuracy: 33%, negative predictive accuracy: 93%). The combination of late potentials and low left ventricular ejection fraction ranked second best in their hands (sensitivity: 25%, specificity: 94%, positive predictive accuracy: 19%, negative predictive accuracy: 94%).

Selected Reading

1. Kempf FC, Josephson ME: Cardiac arrest recorded on ambulatory electrocardiograms. *Am J Cardiol* 1984; 53:1577.
2. Liberthson R, Nagel E, Hirschman J, Nussenfeld S, Blackbourne B, Davis J: Pathophysiologic observations in pre-hospital ventricular fibrillation and sudden cardiac death. *Circulation* 1974; 49:790.
3. Milner PG, Platia EV, Reid PR, Griffith LSC: Ambulatory electrocardiographic recordings at the time of fatal cardiac arrest. *Am J Cardiol* 1985; 56:588.
4. Myerburg RJ and Castellanos A: *Cardiac Arrest and Sudden Cardiac Death.* in Braunwald E (editor) *Heart Disease: A Textbook of Cardiovascular Medicine.* (Philadelphia) W.B. Saunders Company, 1992, 756-789.
5. Myerburg JR, Kessler KM, Castellanos A: Sudden cardiac death. Structure, function, and time-dependence of risk. *Circ* 1992; 85 [suppl I]:I-2-I-10.
6. Panidis IP, Morganroth J: Holter monitoring and sudden cardiac death. *Cardiovasc Rev Rep* 1984; 5 (3): 283-304.

Risk Factors for Sudden Cardiac Death

1. Algra A, Tijssen JPG, Roelandt JCTR, Pool J, Lubsen J: Heart rate variability from 24-Hour electrocardiography and the 2-year risk for sudden death. *Circ* 1993; 88:180-185.
2. Cupples AL, Gagnon DR, Kannel WB: Long- and short-term risk of sudden coronary death. *Circulation* 1992; 85[suppl I]:I-11-I-18.

3. El Maraghi N, Genton E: The relevance of platelet and fibrin thromboembolism of the coronary microcirculation with special reference to sudden cardiac death. *Circ* 1980; 62:936.
4. Josephson ME: (ed.) *Sudden cardiac death.* (Philadelphia) F.A. Davis Company, 1985.
5. Kuller LH: Sudden death: definition and epidemiologic considerations. *Prog Cardio Dis* 1980; 23:1.
6. Marchilinski FE, Buxton AE, Waxman HL, Josephson ME: Identifying patients at risk of sudden death after myocardial infarction: Value of the response to programmed stimulation, degree of ventricular activity, and severity of left ventricular dysfunction. *Am J Cardiol* 1983; 52:1190.
7. Martin GJ, Magid NM et al: Heart rate variability and sudden death secondary to coronary artery disease during ambulatory ECG monitoring. *Am J Cardiol* 1987; 60:86-89.
8. Myerburg JR, Kessler KM, Castellanos A: Sudden cardiac death. Structure, function, and time-dependence of risk. *Circ* 1992; 85 [suppl I]:I-2-I-10.
9. Schwartz JP, La Rovere T, Vanoll E.: Autonomic nervous system and sudden cardiac death, experimental basis and clinical observations for post-myocardial infarction risk stratification. *Circ* 1992; 85[Suppl I]:I77-91.
10. Simson MB: Noninvasive identification of patients at high risk for sudden cardiac death. *Circ* 1992; 85[suppl I] I-145-I-151.

Myocardial Damage/Dysfunction

1. Anderson KP: Sudden death, hypertension, and hypertrophy. *J Cardio Pharm* 1984; 6 (Suppl 3): S498.
2. Anderson KP: Hypertension and sudden cardiac death. *NZ Med J* 1982; 95:33.
3. Cobb LA Baum RS, Alvarez H, Schaffer WA: Resuscitation from out-of-hospital ventricular fibrillation: Four year follow-up. *Circ* 1075; 51-52 (Suppl 3):223.
4. Goldstein S: The necessity of a uniform definition of sudden coronary death: Witnessed death within 1 hour of the onset of acute symptoms. *AHJ* 1982; 103:156.
5. Goldstein S, Landis J, Leighton R, et al.: Characteristics of the resuscitated out-of-hospital cardiac arrest victim with coronary heart disease. *Circ* 1981; 64:977.
6. Gordon T, Kannel WB: Premature mortality from coronary heart disease. The Framingham Study. *JAMA* 1971; 215:1617.
7. Hammermeister K, DeRouen T, Dodge H: Variables predictive of survival in patients with coronary disease. *Circ* 1979; 59:425.
8. Hinkle LE: The immediate antecedents of sudden death. *Acta Med Scand* 1981; 210:207.
9. Lovegrove T, Thompson P: The role of acute myocardial infarction in sudden cardiac death — a statistician's nightmare. *AHJ* 1978; 96:711.
10. Myerburg R, Conde C, Sung R, et al.: Prevention of recurrent sudden cardiac arrest: Role of provocative electrophysiologic testing. *JACC* 1983; 2:418.
11. Moss A: Profile of high risk in people known to have coronary heart disease: A review. *Circ* 1975; 51&52 (Suppl 3):147.
12. Newman WP, Tracy RE, Strong JP et al.: Pathology of sudden cardiac death. *Ann NY Acad Sci* 1982; 382:39.
13. Perper JA, Kuller LH, Cooper M: Arteriosclerosis of coronary arteries in sudden, unexpected deaths. *Circ* 1976; 52 (Suppl 3):27, 1975.
14. Ritchie J, Hallstrom A, Troubaugh G, et al.: Out-of-hospital sudden coronary death: Rest and exercise radionuclide left ventricular function in survivors. *AJC* 1985; 55:645.
15. Schwartz C, Gerrity R: Anatomical pathology of sudden

719

unexpected cardiac death. *Circ* 1975; 51&52 (Suppl 3):18.

16. Weaver W, Lorch G, Alvarez H, et al.: Angiographic findings and prognostic indicators in patients resuscitated from sudden cardiac death. *Circ* 1976; 54:895.

Late Potentials

1. Breithardt G, Borggrefe M, Karbenn V, et al.: Prevalence of late potentials in patients with and without ventricular tachycardia: Correlation with angiographic findings. *Am J Cardiol* 1982; 49:1932.

2. Coto H, Maldonado C, Palakurthy P, et al.: Late potentials in normal subjects and in patients with ventricular tachycardia unrelated to myocardial infarction. *Am J Cardiol* 1985; 55:384.

3. Fintel D, Huang S, Kim K, Abi-Mansour P, Schaad J, Weiss J, Reddy S, Singer D: Late potentials in ventricular fibrillation: Improved detection by visual reanalysis. *JACC* 1991; 17 (2):388.

4. Gomes J, Mehra R, Barreca P et al.: Quantitative analysis of the high-frequency components of the signal-averaged QRS complex in patients with acute myocardial infarction: A prospective study. *Circ* 1985;72:105.

5. Gomes AJ, Winters LS, Stewart D, Horowitz S, Milner M, Barreca P: A new noninvasive index to predict sustained ventricular tachycardia and sudden death in the first year after myocardial infarction: Based on signal-averaged electrocardiogram, radionuclide ejection fraction and holter monitoring. *JACC* 1987; 10:349-357.

6. Kanovsky M, Falcone R, Dresden C et al.: Identification of patients with ventricular tachycardia after myocardial infarction: Signal-averaged electrocardiogram, Holter monitoring and cardiac catheterization. *Circ* 1984; 70:264.

7. Kuchar LD, Thorburn WC, Sammel LN: Prediction of serious arrhythmic events after myocardial infarction: signal averaged electrocardiogram, holter monitoring and radionuclide ventriculography. *JACC* 1987;9:531-538.

8. Simson MB: Noninvasive identification of patients at high risk for sudden cardiac death. *Circ* 1992; 85[suppl I]:I-145-I-151.

9. Simson M: Use of signals in the terminal QRS complex to identify patients with ventricular tachycardia after myocardial infarction. *Circ* 1991; 64:235.

Ventricular Ectopy

1. Bigger JT, Fleiss JL, Kleiger R, Miller JP, Rolnitzky LM and the Multicenter Post-infarction Research Group: The relationships among ventricular arrhythmias, left ventricular dysfunction, and mortality in the two years after myocardial infarction. *Circ* 1984; 69:250.

2. Cardiac Arrhythmia Suppression Trial (CAST) Investigators: Preliminary report: Effect of encainide and flecainide on mortality in a randomized trial of arrhythmia suppression after myocardial infarction. *NEJM* 1989; 321:406.

3. Chiang BN, Perlman L, Ostrander LD, Epstein G: Relation of premature systoles to coronary heart disease and sudden death in the Tecumseh epidemiologic study. *Ann Intern Med* 1969;70:1159.

4. Follansbee WP, Michaelson EL, Morganroth H: Non-sustained ventricular tachycardia in ambulatory patients. Characteristics and association with sudden cardiac death. *Ann Intern Med* 1980; 92:741.

5. Holmes J, Kubo SH, Cody RJ, Kligfield P: Arrhythmias in ischemic and non-ischemic dilated cardiomyopathy; prediction of mortality by ambulatory electrocardiography. *Am J Cardiol* 1985; 55:146.

6. Lown B, Calvert AF, Armington R, Ryan M: Monitoring for serious arrhythmias and high risk of sudden death. *Circ* 1975; 52 (Suppl III):189.

7. Messerli FH, Ventura HO, Elizardi DJ, et al.: Hypertension and sudden death: Increased ventricular ectopic activity in left ventricular hypertrophy. *AJM* 1984;77:18.

8. Moss AJ, Davis HT: Clinical significance of ventricular arrhythmias in patients with and without coronary artery disease. *Prog Cardio Dis* 1980; 23:33.

9. Moss AJ, Davis HT, DeCamilla J, Bayer LW: Ventricular ectopic beats and their relation to sudden death and non-sudden cardiac death after myocardial infarction. *Circ* 1979; 60:998.

10. Panidis IP, Morganroth J: Holter monitoring and sudden cardiac death. *Cardiovasc Rev Rep* 1984; 5 (3):283-304.

11. Pratt CM, Theroux P, Slymen D, et al: Spontaneous variability of ventricular arrhythmias in patients at increased risk for sudden death after acute myocardial infarction: Consecutive ambulatory electrocardiographic recordings of 88 paptients. *AJC* 1987; 59:278.

12. Ruberman W, Weinblatt E, Frank CW, et al.: Repeated 1-hour electrocardiographic monitoring of survivors of myocardial infarction at 6-month intervals: Arrhythmia detection and relation to prognosis. *AJC* 1981; 47:1197.

13. Ruberman W, Weinblatt E, Goldberg JD, et al: Ventricular premature complexes and sudden death after myocardial infarction. *Circ* 1981; 64:297.

14. Vlay SE, Reid PR: Ventricular ectopy: Etiology, evaluation and therapy. *AJM* 1982; 73:899.

Inducibility

1. Benditt D, Benson D, Klein G, et al.: Prevention of recurrent sudden cardiac arrest: Role of provocative electrophysiologic testing. *JACC* 1983; 2:418.

2. Gomes AJ, Hariman RI, Kang PS, El-Sherif N, Chowdhry I, Lyons J: Programmed electrical stimulation in patients with high grade ventricular ectopy: Electrophysiologic findings and prognosis for survival. *Circ* 1984; 70:43.

3. Josephson ME, Horowitz L, Spielman SR, Greenspan AM: Electrophysiologic and hemodynamic studies in patients resuscitated from cardiac arrest. *AJC* 1980; 46:948.

4. Kehoe R, Tommaso C, Zheutlin T, et al: Factors determining programmed stimulation responses and long-term arrhythmic outcome in survivors of ventricular fibrillation with ischemic heart disease. *AHJ* 1988; 116:355.

5. Marchilinski FE, Buxton AE, Waxman HL, Josephson ME: Identifying patients at risk of sudden death after myocardial infarction: Value of the response to programmed stimulation, degree of ventricular activity, and severity of left ventricular dysfunction. *AJC* 1983; 52:1190.

6. Mason JW, Winkle RA: Electrode catheter arrhythmia induction in the selection and assessment of antiarrhythmic drug therapy for recurrent ventricular tachycardia. *Circ* 1978; 58:971.

7. Milner PG, DiMarco JP, Lerman BB: Electrophysiological evaluation of sustained ventricular tachyarrhythmia in idiopathic dilated cardiomyopathy. *PACE* 1988; 11:562-568.

8. Morady F, Scheinman M, Hess D, et al.: Electrophysiologic testing in the management of survivors of out-of-hospital cardiac arrest. *AJC* 1983;51:85.

9. Poole JE, Mathisen TL, Kundenchuk PJ, et al: Long-term outcome in patients who survive out of hospital ventricular fibrillation and undergo electrophysiologic studies: Evaluation by electrophysiologic subgroups. *JACC* 1990; 16:657-665.

10. Roy D, Waxman H, Krienzle M, et al.: Clinical characteristics and long-term follow-up in 119 survivors of cardiac

arrest: Relation to inducibility at electrophysiologic testing. *Am J Cardiol* 1983; 52:969.

11. Ruskin JN, DiMarco JP, Garan A: Out-of-hospital cardiac arrest: Electrophysiologic observations and selection of long-term antiarrhythmic therapy. *NEJM* 1980; 303:607.

12. Stevenson WG, Stevenson LW, Weiss J, Tillisch JH: Inducible ventricular arrhythmias and sudden death during vasodilator therapy of severe heart failure. *AHJ* 1988; 116:1447-1454.

13. Wilber JD, Garan H, Kelly E, et al: Out-of-hospital cardiac arrest: Role of electrophysiologic testing in the prediction of long-term outcome. *NEJM* 1988; 318:19.

14. Zheutlin TA, Roth H, Chua W, Steinman R, Summers C, Lesch M, Kehoe RF: Programmed electrical stimulation to determine the need for antiarrhythmic therapy in patients with complex ventricular ectopic activity. *Am Heart J* 1986;111:860.

Autonomic Dysfunction and SCD: Clinical and Experimental Studies

1. Bannister R, Mathias CJ: *Autonomic Failure: A Textbook of Clinical Disorders of the Autonomic Nervous System.* Third Edition, (Oxford) Oxford University Press. 1992.

2. Bigger JT, Fleiss JL, Rolnitzky LM, Steinman RC: The ability of several short-term measures of RR variability to predict mortality after myocardial infarction. *Circ* 1993; 88:927-934.

3. Bigger JT, Hoffman BF: *Antiarrhythmic drugs.* In Gilman AG, Rall, TW, Nies AS, Taylor, P (Eds): Goodman and Gilman's The Pharmacological Basis of Therapeutics (New York) Pergamon Press. 1990, 840-873.

4. Burch GE, DePasquale NP.: Sudden, unexpected, natural death. *Am J Med Sci* 1965; 249:86.

5. Burrell RJW: *The possible bearing of curse death and other factors in Bantu culture in the etiology of myocardial infarction.* In James TN and Keyes JW (eds.): *The Etiology of Myocardial Infarction.* (Boston) Little Brown, 1963.

6. Campbell BC, Sturani A, Reid JL: Evidence of parasympathetic activity of the angiotensin converting enzyme inhibitor, captopril, in normotensive man. *Clin Sci* 1985; 68:49-56.

7. Campese VM, Romoff MS, Levitan D, Lane K, and Massry SG: Mechanisms of autonomic nervous system dysfunction in uremia. *Kidney Int* 1981; 20:246-253.

8. Cannon WB: "Voodoo" death. *Psychosom Med* 1957; 19:182.

9. The Cardiac Arrhythmia Suppression Trial (CAST) Investigators: Preliminary report: effect of encainide and flecainide on mortality in randomized trial of arrhythmia suppression after myocardial infarction. *NEJM* 1989; 321(6):406-412.

10. Cerati D, Schwartz PJ: Single cardiac vagal fiber activity, acute myocardial ischemia, and risk for sudden death. *Circ Res* 1991; 69:1389-1401.

11. Comi G, Sora MGN, Bianchi A, Bontempi B, et al: Spectral analysis of short-term heart rate variability in diabetic patients. *J Auton Nerv Syst* 1990; 30: S45-S50.

12. Corr PB, Gillis RA: Autonomic neural influences on the dysrhythmias resulting from myocardial infarction. *Circ Res* 1978; 43:1.

13. Coumel P, Rosengarten MD, Leclercq JF, Attuel P: Role of sympathetic nervous system in nonischemic ventricular arrhythmias. *BHJ* 47:137, 1982.

14. Dangman KH, Miura DS: *Proarrhythmic effects of antiarrhythmic drugs;* 375-395, in Dangman KH and Miura DS (editors): *Electrophysiology and pharmacology of the heart.* Marcel Dekker, Inc. 1991.

15. Deal BJ, Miller SW, Scagliotti D, et al.: Ventricular tachycardia in a young population without overt heart disease. *Circ* 1986; 73:1111.

16. De Ferrari MG, Vanoli E, Stramba-Badiale M, Hull SS Jr, Foreman DR, Schwartz JP: Vagal reflexes and survival during acute ischemia in conscious dogs with healed myocardial infarction. *Am J Physiol* 1991; 261:H63-H69.

17. Eckberg DL, Drabinsky M, Braunwald E: Defective cardiac sympathetic control in patients with heart disease. *NEJM* 1971; 285:877.

18. Engel GL: Psychologic stress, vasodepressor vasovagal syncope, and sudden death. *Ann Intern Med* 1978; 89:403.

19. Kjellgren O, Gomes JA: Heart rate variability and baroreflex sensitivity in myocardial infarction. *Am Heart J* 1993;125(1):204-215.

20. Kolman B, Verrier R, Lown B: The effect of vagus nerve stimulation upon vulnerability of the canine ventricle: Role of sympathetic parasympathetic interactions. *Circ* 1975; 52:578.

21. Lown B, DeSilva RA, Lenson R: Role of psychologic stress and autonomic nervous system changes in provocation of ventricular premature complexes. *Am J Cardiol* 1977; 41:979.

22. Lown B, Verrier R: Neural activity and ventricular fibrillation. *NEJM* 1976; 294 (21):1165.

23. Maron BJ, Epstein SE, Roberts WC: Causes of sudden death in competitive athletes. *JACC* 1986; 7:204.

24. Meinertz T, Hoffmann T, Kasper W, et al: Significance of ventricular arrhythmias in idiopathic dilated cardiomyopathy. *Am J Cardiol* 1984; 53:902.

25. Muller JE, Stone PH, Turi ZG, Rutherford J, et al and the Mills Study Group: Circadian variation in the frequency of onset of acute myocardial infarction. *NEJM* 1985; 313:1315-1322.

26. Myerburg RJ, Conde CA, Sung RJ, et al: Clinical, electrophysiologic, and hemodynamic profile of patients resuscitated from prehospital cardiac arrest. *Am J Med* 1980; 68:568.

27. Ori Z, Monir G, Weiss J, Sayhouni X, and Singer D: Heart rate variability: Frequency domain analysis. *Cardiology Clinics* 1992; 10 (3):499-537.

28. Rabinowitz S, Verrier R, Lown B: Muscarinic effects of vagosympathetic trunk stimulation on the repetitive extrasystole (RE) threshold. *Circ* 1976; 53:622.

29. Reichenback DD, Moss NS, Meyer E: Pathology of the heart in sudden cardiac death. *Am J Cardiol* 1977; 39:865.

30. Schwartz PJ: The idiopathic long Q-T syndrome. *Ann Intern Med* 1982; 99:561.

31. Schwartz JP, La Rovere T, Vanoll E.: Autonomic nervous system and sudden cardiac death, experimental basis and clinical observations for post-myocardial infarction risk stratification. *Circ* 1992; 85 [Suppl I]:I77-91.

32. Schwartz PJ, Periti M, Malliani A: The long Q-T syndrome. *Am Heart J.* 1975; 89:378.

33. Sheps DS, Conde CA, Mayorga-Cortes A, et al.: Primary ventricular fibrillation: Some unusual features. *Chest* 1977;72:235.

34. Singer DH, Martin GJ, Magid N, Weiss JS, et al: Low heart rate variability and sudden cardiac death. *J Electrocardiol* 1988; Suppl:S46-S55.

35. Surawicz B: Ventricular fibrilllation. *JACC* 1985; 51(Suppl B):43.

36. Vanoli E, De Ferrari MG, Stramba-Badiale M, Hull SS Jr, Foreman DR, Schwartz JP. Vagal stimulation and prevention of sudden death in conscious dogs with a healed myocardial infarction. *Circ Res* 1991; 68:147-181.

721

37. Vidallet HJ, Pressley JC, Henke E, et al.: Familial occurrence of accessory atrioventricular pathways (preexcitation syndrome). *NEJM* 1987; 317:65.
38. Warren JV: Unusual sudden death. *Cardiol Ser* 1984; 8(4):5.
39. Zuanetti G, Latini R, Neilson JMM, Schwartz PJ, Ewing DJ and the Antiarrhythmic Drug Evaluation Group (ADEG): Heart rate variability in patients with ventricular arrhythmias: effect of antiarrhythmic drugs. *JACC* 1991; 17 (3):604-612.

Cellular Electrophysiologic Studies

1. Bailey JC, Greenspan K, Elizari MV et al: Effects of acetylcholine on automaticity and conduction in the proximal portion of the His-Purkinje specialized conduction of the dog. *Circ Res* 1972; 30:210-216.
2. Baumgarten CM, Fozzard HA: *Cardiac resting and pacemaker potentials.* in Fozzard HA, Haber E, Jennings RB, Katz AM, Morgan HE (eds) *The Heart and Cardiovascular System, Scientific Foundations,* Volume I, (New York) Raven Press, 1991, pp 963-1001.
3. Cranefield PF: Action potentials, afterpotentials and arrhythmia. *Circ Res* 1977; 41:415-423.
4. Ferrier GR: Digitalis arrhythmias: Role of oscillatory afterpotentials. *Prog Cardiovasc Dis* 1977; 19:459-474.
5. Fozzard HA, Arnsdorf MF: *Cardiac electrophysiology.* in Fozzard HA, Haber E, Jennings RB, Katz AM, Morgan HE (eds) *The Heart and Cardiovascular System, Scientific Foundations,* Volume I, (New York) Raven Press, 1991, pp. 63-98.
6. Hoffman BF: *Experiments on abnormal automaticity*, in Rosenbaum MB, Felizari MV (eds): *Frontiers of Cardiac Electrophysiology.* (The Hague) Martinus Nijhoff, 1983, pp 144-157.
7. Hoffman BF, Cranefield PF: *Electrophysiology of the Heart* (New York) McGraw-Hill, 1960.
8. Hoffman BF, Cranefield PF: Physiological basis of cardiac arrhythmias. *Am J Med* 1964; 37:670-684.
9. Hoffman BF, Rosen MR: Cellular mechanisms for cardiac arrhythmia. *Circ Res* 1981; 49:1-15.
10. Lazzara R, El-Sherif N, Hope R, et al: Ventricular arrhythmias and electrophysiological consequences of myocardial ischemia and infarction. *Circ Res* 1978; 42:740-749.
11. McCullough JR, Baumgarten CM, Singer DH: Intra- and extracellular potassium activities and the potassium equilibrium potential in partially depolarized human atrial cells. *J Mol Cell Cardiol* 1987; 19:477-486.
12. McCullough JR, Chua WT, Rasmussen HH, Ten Eick RE, Singer DH: Two stable levels of diastolic potential at physiological K$^+$ concentrations in human ventricular myocardial cells. *Circ Res* 1990; 66:191-201.
13. Noble D: The surprising heart: A review of recent progress in cardiac electrophysiology. *J Physiol* (Lond) 1984; 353:1-50.
14. Panidis IP, Morganroth J: Holter monitoring and sudden cardiac death. *Cardiovasc Rev Rep* 1984; 5 (3):283-304.
15. Rosen MR, Janse MJ, Wit AL: *Cardiac Electrophysiology: A Textbook. In Honor of Brian F. Hoffman.* (Mt Kisco, NY.) Futura Publishing Co. 1990.
16. Sato R, Hisatome I, Wasserstorm JA, Arentzen CE, Singer DH: Acetylcholine-sensitive K+ channel in human atrial myocytes. *Am J Physiol* 1990; 259:H1730-1735.
17. Singer DH, Baumgarten CM, and Ten Eick RE: Cellular electrophysiology of ventricular and other dysrhythmias: studies on diseased and ischemic heart. *Prog Cardiovasc Dis* 1981; 24:97-156.
18. Singer DH and Cohen HC: *Aberrancy: Electrophysiologic mechanisms and electrocardiographic correlates.* In: Mandel WJ, ed. *Cardiac Arrhythmias: Their Mechanisms, Diagnosis, and Management.* (3rd ed) Philadelphia: J.B. Lippincott, 1995: In press.
19. Singer D, Lazzara R and Hoffman B: Interrelationships between automaticity and conduction. *Circ Res* 1967; 21:537-558.
20. Singer D and Ten Eick R: Pharmacology of cardiac arrhythmias. *Prog Cardiovasc Dis* 1969; 11:488-514.
21. Ten Eick RE, Singer DH, Solberg LE et al: Alterations in the electrophysiologic characteristics of diseased human ventricle (abstr). *Circ* 1972; 44:II-9.
22. Ten Eick RE, Singer DH, Solberg LE: Coronary occlusion: Effect on cellular electrical activity of the heart. *Med Clin North Am* 1976; 60: 49-67.
23. Wit AL, Cranefield PF, Gadsby DC: *Triggered activity,* in Zipes DP, Bailey JC, Elharrar V (eds): *The Slow Inward Current and Cardiac Arrhythmias.* (The Hague) Martinus Nijhof, 1980, pp 437-454.
24. Wit A, Friedman P: The basis for ventricular arrhythmias accompanying myocardial infarction. Alterations in electrical activity of ventricular muscle and Purkinje fiber after coronary artery occlusion. *Arch Intern Med* 1975; 135:459-472.

Heart Rate Variability

1. Akselrod S, Gordon D, Ubel FA, Shannon DC, Barger AC, Cohen RJ: Power spectrum analysis of heart rate fluctuation: a quantitative probe beat-to-beat cardiovascular control. *Science* 1981; 213:210-222.
2. Bernardi L, Rossi M, Soffiantino F, et al: Cross relation of heart rate and respiration versus deep breathing. *Diabetes* 1990; 38:589-596.
3. Eckberg DL: Human sinus arrhythmia as an index of vagal cardiac outflow. *J Appl Physiol* 1983; 54 (4):961-966.
4. Ewing DJ, Martyn CN, Young RJ, Clarke BF: The value of cardiovascular autonomic function tests: 10 years experience in diabetes. *Diabetes Care* 1985; 8:491-498.
5. Farrel TG, Paul V, Cripps TR, Malik M, Bennett ED, Ward D, Camm AJ: Baroreflex sensitivity and electrophysiological correlates in patients after acute myocardial infarction. *Circ* 1991; 83:985-952.
6. Furlan R, Guzzetti S, Crivellaro W, et al: Continuous 24-hour assessment of neural regulation of systemic arterial pressure and RR variabilities in ambulant subjects. *Circ* 1990; 81:537-547.
7. Hales S: Statistical Essays. Vol II, *Haemostaticks.* Innings & Manby & Woodward, London, 1733.
8. Hyndman BW, Gregory JR: Spectral analysis of sinus arrhythmia during mental loading. *Ergonomics* 1975; 18(3):255-270.
9. Jose AD, Effect of combined sympathetic and parasympathetic blockade on heart rate and cardiac function in man. *Am J Cardiol* 1966; 18:476-478.
10. Karemaker JM: *Analysis of blood pressure and heart rate variability: theoretical considerations and clinical applicability.* In Low PA (editor) *Clinical Autonomic Disorders: Evaluation and Management,* (Boston) Little, Brown and Company, 1993, 315-329.
11. Katona P, Poitras JW, Barnett GO, Terry BS: Cardiac vagal efferent and heart period in the carotid sinus reflex. *Am J Physiol* 1970; 218 (4):1030-1037.
12. Katona P, Jih F: Respiratory sinus arrhythmia: non-invasive measure of parasympathetic cardiac control. *J Appl Physiol* 1975; 39 (5):801-805.
13. Kitney RI, Rompelman O: *The study of heart rate variability.* (Oxford) Clarendon Press, 1980.
14. Lombardi F, Sandrone G, Pernpruner S, et al: Heart rate

variability as an index of sympathovagal interaction after acute myocardial infarction. *Am J Cardiol* 1987; 60:1239-1245.

15. Malliani A, Pagani M, Lombardi F. and Cerutti S: Cardiovascular neural regulation explored in the frequency domain. *Circ* 1991; 84 (2):482-492.

16. Ori Z, Monir G, Weiss J, Sayhouni X, and Singer D: Heart rate variability: Frequency domain analysis. *Cardiology Clinics* 1992; 10 (3): 499-537.

17. Pagani M, Malfatto G, Pierini S, Casati R, Masu AM, Poli M, Guzzetti S, Lombardi F, Cerutti S, and Malliani A: Spectral analysis of heart rate variability in the assessment of autonomic diabetic neuropathy. *J Auton Nerv Syst* 1988; 23:143-153.

18. Sands KEF, Appel ML, Lilly LS, Schoen FJ, Mudge GH, and Cohen RJ: Power spectrum analysis of heart rate variability in human cardiac transplant recipients. *Circ* 1989; 79:76-82.

19. Sayers B McA: Analysis of heart rate variability. *Ergonomics* 1973; 16 (1):17-32.

HRV Methods of Analysis

1. Akselrod S, Gordon D, Ubel FA, Shannon DC, Barger AC, Cohen RJ: Power spectrum analysis of heart rate fluctuation: a quantitative probe beat-to-beat cardiovascular control. *Science* 1981; 213:210-222.

2. Bigger JT, Albrecht P, Steinman RC, Rolnitzky, Fleiss JKL and Cohen RJ: Comparison of time and frequency domain-based measures of cardiac parasympathetic activity in holter recordings after myocardial infarction. *Am J Cardiol* 1989; 64:536-538.

3. Bigger JT, Kleiger RE, Fleiss JL, Rolnitzky LM, Steinman RC, Miller JP, and The Multicenter Post-Infarction Research Group: Components of heart rate variability measured during healing of acute myocardial infarction. *Am J Cardiol* 1988; 61:208-215.

4. Bloomfield P: Fourier *Analysis Of Time Series: An Introduction.* John Wiley & Sons 1976.

5. Chess GF, Tam RMK, Calaresu FR: Influences of cardiac neural inputs on rhythmic variations of heart rate period in the cat. *Am J Physiol* 1975; 228 (3):775-780.

6. Eckberg DL: Human sinus arrhythmia as an index of vagal cardiac outflow. *J Appl Physiol* 1983:54 (4) 961-966.

7. Ewing DJ: Analysis of heart rate variability and other non-invasive tests with special reference to diabetes mellitus. in *Autonomic Failure: A Textbook of Clinical Disorders of the Autonomic Nervous System.* pp 312-333, Bannister R and Mathias CJ eds. (Oxford) Oxford Medical Publications, 1992.

8. Ewing DJ: *Noninvasive evaluation of heart rate: the time domain.* In Low PA (editor) *Clinical Autonomic Disorders: Evaluation and Management.* (Boston) Little, Brown and Company, 1993, pp 297-312.

9. Ewing DJ, Neilson JM, Shapiro CM, Stewart JA, Reid W: Twenty four hour heart rate variability: effects of posture, sleep and time of day in healthy controls and comparison with bedside tests of autonomic function in diabetic patients. *BHJ* 1991; 65:239-244.

10. Ewing DJ, Neilson JMM, Travis P: New method for assessing cardiac parasympathetic activity using 24-hour electrocardiograms. *BHJ* 1984; 52:396-402.

11. Furlan R, Guzzetti S, Crivellaro W, Dassi S, Tinelli M, Baselli G, Cerutti S, Lombardi F, Pagani M, Maliani A: Continuous 24-hour assessment of neural regulation of systemic arterial pressure and R-R variabilitiy in ambulant subjects. *Circ* 1990; 81:537-547.

12. Hrushesky WJ, Fader D, Schmitt O, Gilbertsen V: Respiratory sinus arrhythmia: a measure of cardiac age. *Science* 1984; 224:1001-1004.

13. Hyndman BW, Gregory JR: Spectral analysis of sinus arrhythmia during mental loading. *Ergonomics* 1975; 18 (3):255-270.

14. Julius S and Randall OS: Role of the autonomic nervous system in mild human hypertension. *Clin Sci Mol Med* 1975; 48:243S-252S.

15. Karemaker JM: *Analysis of blood pressure and heart rate variability: theoretical considerations and clinical applicability.* In Low PA (editor) *Clinical Autonomic Disorders: Evaluation and Management.* (Boston) Little, Brown and Company, 1993, 315-329.

16. Katona P, Poitras JW, Barnett GO, Terry BS: Cardiac vagal efferent and heart period in the carotid sinus reflex. *Am J Physiol* 218 (4):1030-1037, 1970.

17. Kitney RI, Rompelman O: *The study of heart rate variability.* (Oxford) Clarendon Press, 1980.

18. Kleiger RE, Bigger JT, Bosner MS, et al: Stability over time of variables measuring heart rate variability in normal subjects. *Am J Cardiol* 1991; 68:626-630.

19. Kleiger RE, Miller JP, Bigger JT, Moss AJ, the Multicenter Post-Infarct Research Group: Decreased heart rate variability and its association with increased mortality after acute myocardial infarction. *Am J Cardiol* 1987; 59 (4):256-262.

20. Kleiger RE, Stein PK, Bosner MS and Rottman JN: Time domain measurements of heart rate variability. *Card Clinics* 1992; 10 (300):487-498.

21. Kluge KA, Harper RM, Schechtman VL, et al: Spectral analysis assessment of respiratory sinus arrhythmia in normal infants who subsequently died of sudden infant death syndrome. *Pediatr Res* 1988; 24 (6):677-682.

22. Kobayashi M and Musha T: 1/f fluctuation of heartbeat period, *IEEE Tr on Biomed Eng* 1982; 29 (6):456-457.

23. Kolman B, Verrier R, Lown B: The effect of vagus nerve stimulation upon vulnerability of canine ventricle: role of sympathetic parasympathetic interaction. *Circ* 1975; 52:578-585.

24. Korkushko OV, Shatilo VB, Plachinda YuI, Shatilo TV: Autonomic control of cardiac chronotropic function in man as a function of age: assessment by power spectral analysis of heart rate variability. *J Auton Nerv Syst* 1991; 32:191-198.

25. Korner PI, Shaw J, Uther JB, West MJ, McRitchie RJ, Richards JG: Autonomic and non-autonomic circulatory components in essential hypertension in man. *Circ* 1973; 48:107-117.

26. Makhoul J: Linear prediction: a tutorial review. Proc *IEEE* 1975;63:561-580.

27. Malliani A, Pagani M, Lombardi F. and Cerutti S: Cardiovascular neural regulation explored in the frequency domain. *Circ* 1991; 84 (2):482-492.

28. Myers GA, Martin GJ, Magid NM, Barrett PS, Schaad JW, Weiss JS, Lesch M, and Singer DH: Power spectral analysis of heart rate variability in sudden cardiac death: comparison to other methods. *IEEE Tr Biomed Eng* 1986; 33 (12):1149-1156.

29. Ori Z, Monir G, Weiss J, Sayhouni X, and Singer D: Heart rate variability: Frequency domain analysis. *Card Clinics* 1992; 10 (3): 499-537.

30. Pagani M, Lombardi F, Guzetti S, et al: Power spectral analysis of heart rate and arterial pressure variabilities as a marker of sympatho-vagal interaction in man and conscious dog. *Circ Res* 1986; 59:178-193.

31. Perini R, Orizio C, Baselli G, Cerutti S, Veicsteinas A: The influence of exercise intensity on power spectrum of heart rate variability. *Eur J Appl Phys* 1990; 61(1-2):143-148.

32. Pomeranz B, Macaulay RJB, Caudill MA, et al: Assessment of autonomic function in humans by heart rate spectral

analysis. *Am J Physiol* 248 (Heart Circ Physiol) 1985; 17:H151-H153.

33. Saul JP, Arai Y, Berger RD, et al: Assessment of autonomic regulation in chronic congestive heart failure by heart rate spectral analysis. *Am J Card* 1988; 61:1292-1299.

34. Saul JP, Rea RF, Eckberg DL, et al: Heart rate and muscle sympathetic nerve variability during reflex changes of autonomic activity. *Am J Physiol* 258 (Heart Circ Physiol) 1990; 27:H713-H721.

35. Shiavi R: Introduction to applied statistical signal analysis. Aksen Associates Inc, 1991. Van Hoogenhuyze D, Weinstein N, Martin GJ, Weiss JS, Schaad JW, Sahyouni XN, Fintel D, Remme WJ, Singer DH: Reproducibility and relation to mean heart rate variability in normal subjects and in patients with congestive heart failure secondary to coronary artery disease. *Am J Card* 1991; 68:1668-1676.

36. Vybiral T, Bryg RJ, Maddens ME, et al: Effect of passive tilt on sympathetic and parasympathetic components of heart rate variability in normal subjects. Am J Cardiol 1989; 63:1117-1120.

Methodologic Caveats

1. Bloomfield P: *Fourier Analysis of Time Series: An Introduction.* John Wiley & Sons, 1976.

2. DeBoer RW, Karemaker JM Strackee J: Comparing spectra of a series of point events particularly for heart rate variability data. *IEEE Trans Biomed Eng* 1984:31 (4):384-387.

3. Makhoul J: Linear prediction: a tutorial review. *Proc IEEE* 1975; 63:561-580.

4. Ori Z, Monir G, Weiss J, Sayhouni X, and Singer D: Heart rate variability: Frequency domain analysis. *Cardiology Clinics* 1992; 10 (3): 499-537.

5. Perini R, Orizio C, Baselli G, Cerutti S, Veicsteinas A: The influence of exercise intensity on power spectrum of heart rate variability. *Eur J Appl Physiol* 1990; 61(1-2):143-148.

6. Rimoldi O, Pagani M, Pagani MR, Baselli G, and Malliani A: Sympathetic activation during treadmill exercise in conscious dog: assessment with spectral analysis of heart period and systolic pressure variabilities. *J Auton Nerv Syst* 1990; 30:S129-S132.

7. Shiavi R: *Introduction to applied statistical signal analysis.* Aksen Associates Inc, 1991.

8. Xia R., Odemuyiwa O, Gill J, Malik M, Camm AJ: Influence of recognition errors of computerized analysis of 24-hour electrocardiograms on the measurement of spectral components of heart rate variability. *Int J Biomed Comput* 1993; 32 (3-4):223-235.

HRV: Clinical Considerations

1. Abboud FM: The sympathetic system in hypertension. *Hypertension* 1982; 4:(supp II):II208-II225.

2. Alboni P, Paparella N, Cappato R, Candini GC: Direct and autonomically mediated effects of oral flecainide. *Am J Card* 1988; 61 (10):759-763.

3. Arai Y, Saul JP, Albrecht P, Haltley LH, et al: Modulation of cardiac autonomic activity during and immediately after exercise. *Am J Physiol* 1989; 256:H132-H141.

4. Bianchi A, Bontempi B. Cerutti S, Gianoglio P, Comi G, Natali Sora MG: Spectral analysis of heart rate variability signal and respiration in diabetic subjects. *Med & Biol Eng & Comput* 1990; 28:205-211

5. Bigger JT, Albrecht P, Steinman RC, et al: Comparison of time and frequency domain-based measures of cardiac parasympathetic activity in Holter recordings after myocardial infarction. *Am J Cardiol* 1989; 64:536-538.

6. Bigger JT, Kleiger RE, Fleiss JL, et al and The Multicenter Post-Infarction Research Group: Components of heart rate variability measured during healing of acute myocardial infarction. *Am J Cardiol* 1988; 61:208-215.

7. Binkley PF, Nunziata E, Haas GJ, Nelson SD, Cody RJ: Parasympathetic withdrawal is an integral component of autonomic imbalance in congestive heart failure: demonstration in human subjects and verification in a paced canine model of ventricular failure. *JACC* 1991; 18 (2):464-472.

8. Braunwald E, Chidsey CA, Pool PE, et al: Congestive heart failure: biochemical and physiological considerations: combined clinical staff conference at the National Institutes of Health. *Ann Intern Med* 1966; 64:904-941.

9. Cinca J, Moya A, Bardaji A, Rius J, Soler-Soler J: Circadian variation in electrical properties of heart. *Ann NY Acad Sci* 1990; 601:222-233.

10. Comi G, Sora MGN, Bianchi A, et al: Spectral analysis of short-term heart rate variability in diabetic patients. *J of Auton Nerv Syst* 1990; 30:S45-S50.

11. Eckberg DL, Drabinsky M, Braunwald E: Defective cardiac parasympathetic control in patients with heart disease. *NEJM* 1971; 285 (16):877-883.

12. Ewing, DJ, Campbell IW, Clarke BF: Mortality in diabetic autonomic neuropathy. *Lancet* 1976; 601-603.

13. Ewing DJ, Neilson JMM, Shapiro CM, Stewart JA, Reid W: Twenty four hour heart rate variability: effects of posture, sleep and time of day in healthy controls and comparison with bedside tests of autonomic function in diabetic patients. *BHJ* 1991; 65:239-244.

14. Fallen EL, Kamath MV, Ghista DN, et al: Spectral analysis of heart rate variability following human heart transplantation: evidence for functional reinnervation. *J Auton Nerv Syst* 1988; 23:199-206.

15. Furlan R, Guzetti F, Crivellaro W, et al: Continuous 24-hour assessment of neural regulation of systemic arterial pressure and RR variabilities in ambulant subjects. *Circ* 1990; 81:537-547.

16. Guzetti S, Piccaluga E, Casati R, et al: Sympathetic predominance in essential hypertension: a study employing spectral analysis of heart rate variability. *J Hypertens* 1988; 6:711-717.

17. Hayano J, Sakakibara Y, Yamada M, et al: Decreased magnitude of heart rate spectral components in coronary artery disease its relation to angiographic severity. *Circ* 1990; 81:1217-1224.

18. Hellman JB, Stacy RW: Variations of respiratory sinus arrhythmia with age. *J Appl Physiol* 1976; 41(5):734-738.

19. Higgins CB, Vatner FF, Ekberg DL, Braunwald E: Alteration in the baroreceptor reflex in conscious dogs with heart failure. *J Clin Invest* 1972; 51:715-724.

20. Hyndman BW, Gregory JR: Spectral analysis of sinus arrhythmia during mental loading. *Ergonomics* 1975; 18 (3):255-270.

21. Julius S and Randall OS: Role of the autonomic nervous system in mild human hypertension. *Clin Sci Mol Med* 1975; 48:243S-252S.

22. Kjellgren O, Gomes JA: Heart rate variability and baroreflex sensitivity in myocardial infarction. *Am Heart J* 1993; 125 (1):204-215.

23. Kleiger RE, Miller JP, Bigger JT, Moss AJ, the Multicenter Post-Infarct Research Group: Decreased heart rate variability and its association with increased mortality after acute myocardial infarction. *Am J Cardiol* 1987; 59 (4):256-262.

24. Korner PI, Shaw J, Uther JB, et al: Autonomic and non-autonomic circulatory components in essential hypertension in man. *Circ* 1973; 48:107-117.

25. Leclercq JF, Maisonblanche P, Cauchemez B, Coumel P: Respective role of sympathetic tone and of cardiac pauses in

the genesis of 62 cases of ventricular fibrillation recorded during Holter monitoring. *Eur Heart J* 1988; 9:1276-1283.

26. Leimbach WN, Wallin BG, Victor RG, Aylward PE, Sundlof G, Mark LA: Direct evidence from intraneural recordings for increased central sympathetic outflow in patients with heart failure. *Circ* 1986; 73 (5):913-919.

27. Lipsitz LA, Mietus J, Moody GB, Goldberger AL: Spectral characteristics of heart rate variability before and during postural tilt relation to aging and risk of syncope. *Circulation* 1990; 81:1803-1810.

28. Lown B and Verrier R: Neural activity and ventricular fibrillation. *NEJM* 1976; 294 (21):1165-1170.

29. Malliani A, Pagani M, Lombardi F: *Positive feedback reflexes.* p 69-81. In Eds.: Zanchetti A, Tarazi RC: *Handbook of hypertension:* volume 8 Pathophysiology of hypertension. (Amsterdam) Elsevier 1986.

30. Malliani A, Schwartz PJ, Zanchetti A: Neural mechanisms in life-threatening arrhythmias. *Am Heart J* 1980; 100 (5):705-715.

31. Malliani A, Schwartz PJ, and Zanchetti A: A Sympathetic reflex elicited by experimental coronary occlusion. *Am J Physiol* 1969; 217(3):703-709.

32. Masaoka S, Lev-Ran A, Hill LR, Vakil G, Hon EHG: Heart rate variability in diabetes: relationship to age and duration of the disease. *Diabetes Care* 1985; 8:64-68.

33. Meredith IT, Broughton A, Jennings GL, and Esler MD: Evidence of selective increase in cardiac sympathetic activity in patients with sustained ventricular arrhythmias. *NEJM* 1991; 325:618-624.

34. Ori Z, Monir G, Weiss J, Sayhouni X, Singer D: Heart rate variability: Frequency domain analysis. *Cardiology Clinics* 1992; 10 (3): 499-537.

35. Pagani M, Malfatto G, Pierini S, et al: Spectral analysis of heart rate variability in the assessment of autonomic diabetic neuropathy. *J Auton Nerv Syst* 1988; 23:143-153.

36. Parati G, Castiglioni P, Rienzo MD, et al: Sequential spectral analysis of 24-hour blood pressure and pulse interval in humans. *Hypert* 1990; 16:414-421.

37. Rockel A, Hennemann H, Sternagel-Haase A, Heidland A: Ureamic sympathetic neuropathy after haemodialysis and transplantation, *Eur J Clin Invest* 1979;9:23-27.

38. Sands KEF, Appel ML, et al: Power spectrum analysis of heart rate variability in human cardiac transplant recipients. *Circ* 1989; 79:76-82.

39. Saul JP, Arai Y, Berger RD, Lilly LS, Colucci WS, and Cohen RJ: Assessment of autonomic regulation in chronic congestive heart failure by heart rate spectral analysis. *Am J Card* 1988; 61:1292-1299.

40. Schwartz PJ, Stramba-Badiale M: *Parasympathetic nervous system and cardiac arrhythmias.* In: Kulbertus HE and Frank G, Neurocardiology. Futura Pub 1988, 179-200.

41. Schwartz PJ, Zaza A, Locati E, and Moss AJ: Stress and sudden death: the case of the long QT syndrome. *Circ* 1991; 83(suppl II): II71-II80.

42. Shannon DC, Carley DW, Benson H: Aging of modulation of heart rate. *Am J Physiol* 253 (Heart Circ Physiol) 1987; 22:H874-H877.

43. Singer DH, Martin GJ, Magid N, et al: Low heart rate variability and sudden cardiac death. *J Electrocard* 1988; (Suppl):S46-55.

HRV: A Predictor of All Cause Mortality

1. Bigger JT, Albrecht P, et al: Comparison of time and frequency domain-based measures of cardiac parasympathetic activity in Holter recordings after myocardial infarction. *Am J Cardiol* 1989; 64:536-538.

2. Bigger JT Jr, Fleiss JL, et al: Frequency domain measures of heart period variability and mortality after myocardial infarction. *Circ* 1992; 85:164-171.

3. Bigger JT, Hoffman BF: Antiarrhythmic drugs. In Gilman AG, Rall TW, Nies AS, Taylor, P (Eds): *Goodman and Gilman's The Pharmacological Basis of Therapeutics* (New York) Pergamon Press. 1990, 840-873.

4. The Cardiac Arrhythmia Suppression Trial (CAST) Investigators: Preliminary report: effect of encainide and flecainide on mortality in randomized trial of arrhythmia suppression after myocardial infarction. *NEJM* 1989; 321(6):406-412.

5. Cook JR, Bigger JT, Kleiger RE, et al. Effect of atenolol and diltiazem on heart period variability in normal persons. *JACC* 1991; 17:480-484.

6. Cripps TR, Malik M, Farrell TS, et al: Prognostic value of reduced heart rate variability after myocardial infarction: Clinical evaluation of a new analysis method. *BHJ* 1991; 65:14.

7. Dangman KH, Miura DS: *Proarrhythmic effects of antiarrhythmic drugs.* P 375-395 in eds: Dangman KH, Miura DS: *Electrophysiology and pharmacology of the heart.* Marcel Dekker, Inc, 1991.

8. Ewing DJ, Campbell IW, Clarke BF: Assessment of cardiovascular effects in diabetic autonomic neuropathy and prognostic implications. *Ann Intern Med* 1980; 92 (part2):308-311.

9. Ewing DJ, Campbell IW, Clarke BF: Mortality in diabetic autonomic neuropathy. *Lancet* 1976; 1:601.

10. Farrel TG, Bashir Y, Cripps T, Malik M, Polonieci J, Bennett D, Ward DE, Camm JA. Risk stratification for arrhythmic events in postinfarction patients based on heart variability, ambulatory electrocardiographic variables and signal averaged electrocardiogram. *JACC* 1991;8:687-697.

11. Singer DH, Martin GJ, Magid N, et al: Low heart rate variability and sudden cardiac death. *J Electrocardiol* 1988; (Suppl):S46-S55.

12. Van Hoogenhuyze D, Weinstein N, Martin GJ, Weiss JS, Schaad JW, Sahyouni XN, Fintel D, Remme WJ, Singer DH: Reproducibility and relation to mean heart rate variability in normal subjects and in patients with congestive heart failure secondary to coronary artery disease. *Am J Cardiol* 1991; 68:1668-1676.

13. Yusuf S, Peto R, Lewis J, et al: Beta blockade during and after myocardial infarction: An overview of the randomized trials. *Prog Cardiovasc Dis* 1985; 27:335-371.

14. Zuanetti G, Latini R, Neilson JMM, Schwartz PJ, Ewing DJ and the Antiarrhythmic Drug Evaluation Group (ADEG): Heart rate variability in patients with ventricular arrhythmias: Effect of antiarrhythmic drugs. *JACC* 1991; 17 (3):604-612.

HRV: Sudden Cardiac Death

1. Ahmed M, Fintel D, Zhang F, Sahyouni N, Weiss J, Brenauer T, Singer D: Survival post-sudden cardiac death: Predictive value of heart rate variability vs. inducibility. *JACC* 1992; 19:3:167A.

2. Algra A, Tijssen JPG, Roelandt JCTR, Pool J, Lubsen J: Heart rate variability from 24-Hour electrocardiography and 2-year risk for sudden death. *Circ* 88: 180-185, 1993.

3. Bigger JT, Albrecht P, Steinman RC, Rolnitzky, Fleiss JKL and Cohen RJ: Comparison of time and frequency domain-based measures of cardiac parasympathetic activity in Holter recordings after myocardial infarction. *Am J Cardiol* 1989; 64:536-538.

4. Dougherty CM, Burr RL. Comparison of heart rate variability in survivors and nonsurvivors of sudden cardiac arrest. *Am J Cardiol* 1992;70(4):441-448.

HRV: Predictive Value

1. Algra A, Tijssen JPG, Roelandt JCTR, Pool J, Lubsen J: Heart rate variability from 24-hour electrocardiography and 2-year risk for sudden death. *Circ* 88: 180-185, 1993.

2. Bernardi L, Lumina C, Ferrari MR et al: Relationship between fluctuations in heart rate and asymptomatic nocturnal ischemia. *Int J Cardiol* 20:399-51, 1980.

3. Bigger JT, Fleiss JL, Rolnitzky LM, Steinman RC: The ability of several short-term measures of RR variability to predict mortality after myocardial infarction. *Circulation* 88: 927-934, 1993.

4. Bigger JT, Fleiss JL, Steinman RC, Rolnitzky LM, Kleiger RE, Rottman JN: Frequency domain measures of heart period variability and mortality after myocardial infarction. *Circ* 85: 164-171, 1992.

5. Bigger JT Jr, et al. Prediction of death after myocardial infarction with RR variability calculated from 2 to 15-minute ECGs. *JACC* 21:271A, 1993.

6. Coumel P: Modification of heart rate variability preceding the onset of tachyarrhythmias. *Cardiologia* 35: (Suppl): 7-12, 1990.

7. Dougherty CM, Burr RL: Comparison of heart rate variability in survivors and nonsurvivors of sudden cardiac arrest. *Am J Cardiol* 70(4): 441-448, 1992.

8. Farrel TG, Bashir Y, Cripps T, Malik M, Polonieci J, Bennett D, Ward DE, Camm JA: Risk stratification for arrhythmic events in postinfarction patients based on heart variability, ambulatory electrocardiographic variables and signal averaged electrocardiogram. *JACC* 8:687-697, 1991.

9. Furlan R, Guzzetti S, Crivellaro W, Dassi S, Tinelli M, Baselli G, Cerutti S, Lombardi F, Pagani M, Maliani A: Continuous 24-hour assessment of neural regulation of systemic arterial pressure and RR variabilities in ambulant subjects. *Circ* 81:537-547, 1990.

10. Goldberger AL, Rigney DR, Mietus J, Antman EM, Greenwald S: Nonlinear Mechanism in Sudden Cardiac Death Syndrom: Heart rate oscillations and bifurcations. *Experientia* 44: 983-987, 1989.

11. Goldberger AL, Rigney D: *Sudden death is not chaos. Dynamic patterns in complex systems.* Kelso JAS, Mandell AJ, Shlesinger MF (eds) (in press), World Scientific Publishers, Singapore, 1988.

12. Goldberger AL, West BJ: *Chaos in physiology: Health or disease? Chaos in biological systems.* Degn H, Holden AV, Olsen LF (eds) p 1, Plenum Press, New York, NY, 1987.

Combinations of Risk Factors

1. Farrel TG, Bashir Y, Cripps T, Malik M, Polonieci J, Bennett D, Ward DE, Camm JA: Risk stratification for arrhythmic events in postinfarction patients based on heart variability, ambulatory electrocardiographic variables and signal averaged electrocardiogram. *JACC* 1991; 8:687-697.

2. Gomes AJ, Winters LS, Stewart D, Horowitz S, Milner M, Barreca P: A new noninvasive index to predict sustained ventricular tachycardia and sudden death in the first year after myocardial infarction: Based on signal-averaged electrocardiogram, radionuclide ejection fraction and holter monitoring. *JACC* 1987; 10:349-357.

3. Kanovsky M, Falcone R, Dresden C, et al.: Identification of patients with ventricular tachycardia after myocardial infarction: Signal-averaged electrocardiogram, Holter monitoring, and cardiac catheterization. *Circ* 984;70:264.

4. Kuchar LD, Thorburn WC, Sammel LN: Prediction of serious arrhythmic events after myocardial infarction: signal averaged electrocardiogram, Holter monitoring and radionuclide ventriculography. *JACC* 1987; 9:531-538.

5. Multicenter Post-infarction Research Group: Risk stratification and survival after myocardial infarction. *NEJM* 1983; 309:331.

6. Odemuyiwa O, Malik M, Farrell TG, Bashir Y, Staunton A, Poloniecki J, Camm AJ: Multifactorial prediction of arrhythmic events after myocardial infarction. Combination of heart rate variability and left ventricular ejection fraction with other variables. *PACE* 14(11 Pt2): 1986-1991, 1991.

CHAPTER 31

Nonpharmacologic Treatment of Arrhythmias

Ron J. Vanden Belt, M.D.

The frequent failure of drugs to control recurrent tachyarrhythmias, the potential for side effects, the expense and inconvenience of long-term medication administration, the requirement for patient compliance, and the consequences of medication failure when the arrhythmia is life-threatening make surgical or device therapy for arrhythmias a very attractive alternative. The development of clinical electrophysiology over the last 25 years has led to better understanding of the mechanisms of cardiac arrhythmias in general and in the individual patient as well. Drug therapy guided by information derived from electrophysiologic testing represents a quantum step from the empiric drug therapy of the past. With the maturation of electrophysiologic techniques there are now a variety of nonpharmacologic options for treatment of arrhythmias that may result in "cure" of the problem with excellent symptom control and avoidance of long-term medication in some, or a substantial reduction of morbidity and mortality in others.

CARDIAC PEARL

One has to be impressed with the many significant advances that have occurred as well as those that are presently evolving concerning the understanding and management of ventricular arrhythmias and sudden death.

It is obvious that the problem is not a simple one. It is also apparent that a number of serious, often fatal arrhythmias that formerly were untreatable are now being successfully managed.

The amount of research on these arrhythmias is fortunately great and predictably will continue to result in even better management and prevention in the future. The research and patient application of both drugs plus the advances of treatment by implantable devices, pacemakers and surgery give solid support to the fact that prevention and treatment of ventricular arrhythmias (and of course, sudden death) will be better and better.

W. Proctor Harvey, M.D.

Cardiac Pacing

In the late 1950s, the knowledge that the heart could be activated by an electrical stimulus was coupled with available technology leading to development of artificial pacing. Initially, only patients who were markedly symptomatic with Adams-Stokes syncope or had heart failure due to heart block or severe sinus bradycardia received pacemakers, which were extraordinarily crude by contemporary standards. Early experience with cardiac pacing was plagued with component and battery failure as well as electrode fractures. The combination of considerable clinical experience and major technologic advances has all but eliminated the hardware problems and led to greatly expanded applications for cardiac pacing. The electronic sophistication, reliability, longevity and miniaturization of components, and the durability of electrode systems developed over three decades represent a major achievement for physicians, engineers, and industry. Comparison of a contemporary pacemaker with an old, nonprogrammable fixed rate or simple demand pacemaker is astonishing (Figure 1).

The three components of a pacemaker system are electrodes that make contact with the endocardium or myocardium for transmission of the

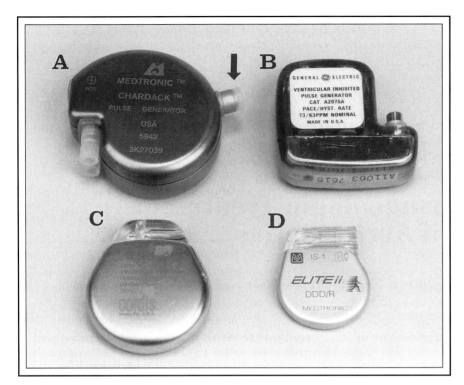

Figure 1. Pacemakers through the years. **A.** Late 60s / early 70s mercury zinc battery powered single chamber-demand pacemaker (weight 210 gm). The projecting nipple at 2:00 o'clock (arrow) provided a means to adjust the rate of this pacemaker. By inserting a specially mounted Keith needle through the skin into the center of the silastic covered projection, seating it securely in the center and then rotating it, the rate of the pacemaker could be adjusted. **B.** Early-mid 70s mercury zinc battery powered single chamber, demand pacemaker (weight 178 gm). **C.** Late 70s era - early lithium powered single chamber demand pacemaker (weight 76 gm). **D.** Contemporary lithium powered rate responsive dual chamber pacemaker with multiple programmability options (weight 27 gm).

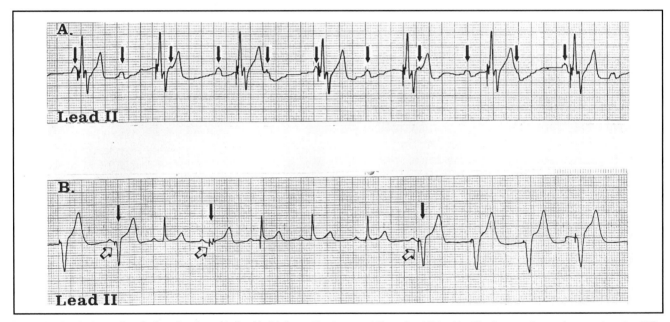

Figure 2. Ventricular pacing. **A.** Complete heart block with AV dissocation is present throughout this strip. The P waves (arrows) occur at a rate of 79 per minute and are completely unrelated to the paced QRS complexes. **B.** Ventricular demand pacing is demonstrated in this strip. With slight changes in the sinus rate, the pacemaker fires (open arrows), capturing the ventricle with a wide QRS complex with LBBB pattern. The three beats indicated by the solid arrows are intermediate in configuration between the sinus and the purely paced beats and represent fusion of a sinus impulse conducted across the AV junction and a paced beat *(Courtesy Susan L. Honoway, RN).*

electrical stimulus into the heart and transmission of electrical impulses from the heart to the pulse generator for sensing, electronic circuitry to sense the heart's electrical activity and time and deliver electric stimuli to the heart, and a power source.

For many years, most cardiac pacing was ven-
tricular (occasionally atrial) in either the fixed rate or demand (standby) mode. The fixed rate pacemaker, rarely if ever used now, fires at a regular preset rate and does not sense or detect the patient's intrinsic cardiac activity. Demand pacemakers have, in addition to pacing circuitry, a sens-

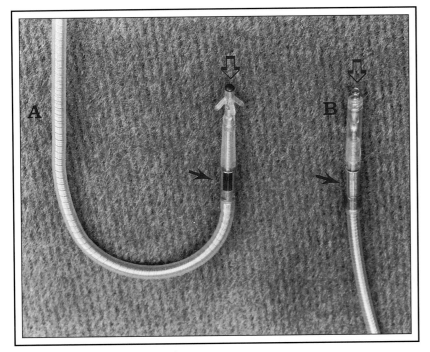

Figure 3. Permanent pacemaker leads. **A.** The J configuration of the distal part of the lead allows ease of placement into the right atrial appendage (see Figure 6). The tines at the tip of the lead hook among the trabeculae and help secure the position of the lead. The distal electrode which appears porous, contains small amounts of steroids which are slowly released, lessening the increase in the pacing threshold that occurs following implant. The shaft of this lead is 7.68°F. **B.** The tip electrode of this bipolar pacing lead is of a retractable corkscrew configuration. The lead is passed into and through the vein with the electrode retracted. When appropriately positioned in the heart, the corkscrew is extended with active fixation of the lead to the endocardium. The body of the lead is 7.08°F.

ing circuit that detects cardiac electrical activity and activates the pacemaker only if the heart rate falls below a preset rate (Figure 2). When the fundamental problem is that of impulse conduction from the atria to the ventricles, ventricular pacing must be used. If atrioventricular conduction is intact and the problem is failure of impulse generation in the SA node, atrial pacing may be used.

Two major technologic advances, stable atrial electrode systems and the ability to noninvasively modify the function of a pacemaker have greatly expanded the options available for optimal management of the patient. A variety of preformed electrodes and active fixation electrodes allow one to achieve a stable electrode position in the right atrium (usually right atrial appendage) in most patients (Figure 3). The programmability feature allows one to modify many parameters of pacing function, such as the mode (Table 1, Figure 4), rate, output, pulse width, and various intervals and refractory periods in the cardiac cycle using an external device with transcutaneous transmission of electromagnetic or radio frequency waves. Programmability allows one to change the pacing mode and other parameters as the condition of the patient changes, and achieve settings which are most economical in terms of battery life. A real-time telemetry function is incorporated in many modern pacemakers that allows the pacemaker to send information back to the programming device. Information about lead impedance and intracardiac electrograms can be acquired, which helps diagnose

pacemaker malfunction when it occurs. Sometimes, repeat procedures can be avoided by reprogramming to correct a malfunction of the pacemaker. The widely used North American Society of Pacing

---

T A B L E 1
Pacing Modes

VVI – **Ventricular demand pacemaker**
(VVT) Does not preserve AV synchrony
  Not rate responsive
  Used for backup when bradycardia is infrequent and brief
  Used in patients with atrial fibrillation

AAI – **Atrial demand pacemaker**
(AAT) Preserves AV synchrony
  Not rate responsive
  Requires intact AV conduction

DVI – **AV sequential pacemaker**
  Does not sense in atrium
  Not rate responsive
  Preserves AV synchrony with atrial rate ≤ pacemaker rate

DDD – **Dual chamber pacing and sensing**
  Atrial sensing allows atrial tracking with rate responsiveness
  Requires intact SA node function for rate increase
  Preserves AV synchrony

VDD – **Atrial tracking pacemaker**
  Preserves AV synchrony and rate responsiveness
  Does not pace atrium at time of atrial slowing

Pacing Modes – The commonly used pacing modes with their principal characteristics and applications are listed. Recall that a rate responsive feature can be added to either a single or dual chamber system if the patient does not have the ability to increase his/her rate appropriately with exercise. If rate responsiveness is incorporated, the pacing code would be changed from VVI to VVIR or DDD to DDDR, etc.

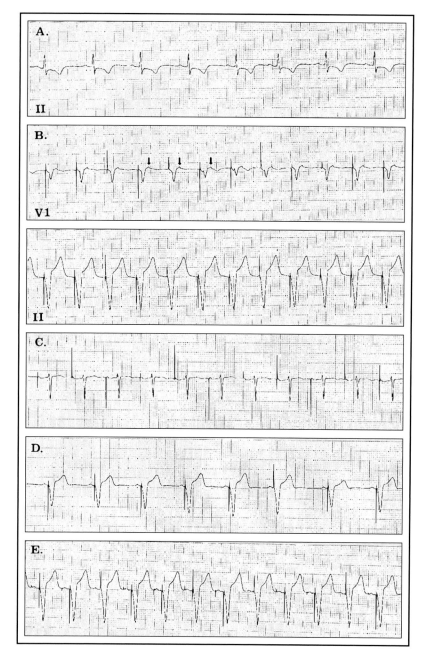

Figure 4. Pacing modes. These rhythm strips were all obtained from a 78 year old woman at follow-up testing of her pacemaker which had been placed for the bradycardia-tachycardia syndrome with intermittent atrial fibrillation. These strips were obtained with the pacemaker in a unipolar mode which results in larger, more easily seen pacemaker spikes. The variation in the vector of the pacing spikes reflects the characteristics of the filtration mechanism in the ECG machine rather than any beat-to-beat alteration in the pacemaker spike.

A. Normal sinus rhythm – Lead II. Normal sinus rhythm at a rate of 60-per-minute with a PR interval of 0.18 seconds. Note the normal appearance of the P waves and the narrow QRS complexes. No pacemaker activity is seen.

B. VVI pacing – Leads V1 and II. The ventricle is now being paced. The paced QRS is wide with an LBBB pattern and the axis is superiorly directed. P waves are not seen in Lead II, but in the V1 lead, P waves are seen in the terminal portion of each QRS complex (arrows). This represents retrograde ventricle to atrium conduction with 1:1 capture of the atria. The rate of the atria is now 88/minute in contrast to the baseline rate of 60/minute. The more usual situation with VVI pacing (AV dissociation) is shown in Figure 2B.

C. AAI – Lead V1. The atrium is now being paced and normal AV conduction occurs with a narrow, normal appearing QRS similar to A above. With the slightly faster rate and the atrial pacing, the PR interval has lengthened to 0.22 seconds.

D. VVD – Lead V1. The native P waves are now being sensed by the pacemaker. At an interval of 0.12 seconds the ventricle is paced. Note that the atrial rate in this strip is nearly the same as the resting atrial rate.

E. DDD – Lead II. In this strip, both the atrium and the ventricle are being paced at a rate of 93 beats per minute with an AV delay (PR interval) of 0.15 sec. Note the difference in the paced P waves in contrast to those in A. The paced QRS complexes are the same as those in B above. *(Courtesy Susan L. Honoway, RN).*

and Electrophysiology/British Pacing and Electrophysiology Group (NASPE/BPEG) pacemaker code is reproduced in Table 2.

For patients with atrial fibrillation (no P waves to track) or sinus node dysfunction (minimal or no increase in heart rate with activity — chronotropic incompetence) rate responsive pacemakers, either single or dual chamber, are commonly implanted. Rate responsive pacemakers sense some physiologic indicator of physical or metabolic activity, such as mechanical activity, blood temperature, respiratory rate, right ventricular dp/dt or right ventricular volume. In response to the sensed indicator of increasing activity, the pacemaker increases its pacing rate.

Incorporation of more than one type of activity sensor may allow for a more physiologic increase in the heart rate with activity. By preserving atrioventricular synchrony, dual chamber pacing provides more physiologic activation of the heart than does single chamber ventricular pacing. Some data suggest improved longevity and decreased morbidity with dual chamber pacing; most patients with intact sinoatrial node function receive dual chamber pacemakers. A programmable dual chamber system allows one to deal with most potential problems of impulse formation and transmission encountered.

Although atrial pacing is satisfactory for pure sinus node dysfunction, the not uncommon occur-

TABLE 2
The NASPE/BPEG* Generic (NBG) Pacemaker Code

POSITION	I	II	III	IV	V
Category	Chamber(s) paced O = None A = Atrium	Chamber(s) sensed O = None A = Atrium	Response to sensing O = None T = Triggered	Programmability, rate modulation O = None P = Simple Programmable	Antitachyarrhythmia function(s) O = None P = Pacing (antitachyarrhythmia)
	V = Ventricle D = Dual (A + V)	V = Ventricle D = Dual (A + V)	I = Inhibited D = Dual (T + I)	M = Multiprogrammable C = Communicating R = Rate modulation	S = Shock D = Dual (P + S)
Manufacturer's designation only	S = Single (A or V)	S = Single (A or V)			

Note: Positions I through III are used exclusively for antibradyarrhythmia function.
* North American Society of Pacing and Electrophysiology/British Pacing and Electrophysiology Group.
Reproduced with permission.

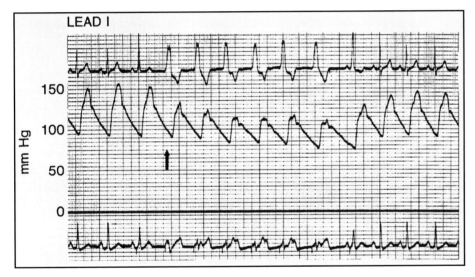

Figure 5. Pacing-induced hypotension. Normal sinus rhythm with a blood pressure of 150/95 is present on the left side of the panel. A ventricular demand pacemaker captures the ventricle with resultant AV dissociation and loss of atrial transport in beats 4-9, at the arrow. Note the prompt fall of blood pressure to levels as low as 110/75. In the supine position at cardiac catheterization, this patient did not experience symptoms, but in the upright position or during physical activity, such a rapid fall in blood pressure can cause symptoms of low cardiac output, clinically manifest as the pacemaker syndrome.

rence of AV block in these patients argues for initial implantation of a dual chamber system. VVI pacing is used in the setting of established atrial fibrillation for prevention of sporadic syncopal episodes in patients who are not expected to be paced for any significant proportion of time or in patients with an extremely poor overall prognosis or with limited activity requirements who only need the pacemaker to avoid consequences of severe bradycardia. It's not uncommon to "upgrade" a perhaps inappropriately implanted single chamber ventricular pacemaker to a dual chamber system for treatment of the pacemaker syndrome (weakness, presyncope, and syncope related to loss of AV synchrony, Figure 5) or at a time when there is evidence of left ventricular dysfunction.

Permanent pacing requires implantation of the entire pacing system. Pacing electrodes are introduced transvenously into the subclavian vein using the Seldinger technique or by direct cutdown and venotomy of the cephalic vein in the deltopectoral groove. Under fluoroscopic control, leads are positioned in the right ventricular apex and /or the right atrial appendage (Figure 6). Mechanical stability and satisfactory pacing and sensing function are confirmed before the leads are secured in position. The electrodes are then attached to the permanent pulse generator, which is implanted beneath the subcutaneous tissue or muscle. Myocardial electrodes are occasionally used when it's difficult to maintain a stable transvenous electrode position (RV enlargement and severe tricuspid regurgitation) when the patient is having other cardiac surgery done, or sometimes in young patients with significant growth potential.

Early permanent pacemakers were powered by conventional mercury zinc batteries. The life expectancy of these early batteries increased from

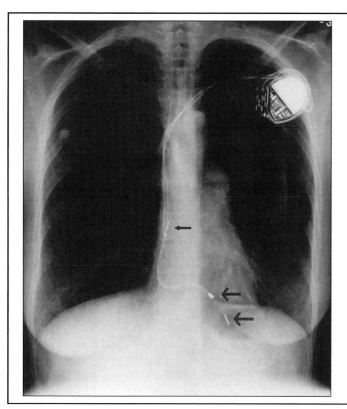
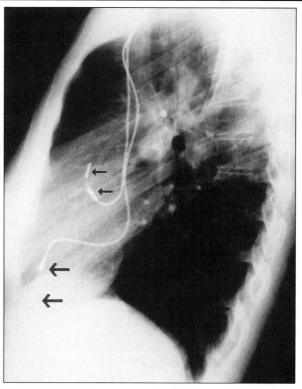

Figure 6. Chest x-ray dual chamber pacemaker. The J shape of the atrial lead (small arrows) which is positioned in the right atrial appendage points medially in the frontal view and anteriorly in the lateral projection. A characteristic swinging motion of a properly positioned J lead in the atrial appendage is seen at fluoroscopy. The ventricular lead (large arrows) is positioned in the right ventricular apex. Note its anterior direction in the lateral view. A right anterior projection, commonly done at the time of implant, projects the tip of the lead more laterally than is apparent in the frontal projection. These are bipolar leads, each having two electrodes at its tip. Both leads are attached to the pacemaker pulse generator in the left infraclavicular location.

18 months to 24 months to up to 3 years to 4 years as technology advanced. Lithium halide (iodide) batteries have improved longevity (4 years to 10 years) at favorable cost and are used in most pacemakers today. Nuclear-powered (plutonium) pacemakers enjoyed some popularity in the 1970s because of the anticipated long duration of the power source. With the advent of lithium batteries, which do not have the inherent disadvantages of a nuclear power supply, and the fact that most patients with pacemakers do not require this long battery life, led to the demise of nuclear-powered pacemakers.

Initially, permanent pacing was used in patients with symptomatic complete heart block. The utility of pacing for treatment of symptomatic sinus bradycardia, usually due to sinus node dysfunction, is readily apparent. More pacemakers are now implanted for this indication than for heart block. In patients with the bradycardia-tachycardia syndrome, a pacemaker will terminate the pauses caused by overdrive suppression that occur at the end of a paroxysm of tachycardia and will accelerate the slow rate that predisposes to development

of the tachycardia. However, most patients with the bradycardia-tachycardia syndrome continue to require some pharmacologic therapy after pacemaker implantation; the pacemaker controls the bradycardia, and the drugs prevent the tachycardia. Carotid sinus hypersensitivity and occasional vasovagal syncope are other clinical problems that lead to pacemaker implantation. These causes of syncope often involve a substantial vasodepressor component in addition to the bradycardia. Pacing will prevent the bradycardia, but some patients will still have intermittent symptoms secondary to the hypotensive element of their underlying disorder. Dual chamber pacing has emerged recently as a promising option for those with hypertrophic cardiomyopathy. The generally accepted indications for cardiac pacing appear in Table 3.

In addition to the recommendation for and the implantation of the permanent pacemaker, management of these patients requires a conscientiously applied system of regular follow-up to be certain of continued satisfactory function of the pacemaker system. Much of this can be accomplished by phone. Some cardiologists have the staff and equipment to

Indications for Permanent Pacemakers

CLASS	ACQUIRED AV BLOCK	AFTER MYOCARDIAL INFARCT	CHRONIC BIFASCICULAR & TRIFASCICULAR BLOCK	SINUS NODE DYSFUNCTION	HYPERSENSITIVE CAROTID SINUS & NEUROVASCULAR SYNDROME
I.	CHB - with: Symptomatic bradycardia. CHF. Condition requiring drugs that suppress automatic pacemaker. Asystole > 3.0 sec or rate < 40/min in asymptomatic patient. 2nd degree AV block with symptomatic bradycardia. Atrial flutter fib with advanced AV block or marked bradycardia, symptomatic, which is not drug-induced.	CHB/advanced second degree AV block with evidence of disease in His-Purkinje system. Transient advanced AV block and associated BBB.	Bifascicular block with intermittent CHB/associated symptomatic bradycardia. Bifascicular/trifascicular block with intermittent second degree AV block without symptoms.	Sinus node dysfunction with symptomatic bradycardia (may be result of essential drug without alternative therapy).	Recurrent syncope with events provoked by CS stimulation (light CS pressure → asystole > 3 sec in absence of cardiac depressant med).
II.	Asymptomatic CHB, with ventricular rate ≥ 40/min. Asymptomatic type II second degree AV block. Asymptomatic type I second degree AV block at His or infra-His levels.	Persistent advanced block at AV junction.	Long H-V interval (> 100 ms). Pacing-induced infra-His block. Bifascicular disease with syncope but without documentation of CHB as cause of symptoms.	SB where association between symptoms and brady not clear.	Syncope without clear provocative events but demonstrated sensitive carotid sinus. Syncope with positive head up tilt table test.
III.	First degree AV block. Asymptomatic type I second degree AV block.	Transient AV conduction disturbance without BBB. Transient AV block with LAH. Acquired LAH without AV block. Persistent first degree AV block in setting of new BBB.	Fascicular block without symptoms or AV block. Fascicular block and first degree AV block without symptoms.	Asymptomatic patients with SB, including those with SB caused by a drug. SB when symptoms shown not to correlate with bradycardia.	Hypersensitive carotid sinus without symptoms. Vague symptoms with demonstrated hypersensitive CS. Recurrent syncope without hypersensitive CS.

Indications for Permanent Pacing – Adapted with modifications from AHA/ACC guidelines. As they have done with other procedures, the AHA and ACC have divided the indications for permanent pacing into three categories. Type I indications are those for which there is general agreement that a pacemaker should be placed. Type II indications are those for which pacemakers are frequently placed but there are divergent opinions about the necessity for their placement. Type III indications are those for which there is agreement that a pacemaker should not be placed. "Symptomatic bradycardia" is defined as symptoms such as near syncope, syncope, light headedness, marked exercise intolerance or congestive heart failure directly attributable to the slow heart rate. In general, the patient should be free of any drug, electrolyte abnormality or condition such as ischemia which when reversed would eliminate the need for the pacemaker. On occasion, a pacemaker may be placed for symptomatic bradycardia caused by some medication for which there is no acceptable alternative. Abbreviations are: AV = atrioventricular; BBB = bundle branch block; CHB = complete heart block; CS = carotid sinus; LAH = left anterior hemiblock; SB = sinus bradycardia; CHF = congestive heart failure.

do this in their office or clinic, while others choose to assign this function to one of several commercially available services. Although infrequent, electrode displacement, random component failure, premature battery depletion, or infection at the site can compromise the system. The ability to change pacing functions with programming has greatly reduced frequency of surgical revisions for problems with pacing and sensing. The prevalence of multiple other medical problems in this population is another reason for careful follow-up.

Temporary pacing is accomplished with an electrode catheter inserted percutaneously from the subclavian, jugular, or femoral vein, usually positioned with fluoroscopic control in the apex of the right ventricle and attached to an external tempo-rary pulse generator. Temporary atrial or AV sequential pacing can be accomplished but usually isn't needed in most clinical settings where temporary pacing is applied. Additionally, maintenance of a stable position of a temporary pacing electrode in the atrium is more difficult than it is in the ventricle. Temporary pacing may be used in selected subsets of patients with acute myocardial infarction, to stabilize patients prior to implantation of a permanent pacemaker; a self-limited bradycardic episode (commonly drug-induced) acts as a therapeutic trial prior to deciding about a permanent pacemaker. Temporary pacing is rarely helpful, even when it can be successfully established, after a period of cardiac resuscitation when the patient has asystole or a very slow idioventricular rhythm.

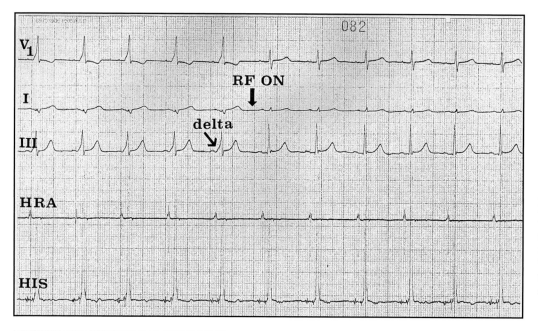

Figure 7. Radiofrequency (RF) ablation of left sided accessory pathway in a 36-year-old woman with the Wolff-Parkinson-White Syndrome. Note the almost immediate loss of delta waves after the RF is applied. *(Courtesy of Stuart A. Winston, DO).*

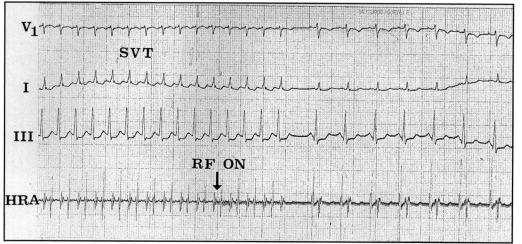

Figure 8. Successful radiofrequency (RF) ablation of left lateral concealed accessory pathway in a 23-year-old student. Note prompt termination of the AV reciprocating SVT after RF application. *(Courtesy Stuart A. Winston, DO).*

External (transcutaneous) pacing used in the early days of pacing was abandoned because of poor reliability and patient discomfort; newer devices have in large part overcome these drawbacks. External pacing may be used for very unstable patients while stable transvenous pacing is established. The most common use of external pacing is the standby mode for patients in whom there is felt to be some significant risk of a serious bradycardic episode. In general, if there is or has been symptomatic or life-threatening bradycardia, most clinicians prefer temporary transvenous pacing.

CARDIAC PEARL

There is no question that the use of cardiac pacing in the treatment of selected patients with heart disease has represented one of the most significant advances of the past several
decades. We are seeing patients who are comfortable and leading productive lives, who certainly would have died a number of years ago had it not been for cardiac pacemakers.

W. Proctor Harvey, M.D.

Ablation

Identification of the anatomic location of various accessory pathways in patients with Wolff-Parkinson-White syndrome led to the development of open surgical techniques to interrupt pathways and control arrhythmias. Other supraventricular arrhythmias were also treated surgically. Open and then later closed His bundle ablation with creation of complete heart block (permanent pacemaker required) was used for patients with uncontrollable rapid ventricular response to atrial fibrillation. Application of a direct current (DC) shock applied through appropriately-positioned intracardiac elec-

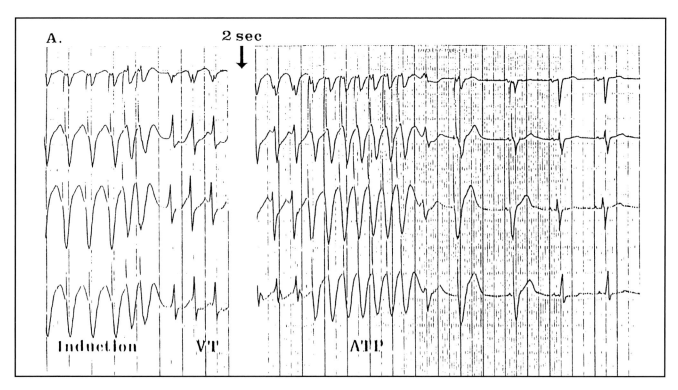

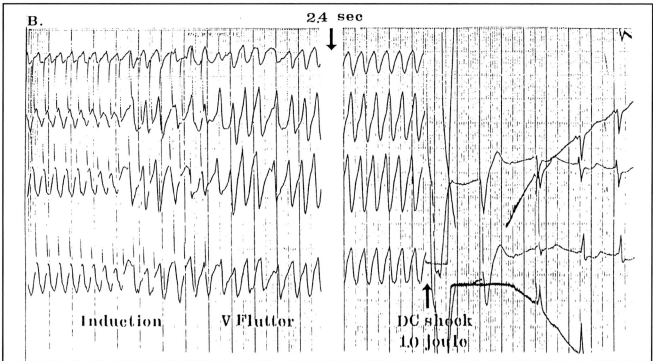

Figure 9. Implanted automatic cardioverter-defibrillator (ICD) with tiered therapy. **(A)** Ventricular tachycardia was induced using the device's non-invasive programmed stimulation feature. The VT was then converted with ramp type anti-tachycardia pacing (ATP). Ventricular paced rhythm follows the conversion. **(B)** Ventricular flutter was then induced. Because it met a higher rate criterion, it was converted with an automatically delivered low energy cardioversion. *(Courtesy Stuart A. Winston, DO).*

trodes has also been used to treat a variety of arrhythmias. The open procedures had the usual morbidity and mortality (up to 5%) associated with cardiac procedures. Although DC shock avoided thoracotomy, general anesthesia was required, there was some release of CK, and occasionally disastrous cardiac or coronary sinus rupture occurred.

Radiofrequency (RF) current application has emerged as the preferred modality for most ablation procedures. RF current can be applied to specific sites in the heart through a catheter without general anesthesia and minimal if any patient discomfort. Lesions created by RF are much more discrete and can be controlled more precisely than those with a DC shock. RF ablation is a highly technical and operator-dependent procedure associated with a significant learning curve. The procedure can be somewhat lengthy and involves exposure to ionizing radiation. In experienced hands, the primary success for ablation in patients with the common supraventricular tachycardias is well over 90%. Success rates for ablation in the atrial tachycardias are about 70%, for idiopathic ventricular tachycardia about 85% to 90% and for ventricular tachycardia due to coronary disease about 50%. Complication rates for RF ablation are under 5%; there is a low recurrence rate of under 10%. In those instances, a second application of RF usually results in long-term success.

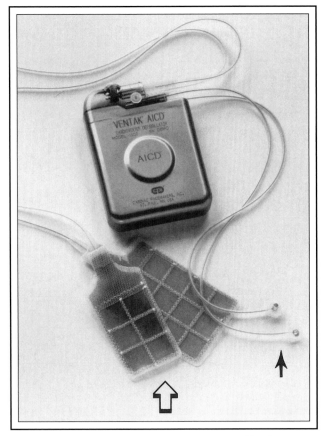

Figure 10. ICD and epicardial electrode patches. This ICD pulse generator is 76 x 100 x 20 mm and weighs 235 gm. Compare the size and weight of this very sophisticated device to some of the early pacemakers (Figure 1). The small screw in electrodes are attached to the myocardium for sensing of the rhythm.

The appeal of a safe, highly effective therapy for symptomatic arrhythmias that avoids the need for long-term medication and that can be done at the time of an initial diagnostic electrophysiologic study is evident, and many patients opt for this. RF is the preferred technique for ablation in the W-P-W syndrome (Figure 7) as well as for atrioventricular nodal reentrant tachycardia (AVNRT) or AV reciprocating tachycardia due to a concealed accessory pathway, two of the common forms of paroxysmal supraventricular tachycardia (Figure 8). RF ablation is also used in some atrial tachycardias and in ventricular tachycardias, especially the idiopathic variety, when there is no underlying structural cardiac disease.

Surgical incision into the ventricular myocardium to isolate segments of scar or fibrosis has been used for treatment of ventricular tachycardia. Resection of a patch of endocardium in the area identified by electrophysiologic mapping as the site of origin of the ventricular tachycardia has been effective. When a left ventricular aneurysm is to be resected because of ventricular tachycardia, it is preferable that the surgical procedure be guided by pre/intraoperative mapping of the arrhythmia. Cryoablation (freezing) has been utilized in some of the open surgical approaches to supraventricular and ventricular arrhythmias. The Maze procedure, a highly technical open surgical procedure, involves a series of incisions and cryolesions in the atria which interrupt the reentrant circuits that sustain atrial fibrillation. It has restored and maintained normal sinus rhythm in highly selected patients with paroxysmal or chronic atrial fibrillation.

Implantable Cardioverter Defibrillator

The implantable cardioverter defibrillator (ICD) is an important therapeutic modality for some patients who have survived cardiac arrest or have malignant ventricular arrhythmias unresponsive to conventional therapy, or whose response to such therapy cannot be assessed. ICDs were initially developed by Michel Mirowski at Johns Hopkins University, who reported the first clinical application in 1980. Mirowski's pioneering efforts were viewed somewhat skeptically, but since the introduction of the ICD, their use has spread rapidly. Many ICDs are now implanted annually in the U.S. But at a cost of more than $20,000 per unit for hardware alone, the overall expense implications of this technology are evident. The ICD has circuitry capable of detecting malignant ventricular arrhythmias and delivering appropriate electrical therapy for the rhythm disturbance (Figure 12). First generation devices were able to detect ventricular fibrillation/tachycardia and deliver shocks of a predetermined magnitude (+/- 30 Joules). These units were not programmable except for being switched from the active to inactive mode. Once the capacitor was charged, the unit was "committed" and the patient received a shock even if the arrhythmia had spontaneously terminated. Second generation devices incorporated anti-bradycardia pacing and some programmable features. The currently available third generation devices are far more sophisticated with extensive programmability for various modes of antitachycardia pacing (ramp and burst), low energy as well as higher energy shocks, different wave forms (monophasic or biphasic), antibradycardia pacing, telemetry function and the ability to perform some electrophysiologic testing noninvasively (Figures 9 A&B). The progression through burst pacing, low energy, then high energy shocks is referred to as "tiered" therapy.

Initially, ICD implantation required thoracotomy with placement of one or more epicardial patches with a superior vena cava electrode being required in some patients (Figures 10 & 11). Electrode systems have been developed which permit transvenous implantation (may require a subcutaneous patch) of the electrode system (Figure 12). In many

centers, the placement of transvenous ICDs is being done by experienced electrophysiologists without the participation of the cardiac surgeons. The mortality rate for thoracotomy placement of ICDs has been in the 3% to 5% vicinity while the mortality rate for transvenous placement has been 1% or slightly less. Perhaps as many as 10% of patients cannot be successfully implanted using the nonthoracotomy approach as defibrillation thresholds may be higher for the transvenous system.

ICDs are indicated for patients with a history of cardiac arrest or malignant ventricular arrhthymias in whom medical therapy is ineffective, cannot be tolerated, or who are noncompliant. Other patients who receive ICDs are those whose clinical arrhythmia is noninducible at EPS testing which limits the ability to assess the efficacy of medical therapy. ICDs are not indicated for patients with arrhythmias caused by reversible and otherwise treatable conditions such as ischemia, infarction, drug effects, or electrolyte disturbances; patients with incessant ventricular arrhythmias, or patients who do not have an otherwise reasonable prognosis. Patients in whom ICDs are placed have an annual incidence of sudden death of under 2%, a substantially lower rate than has been observed in historic

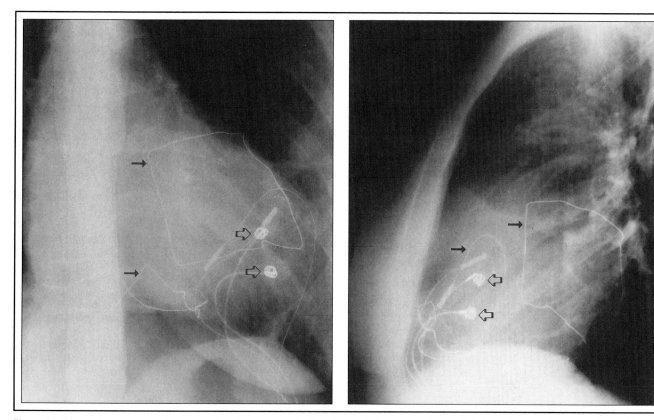

Figure 11. Chest X-Ray – closeup. ICD with epicardial patches. The fine wires (solid arrows) outline the inferior and posterolateral locations of the electrode patches. Their relative locations are best appreciated on the lateral view. The ICD pulse generator in the left flank is out of view. The two corkscrew electrodes (dark arrows) are for sensing the rhythm. The less dense metallic objects are lead connectors.

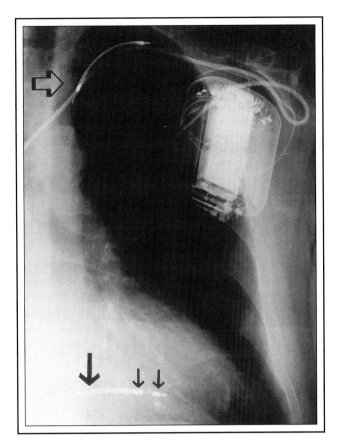

Figure 12. Chest x-ray of transvenous ICD – The electrode for the ICD is positioned in the apex of the right ventricle. The sensing and pacing electrodes are located on the distal portion of the lead (small arrows). The cathode for the delivery of shocks is the heavy part of the electrode (large arrow) located just proximal to the tip electrodes. The anode is adjacent to the pulse generator (open arrow). The pulse generator is 88 x 63 x 18 mm and weighs 132 gm. Compare its size to an early pacemaker in Figure 1.

controls. There are not, however, confirmatory data from a prospective randomized trial comparing effect of ICD placement to best available medical therapy on the rates of sudden death and all cause mortality.

Selected Reading

1. Bernstein AD, Camm AJ, Fletcher RD, Gold RD, Richards AF, Smyth NPD, Spielman SR, Sutton R: NASPE/BPEG generic pacing code for antibradyarrhythmia and adaptive-rate pacing and antitbradyarrythmia devices. *PACE* 1987; l0:794-799.
2. Cox JL, Schuessler RB, D'Agostino HJ Jr., et al: The surgical treatment of atrial fibrillation. III. Development of a definitive surgical procedure. *J Thor Card Surg* 1991; 101:569-83.
3. Dreifus LS, Fisch C, Griffin JC, Gillette PC, Mason JW, Parsonnet V: Guidelines for implantation of cardiac pacemakers and antiarrhythmia devices. A report of the American College of Cardiology/American Heart Association Task Force on Assessment of Diagnostic and Therapeutic Cardiovascular Procedures (Committee on Pacemaker Implantation). *JACC* 1991; 18(1):1-13.
4. Fitzpatrick AP, Lesh MD, Epstein LM, Lee RJ, Siu A, Merrick S, Griffin JC, Scheinman MM: Electrophysiologic laboratory, electrophysiologist-implanted, nonthoracotomy-implantable cardioverter defibrillators. *Circ* 1994; 89:2503-2508.
5. Furman S, Hayes DL, Holmes DR, Jr: *A Practice of Cardiac Pacing,* 3rd Ed. Futura Publishing Company, Inc, Mt Kisco, NY 1993.
6. Jackman WM, Beckman KJ, McClelland JH, et al: Treatment of supraventricular tachycardia due to atrioventricular nodal reentry by radio frequency catheter ablation of slow-pathway conduction. *NEJM* 1992; 327 (5):313-318.
7. Jackman WM, Wang X, Friday KJ, et al: Catheter ablation of accessory atrioventricular pathways (Wolff-Parkinson-White Syndrome) by radiofrequency current. *NEJM* 1991; 324 (23):1605-1611.
8. PCD Investigator Group: Clinical outcome of patients with malignant ventricular tachyarrhythmias and a multiprogrammable implantable cardioverter defibrillator implanted with or without thoracotomy: An international multicenter study. *JACC* 1994; 23 (7):1521-1530.
9. Pinski SL, Trohman RG: Implantable cardioverter-defibrillators: Implications for the non electrophysiologist. *Ann Int Med* 1995; 122:770-777.
10. Zipes DP: Are implantable cardioverter-defibrillators better than conventional anti-arrhythmic drugs for survivors of cardiac arrest? *Circ* 1995; 91:2115-2117.
11. Zipes DP: Implantable cardioverter defibrillator. Lifesaver or a device looking for a disease? *Circ* 1994; 89:2934-2936.

CHAPTER 32

The Optimal Technique of Electrical Cardioversion From Atrial Tachyarrhythmias

Gordon A. Ewy, M.D.

Tachyarrhythmias, ventricular or supraventricular, that produce chest pain, shortness of breath, decreased level of consciousness, low blood pressure, shock, pulmonary congestion, congestive heart failure or acute myocardial ischemia may need emergency cardioversion. Emergency equipment such as oxygen, a suction device, and intubation equipment needs to be at hand. An intravenous line is extremely important, with premedication accomplished whenever possible. For supraventricular tachycardia, the guidelines recommend a sequence of 100J, 200J, 300J and, if necessary, 360J. Shocks should be synchronized; when possible, the same care and technique outlined below for elective cardioversion should be followed. Atrial flutter and fibrillation, even with a controlled ventricular response, may benefit from cardioversion. Chronic atrial flutter and fibrillation predispose the individual to systemic emboli, and cardioversion to sinus rhythm may eliminate the need for chronic anticoagulation. In some patients, especially those with left ventricular diastolic dysfunction, sinus rhythm results in significant hemodynamic and symptomatic benefit. For these and other reasons, electrical cardioversion is indicated in a number of patients with atrial fibrillation or atrial flutter.

Technique of Electrical Cardioversion

Three decades ago, the technique of transthoracic direct current electrical cardioversion from atrial fibrillation was developed by Lown and associates. Perfecting the technique, Lown reported that sinus rhythm was reinstated in 94% of the 456 episodes of atrial fibrillation. External cardioversion success rates vary and were recently reported at only 67%. Why have cardioversion success rates been so different? One possible explanation could be that in some series, many of the patients were in chronic atrial fibrillation of over one year's duration and had failed previous pharmacological attempts at cardioversion. Another possible explanation for the different success rates is the difference in techniques of external cardioversion. Accordingly, it seems appropriate to review the optimal technique of electrical cardioversion of atrial fibrillation and atrial flutter and update information previously published.

Electrical Considerations

When the capacitor of the defibrillator or cardioverter discharges, it delivers energy measured in watt-seconds or joules. This energy is composed of current (somewhat analogous to "flow") and voltage (somewhat analogous to "pressure"). As with the cardiovascular system where the amount of blood flow resulting from blood pressure is dependent upon resistance or impedance, the amount of delivered current resulting from discharge of the voltage in the capacitor depends upon impedance or resistance between the defibrillator electrodes (Figure 1). The higher the impedance, the lower the delivered current, and it is the current that defibrillates. Specifically, it is the current density that traverses the muscle of the chambers to be defibrillated that determines successful defibrillation. Accordingly, different electrode placement is needed for electrical cardioversion of atrial fibrillation than for defibrillation of ventricular fibrillation. To be successful,

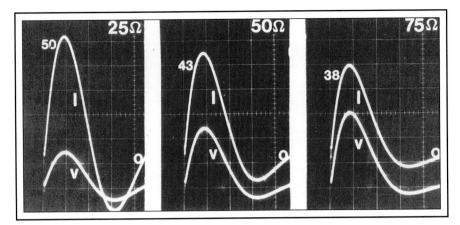

Figure 1. Simultaneous current (I) and voltage (V) waves from a defibrillator with the same stored energy delivered into 25, 50, and 75 ohms of resistance. Delivered peak current decreases with increasing resistance. *(Copyrighted and reprinted with the permission of Clinical Cardiology Publishing Company, Inc., and/or Foundation for Advances in Medicine and Science, Inc., P.O. Box 832, Mahwah, NJ 07430.)*

a critical muscle mass of the appropriate chambers must be defibrillated.

Since the output of present defibrillators in the United States is limited to 360J (delivered energy through 50 ohm resistance) transthoracic impedance is a major factor determining success. Other factors include the underlying heart disease, electrode size and electrode placement.

Transthoracic Impedance

Determinants of transthoracic impedance to DC defibrillator or cardioverter discharge (Table 1) include amount of stored energy, electrode size, electrode composition, interface between electrode and skin, phase of ventilation, pressure on electrodes, distance between electrodes, effect of previous discharges, and time interval between previous discharges. The patient's body build will also influence impedance as a hyperinflated, emphysematous chest will have a higher transthoracic impedance to direct current shock. Kerber and associates reported that a recent sternotomy significantly reduces transthoracic chest impedance. The larger the defibrillator electrode the lower the impedance. If the electrodes are too small, not only is impedance higher, but delivered current is concentrated and myocardial damage is more likely. If the electrodes are too large, the impedance is low but the current density is not great enough for defibrillation. The optimal electrode size for defibrillation is about 12 cm to 13 cm in diameter. In studies of animals of various sizes, the electrode size appears to be optimal if the electrode is about the same size as the cross-section of the heart. The optimal size for cardioversion of atrial fibrillation is unknown, but when both electrodes are 8 cm or less in diameter, electrode size is probably not optimal for a normal size adult.

Electrode composition and interface between the electrodes and skin of the chest wall are important.

Everything that is "gooey" does not conduct electricity well. For example, gels used for echocardiography conduct electricity very poorly. Of the various gels tested as interface for defibrillation or cardioversion, Hewlett-Packard (HP) Redux Paste (not cream) was one of the best. Kerber's group also found HP Redux Paste offered lower impedance than either Littman or Harco disposable defibrillation pads; electrode gels in some disposable electrodes have a higher impedance. In Kerber's study of self-adhesive pre-applied electrode pads for cardioversion, the transthoracic impedance was 75 ± 21 ohms (range 28 ohms to 150 ohms. In Ewy's study, using metal electrodes (8.0 cm anterior and 12.8 cm posterior) and HP Redux Paste, transthoracic impedance was significantly lower at 56 ± 16 ohms. In Ewy's study, the 13 patients successfully cardioverted, had a mean impedance of 50 ± 12 ohms, while the 13 patients who did not cardiovert with the first 100J shock had a mean impedance of

T A B L E   1
Determinants of Transthoracic or Transchest Resistance to DC Defibrillator or Cardioverter Capacitor Discharge
• Stored energy
• Electrode size
• Electrode composition
• Interface between the electrode and the skin
• Distance between electrodes
• Number of previous shocks
• Time interval between previous and present shock
• Pressure on the electrodes
• The phase of ventilation
• Patients body build
• Recent sternotomy

59 ± 10 ohms. As Lown writes, "thick layers of conductive paste is recommended".

The phase of ventilation and pressure applied to paddle electrodes are probably related, as air does not conduct electricity well. Firm electrode pressure with the patient in full expiratory phase of ventilation is important. The presence or absence of previous DC shocks and the time interval between shocks also influences transthoracic impedance, which falls slightly with each DC shock. Finally, for at least a month following the procedure, a sternotomy lowers transchest impedance.

Electrode Positions

Electrode position is critical since the current must traverse a critical mass of the atrial muscle for cardioversion to occur. Lown reported that the anterior-posterior electrode position was more effective for cardioversion of atrial fibrillation than the anterior-anterior electrode position. Lown writes that "anterior paddle is held with pressure over the upper sternum at the level of the third intercostal space. This antero-posterior position, compared with the previously employed antero-lateral placement, shortens the pathway between the electrodes and augments the density of the electrical field which traverses the heart, thereby diminishing by about 50% the energy required for reversion".

In contrast, Kerber and associates reported that the electrode position or size made little difference to cardioversion success. However, in Kerber's study, the 111 patients with atrial fibrillation were divided into four groups, each with high success rates, making a statistical error so it's likely that the study is not definitive. In addition, in Kerber's study of electrode position, the electrode positions recommended by Lown (sternal or right parasternal anterior-left posterior; Figure 2) or Ewy (left parasternal anterior-posterior; Figure 3) for cardioversion of atrial fibrillation were not tested.

Analysis of CT scans of the thorax at the level of the heart provides insight into appropriate electrode positions for defibrillation of the atria (Figures 2, 3). As noted above, for successful cardioversion the current vector must traverse a critical mass of the atrial muscle. The anterior-posterior positions (Figures 2, 3) fulfill this criteria best. The right anterior-left posterior position (Figure 2) or Lown's sternal-posterior is the position of choice if the pathology involves both atria (such as atrial fibrillation due to atrial septal defect or diffuse cardiomyopathy). This position has more of the right atria between the electrodes. The right anterior-posterior electrode position (Figure 2) has the dis-

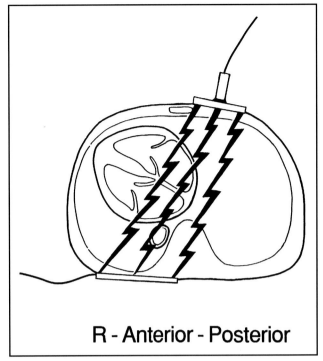

R - Anterior - Posterior

Figure 2. Illustration of right parasternal anterior-posterior electrode placement (8 cm diameter anterior and 12.8 cm diameter posterior electrode). This and the sternal-posterior electrode positions are recommended by Lown. *(Copyrighted and reprinted with the permission of Clinical Cardiology Publishing Company, Inc., and/or Foundation for Advances in Medicine and Science, Inc., P.O. Box 832, Mahwah, NJ 07430.)*

advantage of a greater inter-electrode distance and more lung between the electrode and the heart in the unoperated or emphysematous chest. The left parasternal anterior-posterior electrode position has the advantage of smaller inter-electrode distance and less lung between the electrodes (Figure 3). It is not known whether the right parasternal anterior-left posterior position (Figure 2) is better than the left parasternal anterior-posterior paddle electrode position (Figure 3) that Ewy advocates in patients whose major pathology is left atrial enlargement. The anterior-anterior (Figure 4) or the apical-left posterior positions (Figure 5) are not recommended for electrical cardioversion of atrial fibrillation as these positions probably do not provide optimal current flow through the atria.

With anterior-posterior electrode placement, the greater the anterior-posterior chest diameter, the greater the impedance and the less likely successful cardioversion. In a recent study, the only determinant of successful cardioversion was body weight, which usually correlates with chest diameter. Geddes and associates clearly showed that the electrical dose for ventricular fibrillation was related to body size and weight; when impedance is low and

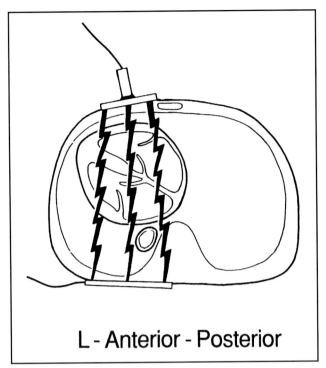

L - Anterior - Posterior

Figure 3. Illustration of left parasternal anterior-posterior (Ewy) electrode placement (8 cm diameter anterior and 12.8 cm diameter electrode). *(Copyrighted and reprinted with the permission of Clinical Cardiology Publishing Company, Inc., and/or Foundation for Advances in Medicine and Science, Inc., P.O. Box 832, Mahwah, NJ 07430.)*

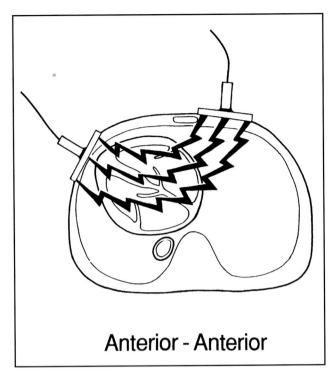

Anterior - Anterior

Figure 4. Illustration of anterior-anterior (standard) electrode position (8 cm diameter electrodes). *(Copyrighted and reprinted with the permission of Clinical Cardiology Publishing Company, Inc., and/or Foundation for Advances in Medicine and Science, Inc., P.O. Box 832, Mahwah, NJ 07430.)*

current delivery is high, the relationship between shock strength and body weight is difficult to show and is not clinically important in adults. However, if current delivery is marginal, this relationship is evident.

Predictors of Long-Term Success

The initial enthusiasm for elective cardioversion following Lown's innovative and important clinical advance was somewhat dampened by the high recurrence rate in some subsets of patients. As Lown emphasized, often the initiating mechanism and sustaining mechanism of atrial fibrillation were different. If the initiating mechanism was no longer present, then cardioversion would have lasting success. If, however, the initiating mechanism was still present, atrial fibrillation would recur. Certain patients were found not to be suitable candidates for cardioversion because of the high recurrence rate. Untreated thyrotoxicosis, significant untreated mitral valve disease or congestive heart failure are obvious examples of situations where the initiating mechanism is still present. Atrial fibrillation of more than one year's duration, first degree heart block greater than 0.24 seconds prior to the onset of atrial fibrillation, and significant left atrial enlargement are markers that the initiating

pathology is still present, since these factors predict early recurrence. Some studies have not shown a relation between left atrial size and post-cardioversion atrial fibrillation recurrence rate. However, those studies that looked at cardioversion success rates and recurrence rates within disease states (such as mitral disease, hypertrophic cardiomyopathy, idiopathic atrial fibrillation) have shown that a large left atrium is one of the contributing factors to atrial fibrillation and failure or high recurrence rates in those with larger left atriums post-cardioversion.

CARDIAC PEARL

Atrial Fibrillation- The unexplained onset of atrial fibrillation in a patient who is 50 years of age or older may be a clue to the presence of underlying coronary artery disease. However, this is not necessarily true, since other conditions can cause this.

One example was President Bush's atrial fibrillation, which apparently was triggered by hyperthyroidism. His hyperthyroidism was treated and in turn the atrial fibrillation has apparently been controlled.

There is still a place for the medical treatment of paroxysmal atrial fibrillation. Too often the first step in management is to have electroconversion, whereas if antiarrhythmic drugs are given under supervision this can be accomplished medically.

It is best to have the patient under supervision in the hospital when attempting conversion to normal sinus rhythm, either with medication or electroconversion.

When it is not possible to control atrial fibrillation after trying several antiarrhythmic drugs, it may be best for both physician and patient to "accept" and live with a chronic atrial fibrillation with a ventricular range in the 60s and 70s.

A patient with heart disease may have no evidence of cardiac decompensation, but acute pulmonary edema can occur with the change from normal sinus rhythm to atrial fibrillation. This also may be the first indication of underlying heart disease in some patients.

W. Proctor Harvey, M.D.

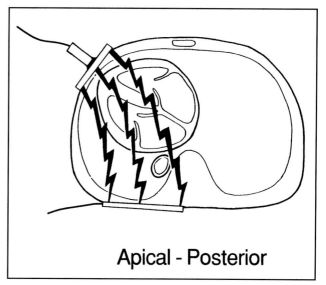

Figure 5. Illustration of apical-posterior electrode position (8 cm diameter anterior electrode and 12.8 cm diameter posterior electrode). *(Copyrighted and reprinted with the permission of Clinical Cardiology Publishing Company, Inc., and/or Foundation for Advances in Medicine and Science, Inc., P.O. Box 832, Mahwah, NJ 07430.)*

Anticoagulation

Should all patients be anticoagulated prior to cardioversion? The landmark study of Bjerkelund and Orning suggested that they should. The study was not randomized since all patients admitted on oral anticoagulation, including all patients with previous emboli, were placed in the anticoagulated group. Incidence of post-cardioversion emboli was 5.3% in the group not anticoagulated and 0.8% in the anticoagulated group. Based on this study, many cardiologists have routinely anticoagulated patients prior to pharmacologic or electrical cardioversion. The importance of anticoagulation was recently emphasized by retrospective review of 454 elective direct-current cardioversions of patients with atrial arrhythmias. Rate of embolic complications was low at 1.32%. All six patients with emboli had atrial fibrillation and none had been on anticoagulation. The duration of atrial fibrillation was less than one week in five of the six patients who had embolic complications. The last American College of Chest Physicians' Conference on Antithrombotic Therapy does not recommend anticoagulation if the duration of atrial fibrillation is less than three days. This recommendation is now questionable since in patients with enlarged atria and low cardiac output, it probably takes fewer than three days to form atrial appendage clots. In the transesophageal study by Dawkin and associates, the incidence of atrial appendage clot was 11% in patients with atrial fibrillation of four days or less and 25% in patients with atrial fibrillation of more than four days duration. In this series, incidence of

new emboli was as frequent in the patients with atrial fibrillation less than four days duration as it was for those with atrial fibrillation longer than four days. Therefore, unless the atrial fibrillation is of very recent onset in a patient with an otherwise normal heart, this author recommends that patients undergo anticoagulation prior to elective cardioversion.

This recommendation applies to atrial flutter as well as atrial fibrillation. Although emboli with atrial flutter are rare, not occurring in some series, the most severe episode of cerebral embolus that this author has ever encountered was a patient with relatively recent onset atrial flutter who had fatal cerebral emboli following non-anticoagulated electrical cardioversion. There was a disturbing trend toward performing a transesophageal echocardiogram and if no atrial thrombi are seen, to proceed with elective cardioversion without anticoagulation. However, a non-anticoagulated patient in one of our affiliated hospitals had a cerebral embolus following elective cardioversion. This patient had transesophageal echocardiography with no evidence of intra-atrial or appendage thrombi, even on intensive review. A recent study from Australia reported thromboembolic complications in four of 66 patients, none of whom had evidence of left atrial thrombus before cardioversion.

There are at least three possible explanations for this phenomenon. The first is that the transesophageal echo is or was not technically satisfactory. The second is that the clot that produces the embolus is too small to be detected by currently available transesophageal echocardiography. The third is that the cardioversion itself predisposes to clot formation. This latter possibility was raised by Grimm, Klein and associates, and by Fatkin, Feneley and associates from Australia. Grimm and associates studied left atrial appendage function with transesophageal echocardiography in 20 patients with atrial fibrillation before and 5 minutes to 15 minutes after successful cardioversion. Organized left atrial appendage function did not immediately return in 20% of their patients. Even in the patients whose atrial appendage function returned immediately, its function was impaired compared with that before cardioversion. Spontaneous echo contrast or "smoke" increased in the left atrium or left atrial appendage in 35%. These observations suggest that stunned left atrial appendage function after cardioversion may play a role in the mechanism involved in the occurrence of embolism after cardioversion. Fatkin and associates who performed transesophageal echo before and during cardioversion also reported transient atrial dysfunction ("stunning") caused by cardioversion. In their study, five patients had new spontaneous echo contrast in the left atrium that appeared within 10 seconds of restoration of sinus rhythm.

Use of transesophageal echocardiography and short term anticoagutation was recently reported. Manning and associates gave intravenous heparin anticoagulation for a mean of 2.1 ± 1.2 days prior to cardioversion. Thus, their recommendation of cardioversion without long-term anticoagulation is not the same as no anticoagulation. Since cardioversion can be performed on an outpatient basis it might be cost effective to use the following approach. If the patient is hemodynamically stable and hospitalization is not required for some other reason, the patient may receive oral anticoagulant therapy for three weeks prior to elective outpatient cardioversion. If hospitalization is necessary for other reasons, and semi-urgent cardioversion is necessary, transesophageal echocardiography to rule out intra-atrial thrombi followed by two days of heparin therapy prior and one day of heparin therapy post cardioversion is recommended. If there is no contraindication, warfarin therapy should be initiated with the heparin. Transesophageal echocardiography may identify very high risk patients with atrial thrombi in which even short term heparin therapy prior to cardioversion would be inadequate, and in whom cardioversion should be postponed to avoid the risk of embolization.

This author's practice is to keep patients on chronic oral anticoagulation therapy for at least three months post cardioversion because of the high recurrence rate during this time. If one were sure that the patient would remain in sinus rhythm, shorter duration of anticoagulation might be justified as Bjerkelund and Orning found in their study that emboli occurred six hours to six days following electrical cardioversion, and the emboli reported by Fatkin and associates occurred within the first week.

CARDIAC PEARL

The incidence of stroke associated with atrial fibrillation can be reduced by the use of anticoagulants such as warfarin.

With life expectancy increasing, more patients will have atrial fibrillation; the above pearl will be even more apropos.

It is of interest that several decades ago there was controversy as to whether anticoagulants were indicated for patients having atrial fibrillation.

However, recent analysis showed that patients who have atrial fibrillation will be less prone to thromboembolic events if they are on warfarin (Coumadin). Of course, contraindications to anticoagulant administration should be checked before use of these drugs.

W. Proctor Harvey, M.D.

The Role of Antiarrhythmic Therapy

Lown instituted quinidine therapy one or more days before attempted electrical reversion stating that quinidine improved the chance of the patient remaining in normal sinus rhythm immediately after cardioversion, decreases by about 40% the energy required, diminishes incidence of post-cardioversion arrhythmias, and obtains a small dividend of reversions "in about 10%" of patients.

A major unanswered question is the role of antiarrhythmic drugs post cardioversion. A meta-analysis of patients treated with quinidine post pharmacologic or electrical cardioversion indicated a higher percentage of patients in normal sinus rhythm, but a higher mortality rate in the quinidine treated group. This and the results of the CAST studies cast doubt on the wisdom of long-term antiarrhythmic therapy in these patients. It is not known, however, whether patients in the randomized quinidine studies were carefully monitored for evidence of QT prolongation following initiation of quinidine therapy. My present recommendation is to hospitalize and monitor all patients started on antiarrhythmic therapy for attempted cardioversion. If the corrected QT interval becomes greater than 485 msec, the drug is discontinued. Antiarrhythmic drugs are frequently discontinued after several days to weeks of therapy. If long term antiarrhythmic drug therapy is not contemplated, outpatient electrical cardioversion might be the most cost effective approach to reversion of atrial fibrillation.

Remember that antiarrhythmic drugs can also be pro-arrhythmic, and ironically produce the same fatal arrhythmia that one is trying to prevent.

Therefore, careful observation and follow-up after initiation of a new antiarrhythmic drug is essential. The possibility of a pro-arrhythmia effect of a drug is not appreciated as well as it should be.

The following is a case in point, which I only learned about recently:

A friend, who is in his late 70's, developed atrial fibrillation. He was anticoagulated as a precaution to prevent emboli coincident or following reversion to normal sinus rhythm. Wisely, he was admitted to the hospital for attempt at medical conversion with quinidine before resorting to electroconversion. On quinidine, he is reported to have developed "torsades de pointes" ventricular arrhythmia and cardiac arrest (Figure A). Fortunately he was immediately and successfully resuscitated.

This is a reminder to us that the drug we use to control arrhythmias can also cause them. It is, of course, important that the possibility of this adverse, sometimes very serious, effect be looked for. This is currently apropos, because many newer drugs are being introduced and advocated for treatment of arrhythmias.

W. Proctor Harvey, M.D.

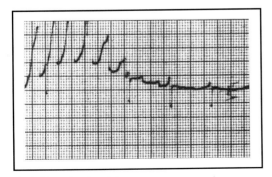

Fig A: Torsades de pointes.

In some patients, for example, patients with hypertrophic or congestive cardiomyopathy, maintenance of sinus rhythm has a significant clinical benefit. In such patients, the role of Class III antiarrhythmic therapy in those who have failed Class I antiarrhythmics is unknown. Levy and associates treated patients whose atrial fibrillation was refractory to Class I antiarrhythmics with one month of amiodarone prior to cardioversion. Although the initial success was encouraging, the high recurrence rate (45% in two months) was not. Sotalol therapy for reversion of atrial fibrillation and maintenance of sinus rhythm is encouraging, but the role of sotalol as well as amiodarone must await further studies.

Shock Strength

For atrial fibrillation, the shock strength for the initial shock should be 200J (stored energy) since only 50% of patients will be cardioverted with 100J. About 85% of those who will electrically cardiovert will do so at 200J; the next shock should be 360J since almost all patients who will cardiovert electrically via the external technique will do so at the maximal setting. If the first 360J shock is not successful, one should wait a full three minutes before delivering a final 360J shock, if the electrode positions are to be unchanged. This three-minute wait allows a greater decrease in transthoracic impedance from the previous DC shock than shocks delivered at 15-second or one-minute intervals. Lower shock strength is needed for cardioversion of atrial flutter, and energies of 25J to 50J are recommended initial shock strengths.

Initial shock strength for elective cardioversion of atrial flutter should be about 50J. Many patients with atrial flutter will cardiovert with less energy, but lower energies are likely to result in the induction of atrial fibrillation. The optimal approach to electrical cardioversion includes appropriate patient selection, anticoagulation, careful selection and monitoring of antiarrhythmic therapy, and proper electrical cardioversion technique. The optimal technique is one that utilizes metal electrodes with one electrode at least 8 cm in diameter, placed in the right or left parasternal anterior position, and the second 12.8 cm diameter electrode placed posteriorly just below the left scapulae, with generous amounts of the appropriate gel (such as Hewlett-Packard Redux Paste) as the electrode-skin interface, and firm pressure to the paddle electrode with the patient in the expiratory phase of ventilation, thus decreasing the anterior-posterior chest diameter and assuring less air between the electrodes. Appropriate energy is selected; shock is synchronized with the electrocardiographic QRS complex.

Selected Reading

1. Arnold AZ, Mick MJ, Mazurek RP, Loop FD, Trohman RG: Role of prophylactic anticoagulation for direct current cardioversion in patients with atrial flutter or fibrillation. *JACC* 1992; 19:851-5.

2. Aylward PE, Kieso R, Hite P, Charbonnier F, Kerber RE: Defibrillator electrode-chest wall coupling agents: Influence on transthoracic impedance and shock success. *JACC* 1985; 6:682-686.

3. Bjerkelund CJ, Orning OM: The efficacy of anticoagulant therapy in preventing embolism related to DC electrical conversion of atrial fibrillation. *AJC* 1969; 23:208-216.

4. Cardiac Arrhythmia Suppression Trial (CAST) Investigators: Effect of encainide and flecainide on mortality in a randomized trial of arrhythmia suppression after myocardial infarction. *NEJM* 1989; 321:406-412.

5. Chan M, Marcus R, Bednarz J, Childers R, Lan R: Contribution of transesophageal echocardiography to cardioversion protocols for atrial fibrillation (abst). *JASC* 1992; 5:308.

6. Connell PN, Ewy GA, Dahl CF, Ewy MD: Transthoracic impedance to defibrillator discharge. Effect of electrode size and chest wall interface. *J. Electrocard* 1973; 6:313-317.

7. Coplen SE, Antman EM, Berlin JA, et al: Efficacy and safety of quinidine therapy for maintenance of sinus rhythm after cardioversion: a meta-analysis of randomized control trials. *Circ* 1990; 82:1106-1116.

8. Dahl CF, Ewy GA, Ewy MD, Thomas ED: Transthoracic impedance to direct current discharge: Effects of repeated countershocks. *Medical Instrum* 1976; 10:151-154.

9. Dahl CF, Ewy GA, Warner ED, Thomas ED: Myocardial necrosis from direct current countershock. *Circ* 1974; 50:956-961.

10. Daniel WG: Should transesophageal echocardiography be used to guide cardioversion? *NEJM* 1993; 328:803-804.

11. Dawkin PR, Stoddard MT, Liddel NE, Longaker RA: Acute vs chronic atrial fibrillation: Incidence of appendage thrombus, spontaneous contrast and embolic events. *Circ* 1992; 19:201A.

12. Ewy GA: The optimal technique for electrical cardioversion of atrial fibrillation. *Circ* 1992; 86:1645-1647.

13. Ewy GA: The optimal technique for electrical cardioversion of atrial fibrillation. *Clin Card* 1994; 17:79-84.

14. Ewy GA: Direct current shock and transcardiac impedance. *AJC* 1980; 45:909 (Letter).

15. Ewy GA: Effectiveness of direct current defibrillation: role of paddle electrode size: *AHJ* 1977; 91:674-675.

16. Ewy GA: Ventricular fibrillation and defibrillation (in) Ewy GA, Bressler (eds) *Cardiovascular Drugs and the Management of Heart Disease* (1st ed) 1982; Raven Press, New York p 331-349.

17. Ewy GA, Haran WJ, Ewy MD: Disposable defibrillator electrodes. *Heart and Lung* 1977; 6:127-130.

18. Ewy GA, Taren D: Comparison of paddle electrode pastes used for defibrillation. *Heart and Lung* 1977; 6:847-850.

19. Ewy GA, Taren D: Impedance to transthoracic direct current discharge: A model for testing interface material. *Medical Instrum* 1978; 12:47-48.

20. Ewy GA, Hellman DA, McClung S, Taren D: Influence of ventilation phase on transthoracic impedance and defibrillation effectiveness. *Critical Care Medicine* 1980; 8:164-1 66.

21. Ewy GA: Cardioversion (in) Ewy GA, Bressler R (eds) *Cardiovascular Drugs and Management of Heart Disease* (1st Ed) Raven Press, 1982; New York p 427-440.

22. Ewy GA, Ulfers L, Hager WD, Rosenfeld AR, Roeske WR, Goldman S: Response of atrial fibrillation to therapy: role of etiology and left atrial diameter. *Electrocardiol* 1980; 13:119-124.

23. Ewy GA: Cardiac arrest and resuscitation: Defibrillators and defibrillation (in) *Current Problems in Cardiology* (ed) Harvey WP. 1978; Year Book Medical Publishers, Inc., Chicago 11; 1-71.

24. Fatkin D, Kuchar DL, Thorburn CW, Fenely M:. Transesophageal echocardiography before and during direct current cardioversion of atrial fibrillation: evidence of "atrial stunning" as a mechanism of thromboembolic complications. *JACC* 1994; 23:307-316.

25. Geddes LA, Tacker, WA, Rosborough JP, Moore AG, Cabler PS: Electrical dose for ventricular defibrillation of large and small animals using precordial electrodes. *J. Clin. Invest.* 1974; 53:310-319.

26. Grimm RA, Stewart WJ, Black IW, Thomar JD, Klein AL: Should all patients undergo transesophageal echocardiography before electrical cardioversion of atrial fibrillation. *JACC* 1994; 23:533-41.

27. Grimm R, Stewart WJ, Maloney JD, et al: Impact of electrical cardioversion for atrial fibrillation on left atrial appendage function and spontaneous echo contrast: Characterization by simultaneous transesophageal echocardiography. *JACC* 1993; 22:1359-1366.

28. Guidelines for Cardiopulmonary Resuscitation and Emergency Cardiac Care. *JAMA* 1992; 268:2171-2302.

29. Henry WL, Morganroth J, Pearlman AS, et al: Relation between echocardiographically determined left atrial size and atrial fibrillation. *Circ* 1976; 53:273-279.

30. Kerber RE, Grayzel J, Hoyt R, Marcus M, Kennedy, J: Transthoracic resistance in human defibrillation: influence of body weight, chest size, serial shocks, paddle size and paddle contact pressure. *Circ* 1981; 63:676-682.

31. Kerber RE, Vance S, Schomer SJ, Mariano DJ, Charbonnier F: Transthoracic defibrillation: Effect of sternotomy on chest impedance. *JACC* 1992; 20:94-97.

32. Kerber RE, Martins JB, Kelley KJ, Ferguson DW, Klouba C, Jensen SR, Newman B, Parke JD, Kieso R, Melton J: Self-adhesive preapplied electrode pads for defibrillation and cardioversion. *JACC* 1984; 3:815-820.

33. Kerber RE, Jensen SR, Grazel J, Kennedy J, Hoyt R: Elective cardioversion: Influence of paddle-electrode location and size on success rates and energy requirements. *NEJM* 1981; 305:658-662.

34. Levy S, Lauribe P, Dolla E, et al: A randomized comparison of external and internal cardioversion of chronic atrial fibrillation. *Circ* 1992; 86:1415-1420.

35. Lown B, Amarasingham R, Neurrkn J: New method for termination of cardiac arrhythmias: Use of synchionized capacitor discharge: *JAMA* 1962; 1B2:548-555.

36. Lown B: Electrical reversion of cardiac arrhythmias. *Heart J* 1967; 29:469-489.

37. Manning WJ, Silverman Dl, Gordon SPF, Krumholz HYM, Douglas PS: Cardioversion from atrial fibrillation without prolonged anticoagulation with use of transesophageal echocardiography to exclude the presence of atrial thrombi. *NEJM* 1993; 328:750-755.

38. Stoddard MF, Longaker RA. Role of transesophageal echo prior to cardioversion in patient with atrial fibrillation. *JACC* 1993; 21 Suppl A:28A.

39. Taren D, Ewy GA: Relative contribution of paddle electrode area and edge length to transthoracic impedance from a DC defibrillator discharge. *Med Instrum* 1979; 13:183-184.

40. Thomas ED, Ewy GA, Dahl CF, Ewy MD: Effectiveness of direct current defibrillation: role of paddle electrode size. *AHJ* 1977; 93:463-467.

CHAPTER 33

Special Considerations in Cardiopulmonary Resuscitation

Gordon A. Ewy, M.D.

Cardiac arrest's dramatic clinical presentation and the widely variable outcome of cardiopulmonary resuscitation (CPR) attempts continues to attract attention and to be of concern to scientific and lay communities alike. Debate continues over many aspects of CPR, perhaps surprising considering the fact that about two decades ago the medical profession was so seemingly sure that it knew almost all that was needed to know about CPR that "Standards" were published. As more questions arose, these became "Standards and Guidelines" and more recently only "Guidelines"; the latter seems to be an admission that there is still much to be learned in the field of CPR. The omission of "Standards" is also a subtle admission that in our litigious society, "Standards" may do more to limit rather than foster progress.

Previous Standards and Guidelines

Previous standards and guidelines on Cardiopulmonary Resuscitation and Emergency Cardiac Care (CPR-ECC) made several changes:

1. Increased the rate of chest compression from 60 to between 80 and 100 per minute.

2. Restored the recommendation for a "chest thump" in witnessed cardiac arrest.

3. Emphasized the importance of early defibrillation using defibrillation energies of 200J, and if necessary 300J, then 360J.

4. Emphasized importance of early use of intravenous epinephrine if initial defibrillatory shocks are ineffective.

5. Stated that sodium bicarbonate is not the first or initial drug to be used in cardiac arrest.

6. Recommended that calcium chloride was not to be used except in special circumstances.

7. Stated that isoproterenol was contraindicated in most arrests.

8. Emphasized importance of the endotracheal route for drug delivery if intravenous access is unavailable.

New Guidelines

Newer guidelines for CPR-ECC left most of the previous guidelines intact. Major changes were:

1. Call 911 before initiating basic cardiac life support (BCLS) in adults.

2. Do not teach "two rescuer CPR" in BCLS.

3. Increase ventilation duration to 1.5 seconds to 2.0 seconds.

4. Teach mouth-to-barrier device use.

5. Confirm importance of early defibrillation and thus the need for wider availability of the automatic external defibrillators (AED).

6. Do not give high-dose epinephrine to adults.

7. Adenosine is drug of choice for paroxysmal supraventricular tachycardia (PSVT) in adults.

8. Intravenous flush is recommended following drug administration to ensure central drug delivery.

Over the last decade CPR research has confirmed importance of bystander-initiated CPR, early defibrillation in arrest secondary to ventricular fibrillation, epinephrine's alpha adrenergic effect, myocardial perfusion during prolonged CPR efforts, and the lack of importance of sodium bicarbonate therapy during the early minutes of unexpected cardiac arrest in a previously stable patient. In addition, CPR research has confirmed the importance of assessing who is and is not a candidate for CPR, and the importance of the Heimlich maneuver or abdominal thrust in patients with aspiration (Cafe Coronary).

The questions that remain, however, are numerous. Four that come to mind are:

1. How can one assure bystander-initiated CPR?

2. How can one assure adequate myocardial perfusion pressure during prolonged CPR attempts?

3. How can one determine effectiveness of CPR during the resuscitation effort?

4. How can one assure early effective defibrillation?

Assuring Bystander-Initiated CPR

Widespread use of CPR classes, CPR television instruction for the general public, more directed CPR training of spouses or companions of high risk patients, and the highly-focused telephone instructed CPR to those who call 911 to report a cardiac arrest have all been advocated and supported by investigations. Lack of knowledge is one barrier to bystander CPR. Another impediment to bystander-initiated CPR is the fear of potentially-lethal infection from mouth to mouth resuscitation, especially in strangers with facial or oropharyngeal injuries from the fall associated with the arrest.

One solution to this problem could be the use of an infection barrier for mouth-to-mouth resuscitation or the accessibility of bag-mouth ventilation devices. This solution, while practical for health care providers, is impractical for the general public. Another possible solution will be performing chest compression without respiration. There is increasing data that in non-airway obstructive cardiac arrest, ventilation for the first several minutes is not necessary. This thought may come as a shock to most physicians. However, there are studies of out-of-hospital cardiac arrest in adults that show no correlation between pH, PO_2 or PCO_2 and CPR outcome.

Animal studies from our laboratory have shown that 24-hour survival from 12 minutes of CPR followed by Advanced Cardiac Life Support (ACLS) is as effective with chest compression alone as it is with chest compression and interposed ventilation (100% survival in each group). In contrast, if bystander CPR was withheld, ACLS at 12 minutes results in less than 20% survival. If chest compression alone in the early minutes of CPR proves effective, it will not only eliminate the barrier to initiation of bystander CPR because of the fear of infection, it will also make teaching of bystander or lay CPR much easier. It is my prediction that this will be one of the major advances in CPR in the next decade. If there is a witnessed arrest in a previously well individual, all that may be needed prior to the arrival of the paramedics or definitive therapy is rapid lower sternal chest compression.

Obviously in a situation where aspiration is probable, such as a "cafe coronary", attention must first be directed to clearing the airway, and if the arrest is respiratory, then "breathing" is vitally important, especially in infants and children where cardiac arrest is usually secondary to respiratory arrest.

Assuring Adequate Myocardial Perfusion Pressure

Fibrillating ventricles will consume adenosine triphosphate, other energy sources, and autoinfarct without adequate myocardial perfusion. Controlled studies in our laboratory have shown that after 15 minutes of inadequate coronary perfusion pressures, restoration of adequate or even supernormal coronary perfusion pressures will not result in myocardial salvage because the heart is irreversibly damaged or the microvasculature is incapable of blood delivery. Myocardial perfusion during ventricular fibrillation and CPR occurs predominantly during compression diastole (release phase of chest compression).

Myocardial perfusion is directly correlated with the aortic diastolic pressure minus the right atrial diastolic pressure (since the coronary sinus empties into the right atrium). Because myocardial hypoxia produces maximal coronary artery dilation, the amount of myocardial perfusion is initially related to coronary perfusion pressure and presence and severity of coronary stenosis. However, a coronary lesion that is non-critical in sinus rhythm becomes critical during cardiac arrest and CPR.

Determining Aortic Diastolic Pressure During CPR

Factors determining aortic diastolic pressure during CPR are force and velocity of chest compression, frequency of chest compression, peripheral vascular resistance, and effective intravascular volume. Force of chest compression should be adequate to displace the sternum by 1.5 to 2.0 inches. Frequency of chest compression is also important. Too slow, and the aortic diastolic pressure drops too low before the next compression. Too fast, and compression diastole is too short for adequate ventricular filling. To date, experience suggests that a compression rate of 100 per minute is probably near optimal. However, our studies have shown that most rescuers, even ACLS certified rescuers, need a guide, such as a metronome to assure optimal compression rates of 100 per minute.

Because three transesophageal echocardiography studies have now shown that the mechanism of blood flow early in CPR is via cardiac (especially right ventricular) compression, it is important that a rapid chest compression rate be maintained to assure optimal cardiac output during CPR. The compression must be applied briskly to assure mitral and tricuspid valve closure. Compression of adequate force but too slowly applied does not result in adequate momentum to result in mitral and tricuspid valve closure. As McCall wrote in Hurst and Logue, "The manner of compression is extremely important; it should not be described as massage, since this gives the impression of a slow, milking action. In order to produce good ejection a vigorous quick compression must be carried out". This valuable lesson, unfortunately, must be relearned nowadays.

CARDIAC PEARL

With regard to cardiac arrest and a thump on the chest, a cardiac pearl: remember to deliver a good thump on the chest with the clenched fist as an early, initial attempt at treatment of cardiac arrest. This chest blow may disturb the fatal ventricular arrhythmia and convert it to normal sinus rhythm. If not successful, of course, standard cardiopulmonary resuscitation techniques should be given promptly. In addition, it is important to remember that infrequently a chest thump can do the opposite- cause ventricular tachycardia and/or fibrillation.

W. Proctor Harvey, M.D.

There are some situations (such as a patient with a barrel chest due to severe emphysema) where mechanism of blood flow during CPR is via thoracic pump or increased intrathoracic pressure mechanism. This mechanism, however, is generally less effective; our studies have shown that 24-hour survival is best in those situations and techniques where cardiac compression is the dominant mechanism of blood flow during CPR.

Peripheral vascular resistance during cardiac arrest and CPR is determined by many factors. It's clear that the beneficial effect of epinephrine is due to its alpha-adrenergic agonist effect resulting in increased vasoconstriction. The vasodilating effect of beta-adrenergic agonists and other vasodilators is deleterious. Epinephrine plus beta blockers is effective during CPR but epinephrine plus alpha blockers is totally ineffective. A major question that has been raised is the need for high dose (0.2 mg/Kg) epinephrine rather than standard dose (0.02 mg/Kg) epinephrine. Although there are anecdotal reports of high dose epinephrine being more effective, both animal and clinical studies have failed to show its effectiveness. In an experimental

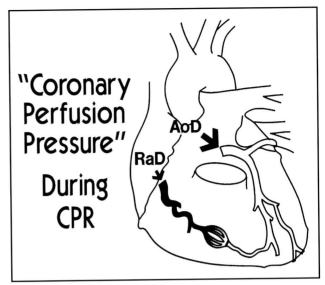

Figure 1. Coronary perfusion pressure during cardiopulmonary resuscitation (CPR) is the aortic "diastolic" (AoD) minus the right atrial "diastolic" (RaD) pressure as the coronary sinus empties into the right atrium. During ventricular fibrillation and CPR, almost all of the coronary blood flow occurs in "diastole", that is the release phase of chest compression.

model with varying degrees of coronary artery stenosis, our laboratory has demonstrated no increase in coronary flow with high-dose epinephrine. In other animal studies, we have failed to demonstrate any survival advantage of high-dose epinephrine. In fact, animals receiving high dose epinephrine were more likely to die in the early hours post resuscitation.

Even when high-dose epinephrine is not used, patients who are difficult to resuscitate may receive several injections of standard doses of epinephrine. The result is often catecholamine-induced tachycardia, increased ischemia, ventricular arrhythmias, and recurrent arrest. If blood pressure is adequate post-defibrillation, intravenous beta-adrenergic blockers to block the excess beta stimulatory affect may be indicated. Ditchey and associates have shown that combined phenylephrine (an alpha agonist) and beta-blockers result in higher coronary perfusion pressures in experimental cardiac arrest than standard dose epinephrine.

Finally, the role of intravascular volume has not been completely elucidated, but adequate intravascular volume is necessary for maintaining cardiac filling, especially with rapid manual chest compression.

Determining Effectiveness of CPR During Resuscitation Attempts

It was previously thought that presence of a palpable arterial pulse with each chest compression was evidence that effective CPR was being per-

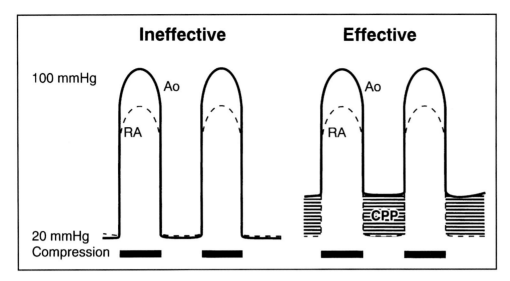

Figure 2. Illustration contrasting the hemodynamics of ineffective with effective cardiopulmonary resuscitation. With chest compression (solid bars) the systolic pressure is 100 mmHg in both. However, effective CPR is that which generates an effective coronary perfusion pressure (CPP); i.e. where the aortic (Ao) "diastolic" or release phase pressures are significantly higher than the right atrial (RA) "diastolic" pressures.

formed. If one does not generate a palpable pulse, the resuscitation effort is obviously inadequate. But presence of a palpable pulse does not guarantee good CPR. It's now known that coronary perfusion pressure (that is, aortic diastolic minus the right atrial diastolic pressure during the release phase of chest compression during CPR) determines coronary flow and thus myocardial perfusion during CPR (Figure 1). As illustrated in Figure 2, one can generate aortic systolic pressures of 100 mmHg or more, but if aortic diastolic and the right atrial diastolic pressures (Figure 1) are not different, there will be no coronary blood flow, and ventricles will become progressively more ischemic. All the while, would-be rescuers think they are doing a great job of CPR because there is a good palpable pulse.

To determine myocardial perfusion pressure during CPR, arterial and central venous or right heart catheters must be in place when the arrest occurs. We have tried to place central venous and aortic catheters during arrest and found that they could not be placed quickly enough. Accordingly, a search for a non-invasive indicator of CPR effectiveness led us and others to measure, in intubated patients, the partial pressure of end-tidal carbon dioxide (PETCO$_2$).

Because carbon dioxide is readily diffusible, and because forward blood flow through the lungs is slow during CPR, all of the carbon dioxide is exhaled. If there is no blood flow there is no exhaled carbon dioxide. If there is a small amount of pulmonary blood flow, there is a small amount of expired carbon dioxide, and if there is a greater amount of pulmonary blood flow, there is a greater amount of expired carbon dioxide. The greater the pulmonary blood flow, the higher the PETCO$_2$. We have shown that patients with PETCO$_2$ less than 10 Torr cannot be resuscitated. Therefore, if during

resuscitation efforts PETCO$_2$ is less than 10 Torr, one should compress the chest at a faster rate, with more force, or change the position of their hands.

Because open chest direct cardiac compression or cardiopulmonary bypass via femoral artery and vein access is more effective than closed chest CPR in selected patients, if one cannot generate more than 10 Torr PETCO$_2$ after 10 minutes of CPR, open chest or cardiopulmonary bypass is indicated. This approach is yet to be proven in humans. These heroic measures should not be instituted unless one is prepared to consider urgent corrective and replacement surgery. In some this will mean an artificial heart as a bridge to cardiac transplantation.

Assuring Early Effective Defibrillation

The new Guidelines for Emergency Cardiac Care recommend that a would-be rescuer notify 911 prior to initiating CPR in adults, saving valuable time. Minutes between the onset of arrest and defibrillation may be the difference between life and death. Early defibrillation will be facilitated by equipping all first responding vehicles with automatic or semi-automatic external defibrillators (AEDs), and assuring presence of AEDs not only in places where a large number of adults congregate, but also in isolated locations such as oil platforms and large airplanes. This approach will require development of less expensive AEDs, and that may require more effective defibrillation wave-forms.

Even earlier defibrillation is assured by the identification of patients with a very high probability of ventricular fibrillation and implanting automatic implantable cardioverter defibrillators (AICDs). Presently, survivors of out-of-hospital cardiac arrest who did not have a Q-wave infarction, who have inducible ventricular tachycardia not suppressible by antiarrhythmic drugs, are candidates for AICDs.

However, immediate defibrillation is not the same as early defibrillation. It is presently recommended that if a defibrillator is available, the patient should be given three shocks prior to epinephrine and chest compression. Studies have shown that this is the best approach if the duration of ventricular fibrilla-

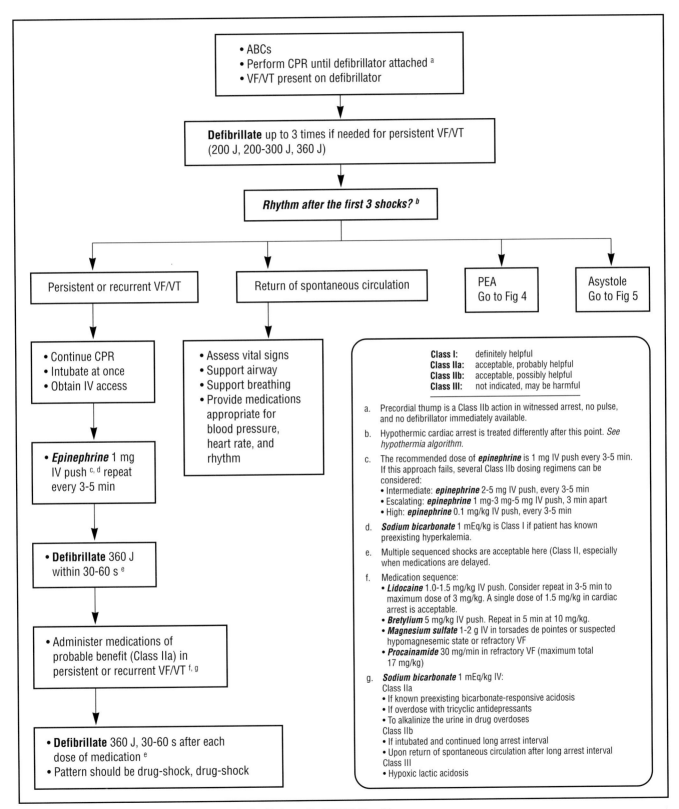

Figure 3. Ventricular Fibrillation/Pulseless Ventricular Tachycardia (VF/VT) Algorithm.
(Modified from Textbook of Advanced Cardiac Life Support, 1994. American Heart Association. Reproduced with permission.)

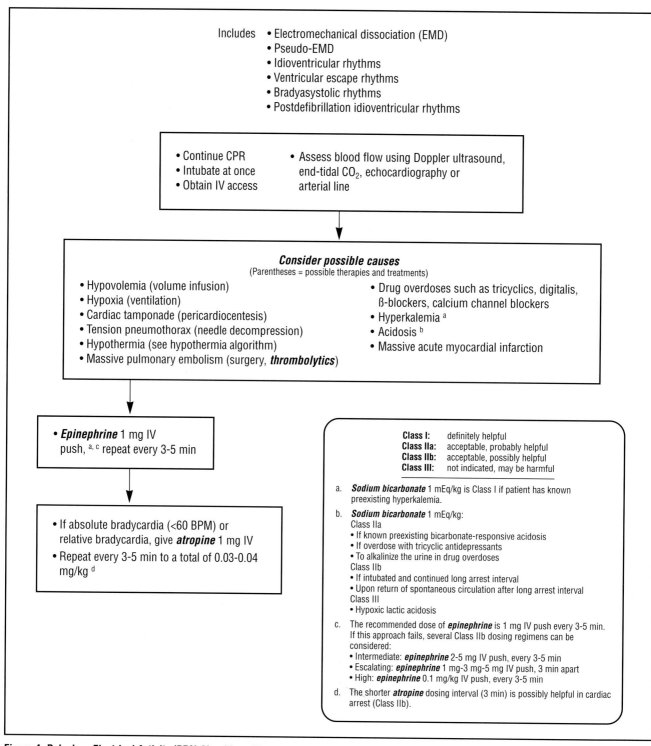

Includes
- Electromechanical dissociation (EMD)
- Pseudo-EMD
- Idioventricular rhythms
- Ventricular escape rhythms
- Bradyasystolic rhythms
- Postdefibrillation idioventricular rhythms

- Continue CPR
- Intubate at once
- Obtain IV access

- Assess blood flow using Doppler ultrasound, end-tidal CO_2, echocardiography or arterial line

Consider possible causes
(Parentheses = possible therapies and treatments)

- Hypovolemia (volume infusion)
- Hypoxia (ventilation)
- Cardiac tamponade (pericardiocentesis)
- Tension pneumothorax (needle decompression)
- Hypothermia (see hypothermia algorithm)
- Massive pulmonary embolism (surgery, *thrombolytics*)

- Drug overdoses such as tricyclics, digitalis, ß-blockers, calcium channel blockers
- Hyperkalemia [a]
- Acidosis [b]
- Massive acute myocardial infarction

- *Epinephrine* 1 mg IV push, [a, c] repeat every 3-5 min

- If absolute bradycardia (<60 BPM) or relative bradycardia, give *atropine* 1 mg IV
- Repeat every 3-5 min to a total of 0.03-0.04 mg/kg [d]

Class I:	definitely helpful
Class IIa:	acceptable, probably helpful
Class IIb:	acceptable, possibly helpful
Class III:	not indicated, may be harmful

a. *Sodium bicarbonate* 1 mEq/kg is Class I if patient has known preexisting hyperkalemia.

b. *Sodium bicarbonate* 1 mEq/kg:
Class IIa
- If known preexisting bicarbonate-responsive acidosis
- If overdose with tricyclic antidepressants
- To alkalinize the urine in drug overdoses
Class IIb
- If intubated and continued long arrest interval
- Upon return of spontaneous circulation after long arrest interval
Class III
- Hypoxic lactic acidosis

c. The recommended dose of *epinephrine* is 1 mg IV push every 3-5 min. If this approach fails, several Class IIb dosing regimens can be considered:
- Intermediate: *epinephrine* 2-5 mg IV push, every 3-5 min
- Escalating: *epinephrine* 1 mg-3 mg-5 mg IV push, 3 min apart
- High: *epinephrine* 0.1 mg/kg IV push, every 3-5 min

d. The shorter *atropine* dosing interval (3 min) is possibly helpful in cardiac arrest (Class IIb).

Figure 4. Pulseless Electrical Activity (PEA) Algorithm. (Electromechanical Dissociation [EMD])
(Modified from Textbook of Advanced Cardiac Life Support, 1994. American Heart Association. Reproduced with permission.)

tion is relatively short. For longer periods of arrest (five minutes in our studies), resuscitation is enhanced if one gives intravenous epinephrine and one minute of chest compression and ventilation prior to defibrillation. These differences in initial approach have yet to be incorporated in the Guide-lines for Emergency Cardiac Care, perhaps because duration of arrest is often difficult to determine.

Further directions in CPR will be based on several important findings. The recent 2D echo Doppler findings that blood flow during early phases of external chest compression is due to cardiac com-

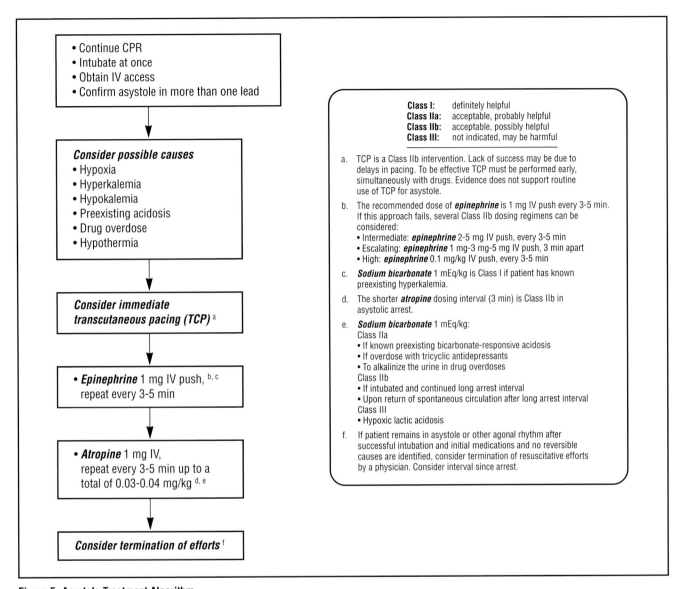

Figure 5. Asystole Treatment Algorithm.
(Modified from Textbook of Advanced Cardiac Life Support, 1994. American Heart Association. Reproduced with permission.)

pression, especially right ventricular compression, is an important observation because it explains why rapid, high impulse CPR is most effective. Studies of active-compression-decompression (ACD) CPR have shown enhanced hemodynamics during cardiac arrest. Studies are ongoing to determine if this mode of CPR is better. Use of intermittent abdominal compression has also been reported to enhance effectiveness of CPR. New studies will clarify the role of ACD and interposed abdominal pressure in our approach to CPR.

CARDIAC PEARL

I participated in a Cardiac Symposium and heard the author speak on cardiopulmonary resuscitation. He presented the following pertinent cardiac pearls:

"The optimal approach to cardiopulmonary resuscitation has changed somewhat over the last several years. Critical factors necessary for successful CPR include the following:

"In all arrests due to ventricular fibrillation, the critical step is defibrillation and if prompt, no other intervention is necessary. If defibrillation is delayed, usually because of the location of the cardiac arrest, then basic CPR techniques are necessary to slow the process of organ deterioration until defibrillation can be applied.

"Accordingly, in out-of-hospital cardiac arrest, one of the major determinants of survival is the time to onset of basic CPR and the time to defibrillation. Time to onset of basic

CPR is shortened with the initiation of bystander CPR. If bystander CPR is initiated within four minutes and definitive therapy within eight minutes, 43% of patients with ventricular fibrillation survive to leave the hospital. If CPR is not initiated by a bystander and is not begun until the ambulance or paramedic arrive, even when the units arrive within eight minutes, survival decreases to 27%. If definitive therapy is delayed by more than eight minutes, survival is rare.

"Surveys indicate that many individuals are reluctant to perform bystander CPR because of the fear of infection from mouth-to-mouth ventilation. Accordingly, we studied the feasibility of performing only chest compression during the first 12 minutes of CPR and found in our experimental model that when promptly initiated, chest compression alone was as effective as basic CPR.

"The new guidelines have made one major change in basic CPR recommendations. Since early defibrillation is critical to survival, the bystander is to call 911 first before initiating CPR. This will help to decrease the delay in arrival of definitive therapy.

"Sodium bicarbonate is not necessary during the first 15 minutes of CPR and calcium carbonate is contraindicated except in rare situations where hypocalcemia is present. Isoproterenol is also contraindicated since the beneficial effect of epinephrine is its alpha adrenergic effect. Epinephrine works well when given with a beta blocker but not at all when given with an alpha blocker, leaving only its beta stimulating properties, like isoproterenol."

W. Proctor Harvey, M.D.

The reader is referred to the current AHA guidelines for CPR and Emergency Cardiac Care. A summary of the guidelines on the treatment of ventricular fibrillation/pulseless ventricular tachycardia, pulseless electrical activity (electromechanical dissociation), and asystole is presented in algorithm form in Figures 3, 4, 5.

Selected Reading

1. Berg R, Otto C, Kern K, Sanders A, Ewy GA: High-dose epinephrine does not improve survival from prolonged cardiac arrest. *Crit Care Med* 1992; 20:510.

2. Cummins RO (ed.): *Textbook of Advanced Cardiac Life Support*. AHA. Dallas, TX, 1994.

3. Feneley MP, Maier GW, Kern KB, Ewy GA, et al: Influence of compression rate on initial success of resuscitation and 24-hour survival after prolonged manual cardiopulmonary resuscitation in dogs. *Circ* 1988; 77:240-250.

4. Guidelines for Cardiopulmonary Resuscitation and Emergency Cardiac Care. *JAMA* 1992; 268:2171-2302.

5. Higano ST, Oh JK, Ewy GA, Seward JB: Mechanism of blood flow during closed chest cardiac massage in humans: transesophageal echocardiographic observations. *Mayo Clin Pro* 1990; 65:1432-1440.

6. Kern KB, Carter AB, Showen RL, et al: CPR-induced trauma: Comparison of three manual methods in an experimental model. *Ann Emer Med* 1986; 674-679.

7. Kern KB, Garewal HS, Sanders AB, Janas W, Nelson J, Sloan D, Tacker WA, Ewy GA: Depletion of myocardial adenosine triphosphate during prolonged untreated ventricular fibrillation: effect on defibrillation success. *Resusc* 1990; 20:221-229.

8. Kern KB, Sanders AB, Janas W, Nelson JR, Badylak SF, Babbs CF, Tacker WA, Ewy GA: Limitations of open-chest cardiac massage after prolonged, untreated cardiac arrest in dogs. *Ann Emer Med* 1991; 20:761-767.

9. Kern KB, Sanders AB, Raife J, Milander MM, Otto CW, Ewy GA: A study of chest compression rates during cardiopulmonary resuscitation in humans. *Arch Int Med* 1992; 152:145-149.

10. Kern KB, Sanders AB, Badylak DVM, Janas W, et al: Long-term survival with open-chest cardiac massage after ineffective closed-chest compression in a canine preparation. *Circ* 1986; 498-503.

11. Kern KB, Ewy GA, Voorhees WD, Babbs CF, Tacker WA: Myocardial perfusion pressure: a predictor of 24-hour survival during prolonged cardiac arrest in dogs. *Resusc* 1988; 16:241-250.

12. Kern KB, Sanders AB, Voorhees WD, Babbs CF, Tacker WA, Ewy GA: Changes in expired end-tidal carbon dioxide during cardiopulmonary resuscitation in dogs: a prognostic guide for cardiopulmonary resuscitation. *JACC* 1989; 13:1184-1189.

13. Kern KB, Lancaster L, Goldman S, Ewy GA: The effect of coronary artery lesions on the relationship between coronary perfusion pressure and myocardial blood flow during cardiopulmonary resuscitation in pigs. *AHJ* 1990; 120:324-333.

14. Otto CW, Yakaitis RW, Ewy GA: Effect of epinephrine on defibrillation in ischemic ventricular fibrillation. *Am J Em Med* 1985; Vol. 3, 4: 285-287.

15. Otto C, Berg R, Milander M, Kern K, Sanders A, Ewy GA: Beta blockade attenuates tachycardia and early death after resuscitation from prolonged cardiac arrest with high dose epinephrine. *Crit Care Med* 1992; 20-574.

16. Raessler KL., Kern KB, Sanders AB, Tacker Jr WA, Ewy GA: Aortic and right atrial systolic pressures during cardiopulmonary resuscitation: a potential indicator of the mechanism of blood flow. *AHJ* 1988; Vol. 115, 5:1021-1029.

17. Sanders AB, Ewy GA, Alferness C, Taft T, Zimmerman M: Failure of a simultaneous chest compression, ventilation and abdominal binding technique of cardiopulmonary resuscitation. *Cr Care Med* 1982; 10; 609-513.

18. Sanders AB, Ogle M, Ewy GA: Coronary perfusion pressure during cardiopulmonary resuscitation. *Am J Emer Med* 1984; Vol. 3, 1:11-14.

19. Sanders AB, Ewy GA, Taft TV: Patterns and significance of arterial blood gases during prolonged cardiopulmonary resuscitation. *Ann Emer Med* 1984; 13:676-679.

20. Sanders AB, Ewy GA, Taft TV: Prognostic and therapeutic importance of the aortic diastolic pressure in resuscitation from cardiac arrest. *Cr Care Med* 1984; 12:871-873.

21. Sanders AB, Kern KB, Ewy GA: Neurologic benefits from the use of early cardiopulmonary resuscitation. *Ann Emer Med* 1987; 16:142-146.

22. Sanders AB, Kern KB, Otto CW, Milander MM, Ewy GA: End-tidal carbon dioxide monitoring during cardiopulmonary resuscitation: a prognostic indicator for survival. *JAMA* 1989; 262:1347-1351.

23. Sanders AB, Meislin MV, Ewy GA: The physiology of cardiopulmonary resuscitation. *JAMA* 1984; Vol.252, 23:3283-3286, 1984.